TEXTBOOK OF DIAGNOSTIC ULTRASONOGRAPHY

TEXTBOOK OF DIAGNOSTIC ULTRASONOGRAPHY

SANDRA L. HAGEN-ANSERT
B.A., RDMS/RDCS

Program Director of Diagnostic Ultrasound,
Department of Radiology;
Clinical and Research Echocardiographic Sonographer,
Pediatric Cardiology Division;
Clinical Neonatal Echoencephalographic Sonographer,
Neonatal Support Center,
University of California, San Diego, Medical Center,
San Diego, California

THIRD EDITION

with 2315 illustrations

The C. V. Mosby Company
ST. LOUIS ▪ BALTIMORE ▪ PHILADELPHIA ▪ TORONTO 1989

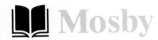 Mosby

Editor: David T. Culverwell
Developmental Editor: Kathryn H. Falk
Design: Elizabeth Fett
Production: Jeanne A. Gulledge, CRACOM Corporation

THIRD EDITION

Printed in the United States of America
The C. V. Mosby Company
11830 Westline Industrial Drive, St. Louis, Missouri 63146

Library of Congress Cataloging-in-Publication Data
Hagen-Ansert, Sandra L.
    Textbook of diagnostic ultrasonography/Sandra L. Hagen-Ansert.—3rd ed.
        p.   cm.
    Bibliography: p.
    Includes index.
    ISBN 0-8016-2446-0
    1. Diagnosis, Ultrasonic.   2. Echocardiology.   I. Title.
    [DNLM: 1. Echocardiography.   2. Ultrasonic Diagnosis.   WS 289
H143t]
RC78.7.U4H33   1989
616.07′543—dc19
DNLM/DLC
for Library of Congress   88-37215
                                                                        CIP

NWST
IADD 7051

C/MV/MV 9 8 7 6 5

Contributors

MARY ALLARE, M.D.

Division of Neonatal Perinatal Medicine, Department of Pediatrics, University of California, San Diego, San Diego, California

KARA L. MAYDEN ARGO, BS, RDMS, RTR

Adjunct Assistant Professor, Department of Obstetrics and Gynecology and Reproductive Biology, College of Human Medicine, Michigan State University, East Lansing, Michigan; Director, Obstetrics and Gynecology Residency Ultrasound Program, Blodgett Memorial Medical Center, Grand Rapids, Michigan; formerly, Department of Obstetrics and Gynecology, The University of Illinois at Chicago College of Medicine, Chicago, Illinois

RAUL BEJAR, M.D.

Division of Neonatal Perinatal Medicine, Department of Pediatrics, University of California, San Diego, San Diego, California

CAROLYN M. CARUSO, BS, RDMS

Department of Obstetrics, Gynecology, and Reproductive Science, The Mount Sinai School of Medicine, New York, New York

FRANK A. CHERVENAK, M.D.

Director, Obstetric Ulrasound and Ethics; Associate Professor, Department of Obstetrics and Gynecology, New York Hospital–Cornell Medical Center, New York, New York

MELANIE G. EZO, RT, RDMS

District Manager, Spectrascan Imaging Services, Inc., Hartford, Connecticut

HECTOR GRAMAJO, M.D.

Division of Neonatal Perinatal Medicine, Department of Pediatrics, University of California, San Diego, San Diego, California

CRIS D. GRESSER, RN, RDMS

Coordinator Echo Doppler Laboratory, Toronto General Hospital, Toronto, Ontario

BECKY LEVZOW, RT, RDMS

Ultrasound Section, Department of Radiology, Madison General Hospital, Madison, Wisconsin

ANNA K. PARSONS, M.D.

Assistant Professor, Division of Reproductive Endocrinology, Department of Obstetrics and Gynecology, University of South Florida College of Medicine, Tampa, Florida; formerly, Department of Obstetrics and Gynecology, The University of Illinois at Chicago College of Medicine, Chicago, Illinois

RICHARD E. RAE II, RT, RDMS, RVT

Technical Director, Indiana Vascular Imaging, Indianapolis, Indiana

JOANNE C. ROSENBERG, BS, RDMS

Chief Sonographer, Division of Maternal-Fetal Medicine, University of Medicine and Dentistry of New Jersey, Robert Wood Johnson Medical School, New Brunswick, New Jersey

JAMES C. RYVA, RDMS

Department of Obstetrics and Gynecology, The University of Illinois at Chicago College of Medicine, Chicago, Illinois

LAURA SCHOERMAN, RT, RDMS

Division of Ultrasound, Department of Radiology, Kaiser-Permanente Medical Center, San Diego, California

GUSTAVO VICCIOCCO, M.D.

Division of Neonatal Perinatal Medicine, Department of Pediatrics, University of California, San Diego, San Diego, California

BARBARA A. WALKER, RN, RDMS

Department of Obstetrics, Gynecology, and Reproductive Science, The Mount Sinai School of Medicine, New York, New York

JAMES A. ZAGZEBSKI, Ph.D.

Professor, Departments of Medical Physics, Radiology, and Human Oncology, University of Wisconsin Medical School, Madison, Wisconsin

LAURA J. ZUIDEMA, M.D.

Assistant Professor, Department of Obstetrics and Gynecology, The University of Illinois at Chicago College of Medicine, Chicago, Illinois

WILLIAM J. ZWIEBEL, M.D.

Associate Professor of Radiology, University of Utah School of Medicine, Salt Lake City, Utah

To our own little sonic boomers,
Rebecca, Alyssa, and *Katrina*

Foreword

I am honored to write a foreword for the third edition of this extremely well known and liked text. Since the second edition, ultrasound has made dramatic advances—both in its technology and its broadened scope of clinical utility. The need for a new edition was self-evident.

Sandra Hagen-Ansert and her colleagues have proved more than equal to the task. This edition includes thorough revision of many older chapters and now also incorporates major changes in physics and cardiology. Pediatric and fetal echocardiography are now stressed, and the latter is an important facet of the updating in obstetrical sections of the book. The role of Doppler ultrasound is acknowledged in an entirely new section on peripheral vascular diseases.

The focus of this text has always been the sonographer actually performing studies. Those who assume this role have a unique relationship with physicians responsible for interpreting sonographic studies. Real-time sonography provides the sonographer with vast amounts of information, most of which is discarded. Final images reaching the physician are a distillation of this information, and in a very real sense the sonographer performs diagnosis during the study. Nowhere else in medicine does this relationship exist. Perhaps the closest analogy is in gastrointestinal fluoroscopy, where spot films are made of real-time images, often sacrificing functional information. In virtually no institutions do technologists perform these studies. Yet curiously, in these same institutions, sonographers daily churn out complex studies of the heart, abdomen, and pelvis—in my view, a far more complex task.

This unique role as physician assistant clearly deserves recognition. It requires high-quality instruction, of which this book is an excellent example. It also requires outstanding and dedicated individuals, of which the book's principal author is an excellent example. She and her co-authors are to be congratulated on their success in once again advancing our knowledge in this discipline.

GEORGE R. LEOPOLD, M.D.

Preface

TO THE FIRST EDITION

Medicine has always been a fascinating field. I was introduced to it by Dr. Charles Henkelmann, who provided me with the opportunity to learn radiography. Although x-ray technology was interesting, it was not challenging enough. It did not provide the opportunity to evaluate patient history or to follow through interesting cases, which seemed to be the most intriguing aspect of medicine and my primary concern.

Shortly after I finished my training, I was assigned to the radiation therapy department, where I was introduced to a very quiet and young, dedicated radiologist, whom I would later grow to admire and respect as one of the foremost authorities in diagnostic ultrasound. Convincing George Leopold that he needed another hand to assist him was difficult in the beginning, and it was through the efforts of his resident, Dan MacDonald, that I was able to learn what has eventually developed into a most challenging and exciting new medical modality.

Utilizing high-frequency sound waves, diagnostic ultrasound provides a unique method for visualization of soft tissue anatomic structures. The challenge of identifying such structures and correlating the results with clinical symptoms and patient data offered an ongoing challenge to the sonographer. The state of the art demands expertise in scanning techniques and maneuvers to demonstrate the internal structures; without quality scans, no diagnostic information can be rendered to the physician.

Our initial experience in ultrasound took us through the era of A-mode techniques, identifying aortic aneurysms through pulsatile reflections, trying to separate splenic reflections from upper-pole left renal masses, and, in general, trying to echo every patient with a probable abdominal or pelvic mass. Of course, the one-dimensional A-mode techniques were difficult for me to conceptualize, let alone believe in. However, with repeated success and experience from mistakes, I began to believe in this method. The conviction that Dr. Leopold had about this technique was a strong indicator of its success in our laboratory.

It was when Picker brought our first two-dimensional ultrasound unit to the laboratory that the "skeptics" started to believe a little more in this modality. I must admit that those early images were weather maps to me for a number of months. The repeated times I asked, "What is that?" were enough to try anyone's patience.

I can recall when Siemens installed our real-time unit and we saw our first obstetric case. Such a thrill for us to see the fetus move, wave his hand, and show us fetal heart pulsations.

By this time we were scouting the clinics and various departments in the hospital for interesting cases to scan. With our success rate surpassing our failures, the case load increased so that soon we were involved in all aspects of ultrasound. There was not enough material or reprints for us to read to see the new developments. It was for this reason that excitement in clinical research soared, attracting young physicians throughout the country to develop techniques in diagnostic ultrasound.

Because Dr. Leopold was so intensely interested in ultrasound, it became the diagnostic method of choice for our patients. It was not long before conferences were incomplete without the mention of the technique. Later, local medical meetings and eventually national meetings grew to include discussion of this new modality. A number of visitors were attracted to our laboratory to learn the technique, and thus we became swamped with a continual flow of new physicians, some eager to work with ultrasound and others skeptical at first but believers in the end.

Education progressed slowly at first, with many laboratories offering a one-to-one teaching experience. Commercial companies thought the only way to push the field was to develop their own national training programs, and thus several of the leading manufacturers were the first to put a dedicated effort into the development of ultrasound.

It was through the combined efforts of our laboratory and commercial interests that I became interested in furthering ultrasound education. Seminars, weekly sessions, local and national meetings, and consultations became a vital part of the growth of ultrasound.

Thus, as ultrasound grew in popularity, more intensified training was desperately needed to maintain its initial quality that its pioneers strived for.

Through working with one of the commercial ultrasound companies conducting national short-term training programs, I became acquainted with Barry Goldberg and his enthusiasm for quality education in ultrasound. His organizational efforts and pioneer spirit led me to the east coast to further develop more intensive educational programs in ultrasound.

Through these experiences the need for a diverse ultrasound textbook was shown. Thus this text was written for the sonographer involved in clinical ultrasound, with emphasis on anatomy, physiology, pathology, and ultrasonic techniques and patterns. Clinical medicine and patient evaluation are important parts of the ultrasonic examination and as such are discussed as relevant to pathology demonstrated by ultrasound.

It is my hope that this textbook will not only introduce the reader to the field of ultrasound but also go a step beyond to what I have found to be a very stimulating and challenging experience in diagnostic patient care.

SANDRA L. HAGEN-ANSERT

Part One

PHYSICS

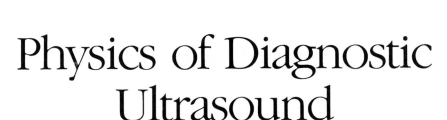

Physics of Diagnostic Ultrasound

JAMES A. ZAGZEBSKI

NATURE OF SOUND WAVES

The passage of sound through a medium involves wave propagation, in which particles within the medium are caused to vibrate about their resting position. Once initiated, an acoustic disturbance propagates through the medium at a speed determined by the properties of the medium. Passage of the wave results in the transfer of energy through the medium. However, there is no net transfer of particles (i.e., after a sound wave has passed through the medium the particles return to their normal equilibrium position; we are assuming that the strength of the wave is low enough to allow this latter statement to be made). Sound waves can be transmitted through many materials, such as air, water, wood, plastic, and biologic tissues. They cannot be transmitted through a vacuum because they require some form of matter for their propagation.

Sound waves are produced by vibrating sources. A simple example of a source of sound is a tuning fork vibrating in air (Fig. 1-1, A). The vibrations of the tuning fork cause adjacent molecules in the air to be compressed together and drawn apart, depending on the direction of movement of the arm of the tuning fork. Molecules that are compressed together push other molecules closer together, which push other farther molecules closer together, and so on; thus the acoustic disturbance propagates outward.

A tuning fork vibrates back and forth in a regular fashion, sometimes referred to as *simple harmonic motion.*

The resultant air compressions are accompanied by increases in the pressure. If it were possible to measure the pressure at different points near the tuning fork at any instant of time, the measurement results would appear as in Fig. 1-1, B. The pressure varies with distance, tracing out a *sine wave,* as shown. Here 0 pressure refers to equilibrium, ambient conditions, usually the atmospheric pressure if we are considering a sound wave in air. Places where particles are squeezed together are referred to as regions of *compression,* and the pressure here is greater than 0. The maximum pressure swing occurring during passage of the wave is called the *pressure amplitude,* also defined in Fig. 1-1. Places where the particles are drawn apart are referred to as regions of *rarefaction,* and the pressure here is less than 0. The distance over which the curve repeats itself is called the acoustic *wavelength,* given by the symbol λ in Fig. 1-1.

Just as the vibrating tuning fork does not remain stationary, so a plot of pressure versus distance also varies from one instant to the next. This is because the sound wave is propagating outward from the source. Fig. 1-2 shows two plots of the pressure versus distance taken at slightly different times. The wave forms are slightly out of phase. A useful way of expressing the temporal behavior of a sound wave is to plot the pressure versus time *at a single point* in the medium. The resultant curve also traces out a *sine wave* (Fig. 1-3). The number of times per second the disturbance is repeated at any point is

Particle vibrations (◀▬▶)

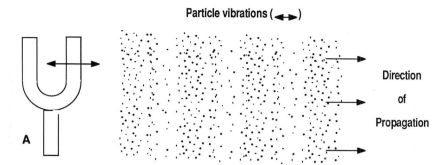

A

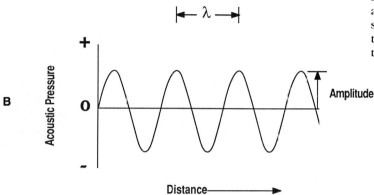

B

FIG. 1-1. Generation of a sound wave by a vibrating tuning fork, depicting the medium, **A**, and the acoustic pressure, **B**, at an instant of time. Motion of the tuning fork results in transmission of longitudinal sound waves. The direction of particle vibrations is along a line parallel to the direction of propagation of the wave.

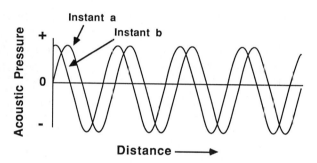

FIG. 1-2. Acoustic pressure versus distance at two different times.

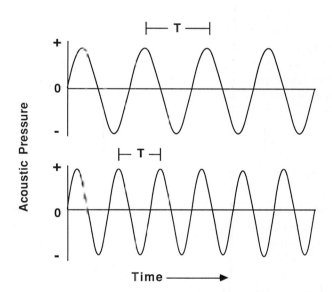

FIG. 1-3. Acoustic pressure versus time at a fixed spot in the medium. The period is T. The bottom waveform depicts a higher frequency than the top. Notice the period is greater in the top waveform.

called the *frequency*. The time it takes for the disturbance to repeat itself is the *period*, labeled T in Fig. 1-3. Frequency, f, and period, T, are inversely related; that is,

$$T = 1/f \qquad (1\text{-}1)$$

Example: Suppose the period of a wave form is 0.5 second. Calculate the frequency.

Solution: You can rearrange Equation 1-1 by multiplying both sides of the equation by f and dividing both sides by T. The result is

$$f = 1/T$$

Substituting gives

$$f = 1/0.5 \text{ s} = 2/\text{s}$$

In other words, if the period is 0.5 second, the frequency is 2 times per second.

Fig. 1-3 also shows that as the period decreases, the frequency increases, and vice versa.

TYPES OF SOUND WAVES

Sound waves are mechanical vibrations that propagate in a medium. In response to the sound wave, particles in the medium are displaced from their resting position and vibrate back and forth. In the example in Fig. 1-1 the particle displacement is in the same direction as the wave propagates. This mode of vibration is referred to as *longitudinal wave* propagation. Other types of vibrations are

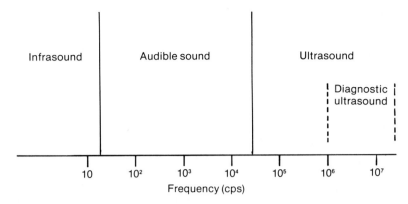

FIG. 1-4. Division of sound into different frequency ranges. Ultrasound refers to a sound wave whose frequency is greater than 20 kHz.

possible, depending on the type of medium. For example, *transverse vibrations* or shear waves may be transmitted through solid materials. These are characterized by particle vibrations perpendicular to the direction of vibration.

In this textbook we are concerned mainly with propagation of sound in the soft tissues of the body. Only longitudinal waves are of interest here because this is the only mode of vibration that can be transmitted through soft tissue.

FREQUENCY

It was mentioned earlier that the sound frequency is the number of oscillations per second that the source or the particles in the medium make as they vibrate about their resting position. The unit for frequency is *cycles per second* or *hertz*. Commonly used multiples of 1 hertz are as follows:

1 cycle per second = 1 hertz = 1 Hz

1000 cycles per second = 1000 hertz = 1 kilohertz = 1 kHz

1,000,000 cycles per second = 1,000,000 hertz
= 1 megahertz = 1MHz

The metric notation will be used consistently in this book. Appendix 1 (pages 15 and 16) gives the more common metric prefixes and their decimal equivalents.

A classification scheme for acoustic waves according to their frequency is given in Fig. 1-4. Most humans can hear sound if it has a frequency in the range of 15 Hz to approximately 20 kHz. This is referred to as the *audible frequency range*. Sound whose frequency is greater than 20 kHz is termed *ultrasonic*. Vibrations whose frequencies are below the audible range are termed *infrasonic*. Examples of infrasonic transmissions include vibrations introduced by air ducts, ocean waves, and seismic waves.

The ultrasonic frequency range is used extensively, both by humans and by animals. Except for therapy ultrasound, most medical applications use frequencies that lie in the 1 MHz to 20 MHz range.

SPEED OF SOUND

The speed with which acoustic waves propagate through a medium is determined by the *characteristics of the me-*

dium itself. (There are slight dependencies on other factors, such as the ultrasonic frequency, but these are so small that they can be ignored completely in our discussion.) Specifically, for longitudinal sound waves in either liquids or body tissues, an expression for the speed of sound, *c*, is

$$c = \sqrt{B/\rho} \qquad (1-2)$$

In this equation B refers to the elastic properties of the medium and is called the *bulk modulus*. The symbol ρ is the density, given in g/cm^3 (grams per cubic centimeter) or kg/m^3 (kilograms per cubic meter). Thus we see that the speed of sound in a medium depends on the elastic properties or "stiffness" of the medium and on the density. Appropriate units for speed are m/s (meters per second). The speed of sound in some nonbiologic materials is as follows[4]:

Material	m/s
Air	330
Silastic materials	950
Ethyl alcohol	1177
Water	1480
Lead	2400
Crown glass	6120
Aluminum	6400

The speed of sound in biologic tissues is an important parameter in imaging applications. Values that have been measured in different human tissues are as follows[1,4]:

Tissue	m/s
Lung	600
Fat	1460
Aqueous humor	1510
Liver	1555
Blood	1560
Kidney	1565
Muscle	1600
Lens	1620
Skull bone	4080

The lowest speed shown is that for lung tissue, due to the presence of air-filled alveoli in this tissue. Most tissues of concern to us (that is, those through which sound can be readily propagated in the megahertz frequency range) have speed-of-sound values in the neighborhood of 1500 to 1600 m/s. Fat is seen to come out on the low end of the range for soft tissue and muscle tissue on the high end. Measurements of the speed of sound in bone tissue result in values two to three times those recorded in most soft tissues.

The average speed of sound in soft tissues (excluding the lung) is 1540 m/s, and range-measuring circuits on many diagnostic ultrasound instruments are calibrated on this basis. Close inspection of the biologic tissue list above reveals that the propagation speed in every soft tissue of concern to us in diagnostic ultrasound is within a few percentage points of 1540 m/s.

WAVELENGTH

The acoustic wavelength (λ), as defined above and illustrated in Fig. 1-1, depends on the speed of sound in the medium, c, and the frequency, f, according to the following relationship:

$$\lambda = c/f \qquad (1\text{-}3)$$

Thus the wavelength is simply the speed of sound divided by the untrasonic frequency. We can see from Equation 1-3 that the higher the ultrasonic frequency the smaller will be the wavelength.

Example: Calculate the wavelength for a 2 MHz ultrasound beam in soft tissue. Assume the speed of sound is 1540 m/s.

Solution: The wavelength can be calculated directly using Equation 1-3, with c = 1540 m/s and f = 2 MHz = 2 × 10^6 cycles/s.

$$\text{Thus } \lambda = \frac{1540 \text{ m/s}}{2 \times 10^6/\text{s}}$$
$$= 0.0077 \text{ m}$$
$$= 0.77 \text{ mm}$$

You may wish to study the material in Appendix 1 (pages 15 and 16) at this stage to review metric conversions. Appendix 1 also contains examples of addition, subtraction, multiplication, and division in which numbers are expressed as exponentials (i.e., 2,000,000 cycles/s = 2 × 10^6 cycles/s). Although to be a successful sonographer may not require mastering problems of this type, nevertheless we will continue to explore examples such as this throughout the first few chapters of this book in an effort to improve our understanding of the physical factors involved in sound transmission through soft tissue.

The wavelength concept is important in ultrasound physics because it is related to imaging factors such as *spatial resolution*. In addition, the physical size of an object (e.g., a reflecting surface or a transducer surface) is significant only when we compare it to the ultrasonic wavelength. It might be said then that the wavelength is our "acoustic yardstick" (Fig. 1-5). Objects are large or small depending on their size relative to it. In soft tissue, wavelengths for diagnostic ultrasound are on the order of 1 mm or less, with 0.77 mm wavelengths for 2 MHz beams and proportionally smaller ones for higher frequencies.

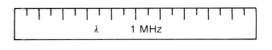

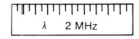

FIG. 1-5. The wavelength is often used as an acoustic yardstick. Wavelength is inversely proportional to frequency.

AMPLITUDE AND INTENSITY

When discussing reflection, attenuation, and scatter, we often must make a quantitative statement regarding the magnitude of a sound wave. One variable that can be used here is the *pressure amplitude*. The acoustic pressure amplitude was illustrated in Fig. 1-1 and was defined as the maximum increase (or decrease) in the pressure relative to ambient conditions in the absence of the sound wave. Other parameters that could have been used in an analogous fashion include the maximum *particle displacement* in the wave and the maximum *particle velocity*.

In some applications, particularly when discussing biologic effects of ultrasound (Chapter 7), it is useful to specify the acoustic intensity. The intensity, I, is related to the square of the pressure amplitude, P, according to the relationship:

$$I = P^2/2\rho c \qquad (1\text{-}4)$$

where, again, ρ is the density of the medium and c the speed of sound.

Acoustic intensity will be discussed in greater detail in Chapter 7.

REFLECTION AND TRANSMISSION AT INTERFACES
Acoustic impedance

The product of the density of a material and the speed of sound in that material is a quantity called the characteristic acoustic impedance or, for our purposes, simply the *acoustic impedance* of a medium. That is,

$$Z = \rho c \qquad (1\text{-}5)$$

where Z is the impedance and ρ and c are as already defined. The significance of this quantity is its role in determining the amplitude of reflected and transmitted waves at an interface. This is discussed in the next section.

Except for the fact that we must concern ourselves with some fairly large numbers and some units that may be difficult to relate to, determining the impedance for materials is just a case of carrying out the simple multiplication involved.

Following is a compilation of acoustic impedance values for both nonbiologic and biologic tissues. The units for expressing these are kg/m²/s (kilograms per square meter per second), which result after multiplying density time speed. Sometimes we find impedance given in *rayls*. One rayl is the same as 1 kg/m²/s:

Tissue	Rayls
Air	0.0004×10^6
Lung	0.18×10^6
Fat	1.34×10^6
Water	1.48×10^6
Liver	1.65×10^6
Blood	1.65×10^6
Kidney	1.63×10^6
Muscle	1.71×10^6
Skull bone	7.8×10^6

Reflection—perpendicular incidence

Whenever an ultrasound beam is incident on an interface formed by two materials having different acoustic impedances, in general, some of the energy in the beam will be reflected and the remainder transmitted. The amplitude of the reflected wave depends on the difference between the acoustic impedances of the two materials forming the interface.

Consider, first, the case of normal or perpendicular beam incidence on a large flat interface (Fig. 1-6). A large smooth interface such as depicted here is termed a *specular reflector*—with dimensions that are much greater than the ultrasonic wavelength. The ratio of the reflected pressure amplitude, P_r, to the incident pressure amplitude, P_i, is called the *amplitude reflection coefficient*— given by R. This ratio depends on the acoustic impedances at the interface according to the expression:

$$R = \frac{P_r}{P_i} = \frac{Z_2 - Z_1}{Z_2 + Z_1} \qquad (1\text{-}6)$$

where Z_2 is the acoustic impedance on the distal side of the interface and Z_1 is the impedance on the proximal side.

Example: Using the values for acoustic impedance just given, calculate the amplitude reflection coefficient for a fat-liver interface.

Solution: The acoustic impedance of fat is 1.34×10^6 rayls, that of liver 1.65×10^6 rayls. From Equation 1-6

$$R = \frac{1.65 \times 10^6 \text{ rayls} - 1.34 \times 10^6 \text{ rayls}}{1.65 \times 10^6 \text{ rayls} + 1.34 \times 10^6 \text{ rayls}}$$

Factoring out 10^6 rayls gives

$$R = \frac{(1.65 - 1.34) \times 10^6 \text{rayls}}{(1.65 + 1.34) \times 10^6 \text{rayls}}$$
$$= \frac{(1.65 - 1.34)}{(1.65 + 1.34)} = \frac{0.31}{2.99} = 0.10$$

We see from the example that the ratio of the reflected to the incident amplitude is quite small. In fact, at most soft tissue—soft tissue interfaces in the body the reflection coefficient is fairly small and most of the sound is transmitted through the interface. If this were not the case, it would be difficult to use diagnostic ultrasound for examining anatomic structures at significant tissue depths.

REFLECTION

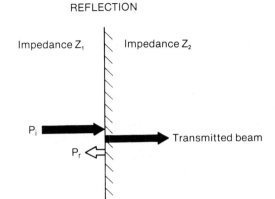

FIG. 1-6. Reflection for perpendicular beam incidence on a specular reflector. The reflector is formed by two materials of differing acoustic impedances, Z_1 and Z_2. P_i is the pressure amplitude of the incident beam and P_r the amplitude of the reflected beam.

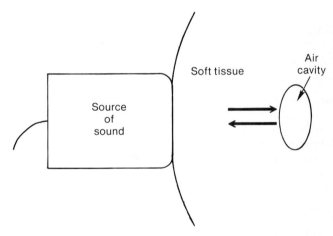

FIG. 1-7. Reflection at a tissue-to-air interface. Essentially all the sound energy is reflected at the interface, and none gets transmitted.

Example: Calculate the reflection coefficient for a muscle-air interface.

Solution: From the acoustic impedances given in the list, calculate

$$R = \frac{0.0004 \times 10^6 - 1.7 \times 10^6}{0.0004 \times 10^6 - 1.7 \times 10^6}$$
$$= \frac{0.0004 - 1.7}{0.0004 + 1.7}$$
$$= -0.99$$

(Notice that several of the mathematical steps illustrated in the previous example were combined into one step.) In this case the beam is almost completely reflected. This example illustrates the difficulty in transmitting ultrasound beyond any tissue-to-air interface (Fig. 1-7). The complete reflection at air interfaces also explains the need for a coupling medium, such as gel or oil, between the ultrasound transducer and the patient during ultrasound examinations. The coupling material ensures that no air is trapped between the transducer and the skin surface, thereby providing good sound transmission into the patient.

Other examples of reflection coefficients (P_r/P_i) calculated for specular reflecting interfaces are as follows:

Muscle-air	−0.99
Fat-liver	0.10
Kidney-liver	0.006
Liver-muscle	0.018
Muscle-bone	0.64

The data presented here show that a soft tissue—to—bone interface also is a fairly strong reflector. In the majority of ultrasound examinations discussed in this text, bone is avoided because of this and other difficulties associated with propagation through it. Most soft tissue interfaces of importance are fairly weakly reflecting, just as we calculated in the first example.

In summary, reflection of a sound beam occurs whenever the beam is incident on an interface formed by two tissues having different acoustic impedances. The acoustic impedance difference could be caused by a change in speeds of sound, a change in densities, or both. The magnitude of the reflected wave, expressed here as the ratio of the reflected wave amplitude to the incident amplitude, is mainly dependent on the acoustic impedance difference at the interface. Interfaces characterized by a large difference in acoustic impedance reflect more of the incident beam than do interfaces where the acoustic impedance difference (mismatch) is small.

One additional note: some authors use the intensity reflection coefficient rather than the amplitude reflection coefficient to quantify the reflection process. The expression for the size of the reflection looks similar to Equation 1-6, except that the quantity involving the acoustic impedances is squared. In other words, if I_r is the reflected intensity and I_i is the incident intensity, then

$$\frac{I_r}{I_i} = \frac{(Z_2 - Z_1)^2}{(Z_2 + Z_1)^2} \qquad (1\text{-}7)$$

The two expressions (Equations 1-6 and 1-7) are not contradictory. Recall from our earlier discussion that the intensity is proportional to the square of the amplitude. Therefore the ratio of the reflected intensity to the incident intensity at an interface is equal to the square of the ratio of the reflected amplitude to the incident amplitude.

Nonperpendicular sound beam incidence

For nonperpendicular beam incidence on a specular reflector the situation changes somewhat.

First, the reflected beam does not travel back toward the source (Fig. 1-8) but instead travels off at an angle, θ_r, that is equal to the incident angle, θ_i, only in the opposite direction. This has an effect on echo detection from interfaces. As we shall see in Chapter 3, in many diagnostic applications of ultrasound the sound beam source is also used to detect echoes from reflectors in the beam. Therefore the amplitude of an echo that is detected depends on

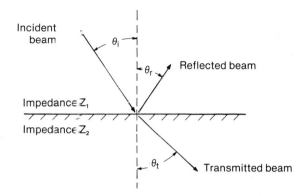

FIG. 1-8. Reflection and refraction for nonperpendicular beam incidence. The incident beam angle, θ_i, reflected beam angle, θ_r, and transmitted beam angle, θ_t, are illustrated.

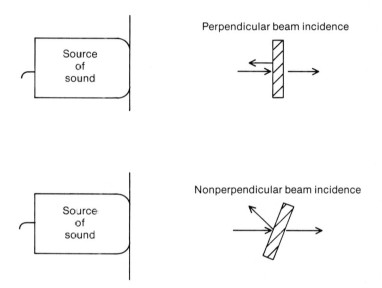

FIG. 1-9. For perpendicular beam incidence at a specular reflector, the echo from a specular reflector returns toward the source. For nonperpendicular incidence the echo travels in a direction that may miss the source.

the orientation of the interface relative to the incident beam (Fig. 1-9). Because of this significant angular dependence on the detection of an echo, specular reflectors are sometimes difficult to pick up by a single-pulse echo transducer.

A second factor that arises when the incident beam is not perpendicular to an interface is the possibility of refraction of the transmitted beam. *Refraction* refers to a bending of the sound beam at the interface, causing the transmitted beam to emerge in a different direction from the incident beam (compare the incident and transmitted beam directions in Fig. 1-8). Most of us are familiar with the effects of refraction of light waves; for example, due to refraction a swimming pool appears shallower than it actually is (Fig. 1-10).

Two conditions are required for refraction of a sound wave to occur:

1. The sound beam must be incident on the interface at an angle that is not perpendicular.

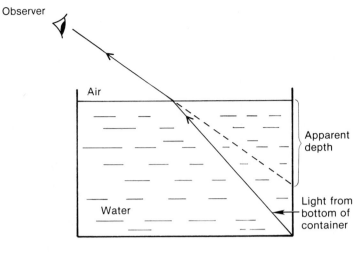

Observer

Air

Apparent depth

Water

Light from bottom of container

FIG. 1-10. Refraction of light at a water-to-air interface. To the observer the container of water appears to be shallower than it actually is.

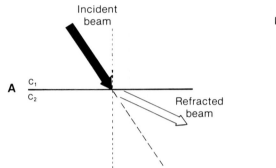
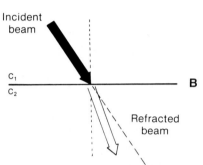

Incident beam

c_1
c_2
A

Refracted beam

Incident beam

c_1
c_2
B

Refracted beam

FIG. 1-11. The direction of the refracted beam depends on the relative sound speed in medium 2 compared to the speed in medium 1. **A,** c_2 greater than c_1; **B,** c_2 less than c_1.

2. The speeds of sound must be different on the two sides of the interface.

Notice what the second condition is saying: it is not sufficient simpy to have a reflecting interface to produce refraction; there also must be a speed of sound change at the interface for refraction to occur.

The direction of the transmitted (not reflected) beam is governed by *Snell's Law.* The direction is related to the speed of sound on the incident beam side of the interface, c_1, to the speed of sound on the transmitted beam side of the interface, c_2, and to the incident beam direction, θ_i, (Fig. 1-8), according to the following relationship:

$$\sin \theta_t = (c_2/c_1) \times \sin \theta_i \qquad (1\text{-}8)$$

The angle θ_t is also shown in Fig. 1-8. Equation 1-8 is a statement of Snell's Law.

The relationship between an angle and its trigonometric sine ("sin") is discussed in Appendix 1 (pages 15 and 16). It is possible to calculate θ_t, given the incident beam direction and the speeds of sound at the interface. We will not do calculations here using Equation 1-8; suffice to say that the sine of any angle between 0 and 90° increases as the angle itself increases. Therefore, if c_2 is greater than c_1, the angle θ_t will be greater than θ_i, and vice versa (Fig. 1-11). Notice, if c_2 equals c_1, θ_t equals θ_i (i.e., there is no refraction).

To help understand the process of refraction, consider the situation of a row of marchers carrying a long banner in a parade (Fig. 1-12, *A*). Suppose the marchers are all walking at the same speed on a concrete pavement as shown. At the end of the pavement is a field of mud, which significantly slows the pace each person can walk upon entering it. The direction of march takes the row towards the concrete-to-mud interface at an angle. When part of the row has passed the interface, the different speeds that can be maintained on either side of the concrete-mud interface result in the situation of Fig. 1-12, *B*, where the row has been bent somewhat. When all marchers have entered the mud field, their direction of travel will have altered.

Refraction results in a change in sound beam direction. Situations in which refraction may occur are those for which a sound beam is incident nonperpendicularly on an interface and the speed of sound changes across the interface. The degree of refraction depends on the difference between the speeds of sound; the greater the difference, the larger the effect. If we reexamine the acoustic properties of soft tissues, it appears that interfaces involving fat (i.e., fat-muscle) offer the best chances for significant (measured) beam refraction. Investigators believe that both fat-nonfat interfaces and sharply curved interfaces (e.g., walls of vessels) provide the best surfaces for refraction to occur.

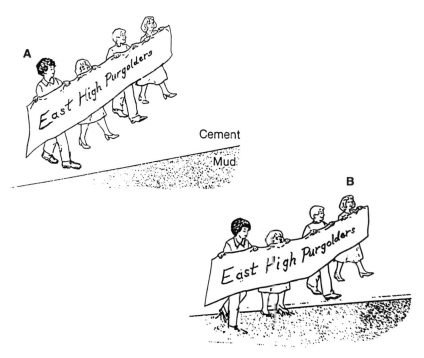

FIG. 1-12.   Simulation of refraction.

GRAZING INCIDENCE

Additional complexity may be introduced if the sound beam is incident on an interface at nearly grazing incident angles. The situations to be described occur only if the speeds of sound on the two sides of the interface are different. Such conditions appear to arise in some diagnostic situations involving, for example, the lateral margins of small cysts and vessels. Therefore we will consider them briefly.

If the speed of sound in the material on the transmitted beam side of the interface, c_2, is greater than that in the material on the incident beam side, c_1, the possibility of *critical angle* refraction exists. This occurs when refraction causes the angle of the transmitted beam, θ_t, to equal 90° (Fig. 1-13). The critical angle is the incident beam angle, θ_i, when this situation occurs. If θ_i is equal to or greater than the critical angle, all the energy is reflected and none is transmitted.

If c_2 is less than c_1, no critical angle exists. However, for grazing incident beam angles the reflected amplitude still increases above the value obtained for perpendicular beam incidence. The reflection coefficient approaches 1 (all the sound reflected and none transmitted) as the incident beam angle approaches 90°.

Both these situations are illustrated by the graphs in Fig. 1-14. In A we graph passage from fat tissue to liver, so c_2 is greater than c_1; therefore a critical angle exists. This angle is about 68°. If the beam were traveling in the opposite direction (from liver to fat, B) there is no critical angle because c_2 is less than c_1. However, near a 90-degree incident angle the beam is deflected because R gets large, as shown in Fig. 1-14. In both A and B we see that with a perpendicular beam incidence, or with modest angles, the reflected wave is of a relatively low amplitude and most of

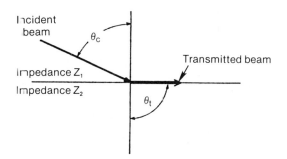

FIG. 1-13.   Demonstration of the critical angle, θ_c, or the incident beam angle, corresponding to a 90-degree transmitted beam when the speed of sound in medium 2 is greater than the speed of sound in medium 1. All the incident sound is reflected for incident angles equal to or greater than the critical angle.

the sound energy is transmitted through the interface. However, at the critical angle or at a grazing incidence the interface becomes a near perfect reflector, not allowing any sound energy through.

Small vessels, ducts, and cysts are examples in which the processes just mentioned could have a significant effect (Fig. 1-15). Considerable disruption of the sound beam at the edge of such a structure leads to a shadow appearance beyond the structure.[3]

DIFFUSE REFLECTION

Many times echo signals are produced in the body from interfaces that are not perfectly specular. For example, small vessels whose dimensions are on the order of the acoustic wavelength fall into this category. So do many larger interfaces, such as the collecting system of the kidney, the walls of the heart chambers, and some organ

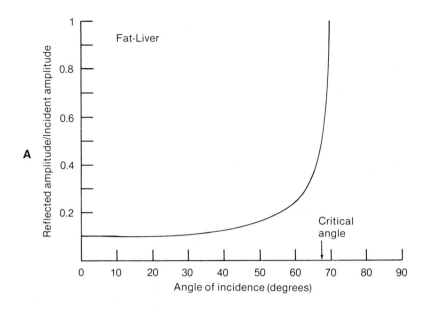

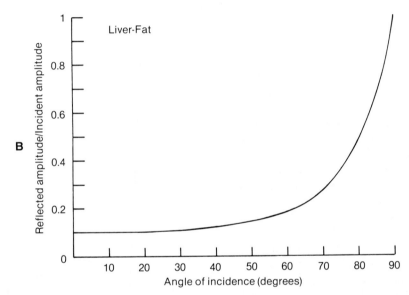

FIG. 1-14. Variation of the amplitude reflection coefficient versus the angle of incidence of the sound beam for two cases. **A,** For a fat-to-liver interface, where c_2 is greater than c_1 and thus a critical angle exists; **B,** for a liver-to-fat interface where c_2 is less than c_1.

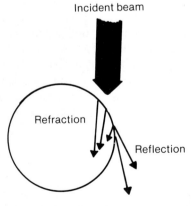

FIG. 1-15. Sound transmission and reflection near the edge of a circular or tubular structure. Very little sound can reach points directly below the edge of the tube because of refraction and reflection.

boundaries, which are generally not perfectly smooth. Interfaces that possess a degree of roughness, as illustrated schematically in Fig. 1-16, are referred to as *diffuse reflectors.* An echo from a diffuse reflector detected with a single pulse-echo transducer is not as sensitive to the orientation of the reflector as an echo from a smooth, specular reflector.

It is likely that most interfaces in the body have both a diffuse and a specular component.

SCATTER

In our discussion of specular and diffuse reflectors we were considering reflections from interfaces that are much larger than the ultrasonic wavelength. Other types of inhomogeneities exist in the body that can give rise to echoes. For structures that are smaller than the wavelength, a process referred to as ultrasonic *scatter* takes

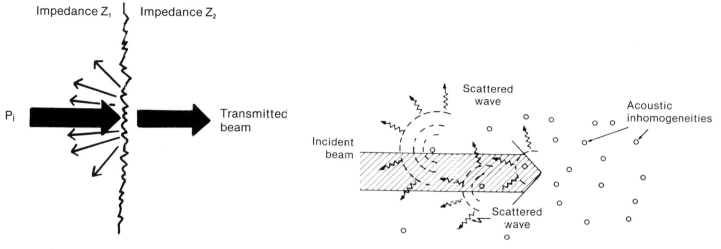

FIG. 1-16. Schema of reflection at a diffuse reflector.

FIG. 1-17. Scattering of sound by small interfaces.

place (Fig. 1-17). In this figure, scatterers are represented as small objects distributed at random locations in the volume of interest. Waves that are scattered tend to travel off in all directions, as suggested in the diagram.

Ultrasonic scattering gives rise to much of the diagnostic information seen in ultrasound imaging. Scattering results in the gray scale texture on images. Changes in scatter result in changes in the brightness of the image and therefore are useful in delineating both normal and abnormal structures. The terms *hyperechoic* and *hypoechoic* are used often in clinical imaging to describe structures on B-mode images. Hyperechoic regions result from increases in the ultrasound scattering level compared to the surrounding tissue. Hypoechoic refers to the opposite condition, where the scattering level is lower than in the surrounding tissue.

Since the scattered waves spread in all directions, echo signals detected from a volume containing small scatterers are not highly dependent on the orientation of individual scatterers. This is in contrast to the strong orientation dependence seen for specular reflectors. For very small scatterers, echo signals depend on the following:
1. The number of scatterers per unit volume
2. The acoustic impedance changes at the scatterer interfaces
3. The size of the scatterer (Scattering usually increases with increasing radius for very small scatterers.)
4. The ultrasonic frequency (Scattering usually increases with increasing frequency for very small scatterers.)

The dependence on frequency can sometimes be used to an advantage in ultrasound imaging. Since specular reflection is frequency independent and scattering increases with frequency, it is often possible to enhance scattered signals over specular echo signals by using higher ultrasonic frequencies.

Red blood cells are sometimes called "Rayleigh scatter-

ers." This term is used when the dimensions of scattering objects is much less than the ultrasonic wavelength. Scattering from Rayleigh scatterers increases with frequency, the intensity being proportional to frequency raised to the fourth power.

DECIBEL NOTATION

Let us digress briefly and discuss a fairly standard method for quantifying amplitudes, intensities, or power levels in ultrasound. The decibel notation provides a comparison of two signal levels, such as two amplitudes or two intensities. It is used primarily to express changes in these quantities resulting, for example, from attenuation, signal amplification, or instrument power control variations.

If we have two different wave amplitudes, A_2 and A_1, we could express their relative amplitudes by simply taking the ratio of one to the other. Alternatively, using decibels, the relationship between A_2 and A_1 is expressed as follows:

$$\text{Signal level (dB)} = 20 \log A_2/A_1 \qquad (1\text{-}9)$$

If the power or intensity is used rather than the amplitude, the expression appears on the surface to be somewhat different:

$$\text{Signal level (dB)} = 10 \log I_2/I_1 \qquad (1\text{-}10)$$

where I refers to an intensity.

In fact, Equation 1-9 can be shown to be equivalent to Equation 1-10. To do this we make use of the fact that the logarithm of a number raised to any power (e.g., $\log 10^2$) is equal to that power times the logarithm of the number alone:

$$\log 10^2 = 2 \times \log 10$$

If we use the expression for decibels employing the intensities (Equation 1-10)

$$\text{Signal level (dB)} = 10 \log I_2/I_1$$

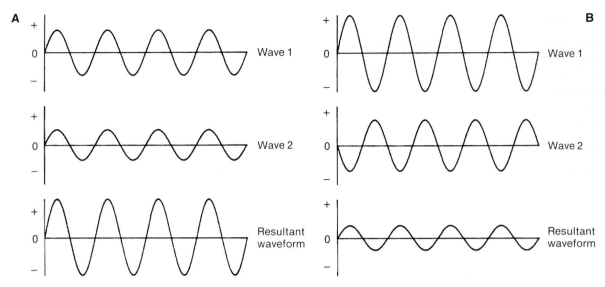

FIG. 1-20. Interference of two sine waves of equal frequency. **A,** When the two waves are in phase; **B,** when the two waves are of opposite phase.

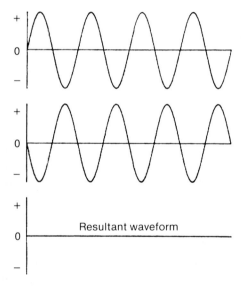

FIG. 1-21. Complete destructive interference. The two waves are of equal amplitude and exactly opposite phases.

SUMMARY

1. A sound wave is a mechanical disturbance propagating through a medium. Longitudinal sound waves are involved in diagnostic ultrasound imaging.

2. The propagation speed depends on properties of the medium; the average speed of sound for soft tissue is 1540 m/s.

3. The wavelength is the speed of sound divided by the frequency. It's importance in acoustics is that it is our "yardstick" for comparing the relative sizes of objects.

4. Ultrasound refers to sound waves whose frequency is above the audible range; medical ultrasound uses frequencies in the 1 to 15 MHz range.

5. The intensity of a sound wave is proportional to the square of the amplitude.

6. The acoustic impedance is the speed of sound times the density.

7. Partial reflection occurs whenever a sound wave encounters an interface formed by two materials of different acoustic impedance. The amount of sound reflected is related to the difference between the acoustic impedances at the interface.

8. A specular reflector refers to a large, smooth interface. The angle of the reflected wave is equal and opposite to the angle of incidence. A diffuse reflector spreads the reflected sound in all directions. A scatterer is a small reflector that scatters sound in all directions.

9. Refraction is a bending of the transmitted beam at an interface. It occurs if the sound beam is incident at an angle that is not perpendicular to the interface and there is a change is the speed of sound across the interface.

10. Decibels are used to quantify the ratio of two amplitudes or two intensities.

11. The reduction in amplitude or intensity as a sound wave propagates through a medium is called attenuation. Attenuation in soft tissue is caused by (1) reflection and scatter losses and (2) absorption.

12. Attenuation in soft tissues is nearly proportional to the ultrasound frequency.

13. Interference describes what happens when waves from two or more sources are present. Interference may be constructive or destructive.

REFERENCES

1. Goss S, Johnston R, and Dunn F: Comprehensive compilation of empirical ultrasonic properties of mammalian tissue, J Acoust Soc Am 64:423, 1978.
2. Ophir J: Measurements of ultrasound attenuation in human liver tissue, Ultrasonic Imaging, 1986.
3. Robinson D, Wilson L, and Kossoff G: Shadowing and enhancement in ultrasonic echograms by reflection and refraction, J Clin Ultrasound 9:181, 1981.
4. Wells PNT: Biomedical ultrasonics, New York, 1977, Academic Press, Inc.

Appendix

REVIEW OF MATH CONCEPTS
Exponential notation

Although perhaps not necessary for a cursory understanding of the material, liberal use of exponentials is made in the examples worked out in the text. It is suggested that the student who wishes more than a brief review of this material consult a textbook on college mathematics.

A quantity is usually expressed in scientific notation as a number between 1 and 10 multiplied by 10 raised to the correct power.

$$25 = 2.5 \times 10^1$$
$$693 = 6.93 \times 10^2$$
$$3200 = 3.2 \times 10^3$$
$$6,000,000 = 6 \times 10^6$$
$$0.25 = 2.5 \times 10^{-1}$$
$$0.003 = 3 \times 10^{-3}$$
$$0.00042 = 4.2 \times 10^{-4}$$

In adding or subtracting two numbers expressed with this notation, it is necessary to express both numbers as the same power of 10 first and then carry on with the operation. Thus

$$1.75 \times 10^6 - 3 \times 10^5$$
$$= 1.75 \times 10^6 - 0.3 \times 10^6$$
$$= (1.75 - 0.3) \times 10^6$$
$$= 1.45 \times 10^6$$

$$0.23 + 4.1 \times 10^{-2}$$
$$= 23 \times 10^{-2} + 4.1 \times 10^{-2}$$
$$= (23 + 4.1) \times 10^{-2}$$
$$= 27.1 \times 10^{-2}$$
$$= 2.71 \times 10^{-1}$$

To multiply or divide numbers expressed as 10 to a power, use the formula

$$\frac{a \times 10^m}{b \times 10^n} = \frac{a}{b} \times 10^{m-n}$$

and

$$(a \times 10^m) \times (b \times 10^n) = (a \times b) \times 10^{m+n}$$

This means that exponential values are *substracted* from each other when you divide and *added* to each other when you multiply.

Sine and cosine functions

The sine and cosine are trigonometric functions used quite often in acoustics and descriptions of wave phenomena. They are defined with the use of the right triangle shown in the following diagram. Let *a*, *b*, and *c* be the sides of this triangle, as shown. For angle B

$$\sin B \equiv \frac{b}{c}$$
$$\cos B \equiv \frac{a}{c}$$

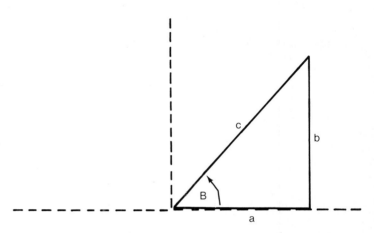

(The notation $\equiv$ means "is defined as.") It is easy to see that when angle B is small, side b is also very small and sin B is nearly 0. If angle B is small, side a is almost equal to side c. It follows then that the cosine for a very small angle is nearly 1. Similarly, as angle B approaches 90 degrees, sin B goes to 1 and cos B goes to 0.

A graph of cos B and sin B when angle B is between 0 and 90 degrees is shown below:

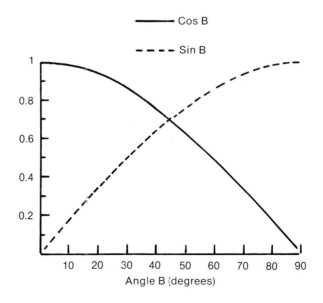

Summary of important units

The units commonly used in ultrasound are as follows:

Quantity	Unit	Abbreviation
Length	meters	m
Mass	kilograms	kg
Time	seconds	s
Speed	meters/second	m/s
Period	inverse seconds	sec^{-1}
Area	square meters or meters squared	m^2
Volume	cubic meters or meters cubed	m^3
Frequency	cycles per second (hertz)	cps(Hz)
Density	kilograms per cubic meter	kg/m^3
Impedance	kilograms per square meter per second	$kg/m^2/s$
Attenuation	decibels	dB
Attenuation coefficient	decibels per centimeter	dB/cm
Power	watts	W
Intensity	watts per square meter	W/m^2
Amplifier gain	decibels	dB

Following are the more commonly used metric system conversions:

Prefix	Meaning	Abbreviation
micro	10^{-6}	μ
milli	10^{-3}	m
centi	10^{-2}	c
deci	10^{-1}	d
kilo	10^3	k
Mega	10^6	M

2

Properties of Ultrasound Transducers

JAMES A. ZAGZEBSKI

The general term *transducer* refers to any device that is used to convert energy from one form to another. In medicine many different types of transducers are used to measure patient or laboratory data. Most of these respond to the parameter of interest (e.g., pressure, electrolyte levels, or movement) by converting energy into electric signals, which can be applied to electronic instruments for processing and display. *Ultrasonic transducers* convert acoustic energy to electric signals and electric energy to acoustic energy. These transducers can be used both as detectors and transmitters of ultrasonic waves.

THE PIEZOELECTRIC EFFECT

The most common type of transducer used in medical ultrasound employs the *piezoelectric effect*. The word piezoelectric originates from the Greek *piezein*, to press. The piezoelectric effect was discovered in the 1880s by Pierre and Jacques Curie. They discovered that when a force is applied perpendicular to the faces of a quartz crystal, an electric charge results (Fig. 2-1). This charge can be detected and amplified, producing a useful electric signal. Thus the crystal can be used to detect the mechan-

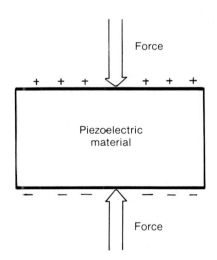

FIG. 2-1. The piezoelectric effect. A force applied to opposite faces of materials that are piezoelectric results in an electrical signal.

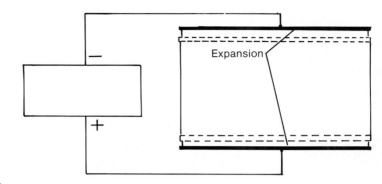

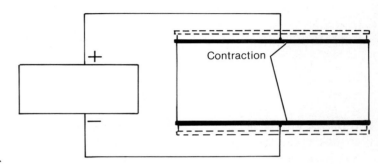

FIG. 2-2. The reverse piezoelectric effect. Application of an electric signal causes the element to contract or expand.

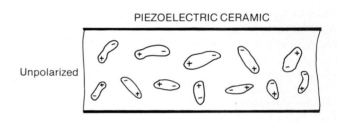

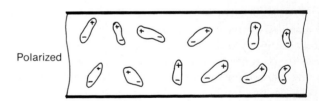

FIG. 2-3. Rough schema of piezoelectric ceramic material. *Top,* before polarization; *bottom,* after polarization. Note the partially aligned microscopic crystals in the polarized material. The dark lines on the top and bottom are electrodes adhered to the element.

ical vibrations of a sound wave. Conversely, if an electric signal is applied to the crystal, expansion or contraction of the crystal takes place, depending on the polarity of the signal (Fig. 2-2). Oscillating signals cause the crystal to vibrate, resulting in propagation of sound waves into the medium with which the crystal is in contact.

A number of substances, including quartz and tourmaline, are naturally piezoelectric and have been used for medical ultrasound transducers. Quartz is still used, especially for precision acoustic measurements in the laboratory and occasionally for high-power applications. However, it has been superseded for the most part by *piezoelectric ceramic* transducer elements.

Ceramic elements, such as *lead zirconate titanate* (PZT), consist of mixtures of microscopic crystals randomly oriented throughout the volume of the element (Fig. 2-3). Mechanically, these materials are somewhat brittle and may be damaged if dropped or pounded. During manufacturing they can be shaped into various configurations, such as rectangular slabs, planar disks, or concave disks. To be useful as medical transducers, these ceramics must first be *polarized,* which is done by heating the material above the Curie temperature (365° C for PZT) and applying a very high voltage across its face. This results in partial alignment, or *polarization,* of the microscopic crystals, as shown in the lower part of Fig. 2-3. The element is then cooled with the voltage still applied. It will now remain polarized with the voltage removed and exhibit piezoelectric properties. The element can lose its piezoelectric properties (become depolarized) if it is inadvertently heated above the Curie temperature.

Besides ceramic elements, two other types of piezoelectric materials should be mentioned at this point. Polyvinylidene diflouride (PVF$_2$) is a piezoelectric material available in thin membranes that look like plastic sandwich wrap. This material is used for constructing miniature *hydrophones,*[1] which are small ultrasound transducers for measuring the acoustic output of medical ultrasound equipment (see Chapter 7). *Composite ceramic* materials are mixtures of ordinary piezoelectric ceramics and an epoxy or rubber-based material. Some researchers have found that composite elements possess advantages over ordinary ceramic elements for efficient transmission of well-defined sound beams into tissue.[2] In the remain-

PLANE DISK TRANSDUCER ELEMENTS

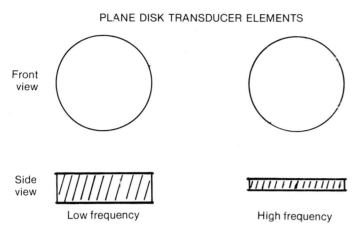

FIG. 2-4. The thickness of the piezoelectric element determines the element's resonance frequency.

der of this chapter, however, we assume ordinary ceramic elements in our examples of ultrasonic transducer construction and operation.

A piezoelectric transducer element has a natural resonance frequency. At this frequency it is most efficient in converting electric energy to acoustic energy and vice versa. The resonance frequency is determined mainly by the *thickness* of the piezoelectric element: thin elements have high resonance frequencies and thick elements have lower resonance frequencies (Fig. 2-4).

TRANSDUCER CONSTRUCTION
Basic components

Different diagnostic ultrasound instruments require different transducer designs. Some general properties of transducer design and performance will be illustrated by considering a specific type of transducer used in pulse-echo work—a single-element nonfocused probe. Focusing techniques, transducer arrays, and transducer designs for continuous wave Doppler applications will be discussed later.

A diagram of a single-element nonfocused transducer is presented in Fig. 2-5. Such a transducer is used both to produce brief pulses (or bursts) of ultrasound and to de-

tect echoes resulting from reflections of the sound pulses as they travel through the medium. The piezoelectric element for this application consists of a flat circular disk. The thickness of the element is selected in accordance with the desired operating frequency of the transducer. The element is mounted coaxially in a cylindrical case, and the ultrasound beam travels to the right in the diagram. Acoustic insulation such as rubber or cork is necessary to avoid coupling ultrasonic energy to the case. A metal electric shield prevents pickup of extraneous electric noise signals by the transducer leads. Such signals are undesirable because they contribute to excessive noise on a display during echo detection. Wires that connect to a tuning coil and then to the external connectors provide electric contact between the transducer element and the instrument.

Damping

Pulsed transducers are excited by a short burst of electric energy from a pulser. In response to this excitation pulse the transducer element "rings," vibrating at its resonance frequency. Alternatively, the transducer may be driven with an oscillating electric signal whose frequency is the same as that of the transducer's. The time required for the ringing to decrease to a negligible level following excitation, the *ring down time,* is referred to as the *pulse duration.* The pulse duration, *PD,* is given by the following expression:

$$PD = N_c \times T \qquad (2\text{-}1)$$

where N_c is the number of cycles of oscillation of the element after it is pulsed, and T is the period (see Equation 1-1). The pulse duration must be kept as low as practical to obtain good axial resolution. This is done by reducing N_c or T or both.

Example: What is the duration of a 5 MHz pulse if the transducer rings for 3 cycles?

Solution: Recall from Equation 1-1 that the period, T, is the inverse of the frequency. Consequently,

$$PD = N_c \times T$$
$$= N_c/f$$
$$= \frac{3}{5 \times 10^6/s}$$
$$= 0.6 \ \mu s$$

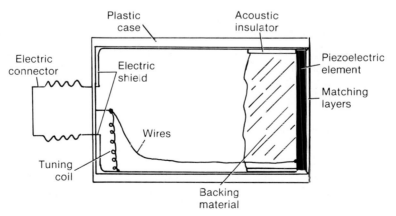

FIG. 2-5. Schema of a single-element nonfocused transducer used in pulse-echo applications. The sound beam emerges toward the right.

Table 2-1 Acoustic Impedances of Materials Relevant to Transducer Design

Material	Impedance (rayls)
Piezoelectric ceramic (lead zirconate titanate)	30×10^6
Backing material (without impedance-matching layers on transducer face)	Matched to that of ceramic element
Matching layers*	7×10^6
Typical soft tissue	1.7×10^6

*Actual values may differ depending on state-of-the-art manufacturing techniques.

It is easy to see that if the frequency *increases* and the number of cycles in the pulse remains the same, the pulse duration *decreases,* and vice versa.

N_c, the number of cycles in the pulse, may be minimized by *damping* the vibration of the transducer as quickly as possible following excitation. The backing material of some transducers plays a major role in *damping* out the transducer vibrations. This material needs to have two properties to facilitate this role. First, its acoustic impedance must be comparable to the impedance of the piezoelectric element (Table 2-1). This reduces reflections at the transducer-to-backing material interface so that any energy propagated in the backward direction is transmitted out of the element. Second, it is filled with a special preparation so that sound waves transmitted into it are completely absorbed. A heavy sound-absorbing backing material serves to damp the vibrations of the piezoelectric element, resulting in short-duration acoustic pulses transmitted into the medium.

Quarterwave and multiple matching layers

Many modern transducers use *impedance-matching layers,* which both improve the sensitivity of the transducer (the ability to detect very weak echoes) and change the requirements for the backing material. Analogous to the optical transmission properties of special coatings on non-glare glass, impedance-matching layers provide efficient transmission of sound waves from the transducer element to soft tissue and vice versa.

Inspection of Table 2-1 shows that the acoustic impedance of piezoelectric ceramics, such as PZT, is about 20 times the impedance of soft tissue. This is a significant mismatch, producing a reflection coefficient of 0.82 if an element is used in contact with the skin surface. (It never is, but let's continue the discussion anyway.) The presence of a plastic *wear face* between the element and the skin surface improves the situation somewhat but does not provide the best results possible.

Transmission of sound into soft tissue is improved when matching layers are attached to the transducer element. These layers make it "appear" to the transducer that the tissue has the same impedance as the piezoelectric element. Hence the term *impedance matching* is used. A single "quarterwave" matching layer has the following properties:

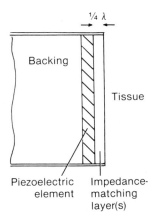

FIG. 2-6. Attachment of impedance matching layers to the front face of the transducer provides more efficient transmission of sound from the transducer into the patient and vice versa.

1. Its acoustic impedance, Z_m, is intermediate between the impedance of the transducer element, Z_t, and the impedance of soft tissue, Z_{st}. (Actually

$$Z_m = \sqrt{Z_{st} \times Z_t}$$

is the appropriate value.)
2. Its thickness exactly equals one fourth of the ultrasonic wavelength in the layer.

If these properties are achieved, there is no reflection at a soft tissue–transducer interface; hence sound transmission is very efficient (Fig. 2-6).

As will be seen later in this chapter, a pulsed transducer emits not a single ultrasonic frequency but rather a *spectrum* of frequencies. A single quarterwave matching layer is exactly one quarter wavelength only for one frequency. Thus all frequencies in a pulsed waveform are not efficiently transmitted with a single matching layer. Transducer manufacturers overcome this problem by designing transducers with *multiple* matching layers adhered to the face of the element. Multiple matching layers provide efficient sound transmission between the piezoelectric element and soft tissue for a range, or spectrum, of ultrasound frequencies.

We saw that a short-duration pulse is produced by damping of the vibrations of the piezoelectric element after it is pulsed. Damping can be achieved by using a heavy absorbing material in contact with the back of the element. This reduces the transducer efficiency somewhat because energy is lost in the backing material. With matching layers, however, it is not always necessary to couple energy out of the back of the transducer to damp the vibrations because the ultrasonic energy is very efficiently transmitted into the patient. This is another way in which matching layers can improve the sensitivity of ultrasound transducers.

TRANSDUCER FREQUENCY CHARACTERISTICS

In pulse-echo ultrasound the transducer is excited with a brief electric signal, after which it oscillates near its *resonance* frequency. As has been pointed out, the resonance frequency of a transducer is determined for the most part by the thickness of the piezoelectric element. Other fac-

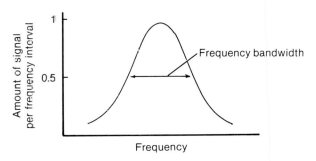

FIG. 2-8. Frequency spectrum and bandwidth of an ultrasound pulsed signal.

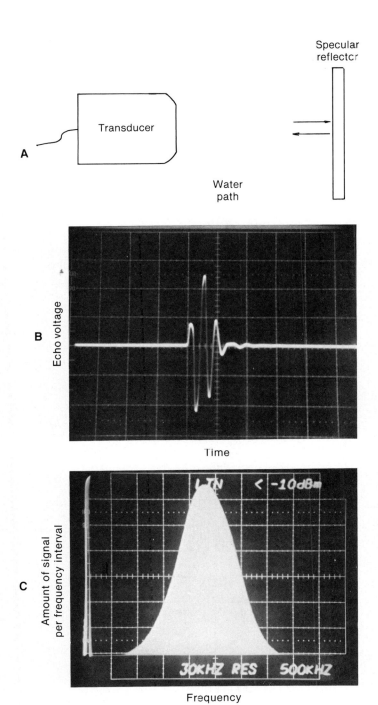

FIG. 2-7. **A,** Arrangement used to study the echo signal waveform for a pulse-echo transducer. **B,** Echo signal waveform obtained from the planar reflector. **C,** Frequency spectrum of the waveform in **B.**

mined by *spectral analysis* of an echo signal obtained from a planar smooth reflector.

For an illustration of how this works, consider the experimental arrangement shown in Fig. 2-7. The beam from a pulsed transducer is directed toward a large smooth reflector. The reflector is so oriented that the largest possible echo signal amplitude is obtained at the transducer. A typical echo signal is shown in Fig. 2-7, *B*. Instruments are available that can be used to measure the relative amount of signal at different frequencies in a pulsed waveform of this type. They are called *spectrum analyzers*. If the signal shown in Fig. 2-7, *B,* is applied to a spectrum analyzer, a record as illustrated in Fig. 2-7, *C,* is obtained.

The spectral display represents a plot of the fraction of signal within a given frequency interval versus the frequency (Fig. 2-8). The curve usually peaks out at or near the resonance frequency of the transducer, with a gradual falloff on either side of the maximum value. A frequency plot of this type is one performance measurement applied to transducers by the manufacturer.

The *frequency bandwidth* is a measure of the spread of frequencies in the plots of Figs. 2-7 and 2-8. It turns out that, for a given resonance frequency, the shorter the pulse duration the wider the frequency bandwidth, and, vice versa, the longer the pulse duration the narrower the frequency bandwidth.* Pulse duration and frequency bandwidth are illustrated for three hypothetical waveforms in Fig. 2-9.

TRANSDUCERS AND SPATIAL RESOLUTIONS
Spatial detail in ultrasound

In an ultrasound examination, spatial resolution refers to how closely positioned two reflectors or scattering regions can be to one another and still be identified as separate reflectors on a display. Generally speaking, we wish to obtain the best possible resolution, since this usually means maximum information and best detail in the examination. In nearly all instances it is the design and operation of the ultrasound transducer that most influences the spatial resolution.

tors—including the mounting of the transducer element in the assembly, the precise thickness of the front surface matching layers, and the electric components within the transducer assembly (e.g., the tuning coil in Fig. 2-5) and the ultrasound instrument—also can affect the frequency characteristics.

A pulse of sound emitted by a transducer contains ultrasonic energy at the resonance frequency of the transducer. It also contains energy at frequencies above and below the resonance frequency, covering a fairly wide spectrum. The frequency range represented in the pulse is described in terms of the *frequency bandwidth* of the ultrasound transducer. The bandwidth may be deter-

---

*Some authors describe the frequency bandwidth using what is referred to as the Q of the transducer. Q stands for "quality factor" and denotes the ease with which the transducer maintains its oscillations. A transducer with a low Q has a short pulse duration and a broad bandwidth.

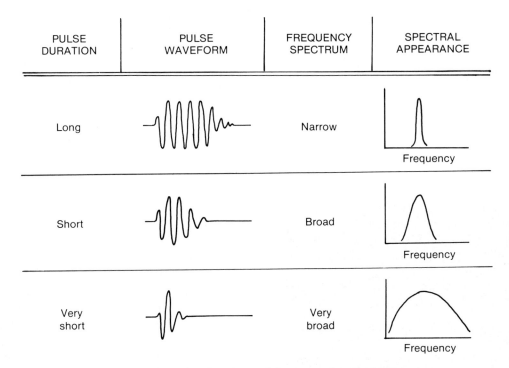

FIG. 2-9.   Relationship between pulse duration and frequency bandwidth for a pulsed waveform.

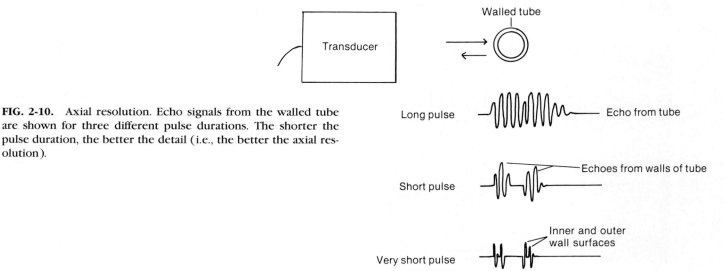

FIG. 2-10.   Axial resolution. Echo signals from the walled tube are shown for three different pulse durations. The shorter the pulse duration, the better the detail (i.e., the better the axial resolution).

For stationary sound beams and within the scanning plane of scanned ultrasound beams we specify both the *axial resolution* and the *lateral resolution.* These are discussed in detail below.

Axial resolution

Axial resolution refers to the *minimum* reflector spacing *along the axis of a sound beam* that results in separate, distinguishable echoes on the display. Axial resolution is determined mainly by the duration of the ultrasonic pulse transmitted into the medium. The longer the pulse duration, the worse will be the axial resolution; and, in general, the shorter the pulse duration the better will be the axial resolution.

The relationship between axial resolution and pulse duration is illustrated schematically in Fig. 2-10, wherein an ultrasound transducer is positioned to obtain echo sig-

nals from a walled tube. In the top waveform the pulse duration is depicted as extremely long, so that it extends simultaneously over the entire tube. A single echo signal is detectable from the tube. In the middle waveform the pulse duration is depicted as short enough that each wall is insonified by the beam at different times. Now separate echo signals are detectable from the two walls of the tube. Finally, the bottom waveform depicts a situation in which the pulse duration is extremely short compared to the other two. The very closely spaced inner and outer margins of the walls are resolved with the short-duration pulse in this schematic representation.

The pulse duration is given in Equation 2-1 above. For a fixed number of cycles in the pulse, short pulse durations are obtained by using high-frequency transducers, resulting in a shorter period (T in the equation). For a given resonance frequency, short pulses are obtained by

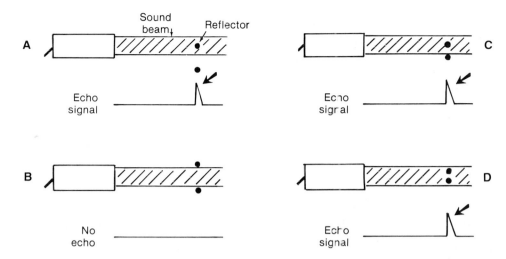

FIG. 2-11. Lateral resolution. When the reflector separation is less than the transducer beam width the reflectors cannot be distinguished. The reflectors are resolved (**A** and **B**) when they are sufficiently far apart that a null in the echo signal is obtained when the beam passes between them. In **C** and **D** the reflectors are too closely spaced to be detected as separate, individual echo sources.

rapidly damping the "ringing" of the transducer after it is excited, thereby making N_c, the number of cycles in the pulse, small. As already mentioned, damping is done by means of heavy absorbing backing material and/or matching layers attached to the front of the element. The relationship between pulse duration, axial resolution, and frequency bandwidth (for a fixed resonance frequency) is illustrated as follows:

Pulse duration	Axial resolution	Frequency bandwidth
Long	Poorer	Narrow
Short	Better	Wide

Lateral resolution

Lateral resolution refers to the ability of the instrument to distinguish two closely spaced reflectors that are positioned *perpendicular* to the axis of the ultrasound beam. For pulse-echo ultrasound the lateral resolution is most closely related to the transducer's displayed *beam width* at the depth of interest. This is illustrated in Fig. 2-11. If the spacing between the two reflectors is greater than the displayed beam width, their separation can be appreciated because of the absence of an echo from the space between. The reflectors are then said to be "resolved." On the other hand, if reflectors are separated by a distance less than the displayed beam width, then echoes from both reflectors are picked up simultaneously and the fact that there are two reflectors rather than a single reflector cannot be established from the echo information. As we will show in the next discussion, the transducer beam width varies with distance from the transducer; hence the lateral resolution also is depth dependent.

TRANSDUCER BEAM CHARACTERISTICS
Beam directivity

In the previous discussion we saw that the displayed beam width effects the lateral resolution of an ultrasound instrument. In this discussion we will examine the sound beam pattern for single-element transducers and study how the width of the beam at different depths depends on the frequency and diameter of the ultrasound transducer.

Many sources of audible sound appear as point sources in that the sound energy emitted radiates outward in all directions. An ultrasound beam produced by a medical transducer, on the other hand, is very *directional*. Most of the acoustic energy in the beam is confined to a region close to the axis of the transducer. This directionality is a result of the dimensions of the transducer face being large compared to our "acoustic yardstick," the ultrasound wavelength. Typically the diameter of the face is 20 or more wavelengths at the frequencies used.

Near field versus far field

The beam produced by an unfocused circular transducer may be modeled as shown in Fig. 2-12, wherein two distinct regions are identified. The *near field*, or Fresnel zone, extends from the transducer face outward approximately to the distance:

$$NFL = a^2/\lambda \qquad (2\text{-}2)$$

where *NFL* stands for near field length, a is the transducer radius, and λ is the ultrasonic wavelength.

The near field is characterized by point-to-point fluctuations in the amplitude and intensity of the ultrasound beam, both along and perpendicular to the axis of the beam. This can be demonstrated with the help of *lateral beam profiles* illustrated in Fig. 2-13. Each profile is recorded by measuring the amplitude of an echo from a small reflector at various points as the reflector is translated perpendicular to the axis of the transducer beam. One then plots the echo amplitude versus distance from the axis. Five such plots make up the lateral beam profile set in Fig. 2-13.

The two profiles closest to the transducer in Fig. 2-13 illustrate the point-to-point fluctuations in beam strength

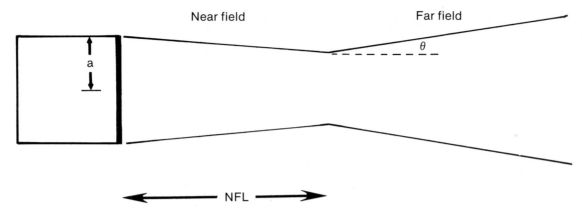

FIG. 2-12. Schema of the beam from an unfocused circular transducer, showing the near field length, *NFL*, and the angle of beam divergence, θ, in the far field.

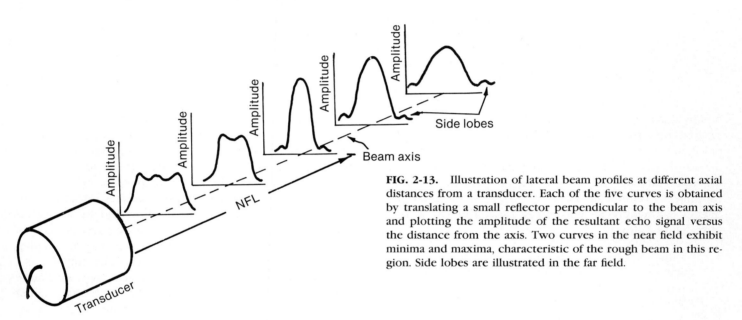

FIG. 2-13. Illustration of lateral beam profiles at different axial distances from a transducer. Each of the five curves is obtained by translating a small reflector perpendicular to the beam axis and plotting the amplitude of the resultant echo signal versus the distance from the axis. Two curves in the near field exhibit minima and maxima, characteristic of the rough beam in this region. Side lobes are illustrated in the far field.

mentioned earlier. Thus the beam within the near field appears rough with peaks and valleys. As the axial distance approaches the near field length, the profiles are smooth with a maximum along the beam axis.

The region of the beam beyond the *NFL* is called the *far field* or Fraunhofer zone of the ultrasound transducer. Beam profiles obtained in this region exhibit smooth curves, as illustrated in Fig. 2-13. In the far field the beam gradually becomes weaker and begins to diverge with increasing distance from the transducer. This is shown by the central peak of the profiles becoming progressively smaller and each profile widening. The divergence angle, shown by θ in Fig. 2-12, depends on the wavelength and transducer size. It is given by the relationship

$$\sin \theta = 0.61 \, \lambda/a \qquad (2\text{-}3)$$

where λ and *a* are the same as in Equation 2-2. This could also be written as

$$\sin \theta = (0.61 \, c)/fa \qquad (2\text{-}4)$$

by substituting the now familiar expression for the wavelength into Equation 2-3.

Dependencies on transducer frequency and size

We will illustrate important properties of the transducer beam parameters with some examples.

Example: What is the near field length for a 2.25 MHz 13 mm diameter transducer?

Solution: You are given the diameter and hence the transducer radius, *a*, which is 6.5 mm. You need to know the wavelength, λ, before computing the *NFL*. From Chapter 1,

$$\lambda = c/f$$

where *c* is the speed of sound and *f* the frequency. First, find

$$\lambda = \frac{1540 \text{ m/s}}{2.25 \times 10^6/\text{s}}$$
$$= 6.8 \times 10^{-4} \text{ m}$$
$$= 0.68 \text{ mm}$$

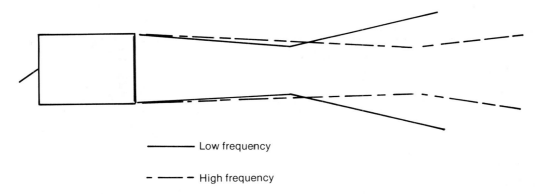

FIG. 2-14. Changes in the near field length and the far field divergence angle with changes in frequency for an unfocused transducer.

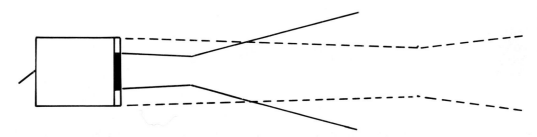

FIG. 2-15. Changes in the near field length and the far field divergence angle with changes in the radius or diameter of the transducer face. (This assumes the same frequency.)

Then, from Equation 2-2,

$$NFL = \frac{a^2}{\lambda}$$
$$= \frac{(6.5 \text{ mm})^2}{0.68 \text{ mm}}$$
$$= 62 \text{ mm}$$
$$= 6.2 \text{ cm}$$

The near field for this transducer extends out to a distance of 6.2 cm. Now consider a similar situation, only one in which the ultrasound frequency is greater.

Example: What is the near field length for a 5 MHz 13 mm diameter transducer?

Solution: First, compute the wavelength.

$$\lambda = \frac{1540 \text{ m/s}}{5.0 \times 10^6/\text{s}}$$
$$= 3 \times 10^{-4} \text{ m}$$
$$= 0.3 \text{ mm}$$

Again, from Equation 2-2,
$$NFL = (6.5 \text{ mm})^2/0.3 \text{ mm}$$
$$= 140 \text{ mm}$$
$$= 14 \text{ cm}$$

From these two examples we see that the *NFL* increases with increasing frequency.

Equation 2-4 above illustrates that the divergence angle also depends on the transducer frequency. The sine of the divergence angle is inversely proportional to the frequency. Since the sine of an angle *increases* with increasing angle (if the angle is between 0 and 90°, as shown in the figure in Appendix 1, pages 15 and 16), as frequency *increases,* the divergence angle *decreases.*

Thus, for a given transducer size:
1. The *NFL* increases with increasing frequency.
2. Beam divergence is less for higher frequencies.
The dependence of these two beam characteristics on transducer frequency is illustrated in Fig. 2-14.

The *NFL* also increases with increasing transducer size. This is readily seen upon inspection of Equation 2-2. Since *NFL* is proportional to the square of the radius, doubling the transducer radius quadruples the *NFL*. The divergence angle in the far field, on the other hand, **decreases** with increasing transducer radius, as shown in Equation 2-3. The dependence on transducer diameter may be summarized as follows:
1. For a given frequency, the *NFL* extends farther for larger diameter transducers.
2. For a given frequency, beam divergence in the far field *decreases* with *increasing* transducer size.

The beam patterns shown in Figs. 2-14 and 2-15 give some hints as to how the lateral resolution behaves with frequency and transducer size. The smaller divergence angle with higher frequencies indicates that lateral resolution would generally be improved if higher frequencies were used. Also, at large distances from the transducer (Fig. 2-15) a larger-diameter transducer results in better lateral resolution than does a smaller-diameter transducer.

Side lobes

In the data in Fig. 2-13, *side lobes* in the transducer beam profile are evident. Side lobes are energy in the sound beam that falls outside the main lobe (or main beam). Generally speaking, strong side lobes are not desirable because this would degrade lateral resolution.

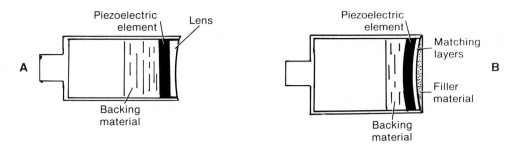

FIG. 2-16.   Single-element transducer focusing. **A,** With a lens; **B,** with a curved transducer element.

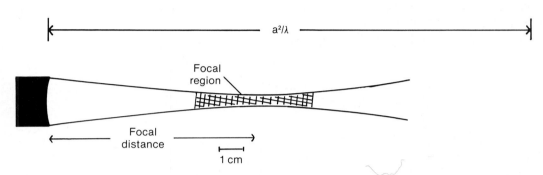

FIG. 2-17.   Schema of a focused transducer beam. The sketch is taken from data for a 3.5 MHz, 19 mm diameter transducer, and the focal distance is 8 cm. The focal region, where the beam cross-sectional area is less than or equal to two times the area at the focal distance, is the crosshatched region.

Side lobes are cut down considerably in pulse-echo ultrasound because of the presence of broad bandwidth pulses. The position of a side lobe differs for each frequency component in the pulse, so they smear each other out. For single-element weakly focused transducers, the side lobes usually are suppressed as a result of the pulsing characteristics. Thus under normal circumstances they are probably inconsequential to the image.

Sidelobes can be reduced further by *apodization.* In this process the amplitude of vibration of the transducer surface is made to decrease gradually from the center to the edge, rather than remaining uniform over the surface and ending abruptly at the edge. It applies mainly to some array transducers. (See Apodization of Arrays, p. 30.)

FOCUSED TRANSDUCERS

Single-element transducers may be focused by using an acoustic lens along with a planar piezoelectric element or by using an element that is curved. Both techniques are illustrated in Fig. 2-16. The curved element is the more common approach employed with single-element pulse-echo transducers. As shown in Fig. 2-16, both the transducer element and the matching layers are curved. The latter is done so the correct matching layer thickness can be maintained over the face of the transducer. Usually the concave center is filled in with material to help maintain transducer contact with the skin.

Focusing has the effect of narrowing the beam profile and increasing the amplitude of echoes from reflectors over a limited axial range in comparison to an equivalent unfocused transducer (here equivalent refers to one having the same diameter and frequency).

The beam margins* for a focused transducer are illustrated schematically in Fig. 2-17. Also shown is the distance, a^2/λ, for this transducer; it would be the *NFL* if the beam were not focused. The *focal distance* is the distance to the plane where the beam width is narrowest. The *focal zone* corresponds to the region over which the width of the beam is less than two times the width at the focal distance.

The lens or the element curvature plays a major role in aiming the focal distance to a particular depth. However, most focused transducers used for scanning are "weakly focused." This means that their beam patterns depend on the transducer diameter and frequency as well as the curvature of the element. The following general principles apply to weakly focused transducers:

1. Focusing, or beam narrowing, always occurs in the near field of an equivalent unfocused transducer. If the curvature of the element or lens were such as to aim the focal distance into the far field, focusing would still take place in the near field.
2. The actual focal distance falls short of the aimed at focus, the latter determined by the element or the lens curvature.
3. Identical transducers (same diameter, same curvature) with different frequencies have slightly different focusing properties. Higher frequencies tend to focus closer

---

*The beam, of course, does not end abruptly at the sketched boundaries in any of these diagrams; the amplitude varies with distance from the axis, as the beam profiles in Fig. 2-13 indicate. The sketched boundaries in Figs. 2-12, 2-14, and 2-15 are useful for indicating the general shape of the beam.

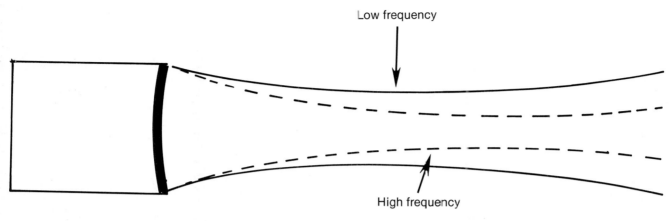

FIG. 2-18. Comparisons of focusing effects for transducers of the same diameter and curvature, but different frequency. The higher frequency transducer has a narrower beam in the focal region than the lower frequency transducer.

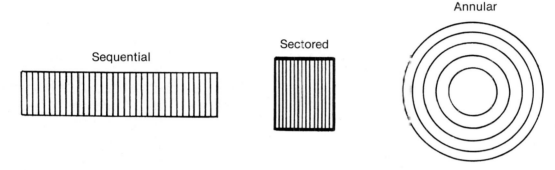

FIG. 2-19. Three commonly used transducer array geometries. Each view is from the surface of the array, with the sound beam emerging out of the plane of the figure. (Note linear and phased arrays usually have thinner elements than presented in the illustration.)

to the aimed at focus; lower frequencies tend to focus at a point falling farther short of the aimed at focus.

4. For identically shaped transducers (same diameter, same curvature) with different frequencies, the higher-frequency transducers have narrower beams in the focal region than do lower-frequency probes (Fig. 2-18). With a single-element transducer the focal distance is fixed during the manufacturing process. Therefore in a clinical situation a transducer's frequency and dimensions must be chosen carefully to optimize the resolution over the region of interest. In the next section we will see that transducer arrays can provide more flexibility in terms of focusing characteristics of transducers.

TRANSDUCER ARRAYS
Types of arrays

In some instruments transducer arrays are used rather than single-element transducers. An array transducer assembly consists of a group of piezoelectric elements, each of which can be excited individually and whose echo signals can be detected and amplified separately.

Three types of arrays are shown in Fig. 2-19. Sequential (linear) arrays and electronically sectored (phased) arrays consist of a group of rectangularly shaped piezoelectric elements arranged side by side as shown. Annular arrays consist of a circular target and bull's eye arrangement of elements.

Advantages offered by arrays, depending on the configuration, include their potential for electronically varying the focal distance and for automatic variations in the aperture size. These two features enhance the spatial resolution capabilities of an ultrasound instrument. In addition, both linear and phased arrays provide the capability for electronically sweeping a sound beam during scanning. Thus scanning can be done without mechanical movement within a transducer assembly or scan head. This is discussed in Chapter 3.

Beam formation with an array

A sound beam is produced by a transducer array by sending individual electrical excitation signals to each element used to form the beam. With linear arrays a small group of elements is involved for each beam, but with sectored and annular arrays all elements usually are involved in transmitting and detecting echoes for every beam. The emerging sound beam is the sum of individual beams from each of the elements (Fig. 2-20). Since the width of an individual element may be quite small, often less than a half wavelength, the transmitted beam from a single element by itself would be broad. The wider aperture formed by a group of elements produces a narrower sound beam in the patient. This beam may be focused by manipulation of individual signals applied to different elements.

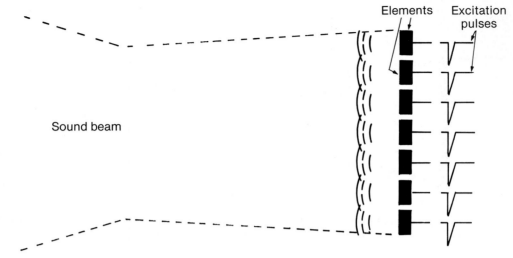

FIG. 2-20.   Formation of a sound beam by a group of elements in an array.

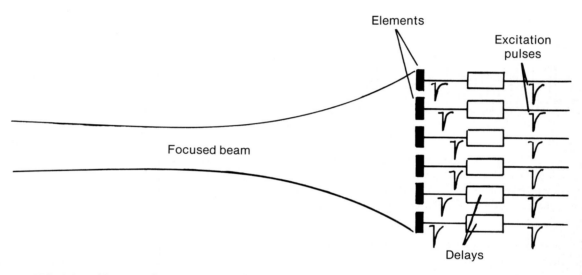

FIG. 2-21.   Transmit focusing applied to an array. Time delays applied to signals for individual elements have the same effect on the emerging beam as a curved element.

Transmit focus

When all elements in an array or group are excited precisely at the same time, the effect is analogous to the situation in which a planar unfocused transducer element is pulsed. The resultant beam is directional but unfocused. Electronic focusing can be achieved by introducing time delays in the application of the excitation pulses to the separate elements (Fig. 2-21). In this case the wavefronts emerging from the transducer converge toward the focal position, producing a narrower sound beam over a selected region than when no focusing is used. With the time delays in action, the situation is as though a focusing lens or a curved piezoelectric element were producing the beam.

Time delays are produced by electronic delay lines, which hold an electric signal for a fixed time, depending on the delay line setting, before passing the signal on. If the delays are such that the inner elements of a cluster are excited a bit later than the outer elements in the sequence suggested in Fig. 2-21, the beam emerging from the transducer will converge toward a focal position.

Unlike the focal distance of a single-element transducer, the focal distance of an array may be varied electronically by changing the electronic delay sequence. Thus arrays allow user selection of the *transmit focal zone.*

Some arrays provide simultaneous *multiple transmit focal zones,* greatly expanding the effective focal region. Multiple transmit focal zones are obtained by transmitting a sound beam with the focal zone at a particular depth setting, receiving echo signals from that depth setting only by rejecting echo signals from other depths, transmitting another sound beam along the same beam axis as the first but with a different focal zone, and so on. When multiple transmit zones are applied, individual acoustic pulses must be transmitted into the body for each transmit focal distance or zone. That is, an individual outgoing sound pulse produced by an array may only be focused at a single depth; thus simultaneous multiple transmit focal zones are obtained at the expense of increased scanning times for a single image. Although it takes several acoustic pulses transmitted along the beam

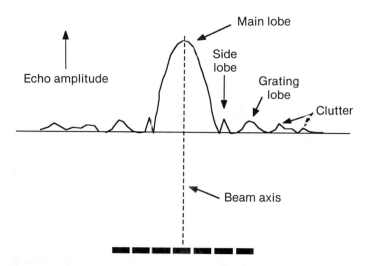

FIG. 2-25. Schema of lateral beam profile for an array transducer assembly. Just as in Fig. 2-13, the plot is the amplitude of an echo versus distance from the beam axis. Besides side lobes, additional off-axis sensitivity is depicted, due to grating lobes and clutter.

Performance differences

Both annular arrays and rectangularly shaped arrays can provide multiple transmit focal zones, dynamic receive focusing, and dynamic aperture. However, there are potential differences in the performances of annular and rectangularly shaped arrays because of the nature of the two types of beams. With most current linear and phased arrays, beam focusing in the slice thickness direction is done by using a fixed focal length acoustic lens. Thus the extended focal region provided by electronic focusing only applies in the image plane. In Fig. 2-26, A, the slice thickness direction is vertical on the diagram. The diagram depicts the slice thickness as quite wide at the transducer face, narrowing considerable at a midrange, corresponding to the focal length of the above-mentioned acoustic lens, and widening out at more distant ranges. For this array the slice thickness may change with distance much more extensively than the lateral resolution changes.

On the other hand, for annular arrays the electronic beam formation processes apply both in the image plane and perpendicular to the image plane because the beam is symmetric about its axis (Fig. 2-26, B). Thus the slice thickness improves (gets smaller) to the same degree that lateral resolution improves when electronic focusing is present.

TRANSDUCER SELECTION

The label printed on most transducers or transducer assemblies provides information relevant to their suitability for specific diagnostic applications.

Important information includes, in most cases, the following:
1. Transducer frequency (sometimes referred to as the center frequency)
2. Element dimensions

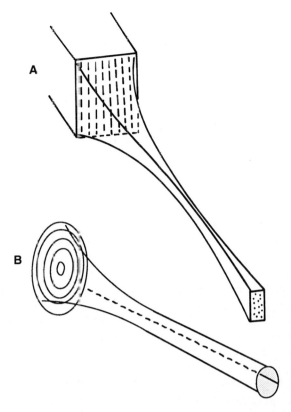

FIG. 2-26. A, Focusing a rectangular array in to narrow the slice thickness over a limited range. B, Focusing an annular array, where the slice thickness and the lateral resolution are the same.

3. Focal distance
4. Focal region

For instruments having interchangeable transducers, significant improvements in image quality and diagnostic information can be realized by optimizing the transducer for the study at hand. It should go without saying that a transducer whose focal region encompasses the region of interest in the patient is the best one to use for any study. Notice that this usually requires a narrow-diameter high-frequency transducer for structures located close to the probe and a large-diameter probe for deep-lying structures. Although lateral resolution is better at higher frequencies, attenuation may cause difficulty in picking up a deeper-lying structure.

Experience has shown that the detail obtained regarding contrast between different reflectors (differences in echo amplitude) can sometimes be improved by using higher frequencies. Scattering from many structures increases with frequency while reflections from specular interfaces usually do not change with frequency. Thus one effect of using higher-frequency transducers may be to enhance signals from scatterers over echo signals from specular interfaces.

ULTRASOUND TRANSDUCER BEAM FORMATION*

The beam of an ultrasound transducer is somewhat complicated—with minima and maxima in the near field, a

---

*This section may be skipped during the first reading of the chapter.

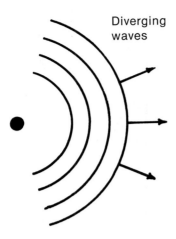

Diverging waves

FIG. 2-27. Wavefront for a point source.

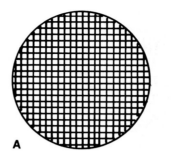
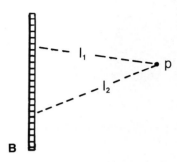

FIG. 2-28. **A,** A transducer can be modeled as a large number of point sources uniformly distributed over its surface. **B,** Side view; the distances l_1 and l_2 could be such that the waves from the two point sources indicated arrive at point p out of phase.

near field length depending on factors such as the transducer radius and the wavelength, and a far field in which the beam gradually diverges with distance. These characteristics are part of the normal diffraction pattern of an ultrasound transducer. *Diffraction* refers to the pattern obtained when waves from different regions of an obstacle or source add up at different points in the beam.

A rather simple source of sound from the point of view of the beam pattern is a point source. This source has dimensions that are small compared to the wavelength. We can simulate a point source by dropping a small stone into a quiet pond of water. Waves produced by this disturbance in the water radiate in all directions, somewhat like the situation shown schematically in Fig. 2-27.

The radiating surface of most diagnostic ultrasound transducers is large compared to the ultrasonic wavelength. Engineers and physicists sometimes describe the sound beam mathematically by conceptually dividing the transducer face into an array of small point sources (Fig. 2-28). A diverging wave, analogous to that shown in Fig. 2-27, emanates from each source. The strength of the beam at any position in the transducer field can be found by adding together the contributions from each point source on the transducer surface. The point sources are sometimes referred to as Huygen sources, and the individual diverging waves as Huygen wavelets.

In Chapter 1 the phenomenon of interference of waves produced by two different sources was discussed. It was mentioned that when both waves reach a spot in space in phase the resultant amplitude at that spot is the sum of the individual wave amplitude. If the waves are out of phase, destructive interference occurs, with the signals partially or totally canceling each other, depending on their relative amplitudes and phases.

We have just seen an ultrasound transducer model described as a distribution of point sources. The amplitude of the beam at any spot in the field is equal to the total effect (or superposition) of waves emitted from all the point sources. Although the diverging waves start from all the point sources in phase, any given spot close to the ultrasound transducer is usually an unequal distance from the various point sources. Therefore the individual wavelets do not necessarily arrive at that spot in phase (Fig. 2-

28). When we sum up the contributions from the entire transducer, we find that the amplitude in the near field of the beam is strongly dependent on the position. At some spots the summation yields a large amplitude whereas at others a smaller net amplitude is obtained. The minima and maxima in the near field of an ultrasound transducer are a result of constructive and destructive interference among waves emanating from different points of the surface of the transducer.

In the far field the beam pattern is smooth, exhibiting none of the minima and maxima found in the near field. This is because the phase differences, due to the different paths from the field pointing to separate regions of the transducer face, are never very great. The far field of a transducer is sometimes characterized as a region where the transducer itself begins to look like a point source as we move farther and farther away.

EFFECTS OF THE FREQUENCY SPECTRUM*

For pulsed transducers a spectrum of frequencies is emitted, and this adds some complexity to our simple beam models. The different components of the frequency spectrum of a pulsed transducer (Fig. 2-7) have slightly different beam-forming characteristics. This follows from reasoning presented for single frequencies. The resultant beam in this case is the net effect of all frequencies available in each pulse—illustrated schematically in Fig. 2-29 for a hypothetical 3.5 MHz center-frequency transducer. Fig. 2-29 illustrates the fact that in the far field the higher-frequency components of a pulsed beam are more directional; that is, they lie closer to the central axis of the beam than do the lower-frequency components. Although the illustration is presented for an unfocused transducer, the same principle applies to focused transducers. During clinical scanning, attenuation in soft tissues modifies the frequency spectrum since higher frequencies in the pulse are attenuated to a greater degree than are lower frequencies. This leads to some loss of resolution in tissue during clinical scanning.[6]

DAMAGE TO TRANSDUCERS

Ultrasound transducers should not be heat sterilized, since this can damage the probe severely. One manifesta-

---

*This section may be skipped during the first reading of the chapter.

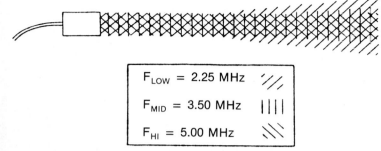

$F_{LOW} = 2.25\ MHz$

$F_{MID} = 3.50\ MHz$

$F_{HI} = 5.00\ MHz$

FIG. 2-29.   Schema of a 13 mm diameter broadband transducer beam.

tion of heat damage is depolarization if the transducer is heated above its Curie temperature. Transducer damage due to heat actually occurs at elevated temperatures that are lower than the Curie temperature, for the different bonding joints and cements in the probe are susceptible to thermal damage.

If a transducer is dropped or sustains an impact, damage to the interior of the probe may occur. A cracked transducer surface can lead to a dangerous situation involving electric shock. This is especially true with the use of acoustic coupling materials, since they also tend to be good conductors. A transducer that has a cracked face should be replaced immediately.

A frequent source of transducer malfunction, especially with probes having built-in cables, is damage to the cable assembly. Twisting and bending that take place quite naturally during handling may cause cable damage and lead to loss of sensitivity, intermittent operation, or excessive electric noise on the display.

Damage to the transducer of static scanners (see next chapter) can also result from excessive wear when it is being attached to the ultrasonic scanner arm, particularly if it is heavily "torqued" to assure good electric contact. Besides damaging the transducer itself, excessive force can damage the connections in the scanner arm. When attaching transducers to threaded connectors, try to obtain a firm snug fit, but avoid excessive force when tightening the probe.

SUMMARY

1. The most common transducer used in medical ultrasound employs the *piezoelectric effect*.

2. The resonance frequency of a piezoelectric transducer is determined mainly by the thickness of the piezoelectric element.

3. The pulse duration is minimized by damping the vibration of the transducer as quickly as possible following excitation.

4. Impedance-matching layers provide efficient transmission of sound waves from the transducer element to soft tissue.

5. Axial resolution is the minimum reflector spacing along the axis of a sound beam resulting in separate, distinguishable echoes on the display. It is closely related to the pulse duration.

6. Lateral resolution is the minimum reflector spacing perpendicular to the axis of the sound beam resulting in separate distinguishable echoes on the display. It is most closely related to the beam width.

7. The near field, or Fresnel zone, extends from the transducer face outward approximately to the distance a^2/λ. The region beyond this distance is the Fraunhofer zone or far field.

8. Single-element transducers are focused using an acoustic lens along with a planar piezoelectric element or using an element that is curved.

9. For identically shaped transducers (same diameter, same curvature) but with different frequencies, higher frequency transducers have narrower beams in the focal region than do lower frequency probes.

10. An array transducer assembly consists of a group of piezoelectric elements, each of which can be excited individually and whose echo signals can be detected and amplified separately.

11. Arrays provide capabilities of electronic focusing during transmission and reception. This is done using time delays in the transmission and/or reception circuitry.

12. Multiple transmit focal zones are produced by an array using a sequence of pulsed beams electronically focused at different depths along each beam line. It takes longer to gather the echo signals when multiple zones are present than when a single transmit focal zone is used.

13. Dynamic receive focusing is done during echo detection with an array using a real-time variation of the electronic time delays applied to signals from individual elements. The process is sometimes referred to as a *tracking lens*.

14. Elevational focus is related to image slice thickness. Current linear and electronically sectored (phased) arrays use fixed focal length lenses to focus in the elevational (slice thickness) direction. For most annular arrays elevational focus is the same as beam focusing in the image plane because the beam is symmetric about its axis.

REFERENCES

1. Lewin P: Miniature piezoelectric polymer ultrasonic hydrophone probes, Ultrasonics 19:213, 1981.
2. Madhaven C, Gururaja T, Srinivassan T, Xu Q, and Newnham R: Fired 0-3 piezoelectric composite materials for biomedical ultrasonic imaging applications. IEEE Ultrasonics Symposium Proceedings, 1987, IEEE, Piscataway, N.J., p. 645.
3. Banjavic R, Zagzebski J, Madsen E, and Goodsitt M: Distortion of ultrasound beams in attenuating media, Acoust Imag Holog 1:165, 1979.
4. Kossoff G: Analysis of focusing action of spherically curved transducers, Ultrasound Med Biol 5:359, 1979.
5. Wells, PNT: Biomedical ultrasonics, New York, 1977, Academic Press, Inc.
6. Zagzebski J, Banjavic R, Madsen E, and Schwabe M: Focused transducer beams in tissue-mimicking material, J Clin Ultrasound 10:159, 1982.

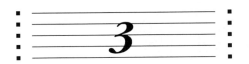

3

Pulse-Echo Ultrasound Instrumentation

JAMES A. ZAGZEBSKI

PULSE-ECHO ULTRASOUND: RANGE EQUATION

This chapter describes instrumentation that uses pulse-echo ultrasound to localize the image structures in the body. In these techniques an ultrasound transducer transmits a short-duration acoustic pulse that propagates in a direction determined by the transducer and at a speed determined by the properties of the medium. Echo signals resulting from scatter and reflection at interfaces in the medium are detected, usually by the same transducer. The time delay between pulse propagation and echo signal detection is used to determine the transducer-to-reflector distance.

The principle is illustrated in Fig. 3-1. A reflector is positioned a distance, d, from the transducer. The time, t_1, it takes for a pulse of sound to travel to the interface is given by

$$t_1 = d/c \qquad (3\text{-}1)$$

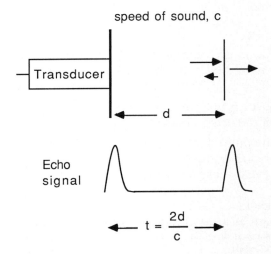

FIG. 3-1. Demonstration of pulse-echo ultrasound. The time, t, required to pick up an echo is related to the reflector distance, d, and the speed of sound, c.

where c is the speed of sound in the medium. We assume the interface reflects part of the incident pulse; it takes an additional time t_1 for the echo signal to travel back to the transducer. The total delay time between pulse transmission and echo detection, t, is therefore

$$t = 2d/c \qquad (3\text{-}2)$$

So, if the speed of sound, c, and the reflector distance, d, are known, the delay time can be determined.

Example: If the speed of sound is 1540 m/s and a reflector is positioned 1 cm from the transducer, how long does it take a pulse of sound to propagate 1 cm, be reflected, and return to the transducer?

Solution: The time required is that needed for the pulse to propagate to and from the interface. From Equation 3-2,

$$t = 2d/c$$
$$= \frac{2 \times 1 \text{ cm}}{1.54 \times 10^5 \text{ cm/s}}$$
$$= 1.3 \times 10^{-5} \text{ s}$$
$$= 13 \ \mu s$$

It is also possible to compute the reflector distance if the delay time, t, and the speed, c, are known.

Example: If the delay time is 130 μs and the speed of sound is 1540 m/s (1.54×10^5 cm/s), what is the reflector distance?

Solution: First, isolate d on one side of Equation 3-2.

$$t = 2d/c$$
$$2d = ct$$
$$d = ct/2$$

Then

$$d = 1.54 \times 10^5 \text{ cm/s} \times 130 \times 10^{-6} \text{ s}/2$$
$$= 10 \text{ cm}$$

The expression given by Equation 3-2 is sometimes referred to as the *range equation*.[6] This relationship between echo transit time, t, and reflector depth is implicitly built into pulse-echo imaging instruments. For a pulse traveling with a propagation speed of 1540 m/s in tissue, the round trip transit time is 13 μs/cm of tissue path.

INSTRUMENTATION—THE PULSER-RECEIVER

A simplified block diagram showing principal components of a pulse-echo instrument is presented in Fig. 3-2. We will begin our discussion of instrumentation by considering each of the components and their related function.

Pulser

The function of the pulser is to provide signals for driving the piezoelectric transducer. In response to the excitation signals from the pulser the transducer surface vibrates, producing an ultrasonic pulse that propagates through the tissue. This is done at a rate called the *pulse repetition frequency* (PRF). The PRF varies for different instruments and operating modes. (Operating modes are discussed later in this chapter.) It is usually set high enough that the display of echo signals appears to be continuous. There is,

however, an upper limit to the PRF, which will be discussed below in conjunction with rapid-scanning instruments.

The amplitude of the electric signal applied by the pulser to the transducer is a factor in determining the output *acoustic power* emitted by the instrument (see Chapter 7). Some instruments allow operator adjustable control of the *output acoustic power* to vary the sensitivity of the unit (Fig. 3-3). Sensitivity refers to the weakest echo signals that the instrument is capable of detecting and displaying. By increasing the output power to the transducer we produce higher-intensity transmit pulses and larger-amplitude echoes, and in so doing allow echo signals from weaker reflectors and scatterers to be visualized on the display. This is done at the expense of increased acoustic exposure to the patient.

Array transducer systems may require separate pulser circuits for each element in the array. As was mentioned in Chapter 2, some array transducer systems allow user selection of the transmit focal region or focal zone. The transmit focal zone of an array is determined by time delays between the excitation pulses applied to individual elements. There may be a single zone or multiple zones for each acoustic line.

The product of the PRF (number of pulses per second) and the time duration of each pulse (seconds per pulse) is a dimensionless quantity called the *duty factor*. The duty factor is the fraction of time that the transducer is actually emitting sound. In a typical single-element transducer system the PRF is 500/s and the pulse duration is 1.0 second or less (1×10^{-6} s). The duty factor here is (5.00×10^{-2}/s) $\times$ (1×10^{-6} s) = 0.5×10^{-3}. Expressed as a percentage, the duty factor, or the fraction of time the transducer is transmitting is only 0.05%; most of the time it is "listening" for echo signals reflected from interfaces. In real-time scanners the duty factor may be 10 times the value just mentioned; still, most of the operational time of such instruments is occupied in echo detection.

Receiver

Echo signals detected by the transducer are applied to the receiver, where they are processed for display. The first part of this processing involves echo signal *amplification* and *compensation* for attenuation losses in tissue.

Signal amplification is necessary since the amplitudes of echo signals at the transducer are generally too low to allow visualization on the display. The degree of amplification is called the *gain* of the receiver, which is the ratio of the output signal amplitude to the input signal amplitude (Fig. 3-4). The gain may be expressed as a simple ratio (say 10 or 100). More commonly it is expressed in decibels, whereby a gain of 10 is equivalent to a gain of 20 dB and a gain of 100 translates into one of 40 dB (see Table 1-1). Depending on the instrument, the maximum gain available in the receiver of a pulse-echo instrument may exceed 80 dB.

A significant fraction of this available gain is taken up by *swept gain* or *time gain compensation* (TGC) circuitry. Echoes returning to the transducer from structures

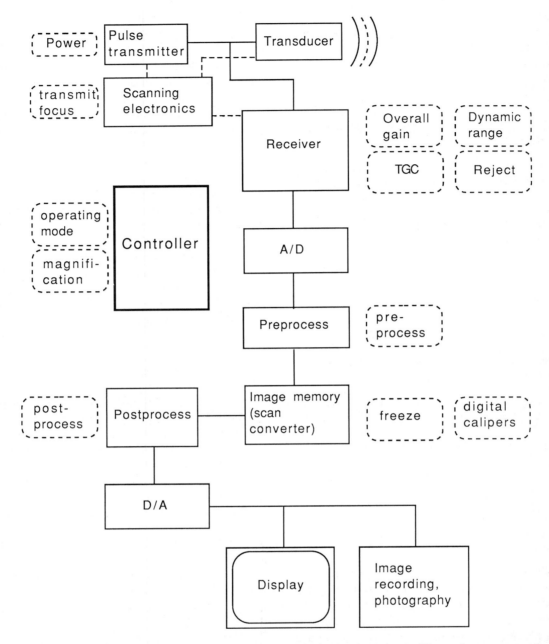

FIG. 3-2. Block diagram of a pulse-echo ultrasound imaging instrument. The major components of a typical system are enclosed in solid lines, and their principal controls are shown alongside, enclosed in dashed lines.

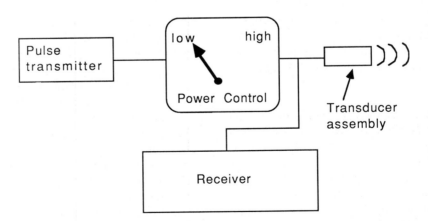

FIG. 3-3. Location of acoustic power output controls. This control may be labeled differently on different instruments. Examples of labels include "Transmit," "Power," and "Output."

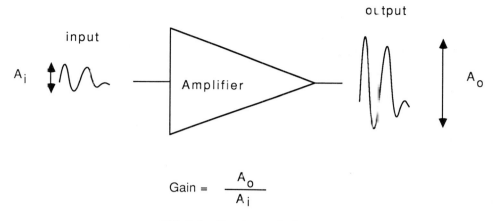

$$\text{Gain} = \frac{A_o}{A_i}$$

FIG. 3-4.   Receiver gain function.

situated at large distances generally are weaker than echoes returning from nearby structures. This is a result of sound beam attenuation in the medium. The situation is depicted schematically in Fig. 3-5, *A.* If the reflection coefficients of the interfaces giving rise to the echo signals shown were all the same and if there was no source of amplitude change other than attenuation (e.g., transducer beam focusing), a gradual weakening of the echo signals with increasing reflector distance would result from attenuation. Effects of attenuation are compensated for using swept gain, a process whereby the receiver amplification is increased with time following the transmit pulse so that echo signals originating from distal reflectors are amplified more than echo signals originating close to the transducer. Fig. 3-5, *B* and *C,* illustrates this process. In *C* the receiver gain is graphically portrayed as it might be adjusted to increase gradually with time after each transmit pulse. Before the transmit pulse the gain is reduced as shown. Proper application of the swept gain function has the effect of equalizing echo signals from similar reflectors, as shown in *B.*

Swept gain controls are available on nearly every pulse-echo instrument, although the form these controls take may differ considerably among instruments. Two commonly followed approaches are shown in Figs. 3-6 and 3-7. In Fig. 3-6 the principal operator controls are labeled initial, slope, and far, and their actions on the receiver gain are illustrated with the aid of the swept "gain curves." The initial setting adjusts the receiver gain at the time of pulse transmission by the transducer. The slope control adjusts the rate of compensation. Ordinarily the slope is adjusted to reflect the rate of sound beam attenuation in soft tissue. Thus, as the ultrasonic frequency is increased by, for example, switching to a higher-frequency transducer, the slope should also be increased. The far gain control adjusts the height of the knee of the curve, and thus the maximum receiver gain applied following each ultrasound transducer pulse.

As mentioned, the slope sensitivity control should reflect the rate of attenuation of the sound beam in tissues. For many imaging situations the ultrasound beam undergoes a fairly significant amount of attenuation just while traversing the body wall (i.e., the skin, connective tissue,

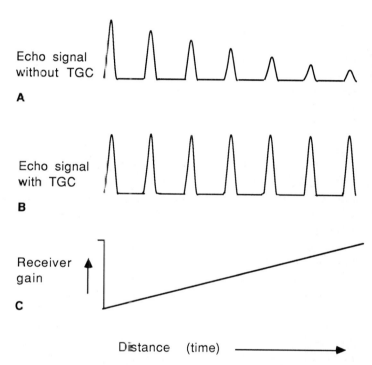

FIG. 3-5.   Demonstration of swept gain. **A,** Echo signal versus time in the presence of attenuation, with no swept gain. **B,** Echo signals after application of swept gain. **C,** Display of swept gain function. Increasing gain is upward on this diagram.

fat, and muscle interfaces overlying internal organs). Some instrument manufacturers have found it useful to add additional controls for the swept gain curve to compensate for these losses. The addition of a body wall correction (Fig. 3-6, *B*) facilitates use of a gradual slope for the compensation through the organ parenchymal path while a steeper slope, compensating for the more highly attenuating body wall, is used for the first few centimeters of tissue. Additional controls are available to adjust the slope of the body wall compensation and the distance over which this compensation takes place.

Some instruments provide a control to vary the depth at which the increase in swept gain begins. This variable delay (Fig. 3-6. *C*) may be positioned to different depths, providing further control of the swept gain function.

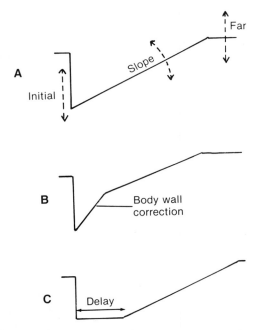

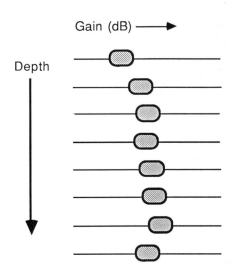

FIG. 3-7. TGC controls consisting of multiple gain potentiometers, each adjusting gain over a particular depth range.

FIG. 3-6. A, Effect of principal swept gain controls on swept gain function. **B,** Swept gain function with body wall correction. **C,** Function of slope delay.

For the form of swept gain control illustrated in Fig. 3-7, individual gain controls adjust the sensitivity, each controlling the gain over a specific depth range. The advantage of this system is that virtually any swept gain function, including compensation for body wall attenuation, can be achieved if fine enough control (sufficient number of control knobs) is provided.

In addition to operator-adjusted gain controls, many instruments provide automatic internal control of the swept gain. This feature can both correct for changes in sensitivity versus depth for transducers and can provide an average swept gain compensation rate. The instrument can be made to sense whatever transducer assembly is connected to the pulser-receiver, and adjust the swept gain according to the frequency and focal properties. Operator adjustments, though still necessary, are reduced somewhat by this feature.

Narrow-band versus wide-band amplifiers

In Chapter 2 we discussed the frequency bandwidth of an ultrasonic transducer; you may wish to review that material at this time. Just as the response of a transducer is not equal at all frequencies, so the gain of the amplifier in a receiver may not be the same at all frequencies. The frequency bandwidth of a receiver refers to the range of ultrasound signal frequencies that the receiver can amplify with maximum or nearly maximum gain.

Two types of amplifiers are in common use in pulse-echo work, and they are referred to as wide-band or narrow-band, depending on their frequency characteristics.

A wide-band amplifier's frequency characteristics are illustrated in Fig. 3-8. The amplifier is designed to respond to all ultrasonic echo signals over a large frequency range (Fig. 3-8, *B*). A wide-band amplifier will usually respond equally to all frequencies produced by the different transducers that can be used with the system.

A narrow-band amplifier (Fig. 3-9) amplifies a smaller frequency range of signals than does the wide-band amplifier. To accommodate transducers of different frequencies, it is sometimes necessary to adjust a frequency control switch on such instruments; other instruments sense which transducer is in use and adjust the receiver's frequency range accordingly. The response is designed to amplify only frequencies available from the transducer being employed, discriminating against other frequencies. This often is advantageous for reducing effects of spurious electronic noise signals on the echo display.

A *dynamic frequency tracking* feature is provided on some modern instruments. Its use has to do with the fact that not all ultrasound frequencies contained in the pulse emitted by a transducer are attenuated at the same rate in tissue. As mentioned in Chapter 1, higher frequencies are attenuated more readily and penetrate less deeply than lower frequencies. The receiver can be set up so that, for echo signals arriving from shallow regions, it responds most effectively to the higher frequencies in the pulse bandwidth. Then, as the high frequencies are preferentially attenuated, the response can be shifted gradually to favor the lower frequencies for signals from deeper structures. This makes most efficient use of the ultrasound frequencies available from the transducer.

Dynamic range and compression

A large range of echo signal amplitudes are picked up by the transducer of a pulse-echo instrument, and the receiver must be capable of responding to this large range. We use the term *dynamic range* to specify the ratio of the largest to smallest signals that an instrument or a part of an instrument can respond to without distortion.

Let's consider typical dynamic range characteristics with the help of Fig. 3-10. Here we have graphed a hypothetical response curve for an amplifier. The amplifier accepts low-level input signals, say in the millivolt ampli-

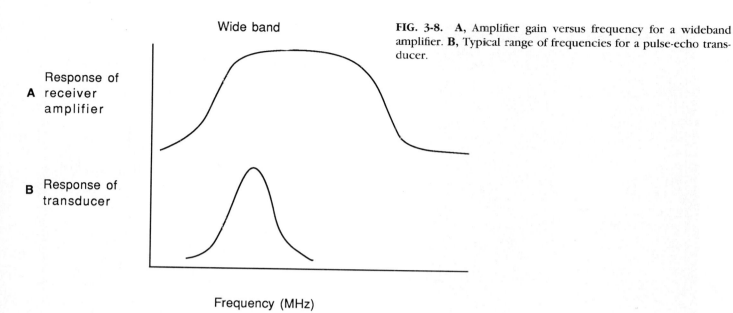

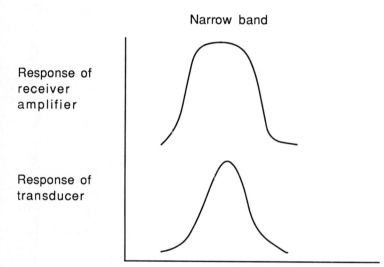

FIG. 3-9.   Narrowband amplifier frequency response characteristics. The amplifier must be tuned to respond to the transducer used.

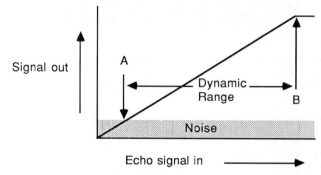

FIG. 3-10.   Hypothetical response curve for a receiver amplifier, illustrating the local dynamic range.

put, which remains at the maximum level. The dynamic range, shown in Fig. 3-10, is a measure of the total range of signals to which the amplifier can respond.

Different parts of the ultrasound instrument have different dynamic range capabilities. The total dynamic range at the input to the receiver can easily exceed 120 dB. However, other instrument components, such as the scan converter memory and the image display, usually cannot respond to signals over this range. One task faced by an instrument manufacturer is that of adjusting the signal levels present at various stages of an instrument so that the maximum amount of echo information desirable is available at the display. This is done in part in the receiver by a process called *signal compression*, or *logarithmic compression*, reducing the difference between signals from large amplitude echoes and signals from low amplitude echoes (hence the term *compression*). This enables components that handle the signals after the receiver to accommodate all echo signals of interest. Logarithmic compression is frequently employed since it enables variations in signal amplitude of both weakly reflecting and strongly reflecting interfaces to be visualized on the same display.

tude range. Its function is to boost these signals in magnitude while preserving the relative amplitude information between signals of different size. However, this can only be done for input signals within a certain range. In Fig. 3-10, if the input signals are below level *A* there is no response at the output—the amplifier does not respond to the input signals below this level, or the signals are below the level of electronic noise. If the input signal amplitude is between level *A* and level *B*, the amplified output signal level varies in proportion to the relative level of the input. This is the useful operating region of the device. Above level "B" the amplifier is no longer capable of responding to signal changes because the output has reached a maximum level. We say the amplifier is "saturated"; increasing the amplitude of the input signal has no effect on the out-

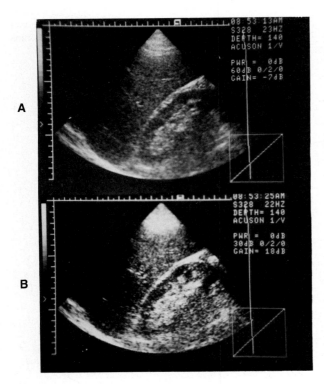

FIG. 3-11. Ultrasound B-mode images of an adult liver recorded with a 60 dB dynamic range, **A,** and a 30 dB dynamic range, **B.** Note the system sensitivity was increased about 25 dB for the lower scan.

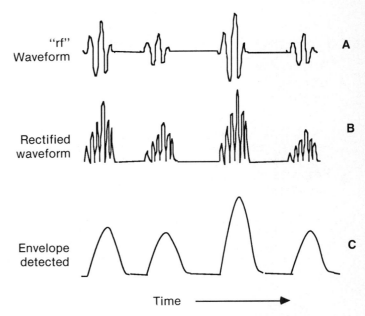

FIG. 3-12. Echo signal rectification and detection. **A,** Original signal waveform. **B,** Rectified signal. **C,** Smoothed, filtered signal.

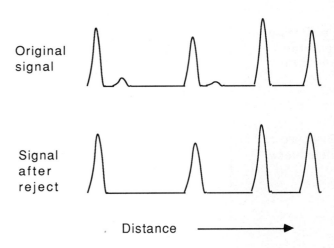

FIG. 3-13. Effect of increasing the reject control.

As shall be discussed below, a common form of echo display uses the amplitude of the echo signal to vary the brightness of a spot on the display screen. This is called *gray scale* processing. The *local dynamic range,* also called the *displayed dynamic range,* is the echo signal level change causing the display to go from a just noticeable echo signal (lowest gray level) to an echo of maximum brightness. The compression circuitry of many instruments allows the operator to vary the local dynamic range. Fig. 3-11 illustrates this for ultrasound images of a normal adult liver, where both a 30 dB and a 60 dB dynamic range were used in forming the image. The lower the dynamic range, the smaller the echo amplitude range needed to vary the brightness from black to white and the higher the image contrast. Many instruments allow up to a 65 or 70 dB local dynamic range setting.

Rectification and rejection

The oscillating type of echo signal waveforms (Fig. 3-12, *A*) are referred to as radio-frequencies or rf signal waveforms. Echo signals are seldom displayed in this format in clinical instruments. More commonly the rf waveform is first *rectified* (Fig. 3-12, *B*), resulting in oscillations in one direction only with respect to the 0 volts line. Additional electronic smoothing, or envelope detection, applied to this signal produces a single spike (Fig. 3-12, *C*) for each echo signal.

Some instruments also provide *rejection* controls at this stage of signal processing. This control and the associated circuitry eliminates low-level (very small ampli-

tude) signals from being displayed (as shown in Fig. 3-13). This may be helpful in discriminating against electronic noise on the display. The circuitry eliminates all signals (echo signals and noise) below a threshold signal level determined by the reject control setting. Caution should be exercised because if a reject control exists on an instrument, it can also reduce the displayed echo dynamic range.

PULSE-ECHO DISPLAY METHODS
A-mode (amplitude mode)

There are two commonly used echo signal display modes in pulse-echo ultrasonography (Fig. 3-14). The A-mode, or amplitude mode, display is a trace that shows the instantaneous echo signal amplitude versus time after transmission of the acoustic pulse. In pulse-echo ultrasound, the time after transmission of the pulse is used to infer reflec-

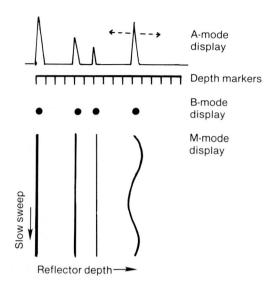

FIG. 3-14. A-mode, B-mode, and M-mode displays.

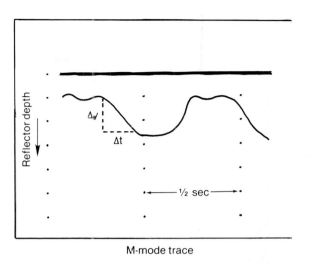

FIG. 3-15. Computing the velocity of a moving reflector using an M-mode display. Δy (the distance moved in time) divided by Δt (time) is the velocity.

tor distances, so the A-mode display also shows echo amplitude versus distance. A pulse propagation speed of 1540 m/s generally is assumed in the instrument's calibration for determining reflector distance from the transit time.

In some instruments, for example, some of those used in ophthalmology, this may be the only echo display format provided. It enables precise transducer-to-reflector distance measurements; it also allows studies of the relative echogenicity or scatter level of structures within the transducer beam. However, in most ultrasound instruments, if an A-mode trace is present, it is only as an ancillary display that may be used by the operator to assist the setting of the gain controls and other operating conditions.

Many instruments provide distance markers along with the echo signal. These markers are derived internally within the instrument, usually from a stable electronic "clock" circuit.

B-mode (brightness-mode)

In a B-mode, or brightness mode, display echo signals are electronically converted to intensity-modulated dots on the screen, as shown by the B-mode trace in Fig. 3-14. The distance between a dot position and the start of the trace (extreme left of graph) represents the distance from the transducer to the reflector. The B-mode display is used for displaying echo signals in pulse-echo scanning systems. It is also used in M-mode instruments to view moving reflectors. Both modes will be described later.

Several choices are available regarding the nature of the brightness modulations that form the B-mode display. In older ultrasound scanning instruments and in certain special-purpose scanners and M-mode units, a *"leading-edge"* display scheme is employed. Any echo signal whose amplitude is above some threshold level established internally in the instrument appears as a dot on the display. All dots are of the same brightness, regardless of the amplitude of the echo signal that they represent. The leading

edge processing results in a very contrasty echo signal presentation on the display.

As already mentioned, *gray scale* refers to modulating the brightness of the B-mode display according to the amplitude of the individual echo signals.[5] For a "white echo on black background" format, the greater the amplitude of the echo the brighter is the displayed dot at the corresponding spot. Gray-scale processing is commonly used in all types of pulse-echo ultrasound imaging.

M-mode (motion mode)

Also shown in Fig. 3-14 is the production of an M-mode display. An M-mode display is generated by slowly sweeping a B-mode trace across a screen, as shown. The resultant display is one illustrating reflector depth on one axis and time on an orthogonal axis. (Note "time" in this latter context is generally on the order of seconds; it should not be confused with echo return time, already discussed.) Stationary reflectors trace out a straight line on such a display, whereas moving reflectors (the dashed arrow on the A-mode signal) trace out a curved line. The M-mode is applied most frequently in echocardiography, where the movement patterns of walls and valves of the heart may be recorded and studied.

Most M-mode instruments have a variable sweep speed, allowing the time representation to be magnified or compressed. The time calibration is usually achieved by internal markers multiplexed on the echo display line at prescribed intervals, such as every ½ second. The markers also can be made to provide echo depth information by being produced to correspond to 1 cm distance intervals. Since the velocity is the displacement per unit time, the velocity component of a reflector along the line of site of the transducer can be computed from the slope of the M-mode trace. The slope is given by $\Delta y/\Delta t$, where Δy and Δt are as shown in Fig. 3-15. (Do not confuse this method of computing reflector velocity with the Doppler effect discussed in Chapter 5.)

Sound beam
orientation

B-mode
display
line

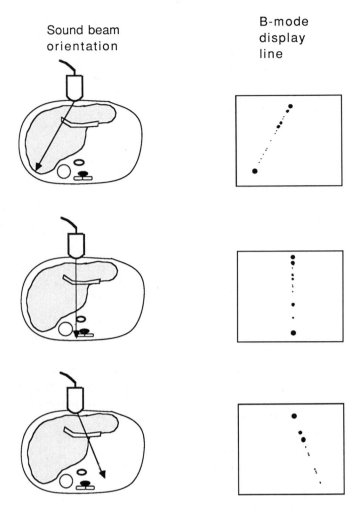

FIG. 3-16. Principle of B-mode imaging. The B-mode display line tracks the position and orientation of the ultrasound beam as it is swept across the region to be imaged.

ULTRASOUND B-MODE SCANNING

Both "real-time" and "static" ultrasound B-mode scanning is done by sweeping an ultrasound beam over the volume of interest and displaying echo signals using the B-mode (Fig. 3-16). An image is progressively built up as the beam is swept. Echo signals are positioned on the display in a location that corresponds to the reflector position in the body. The location of each reflector is obtained from:

1. The position and orientation of the sound beam axis; as the ultrasound beam is swept over the region being scanned, detected echo signals are placed along a line on the display that corresponds to the axis of the sound beam.
2. The delay time between launching of the acoustic pulse by the transducer and reception of an echo signal; from the delay time and the assumed sound propagation speed (1540 m/s) the distance from the reflector to the transducer is known by applying the range equation.

Thus two assumptions are implicitly made when building an ultrasound B-scan image:

1. Echo signals are assumed to originate from along the axis of the sound beam.

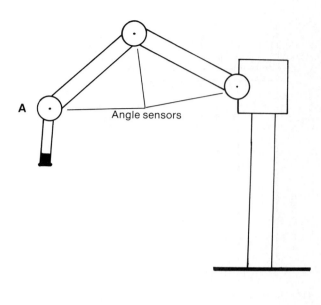

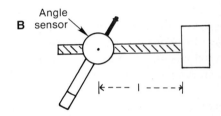

FIG. 3-17. Manual or "static" B-mode scanning arm.

2. The sound pulse always propagates at the assumed speed of sound in the medium.

If these two assumptions are met to a reasonable degree, the resultant image provides a representation of the anatomic positions of reflectors in a plane in the body.

Both static and real-time scanning instruments are described in the next sections.

MANUAL ("STATIC") SCANNERS
The scanning arm

Manual scanning instruments employ a scanning arm (as shown in Fig. 3-17) to facilitate image formation. The operator manipulates the ultrasound transducer so that the ultrasound beam is slowly swept over the region of interest. An image is formed by storing the B-mode echo data during the scan. The scanning arm carries out two functions:

1. It provides signals that enable the instrument to track the position and orientation of the ultrasonic transducer. This information, along with the echo return time, is required to place echo signals in their proper position on the display.
2. It constrains the transducer to a single plane during scan operations. This enables definition of the image scanning plane to be made in the patient.

Function 1 above is performed by sensors at the various arm joints that track the relative angle each arm section makes with other sections. In the case of the three-section scanning arm (Fig. 3-17, *A*) the angles along with the

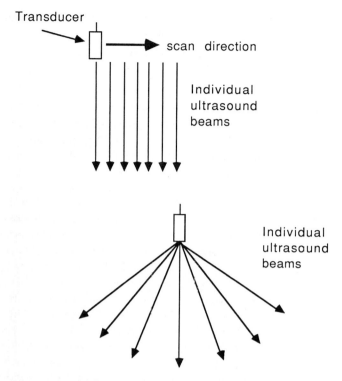

FIG. 3-18.   Linear and sector scanning formats.

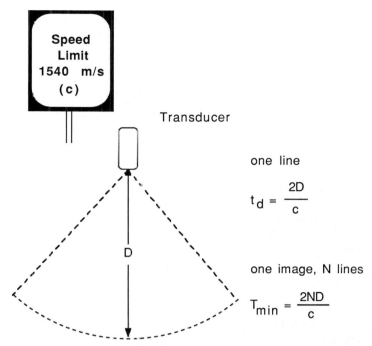

FIG. 3-19.   Scanning speed of real-time imagers is limited by c, the propagation speed of ultrasound pulses in tissue. t_d is the amount of time required to pick up echo signals from one line to a depth, D. T_{min} is the time required to form a complete image consisting of N lines.

arm section lengths are required for the instrument to keep track of the transducer coordinates. The accuracy with which the transducer coordinates are determined forms one part of the *compound registration accuracy* of scanning instruments. This is discussed in detail in Chapter 6.

Types of scan motions

Common transducer or sound beam scanning motions employed in static and real time B-mode imaging are illustrated in Fig. 3-18. If the transducer is swept in a straight line, the operation is referred to as a *linear scan*. A scan obtained by pivoting the transducer about its face or electronically sweeping the sound beam in the same resultant motion is called a *sector scan*. A *compound scan* is obtained by combining the basic motion patterns.

AUTOMATIC ("REAL-TIME") SCANNERS

Manual scanners have for the most part been replaced by automated real-time scanners in most ultrasound imaging centers. Their use provides performance capabilities not attainable with manual scanners—including the ability to visualize the chambers and valves of the heart in echocardiography studies, the ability to locate rapidly important anatomic landmarks and internal organs of interest, and for some units relatively low cost and portability of the instrument.

Scanning speed limitations

Scanning speed, or image frame rate, is an important performance characteristic in some applications of real-time scanners. As it turns out, the maximum speed with which

a real-time instrument can build up images is limited by the finite travel time of sound pulses in tissue.

The principle behind this limitation is straightforward: the separate transducer beam lines used to form an image (see Fig. 3-16) each require a small time interval to detect all echoes emerging from that line. This introduces a minimum required time delay between sound pulses transmitted along separate lines and, hence, a maximum pulse repetition frequency (PRF). The time delay required between pulses depends on the speed of sound in the medium and the maximum visualization depth, as outlined in more detail in the next paragraph.

Consider the sector scan arrangement in Fig. 3-19. The transducer assembly could be one of several types that will be discussed later. An image is produced by separate ultrasound beams distributed evenly over the sector angle. The number of separate beam lines needed for a complete image is dictated by factors such as image quality requirements and size of the sector. For simple scanning arrangements such as shown here, it might be useful to employ 120 or more individual lines to form an image that covers a 90-degree sector angle. Fewer lines could be used, but only at the cost of larger gaps between individual lines, which might be undesirable. If the field of view setting in Fig. 3-19 results in a maximum visualization depth of D, the delay time, t_d, needed to collect all echoes from any single line is given by

$$t_a = 2D/c \qquad (3-3)$$

where c is the speed of sound in the medium. Notice that this equation is identical to the pulse-echo range equation

(3-2) above. The minimum time required to produce a complete image consisting of N such lines is simply $N \times t_d$ or

$$T_{\min} = Nt_d = (2 \times N \times D)/c. \qquad (3\text{-}4)$$

The maximum allowable frame rate, $FR_{\max}$ is just the reciprocal of the time needed for a single complete image. That is,

$$FR_{\max} = 1/T_{\min} \qquad (3\text{-}5)$$
$$= c/(2 \times N \times D)$$

Example: Suppose the field of view of a sector scanner was set for a maximum echo depth of 20 cm. Furthermore, N is 120 lines. Calculate $T_{\min}$; also compute the maximum frame rate.

Solution: Using Equation 3-4,

$$T_{\min} = (2 \times 120 \times 20\text{ cm})/(1.54 \times 10^5\text{ cm/s})$$
$$= 0.031\text{ s}$$

In this example the minimum required time to produce a single image is 0.03 second. (In practice slightly longer times are allowed, so the chances of producing an artifact by overlapping of pulses will be minimized.) The maximum frame rate possible, $FR_{\max}$ is

$$FR_{\max} = 1/T_{\min}$$
$$= 1/0.031\text{ s} = 32/\text{s}$$

Consider one more example. The purpose is not to dazzle the less mathematically inclined reader with algebra but to demonstrate that some practical consequences of a simple although very important concept can be approached through reasoning.

Example: Show that if the distance, D, in Equation 3-3 is expressed in centimeters (i.e., $D = d$ cm) then the maximum frame rate can also be expressed as

$$FR_{\max} = 77,000/\text{s}/Nd \qquad (3\text{-}6)$$

where N is the number of acoustic lines per frame and d is the centimeters of distance.

Solution: As stated earlier, the maximum frame rate, $FR_{\max}$, may be expressed as

$$FR_{\max} = 1/T_{\min}$$

Now plug in the expression for $T_{\min}$ (Equation 3-4) to get

$$FR_{\max} = c/2ND$$

The expression then pops right out after substituting for c and letting D be d cm:

$$FR_{\max} = (1.54 \times 10^5\text{ cm/s})/(2 \times N \times d\text{ cm})$$
$$= \frac{77,000/\text{s}}{N \times d}$$

It is not necessary (nor is it desirable) to memorize expressions such as Equation 3-6 to grasp the principles being discussed. If you understand that the scan speed is limited by the time required for echo signals to return from the maximum image depth along each acoustic line, then it is fairly easy to reason out some important design tradeoffs in rapid-scanning instruments. Scanners employing a large field of view (e.g., 21 cm depth) are somewhat limited in frame rate if a sufficient line density is employed for a reasonable image quality. Reduced fields of view, such as employed in some high-frequency small parts scanners, allow significantly higher frame rates. Most instruments that provide variable magnification decrease the frame rate or decrease the number of lines in the image when the field of view is increased.

Results calculated using Equations 3-5 and 3-6 are for imaging with a single transmit focal zone. Instruments that allow simultaneous multiple transmit focal zones must decrease the image frame rate when these conditions are present; this is because of the longer time required to form each acoustic line with multiple transmit focal zones.

Sequential (linear) array scanners

Transducer arrays were introduced in Chapter 2. Sequential linear arrays, sequential "curvilinear" convex (or radial) arrays, and phased arrays are used for electronic real-time scanning where no mechanical motion is required to build up images.

Sequential linear array scanners consist of arrays of small rectangular elements lined up side by side. They produce images by transmitting sound beams parallel with one another, beginning at one end of the array and continuing along to the opposite end (Fig. 3-20), after which the sequence is repeated.

Typical sequential arrays use 120 or more rectangular piezoelectric elements arranged side by side as shown in Fig. 3-21. The element width, W, is usually about one wavelength, and the length, L, is sufficient to provide a

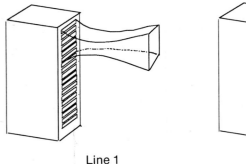
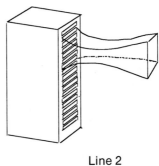
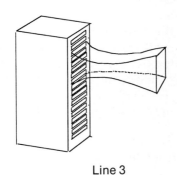

Line 1   Line 2   Line 3

FIG. 3-20. Scanning arrangement of a linear sequential array scanner. Schema is of sound beams for the first three acoustic lines forming the image.

reasonably collimated sound beam in a direction perpendicular to the scan plane. The choice of a small element width provides the ability to produce closely spaced ultrasound beams, as we shall see below; this is necessary so that fine spatial detail of anatomic structures will be obtained.

Individual ultrasound beams are produced by exciting a group or cluster of elements in the array, after which the same elements are used to detect echo signals. Received signals from individual elements are added together electronically, forming a net echo signal that is amplified and processed for display. Subsequent beams are produced by dropping the top element and picking up the next lower element and exciting this new cluster (see

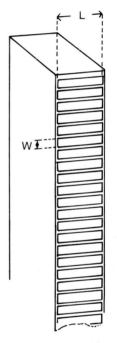

FIG. 3-21. Transducer assembly arrangement in a linear sequential array scanner.

Fig. 3-20). The effect is to move the central region of the beam down one element. The process continues along the array, producing a single ultrasonic B-scan.

The use of a cluster of perhaps seven elements rather than a single element is dictated both by sensitivity and by lateral resolution requirements. The effectively larger aperture formed by the element cluster is more sensitive than the aperture formed by a single element. Also, the cluster provides a narrower sound beam at large distances from the transducer than does an individual element (Fig. 3-22). Consequently, it is possible to obtain better lateral resolution with a cluster than with an individual element. In addition, the cluster of elements enables use of electronic focusing applied both during pulse transmission and echo reception. Other features mentioned in Chapter 2, including dynamic aperture size and dynamic apodization, can be done with an array cluster.

Individual acoustic lines forming the B-mode image are separated by one element width. Finer spacing of the ultrasound beams can be obtained if a process referred to as even-odd element firing is employed. With an odd number of elements the center of the beam corresponds to the middle of the central element (Fig. 3-23). With an even number the center of the beam is situated along a line that cuts between the central two elements in the cluster. If a beam is formed with an odd number of elements, followed by another formed with an even number, followed by another with an odd number, and so on, there are half-element spacings between individual scan lines forming the image.

Another method used to provide higher line densities is to construct additional echo data lines by interpolation. Data for an interpolated line, situated halfway between two actual lines, are calculated by taking the average values of data from points along the neighboring lines.

Convex arrays

A sequential convex array operates on the same principles as a linear array (Fig. 3-24). Individual ultrasound beams are produced by separately exciting clusters of elements in the array. Rather than parallel beams as in the linear ar-

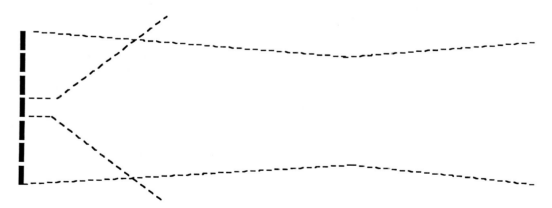

FIG. 3-22. Production of individual acoustic scan lines using a sequential array. A cluster of elements is involved, providing better sensitivity and resolution than with an individual element. Use of a cluster also allows electronically controlled focusing of the transmitted and received beams.

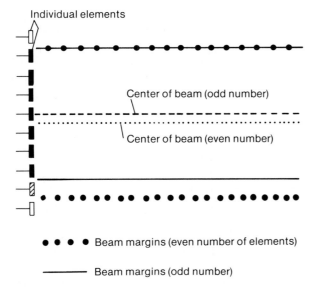

FIG. 3-23. Even-odd element firing to provide beam spacing of one-half element width rather than a complete element width.

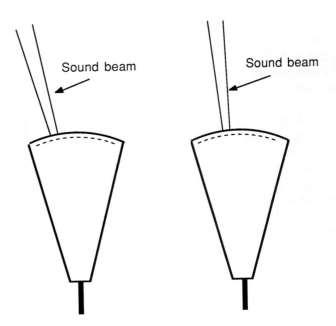

FIG. 3-24. Convex sequential array.

ray, beams from the convex array travel at different angles—like the spokes of a wheel. For each ultrasound beam, echo signals picked up by elements in the cluster are added together and then applied to the display, as in the previous example. The scan format traces out a section of a sector; the exact shape of the sector varies with the radius of the array and the angle over which elements are placed.

The region of a transducer assembly through which sound is coupled to the patient is sometimes referred to as the *entrance window.* The convex shape of this array provides better transducer-to-patient coupling along the entrance window than is provided by the simple linear scanning array. Also, the sector scan format enables larger imaged fields from a smaller entrance beam area than the linear array. Multiple transmit focusing and dynamic focus of received echo signals are important design features in these arrays as well.

In comparison to a phased array (see below), a convex array requires a larger entrance window. However, a possible advantage over the phased array is that the convex elements surface is nearly always perpendicular to the acoustic beam axis. In other words, the convex array elements are always directing their sound beams "forward"; in contrast, a phased array must steer beams off to the side to pick up echoes from structures near the edges of the imaged field. There may be some fall off in the sensitivity of elements in an array for directions that are not perpendicular to the array surface. This fall off depends on the number of elements in the array and the size of individual elements.[3] (Thus very small, closely spaced elements in a phased array would not necessarily suffer from such a decrease in sensitivity.)

Electronic (phased-array) sector scanners

The transducer assembly of a phased array sector scanner consists of a tightly grouped array of elements. Unlike the

previous two types of arrays, all elements are involved in producing the sound beam and receiving echoes for each acoustic line. The sound beam produced by a phased array is electronically steered off at an angle with respect to a line perpendicular to the array surface (Fig. 3-25, *A*). This is done by introducing appropriate time delays in the excitation pulses applied to individual elements in the array. The direction in which the sound beam is steered is dependent on the exact time delay settings and is varied from one transmit pulse to the next, steering the beam in different directions (Fig. 3-25, *B*).

Electronic focusing may be done by programming delay settings for focusing, similar to those described in Chapter 2, along with the beam-steering delays. Both single and multiple transmit focal zones and dynamic receiver focusing are used in phased arrays.

An advantage of electronically sectored arrays is their relatively small entrance window, permitting coupling through the intercostal space. Electronically sectored arrays may have 60 or more individual piezoelectric elements packed into a 1 to 2 cm row. Thus they may be used effectively in pediatric and adult cardiac imaging.

An advantage of phased array electronic sector scanners over mechanical scanners (see below) is the flexibility introduced in the scanning format. It is easy to share a scanning beam with one or more static M-mode lines, for example, enabling multiple-trace M-mode displays to be produced along with a two-dimensional image. Also, since there are no mechanical movements involved in producing the scan, it is easy to synchronize scanning movements to external triggers, such as derived from ECG signals. Both these features have been employed in some electronic sector scanning instruments.

Mechanically scanned real-time instruments

Conceptually the simplest type of rapid autoscanners are mechanical systems. These usually employ one or more

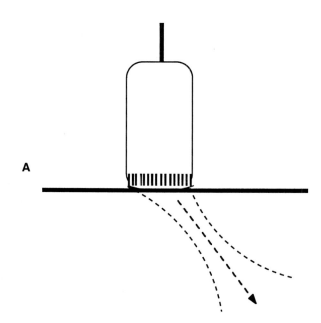

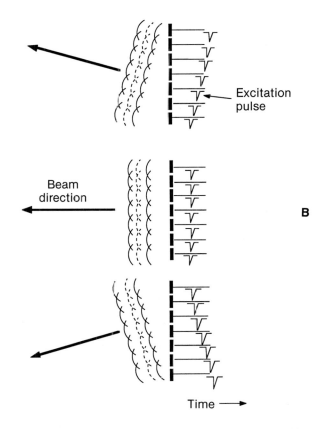

FIG. 3-25. Electronically sectored phased array scanner. The array consists of a dense arrangement of elements. In **A** the beam is shown swept toward one side. **B,** Details of beam steering. Transmitted sound beams and receiving sensitivity patterns are steered at an angle by using time delays. Three different beam directions are illustrated.

single-element transducers to transmit and receive ultrasound signals. They have been designed in many different scanning arrangements. Several examples are shown in Fig. 3-26.

In Fig. 3-26, *A,* a single-element transducer is shown oscillating about a pivot point. On some units the operator can control the sector angle as well as the sector speed. Special servodrive circuits help reduce effects of mechanical vibration.

The multiple transducer rotating wheel (Fig. 3-26, *B*) has proved to be very effective in mechanical sector scanners. This arrangement employs from two to four separate transducers on the rim of a rotating wheel. Transducers are pulsed only during the time they sweep past the scanning window, as shown. The transducer assembly housing must be filled with a fluid to assure acoustic coupling between the transducer element and the window. (The type of fluid used and whether it is user replenishable if, for example, air bubbles are formed should be explained in the accompanying owner's manual.)

Another system (shown in Fig. 3-26, *C*) uses a stationary element to generate sound beams. Beam deflection is done with an oscillating acoustic mirror housed in the transducer assembly.

Some mechanical scanners incorporate annular array transducers rather than single-element transducers. When this is the case, multiple transmit focusing, dynamic receiving focusing, and dynamic aperture control are possible with these units as well.

Unlike sequential linear arrays and electronically sectored arrays, mechanical scanners contain moving parts to generate the scan. The parts may consist of gears, pulleys,

wheels, or oscillating shafts, depending on the design. Normal wear and tear on the drive mechanism can be reduced by placing the transducer assembly in a nonscanning mode when not in use. Again, consult the owner's manual for the recommended transducer assembly standby mode between patient scans.

Special purpose automatic scanners

Most of the real-time scanning arrangements just described have also been used in various special purpose scanners. *Special purpose* transducer assemblies or scanning instruments are those designed mainly for a single imaging application. For example, *transrectal scanners* are used effectively for imaging the prostate. Linear, phased array as well as mechanically scanned probes are used in this application. Some configurations provide simultaneous scanning of two planes perpendicular to each other. This is referred to as "biplane imaging" and has been found advantageous for determining the extent of disease in the prostate.

Transvaginal scanners consist of either mechanical or phased array sector scanning transducer assemblies formed into a special shape for this application. Just as is the case with transrectal probes, distinct advantages provided with use of such transducer assemblies include use of higher frequency probes for better spatial resolution, since the attenuating path to the scanned region is reduced significantly, making this possible and eluding any beam distorting attenuating tissue layers making up the abdominal wall.

Several special purpose scanning conurations have been employed for imaging the breast. One type of scan-

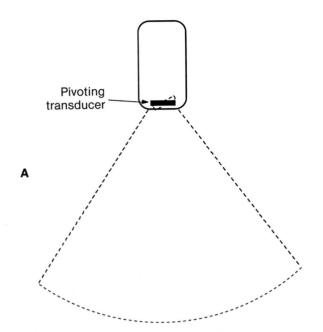

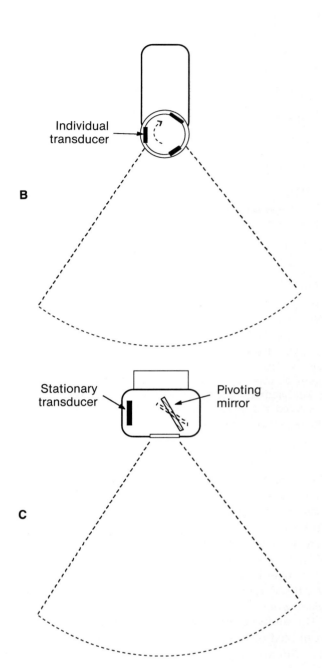

FIG. 3-26. Three arrangements employed in mechanical scanners.

ner uses a water bath standoff between the transducer and the patient. Coupling is done either with the breast submersed or through a water-filled bag. The latter arrangement results in the breast tissue being compressed, reducing the total tissue path the sound beam must penetrate for effective imaging.

ECHO DATA STORAGE AND DISPLAY
Oscilloscope displays

An oscilloscope is an effective instrument for displaying echo signals picked up by an ultrasound scanner. The operation of a standard cathode ray tube (CRT) oscilloscope is illustrated in Fig. 3-27. Electrons (or "cathode rays") are produced in an electron gun by heating a filament. The electrons are focused into a beam and accelerated toward a phosphor screen. Upon striking the phosphor they cause the phosphor to emit light, which is visible to anyone observing the screen from the outside.

The usefulness of the device lies in the fact that the electron beam can be swept or steered across the screen by applying electric signals to horizontal and vertical deflection plates inside the tube. For example, it may be swept from left to right on the screen, tracing out a straight line. If a sinusoidally oscillating signal waveform of sufficient amplitude is applied to the vertical deflection plates at the same time that the left to right sweep is applied, this waveform will be traced out in time (as shown in Fig. 3-28).

An A-mode display may be produced by synchronizing the oscilloscope sweep to the transmit pulse applied to the ultrasound transducer and applying the echo signal waveform from Fig. 3-14, *A,* to the vertical axis. Thus echo signals are represented as deflections on the display, the actual deflections (or height of the spike) being related to the amplitude of the individual echo signals.

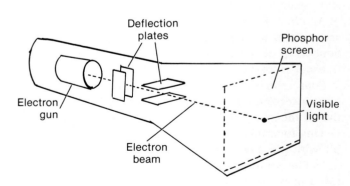

FIG. 3-27. Diagram of an oscilloscope.

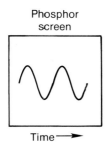

Phosphor
screen

Time →

FIG. 3-28. Application of a sinusoidal signal to the vertical deflection plates of an oscilloscope while a sweep signal is applied to the horizontal deflection plates. The trace on the screen shows the sine wave over time.

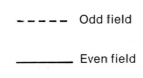

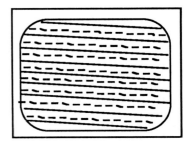

– – – – – Odd field

───── Even field

FIG. 3-29. Sweep operation of a 512-line 2-field video monitor. The view is from the phosphor screen.

In early ultrasound scanners the oscilloscope was also used for displaying M-mode data and ultrasound B-mode images. The oscilloscope was useful in these applications because its electron beam can be deflected in any direction and brightened at any spot on the phosphor screen. In imaging this permits actual tracking of the sound pulse position as it is reflected from interfaces at different depths. The sweep of the electron beam on the screen can be made to follow the sound beam for any scan motion. A special-purpose memory oscilloscope, or storage oscilloscope, allowed the image to be viewed directly during and after image buildup. Ultrasound images built up on storage oscilloscopes most often employed leading-edge signal processing along with a *bistable* storage screen. This produces a very high contrast image on which each section of the display is either white or black, depending on whether an echo signal happens to be detected from the corresponding point in the patient.

In gray scale processing, echo signal amplitudes are encoded in display intensity. Early gray-scale scanning consisted of building up the image on photographic film, which was continuously exposed by the oscilloscope screen during scanning. This has been superseded by television monitor displays and digital memory scan converters.

Television (video) monitors

TV monitors also function somewhat like oscilloscopes, having an electron beam that is accelerated and directed toward a phosphor screen. The screen emits light in response to the electron beam, the brightness of the light being controlled by the intensity of the electron current. In contrast to an oscilloscope display, the electron beam scanning arrangement of most TV monitors is *fixed* in a repeating, horizontal raster format (Fig. 3-29). Ordinary 512-line monitors sweep the electron beam over the screen in two passes, referred to as *fields*. In the first field the raster scan arrangement traces out 256 lines on the screen, the process taking 1/60 of a second. In the second field the electron beam is swept so that it fills in between the lines of the first field, again taking 1/60 of a second. (A completed frame consists of both fields and requires 1/30 of a second.)

Television monitors are advantageous for gray-scale im-

aging because they can produce a large number of distinct brightness levels or gray levels. This is done with very good spatial detail or resolution. (Even higher resolution monitors, with more than 512 raster scanned TV lines, are available and are used in some areas of medical imaging.)

Scan converter memory

A scan converter accepts echo signal data from the ultrasonic scanner, stores these signals in an internal memory, and reads out the data to a TV monitor (see Fig. 3-2). Signal data may be echo amplitude and position information in scanning mode, echo signal versus time data in M-mode, and, if available, Doppler signal information. Image and echo data are displayed and photographed from the monitor screen.

The memory is "written" to with signals from the ultrasound instrument. Data are read out synchronized to the TV monitor sweep and are converted to a brightness variation on the TV display screen. The device is called a scan converter because of the different formats the input and output data have. Although early scan converters used analog components, current instruments use digital technology for storage and control of data. Characteristics of digital devices are discussed in the next section.

Digital representation of values

Most modern ultrasound instruments are controlled by dedicated microcomputers. Onboard computers often provide a readout of the current operational status of the instrument (such as the display magnification, transducer assembly identification, power and gain settings) and adjust the operating conditions of the instrument in response to operator control adjustments. Computers use digital circuitry to manipulate and store data. An important role of digital circuitry in an ultrasound scanner is that of echo signal storage and image formation in the scan converter. In this section basic concepts regarding representation and storage of digital data are introduced.

Any parameter, such as echo signal amplitude, may be represented and displayed in either an analog or a digital format. In an analog format the values of a quantity vary continuously between a minimum and a maximum level. In digital format instantaneous values are represented as

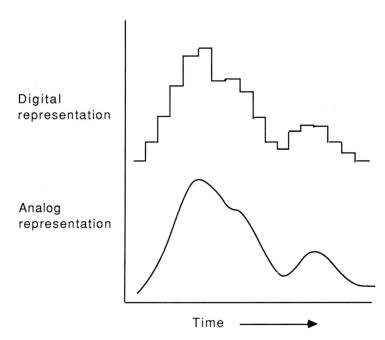

FIG. 3-30.   Analog and digital representations of a signal waveform.

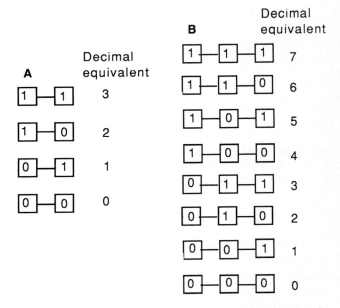

FIG. 3-31.   **A**, A 2-bit word can represent any of four signal levels. Each bit may be in the 0 or the 1 state. **B**, A 3-bit word can represent eight different values.

discrete levels, with fixed steps between the levels (Fig. 3-30).

Digital systems offer advantages over analog devices in terms of stability and immunity to electronic noise. These properties stem from the fact that all digital systems employ as a basic unit a stable electronic circuit, referred to as a *bit*. The circuit comprising a single bit can be electronically switched into either of two states: high or low. The output signal level of the circuit indicates which state it is in. The two states may be used to represent the numbers 1 and 0, respectively. Thus a single bit could represent a quantity as being either of two different levels.

Additional signal level representations for a quantity are obtained by stringing a number of bits together to form a *multibit word*. The number of bits used to represent the word determines the amount of information that can be represented or stored at that location. Consider the very simple situation of a word that consists of two bits. How many discrete values could that word represent? If we allow each bit to be in its 0 or its 1 state, there are four different possibilities or four signal levels that can be represented. These are illustrated in Fig. 3-31, *A.* If we add an additional bit, giving us a 3-bit word, it can readily be seen that now eight different combinations are possible (Fig. 3-31, *B*). In fact, we can generalize by saying that the number of discrete levels, *L,* possible from a word consisting of *n* bits is equal to 2 raised to the power of the number of bits. That is,

$$L = 2^n \qquad (3\text{-}7)$$

The following list gives the number of discrete signal levels that can be represented for different digital word sizes. This information is useful, for example, in comparing the memory size of digital scan converters commonly used.

Bits	Discrete levels
1	2
2	4
3	8
4	16
5	32
6	64
7	128
8	256
10	1024

Appropriate coding applied to the string of bits forming a multibit word allows these words to represent numbers. Computers employ the *binary number* system as a basis for representing numbers and carrying out mathematical computations. Analogous to the decimal number system, employing 10 as a base and using the digits 0 through 9 to represent numbers, the binary number system employs 2 as a base and uses only the digits 0 and 1 to represent numbers. The more bits available in a single word, the larger the integer number that can be represented, as can be seen from the material just presented. Texts on computer architecture can be consulted to learn more about mathematical manipulation of data in the binary number system.

Operation of the digital scan converter

A functional block diagram listing essential components of a digital scan converter and their relationships to the scanning instrument and display electronics are shown in Fig. 3-32. The scan converter accepts echo signals from the receiver of the instrument and stores these in a digital memory at an "address" that corresponds to the location of the echo source. The contents of the memory are read out on a TV monitor, forming an image. Echo signals are in analog format as they emerge from the receiver; they are transferred to a digital format by an analog-to-digital

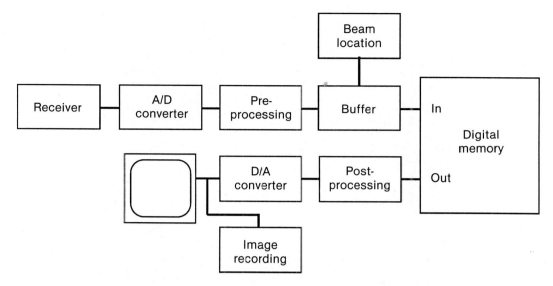

FIG. 3-32. Schema of a digital scan converter and its relationship to other components of an ultrasound imaging system.

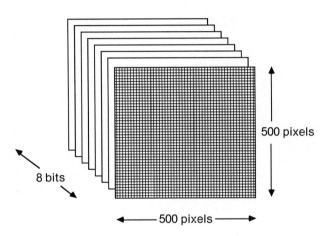

FIG. 3-33. Schema of pixels in a digital scan converter.

(A/D) converter. Here continuously varying analog signals are transferred into digital format, where they are represented as discrete, quantized levels, as in Fig. 3-30.

The digital scan converter memory is divided into discrete and separately addressable elements, referred to as picture elements or *pixels* (Fig. 3-33). The memory size may be as large as 500 to 600 pixels wide by 500 pixels high. In scanning, mode echo signals are inserted into the memory at pixel locations corresponding to reflector positions in the body by using the echo delay time and the transducer beam coordinates to compute the correct *address.* Most instruments use 6 or 8 bits to represent the echo value in each pixel location. Examination of the tabular material above shows that 6 bits provides 64 distinct echo levels at each location, while 8 bits provides 256 distinct levels.

If M-mode processing is available, these data also are processed in the memory, giving a continuous trace depicting reflector positions versus time for one or more acoustic beam lines.

The memory is continuously refreshed with new echo data as the ultrasound beam is swept over the volume be-

ing scanned. Simultaneously, the ultrasound B-mode information is read out to a monitor, providing real-time visualization of the scanned plane. Buffer registers allow transfer of data in and out of the memory at a rate not visible on the display. An *image freeze* enables the echo data to be stored in memory for examination and/or photography as well as video recording. The digital memory is read by transference of pixel values to a digital-to-analog (D/A) converter, providing signals for intensity modulating a screen or a TV monitor. The signal is transferred in raster scanned television format to multi-image cameras and other image recording devices. A multi-image camera contains an internal video monitor that exposes photographic film, producing hard copy images.

Preprocessing and postprocessing

It was mentioned earlier that one of the steps involved in signal processing consists of compression of the echo amplitudes. At that point only reduction of the amplified echo signal amplitude range corresponding to a given echo level range was discussed. Whereas echo signals spanning a 60 dB dynamic range might have amplitudes of, say 0.005 to 5 V in the receiver before compression, this same echo range might have a signal amplitude range of 0.1 to 1 V after compression.

Additional signal processing is provided in some instruments. Depending on whether this processing occurs before or after echo data storage in memory, the signal processing is referred to as *preprocessing* or *postprocessing.*

Some instruments allow selection of signal processing schemes through choice of *preprocessing* controls. Preprocessing here refers to manipulation of digitized echo signals prior to their storage in the memory. Examples of preprocessing functions carried out by various instruments include the following:

1. Selection of different forms of echo signal compression to enhance echo signals within a particular amplitude range.

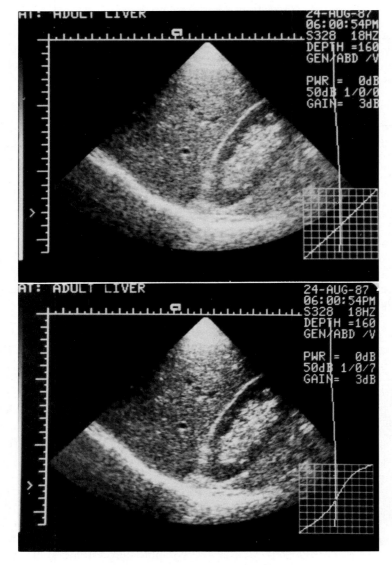

FIG. 3-34.   These two ultrasound B-mode images depict the same information stored in the scan converter memory. Two different postprocessing functions were used to display the images.

2. Echo signal edge enhancement, producing sharper echo signals on a B-mode display.
3. Correction for changes in transducer assembly sensitivity with depth.
4. Automatically programmed TGC.

The assignment of stored digital echo values to brightness levels on the TV monitor can be varied if *postprocessing* control options are provided. In contrast to preprocessing, postprocessing can be done on an image already frozen in memory. Fig. 3-34 is an example of such manipulation of echo signal data by postprocessing. The same B-mode image of an adult liver and kidney was photographed using two different postprocessing settings. The relationship between image brightness and signal level in the image memory is shown graphically by the insert in the lower right of each image. (The horizontal axis of the inserted graphs represents the level stored in memory, and the vertical axis depicts dot brightness.)

Operating modes

We have seen that there are a number of echo display modes available in pulse echo ultrasonography. We often refer to the term "operating mode"[1] to distinguish the distinct method being used to acquire and display ultrasound information. Thus we have already discussed A-mode, M-mode, static B-mode imaging, and real-time B-mode imaging; these are all used in pulse-echo ultrasound. In the next chapter we will discuss Doppler ultrasound instruments and additional operating modes will be described. These include continuous-wave (CW) Doppler, pulsed Doppler, and Doppler flow imaging.

Many instruments have the capability of combined operating modes, which, of course, is any combination of two or more of the discrete operating modes already mentioned.

IMAGE RECORDING
Photographic film

The most common method of obtaining hard copy of ultrasound images is to photograph a monitor that is continuously viewing the image stored in the scan converter. This can be done with any type of photographic negative film, Polaroid positive film, or image-recording transpar-

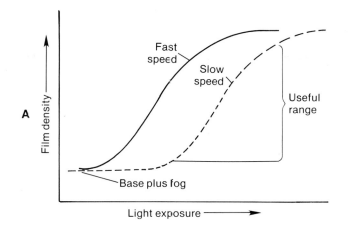

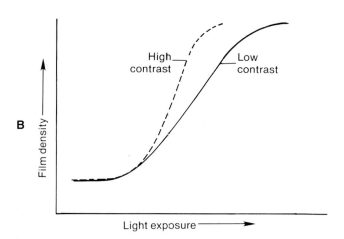

FIG. 3-35. **A,** Characteristic curves for two photographic films that have different speeds. **B,** Characteristic curves for two films that have different contrast.

ency film. In addition, special copying techniques such as thermal printing and ultraviolet-sensitive paper are sometimes used; these are especially handy in systems designed for M-mode recording because they can provide long, continuous records. No matter what the image-recording process, the hard-copy materials and camera settings all require proper matching to optimize the end results. A basic comprehension of the principles of these recording techniques is especially useful in understanding the tradeoffs in this matching process and helping to pinpoint problems in image recording when they exist.

The ensuing discussion deals with the principles underlying recording images on photographic film, since many of these also apply in the other recording medium mentioned. Photographic film contains small grains of silver bromide crystals suspended in a gelatin and supported on a cellulose acetate sheet. When light strikes the crystals, they form a latent image and are very susceptible to chemical change upon development. During the development process the crystals that absorbed light are converted to silver grains. Any unexposed crystals are removed from the film during the fixing stage, leaving behind the exposed silver grains, which form an image.

Several types of film are used in medical image recording. Their properties can be compared with the aid of characteristic curves (examples shown in Fig. 3-35). These curves are obtained by exposing patches of a film and then determining the optical density, a measurement of the opacity of the exposed part of the film. The density is plotted against the relative exposure, the latter being the product of the intensity of the light and the exposure time.

The base plus fog refers to a slight opacity of the film, found upon developing without any exposure. There is a threshold exposure required before any additional film darkening occurs, this threshold level varying for different films. There also is a maximum exposure, above which no additional exposure can cause film darkening. The useful exposure range is situated between these extremes, wherein a change in the light level will be recorded as a change in the developed film density.

The curves in Fig. 3-35, *A,* are for two films having different speeds. The higher-speed film requires less light exposure to cause film darkening than does the low-speed film. The two curves in Fig. 3-35, *B,* are for films with different contrast. The steeper curve is for a high-contrast film, which takes only a small exposure variation to go from minimum to maximum optical density. Low-contrast film has a wider latitude, accommodating a much wider light exposure range.

For optimal results the monitors used for exposing film must be matched in terms of brightness, contrast, and exposure time; so the particular film used is exposed to a level corresponding to its useful range on its characteristic curve. Ideally exposure settings should be such that variations in image brightness caused by amplitude changes among high-level echo signals are successfully recorded at the same time that the weakest echo signals (e.g., recorded from organ parenchyma) are detected on the film image. This can usually be achieved with proper exposure and camera monitor control settings. It often requires an experienced serviceman or sonographer to determine the correct settings.

The results of the developing process are highly dependent on the developing time and the temperature of the processor and the condition of the processing chemicals. Most medical imaging facilities regularly test the photography performance and maintain quality assurance notebooks in which important processing parameters are logged on a daily basis. In addition, it is important to keep in mind that photographic films can be adversely affected by storage conditions of high temperature and humidity. To assure consistent clinical results, one should always follow the film manufacturer's instructions for film handling and processing.

Fiberoptic recorders

At the present time the most practical M-mode displays are those employing a fiberoptic CRT face along with movement of the recording paper across the stationary B-mode display (Fig. 3-36). One process uses ultraviolet light to expose the paper, forming a latent image. The pa-

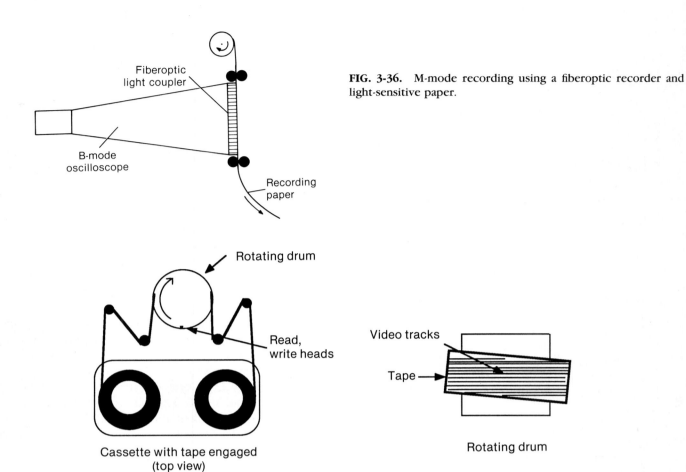

FIG. 3-36. M-mode recording using a fiberoptic recorder and light-sensitive paper.

FIG. 3-37. Operation of a video cassette recorder.

per is developed by exposure to visible light. Another type of recorder uses dry silver paper as the recording medium. The latent image is developed in a thermal processor housed in the recorder. The chief advantage of the latter technique is that better gray scale can be obtained on hard-copy records.

Video copy processors

Video copy thermal processors produce reasonably high-resolution hard copy with sufficient gray scale to yield acceptable quality B-mode image and M-mode records for some applications. These devices accept standard video signals from the image memory of the ultrasound instrument and store the image in their own internal digital memory. The information is transferred to a thermal printing mechanism that exposes the paper. The paper is exposed slowly as it is drawn past the thermal printhead.

Video tape recording

Video cassette tapes are finding increasing use in ultrasound imaging departments. They are used commonly in cardiology studies and other applications of real-time scanners. The basic operation of a VCR is illustrated in Fig. 3-37.[2] The recording medium itself is a continuous acetate tape that has microscopic magnetic oxide particles deposited. These magnetic particles behave like tiny bar magnets and may be aligned in a preferential direction if the tape is placed in a magnetic field. The degree of

alignment is directly related to the strength of the magnetic field. Any such magnetized regions retain this magnetization until it is placed in a different magnetic field.

A video image may be stored on magnetic tape by transporting the tape past magnetic recording *heads*, which align the magnetic particles in the tape as it flies by. The heads consist of small electromagnets, which convert an electric signal into a fluctuating magnetic field when the unit is in record mode. The magnetic field strength is made proportional to the signal strength corresponding to pixels in the image. Thus the recorded image consists of *tracks* of varying amounts of magnetization. To record signals at a fast enough speed both the read/write heads and the tape move. Head movement is done by placing them on a rotating drum, against which the video tape travels by.

The recorded image is played back by transporting the tape past the read/write heads, which now act as pick-up coils. As the tape moves past the heads the induced signal in the reading head is amplified and routed to a video monitor. Because the heads reside on a spinning drum it is possible to stop the motion of the tape and continuously read the signal from a single track (called "pause"). Most tape machines have protection mechanisms that stop the reading process and disengage the stationary tape from the spinning head if the pause feature is activated for more than a few minutes.

Sonographers should follow recommended procedures

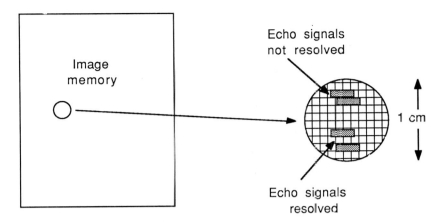

FIG. 3-38.   Spatial resolution limitations introduced by the scan converter memory matrix.

when handling and storing video tapes. In addition, the VCR recording and playback heads should be cleaned at intervals recommended by the manufacturer.

SPATIAL RESOLUTION LIMITATIONS INTRODUCED BY IMAGE STORAGE AND DISPLAY DEVICES

In Chapter 2 there is a discussion of ways in which the spatial resolution of an ultrasound instrument is limited by the transducer. It is not always appreciated that the spatial resolution may be limited also by the image memory and the image display device. These components usually are limiting factors when small image magnifications (i.e., large fields of view) are employed.

In the following discussion we will consider spatial resolution limitations introduced by the digital memory of an ultrasound imaging system. The general principles also apply to other devices (e.g., television monitors).

Consider an image stored in a digital scan converter memory in which a large field of view (say, 24 cm) is used (Fig. 3-38). Assume that the memory consists of 240 rows of pixels, with 240 pixels in each row—a reasonable size. If there are 240 pixels shared over a 24 cm field of view, each centimeter increment in the patient is represented by

$$240/24 \text{ cm} = 10 \text{ pixels/cm}$$

Recall that when we first considered spatial resolution it was described as the ability to distinguish closely spaced reflectors as being individual echo sources. Suppose we have reflectors so close to each other that their imaged positions overlap in memory (see insert in Fig. 3-38). Whether or not these reflectors are distinguishable by the transducer, they cannot be resolved by the imaging system because they fill adjacent pixels in the scan converter. There is no way for the observer to distinguish one reflector from another.

On the other hand, if there is a gap between pixels storing echo signals from two separate reflectors, the reflectors can be distinguished on the image. This gives us a rough idea of the spatial resolution limitations introduced by the scan converter. Assume now that the closest that two reflectors can be and still be "resolved" is a separation corresponding to a 2 pixel spacing in the scan con-

verter. What does this spacing translate into as far as patient dimensions if a 24 cm field of view is used?

As mentioned above, if there are 240 pixels representing a 24 cm range, this means there are 10 pixels for every 1 centimeter in the patient. If the minimum resolved reflector spacing is that corresponding to a 2 pixel separation, this translates into

$$2 \text{ pixels/10 pixels/cm} = 0.2 \text{ cm}$$

or a 2 mm spacing, which usually is worse than the axial resolution limitation introduced by a typical ultrasonic transducer. The resolution will, of course, be better if the scan converter memory has a higher pixel density than in the example presented here.

With the present system we could improve the situation by using a large image magnification (and smaller field of view) when scanning. For small fields of view we usually find transducer performance (displayed beam width, pulse duration, and slice thickness) to be the limiting factor in the spatial resolution.

SUMMARY

1. The range equation relates reflector distance to pulse-echo propagation time. For a pulse traveling with a propagation speed of 1540 m/s in tissue the round trip transit time is 13 μs/cm of tissue path.

2. The pulser of an ultrasound instrument provides signals for driving the piezoelectric transducer.

3. Echo signals detected by the transducer are applied to the receiver, where they are processed for display.

4. Effects of attenuation are compensated for using swept gain, a process whereby the receiver amplification is increased with time following the transmit pulse.

5. The term *dynamic range* is used to specify the ratio of the largest to smallest signals that an instrument or a part of an instrument can respond to without distortion.

6. Signal compression reduces the difference between signals from large amplitude echoes and signals from

low amplitude echoes, allowing a greater echo dynamic range to be displayed.

7. Rectification and smoothing are signal processing steps involved in conditioning echo signals for display.

8. Common pulse-echo display methods include A-mode, B-mode, and M-mode. B-mode is used for both static and real-time scanning.

9. Gray scale refers to modulating the brightness of the B-mode display according to the amplitude of the individual echo signals.

10. Both "real-time" and "static" ultrasound scanning are done by sweeping an ultrasound beam over the volume of interest and displaying echo signals using the B-mode.

11. The maximum speed with which a real-time instrument can build up images is limited by the finite travel time of sound pulses in tissue.

12. Sequential linear array scanners produce images by transmitting sound beams parallel with one another, beginning at one end of the array and continuing along to the opposite.

13. A sequential convex array operates on the same principle as a linear array except the scan head is curved.

14. The sound beam produced by a phased array and the directionality of the array during reception of echoes is electronically steered off at an angle with respect to a line perpendicular to the array surface.

15. Mechanical transducer assemblies generate images by physically scanning a transducer over the region of interest.

16. Video (TV) monitors are used to display image data in pulse-echo ultrasonography. They are a form of CRT that uses a fixed, raster format to scan an electron beam across a phosphor screen.

17. A scan converter accepts echo signal data from the ultrasonic scanner, stores these signals in an internal memory, and reads out the data to a TV monitor.

18. In an analog format the values of a quantity vary continuously between a minimum and a maximum level. In digital format instantaneous values are represented as discrete levels, with fixed steps between the levels. Digital systems offer advantages over analog devices in terms of stability and immunity to electronic noise.

19. Depending on whether echo signal processing occurs before or after data are stored in memory, the signal processing is referred to as *preprocessing* or *postprocessing*.

20. For large fields of view the spatial resolution in an ultrasound image may be limited by the resolution of the image memory or by the resolution of the TV monitor. For smaller fields of view resolution is ultimately limited mainly by transducer performance.

REFERENCES

1. Acoustic output measurement standard, (Draft) American Institute of Ultrasound in Medicine, Bethesda, Md.
2. Curry T, Dowdey J, and Murray R: Christiansen's introduction to the physics of diagnostic radiology, Philadelphia, 1984, Lea & Febiger, pp 238-242.
3. Dick D and Carson P: Principles of auto scan ultrasound instrumentation. In Fullerton G and Zagzebski J, editors: Medical physics of CT and ultrasound, New York, 1980, American Association of Physicists in Medicine.
4. Iinuma K, Kidokora T, Ogura I, et al: High resolution electronic-linear-scanning ultrasonic diagnostic equipment, Ultrasound Med Biol 5:51, 1979.
5. Kossoff G, Garrett W, Carpenter D, et al: Principles and classification of soft tissues by gray scale echography, Ultrasound Med Biol 2:89, 1976.
6. Kremkau F: Diagnostic ultrasound principles instrumentation and exercises, ed 2, Orlando, 1984, Grune & Stratton.

Images and Artifacts

JAMES A. ZAGZEBSKI

An ultrasound B-scan image is produced by exciting a transducer that is in acoustic contact with a patient, detecting echo signals, and displaying these signals on the B-mode display. The displayed echo position corresponds to its anatomic origin in the body. The separate aspects of this imaging process have been discussed in Chapters 1 to 3. The interactions between acoustic waves and tissues, including the speed of sound, ultrasonic attenuation, and reflection and scatter, are patient-based factors contributing to the process. Communication between the anatomic region of interest and an instrument that can process echo information and display this information in a fashion that may be understood by human observers is the function of the ultrasound transducer. The transducer adds its own "signature" to the echo information in the form of beam width effects, axial resolution limitations, and frequency characteristics. Finally, the options available for amplification signal processing and echo signal display as well as the number of operator choices available for control of the related instrumentation can lead to significant differences in the displayed appearance of otherwise similar echo data.

Our overall task in this chapter is to examine ultrasound pulse-echo images in more detail than we did in previous examples by studying the information the images convey and the artifacts they contain. Those who understand the physical basis for production of signals displayed on ultrasound images are in a better position to judge the adequacy of a clinical scan, avoid or minimize artifacts on images, and interpret the results of studies.

SPECULAR VERSUS DIFFUSE REFLECTION AND SCATTERING

Longitudinal scans of the liver or spleen and kidneys contain many practical examples of the tissue—sound beam interactions that were considered earlier from a conceptual point of view. Proper scanning techniques for imaging the liver with B-mode ultrasonography is discussed in Chapter 12.

With a sector scanner images depicting sagittal planes within the liver are obtained by scanning from an anterior subcostal window. The liver-to-kidney interface (Fig. 4-1), seen partially as a bright, smooth surface, has the characteristics of a *specular reflector*. The amplitude of an echo picked up from this interface and displayed on the monitor as a shade of gray is highly dependent on the angle between the incident sound beam and the reflector. The scanning technique used resulted in perpendicular beam incidence over a limited region of the liver-kidney interface. That region (see Fig. 4-1, *B*) is accompanied by a large amplitude echo returning to the transducer and appears as a bright area on the image. However, other parts of the interface are not visualized clearly because the incident sound beam was not perpendicular during scan buildup. As Fig. 4-1, *B*, illustrates, for nonperpendicular ultrasound beam incidence, the reflected wave travels in a direction that is not back toward the transducer.

Interfaces that reflect sound in all directions are referred to as diffuse reflectors while very small reflectors are referred to as scatterers. The parenchyma of most organs, including the liver and kidneys, contains a large

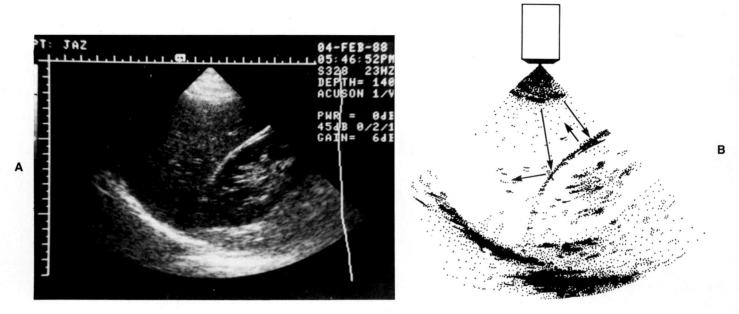

FIG. 4-1. **A,** B-mode image depicting a sagittal section of the liver. **B,** Beam paths when two different aspects of the liver-to-kidney interface are imaged.

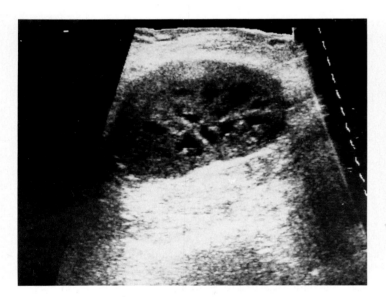

FIG. 4-2. Ultrasound B-mode image of the kidney, where renal pyramids are visualized because of local variations in ultrasound scattering.

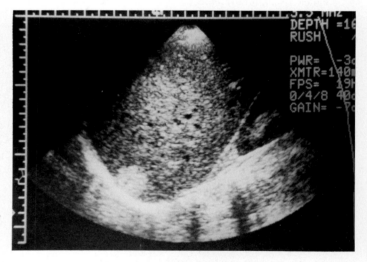

FIG. 4-3. Hyperechoic mass in the liver.

number of acoustic scatterers. Echo signals from scattering regions are much less dependent on the transducer beam orientation than are echoes from specular reflectors. Thus the brightness of displayed echo signals from different regions of the liver does not vary greatly, no matter what transducer angle is needed to visualize that region, and the liver appears uniform on the B-mode image in Fig. 4-1, *B.*

As mentioned in Chapter 1, ultrasonic scattering gives rise to much of the diagnostic information seen in ultrasound imaging. Regional variations in the scattered signal amplitude sometimes provide diagnostic information or added anatomic detail. With a gray-scale display these am-

plitude variations are transformed into changes in displayed echo brightness. An example is the visualization of the kidney pyramids (Fig. 4-2) as a result of scatter level changes. Focal lesions in the liver (Fig. 4-3) are often partly diagnosed by either an increased or a subdued ultrasound scatter level in comparison to the normal surrounding parenchyma. Regions where the acoustic scattering is greater than that of the surrounding tissue are referred to as "hyperechoic," and lower scattering regions are termed "hypoechoic."

TEXTURE IN AN ULTRASOUND B-SCAN IMAGE

The arrangement of dots or B-mode marks on an ultrasound image of an organ or tissue site is referred to as image "texture." Texture in an ultrasound image results from scattered and reflected waves from sites distributed

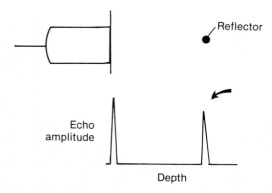

FIG. 4-4. Echo signal from a single reflector.

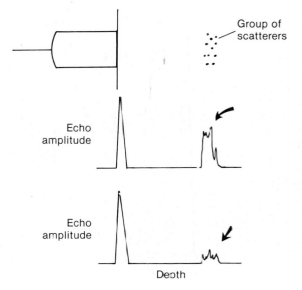

FIG. 4-5. Echo signals from a group of reflectors. An isolated echo signal could be of different magnitudes, depending on the exact number and spatial arrangement of the scatterers contributing to the signal at any instant of time. Two possible A-mode signals for the group of scatterers at the top of the diagram are shown.

throughout an organ. At present the interfaces and scattering sites giving rise to these scattered signals are not precisely known for many anatomic regions that are imaged. This is the subject of ongoing research studies in a number of laboratories.

A dominant source of image texture in B-mode ultrasonography is that due to interference of waves originating from multiple scatterers in the sound beam. These scatterers are so closely positioned that none can be resolved individually with conventional equipment. The collective effects of groups of such scatterers results in a granular, "noisy" background on B-mode images (Fig. 4-3). This is discussed in more detail below.

Interference between waves was discussed in Chapter 1, and it may be useful to review that material here. It was indicated there that when sound waves are received simultaneously from two or more separate sources, the waves can partially or completely cancel, or partially or completely reinforce, depending on the relative phases of the waves from the different sources.

A single reflector in the beam of a pulse-echo transducer will yield an echo signal whose magnitude depends in part on the position of the reflector in the beam (Fig. 4-4). If a group of very closely spaced reflectors is positioned in the beam, the *average* signal obtained depends on factors discussed in Chapter 1 (i.e., the scatterer size, number of scatterers per unit volume, the acoustic impedance difference between the scatterer and the surrounding medium, and the ultrasonic frequency). However, any *isolated* echo signal originating from this group could be of any magnitude, depending also on the relative spatial distribution of the reflectors. For example, the reflectors could be so arranged (by chance) that due to *constructive* interference a relatively large amplitude echo signal is obtained; or they also could be arranged that *destructive* interference of the scattered waves would occur, resulting in a low amplitude echo from the group (Fig. 4-5). When a pulsed sound beam is scanned over a volume of tissue that contains a fairly large number of closely spaced scatterers which are too close together to be resolved individually, the echo signal amplitude at any depth will fluctuate from one beam position to another (Fig. 4-6). The fluctuations result from random variations in the number and positions of scatterers contributing to the echo signal at any instant of time and are dominated by

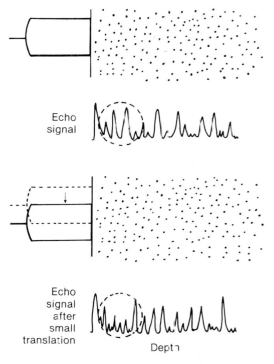

FIG. 4-6. Fluctuations in the echo signal amplitude as an ultrasound beam is scanned over a volume of tissue containing many closely spaced scatterers. These fluctuations result in texture on a B-mode image.

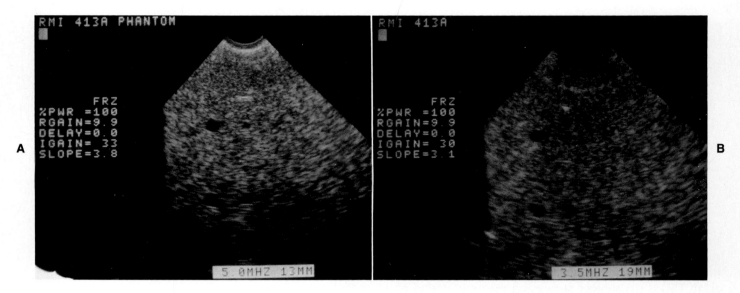

FIG. 4-7. B-mode images of a tissue-mimicking phantom using a mechanical sector scanner with a 5 MHz, **A**, and a 3 MHz **B**, probe. Notice the different appearances of the texture for different transducers and the variation in texture with depth, even though the phantom is uniform.

interference effects. These fluctuations in echo signal amplitude as the sound beam is scanned produce the texture pattern on a B-mode image. Although individual B-scan marks resemble those from individual discrete reflectors, in fact, collections of scatterers contribute to each texture dot, and the dot appearance is statistical.

When scanning tissue that has closely spaced, unresolvable scatterers, the spatial characteristics of the texture pattern, including the size of individual B-scan marks and the number of marks or dots per unit area on the image, turn out to be strongly dependent on the imaging system itself. In other words, for the situation described, the texture's spatial arrangement may convey little if any information regarding the arrangement of reflectors, but will simply make up a granular "noisy" background illustrated earlier. This granular texture is sometimes referred to as "speckle," and methods for reducing the amount of speckle are currently being pursued in some laboratories.[18] With single-element transducers the texture pattern is quite fine for positions near the transducer face, less so near the focal region, and smeared out beyond the focal region. Transducers of different nominal frequency and size may result in different texture patterns for the same scatterers (Fig. 4-7). With array transducers and employing dynamic focusing, the texture from organ parenchyma appears to be more consistent at different depths in the same organ, although subtle changes are still observed.

Several conclusions regarding this aspect of image texture can be made:

1. The pattern results from groups of unresolvable scatterers rather than from individual reflectors imaged separately.
2. For a given anatomic site the pattern obtained is dependent on the transducer frequency, diameter, and focusing properties and on the distance from the transducer.

3. Differences in texture have also been noted to be due to anatomic variations. We often use terms such as "coarse echoes" in describing such differences; however, it must be kept in mind that these patterns are influenced by the instrument also.
4. Individual dot sizes on images from such scatterers are not necessarily good indicators of spatial resolution. In fact, with single-element transducers the texture pattern is finest in the near field of the transducer, where the spatial resolution is worse.

IMAGE ARTIFACTS

An artifact is any echo signal whose displayed position does not correspond to the position of a reflector in the body.[16] It could also refer to displayed signal amplitude variations that are not due to properties of reflectors being displayed but to properties, for example, of intermediate tissues. The first type of artifact to be considered is related to the width of ultrasound transducer beams used for scanning.

Implicit assumptions in B-mode imaging

When an ultrasound pulse-echo image is produced, two assumptions are implicitly built into the instrument to place echo signals in their proper position on the display:

1. Echo sources are assumed to lie along the axis of the ultrasonic transducer beam.
2. The delay time between transmission of an acoustic pulse by the transducer and reception of an echo signal is assumed to be directly proportional to the reflector distance.

We have seen in Chapter 3 (Fig. 3-19) how using these assumptions leads to production of a B-mode image with static and real-time scanners. Significant deviations from the assumed conditions can give rise to image artifacts on a display.

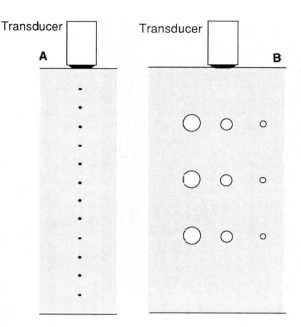

FIG. 4-8. **A,** Column of reflectors for studying displayed beam widths. **B,** Schema of part of a tissue-mimicking phantom containing echo-free vessels of different diameter and depth from the scanning window.

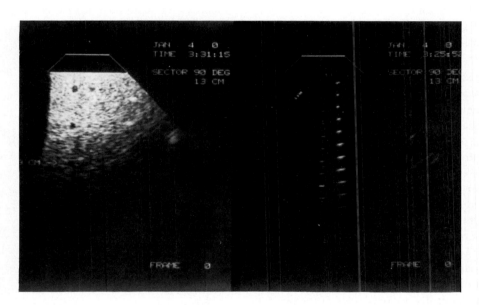

FIG. 4-9. Side-by-side images of the column of point reflectors and the vessel phantom, both scanned using a fixed-focus mechanical sector scanner with a 3 MHz, 13 mm diameter medium-focus probe. The displayed beam width at different depths may be inferred from the width of the reflector images.

Beam width effects

When an ultrasound beam is scanned over a small reflector, the resultant B-scan image of the reflector is a line. The generation of this line is rather straightforward. An echo will be detected from the reflector whenever it is within the margins of the ultrasound beam. However, the displayed position of the echo always corresponds to the beam axis. As the beam sweeps past the reflector, the displayed position of the echo moves, always coinciding with the beam axis, resulting in a line on the display. The length of the line may be called the "displayed beam width" for this target and the imaging conditions employed. The displayed beam width depends on numerous factors, including the actual transducer beam pattern; the attenuation in the medium; the dimensions, orientation, and reflection coefficient of the reflector; the instrument's pulser power; the gain and signal processing of the receiver; and even the characteristics of the echo display.

The displayed beam width can be studied by scanning line reflectors in a test object or phantom. (We will talk more about specific test object configurations in Chapter 6.) An example is shown in Fig. 4-8, wherein a column of thin nylon fibers each separated by a distance of 1 cm is present. The effects of the displayed beam width on ultrasound images can be studied more directly using the vessel phantom also shown in Fig. 4-9. This phantom has three sets of simulated vessels at depths of 3, 6, and 9 cm from the scanning window. At each depth there are three sizes of vessels: 6, 4, and 2 mm. The vessels do not contain scatterers and therefore may be visualized on a B-mode image of the phantom as an echo free zone.

Fig. 4-9 presents side-by-side images of both the col-

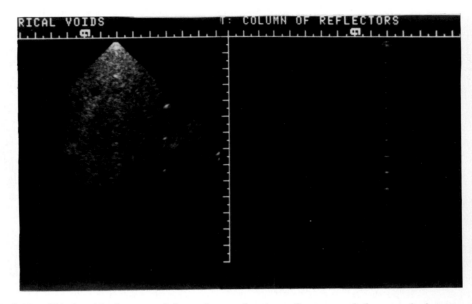

FIG. 4-10. Side-by-side images of the column of point reflectors and the vessel phantom, both scanned using a 3.5 MHz phased array with dynamic focusing. Notice the displayed beam width for the dynamically focused array is much more uniform with depth than that for the single-element transducer in the mechanical scanner used for the scans in Fig. 4-9.

umn of reflectors and the vessel phantom. The images were obtained by scanning with a 3 MHz mechanical sector scanner instrument. Notice from the image of the column of reflectors that the displayed beam width appears narrowest at about 3 cm depth, after which it gradually widens out. Examining the images of the vessels, one sees the sharpest outline of these structures also at 3 cm, with the 6 mm and 4 mm vessels crisply delineated and even a hint of the 2 mm vessel appearing. However, the details begin to fade at 6 cm, where the corresponding displayed beam width also is noticeably wider than at 3 cm. At 9 cm, where the displayed beam width is quite wide, the vessels are hardly visualized.

Similar information is conveyed on images obtained with a 3.5 MHz dynamically focused electronically sectored array, shown in Fig. 4-10. All vessels at 3 cm are visualized, perhaps with better clarity than appears in Fig. 4-9. At this depth the displayed beam width appears narrower than for the previous system. Moreover, the displayed beam width varies much less drastically with depth than with the fixed-focus mechanically scanned probe. This helps explain the presence of crisp, clear images of both the 4 mm and the 6 mm vessels at both 6 and 9 cm.

The narrower the beam width, the sharper and crisper are the echo signals displayed from any region and the better the spatial resolution. This contributes to imaging finer detailed anatomic structures. You should be able to see the correlation between narrow displayed beam widths in Figs. 4-9 and 4-10 and the spatial detail seen on the B-mode images of the vessels in the same figures. Fill-in of the echo-free regions is depicted schematically in Fig. 4-11. When the beam is larger than the echo-free region, echo signals are picked up lateral to the margins; of course, these signals are displayed along a line corre-

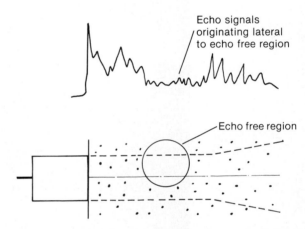

FIG. 4-11. Fill-in of echo-free structures because of beam width effects.

sponding to the beam axis, which for the example illustrated falls in the middle of the vessel!

Slice-thickness artifacts

Structures contributing to fill-in of echo-free regions do not necessarily have to be located in the plane of the scan, as in the previous examples. In the longitudinal scan shown in Fig. 4-12 partial fill-in of the aorta can be seen. In this case, fill-in was probably due in part to echo signals arising from structures lateral to the vessel, out of the indicated plane of the image. This is a manifestation of "slice thickness" effects.[5]

Fill-in of echo-free objects such as small cysts is illustrated in Fig. 4-13. The figure shows the scan plane of a real-time scanner cutting through three spherical objects. The actual scan plane extends in and out of the plane of the diagram. When the slice margins are significantly

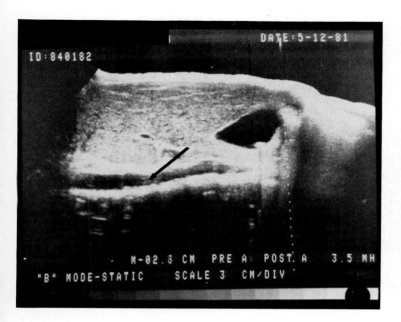

FIG. 4-12. Echo signals appearing within the aorta, probably due to slice-thickness effects.

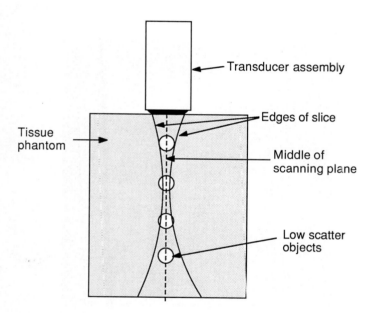

FIG. 4-13. Origin of fill-in of echo-free cysts due to slice-thickness effects. This is an edge view of the middle of the scanning plane; the projection of the scanning plane is shown by the dashed line.

greater than the size of the spherical objects, echo signals picked up from the depth of an object but outside the scanning plane are displayed in the image plane at a position corresponding to that of the spherical objects. In Fig. 4-14 a B-mode image of a phantom that has many small spherical objects is presented. The scan was done using a 3.5 MHz linear array transducer; this transducer is dynamically focused within the image plane but has a fixed focal length lens to focus perpendicular to the plane. Notice that for distances closer than 4 cm and greater than 12 cm no cystlike objects can be seen on this image; this is due mainly to the slice thickness being greater than the 4 mm spherical objects for these ranges. (Of course, beam width effects also contribute to the fill-in here as well.)

A task illustrated by the foregoing situations is differentiating artifactual echo signals from signals due to actual ultrasonic scatterers in the region of concern. We see that not every apparent echo signal on a display corresponds to an actual reflector. Conversely, we must exercise caution to avoid judging actual reflectors and scatterers as simple artifacts. It is necessary to consider all possible sources of signals, both artifactual and actual, when attempting to determine the acoustic properties of a particular region. A knowledge of the physical principles underlying the imaging process and experience with one's own equipment certainly aid in this differentiation process.

Reverberation artifacts

Many tissue interfaces in the body can produce a relatively large-amplitude echo. This could, in turn, lead to reverberation artifacts on an A-mode, M-mode, or B-mode display.

Consider the situation shown schematically in Fig. 4-15. The reflector could be, for example, a fat-muscle interface just below the skin surface. In the figure a reflected wave (solid arrow) from this interface is shown directed back toward the transducer, where it is detected, amplified, and displayed. If the echo is of significant magnitude, it will be partially reflected at the transducer surface and redirected back toward the interface. Reflection of this reverberation pulse back to the transducer produces a reverberation echo signal. The reverberation echo results from a pulse that has traveled the round trip distance between the transducer and interface twice. Thus it is displayed in a position corresponding to twice the reflecting interface distance (echo 2 in Fig. 4-15). Additional reverberations, such as echo 3 in Fig. 4-15, corresponding to three round trips of the sound pulse between the transducer and the interface, are sometimes observed. Reverberations produce artifactual echo signals that can partially mask actual echo signals on a display. They also contribute additional "acoustic noise" on an image. This

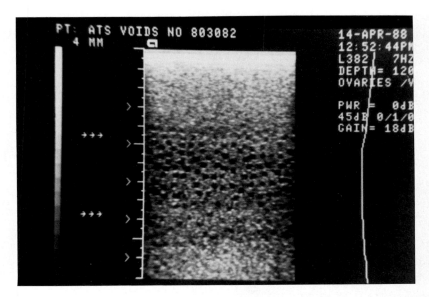

FIG. 4-14. B-mode image of a phantom containing echo-free spherical objects. No spheres are visualized in the first 4 cm of the image and beyond 11 cm because of slice-thickness effects causing fill-in.

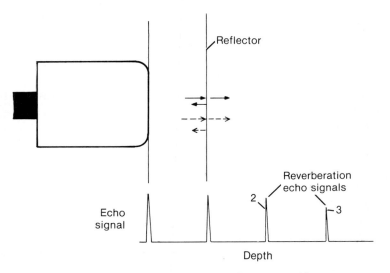

FIG. 4-15. Production of reverberation artifacts.

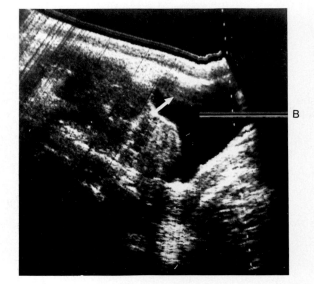

FIG. 4-16. B-mode image of a urine-filled bladder, *B*, with reverberation echoes (*arrow*).

sometimes makes it difficult to view clearly an echo-free structure, such as the aorta, or abnormal fluid collections like abscesses, by contributing to artifactual fill-in of these structures. This often leads to difficulties in identifying and/or diagnosing such structures echographically.

Examples of reverberation artifacts appearing on a B-mode display appear in Figs. 4-16 and 4-17. In the case of the urine-filled bladder (Fig. 4-16), ghost images of superficial structures are easily identifiable because of the echo-free void usually obtained during scanning of fluid-filled volumes. The ghost images of superficial tissue layers are produced by sound pulse reverberations as the transducer beam is scanned over the anatomic regions shown. Reverberations and similar ghost images are seen also in the gall bladder image in Fig. 4-17.

Echoes beyond the diaphragm

On many B-mode images of the liver one detects echo signals that appear to arise from beyond the tissue-air interface of the diaphragm (Fig. 4-18). This appears to be the result of both a reverberation artifact involving both the diaphragm and scatterers within the liver; sometimes it also involves slice-thickness effects.

An ultrasound B-mode image of a tissue phantom helps explain the reverberation contribution to this artifact (Fig. 4-19). Echo signals appear to originate beyond the end of the phantom, although the sound beam is completely reflected at this interface. The origin of this artifactual pattern is as follows: As the incident beam traverses

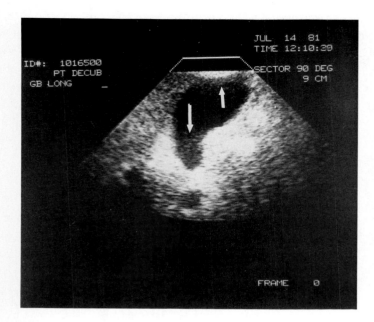

FIG. 4-17. B-mode image of the gallbladder, *G*, with reverberation echoes *(upward arrow)*. Echo signals that were from actual scatterers *(downward arrow)*.

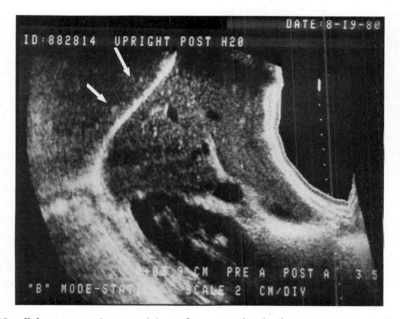

FIG. 4-18. Echoes appearing to originate from past the diaphragm as seen on a liver scan.

the medium, scattering occurs, producing the texture echoes seen on the display (Fig. 4-20, *A*). The beam is shown striking the bottom surface of the phantom, where a large fraction of the energy is reflected. Analogous to scattering of the incident beam, scattering of the reflected beam may also occur (Fig. 4-20, *B*). Scattered waves from the reflected beam path may themselves reflect off the bottom surface and trail the main reflection back toward the transducer (Fig. 4-20, *C*). Since these latter echo signals return to the transducer after the echo from the bottom surface is detected, they appear to originate from beyond this surface.

In Fig. 4-21 the tissue-air interface of the diaphragm of

a normal adult represents a highly reflective surface analogous to the bottom of the phantom in the example above. Sound waves reflected from the diaphragm can be partially scattered by reflections in the liver. A portion of these scattered waves returns to the diaphragm and is reflected back to the transducer. The longer echo transit time, of course, results in their position on the display beyond the echo from the diaphragm.

As illustrated in Fig. 4-22, slice thickness also may contribute to these artifactual signals. We are viewing a scanner from the side, with the dashed line depicting the image plane cutting the plane of the figure. The slice thickness results in energy being picked up from reflectors out-

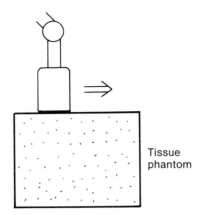

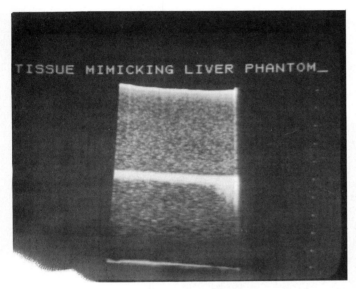

FIG. 4-19. On a scan of a liver-mimicking phantom (top), echo signals appear to originate from beyond the margin of the phantom (*arrows in image*), similar to echo signals appearing to originate from beyond the diaphragm in Fig. 4-18.

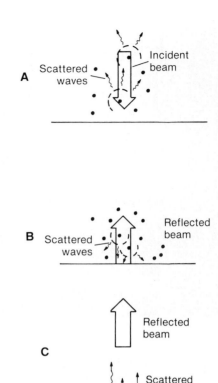

FIG. 4-20. Steps in the production of the artifactual echo signals displayed past the margin of the phantom in Fig. 4-19.

side of the image plane. Echoes picked up from the scatterers schematically shown in the lower right part of the figure must travel a greater distance than a direct echo from the diaphragm. Consequently, they appear to originate from distal to the diaphragm on an ultrasound B-mode image.

Reverberations from metallic objects

When a metallic object such as a foreign body or a biopsy needle appears in an ultrasound image, the object often leaves a clear pattern that allows it to be distinguished from soft tissue interfaces.[1,7,15,19,22] For example, the B-mode image in Fig. 4-23 illustrates a reverberation pattern obtained from a fetoscope shaft during a biopsy procedure.[15] Such artifacts are the result of reverberations and ringing of the sound pulse within the metallic object. In the example the reverberation pattern assists the operator because it helped identify the position of the tip of the fetoscope. Similarly, ringing and reverberations of pulses within metallic objects, and the resultant "tail" sign, assist in identifying such objects[19,22]

Shadowing and enhancement

If output power controls and receiver sensitivity controls are properly adjusted, a uniform echo signal brightness level can be obtained on ultrasound scans of homogeneous tissue volumes. In particular, adequate setting of the swept gain controls on the receiver can result in a uniformly displayed echo level versus depth, even when sound beam attenuation takes place in the medium. The requirement for this condition is that the attenuation rate not vary significantly from one area to another. Variations in the ultrasonic attenuation are detected on pulse-echo scans because of partial or total "acoustic shadowing" or because of distal echo enhancement. The resultant artifacts actually provide useful diagnostic information.[3,13]

Partial shadowing is a reduction in the amplitude of echo signals detected from regions distal to a mass whose attenuation is greater than that of the surrounding region. This is illustrated in Fig. 4-24. We assume the operator controls on the B-mode scanner have been adjusted for a uniform texture pattern from the region being scanned. If a mass whose attenuation coefficient is significantly higher than that of the surrounding material is situated in the scanned region, echo signals for beams traversing this mass will be comparatively weaker than echo signals traversing the same distance but through the homogeneous path. Thus there is a change in gray-scale brightness for echoes from the background material picked up after the sound beam traverses this mass. The mass partially "shadows" the region distal to it. The opposite effect takes place when a low attenuating mass, such as a cyst, is en-

FIG. 4-21. Steps in the production of the artifactual echo signals from beyond the diaphragm.

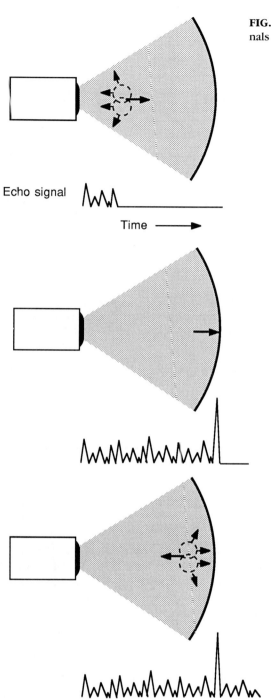

Echo signal

Time ⟶

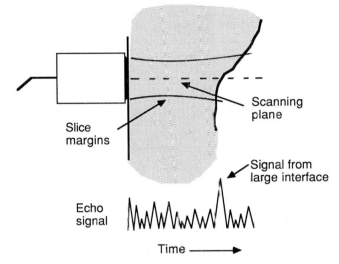

Scanning plane

Slice margins

Signal from large interface

Echo signal

Time ⟶

FIG. 4-22. Side view of a transducer assembly scanning an inclined interface, illustrating how slice thickness contributes to an apparent echo signal from beyond the diaphragm. The dashed line represents the image plane, and the solid lines represent the imaged slice.

FIG. 4-23. Real-time B-mode image of the uterus when a fetoscope is present. A curvilinear series of short echoes, *C*, leads to the location of the fetoscope tip, *T.* Additional artifactual echoes, *E*, are seen arising from the shaft of the fetoscope, S. *P*, placenta; *AC*, amniotic cavity; *S*, shaft of the fetoscope cannula. (From Schwartz D, Zweibel W, Zagzebski J, et al: J Clin Ultrasound 11:161, 1983.)

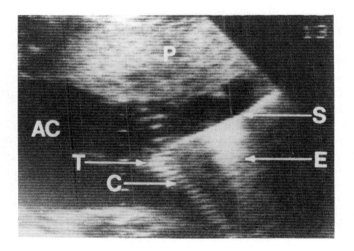

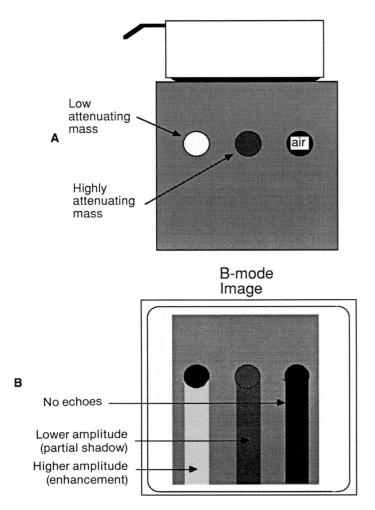

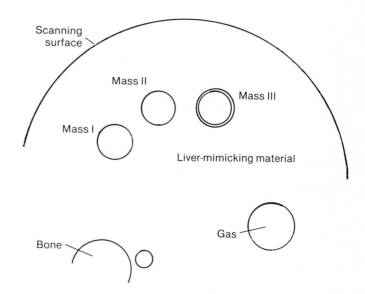

FIG. 4-25. Phantom used for demonstrating partial shadowing and echo enhancement due to differences in attenuation between masses and background material.

FIG. 4-24. Schema of partial and total acoustic shadowing and echo enhancement. **A,** Experimental setup. **B,** Possible B-mode image.

Table 4-1   Ultrasonic Properties of Masses in Fig. 4-25 (Compared to the Background)

Mass	Scatter level	Attenuation level
I	Lower	Slightly lower
II	Lower	Higher
III	Lower	Lower

countered in a similar situation (Fig. 4-24). Echo signal "enhancement" is said to take place because of the increased amplitude of the displayed signals beyond the cyst. Occasionally we say that the mass has good "through-transmission" properties. As the diagram suggests, echo enhancement is seen for all echoes detected distal to the low attenuating mass.

The presence of either of these features provides clues[17] regarding the nature of masses visualized on an ultrasound scan. To see how this occurs, consider the phantom diagrammed in Fig. 4-25. This is a section of a larger teaching phantom for sonographers.[20] It contains three spherical masses (masses I to III) whose acoustic properties compared to the background material are described in Table 4-1.

Ultrasound B-scan images of these masses are presented in Fig. 4-26. Both images were obtained with a single scan motion of the manual scanner, a technique that helps emphasize the partial shadowing and enhancement features of an image.

The walled cyst yields typical image features of a cystic structure, including an echo-free interior and excellent

through-transmission properties, the latter being indicated by the echo enhancement distal to the margins of the mass. Partial shadowing is seen in Fig. 4-26, *A,* for the highly attenuating mass. It is difficult to visualize any enhancement distal to mass *I;* apparently its attenuation coefficient is too close to that of the background material.

How would enhancement and partial shadowing be affected by changes in the ultrasonic frequency? In Chapter 1 it was stated that ultrasonic attenuation in soft tissues is proportional to the frequency. Therefore differences in the attenuation between two regions are also frequency dependent. If we reduce the ultrasonic frequency (by using a lower-frequency transducer), adjust the sensitivity controls to provide a uniform display of the background, and scan the phantom section again, the image shown in Fig. 4-26, *B,* results. Echo enhancement and partial shadowing are much less pronounced in this case. In essence, we see that partial acoustic shadowing and echo enhancement distal to masses are both more pronounced for higher-frequency sound beams.

Some interfaces in the body produce nearly complete acoustic shadowing on an image. Tissue-air interfaces (e.g., loops of gas-filled bowel or airways) are completely impenetrable because of the large impedance mismatch associated with them. Nearly complete shadowing is also

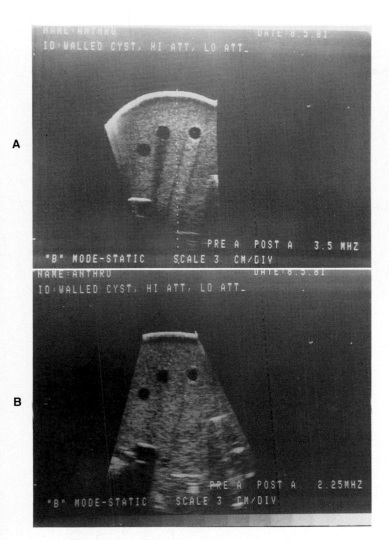

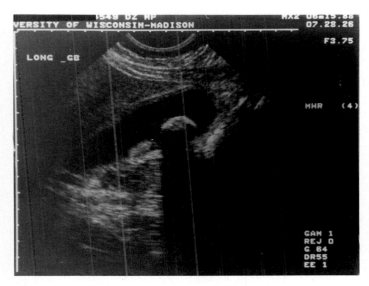

FIG. 4-27. Complete shadowing of distal structures by gallstones.

FIG. 4-26. B-mode scan images of the phantom in Fig. 4-25. **A,** With a 2.25 MHz transducer; **B,** with a 3.5 MHz transducer.

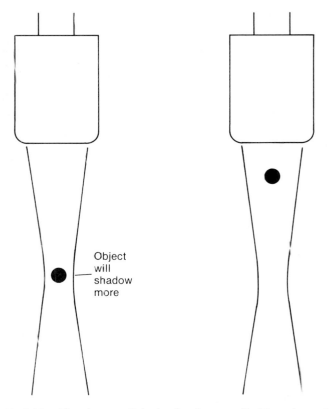

FIG. 4-28. The degree of shadowing by a small object depends on where the object is with respect to the ultrasound beam. Maximum shadowing is, of course, obtained when the object is in the focal region of the transducer.

obtained from gallstones and other calcified objects (Fig. 4-27). Manifestation of such shadowing from small objects is somewhat dependent on the objects' positions in the ultrasound beam. If a small shadowing object is nearly in the focal region of the transducer, it stands a better chance of interrupting a significant fraction of the sound beam than if it is placed in other regions of the beam (Fig. 4-28).

Sound beam deflection

Occasionally all or part of the energy within the sound beam will be deflected at a significant angle relative to the original sound beam axis. Sources of beam deflection include refraction and reflections at specular interfaces. Since the displayed echo position (Fig. 4-29) is along the line of sight of the transducer beam axis, echo signals could appear on a B-scan image in a position quite remote from their actual anatomic origin.

Refraction of a sound beam takes place when the beam strikes an interface at an angle and the speed of sound is different on each side of the interface. The larger the difference in the speeds of sound, the greater the refraction

effect will be. The greatest speed-of-sound difference where refraction can occur is at a soft tissue-bone interface. However, refraction here is usually of little practical consequence because in most instances we do not image through bone interfaces. (In fact, the significant refraction effect contributes to the problem of transmission through bone.). The major exception of clinical interest is imaging

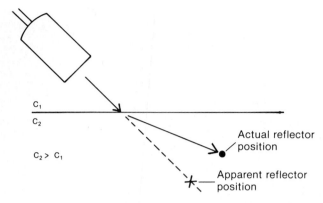

FIG. 4-29. If sound beam deflection or refraction occurs, echo signals are displayed as though they originate along the original (undeflected) beam axis. The speed of sound in the two materials is represented by c_1 and c_2 forming the interface, and c_2 is assumed greater than c_1 to get refraction in the direction shown.

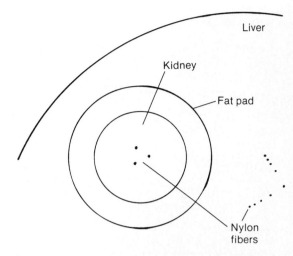

FIG. 4-30. Section of a torso-section phantom containing a simulated kidney and fat pad. Also shown is an L-shaped set of reflectors.

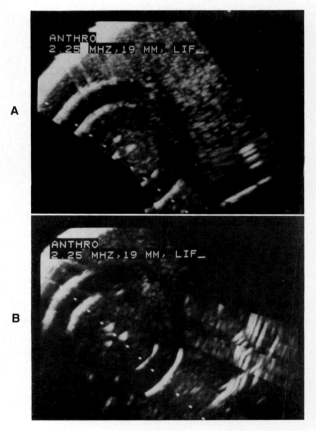

FIG. 4-31. Static B-mode image of the torso-section phantom shown in Fig. 4-30. **A,** Simple, single-pass scan. **B,** Compound scan where the reflectors were imaged with beams passing through the kidney and fat pad region. (From Madsen E et al: Med Phys 7:43, 1980.)

and Doppler examining through the skull, where ultrasound has some (although limited) use.

Soft tissue interfaces that can cause significant refraction artifacts include those formed with the lens of the eye[8] plus those formed with fat.

Because of the relatively high speed of sound in the lens and the curvature of the tissue surfaces, this structure can significantly distort and deflect a sound beam. Excellent demonstrations of this effect using Schlieren photography have been published.[8] For this reason imaging the eye with ultrasound usually involves the use of windows that exclude the lens, unless one is specifically interested in this structure in the examination.

Fat can also result in substantial refraction artifacts. The speed of sound through fat is significantly lower than that through most soft tissues. Moreover, fat is often found in abundance in planes throughout the body. These planes could be imaged with sharp angles of the incident sound beam.

Refraction and beam deflection artifacts involving fat have been demonstrated by Madsen et al.[9] using an abdominal tissue phantom. The phantom contains various structures embedded in a liver-mimicking material. Included in this phantom is a simulated kidney with a surrounding fat pad (Fig. 4-30) in turn surrounded by liver-mimicking material. The speed of sound through the fat pad material is 1450 m/s, whereas through the simulated liver and kidney it is 1560 m/s; this is sufficient difference to produce refraction for the curvature of the interfaces involved.

Images through a section of this phantom, obtained with a manual (static) scanner, are shown in Fig. 4-31. The structures seen to the right of the kidney and fat pad are images of a set of thin nylon fibers whose axes are perpendicular to the plane of the image. Several fibers forming a backward L make up the set. The scan in Fig. 4-31, *A,* was obtained with a simple scan technique, no compound scan motion being employed. That in Fig. 4-31, *B,* from the same region of the phantom, shows significant distor-

tion of the fiber images, due to transmission through the kidney and fat pad. It was produced by sectoring the transducer beam from several positions on the surface, including positions above the fat pad region. The effects on the fiber images are quite dramatic. With this simple phantom it was possible to account for the reflections and

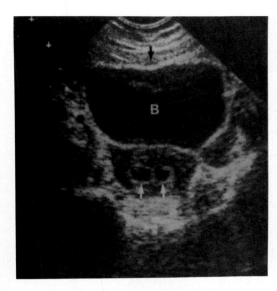

FIG. 4-32. Transverse sector scan of the pelvis with transducer placed on the midline of the abdominal wall. The image suggests two gestational sacs *(arrows)* within the uterus. Scans from other orientations failed to reveal two sacs. (From Sauerbrei E: J Ultrasound Med 4:29-34, 1985.)

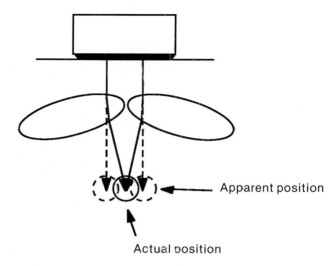

FIG. 4-33. Beam deflection paths possibly accounting for the split-image artifact in Fig. 4-32.

refraction that make up the distorted image. The case presented shows the effects that beam deflection and refraction can have on a B-scan image.

Under most clinical circumstances the geometry and complexity of the patient's anatomy make it difficult to recognize such artifacts, if indeed they exist, in clinical scans. Occasionally, however, effects as striking as that just presented are seen. An example is a double gestational sac sign early in pregnancy, giving the clinical impression of twins (Fig. 4-32), even though other ultrasound images from different orientations proved that only a single fetus was present.[14] This artifact will be seen occasionally when a transverse echogram is obtained through the lower abdomen.[2,11] Sound beams traveling through the underlying muscle fat and connective tissue layers may be deflected, resulting in the beam sweeping past the gestational sac from more than one beam axis position in the scan (Fig. 4-33).

Additional examples of beam deflection, shadowing, and enhancement

An intriguing artifact is frequently observed distal to the lateral margins of some cysts and vessels, including the gallbladder (Fig. 4-34). It is a shadowing effect below these areas. This also is a useful artifact since it sometimes aids in characterizing these structures.

Depending on the characteristics of the medium, the artifact may be related to attenuation of the sound beam through beam deflection and refraction at the vessel interface; it may also be partially due to attenuation in the vessel walls. If the speed of sound through a circular object is lower than through the surrounding material, a sound beam incident on the edge of the object will be deflected in the manner shown in Fig. 1-17.[13] Beam spreading of

this type is accompanied by significant attenuation. Reflectors situated distal to regions where beam spreading occurs will yield lower-level echo signals than if the beam is unperturbed. Thus the apparent partial shadow occurs.

Robinson et al.,[13] Madsen et al.,[9] and Ziskin et al.[21] have demonstrated that circular objects through which the speed of sound is lower than through the surrounding material also focus the acoustic energy transmitted directly through the object. This focusing contributes to echo enhancement beyond these structures. An important clinical example is the bile ducts distributed in the liver, which result in significant echo enhancement distal to them.

Another source of beam attenuation along the margins of cystic regions may be the walls of these structures. It is easy to see from Fig. 4-34 that the thickness of the wall material that must be traversed by the beam is greater at the periphery of the structure. If the attenuation coefficient of the wall is greater than that of the surrounding tissues, the increased path length will result in greater attenuation at the lateral margins than through the near and far walls of the structure.

In any case the edges of many cysts and vessels produce a so-called lateral shadow sign. A combination of the lateral shadow sign and the echo enhancement accompanying the transmission of sound through low-attenuating masses has come to be called the "tadpole tail sign." This is evident in the image of the simulated walled cyst in Fig. 4-26, A.

Speed of sound artifacts

If the sound propagation path to a reflector is partially through bone, wherein the speed of sound is greater than in the average soft tissue (assumed in the calibration of an instrument), echo "position registration" artifacts will be produced. Reflectors appear closer to the transducer than their actual distance because of this greater speed of sound, resulting in a shorter echo transit time than for paths not containing bone.

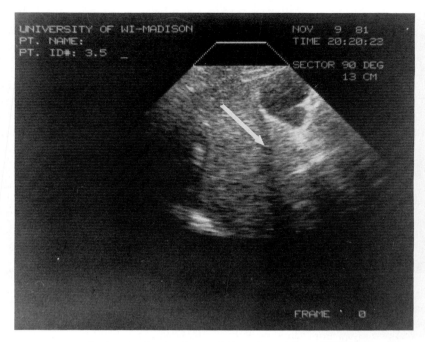

FIG. 4-34. Shadowing beyond the edge of the gallbladder.

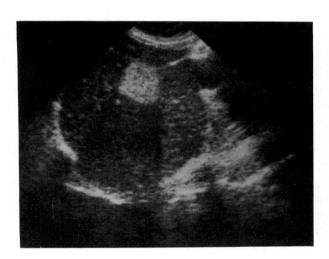

FIG. 4-35.   B-mode image of a hyperechoic mass adjacent to the diaphragm. The displayed position of the diaphragm is displaced because of the lower speed of sound within the mass than in the liver. (From Richman T, Taylor K, and Kremkau F: J Ultrasound Med 2:45, 1983.)

The opposite effect is seen in Fig. 4-35. This is a B-mode image of the liver containing a hyperechoic mass. The speed of sound within the mass appears to be lower than the speed in the surrounding liver tissue.[12] This is evident because of the distorted position of the diaphragm, as demonstrated in Fig. 4-35, indicating a longer echo transit time through the mass than through corresponding liver tissue.[10] Fatty tissues with a lower speed of sound are believed to be present in this mass. Another common example of this artifact occurs when scanning a breast implant involving silicone, which has a lower speed of sound than does soft tissue. All structures distal to this material will appear distal with respect to their anatomic position because of this longer echo transit time.

DISTANCE, AREA, AND VOLUME COMPUTATIONS
Distance measurements

Accurate measurements of organ and structure dimensions are possible in diagnostic ultrasound because the speed of sound in most soft tissues is known to within about 1%. By using an instrument's internal depth markers whose spacing corresponds to a known distance in tissue when a speed of sound of 1540 m/s is assumed, a measurement accuracy to within 1% or 2% is possible. Even greater measurement accuracy can be obtained in ophthalmologic applications because of the use of high frequencies, careful scanning, and well-known speeds of sound in the media traversed.

Careful choice of measurement reference positions is necessary to realize maximum accuracy for distance measurements. On A-mode or B-mode displays the leading edge of the reflector echo signal is usually the best choice (Fig. 4-36). This point is least affected by variations in echo signal amplitude stemming from the reflectors themselves or the settings and characteristics of the instrument.

Distance measurements are always more accurate if the direction over which the measurement extends corresponds to an ultrasonic beam axis orientation at the time the scan was done (Fig. 4-37) rather than perpendicular to the beam axis. This is because the reflector position can be pinpointed more accurately since the axial resolution of a pulse-echo imaging system is generally better than the lateral resolution. In addition, any errors due to scan position registration inaccuracy (discussed in Chapter 6) will not contribute to the distance measurement er-

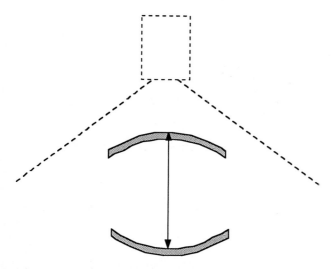

FIG. 4-36. Arrows illustrate the best choice of echo signal reference spots for distance measurements on echograms. The leading edge (with respect to the transducer position) of the echo signal is preferred.

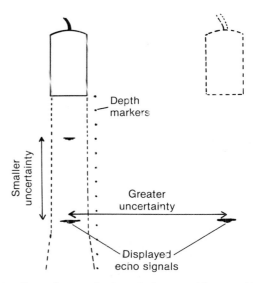

FIG. 4-37. From the standpoint of ultrasound beam width considerations, distance measurements along a beam line are more accurate than measurements perpendicular to a beam line.

ror if distances are measured along a sound beam axis. However, for many types of measurements the measured direction must be perpendicular to the beam direction; care must be exercised in being certain that the points of reference to be measured from are properly viewed on the image.[4]

Depth markers can be used reliably since these are produced by stable electronic circuitry and usually correspond to 1 cm depth intervals in tissue. Care required in proper use of depth markers requires that their calibration be checked routinely. This can be done as part of a normal quality assurance program for ultrasound equipment (Chapter 6). Also, primarily for manual scanners in which the depth markers can be produced at different orientations on the screen, caution must be exercised to avoid measurement inaccuracies due to TV monitor distortion. A common source of distortion is unequal display magnification in the horizontal and vertical directions. The distance on hard copy between two reflectors may appear different when measurements are obtained by means of depth markers produced in the vertical and the horizontal directions. Errors resulting from possible TV monitor distortion can be minimized if the depth markers are generated as closely as possible and in the same orientation as the line segment connecting the points to be measured.

Measurements can also be done with digital calipers on most units. Operationally the digital calipers in many instruments determine the pixel separation between two specified points on the image and convert this to a distance. The user merely places the cursors on the two points between which a measurement is desired. The instrument determines the number of pixels separating the two cursors, multiplies this number by an appropriate magnification factor depending on the field of view, and provides a numeric readout of the distance in the patient.

Digital caliper circuitry is also subject to error, and its calibration should be assessed routinely (Chapter 6).

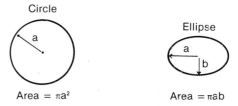

FIG. 4-38. Formulas for computing the area of a circle and an ellipse.

Areas

In certain situations the cross-sectional area of a structure viewed on an echogram provides diagnostic information. Often the area can be estimated by assuming a shape and applying appropriate formulas to the area measurement. For circles and ellipses the areas are presented in Fig. 4-38. Some instruments have built-in programs requiring operator input of structure axes from which the circumference and area are computed internally.

For complex shapes some instruments provide area analysis programs that require tracing the region of interest using a joystick or cursor; once this is carried out, the system can first count the number of pixels enclosed by the outlined region. Each pixel can be thought of as a tiny piece of the area of the entire contour. That is when the number of pixels within the contour is multiplied by an area magnification factor, the area enclosed by the contour may be estimated. Software such as this is available in many instruments.

Volumes

Ultrasound images can also be used to estimate the volumes of structures and organs. Such measurements may provide more sensitive indications of changes in structure dimensions than simple distance or area measurements.[6]

Volume estimates are sometimes made by assuming a

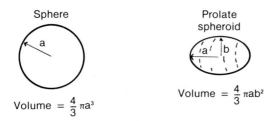

FIG. 4-39. Formulas for computing the volumes of a sphere and a prolate spheroid.

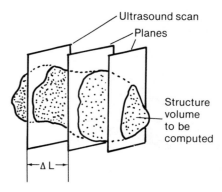

FIG. 4-40. "Bread slice" approach to computing the volume of a structure from serial scans.

simple shape and using ultrasound scans to obtain the necessary dimensions to plug into equations for the volumes. In certain cases, for example, it is reasonable to estimate the volume by assuming that the shape is a sphere (Fig. 4-39). In this case the volume is that shown in the figure. Another common shape is a prolate spheroid, also shown in the figure.

For irregularly shaped structures in which a sphere or spheroid is not appropriate for estimating the volume, a serial scan approach can be followed. This technique, outlined in Fig. 4-40, is sometimes referred to as the "read-slice approach." Serial scans a known separation apart, ΔL, are obtained through the region of interest. Then the area of the structure in question is estimated for each echogram on which the structure is included. The area can be estimated by any of the methods just outlined.

The area multiplied by the distance between echograms represents a section of the volume, or one slice of the loaf of bread. Summing all the volume sections corresponding to each scan that cuts through the structure provides an estimate of the volume.

SUMMARY

1. Echo signal amplitudes from specular reflectors are dependent on the orientation of the reflector with respect to the ultrasound beam. Signals from diffuse reflectors and scatterers are much less dependent on orientation.

2. Regional variations in ultrasound scattering are recognized on gray-scale images and help delineate normal and abnormal structures.

3. Much of the gray-scale texture on ultrasound images is the result of interference of waves from small, unresolvable scatterers.

4. An artifact is any echo signal whose displayed position does not correspond to the position of a reflector in the body.

5. The displayed beam width for a reflector depends on the transducer beam pattern; the attenuation in the medium; the dimensions, orientation, and reflection coefficient of the reflector; the instrument's pulser power; the gain and signal processing of the receiver; and the characteristics of the display.

6. The narrower the beam width, the better the spatial resolution and the finer the details of anatomic structures.

7. Slice thickness contributes to fill-in of scatter-free regions in the image plane.

8. Reverberation artifacts are caused by sound pulses reflecting back and forth between highly reflective surfaces.

9. Ringing and reverberations of pulses within metallic objects produce a "tail" sign, assisting in identifying such objects.

10. Variations in ultrasonic attenuation are detected on B-mode images because of partial or total "acoustic shadowing" or because of distal "echo enhancement."

11. Fat can result in significant refraction artifacts because the speed of sound is significantly lower than that through most soft tissues.

12. Circular objects through which the speed of sound is lower than through the surrounding material focus the acoustic energy transmitted directly through the object.

13. If the sound propagation path to a reflector is partially through a structure whose speed of sound differs from 1540 m/s (or the value assumed in the calibration of the instrument), echo "position registration" artifacts will be produced.

14. Accurate measurements of organ and structure dimensions are possible in diagnostic ultrasound because the speed of sound in most soft tissues is known to within about 1%.

15. Distance measurements are always more accurate if the direction over which the measurement extends corresponds to an ultrasonic beam axis orientation at the time the scan was done.

REFERENCES

1. Avruch L and Cooperberg P: The ring-down artifact, J Ultrasound Med 4:21-28, 1985.

2. Buttery B and Davison G: The ghost artifact, J Ultrasound Med 3:49-52, 1984.

3. Filly R, Sommer F, and Minton M: Characterization of biological fluids by ultrasound and computed tomography, Radiology 134:167, 1980.

4. Goldstein R, Filly R, and Simpson G: Pitfalls in femur length measurements, J Ultrasound Med 6:203-207, 1987.

5. Goldstein A and Madrazo B: Slice thickness artifact in gray-scale ultrasound, J Clin Ultrasound 9:365, 1981.

6. Jones T, Riddick L, Harpen M, et al: Ultrasonographic determination of renal mass and volume, J Ultrasound Med 2:151-154, 1983.

7. Lewandowski B, French G, and Winsberg F: The normal post-cholecystectomy sonogram; gas vs clips, J Ultrasound Med 4:7-12, 1985.

8. Lizzi F, Burt W, and Coleman D: Effects of ocular structures on the propagation of ultrasound in the eye, Arch Ophthalmol 84:635, 1970.

9. Madsen E, Zagzebski J, and Ghilardi-Netto T: An anthropomorphic torso phantom for ultrasonic imaging, Med Phys 7:43, 1980.

10. Mayo J and Cooperberg P: Displacement of the diaphragmatic echo by hepatic cysts: a new explanation with computer simulation, J Ultrasound Med 3:337, 1984.

11. Muller N, Cooperberg P, Rowley V, et al: Ultrasonic refraction by the rectus abdominus muscles: the double image artifact, J Ultrasound Med 3:515-519, 1984.

12. Richman T, Taylor K, and Kremkau F: Propagation speed artifact in a fatty tumor (myelolipoma): significance for tissue differential diagnosis, J Ultrasound Med 2:45-47, 1983.

13. Robinson D, Wilson L, and Kossoff G: Shadowing and enhancement in ultrasonic echograms by reflection and refraction, J Clin Ultrasound 9:181, 1981.

14. Sauerbrei E: The split image artifact in pelvic ultrasonography: anatomy and physics, J Ultrasound Med 4:29-34, 1985.

15. Schwartz D, Zweibel W, Zagzebski J, et al: The use of real-time ultrasound to enhance fetoscopic visualization, J Clin Ultrasound 11:161-164, 1983.

16. Skolnick M, Meire H, and Lecky J: Common artifacts in ultrasound scanning, J Clin Ultrasound 3:273, 1975.

17. Skwarok D, Goiney R, and Cooperberg P: Hepatic pseudotumors in patients with ascites, J Ultrasound Med 5:5-8, 1986.

18. Sommer F and Sue J: Image processing to reduce ultrasonic speckle, J Ultrasound Med 2:413-416, 1983.

19. Wendell B and Athey P: Ultrasonic appearance of metallic foreign bodies in parenchymal organs, J Clin Ultrasound 9:133, 1981.

20. Zagzebski J, Madsen E, Frank G, et al: A teaching phantom for ultrasonographers. Program and abstracts, Twenty-sixth annual meeting of the American Institute of Ultrasound in Medicine, San Francisco, August 1981.

21. Ziskin M, Lafollette P, Radecki P, and Villafana T: The retrolenticular afterglow: an echo enhancement artifact, J Ultrasound Med 5:385-389, 1986.

22. Ziskin M, Thickman D, Goldenberg N, et al: The comet-tail artifact, J Ultrasound Med 1:1, 1982.

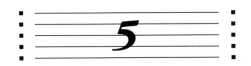

5

Doppler Instrumentation

JAMES A. ZAGZEBSKI

The Doppler effect is used in medical ultrasound to detect moving reflectors and to measure and characterize blood flow in different sites. In this chapter we will describe the Doppler effect and outline principles and limitations of Doppler instruments.

Whenever there is relative motion between a sound source and a listener, the frequency heard by the listener differs from that produced by the source. The perceived frequency is either greater or less than that transmitted by the source, depending on whether the source and the listener are moving toward or away from one another. This change in the perceived frequency relative to the transmitted frequency is called a *Doppler shift*. In general, a Doppler frequency shift can occur for a moving source and stationary listener, a moving listener and stationary source, or a moving source and moving listener.

Most of us are familiar with the Doppler effect occurring when an automobile, truck, or other motor vehicle sounds its horn as it passes by. If the horn is sounding continuously, its pitch seems to drop abruptly just as the vehicle passes. As the vehicle approaches the listener the Doppler shift results in the perceived pitch of the horn being higher than that actually transmitted. Similarly the perceived frequency is lower than that transmitted as the vehicle recedes. The very noticeable drop in pitch as the vehicle passes is just the transition between the two conditions.

The origin of a Doppler shift is depicted schematically in Fig. 5-1. The impatient motorist's car horn in *A* represents a stationary sound source, transmitting diverging sound waves. The circles can be taken as individual cycles of the sound wave, each separated by one wavelength. The sound frequency heard by the listener is the same as that transmitted. (It is assumed that no movement of the medium occurs, such as caused by wind and so on.)

If the source is moving toward the listener (Fig. 5-1, *B*), the appearance of the wave fronts changes. The motion causes wave fronts between the source and the listener to be "squeezed together" somewhat. Likewise, if the movement is away from the listener, the wave fronts are spread apart somewhat. For movement toward the listener a greater number of cycles is heard per second than for the stationary source and listener. Hence there is an increase in the perceived sound frequency relative to the transmitted frequency. The opposite is true for movement away from the listener—the frequency heard by the listener is less than the frequency transmitted by the source. In both cases the magnitude of the difference between transmitted and perceived sounds is proportional to the speed of the source.

DOPPLER EQUATION FOR MOTION ALONG THE BEAM AXIS

The ultrasound Doppler effect is employed in medicine using the general scheme shown in Fig. 5-2. The ultrasound transducer produces a sound beam whose fre-

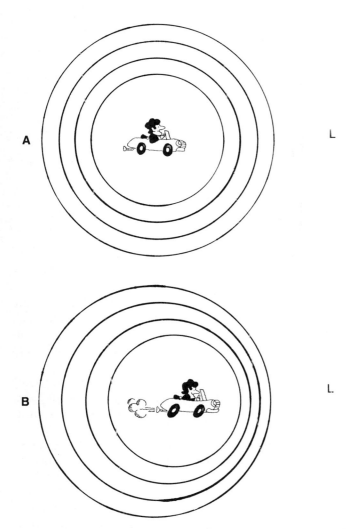

FIG. 5-1. Schema of the origin of the Doppler effect. Wavefronts are shown for a stationary sound source, **A**, and a moving source, **B**, **L** corresponds to the position of a listener.

quency is f_o. The beam is shown reflecting from an interface that is moving toward the transducer. Because of this movement the frequency of the reflected sound, given by f_r in the figure, is somewhat greater than that of the transmitted beam. The Doppler shift frequency, f_D, is the *difference* between the received and the transmitted frequencies and is given by

$$f_D = f_r - f_o \qquad (5\text{-}1)$$
$$= 2f_o v/c$$

where v is the velocity of the reflector and c is the speed of sound in the medium.

Example: Suppose $f_o = 2$ MHz and v $= 5$ cm/s. What is the Doppler frequency? Assume the speed of sound is 1540 m/s.

Solution: Simply substitute the given values into Equation 5-1. Notice that 2 MHz = 2×10^6 cycles per second (cps).

$$f_D = \frac{2 \times 2 \times 10^6 \text{ cps} \times 0.05 \text{ m/s}}{1.54 \times 10^3 \text{ m/s}}$$

The units m/s in the numerator and denominator cancel. Simplifying gives

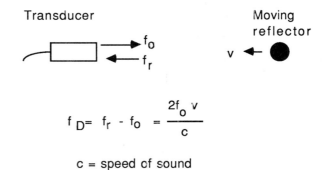

$$f_D = \frac{2f_o v}{c}$$

$$c = \text{speed of sound}$$

FIG. 5-2. Doppler effect brought about by a moving reflector. The frequency of the transmitted sound beam is f_o, and the frequency of the echo signal from the reflector is f_r.

$$f_D = \frac{0.2 \times 10^6 \text{ cps}}{1.54 \times 10^3}$$
$$= 1.3 \times 10^2 \text{ cps}$$

or

$$f_D = 130 \text{ Hz}$$

For the example presented, the frequency of the transmitted wave was said to be 2.0 MHz. The received ultrasound frequency is very close to the same value, 2.00013 MHz. The Doppler frequency, being the difference between the received and transmitted frequencies, is in the audible frequency range for this example. (In fact, it is in the audible range for most situations of interest in this chapter, and medical ultrasound instruments present the Doppler signals in the form of audio signals for interpretation.)

The Doppler frequency shift is directly proportional to the reflector velocity. In other words, the shift in frequency can be used to measure the speed of a reflector, as illustrated in the following example.

Example: If a 2000 Hz Doppler signal is detected using a 5 MHz transducer, how fast is the reflector moving? (Assume the direction of motion is directly toward the transducer.)

Solution: We must solve Equation 5-1 for v. This is done by multiplying both sides of the equation by c and then dividing both sides by $2f_o$. The result is

$$v = \frac{c f_D}{2f_o}$$
$$= \frac{1540 \text{ m/s} \times 2000/\text{s}}{2 \times 5,000,000/\text{s}} \qquad (5\text{-}2)$$
$$= 0.3 \text{ m/s}$$
$$= 30 \text{ cm/s}$$

DOPPLER EQUATION FOR MOTION AT AN ANGLE TO THE BEAM AXIS

Doppler equipment is commonly used for detecting and evaluating the characteristics of blood flow in arteries and veins. Here the usual situation is that depicted schematically in Fig. 5-3, where the ultrasonic transducer is placed in contact with the external skin surface and the ultrasound beam directed toward the vessel of interest. The beam is at an angle θ with respect to the axis of the vessel. Red blood cells flowing in the vessel are small-sized

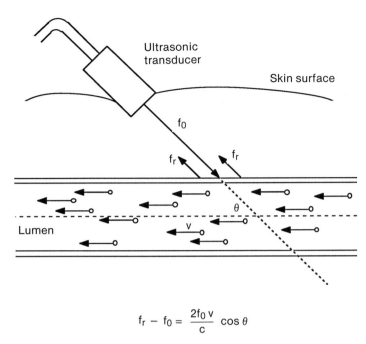

$$f_r - f_0 = \frac{2f_0\,v}{c}\cos\theta$$

FIG. 5-3. Doppler frequency shift for echo signals detected when the transducer beam is at an angle *A* with respect to the direction of flow.

inhomogeneities, which scatter ultrasound in the manner discussed in Chapter 1. In most instruments the scattered echo signals are detected by the same ultrasonic transducer assembly used to produce the incident beam. Because the scatterers are moving, the frequency of the return echo signals are Doppler shifted. The Doppler shift in this situation is given by:

$$f_D = (2f_0 v/c)\cos\theta \qquad (5\text{-}3)$$

This equation is identical to Equation 5-1, except for the cos θ term, where the angle θ is shown in Fig. 5-3.

Let's look at how the angle term (cos θ) affects the Doppler equation. The function cos θ plotted in Fig. 5-4, varies between 1.0 and 0 for angles between 0 and 90 degrees. If the sound beam propagates directly toward the direction of blood flow, θ is 0 degree, cos θ is 1, and Equation 5-3 simplifies to the expression in Equation 5-1. For the sound beam incident at an angle other than 0 degree, the detected Doppler frequency shift is reduced according to the cos θ term. Notice that for perpendicular beam incidence, θ = 90 degrees and cos θ = 0; therefore there is no detected Doppler shift! (Thus the transducer beam orientation that provides the best B-mode image detail of a vessel wall, that is, perpendicular beam incidence, results in the least favorable Doppler signals from within the vessel.) In practice the transducer beam is usually oriented to make a 30- to 60-degree angle with the lumen of the vessel when the vessel runs nearly parallel to the skin surface. For certain situations, such as those that may be encountered in echocardiology, it is possible to align the sound beam almost in the same direction as the flow. Then cos θ is approximately 1.

If the incident beam angle is greater than 90 degrees

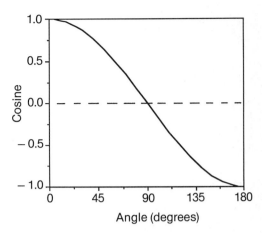

FIG. 5-4. Plot of the cosine function versus angle for 0 to 180 degrees.

with respect to the direction of flow, the cosine of the angle is negative. This corresponds to flow directed *away* from the transducer; the frequency, f_r, of echo signals from within the vessel is now *lower* than f_0, the transmitted frequency. As we shall see below, "directional" Doppler instruments detect whether the received frequency is greater than or less than the transmitted frequency and, hence, display whether flow is directed toward or away from the transducer.

The Doppler angle will be discussed later in this chapter when pulsed Doppler instrumentation is described.

CONTINUOUS-WAVE DOPPLER INSTRUMENTS

Continuous-wave (CW) Doppler instruments are the simplest and often the least expensive Doppler devices available. A simplified block diagram of such an instrument is presented in Fig. 5-5. A transmitter continuously excites the ultrasonic transducer with a sinusoidal electric signal, producing a sound wave of frequency f_0. Echo signals resulting from reflection and scattering return to the transducer, creating an electric signal that is applied to the receiver amplifier. Within the amplifier the signal is boosted in strength and applied to a detector. In the detector the return echo signal is "mixed" with a reference signal derived from the transmitter (this usually is done by multiplying the return signal by the reference signal), producing a complicated product; the product contains a mixture of signals, one whose frequency is equal to the *sum* of the reference frequency and the return echo signal frequency and another that is equal to the *difference* between the reference frequency and the return frequency. The "difference frequency" signal is the Doppler shift signal; it is isolated by electronically filtering away all of the high frequencies in the complicated product. The result is that only low-frequency Doppler shift signals—say 20 kHz and less— emerge in the output.

Further filtering is done at this stage to remove signals originating from slowly moving reflectors, such as vessel walls. The upper frequency end of these latter filtered signals usually is adjustable by the operator using a "wall filter" or similar control on the instrument.

The output of the device is a complex signal whose fre-

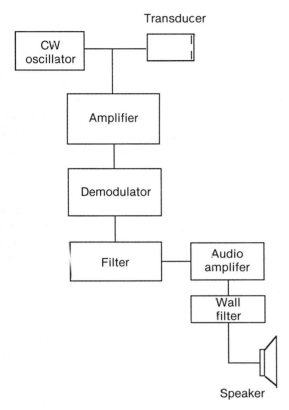

FIG. 5-5. Continuous-wave Doppler instrument.

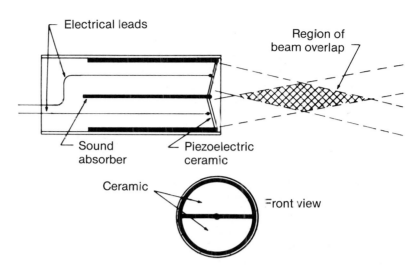

FIG. 5-6. Typical construction of a continuous-wave Doppler transducer. (From Zagzebski J: Ultrasound Dec. 1981, Fig. 6.)

quency is related to the velocity of all reflectors and scatterers within the sound beam.

The filtered-output Doppler signal usually is applied to a loudspeaker or headphones for interpretation. The signals also can be recorded on audio tape or applied to a spectral analysis system (see above). Real-time spectrum analyzers indicate the distribution of signal frequencies, and hence, reflector velocities, contributing to the Doppler signal.

Continuous-wave Doppler instruments range in complexity from simple, pocket-type instruments to units that are part of large, "duplex" scanners (see above). Operator controls available on a continuous-wave Doppler instrument vary with the degree of complexity of the unit. Typically the following are available:

1. Transmit power control; this varies the electrical power applied to the ultrasound transducer and, hence, varies the amplitude of the transmitted beam. Higher power output settings result in larger amplitude echo signals picked up by the transducer. Of course, they also result in greater acoustic exposure to patients.

2. Receiver sensitivity control; this adjusts the amount of amplification or gain of the receiver amplifier.

3. Loudness or volume control; this allows adjustments of the gain of the audio amplifier section of the instrument.

4. Wall filter control; adjusts the low frequency cutoff of the output Doppler signals. Signals whose frequencies are lower than this cutoff are eliminated from the display.

Some combination of controls 1 to 3 generally are available to allow the operator to vary the sensitivity of the Doppler instrument. Most Doppler units have a wall filter adjustment also.

CONTINUOUS-WAVE DOPPLER TRANSDUCERS

Most continuous-wave Doppler instruments employ separate transducer elements for transmitting and receiving. The reason for this is that since the transducer transmits sound waves continuously, weak echo signals picked up by the transducer would be overwhelmed by the transmit signal if the same element were used for both transmitting and receiving. Thus one element is used for continuous transmitting while the other is used for receiving. This could be done using separate elements in the array of a duplex (see below) scanner. More commonly, stand-alone transducers are used in continuous-wave Doppler instruments.

A typical stand-alone transducer design for continuous-wave Doppler is illustrated in Fig. 5-6. Each element is cut in the shape of a semicircle and the elements are tilted slightly, as shown in the figure. The beam patterns of the transmitting and receiving transducers are thus made to cross. The region of beam overlap is the most sensitive area of this type of transducer, and scatterers that happen to be within this region yield the largest amplitude Doppler signals. Transducers may be designed to emphasize signals from any depth by appropriate choice of beam overlap or beam focal distance.

Since a continuous-wave Doppler transducer does not produce short duration pulses, steps taken to dampen the ringing of the element that are common to pulsed transducers do not need to be taken. It may be advantageous, however, to add quarterwave matching layers to improve the sensitivity of the probe.

CHOICE OF ULTRASOUND OPERATING FREQUENCY

In our discussions of pulse-echo imaging we indicated that the choice of operating frequency for that modality was the result of a tradeoff between the desire to obtain high resolution (which improves with increasing frequency) and the need to obtain adequate penetration of the ultrasound beam (which decreases with increasing frequency). These tradeoffs also are factors in determining the best frequency for specific applications of Doppler instruments.

However, factors besides attenuation play a role in the signal strength in Doppler ultrasound. Since the source of ultrasound signals is blood, the scatterers are small, Rayleigh scatterers. The intensity of scattered signals for Rayleigh scatterers increases with the frequency raised to the fourth power. It would thus seem reasonable to use a high ultrasound frequency to increase the intensity of echo signals scattered from blood. As the frequency increases, however, the rate of beam attenuation also increases. In selecting the optimal frequency for detecting blood flow, these competing processes must be balanced, and the choice is related to the depth of the vessel of interest. For small, superficial vessels, where attenuation from overlying tissues is not significant, Doppler probes operating in the 8 to 10 MHz frequency range are common. Frequencies as low as 2 MHz are used where significant ranges and large amounts of attenuation are present.

DIRECTIONAL DOPPLER

In a simple, "nondirectional" Doppler instrument, the output Doppler signals are identical for reflectors moving toward the transducer or away from the transducer. In other words, a nondirectional Doppler instrument cannot distinguish whether the Doppler shift is positive or nega-

tive. In some applications only the presence of flow or the relative speed of reflectors needs to be detected, and simple processing with no directional information will do. However, in many situations the direction of flow also is important, requiring directional Doppler circuitry.

Special signal processing is required in an instrument that displays the direction of flow. Ordinarily this is done in two stages: (1) Doppler signals are generated that have the directional information encoded, and (2) the directional information is displayed using loud speakers, spectral analyzers, or velocity waveform circuits.

A commonly used signal processing method in directional Doppler instruments is known as "quadrature detection"[1,3,8,9] (Fig. 5-7). After the received signal is amplified it is sent to two separate channels or circuits within the instrument. In each channel the signal is mixed with a reference signal derived from the transmitter, similar to nondirectional processing outlined earlier. Filtering out all but the audible Doppler signals yields two nearly identical Doppler signals, v_a and v_b, in the separate channels. Processing in the two channels is the same except for a slight difference in the reference signals. These differ in phase by exactly one fourth the period of the reference frequency, hence the term "quadrature detectors." Although not obvious unless one works through the mathematics involved in multiplying the signals together in each of the channels, the output Doppler signals, v_a and v_b, will also differ in phase: their relative phase depends on whether the received echo signal frequency is greater or less than the transmitted signal frequency. Hence the phase relationship of the output quadrature signals de-

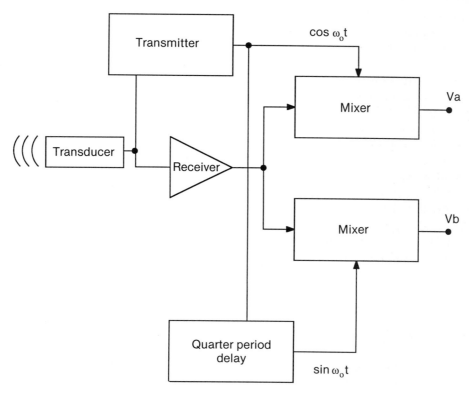

FIG. 5-7. Quadrature detection circuitry for determining whether movement is toward or away from the transducer.

pends on whether the scatterers are moving toward or away from the transducer (Fig. 5-8). This can be used to determine the flow direction.

The two quadrature signals sound identical when applied individually to loudspeakers. They are processed further to derive directional information. A commonly used method to present flow direction is with stereo speakers, each speaker being made to respond to flow in one direction only. This can be done by combining the signals from the quadrature channels as illustrated in Fig. 5-9.[1] Before combining, if v_a is *delayed* by exactly one-fourth cycle, it is brought directly into phase with v_b when flow is forward and directly opposite (that is, out of phase) when flow is reversed. The signal for the forward speaker is obtained by *adding* the two signals, $v_{a'}$ and v_b. That for the reverse speaker is obtained by *subtracting* $v_{a'}$ from v_b. When this is done, the desired effect of forward flow signals assigned to one speaker and reverse flow to the other is obtained.

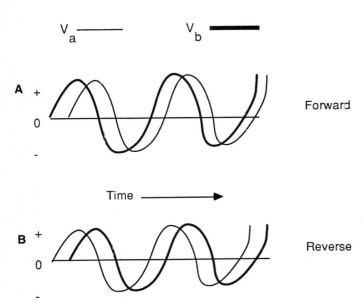

FIG. 5-8. Representative output signals of the two quadrature channels when flow is toward, **A**, and away from, **B**, the transducer.

The quadrature signals are also used in spectral analysis displays. This is discussed later in this chapter.

DIRECTIONAL DISCRIMINATION CAPABILITY

The purpose of directional Doppler is, of course, to provide the operator a display that indicates whether flow is toward or away from the ultrasonic transducer. A delicate balance must be maintained between the two quadrature channels within the Doppler instrument for this directional discrimination to take place. If this balance is inadequate, "leakage" of signals corresponding to flow in one direction will occur, giving the impression of flow also in the opposite direction (Fig. 5-10). This leakage often occurs, even on well-balanced units, with very strong Doppler signals. However, on units that are functioning poorly, the leakage is strong enough to make it difficult to discriminate whether flow actually exists in both directions or whether the instrument is producing an erroneous display.

Inadequate directional discrimination, a fault of the instrument, should not be confused with *aliasing*, a physical limitation in pulsed Doppler systems, discussed later.

PULSED DOPPLER

With continuous-wave Doppler instruments, reflectors and scatterers anywhere within the beam of the transducer can contribute to the instantaneous Doppler signal. Pulsed Doppler provides discrimination of Doppler signals from different depths, allowing for the detection of moving interfaces and scatterers from within a well-defined "sample" volume (Fig. 5-11). In this modality a pulse of sound is transmitted into the body, and echoes from scattering and reflecting interfaces are detected. The Doppler detection part of the instrument can be made sensitive to signals arriving during a fixed time interval following the transmit pulse, thus defining the sample volume. The sample volume can be positioned anywhere along the axis of the Doppler ultrasound beam.

A schema of a pulsed Doppler instrument is presented in Fig. 5-12. The drawing illustrates use of a single-element transducer, although array transducer assemblies

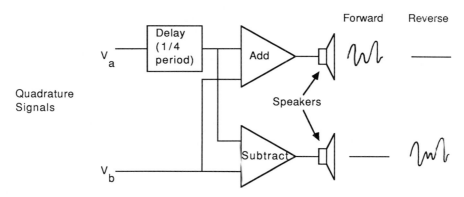

FIG. 5-9. Method for combining quadrature signals so that a signal is applied to one stereo speaker for flow in one direction and a second speaker for flow in the opposite direction.

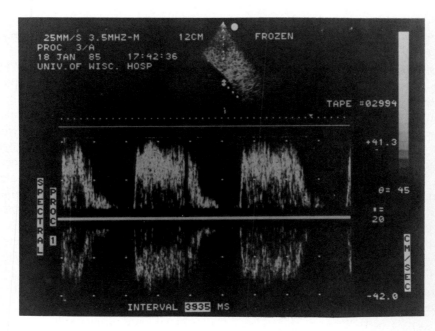

FIG. 5-10.   Doppler signal spectral display, illustrating inadequate directional discrimination.

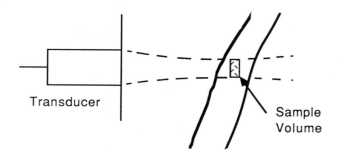

FIG. 5-11.   Principle of pulsed Doppler. Doppler signals from a sample volume may be isolated on the display.

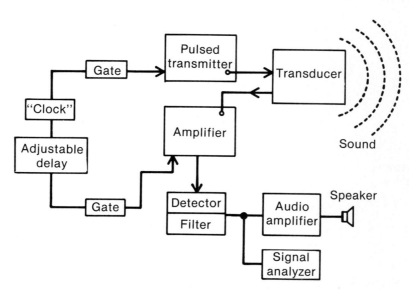

FIG. 5-12.   Pulsed Doppler instrumentation.

and other real-time scanning configurations also are used. The transducer is driven with short bursts of electrical energy, very similar to the way it is excited in pulse-echo imaging. However, in pulsed Doppler mode there usually is a fairly narrow frequency band in the sound pulse rather than the broad band pulse used in pulse-echo imaging. Some pulsed Doppler instruments allow the operator to vary the burst duration, that is, the number of cycles in the pulse, in order to vary the sensitivity. More cycles in the burst results in improved sensitivity and better performance of the Doppler circuitry. This is done at the expense of greater acoustic exposure to the patient and poorer axial resolution.

The region of interest from which Doppler signals are displayed over a speaker or on a spectral display is selected by gating on the receiver or the display at the appropriate delay time following transmission of the burst. The relation between the delay time and the Doppler "sample gate" is given by the range equation in Chapter 3. Only signals originating from scatterers and reflectors within the sample gate are displayed. On most instruments the size of the sample gate may be adjusted, allowing selection of signals from a very narrow region if desirable. Increasing the sample gate expands the region from which Doppler signals are picked up.

Operator controls on pulsed Doppler instruments, in addition to those already mentioned for continuous-wave Doppler units, include the following:
1. Range gate position
2. Gate or sample volume size
3. Flow angle cursor (for duplex instruments—see below)
4. Burst duration (on some instruments)

DUPLEX SCANNERS

A pulse-echo scanner and a Doppler instrument provide complimentary information in that the scanner can best outline anatomic details whereas a Doppler instrument yields information regarding flow and movement patterns. "Duplex" ultrasound instruments are real-time B-mode scanners with built-in Doppler capabilities. In typical applications the pulse-echo B-mode image obtained with a duplex scanner is used to localize areas where flow will be examined using Doppler. The area to be studied in pulsed Doppler mode may be identified on the B-mode image with a "sample volume" or "sample gate" indicator (Fig 5-13). The cursor position is controlled by the operator, greatly facilitating positioning the Doppler sample volume over the region of interest. Many duplex instruments allow the operator to indicate the direction of flow with respect to the ultrasound beam direction by adjusting an angle cursor. This is necessary to estimate the reflector velocity from the frequency of the Doppler signal.

During duplex scanning the ultrasound transducer assembly and the instrument "time-shares" between pulse-echo and Doppler mode. The extent of this time-sharing is often under operator control directly or indirectly. Thus some instruments allow the operator to specify the rate at which the B-mode image is updated while in Dop-

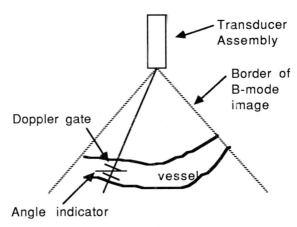

FIG. 5-13. Schema of a duplex scanner, showing placement of the pulsed Doppler sample gate.

pler mode. This may range from 7 to 10 times per second to no updating at all. Of course, the more frequently the B-mode image is updated, the more certain the operator is of the exact location of the sample volume during a Doppler study, an important consideration especially for smaller vessels. However, as we will discuss below, pulsed Doppler sometimes is very demanding in terms of the fraction of time the instrument must launch Doppler mode pulses into the sample volume, especially if reflectors are moving very rapidly. This usually limits the frequency of image updating.

Both mechanical scanners and array transducer assemblies are used as duplex scanners. Mechanical sector scanners provide the ability to incorporate annular array transducers (see Chapter 2) for an improved slice thickness over the image. Phased and linear arrays offer other advantages for duplex scanning, especially in terms of the flexibility in switching between Doppler and real-time B-mode. Because there are no moving parts in the transducer assembly the array scanning instrument can quickly and automatically shift between steering the beam toward the sample volume in Doppler mode and then back to B-mode to build up part of the B-mode image, then back to Doppler mode, and so on. Thus B-mode image updating may be more rapid when studies are done in a combined B-mode scan and pulsed Doppler mode.

DOPPLER SPECTRAL ANALYSIS

Doppler signals from flowing blood may be complicated because of the nature of the flow patterns encountered by the sound beam. Sometimes the flow is *parabolic*, as shown in the top of the diagram in Fig. 5-14. Blood cells move faster along the axis of the vessel than near the walls. The length of the arrows schematically illustrates the relative speed of blood cells at a particular distance from the axis of the vessel for parabolic flow.

In large vessels, such as the aorta, the flow may take on a more blunt profile (Fig. 5-14, *B*). Here the flow profile is nearly constant across the vessel; near the wall the flow decreases to zero again.

The actual velocity profile across any vessel depends on a number of factors, including the diameter of the ves-

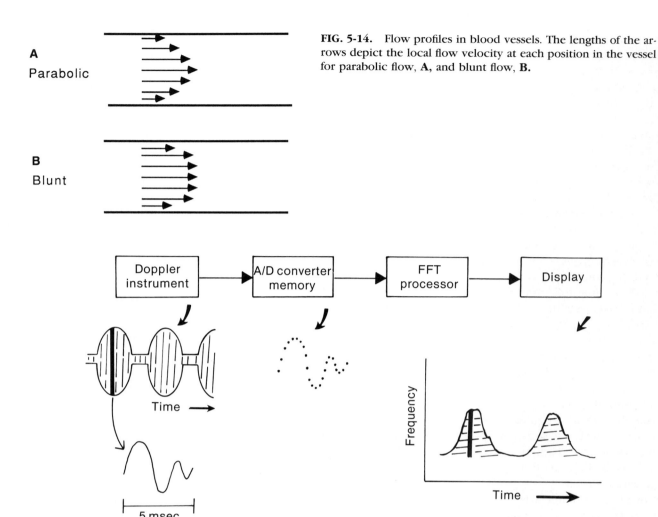

FIG. 5-14. Flow profiles in blood vessels. The lengths of the arrows depict the local flow velocity at each position in the vessel for parabolic flow, **A**, and blunt flow, **B**.

FIG. 5-15. Frequency analysis of the Doppler signal using a digitally controlled FFT analyzer.

sel, the mechanical properties of blood, the flow velocity, and the time. If echo signals are detected simultaneously from different locations in the vessel, different Doppler frequencies may be present in the signal. The number of different frequencies depends on the distribution of velocities present, the transducer beam width, and the size of the Doppler sample volume if pulsed Doppler is employed.

Because the beam is reflected from scatterers moving at different speeds, the instantaneous Doppler signal consists of many different frequencies. The frequencies present in the signal result in the characteristic "swish" sounds heard for blood flow during the cardiac cycle. A quantitative analysis showing the distribution of frequencies is done by *spectral analysis.*

Spectral analysis is a process by which a complex signal is broken down or analyzed into simple frequency components. In physics and engineering the most common way to do spectral analysis is to use a process called Fourier analysis. A commonly used device that performs the spectral analysis in ultrasound instruments is a fast Fourier transform (FFT) analyzer. The FFT instrument, along with a display screen, allows the amount of Doppler signal present at different frequencies to be displayed as a function of time.

The FFT analyzer (Fig. 5-15) operates serially on small, 1 to 5 ms, segments of the quadrature Doppler signals. The signal segment is converted to digital format ("digitized") in an analog-to-digital (A/D) converter and is then sent to the analyzer. The analyzer produces a record showing the relative amount of signal within each of a number of discrete frequency bins. It then operates on another signal segment, and so on, producing a continuous display.

The result of the FFT's operation is illustrated schematically in Fig. 5-16. In this figure the horizontal axis represents time and is broken into small intervals to correspond to the signal segments mentioned earlier. The vertical axis represents frequency and is divided into discrete frequency bins. The higher the bin on the vertical scale, the greater the signal frequency. The FFT analyzer fills each frequency bin with a density or shade of gray that represents the amount of signal with that frequency during the time segment. By operating on successive signal segments it produces a continuous spectral display.

As mentioned above, one axis of the Doppler signal spectral display represents time. The other axis represents frequency; since the Doppler frequency also is proportional to reflector velocity, the Doppler equation (Equation 5-3) can be employed to convert this axis to read ve-

Frequency
(Velocity)
Bins

FIG. 5-16. Schema of the output of a Doppler signal spectral analyzer.

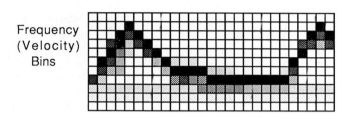

Frequency
(Velocity)
Bins

Time Increments

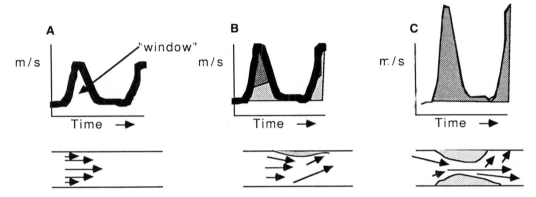

FIG. 5-17. Some characteristics of the Doppler signal spectral display for different flow conditions. **A,** Normal spectrum with a very narrow band of frequencies contributing to the signal. The open region within the spectral envelope during peak flow conditions is sometimes referred to as a spectral window. **B,** This spectral window begins to become filled in the presence of turbulence. **C,** Detection of flow from a region of stenosis, illustrating high velocities and absent spectral window. (Adapted from Burns P: J Clin Ultrasound 15:567-590, 1987.)

locity directly. When this is done it generally is necessary to provide an estimate of the angle of the vessel lumen with respect to the direction of the ultrasound beam. This estimate is provided by the operator by orienting a "sample volume cursor" so that the cursor points in the direction of the vessel axis. The accuracy of the velocity representation of the Doppler signals is then related to how correctly the operator positions the angle cursor to lie along the direction of flow.

The Doppler spectral display provides a readout of the distribution of frequencies—and hence, reflector velocities—contributing to the signal. Other important characteristics of the flow pattern may also be gleaned from the spectral display. For example, with a narrow pulsed Doppler sample gate positioned in the center of a vessel the presence of obstructions may sometimes be detected from the spectrum. If the vessel is large compared to the sample volume, a fairly narrow velocity range is sampled. This results in a narrow frequency band and the "spectral window" (Fig. 5-17) on the display. In the presence of mild or severe turbulence caused by obstructions, this

spectral window is filled in partially or entirely (Fig 5-17, A and B).

Various parameters have been derived from the Doppler signal spectrum to quantify important properties of the flow. For example, the pulsatility index, PI, is defined by:

$$PI = \frac{A - B}{Mean}$$

where A and B refer to the peak systolic and minimum diastolic velocities, respectively, during the cardiac cycle and mean is the average flow during the cycle. These quantities are obtained from the spectral display as shown in Fig. 5-18. An advantage of these parameters is that they provide data on the relative resistance to flow of the vascular bed; they do this without the need to quantify velocities and flow absolutely. Absolute quantification may be impossible, especially in situations where the vessel lumen cannot be visualized, such as in the kidney.[2] Many other parameters, for example, the resistivity index, RI,

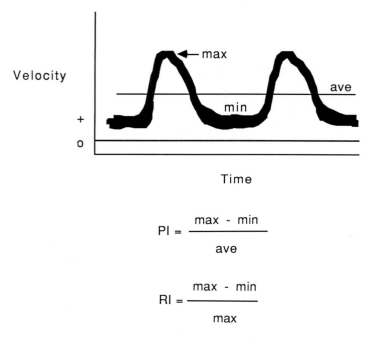

$$PI = \frac{max - min}{ave}$$

$$RI = \frac{max - min}{max}$$

FIG. 5-18. Parameters used to compute the pulsatility index, PI, and resistivity index, RI.

have been defined by various researchers to describe flow patterns. However, it is beyond the scope of this chapter to provide an extensive review. The reader who is interested in using these should consult the references.[2,3]

ALIASING AND THE NYQUIST FREQUENCY

With a pulsed Doppler instrument the output Doppler signal is built up in discrete "pieces," one piece being added each time a pulse is launched and echo signals are detected. We sometimes say that the Doppler signal is "sampled."[2] The signal sampling frequency of a pulsed Doppler instrument is equal to the pulse repetition frequency (PRF) in Doppler mode.

In any situation where sampling occurs, the greater the sampling frequency in comparison to the actual frequencies present, the better the rendition of that signal after it has been sampled. This is illustrated in Fig. 5-19, where a sine wave signal (solid line) is shown sampled at a fairly high rate (arrows). The lower curve is the resultant sampled version of the signal. It is fairly easy to appreciate the original signal with the sampling conditions in this example. To carry the example over to the pulsed Doppler case, the sine wave corresponds to the actual Doppler signal, the arrows to individual pulses transmitted and echoes picked up by the transducer, and the dotted line to the output Doppler signal.

In a practical ultrasound system we usually reach an upper limit on the PRF, limiting the sampling frequency. For pulsed Doppler instruments the upper limit of the PRF is established by two conditions. The first is the desire to minimize the acoustic exposure to the patient since a higher pulse repetition frequency results in more acoustic energy transmitted into the patient. Thus the PRF should be as low as possible, consistent with obtaining adequate Doppler signals. The second limitation on the

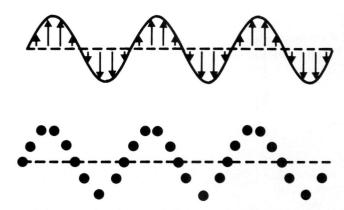

FIG. 5-19. "Sampling" a signal. The solid line at the top traces out a sine wave. The arrows correspond to discrete samples of the wave. The higher the sampling rate, the better the rendition of the sampled signal (*lower curve*).

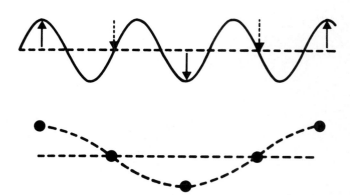

FIG. 5-20. Production of aliasing when the sampling rate is less than two times the signal frequency (*upper curve and arrows*). The resultant signal (*lower curve*) is of lower frequency than the original.

pulse repetition rate is related to the fact that a sound pulse takes a small but measurable amount of time to travel to the sample volume and return. Before a pulse is launched by the instrument, it is necessary to wait for echoes from all previous pulses to return from the sample volume; if the waiting time between pulses is insufficient, "range ambiguities" will arise. This means that there will be uncertainties in the actual range from which Doppler signals occur.

At the very least, the pulse repetition frequency (PRF) on the instrument must be great enough to sample the Doppler signal at least two times for each cycle of the Doppler signal. If the PRF is less than twice the frequency of the maximum Doppler signal frequency, then *aliasing* will occur. Aliasing is the production of artifactual, lower-frequency components in the signal spectrum when the pulse repetition frequency of the instrument is less than two times the maximum frequency of the Doppler signal. The *Nyquist frequency* is defined as the maximum possible frequency that can be sampled and is half the PRF for pulsed Doppler applications.

The production of aliasing is illustrated in Fig. 5-20. This is the same as in the previous figure, only now the Doppler signal (top solid curve) is sampled (arrows)

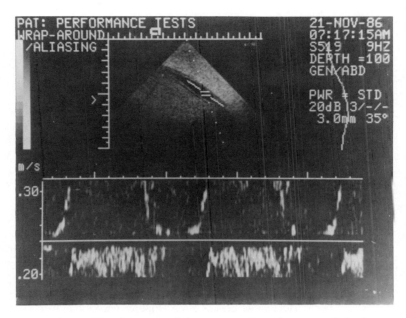

FIG. 5-21. Manifestation of aliasing on a Doppler spectral display.

once every cycle and a quarter, a rate that is less than two times the Doppler frequency. The solid dots illustrate the sampled signal, and a dashed curve is drawn to assist the reader in visualizing the resulting sampled signal shape. It clearly is lower in frequency than that of the actual signal. The actual signal can only be recovered if the PRF of the instrument is increased so that it is at least twice the frequency of the Doppler signal.

Some Doppler instruments allow the operator to adjust the PRF directly; however, most vary the PRF internally according to other operator-adjusted settings on the instrument. Typical controls that also affect PRF include the following:

1. The scale on the spectral display
2. The Doppler sample depth
3. Interleaving Doppler mode with imaging mode on a duplex instrument

Thus when the sample depth is increased, the PRF usually is decreased automatically; when the spectral display scale is increased to allow higher-frequency Doppler signals or greater velocities to be displayed, the PRF may also be increased.

One way that aliasing is manifested on a spectral display is shown in Fig. 5-21. The velocity peaks in the spectral display appear to be cut off on the top and "wrapped around," appearing on the bottom of the record.

One can easily appreciate the loss of higher signal frequencies as the flow speed in the phantom is increased simply by listening to the signals. The frequencies increase with flow speed until the Nyquist frequency is reached. Then the Doppler frequencies seem to decrease with increasing flow speed. The effect frequently is heard during clinical studies when an instrument is operating in combined imaging and pulsed Doppler mode. The Doppler PRF in this mode must be low to allow the instrument to switch rapidly back and forth between imaging and pulsed Doppler. Usually the quality of Doppler signals

improves dramatically when the image frame rate is slowed down or even stopped, allowing the Doppler mode PRF to increase.

Aliasing may sometimes be reduced or eliminated by using a lower-frequency ultrasound transducer, using a high PRF mode, if available, using continuous-wave rather than pulsed Doppler, or locating a window to the region of interest for which the incident sound beam angle is closer to 90 degrees.

MAXIMUM VELOCITY DETECTABLE WITH PULSED DOPPLER

We have seen that to avoid aliasing of the Doppler signal the pulse repetition frequency (PRF) of a pulsed Doppler instrument must be at least two times the maximum frequency in the signal. This requirement establishes a lower limit on the PRF, depending on the frequencies present in the Doppler signal.

An upper limit to the PRF also exists. The upper limit is related to the travel time for a sound pulse in tissue. Each time an ultrasound pulse is produced by the transducer, another pulse cannot be transmitted until echo signals down to the sample volume depth are detected. If insufficient time is allocated between pulses, range ambiguities may occur; this results in simultaneous detection of signals from two or more depths, an undesirable condition—unless steps are followed to take them into account.

Let f_m be the maximum detectable frequency of Doppler signals when the sample volume is at the depth D; also, let T be the delay time between transmitting a pulse and detecting echo signals from that depth. To avoid aliasing, the PRF must be *at least* $2f_m$. On the other hand, the PRF must be *no greater than* $1/T$ to avoid range ambiguities. These two conditions establish v_m, the maximum velocity detectable from depth D.

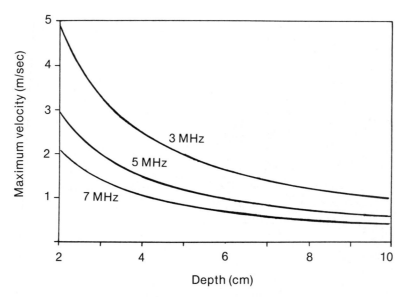

FIG. 5-22. Maximum velocity detectable using pulsed Doppler versus depth of sample volume. Curves are shown for three different ultrasound frequencies. It is assumed that the angle θ in Equation 5-3 and Fig. 5-3 is 0 degrees.

We can find v_m by equating the maximum and the minimum PRF conditions; that is,

$$\text{PRF}_{min} = \text{PRF}_{max}$$

or,

$$2f_m = \frac{1}{T}$$

Using the range equation, we can set $T = 2D/c$, where c is the speed of sound. Also, if we substitute for f_m using the Doppler equation (Equation 5-1), we obtain

$$2\frac{2f_0 v_m}{c} = \frac{c}{2D}$$

where v_m is the maximum detectable reflector velocity. Solving for v_m,

$$v_m = \frac{c^2}{8f_0 D} \qquad (5\text{-}4)$$

Example: What is the maximum detectable velocity in soft tissue if the ultrasound operating frequency is 5 MHz and the reflector depth is 5 cm?

Solution: Use 1540 m/s for the speed of sound; first convert D to meters so all units are the same. Then apply Equation 5-4.

$$v_m = \frac{(1540 \text{ m/s})^2}{8 \times 5 \times 10^6/\text{s} \times 0.05 \text{ m}}$$
$$= 1.18 \text{ m/s} = 118 \text{ cm/s}$$

If the reflector were deeper than 5 cm, the maximum detectable velocity would decrease. A family of curves illustrating the maximum detectable reflector velocity for several different ultrasound operating frequencies is provided in Fig. 5-22. Notice that as the reflector depth increases, the maximum detectable Doppler signal frequency, and hence the maximum detectable reflector velocity, decreases. At any depth lower ultrasound frequencies permit detection of greater reflector velocities than higher operating frequencies, because lower frequencies result in lower-frequency Doppler signals for the same velocity.

HIGH PRF MODE

To overcome the maximum velocity limitations some instruments provide a "high PRF" option. When high velocities need to be detected at large depths, the instrument can be placed in a mode where the Doppler PRF is higher than that allowed to avoid range ambiguity; the presence of the range ambiguities may be recognized by the existence of multiple gates on instruments displaying the Doppler sample volume position. This is illustrated in Fig. 5-23. Although Doppler signals could be picked up from any of these sample volumes, this usually poses no problem since the operator usually has already isolated the vessel of interest and thus can pretty well determine that the Doppler signals are originating from the gate positioned at maximum depth.

COLOR DOPPLER AND COLOR FLOW IMAGING

Until now our discussion of pulsed Doppler instruments has involved the use of a single time gate to pick out Doppler shifted signals from a specific depth range in the field of the transducer. The human ear, a single-channel spectrum analyzer, and simple audio recorders process one Doppler signal at a time, and therefore simultaneous acquisition of signals from within multiple time gates would not be necessary if there were no other means to display the signals. However, recent innovations in Doppler signal acquisition and display have resulted in practical multiple-gated Doppler instruments and Doppler imaging devices. Of special clinical significance here are instruments commonly called *color flow* imaging instruments.

The basic scheme for color flow imaging[3-6] is illustrated in Fig. 5-24. The imaged field can be thought of as

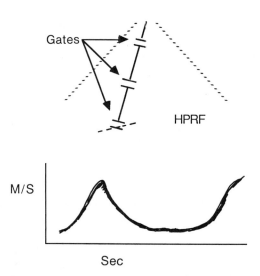

FIG. 5-23. Multiple sample gates present in a "high PRF mode," available on some pulsed Doppler instrument.

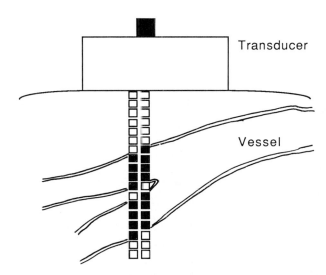

FIG. 5-24. Scheme used to produce color flow images. Signals are sampled along each beam line to detect the average flow velocity. This information is displayed in color, yielding both flow direction and mean velocity within each pixel.

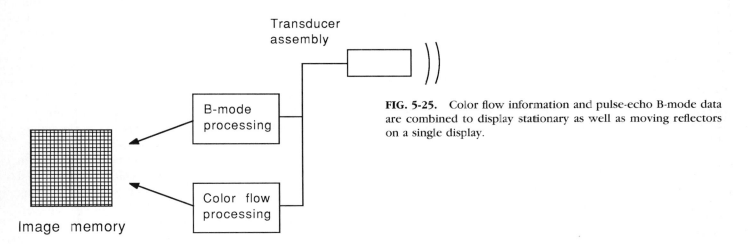

FIG. 5-25. Color flow information and pulse-echo B-mode data are combined to display stationary as well as moving reflectors on a single display.

segmented into beam lines, and each beam line is further divided into contiguous gated regions. An average Doppler shift is then determined and displayed in color for each of these gated regions. The flow information is combined with pulse echo data from stationary reflectors (Fig. 5-25) in the final display, yielding a combined B-mode gray-scale image and color flow image.

Properties of color displays

There are several terms used to describe the attributes of a color display. It is well known that any color in the visible range of the electromagnetic spectrum may be formulated by suitable mixing of the three *primary colors:* red, blue, and green. If all three colors are added together in equal amounts, the perceived color is white. Any single color in the visible spectrum can be produced by mixtures of two of the primary colors in the right proportion. This property of color perception is used advantageously in color television and video monitors. Each small element within the screen of a color monitor consists of three phosphors, one producing red light, one blue, and one green. Three separate electron guns provide the elec-

tron current to modulate the intensity of each phosphor, and hence of the primary colors at every addressable location on the screen. Thus different mixtures of the primary colors result in our perception of different colors on the screen.

We use the terms *hue, saturation,* and *intensity* to describe properties of an image related to the psychophysical perception of color. Hue is the attribute of colors that permits them to be classified as red, yellow, green, blue, or an intermediate between any contiguous pair of colors. The hue is associated with the wavelength of the light. In color flow instruments a red hue might be chosen to represent flow moving toward the ultrasound transducer, while a blue hue could be used to display flow signals from reflectors moving away from the probe. (Obviously, different schemes are also possible.) Saturation has to do with the fact that mixtures involving all three primary colors turn out partially or totally white. Saturation is a measure of the chromatic purity, that is, the freedom from dilution with white light. A completely saturated color has only one wavelength associated with it. It is a pure hue. On the other hand, white light is made up of many wave-

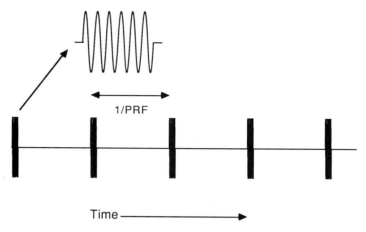

Time ⟶

FIG. 5-26. Typical transmitted pulse packet to compute and display the average flow velocity along each beam line in color flow imaging. Five such pulses are shown; one of these is enlarged in the insert. PRF is the pulse repetition frequency and 1/PRF is the time between successive transmit pulses.

lengths, so the more white there is, the *less* saturated is the color. If we see a color flow display in which higher flow rates, for example, appear whiter than lower flow rates, we know that this is done by varying the saturation of the colors according to the detected flow rate. A third attribute used to describe color in an image is the intensity or brightness; this is similar to the corresponding property of a gray-scale B-mode image. Intensity also is used in some color flow instruments to indicate flow rate.

Color flow signal processing

Determining the flow velocity for each pixel in the color flow image requires special signal processing circuitry. In their present configuration, spectral analysis devices described earlier in this chapter are too slow to permit detection and analysis of signals from multiple pixels at speeds needed for real-time imaging. Alternative techniques have been chosen by instrument manufacturers to provide estimates of flow at each location in a color flow image.

One method of color flow signal processing uses what are termed "correlation detectors,"[5] displaying within each pixel in the color flow image the *average flow velocity* relative to the transducer beam direction. A series of ultrasound pulses, sometimes called a pulse packet (Fig. 5-26), is transmitted in each beam direction. After each transmit, pulse-echo signals from moving as well as stationary reflectors are detected. The color flow detector compares the phases of signals from one pulse with phases of signals from the previous pulse to produce a signal at each pixel depth that is proportional to the mean or average Doppler signal, and hence, the average reflector velocity. Because of noise and other variations in the returning signal it is necessary to use multiple pulse packets for each line to obtain a good estimate of the average velocity and direction of flow within each sample gate along the beam line. Fig. 5-26 illustrates five individual pulses transmitted into the body; one of these is enlarged, shown

in the insert. The PRF is the pulse repetition frequency and 1/PRF is the time between individual pulses. The actual number of pulses within a packet may vary between instruments and for different applications. When phased or linear array transducer assemblies are used, these pulses are transmitted with the ultrasound beam dwelling along the beam line; with mechanical transducer assemblies the scanning motion cannot be started and stopped abruptly, so the beam is actually scanning during the process.

Because several pulses must be launched along each acoustic line to compute an average flow rate for each pixel, color flow imaging frame rates are somewhat lower than real-time B-mode imaging frame rates. To speed up the frame rate the operator usually can reduce the size of the imaged field in color mode. An entire scan can be done in a fraction of a second, allowing 10 or 15 frames per second image rates. Even higher rates are possible with reduced color image fields to accommodate, for example, cardiac applications. The Doppler scan can be mixed with pulse-echo data from stationary reflectors, providing a complete two-dimensional image of moving as well as stationary structures. When setting up the combined color flow B-mode display, different choices are available to the manufacturer when deciding whether a particular pixel should display color flow data or B-mode data. These choices influence the sensitivity of an instrument to low flow rates and the degree of immunity to spurious motion accompanying heart beats, breathing, and probe movements.

An operator-controlled gate may be manipulated on the display of most units to allow detailed Doppler signal spectral analysis from selected regions. Signals originating from the gated region may be applied to an FFT analyzer in the manner discussed previously.

Some aspects of the directional flow information

It is important to understand that a color flow instrument (as well as an ordinary directional continuous-wave or pulsed Doppler instrument) displays flow direction *with respect to the direction of the incident ultrasound beam,* and not with respect to an anatomic reference. Changing the orientation of the ultrasound beam with respect to the flow direction may change the apparent direction of flow within a vessel and hence the displayed color. This is brought out vividly by imaging a flow phantom or a vessel with the axis of the vessel in the plane of the image oriented as shown in Fig. 5-27. When using a display scheme that depicts flow toward the transducer with a red hue and flow away from the transducer with a blue hue, the vessel image would appear somewhat like that illustrated in the bottom of the figure. For the vessel orientation shown, the flow within the right half of the image is directed slightly toward the ultrasound source and the direction of the incident ultrasound beam, and that on the left half of the image is directed slightly away from the ultrasound source. Hence the vessel image is divided into two regions: a red section and a blue section. Notice that for the image shown we are assuming a sector sweep of

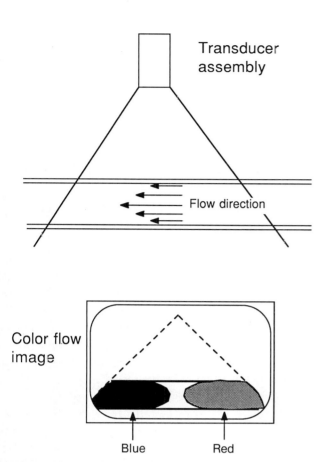

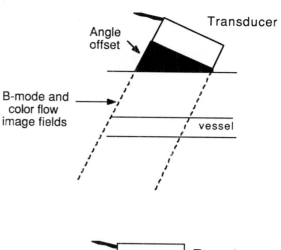

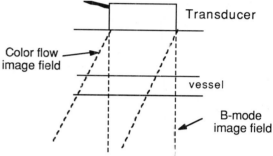

FIG. 5-27. Schema of possible image from a flow phantom (bottom), obtained with a sector scanner oriented as shown in the top of the illustration. The flow display is discontinuous in the region where the incident sound beam is perpendicular to the direction of flow.

FIG. 5-28. Arrangements used to produce simultaneous color flow and B-mode images of vessels that are parallel to the skin surface when a linear array system is used for color flow studies. The top scheme illustrates use of an angle offset; the bottom technique has beams used for flow imaging transmitted in a different direction than beams used for B-mode imaging.

the ultrasound beam across the vessel. When the beam is perpendicular to the direction of flow, there is no detected Doppler shift; hence we see a discontinuity in the flow image.

In some applications one wishes to obtain images of vessels running parallel to the surface of the skin using linear array transducers, and it is not desirable to have the vessel appear discontinuous and split into two colors as the previous example. Two methods have been developed to provide a continuous color flow image of a vessel when using a linear array (Fig. 5-28). In one a transducer offset cut at an angle is used so that the ultrasound beams producing the color flow image always are incident on the vessel at an angle other than 90 degrees with respect to the direction of flow. B-mode image information and Doppler flow information are obtained along the same acoustic lines. In another method the Doppler beams are steered at an angle with respect to the direction of the B-mode imaging beams. This can be done using phased array techniques analogous to those described in Chapter 3. The B-mode image information is still obtained in the usual manner by directing sound beams perpendicular to the surface of the transducer; however, the Doppler flow information is picked up with the beams that are steered off at an angle.

Aliasing

A color flow examination is subject to the effects of aliasing, just as a single-channel pulsed Doppler study is. When aliasing is present, the displayed Doppler signals tend to "wrap around," appearing as high velocities but in the wrong direction. In color flow imaging this wrap around results in an erroneous color, appearing as though a reversal of the flow direction occurred. Aliased signals originating from flow toward the probe begin to be displayed as though originating from reflectors moving away from the probe, and vice versa. The reversal can usually be identified because it occurs first in the region of an image corresponding to that part of a vessel where the highest velocities are present. Most color flow instruments provide controls to adjust the displayed velocity scale. If the PRF of the instrument is linked to the velocity scale setting, increasing the velocity detectably increases the PRF. In addition to this, some color flow instruments allow the region from which flow signals are displayed to be expanded or reduced. Reducing the color flow imaged region reduces the total number of acoustic lines needed to form the color flow image and allows higher PRFs. This in turn allows detection of higher flow velocities.

Variance

Another attribute of the flow that is displayed on most color flow instruments is called "variance." This is a measure of the variation of Doppler frequencies within each pixel on the image during the brief time period associated with a pulse packet. It may be an effective method to detect turbulent flow, such as caused by obstructions, since there are many velocities present from regions when turbulence is present. Either the hue or the color saturation or both can be used to encode the output of variance estimators for detecting the presence of turbulence.

ACOUSTIC OUTPUT LEVELS FROM DOPPLER EQUIPMENT

The topic of acoustic output levels from ultrasound equipment is considered in Chapter 7. One aspect of these data is the relatively high time average intensity from some pulsed Doppler instruments compared to intensities from real-time B-mode imaging equipment. This is due in part to the large duty factors (discussed in Chapter 7) during pulsed Doppler mode, and the effect of having beams with such large duty factors dwell along a single acoustic line. Users should be aware of the relative intensities produced in each of the operating modes of their instruments and how changing the operating conditions, such as varying the output power level, affect the acoustic intensities. Consult the operator's manual or contact the equipment manufacturer to find out the actual intensities produced by your equipment! If an output power control is provided in Doppler mode, use a low output power setting if practical, especially when examining potentially sensitive tissue, such as a fetus. Also, consider the guidelines presented at the end of Chapter 7.

SUMMARY

1. The Doppler effect is used in medical ultrasound to detect moving reflectors and to measure and characterize blood flow.

2. The Doppler shift is the change in the perceived frequency of a sound source relative to the transmitted frequency whenever there is relative motion between a sound source and a listener.

3. The Doppler shift frequency, f_D, is the *difference* between the received and the transmitted frequencies. When the reflector is moving toward the transducer, the Doppler shift frequency is given by

$$f_D = 2f_0 v/c$$

where f_0 is the ultrasound operating frequency, v is the velocity of the reflector, and c is the speed of sound in the medium.

4. The angle between the sound beam direction and the direction of motion must be taken into account for accurate measurements of reflector velocity.

5. Special signal processing may be provided on a continuous-wave or pulsed Doppler instrument to display the direction of flow.

6. Pulsed Doppler provides discrimination of Doppler signals from different depths, allowing for the detection of moving interfaces and scatterers from within a well-defined "sample" volume.

7. "Duplex" ultrasound instruments are real-time B-mode scanners with built-in Doppler capabilities.

8. A quantitative analysis showing the distribution of frequencies (or velocities) in a Doppler signal is done by *spectral analysis.*

9. Aliasing is the production of artifactual, lower-frequency components in the signal spectrum when the pulse repetition frequency (PRF) of a pulsed Doppler instrument is less than two times the maximum frequency of the Doppler signal.

10. The maximum detectable reflector velocity for a pulsed Doppler instrument is established by the need to avoid aliasing while also avoiding range ambiguities.

11. To overcome the maximum velocity limitations some instruments provide a "high PRF" option.

12. Color Doppler provides images depicting the average velocity and the direction of flow within multiple sample gates distributed over the image.

13. Many pulsed Doppler instruments produce spatial peak time average intensities that are significantly greater than spatial peak time average intensities for other operating modes. Users should be aware of which controls affect the power and intensity on their instrument.

REFERENCES

1. Beach K and Phillips D: Doppler instrumentation for the evaluation of arterial and venous disease. In Jaffe C, editor: Clinics in diagnostic ultrasound, vol 13, Vascular and Doppler ultrasound, New York, 1984, Churchill Livingstone.

2. Bom N, deBoo J, and Rijsterborgh H: On the aliasing problem in pulsed Doppler cardiac studies, J Clin Ultrasound 12:559-567, 1984.

3. Burns P: The physical principles of Doppler and spectral analysis, J Clin Ultrasound 15:567-590, 1987.

4. Kisslo J, Adams D, and Belkin R: Doppler color flow imaging, New York, 1988, Churchill Livingstone, pp 25-46.

5. Omoto R and Kasai C: Basic principles of Doppler color flow imaging, Echocardiography 3:463-473, 1986.

6. Reid J: Doppler ultrasound, IEEE Engrg Med Biology 6:14-17, 1987.

7. Taylor K, Burns P, Woodcock J, and Wells P: Blood flow in deep abdominal and pelvis vessels: ultrasonic pulsed Doppler analysis, Radiology 154:487-493, 1985.

8. Wells P: Ultrasonic Doppler equipment. In Fullerton G, and Zagzebski J, editors: Medical physics of CT and ultrasound, New York, 1980, American Institute of Physics, pp 343-366.

9. Zagzebski J: Physics and instrumentation in Doppler and B-mode ultrasonography. In Zwiebel W, editor: Introduction to vascular ultrasonography, ed 2, Orlando, Fla., 1986, Grune & Stratton, Inc, pp 21-51.

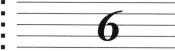

Instrument Quality Assurance

JAMES A. ZAGZEBSKI

In diagnostic ultrasound *quality control* refers to steps taken to assure that an instrument is operating consistently at its expected level of performance. In a general sense quality control encompasses many checks and assessments of ultrasound image data during the routine operation of an ultrasound department. In this chapter one aspect of a quality control program will be discussed: objective tests for evaluating the performance of ultrasound instruments. When done routinely, such tests help document gradual deterioration of instrument performance and provide a more objective means of assessing operating consistency than can be obtained, for example, from impressions of image quality on clinical scans.

A well-planned quality assurance program requires routine performance measurements, careful analysis of results, record keeping, and follow-through on corrective action. This chapter should assist readers who are interested in setting up a program in their own department.

TEST OBJECTS AND PHANTOMS

Phantoms and test objects have been developed for performance measurements of ultrasound scanners. These devices are meant to provide stable sources of echo signals in known geometric configurations and in a well—characterized medium. Two examples are presented, the AIUM standard 100 mm test object and a tissue-mimicking phantom.

AIUM standard 100 mm test object

Although quality control on modern ultrasound imaging instruments is more readily carried out using tissue-mimicking phantoms, we will first describe the standard AIUM 100-mm test object, illustrated in Fig. 6-1. It consists of a series of stainless reflectors arranged as targets for geometric tests of ultrasound pulse-echo instruments. The reflectors are immersed in a liquid medium in which the speed of sound is 1540 m/s. Both an open and an enclosed version of the test object are available.

The important features of the AIUM standard 100 mm test object are summarized as follows:
1. Standardized reflectors; 0.75 mm diameter stainless steel rods are specified.
2. A standard geometric arrangement for reflectors; the arrangement illustrated in the figure must be followed if the test object follows the standard.
3. A speed of sound of 1540 m/s in the medium.

The speed of sound of 1540 m/s is obtained using water plus an additive. For example, 8% ethyl alcohol (by volume) added to ordinary water at 22° C (approximately room temperature) results in the correct speed of sound.[1] Plain tap water alone will not do and should not be used to fill the test object. The speed of sound in water is only 1480 m/s, a value that is 3% too low; on tests of distance measurement accuracy this could lead to significant errors. Small temperature variations are no problem since speed of sound variations of only about 0.1% per degree

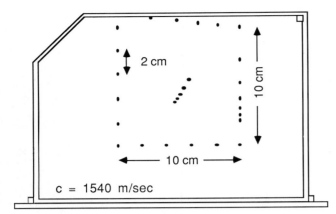

FIG. 6-1. Enclosed version of the standard AIUM 100 mm test object.

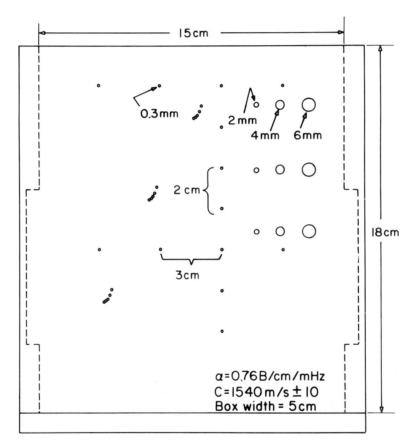

FIG. 6-2. One version of a tissue-mimicking phantom for routine performance measurements of ultrasound scanners. The objects with 2, 4, and 6 mm diameters are scatter-free cylinders. The dots are nylon reflectors spaced as shown. (Courtesy Radiation Measurements, Inc., Middleton, Wis.)

Celsius are typical. If a test object is purchased that is already filled with an appropriate liquid, one need only verify that the speed of sound in the liquid is indeed 1540 m/s. Consult the manufacturer of the test object to assure that this is the case. If a test object requires filling, this can be done following a formula supplied with the test object or available in the references.[6]

Tissue-mimicking phantoms

The use of tissue-mimicking material[3,10,14] in a phantom provides the capability of testing equipment performance under conditions that more closely simulate clinical scanning conditions than do liquid-filled test objects. For example, some tissue phantoms contain material that attenuates sound waves similarly to the way soft tissues attenuate. Therefore when the phantom is scanned, it is necessary to use instrument sensitivity settings that are similar to settings used for scanning patients.

The ultrasound phantom shown in Fig. 6-2, as well as similar versions of this phantom, are used commonly for performance tests of real-time ultrasound scanners. Its design and use will be presented as an example. The tissue-mimicking material consists of a water-based gelatin in which microscopic graphite particles are mixed uniformly throughout the volume. The speed of sound within the phantom material is 1540 m/s. A characteristic of the gel-graphite material is that its ultrasonic attenuation coefficient is controllable. Commonly used values for attenuation in quality control phantoms are in the range 0.5 to 0.7 dB/cm/MHz. Very importantly, the ultrasonic attenuation in this material has nearly the same frequency dependence as that in most soft tissues. Having the same frequency dependence allows a phantom to be used effectively with different-frequency transducers. Moreover, it distorts ultrasonic pulses and sound beams similarly to soft tissues.[13]

Small scatterers are distributed throughout the tissue-mimicking material. Therefore the phantom appears echogenic when imaged with static or real-time B-mode scanners. The simulated cysts are low-attenuating, scatter-free cylinders. These should appear echo free on B-mode images, as discussed in Chapter 4. Discrete reflectors consisting of nylon fibers are distributed in arrangements for geometric tests of scanners and for resolution checks. In the phantom illustrated, a column that has reflectors spaced every 2 cm and two horizontal rows with reflectors spaced every 3 cm are available.

Some tissue phantoms provide image contrast[12] from one region to another by having simulated masses of varying echogeneicity. This is done by varying the scatter level, the ultrasonic attenuation, or both.

SETTING UP PERFORMANCE TESTS
Performance test worksheet

A worksheet I have found useful for keeping records of performance tests of scanners is illustrated in the box opposite. It contains blank spaces for entering scanner setup information, lists various system measurements that can be done easily, and may be used as a checklist for different steps in the process of testing scanners. The worksheet also has spaces for recording the results of the different measurements and thus could be included in the quality control notebook, discussed later in this chapter.

Transducer choice

Results of some test procedures depend on which transducer assembly is used with the instrument. On systems where several transducer assemblies are available it may be inconvenient to do routine tests with more than one probe. If this is the case, choose a transducer assembly that will become a standard for all test procedures. A good choice would be the transducer assembly used most frequently in clinical scanning. Be sure to record all necessary transducer assembly identification information, including the frequency, size, and serial number, so future tests will be conducted with the same probe. Space is available on the worksheet (opposite) to record this.

Instrument sensitivity controls

If a liquid-filled test object (e.g., the AIUM 100 mm) is used, sensitivity controls, including those adjusting the output power and the receiver gain, should be set fairly low. Usually no swept gain (TGC) is applied because there is very little sound beam attenuation in the test object liquid. Also the stainless steel rod reflectors produce very large—amplitude echo signals, requiring little if any amplification for their visualization on a display.

Ultrasound Quality Control Results

Machine: <u>Acuson 128</u>   Room: <u>E3 315</u>
Transducer assembly: I.D.: <u>L 382</u>   Serial no: <u>555-1212</u>
Date: <u>1/18/88</u>   Phantom: <u>RMI 413/A—No</u>
Instrument settings: Power <u>0</u>   dB
                 Dynamic range <u>50</u>dB Pre<u>1</u>/Persis<u>3</u>/Post<u>7</u>
                 Gain <u>4</u> dB
                 Transmit focus: <u>11 cm</u>
                 Image magnification: <u>16 cm</u>

1. Depth measurement accuracy
   Marker grids
       Measured distance . . . . <u>101</u> mm
       Actual distance . . . . <u>100</u> mm
       Error . . . . <u>1</u> mm
   Electronic calipers
       Measured distance . . . . <u>100.2</u> mm
       Actual distance . . . . <u>100</u> mm
       Error . . . . <u>0.2</u> mm
2. Horizontal measurement accuracy
   Electronic calipers
       Measured distance . . . . <u>61</u> mm
       Actual distance . . . . <u>60</u> mm
       Error . . . . <u>1</u> mm
3. Depth of penetration
       Measured distance . . . . <u>133</u> mm
       Baseline distance . . . . <u>140</u> mm
       Variation from baseline . . . . <u>7</u> mm
4. Image uniformity
   Significant *non*uniformity   Excellent uniformity
   1   2   3   4   5
5. Photography
   Gray bars
       Number of gray bars visible . . . . <u>14</u>
       Number of gray bars visible on baseline . . <u>15</u>
       Variation . . . . <u>1</u>
   Low-level echoes
       All echoes displayed on viewing monitor also
       seen on film: Yes <u>x</u> No__
   Contrast and brightness
       Level of agreement between contrast and brightness on viewing monitor and film:
   Poor   Excellent
   1   2   3   4   5
6. Filters
   Clean_____   Dusty_____

If a tissue phantom is employed, sensitivity control settings similar to those employed during patient scans will be necessary, including swept gain to compensate for attenuation. It is convenient to keep a record of the sensitivity control settings used for performance tests to help assure reproducibility of results (see above).

TESTS OF DISTANCE MEASUREMENT ACCURACY OF SCANNERS

Instruments used for measuring structure dimensions, organ sizes, and so on should be tested periodically for accuracy of distance indicators. Distance indicators usually

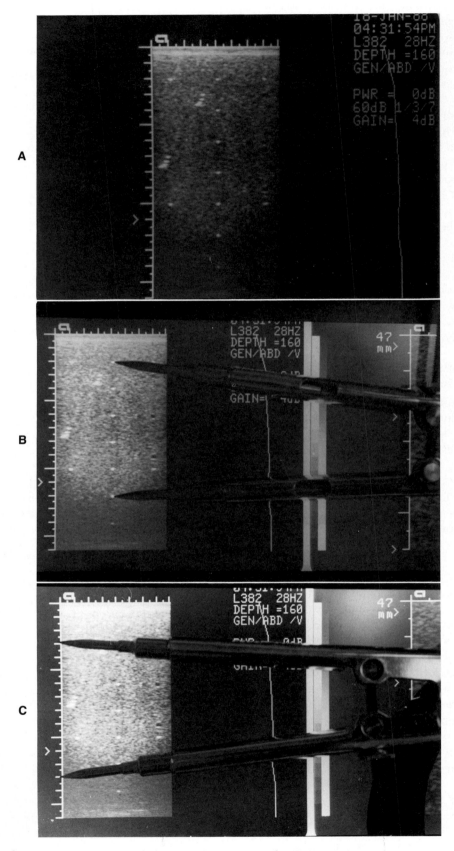

FIG. 6-3.   A, B-mode image of phantom shown in Fig. 6-2. **B,** Dividers set up to measure distance between reflectors that are 8 cm apart. **C,** Verifying distance marker accuracy by comparing with the 8 cm distance.

include 1 cm depth markers on A-mode, M-mode, and B-mode scanning displays, and digital calipers and cm markers on real-time and static B-mode scanning systems.

Our principal distance measurement tests are separated into two parts: one for measurements along the sound beam axis, referred to as the "depth calibration accuracy test," and a second for measurements taken perpendicular to the sound beam axis, called a "horizontal distance measurement test."

Depth calibration accuracy

To evaluate a scanner's depth calibration accuracy a scan of the phantom is obtained with a vertical column of reflectors in the phantom clearly imaged (Fig. 6-3). With the aid of a set of dividers the distance between any two reflectors in this column (Fig. 6-3, *B*) is measured by comparing against the cm scale on the hard copy image (Fig. 6-3, *C*). When testing general-purpose scanners, choose reflectors separated by at least 8 to 10 cm for this test. The measured distance should agree with the actual distance given by the phantom manufacturer to within 1 to 2 mm or 1.5%, whichever is greater. If a larger discrepancy occurs, consult with the ultrasound scanner manufacturer for corrective measures.

With manual scanning instruments, 1 cm depth markers can be positioned along any direction on the image. Dimensions of objects are determined by comparing the distance to be measured with the depth markers. For accurate distance measurements in those cases, the depth markers should always be positioned on the image as closely as possible and in the same orientation as the line joining the two points being measured. This is to avoid introducing errors from distortions on video monitors. The accuracy of distance measurements in the vertical direction taken with depth marker dots should be checked by

imaging a vertical column of reflectors in the phantom and then using the same procedure described above.

The digital caliper readout in the acoustic beam direction should be checked by comparing its reading of the distance between any two reflectors separated vertically on the B-mode image with the known distance between these reflectors (Fig. 6-4). Notice the position of caliper cursors along side-imaged reflectors in this figure. The distance readout is 100.2 mm and corresponds nearly exactly with the 10 cm reflector separation specified for the phantom. For this test, measurements should yield results that agree to within 1.5% or 1 to 2 mm, whichever is greater, of the actual distance.

Horizontal distance measurements

Horizontal measurement accuracy should be checked similarly. Measurements obtained in this direction (Fig. 6-5) are frequently less accurate because of beam width effects and scanner inaccuracies. Nevertheless, results should agree with in-phantom distances to within 3 mm or 3%, whichever is greater. For the example in Fig. 6-5, measurement results are within 1 mm of the actual distance between the reflectors examined. This is well within the expected level of accuracy.

Measurement accuracy may be checked in other directions as well. For example, from the specifications supplied by the phantom manufacturer, the two reflectors whose separation is being measured in Fig. 6-6 are actually 5 cm apart. Notice the digital caliper readout is 50.6 mm, in excellent agreement.

Distortion on video monitors used for photographing images can cause slight differences between the magnification scale factors in the horizontal and vertical directions. (We would expect these magnification factors to be the same.) One way to test for distortion is to use the tar-

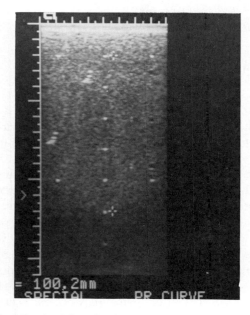

FIG. 6-4. Check of digital calipers in the beam (vertical) direction.

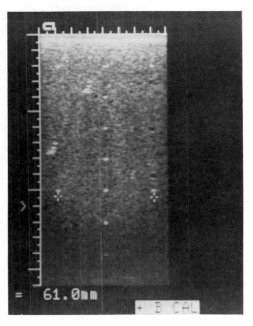

FIG. 6-5. Checking digital calipers in the horizontal direction.

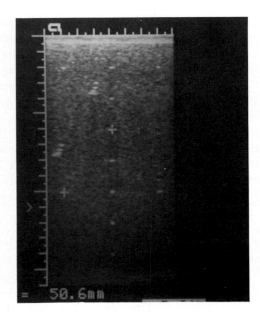

FIG. 6-6. Checking measurement accuracy along other directions.

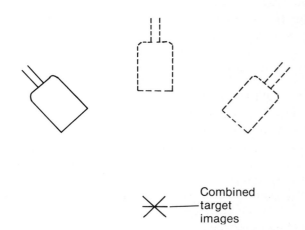

FIG. 6-7. Compound scan position registration accuracy.

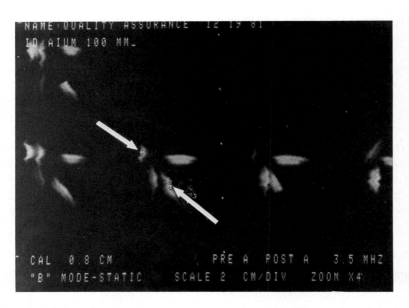

FIG. 6-8. Magnified B-mode image to assess compound scan position registration accuracy. The error to quote in this example is 8 mm, corresponding to the maximum separation of centers of target images from a single reflector (*arrows*).

get spacing employed above (Fig. 6-3) and compare it with distances as indicated by orthogonally positioned depth markers. Differences in the indicated distances greater than 3% should be noted.

Compound scan position registration accuracy

When a very small target is scanned from different directions with a manual scanner, the resultant B-mode image of the target should consist of a series of crossing lines (Fig. 6-7). When the instrument is performing properly, the centers of individual images of the target will coincide, forming an asterisk, as shown in the figure. The accuracy with which a manual scanning instrument positions echo signals from a single reflector on the display,

when the reflector is scanned from different transducer orientations in a fixed scanning plane, is referred to as the *compound scan position registration accuracy*.

Compound scan position registration accuracy is assessed by scanning test object targets from several directions and observing how well the separate registrations of individual targets on the same image coincide. A phantom or test object that has multiple windows, as the one shown in Fig. 6-1, is used. Caution should be exercised to assure that the test object remains perfectly stationary as the transducer is manipulated over the different windows. On the resultant B-mode image, pick out the reflector for which individual image lines appear farthest apart. Measure the distance between the centers of the individual lines and report the registration error as the largest distance between rod image centers (Fig. 6-8).

Any error in the speed of sound in the test object medium would contribute to apparent compound-position registration errors.[6] Therefore it is necessary to be sure that the acoustic properties of the test object are within specification.

SENSITIVITY AND PENETRATION

The sensitivity of an instrument refers to the weakest echo signal level that can be detected and displayed clearly enough to be discernible. Most instruments have controls that vary the receiver amplification and the output power. These are used to adjust the sensitivity during clinical examinations. When the controls are positioned for their maximum practical settings, we refer to the *maximum sensitivity* of the instrument. Often the maximum sensitivity is limited by electric noise appearing on the display when the receiver gain is at maximum levels. The noise may be generated externally, for example, by electronic communication networks or computer terminals. More commonly it arises from within the instrument itself, such as in the first stages of the receiver amplifier.

To allow use of higher-frequency ultrasound transducers for imaging large structures and organs, various steps have been taken to improve the maximum sensitivity on instruments. For example, in Chapter 2 it was pointed out that the use of quarterwave matching layers on the transducer assembly improves the sensitivity. Other instrument components that affect the maximum sensitivity include the pulser and the receiver.

Concern during quality control tests are usually centered around whether any notable *variations in sensitivity*, such as might result from damaged transducers or pulser-receiver components, have occurred. One way of detecting variations in maximum sensitivity is to measure the *maximum depth of visualization* for signals from scattered echoes in a tissue-mimicking phantom. Output power levels and receiver sensitivity controls are adjusted so that echo signals will be obtained from as deep as possible into the phantom. This means that the output power control is positioned for maximum output and the receiver gain adjusted for the highest values without excessive noise on the display. (Experience helps in establishing these control settings; they should be recorded in the quality control worksheet.) The phantom is scanned and the maximum depth of visualization of texture echo signals estimated (Fig. 6-9). Two scans are shown in Fig. 6-9, one done on the phantom and a second with the transducer assembly not coupled to any object. The latter illustrates electronic noise near the bottom of the image and helps the user judge where echo signals from within the phantom become weaker than electronic noise. In this example the maximum depth of visualization is 13.3 cm. A comparison is then made with maximum visualization results from a previous test. Results should agree to within 1 cm.

In addition to doing this measurement using the standard transducer, it may be useful to perform the test oc-

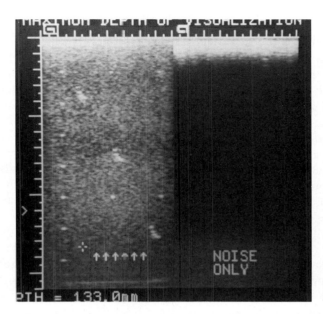

FIG. 6-9. Assessing variations in maximum sensitivity of a B-mode scanner by measuring the maximum depth of visualization of scatterers in a tissue-mimicking phantom.

casionally using different transducers. For example, they could be done with all transducers that are available for each instrument when quality control tests are first established and semi-annually thereafter. This would then help to pinpoint the source of any decrease in the maximum sensitivity or at least determine whether the standard transducer was at fault.

SETTING UP IMAGE PHOTOGRAPHY

Perhaps the most frequent source of instrument variability over time is related to image photography. All too often drift in the imaging instrument, in the hard copy cameras, or in film processing reduces image quality to the point that significant amounts of detail related to echo signal amplitude variations are lost on hard copy B-mode images. However, if image viewing and recording monitors are set up properly, and if sufficient detail is given to photography during routine quality control, these problems can be reduced.

Most instruments provide a separate image display monitor, which is viewed during scan buildup, along with an image recording device. As a general rule, the display monitor should be set up properly first, and then adjustments made, if necessary, to multiformat cameras or other hard copy recording devices to produce acceptable grayscale on hard copy images.

An effective method for setting up both viewing and hard copy monitors has been described by Gray.[8] This author recommends that adjustments be done using an image containing a clinically representative sampling of gray shades. Attention is first directed to the display monitor viewed during scan buildup. With the contrast settings of this monitor initially set at minimum settings, the brightness is adjusted to a level that just allows TV raster lines to be discernible. Once this is done the monitor contrast is adjusted until a clinically acceptable image is obtained.

After the viewing monitor is properly adjusted it is recommended that provisions be made which will prevent any casual changes in settings by department personnel.

The image recording device is then adjusted to obtain the same image gray shades as appear on the display monitor. This may require several iterations, varying the contrast and the overall brightness, until satisfactory results are obtained.

Routine checks should be done of the quality of gray-scale photography or other hard copy recording media. Photography and processing should always be such that all brightness variations in the viewing monitor image are successfully recorded on the hard copy image.

Images of a tissue-mimicking phantom, along with the gray-bar pattern appearing on the edge of most image displays can be used for routinely assessing photography settings. On an image of a tissue-mimicking phantom, check to see whether weak echo signals are successfully recorded at the same time that brightness variations between gray bars associated with large—amplitude signals are distinguishable. When the photography controls are adjusted properly, the weak echo signals will be visible above the background at the same time that brightness changes produced by variations of large-amplitude echoes are detectable.

OTHER HINTS

During routine performance testing it is a good idea to perform other equipment-related chores that require occasional attention. These include cleaning air filters on instruments requiring this service, checking for loose and frayed electric cables, noting any loose handles or control arms on the scanner, and performing recommended preventive maintenance of photography equipment. The last may include dusting or cleaning of photographic monitors and cleaning the developing rollers in Polaroid cameras.

THE QUALITY ASSURANCE NOTEBOOK

The quality assurance tests outlined above form a useful battery of procedures that can be done routinely and the results analyzed fairly quickly. To document the results of performance checks it is best to maintain a quality control notebook, in which a log of the test results, along with relevant images, can be kept. It may be desirable to insert a worksheet, such as the one shown at the beginning of this chapter, to serve as a reminder of the data that should be recorded, provide guidance on fields of view (display magnifications) and sensitivity controls appropriate for a given test, and furnish space for recording results.

It is also useful to maintain a log of equipment malfunctions and equipment service calls in the quality control data book for each instrument. This information provides fairly complete documentation of the operating and performance characteristics of an instrument over a time.

SPATIAL RESOLUTION TESTS

Measurements of spatial resolution generally require more exacting techniques to acquire meaningful results that allow intercomparisons of scanners. Therefore many

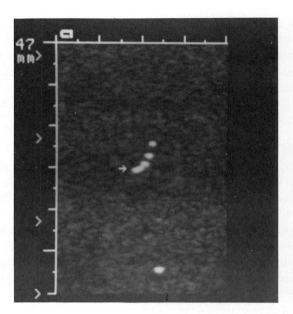

FIG. 6-10. Axial resolution test, consisting of scanning closely spaced reflectors in a phantom.

centers do not do such performance tests routinely, but may do so during equipment acceptance tests.[5]

There are many different methods used by ultrasound physicists and engineers for measuring resolution characteristics of scanners.[11] One approach that has been used for resolution tests is to measure the displayed spot size of point targets within a phantom or test object. For example, Figs. 4-9 and 4-10 present B-mode images of a column of fibers in a phantom. The displayed response width of each point target is related to the lateral resolution at that depth. Notice how the lateral resolution varies with depth for the two scanners.

Another approach is to arrange targets at progressively closer separations and determine the minimal target separation that can be "resolved" on the B-mode image. Fig. 6-10 illustrates this method for evaluating the axial resolution. The phantom scanned is the one shown in Fig. 6-2, and the B-mode image is of a group of targets at a depth of 7 cm. The axial separation between individual pairs of targets in this group are 3, 2, 1, and 0.5 mm. Notice the 0.5 mm pair cannot be resolved.

A phantom intended for detailed evaluation of lateral resolution characteristics is shown in Fig. 6-11. It consists of a planar sheet of scatterers arranged so that the central beam axis of a real-time B-mode scanner passes through the plane. A scan of this phantom (Fig. 6-12) yields a graphic illustration of the entire beam profile. In the example shown the displayed beam width is 3 mm at 6 cm depth and 4 mm at about 9 cm.

In Chapters 2 and 4 we also discussed "slice thickness," distinguishing it from lateral resolution on systems that use rectangular array transducer assemblies. A phantom for assessing slice thickness[7] as a function of depth is illustrated in Fig. 6-13. It consists of a planar sheet of scatterers at a 45-degree angle to the scanning window. The plane is so arranged so that aspects of the beam near a

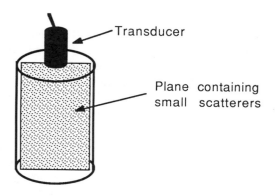

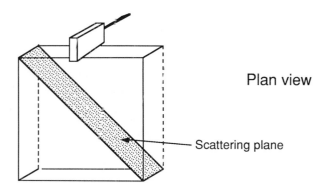

Plan view

Scattering plane

FIG. 6-11. "Beam" profile phantom. (Courtesy ATS Laboratories, Bridgeport, Conn.)

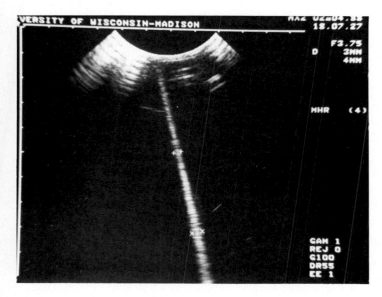

FIG. 6-12. B-mode image of the beam profile phantom, obtained with a real-time scanner. The width of the displayed beam at two different depths is shown. The width at the distance indicated by the pair of plus signs is 3 mm; the width indicated by the pair of *x*'s is 4 mm.

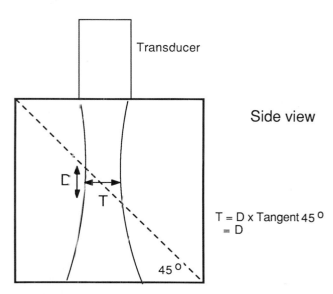

Transducer

Side view

$$T = D \times \text{Tangent } 45^\circ$$
$$= D$$

45°

FIG. 6-13. Slice-thickness phantom. The transducer assembly is shown from the side, with the B-mode image plane cutting in and out of the plane of the figure. The axial extent of the displayed image of the scattering surface is translated directly into slice thickness.

particular depth zone travel different distances from the transducer assembly to the plane. Thus they appear at different depths. For a 45-degree plane the resultant axial thickness of the image of this plane is equal to the slice thickness within that same zone.

Fig. 6-14 presents images of the slice-thickness phantom for a linear array transducer assembly. Results are shown for two different depths, 4 and 8 cm. Notice that the image of the scatterers appears thicker at 4 than at 8 cm, indicating that the slice thickness is much narrower at the greater depth.

Quantitative results for any of the above methods can be obtained if we define the resolution with respect to a threshold level on the B-scan display.[5] One requirement for quantitive resolution tests is a calibrated sensitivity control on the instrument. If this is not available, you should consult the instrument manufacturer or physicist or engineer who may be able to provide such a calibration. Reflectors are imaged at a sensitivity level for which

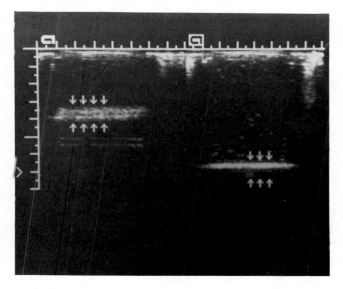

FIG. 6-14. B-mode images of the slice-thickness phantom for two different distances from the transducer assembly. The slice thickness varies in this image.

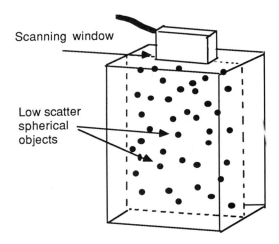

Scanning window

Low scatter
spherical
objects

FIG. 6-15. Spherical void phantom.

they are just barely discernible on the display. Then a calibrated control is adjusted to increase the sensitivity by a fixed amount (e.g., 20 dB) and the scan is repeated. On the resultant image the reflector spacing that can be resolved is quoted as the axial resolution at the level below threshold corresponding to the sensitivity control increase above.

Another type of phantom becoming increasingly popular for spatial resolution tests is one that has low scattering "voids" embedded within echogenic tissue-mimicking material. Voids may be cylindrical, such as those shown in Fig. 6-2. Another handy arrangement is for voids to be spherical,[11] as in the phantom illustrated in Fig. 6-15. An image of a spherical void phantom was presented in Fig. 4-14. A test of the ultrasound imaging system is to determine the "imaging zone" for detection of voids of a given size. A 3.5 MHz linear array may allow detection of 3 mm voids from depths of 4 to 8 cm, for example, while a 5 MHz array may provide imaging from 2 to 5 cm for this size structure. A useful aspect of phantom is that it presents a realistic imaging task that readily demonstrates imaging capabilities that are limited by limited resolution of ultrasound imaging instruments. For spherical targets the resolution is a combined, effective resolution, made up of axial and lateral as well as elevational dimensions. If cylindrical voids are used, as in Fig. 6-2, then only two dimensions, usually axial and lateral, are involved.

Electronic burst generators[4] may be used to evaluate an ultrasound imaging system's gray-scale display characteristics. Such devices also allow calibration of amplifier gain control knobs on the receiver of a pulse-echo instrument. Once this is done, it is possible to obtain quantifiable measurements of displayed beam widths.[5] Original electronic burst generators connect to the pulser-receiver circuit of the scanner. Such connections are no longer available, particularly on instruments employing array transducers. However, similar calibrations can be made using burst generators that use acoustic coupling between the generator and the transducer assembly. A small piezoelectric transducer couples acoustic signals from the transducer of the instrument under test to the generator.

The small transducer also couples signals from the generator back to the transducer. With such a generator it is possible to measure the gray-scale displayed dynamic range, that is, the echo signal range needed to drive the image monitor from full black to full white.

SUMMARY

1. Routine quality control tests help document gradual deterioration of instrument performance and provide a more objective means of assessing operating consistency than can be obtained from impressions of image quality on clinical scans.

2. The standard 100 mm test object consists of a series of stainless reflectors arranged as targets. It is mainly used for geometric tests of ultrasound pulse-echo instruments.

3. Tissue-mimicking phantoms provide the capability of testing ultrasound equipment performance under conditions that more closely simulate clinical scanning conditions than do simple liquid-filled test objects.

4. Tissue phantoms mimic tissues in speed of sound propagation, attenuation characteristics, and ultrasound scatter.

5. Geometric tests of scanners include depth calibration (also called vertical calibration in this chapter) accuracy, horizontal measurement accuracy, and compound registration accuracy for compound scanners.

6. The maximum sensitivity of an instrument refers to the weakest echo signal level that can be detected and displayed clearly enough to be discernible above noise.

7. Quality control assessments of variations in sensitivity are done by noting changes in the maximum depth of visualization of volumetric scatterers in a tissue-mimicking phantom.

8. When the photography controls are adjusted properly, the weak echo signals will be visible above the background at the same time that brightness changes produced by variations of large-amplitude echoes are detectable.

9. A quality control notebook, along with record sheets for documenting the results of tests, should be part of the quality control records for an instrument.

10. During routine performance testing it is a good idea to clean air filters, check for loose and frayed electric cables, check mechanical integrity of the instrument, and perform recommended preventive maintenance of photography equipment.

11. Spatial resolution tests include measurement of lateral, axial, and slice thickness.

REFERENCES

1. AIUM standard 100 mm test object, and recommendations for its use, Reflections 1:74, 1975.
2. AIUM-NEMA standard for measuring performance of ultrasound pulse echo equipment. Draft available from the American Institute of Ultrasound in Medicine, 4405 East West Highway, Bethesda, Md.
3. Burlew M, Madsen E, Zagzebski J, et al: A new ultrasound tissue-equivalent material with a high melting point and extended speed of sound range, Radiology 134:517, 1980.
4. Carson P: Rapid evaluation of many pulse echo system characteristics by use of a triggered pulse burst generator with exponential decay, J Clin Ultrasound 4:259, 1976.
5. Carson P and Zagzebski J: Pulse echo ultrasound imaging systems: performance tests and criteria, AAPM report no 8, New York, 1980, American Institute of Physics.
6. Goldstein A: Quality assurance in diagnostic ultrasound, Washington, DC, 1980, American Institute of Ultrasound in Medicine.
7. Goldstein A: Slice thickness test object, Program and abstracts of the thirty-second meeting of the American Institute of Ultrasound in Medicine, Bethesda, Md, The Institute.
8. Gray J: Test pattern for video display and hard copy cameras, Radiology 154:519-528, 1985.
9. Lopez H and Smith S: Implementation of a quality assurance program for ultrasound B-scanners, HEW Pub No 80-8100, Washington, DC, 1979.
10. Madsen E, Zagzebski J, Banjavic R, and Jula R: Tissue mimicking material for ultrasound phantoms, Med Phys 5:391, 1978.
11. Madsen E, Zagzebski J, and Frank G: Phantoms for assessing the ability of ultrasound scanners to resolve small, low echogenic masses, Program and abstracts of the thirty-second meeting of the American Institute of Ultrasound in Medicine, Bethesda, Md, The Institute.
12. Smith S and Lopez H: Contrast detail analysis of diagnostic ultrasound imaging, Med Physics 9:4-12, 1982.
13. Zagzebski J, Banjavic R, Madsen E, and Schwabe M: Focused transducer beams in tissue-mimicking material, J Clin Ultrasound 10:159, 1982.
14. Zagzebski J and Madsen E: Tissue equivalent materials and phantoms. In Wells P, and Ziskin M, eds: New techniques and instrumentation in ultrasonography, vol 5, New York, 1979, Churchill-Livingstone.

Table 7-1   Power and Intensity Levels Measured for a Mechanical Sector Scanner in Three Different Operating Modes

	Power (mW)	I(SPTA) (mW/cm²)	I(SPPA) (W/cm²)
Scan mode	10	7	35
M-mode	5.2	125	94
Pulsed Doppler	64	1460	43

From American Institute of Ultrasound in Medicine: Acoustic output levels from diagnostic ultrasound equipment, 1988.

multaneously to indicate which measure of intensity is being referred to. Intensity values commonly measured for diagnostic instruments are as follows:

I(SATA): Spatial average—time average intensity; often it is specified at the transducer surface or at the surface of a transducer assembly where the sound beam enters the patient. It may be estimated using Equation 7-1.

I(SPTA): Spatial peak—time average intensity.

I(SPPA): Spatial peak—pulse average intensity.

The ranking from top to bottom is the same as if one were ranking these intensities from low to high. In addition, you will sometimes still see mention of the spatial peak—temporal peak intensity:

I(SPTP): Spatial peak—temporal peak intensity.

The peak positive (or peak compressional) as well as the peak negative (or peak rarefactional) acoustic pressures are indicated in the top waveform in Fig. 7-5. These quantities also are being used by some researchers to help characterize the output of ultrasound scanners.

Values for the acoustic power and intensities measured for one type of diagnostic ultrasound instrument are presented in Table 7-1. The example is for a mechanical sector scanner having a single-element fixed-focus transducer in the scan head. The system operates in three different modes—scan mode, pulsed Doppler mode, and M-mode—and values are presented for each mode.

Notice the difference in intensities between the various operating modes. For example, the M-mode I(SPTA) value is greater than the I(SPTA) in scanning mode, even though in this example the ultrasonic power is lower. This is because the beam is stationary in M-mode, always directed toward the measurement point, whereas it is always scanning in B-scan mode. The much higher spatial peak time average intensity in pulsed Doppler mode should be noted! This is typical for Doppler systems intended mainly for vascular imaging. Stationary pulsed Doppler involves large amplitude acoustic pulses and duty factors that are much greater than in other operating modes. Consequently, the time average intensity at the focal point of the beam is unusually high. Finally, you can see that the pulse average intensity is much larger than the time average values in every mode—the units for pulse average intensity are W/cm², while those for time average intensities are mW/cm².

For any operating mode there is a large variation of output powers and intensities produced by different types of instruments, either different transducer assemblies from a given manufacturer or instruments from different manufacturers. The values quoted in Table 7-1, therefore, only give an indication of the levels involved and the differences that might be encountered for different operating modes. Instruments are available whose powers and intensities are much lower than the values given in the table; some units are available that produce even greater intensities than those shown. Ultrasound equipment manufacturers will usually provide users with output data for their own instruments if requested.

MODES OF PRODUCTION OF BIOLOGIC EFFECTS

At sufficiently high intensities and long enough exposure times, ultrasound is capable of producing a measurable effect on tissues. The effect may be a small temperature elevation or complete destruction of tissue depending on the acoustic exposure. We shall consider briefly some of the modes whereby a sound beam can produce a biologic effect. These have been documented *mainly* for acoustic exposure conditions that exceed those of diagnostic ultrasound.

Heating

As a sound beam propagates through tissue, it undergoes attenuation. A significant fraction of this attenuation is due to absorption or, essentially, conversion of the ultrasonic energy into heat. For very low ultrasonic power levels, any heat that is deposited by the sound beam is quickly dissipated. Therefore no measurable temperature increase occurs. On the other hand, ultrasound therapy devices producing beams with areas of several square centimeters and higher and operating at spatial average—time average intensities of 1000 mW/cm² or greater can cause significant temperature elevations in tissue. In fact, deep heating is one of the beneficial effects of this mode of therapy.[8]

Cavitation

Intense ultrasound beams in a fluid can generate tiny bubbles from dissolved gases in the fluid. This process is called cavitation.[11] In the presence of the sound beam the bubbles can grow in size and produce an effect on the medium. The cavitation bubbles expand and contract synchronously with pressure oscillations in the sound field. This, in turn, causes particle displacements and stresses in excess of those resulting from the sound beam alone. Some experimentally induced biologic effects have been attributed to this cavitation process.

Two types of cavitation may exist.[11] *Stable cavitation* refers to the creation of bubbles that oscillate with the sound beam, as mentioned. In contrast, *transient cavitation* is a process in which the oscillations grow so strong that the bubbles collapse, producing very intense, localized effects. Transient cavitation has been detected at acoustic pressure amplitudes well above those produced by diagnostic instruments.[11] It may be possible to produce cavitation with some clinical instruments if the conditions in the medium are favorable; in fact, cavitation is believed to be responsible for some *in vitro* biologic effects involving single-cell suspensions exposed to diagnostic ultrasound.[10] Whether either form of cavitation is responsible for damage to tissues exposed *in vivo* to diagnostic ultrasound beams has not been demonstrated. Thresholds for cavitation are believed to be closely related to the acoustic pressure amplitudes in the medium. Therefore, instrument manufacturers measure and report peak rarefactional and peak compressional pressures in the field of their instruments.

Direct mechanical effects

Sound transmission is associated with displacements, accelerations, and stresses on particles in the medium. Thus it is possible that the perturbations caused by passage of sound waves will lead directly to "bioeffects." Biologic effects have been produced in some experimental studies on plants and cells in which no temperature rise could have occurred and cavitation was known to be absent. When these two mechanisms are ruled out as the cause of a biologic effect accompanying exposure to ultrasound, direct mechanical effects of the ultrasound beam are usually thought to have occurred.

IS THERE A RISK?

Nearly every clinical study and therapeutic action involves some calculated risk to patients. In many of these cases the level of risk is well known. In making a decision to do a procedure on a patient, clinicians must weigh the risk against the expected benefit.

For diagnostic ultrasound we must presume that there is some element of risk to ultrasound exposures, no matter how low it may be. What researchers are attempting to obtain, and will probably be seeking for a long time, are data that will enable them to better quantify the risk level for different ultrasound exposure conditions. Out of perhaps hundreds of thousands of individuals already insonified during diagnostic ultrasound examinations, no known ill effects have been suffered from these exposures. This information, though certainly very comforting, also indicates that the task of determining a risk factor for diagnostic ultrasound is a difficult one.

A number of different approaches are being followed in these investigations. Epidemiologic studies[18] are aimed at determining whether previous diagnostic ultrasound examinations of fetuses (in utero) may have resulted in any ill effects. Such investigations involve comparisons of medical records and present physical condition of groups of individuals insonified in utero and presumably identical groups of individuals who were not insonified. The idea is to attempt to determine whether factors such as abnormal size and weight, prevalence toward illness, and others are more evident in the group that was exposed. The work is time consuming, because to obtain valid results investigators must study large numbers of patients.

In addition to epidemiologic investigations, numerous studies have been and continue to be performed on animals in vivo and on mammalian cells in vitro. Excellent reviews of the recent literature on bioeffects[13,14] have

been published. When diagnostic ultrasound instruments are used in these studies, equivocal results often appear. A positive finding of an effect in one laboratory may be impossible to duplicate in another laboratory (and sometimes in the same laboratory). Experiments have been done in which small animals were insonified for an extensive time (hours) by diagnostic instruments and no effects were observed.[15] Recently, however, several studies using ultrasound at diagnostic intensities have produced positive effects. For example, Liebeskind et al.[10] used a diagnostic instrument and demonstrated that ultrasound appeared to cause detectable effects on DNA and growth patterns of animal cells in vitro. Recently, effects of ultrasound on cell suspensions have received considerable attention by researchers,[7] still with inconclusive results as far as exposures to diagnostic ultrasound beams are concerned. Perhaps as biologic indicators and assay techniques become more sensitive, it will be possible to obtain a quantifiable indication of risk factors associated with diagnostic ultrasound exposures.

Definitive evidence for biologic effects has been obtained in investigations in which small animals were insonified, usually at spatial peak−time average intensities and exposure times that in most cases could not be obtained with diagnostic equipment.[13] At such intensity levels fetal weight reductions in rats, death of rat fetuses, and altered mitotic rates were observed. For these effects to be produced, it was usually necessary to expose the animal to some minimal intensity for a given time. If the intensity was reduced, the exposure time had to be increased to compensate for the reduced acoustic energy.

This last statement is illustrated in Fig. 7-6 for mammalian tissues exposed to high-intensity ultrasound. Curves such as the one shown have been produced by researchers in an attempt to place the vast amount of experimental data on bioeffects research into perspective. The line divides the data into a region where exposure conditions were sufficient to produce the effect investigated, such as fetal weight reduction (above the line), and a region where the effect being studied could not be found (below the line). In some experiments with high spatial peak intensities, only a brief exposure resulted in an effect. To produce the same effect at a lower intensity level, it was necessary to expose the animal for a longer time. For spatial peak−time average intensities greater than 100 mW/cm^2 the demarcation line follows a curve in which the product of the intensity, I, and the exposure time, T, is given by

$$I \times T = 50(\text{W/cm}^2)\text{s} \qquad (7\text{-}6)$$
$$= 50 \text{ joules/cm}^2$$

(A *joule* is a unit of energy; it is the product when watts are multiplied by seconds.)

Below 100 mW/cm^2 these data indicate that none of the effects for which the researchers were looking could be produced—no matter how long the exposure.

To help clarify these data, a committee of the American

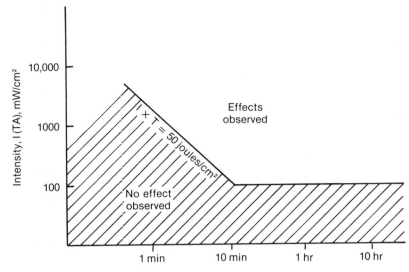

FIG. 7-6. Intensity versus time curve relevant to production of biologic effects in mammalian tissue. Exposure conditions that resulted in positive biologic effects are separated from conditions for which no effects were observed for animal studies. (Derived from Nyborg W: HEW Pub No FDA 788062, 1978.)

Institute of Ultrasound in Medicine issued the following statement[16]:

A review of bioeffects data supports the following statement:
In the low megahertz frequency range there have been (as of this date) no independently confirmed significant biological effects in mammalian tissues exposed in vivo to unfocused ultrasound with intensities* below 100 mW/cm². Furthermore, for exposure times† greater than 1 second and less than 500 seconds, such effects have not been demonstrated even at higher intensities, when the product of intensity and exposure time is less than 50 joules/cm².

This statement was prepared by the AIUM Bioeffects Committee after careful examination of all pertinent literature. It provides some information relative to the current knowledge of risk factors for diagnostic ultrasound. If the acoustic intensities (spatial peak–time average) can be kept substantially below 100 mW/cm², it would appear from the statement that the risk factor is low. For situations in which the spatial peak–time average intensity approaches or even exceeds 100 mW/cm², we may be dealing with ultrasonic exposures that carry a higher risk of producing some effect on tissues.

It should be pointed out once again that the data on which the statement was based were for ultrasonic exposures in small animals. The statement does not offer absolute safe levels, or even state permissible levels; nor does it suggest upper intensity limits for ultrasound equipment.

The data in Fig. 7-6 also suggest that if the *exposure time* is kept low, the possibility of biologic effects will be minimized. The insonification schemes (e.g., the duty factor and the pulse duration) used by the researchers in generating the data summarized in Fig. 7-6 are not the same as those used in pulsed ultrasound. Nevertheless,

the principle would seem to apply to all modes of diagnostic ultrasound.

Most experiments leading to the statement were done by using large beams from unfocused transducers, and researchers believe the bioeffects were due to heating of tissue. However, for focused transducers (the ones used in nearly all diagnostic procedures) greater time average intensities are tolerated because any heat deposited over a small focal area is dissipated easily to the surrounding, unexposed tissue. Taking this into account and considering additional experimental results, the AIUM has revised the statement, claiming that intensities as high as 1 W/cm² have led to no observed effects in mammalian tissues exposed to highly focused* sound beams.[3a] Although all diagnostic beams are not as highly focused as those considered by the AIUM, it is comforting to know that time average intensities higher than 100 mW/cm² may be okay in some instances.

A RATIONAL APPROACH

No matter what the outcome of bioeffects studies, prudence dictates that the lowest possible acoustic exposures be used during ultrasound examinations. The following points are offered in accordance with this philosophy:

1. One should not hesitate to use diagnostic ultrasound when the situation warrants. However, diagnostic ultrasound should be used only when there is a valid medical reason. For example, it seems difficult to justify ultrasound exposures of individuals during commercial demonstrations.

Responsible individuals will not treat ultrasound as a novel plaything but will use it to obtain an anticipated benefit such as diagnostic information or research results.

---

*I(SPTA).
†Total time; this includes off-time as well as on-time for pulse regimes

*Quarter-power (−6 dB) beam width smaller than four wavelengths or 4 mm, whichever is less at the exposure frequency.

2. Users should familiarize themselves with their equipment so they can recognize which operating modes and which control settings result in high or low acoustic intensities. Thus they can avoid using high acoustic intensities, except when the examination warrants. They should avoid using an instrument for the purposes for which it may not have been designed. Table 7-1 shows that the spatial peak–temporal average intensity for different classes of instruments and different operating modes may vary significantly.

Information on acoustic exposure from ultrasound instruments is beginning to be provided by ultrasound equipment manufacturers. Some of this data has been compiled in a single document.[1] Acoustic exposure data are also sometimes available in the operator's manual accompanying the equipment.

3. Many instruments have controls that vary the acoustic power. On such instruments as a general rule, **Use a high receiver gain setting and a low power setting, not vice versa!**

Start an examination with power settings initially adjusted for low power output. Increase the power only when adequate sensitivity cannot be attained with the receiver gains peaking out at their maximum values, or when there is insufficient penetration because of electronic noise on the display. You should be aware that a 10 dB reduction in the output power means a factor of 10 reduction in the acoustic intensity (see Table 1-1). A 20 dB reduction means a factor of 100 reduction in intensity!

4. **Reduce the exposure time** by avoiding repeat scans if possible and avoiding holding the transducer stationary in contact with the patient unless the examination warrants this.

Ultrasound instrument manufacturers are expected to design their equipment so it will deliver the lowest possible acoustic exposure consistent with the diagnostic expectations of that equipment.[3] However, as the foregoing points indicate, user awareness and responsibility are major elements in assuring patient safety during an ultrasound examination.

SUMMARY

1. Experience that has been gained with clinical ultrasound equipment has been accompanied by no known tissue damage. Thus we are led to believe that diagnostic ultrasound poses a low risk for producing biologic effects.

2. Insufficient experimental data exist at present to satisfactorily define this risk factor.

3. Power is the rate at which energy is transmitted from the transducer into the medium; it is expressed in watts or milliwatts.

4. Intensity is the ultrasonic power per unit area. It is expressed in watts per square meter (W/m^2) or,

more commonly, milliwatts per square centimeter (mW/cm^2).

5. A hydrophone consists of a small-diameter probe with a piezoelectric element, usually 0.5 to 1 mm in diameter, at one end. When placed in an ultrasound beam, a hydrophone produces an electric signal whose amplitude is proportional to the acoustic pressure amplitude.

6. Intensity values commonly measured for diagnostic instruments (ranked in approximate order from low to high) are I(SATA), the spatial average–time average intensity; I(SPTA), the spatial peak–time average intensity; and I(SPPA), the spatial peak–pulse average intensity.

7. The peak rarefactional pressure and the peak compressional pressure are also used to characterize the strength of the sound beam.

8. There are differences in intensities between the various operating modes of an ultrasound scanner. There also is a range of intensities and power levels produced by different instruments operating in the same mode.

9. Biologic effects due to exposure to ultrasound beams are usually attributable to heating, cavitation, or direct mechanical effects.

10. For diagnostic ultrasound we must presume that there is some element of risk to ultrasound exposures, no matter how low it may be.

11. Epidemiologic studies are retrospective studies aimed at determining whether previous diagnostic ultrasound examinations of fetuses (in utero) may have resulted in any ill effect.

12. Evidence for biologic effects has been obtained in investigations in which small animals were insonified, usually at average intensities and exposure times that in most cases could not be obtained with diagnostic equipment.

13. The 1978 AIUM Statement on Biologic Effects summarizes results of experimental exposures of mammalian tissue. The data on which the statement was based were for ultrasonic exposures in small animals. The statement does not offer absolute safe levels, or even state permissible levels; nor does it suggest upper intensity limits for ultrasound equipment.

14. Operators of ultrasound equipment should be aware of the acoustic output levels produced by their equipment for the various operating modes of the equipment. They should use a minimum output power setting consistent with obtaining useful clinical results and should use the minimum exposure time.

REFERENCES

1. American Institute of Ultrasound in Medicine: Acoustic output levels from diagnostic ultrasound equipment, Bethesda, Md, 1985 and 1988, The Institute.
2. American Institute of Ultrasound in Medicine: AIUM/NEMA acoustic output measurement standard, Bethesda, Md, 1988, The Institute.
3. American Institute of Ultrasound in Medicine: AIUM/NEMA ultrasound safety standard, Washington, DC, 1981 The Institute.
3a. American Institute of Ultrasound in Medicine: Bioeffects considerations for the safety of diagnostic ultrasound, J Ultrasound Med 7(9)(suppl), 1988.
4. American Institute of Ultrasound in Medicine: Safety considerations for diagnostic ultrasound, Bethesda, Md, 1980, The Institute.
5. Carson P: Diagnostic ultrasound emissions and their measurement. In Fullerton G, and Zagzebski J, editors: Medical physics of CT and ultrasound New York, 1980, AAPM.
6. Carson P, Fischella P, and Oughton T: Ultrasound power and intensities produced by diagnostic ultrasound equipment, Ultrasound Med Biol 3:341, 1978.
7. Cell exposures. In Nyborg W and Ziskin M, editors: Clinics in diagnostic ultrasound, vol 16, Biological effects of ultrasound, New York, 1985, Churchill-Livingston, pp 23-33.
8. Dyson M: Therapeutic Applications of Ultrasound. In Nyborg W and Ziskin M, editors: Clinics in diagnostic ultrasound, vol 16, Biological effects of ultrasound, New York, 1985, Churchill-Livingston, pp 121-133.
9. Lele P: "Local hyperthermia by ultrasound for cancer therapy. In Nyborg W and Ziskin M: Clinics in diagnostic ultrasound, vol 16, Biological effects in ultrasound, New York, 1985, Churchill Livingston, pp 135-155.
10. Liebeskind D, Bases R, Elequin F, et al: Diagnostic ultrasound: effects on the DNA and growth patterns of animal cells, Radiology 131:177, 1979.
11. Nyborg W: Mechanisms for biological effects of ultrasound. In Nyborg W and Ziskin M: Clinics in diagnostic ultrasound, vol 16, Biological effects of ultrasound, New York, 1985, Churchill Livingston, pp 23-33.
12. Nyborg W: Physical mechanisms for biological effects of ultrasound, HEW Pub No (FDA) 78-8062, Washington, DC, 1978, Food and Drug Administration.
13. O'Brien W: Biological effects of ultrasound. In Fullerton G and Zagzebski J, editors: Medical physics of CT and ultrasound, New York, 1980 AAPM.
14. O'Brien W: Safety of ultrasound. In de Vleger M et al, editors: Handbook of clinical ultrasound, New York, 1978, John Wiley & Sons, Inc.
15. Smythe M: Animal toxicity studies with ultrasound at diagnostic power levels. In Grossman CC et al, editors: Diagnostic ultrasound, New York, 1966, Plenum Press.
16. Statement of mammalian in vivo ultrasonic biological effects, Reflections 4:311, 1978.
17. Taylor KJW: Current status of toxicity investigations, J Clin Ultrasound 2:149, 1974.
18. Ziskin M: Epidemiology and human exposure. In Nyborg W and Ziskin M: Clinics in diagnostic ultrasound, vol 16, Biological effects of ultrasound, New York, 1985, Churchill Livingston, pp 111-120.

Part Two

ABDOMINAL AND RETROPERITONEAL CAVITIES

Cross-sectional and Sagittal Anatomy

SANDRA L. HAGEN-ANSERT

The ability of the sonographer to understand anatomy as it relates to the cross-sectional, coronal, oblique, and sagittal projections is critical in performing a quality sonogram. Normal anatomy has many variations in size and position, and it is the responsibility of the sonographer to be able to demonstrate these findings on the sonogram. To complete this task the sonographer must have a thorough understanding of anatomy as it relates to the anterior-posterior relationships, as well as the variations in sectional anatomy. This chapter will provide a background for these anatomic relationships.

INTRODUCTION TO ANATOMIC TERMS

Several anatomic terms that relate to the human body are described below:

anatomic position   (Fig. 8-1) The individual is standing erect, the arms are by the side with the palms facing forward, the face and eyes are directed forward, and the heels are together, with the feet pointed forward.

median plane   A vertical plane that bisects the body into right and left halves.

sagittal plane   Any plane parallel to the median plane.

coronal plane   (Fig. 8-2) Any vertical plane at right angles to the median plane.

transverse plane   Any plane at right angles to both the median and coronal planes.

supine   Lying face up.

prone   Lying face down.

anterior (ventral)   (Fig. 8-2) Toward the front of the body.

posterior (dorsal)   (Fig. 8-2) The back of the body, or in back of another structure.

medial   Nearer to or toward the midline.

lateral   Farther from the midline or to the side of the body.

proximal   Closer to the point of origin or closer to the body.

distal   Away from the point of origin or away from the body.

internal   Inside.

external   Outside.

superior   Above.

inferior   Below.

cranial   Toward the head.

caudal   Toward the feet.

THE ABDOMEN IN GENERAL

The abdominal cavity, excluding the retroperitoneum and the pelvis, is bounded superiorly by the diaphragm, anteriorly by the abdominal wall muscles, posteriorly by the vertebral column, ribs, and iliac fossa, and inferiorly by the pelvis.

Regions of the abdomen

The abdomen (Fig. 8-3) is divided into nine different regions: (1) left hypogastrium, (2) epigastrium, (3) right hypogastrium, (4) left lumbar, (5) umbilical, (6) right lumbar, (7) left iliac, (8) hypogastric, and (9) right iliac.

Horizontal planes of the abdomen

In addition there are two horizontal planes in the abdomen the sonographer should be familiar with (Fig. 8-4).

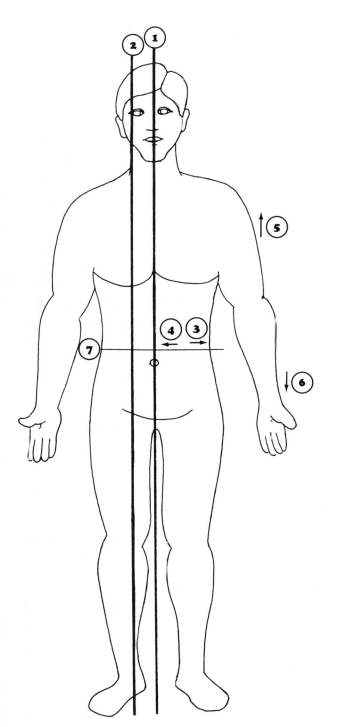

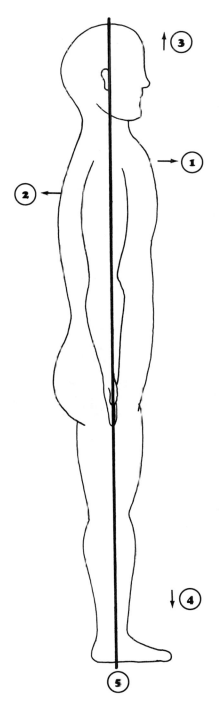

FIG. 8-1. Anterior view of the body in the anatomic position. Median sagittal plane, *1;* paramedian plane, *2;* lateral, *3;* medial, *4;* proximal, *5;* distal, *6;* and transverse plane, *7.* (From Hagen-Ansert SL: The anatomy workbook, Philadelphia, 1986, JB Lippincott Co.)

FIG. 8-2. Lateral view of the body. Anterior, *1;* posterior, *2;* superior, *3;* inferior, *4;* coronal plane, *5.* (From Hagen-Ansert SL: The anatomy workbook, Philadelphia, 1986, JB Lippincott Co.)

The transpyloric plane runs through the level of L1. The subcostal plane runs through L3 and joins the lowest portion of the thoracic cage on the left to the lowest portion of the thoracic cage on the right.

Vertical planes of the abdomen

The two vertical planes are the midclavicular lines. Each of these joins the midpoint of the clavicle with the midlin-guinal point (i.e., the midpoint of a line joining the anterior-superior iliac spine and the pubic symphysis).

Quadrants of the abdomen

Another way of dividing the abdomen is with quadrants. Equal parts of the abdomen may be separated into the left upper quadrant, right upper quadrant, left lower quadrant, and right lower quadrant.

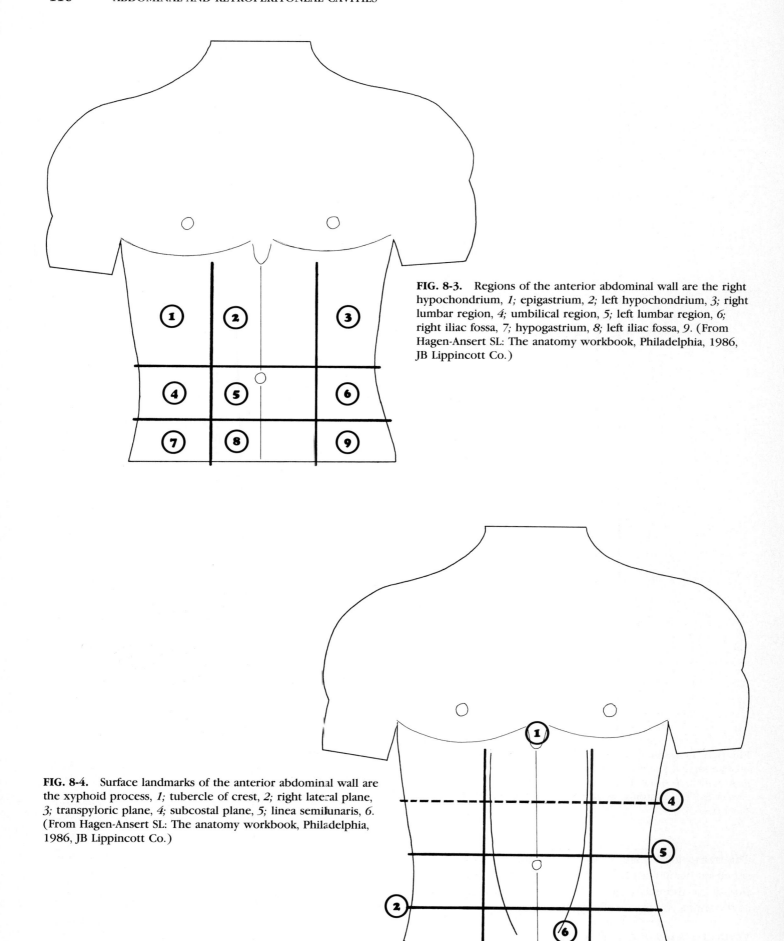

FIG. 8-3. Regions of the anterior abdominal wall are the right hypochondrium, *1;* epigastrium, *2;* left hypochondrium, *3;* right lumbar region, *4;* umbilical region, *5;* left lumbar region, *6;* right iliac fossa, *7;* hypogastrium, *8;* left iliac fossa, *9.* (From Hagen-Ansert SL: The anatomy workbook, Philadelphia, 1986, JB Lippincott Co.)

FIG. 8-4. Surface landmarks of the anterior abdominal wall are the xyphoid process, *1;* tubercle of crest, *2;* right lateral plane, *3;* transpyloric plane, *4;* subcostal plane, *5;* linea semilunaris, *6.* (From Hagen-Ansert SL: The anatomy workbook, Philadelphia, 1986, JB Lippincott Co.)

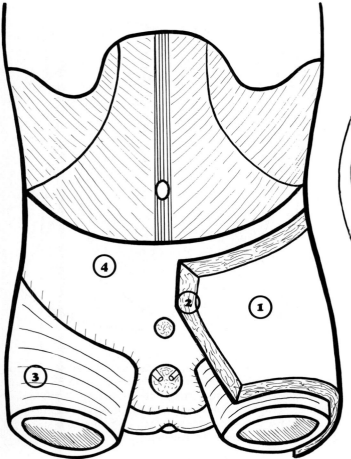

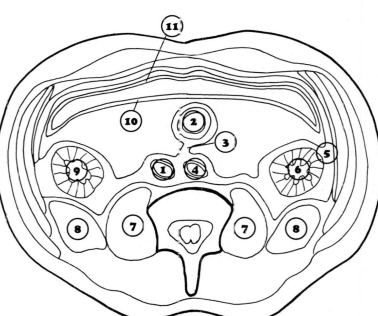

FIG. 8-6. Transverse section of the abdominal cavity showing the reflections of the peritoneum. Inferior vena cava, *1;* small intestine, *2;* mesentery of the small intestine, *3;* aorta, *4;* peritoneum, *5;* descending colon, *6;* psoas major muscle, *7;* quadratus lumborum muscle, *8;* ascending colon, *9;* posterior layers of the greater omentum, *10;* and anterior layers of the greater omentum, *11.* (From Hagen-Ansert SL: The anatomy workbook, Philadelphia, 1986, JB Lippincott Co.)

FIG. 8-5. Superficial fascia of the lower anterior abdominal wall include the superficial fascia, *1;* fatty layer (Camper's fascia), *2;* fascia lata, *3;* membranous layer (Scarpa's fascia), *4.* (From Hagen-Ansert SL: The anatomy workbook, Philadelphia, 1986, JB Lippincott Co.)

THE ANTERIOR ABDOMINAL WALL

The anterior abdominal wall is composed of several layers of muscles: the rectus abdominis, the external oblique, internal oblique, and transversus abdominis. The linea alba is a fibrous band that stretches from the xyphoid to the symphysis pubis. It is wider at its superior end and forms a central anterior attachment for the muscle layers of the abdomen. It is formed by the interlacing of fibers of the aponeuroses of the right and left oblique and transversus abdominis muscles.

Fascia

The fascia of the abdominal wall is divided into superficial and deep fascia (Fig. 8-5). The superficial fascia may be further divided into two layers: the superficial layer contains fatty tissue (Camper's fascia) while the deep layer is mostly membranous with little fat (Scarpa's fascia).

PERITONEUM

The peritoneum (Figs. 8-6 to 8-8) is formed by a single layer of cells called the mesothelium, resting on a thin layer of connective tissue. If the mesothelium is damaged or removed in any area (such as surgery), there is danger

that two layers of peritoneum may adhere to each other and form an adhesion. This adhesion may interfere with the normal movements of the abdominal viscera.

The peritoneum is further divided into two layers; the parietal peritoneum is that portion of the peritoneum which lines the abdominal wall but does not cover a viscus, the visceral peritoneum is that portion of the peritoneum that covers an organ. The peritoneal cavity is the potential space between the parietal and visceral peritoneum. This cavity contains a small amount of lubricating serous fluid to help the abdominal organs move upon one another without friction. Under certain pathologic conditions, the potential space of the peritoneal cavity may be distended into an actual space containing several liters of fluid. This accumulation of fluid is known as ascites. Other fluid substances, such as blood from a ruptured organ, bile from a ruptured duct, or fecal matter from a ruptured intestine, also may accumulate in this cavity.

The peritoneum lines the walls of the abdominal cavity. It forms a completely closed sac (except in the female where the mouths of the fallopian tubes open into it). Retroperitoneal organs remain posterior to the sac and are covered anteriorly with peritoneum. This primarily applies to the urinary system. The other abdominal organs are located within the peritoneal cavity.

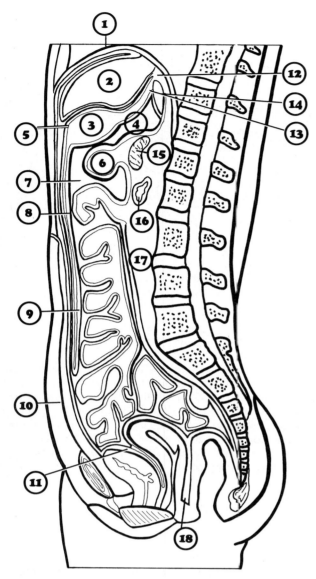

FIG. 8-7. Sagittal section through the abdomen and pelvis: Diaphragm, *1;* liver, *2;* stomach, *3;* omental bursa, *4;* gastric ligament, *5;* transverse colon, *6;* peritoneal cavity, *7;* greater omentum, *8;* parietal peritoneum, *9;* linea alba, *10;* vesicouterine pouch, *11;* subphrenic space, *12;* lesser omentum, *13;* caudate lobe of the liver, *14;* pancreas, *15;* duodenum, *16;* retroperitoneum, *17;* rectouterine pouch, *18.* (From Hagen-Ansert SL: The anatomy workbook, Philadelphia, 1986, JB Lippincott Co.)

Mesentery

The mesentery is a double fold of peritoneum connecting an organ to the abdominal wall. An organ without a mesentery is retroperitoneal (e.g., kidney).

Omentum

The omentum is a double layer of peritoneum running to the stomach. The lesser omentum attaches to the lesser curvature of the stomach, and the greater omentum attaches to the greater curvature of the stomach. The greater omentum runs inferiorly from the greater curvature of the stomach and loops back upon itself to attach to the transverse colon, which runs across the abdomen just inferior to the stomach. The greater omentum is con-

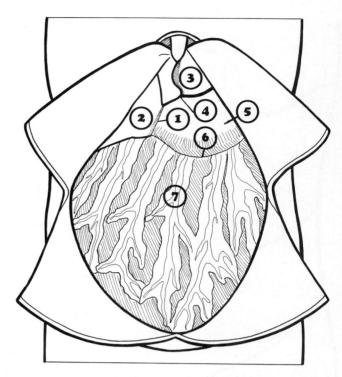

FIG. 8-8. Greater omentum is often referred to as an apron hanging between the small intestine and the anterior abdominal wall. Falciform ligament, *1;* right lobe of the liver, *2;* left lobe of the liver, *3;* ligamentum teres, *4;* stomach, *5;* greater curvature of the stomach, *6;* greater omentum, 7. (From Hagen-Ansert SL: The anatomy workbook, Philadelphia, 1986, JB Lippincott Co.)

sidered an "apron of tissue" that hangs down from the stomach anterior to the intestine (Fig. 8-9).

Lesser sac

The posterior surface of the lesser omentum is continuous over the posterior surface of the stomach with the inner layer of the ligaments to the stomach and kidneys and with the upper layer of the transverse colon. These surfaces form the boundaries of the omental bursa, or lesser sac.

Epiploic foramen

The only entrance to the lesser sac is through a small opening of the epiploic foramen. This foramen is bordered anteriorly by the hepatoduodenal ligament (with the portal triad within to include the common bile duct, hepatic artery, and portal vein); posteriorly to the peritoneum, the inferior vena cava; superiorly and inferiorly the posterior parietal peritoneum is reflected onto the quadrate lobe of the liver and the duodenum.

Ligament

In some cases the folds of peritoneum running from one organ to another is called a ligament (Fig. 8-10). Their names are related to the organs to which they are attached.

Hepatorenal recess

The hepatorenal recess, or pouch of Morrison, is the lowest point in the peritoneal cavity when the patient is lying

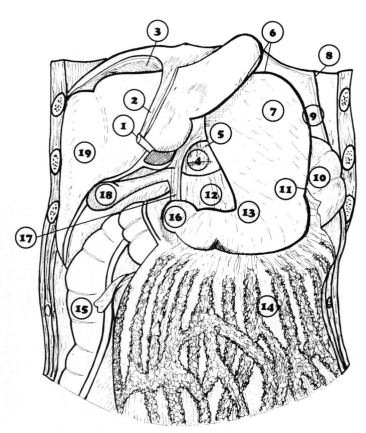

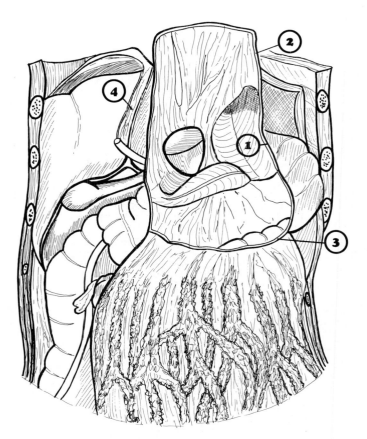

FIG. 8-9. Anterior view of the abdominal viscera with the liver pulled upward. Ligamentum teres, *1;* falciform ligament, *2;* hepatic coronary ligament, *3;* caudate lobe of the liver, *4;* hepatogastric ligament, *5;* cardiac ligament, *6;* fundus of the stomach, *7;* diaphragm, *8;* parietal peritoneum, *9;* spleen, *10;* gastrosplenic ligament, *11;* lesser omentum, *12;* lesser curvature of stomach, *13;* greater omentum, *14;* ascending colon, *15;* pylorus, *16;* epiploic foramen, *17;* gallbladder, *18;* liver, *19.* (From Hagen-Ansert SL: The anatomy workbook, Philadelphia, 1986, JB Lippincott Co.)

FIG. 8-10. Upper abdomen with the greater curvature of the stomach lifted. Gastrosplenic ligament, *1;* phrenic gastric ligament, *2;* gastrocolic ligament, *3;* faciform ligament, *4.* (From Hagen-Ansert SL: The anatomy workbook, Philadelphia, 1986, JB Lippincott Co.)

supine. It is in the greatest sac just to the right of the epiploic foramen. The right kidney is the medial margin, while the liver forms the superior boundary. The right paracolic gutter drains fluid from this pouch.

Peritoneal recesses

The omental bursa normally has some empty places, parts of the peritoneal cavity near the liver are so "slit-like" that they are also isolated. These areas are known as peritoneal recesses and are clinically important because infections may collect in them. Two common sites are where the duodenum becomes the jejunum, and where the ileum joins the cecum.

Peritoneal gutters

The mesentery of the small intestine, ascending colon, and descending colon is attached to the posterior abdominal wall. As a result, four gutters exist that can conduct fluid materials (e.g., ascites, abscess, blood, or bile) from one point of the peritoneal cavity to another. The right lateral paracolic gutter is to the right of the ascending colon; it may conduct fluid from the omental bursa via the hepatorenal pouch into the pelvis. The left lateral para-

colic gutter is to the left of the descending colon. There are two gutters to the right and left of the mesentery that open into the pelvic cavity.

THE PELVIS IN GENERAL

The pelvis is divided into two sections: the major and minor. The major or false pelvis is that portion of the pelvis found above the brim of the pelvis; its cavity is that portion of the abdominal cavity cradled by the iliac fossae. The minor or true pelvis is found below the brim of the pelvis. The cavity of the pelvis minor is continuous at the pelvic brim with the cavity of the pelvis major.

The peritoneal cavity invests several pelvic organs; the rectum, bladder, and uterus (Fig. 8-11 and 8-12). In the female the peritoneum descends from the anterior abdominal wall to the level of the pubic bone onto the superior surface of the bladder. It passes from the bladder to the uterus to form the vesicouterine pouch. It covers the fundus and body of the uterus and extends over the posterior fornix and the wall of the vagina. Between the uterus and the rectum the peritoneum forms the deep rectouterine pouch.

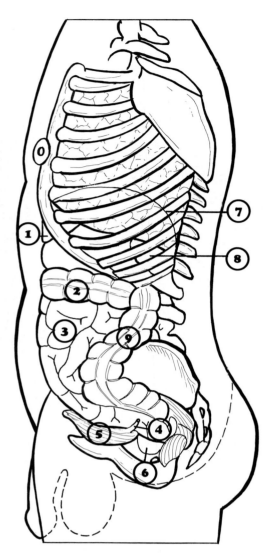

FIG. 8-11. Sagittal view of the abdomen and pelvis in the male. Liver, *1;* transverse colon, *2;* intestine, *3;* ureter, *4;* bladder, *5;* prostate, *6;* diaphragm, *7;* spleen, *8;* descending colon, *9.* (From Hagen-Ansert SL: The anatomy workbook, Philadelphia, 1986, JB Lippincott Co.)

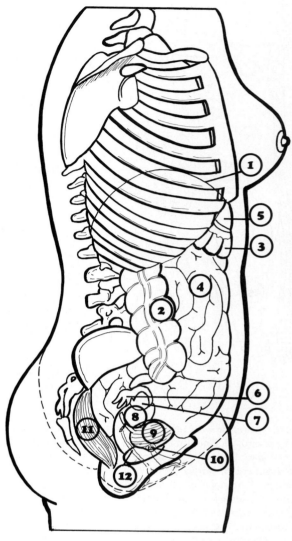

FIG. 8-12. Sagittal view of the abdomen and pelvis in the female. Diaphragm, *1;* ascending colon, *2;* transverse colon, *3;* intestine, *4;* stomach, *5;* fallopian tube, *6;* ovary, *7;* uterus, *8;* bladder, *9;* urethra, *10;* rectum, *11;* vagina, *12.* (From Hagen-Ansert SL: The anatomy workbook, Philadelphia, 1986, JB Lippincott Co.)

INTRODUCTION TO CROSS-SECTIONAL AND SAGITTAL ANATOMY

The sonographer must have a solid knowledge of gross anatomy, sectional anatomy, sagittal anatomy, and the various obliquities of anatomic sections. Although "normal" anatomy is often shown in numerous line drawings and anatomic sections, the sonographer must keep in mind the normal variations that can occur in the anatomic structure. Thus organ and vascular relationships to neighboring structures should be carefully evaluated rather than a memorization made of where in the abdomen a particular structure ought to be. For example, it is better to recall the location of the gallbladder as anterior to the right kidney and medial to the liver than to remember that it is usually found 6 to 8 cm above the umbilicus.

Fig. 8-13 to 8-41 represent a combination of cross-sectional and sagittal anatomic sections of the abdominal and pelvic cavity. These are presented in order from the diaphragm to the symphysis pubis to help the sonographer understand the relationships between vascular structures and organs as one proceeds by small increments through the abdominal and pelvic cavity.

In Fig. 8-13, this transverse section is made at the level of the tenth intervertebral disc. The lower portion of the pericardial sac is seen. The splenic artery enters the spleen, and the splenic vein emerges from the splenic hilum. The abdominal portion of the esophagus lies to the left of the midline and opens into the stomach through the cardiac orifice. The liver extends to the left mammillary line. The falciform ligament extends into the section above this. The upper border of the tail of the pancreas is seen. The spleen is shown to lie alongside the ninth rib.

Fig. 8-14 shows a transverse section at the level of the eleventh thoracic disc and the superior border of the

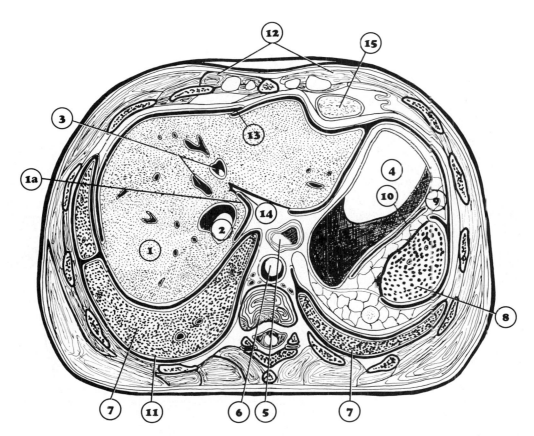

FIG. 8-13. Cross-section of the abdomen at the level of the tenth intervertebral disc. Right lobe of the liver, *1;* caudate lobe, *1a;* inferior vena cava, *2;* hepatic veins, *3;* stomach, *4;* esophagus, *5;* abdominal aorta, *6;* pleural cavity, *7;* spleen, *8;* gastrosplenic ligament, *9;* omental bursa, *10;* pleural sac, *11;* rectus abdominis muscle, *12;* falciform ligament, *13;* ligamentum venosum, *14;* pericardial sac, *15.* (From Hagen-Ansert SL: The anatomy workbook, Philadelphia, 1986, JB Lippincott Co.)

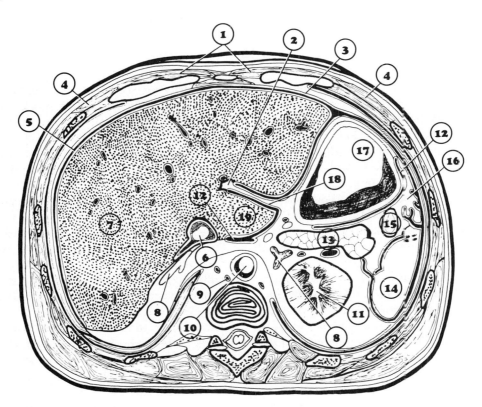

FIG. 8-14. Cross-section of the abdomen at the level of the eleventh thoracic disc. Rectus abdominis muscle, *1;* ligamentum venosum, *2;* diaphragm, *3;* external oblique muscle, *4;* peritoneal cavity, *5;* inferior vena cava, *6;* right lobe of the liver, *7;* suprarenal glands, *8;* azygos vein, *9;* aorta, *10;* kidney, *11;* omental bursa, *12;* pancreas, *13;* spleen, *14;* colic flexure, *15;* gastric ligament, *16;* stomach, *17;* hepatogastric ligament, *18;* caudate lobe, *19.* (From Hagen-Ansert SL: The anatomy workbook, Philadelphia, 1986, JB Lippincott Co.)

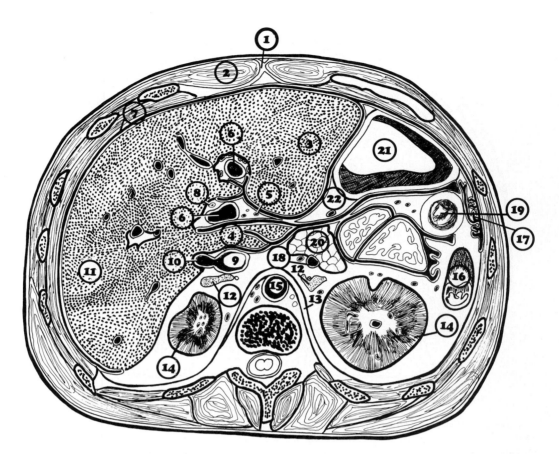

FIG. 8-15. Cross-section of the abdomen at the level of the twelfth thoracic vertebra. Linea alba, *1;* rectus abdominis muscle, *2;* left lobe of the liver, *3;* caudate lobe, *4;* hepatic artery, *5;* portal vein, *6;* diaphragm, *7;* hepatic duct, *8;* inferior vena cava, *9;* hepatic vein, *10;* right lobe of the liver, *11;* suprarenal gland, *12;* crus of the diaphragm, *13;* kidney, *14;* aorta, *15;* descending colon, *16;* peritoneal cavity, *17;* splenic vein, *18;* transverse colon, *19;* pancreas, *20;* stomach, *21;* omental bursa, *22.* (From Hagen-Ansert SL: The anatomy workbook, Philadelphia, 1986, JB Lippincott Co.)

twelfth vertebra. The hepatic vein is shown to enter the inferior vena cava. The renal artery and vein of the left kidney are shown. The left branch of the portal vein is seen to arch upward to enter the left lobe of the liver. The upper part of the stomach is shown with the hepatogastric and gastrocolic ligaments. The lesser omental cavity is posterior to the stomach. The upper border of the splenic flexure of the colon is seen. The caudate lobe of the liver is in this section. The tail and body of the pancreas are shown anterior to the left kidney. The spleen is shown to lie along the left lateral border. The adrenal glands are lateral to the crus of the diaphragm.

Fig. 8-15 is taken at the level of the twelfth thoracic vertebra. The celiac axis arises in the middle of this section from the anterior abdominal aorta. The right renal artery originates at this level. The hepatic vein is shown to enter the inferior vena cava. The greater curvature of the stomach and the pylorus are shown. The transverse and descending colon are shown inferior to the splenic flexure. The caudate lobe of the liver is well seen. The body of the pancreas, both kidneys, and the lower portions of the adrenal glands are shown.

Fig. 8-16 is taken at the level of the first lumbar vertebra. The psoas major muscle is seen. The crura of the diaphragm are shown on either side of the spine. The right

renal artery is seen. The left renal artery arises from the lateral wall of the aorta. Both renal veins enter the inferior vena cava. The portal vein is seen to be formed by the union of the splenic vein and the superior mesenteric vein. The lower portion of the stomach and the pyloric orifice are seen, as is the superior portion of the duodenum. The duodenojejunal flexure and descending and transverse colon are shown. The greater omentum is very prominent. The small, nonperitoneal area of the liver is shown anterior to the right kidney. The round ligament of the liver and the umbilical fissure, which separates the right and left lobes of the liver, are seen. The neck of the gallbladder (not shown) is found just inferior to this section, between the quadrate and caudate lobes of the liver. The cystic duct is cut in two places. The hepatic duct lies just anterior to the cystic duct. The cystic and hepatic ducts unite in the lower part of the section to form the common bile duct. The pancreatic duct is found within the pancreas at this level. Both kidneys are seen just lateral to the psoas muscles.

Fig. 8-17 is taken at the level of the second lumbar vertebra. The superior pancreaticoduodenal artery originates in Fig. 8-16 and shows some of its branches in this section. The lower portion of the stomach is found in this section, and the hepatic flexure of the colon is seen.

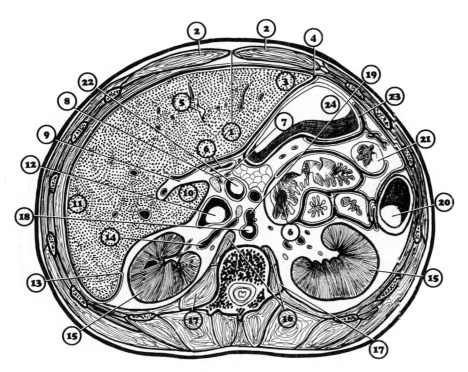

FIG. 8-16.   Cross-section of the abdomen at the first lumbar vertebra. Linea alba, *1;* rectus abdominis muscle, *2;* left lobe of the liver, *3;* peritoneal cavity, *4;* ligamentum teres, *5;* duodenum, *6;* gastroduodenal artery, *7;* hepatic duct, *8;* epiploic foramen, *9;* caudate lobe, *10;* right lobe of the liver, *11;* inferior vena cava, *12;* hepatorenal ligament, *13;* renal artery, *14;* kidney, *15;* crus of the diaphragm, *16;* psoas major muscle, *17;* aorta, *18;* superior mesenteric artery, *19;* descending colon, *20;* transverse colon, *21;* splenic vein, *22;* omental bursa, *23;* stomach, *24.* (From Hagen-Ansert SL: The anatomy workbook, Philadelphia, 1986, JB Lippincott Co.)

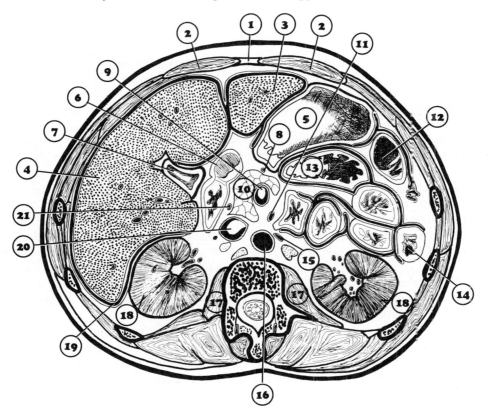

FIG. 8-17.   Cross-section of the abdomen at the level of the second lumbar vertebra. Linea alba, *1;* rectus abdominis muscle, *2;* left lobe of the liver, *3;* right lobe of the liver, *4;* stomach, *5;* duodenum, *6;* gallbladder, *7;* gastroduodenal artery, *8;* superior mesenteric vein, *9;* pancreas, *10;* superior mesenteric artery, *11;* transverse colon, *12;* jejunum, *13;* descending colon, *14;* left renal vein, *15;* aorta, *16;* psoas major muscle, *17;* kidney, *18;* peritoneal cavity, *19;* inferior vena cava, *20;* common bile duct, *21.* (From Hagen-Ansert SL: The anatomy workbook, Philadelphia, 1986, JB Lippincott Co.)

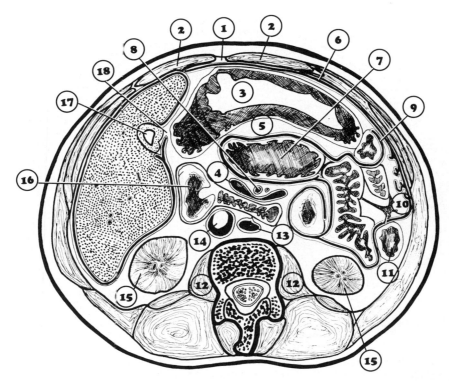

FIG. 8-18. Cross-section of the abdomen at the level of the third lumbar vertebra. Linea alba, *1;* rectus abdominis muscle, *2;* transverse colon, *3;* superior mesenteric vein, *4;* transverse mesocolon, *5;* parietal peritoneum, *6;* jejunum, *7;* superior mesenteric artery, *8;* peritoneal cavity, *9;* greater omentum, *10;* descending colon, *11;* psoas major muscle, *12;* aorta, *13;* inferior vena cava, *14;* kidney, *15;* duodenum, *16;* gallbladder, *17;* hepatocolic ligament, *18.* (From Hagen-Ansert SL: The anatomy workbook, Philadelphia, 1986, JB Lippincott Co.)

The lobes of the liver are separated by the round ligament. The left lobe of the liver ends at this level. The head and neck of the pancreas drape around the superior mesenteric vein. Both kidneys and the psoas muscles are shown.

Fig. 8-18 is taken at the level of the third lumbar vertebra. The inferior mesenteric artery originates from the abdominal aorta at this level. The greater omentum is shown mostly on the left side of the abdomen. The descending and ascending portions of the duodenum lie between the aorta and the superior mesenteric artery and vein. The fundus of the gallbladder lies in the lower portion of this section. The lower poles of both kidneys lie lateral to the psoas muscles.

Fig. 8-19 is taken through the third lumbar disc. The lower portion of the duodenum is shown. The lower margin of the right lobe of the liver is seen along the right lateral border.

Fig. 8-20 is taken at the level of the fifth lumbar vertebra. It cuts the ilium through the upper part of the iliac fossa and passes just above the wings of the sacrum. The gluteus medius and iliacus muscles are shown. The right common iliac artery bifurcates into the external and internal iliac arteries. The common iliac veins are shown to unite to form the inferior vena cava. The lower part of the greater omentum is shown in this section.

Fig. 8-21 is taken at the lower margin of the fifth lumbar vertebra and disc. The gluteus minimus muscle is shown on this section as are the right external and internal iliac arteries. The left common iliac artery branches into the external and internal arteries. The ileum is seen throughout this level, and the mesentery terminates at this level.

Fig. 8-22 is taken at the level of the sacrum and the anterior superior spine of the ilium. The gluteus maximus muscle appears on both sides. The internal and external iliac veins have united to form the common iliac vein. The ileum is seen throughout this section.

Fig. 8-23 passes through the third sacral vertebra near the upper margin of the third anterior sacral foramina. The pyramidalis, obturatorius internus, and piriformis muscles are shown. The cecum is also seen in this section. The lower portion of the descending colon passes over the sigmoid colon, and the sigmoid colon passes over into the rectum.

Fig. 8-24 passes through the sacrum above the margins of the fifth anterior pair of sacral foramina, through the acetabulum and the head of the femur. The external iliac arteries become the femoral arteries in this section. The femoral veins become the external iliac veins. The cecum and rectum are seen. The upper surface of the bladder, the ureters, the seminal vesicles, and the spermatic cord are well visualized.

Fig. 8-25 passes through the coccyx, the spine of the ischium, the acetabulum, the head of the femur, the greater trochanter, the pubic symphysis, and the upper

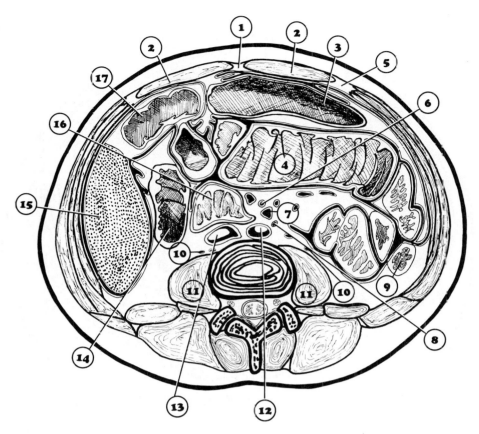

FIG. 8-19. Cross-section of the abdomen at the level of the third lumbar disc. Linea alba, *1;* rectus abdominis muscle, *2;* transverse colon, *3;* jejunum, *4;* linea semilunaris, *5;* superior mesenteric artery, *6;* superior mesenteric vein, *7;* inferior mesenteric artery, *8;* descending colon, *9;* ureter, *10;* psoas major muscle, *11;* aorta, *12;* inferior vena cava, *13;* ascending colon, *14;* right lobe of the liver, *15;* duodenum, *16;* ileum, *17.* (From Hagen-Ansert SL: The anatomy workbook, Philadelphia, 1986, JB Lippincott Co.)

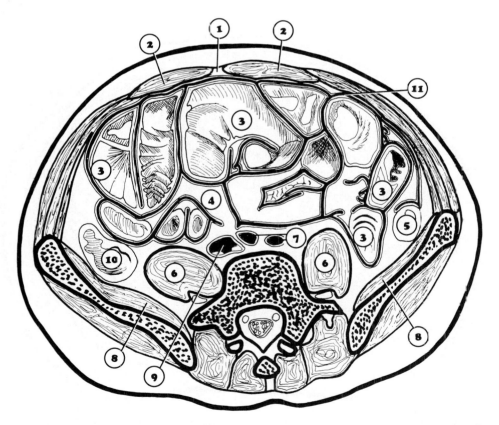

FIG. 8-20. Cross-section of the abdomen at the level of the fifth lumbar vertebra. Linea alba, *1;* rectus abdominis muscle, *2;* ileum, *3;* mesentery, *4;* descending colon, *5;* psoas major muscle, *6;* iliac artery, *7;* iliacus muscle, *8;* inferior vena cava, *9;* ascending colon, *10;* peritoneal cavity, *11.* (From Hagen-Ansert SL: The anatomy workbook, Philadelphia, 1986, JB Lippincott Co.)

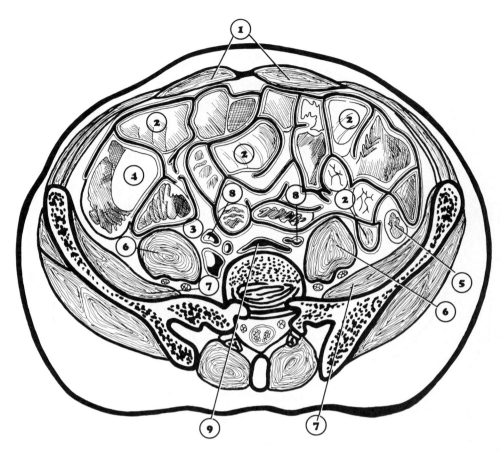

FIG. 8-21. Cross-section of the pelvis taken at the lower margin of the fifth lumbar vertebra and disc. Rectus abdominis muscle, *1;* ileum, *2;* mesentery, *3;* ascending colon, *4;* descending colon, *5;* psoas major muscle, *6;* iliacus muscle, *7;* external iliac artery, *8;* iliac vein, *9.* (From Hagen-Ansert SL: The anatomy workbook, Philadelphia, 1986, JB Lippincott Co.)

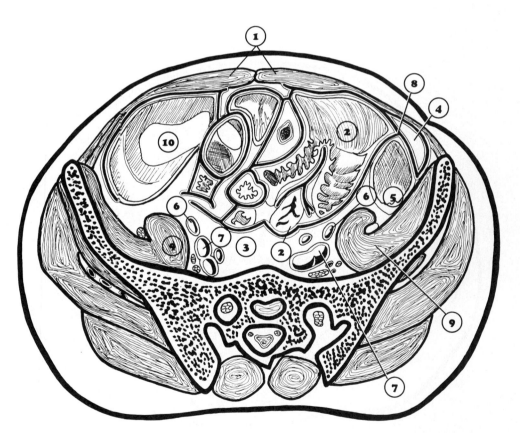

FIG. 8-22. Cross-section of the pelvis taken at the level of the sacrum and the anterior superior spine of the ilium. Rectus abdominis muscle, *1;* ileum, *2;* mesentery, *3;* greater omentum, *4;* descending colon, *5;* external iliac artery, *6;* external iliac vein, *7;* peritoneal cavity, *8;* iliopsoas muscle, *9;* ascending colon, *10.* (From Hagen-Ansert SL: The anatomy workbook, Philadelphia, 1986, JB Lippincott Co.)

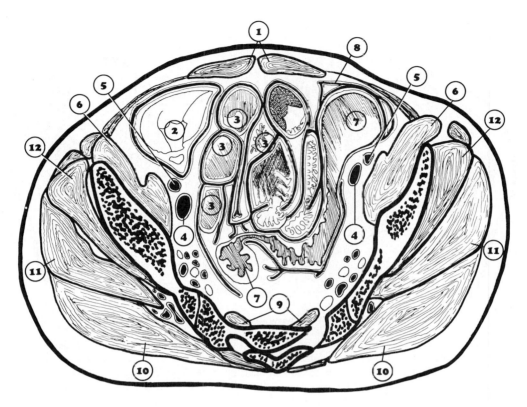

FIG. 8-23. Cross-section of the pelvis taken through the third sacral vertebra near the upper margin of the third anterior sacral foramina. Rectus abdominis muscle, *1;* cecum, *2;* ileum, *3;* external iliac vein, *4;* external iliac artery, *5;* iliopsoas muscle, *6;* sigmoid colon, *7;* peritoneal cavity, *8;* piriformis muscle, *9;* gluteus maximus muscle, *10;* gluteus medius muscle, *11;* gluteus minimus muscle, *12.* (From Hagen-Ansert SL: The anatomy workbook, Philadelphia, 1986, JB Lippincott Co.)

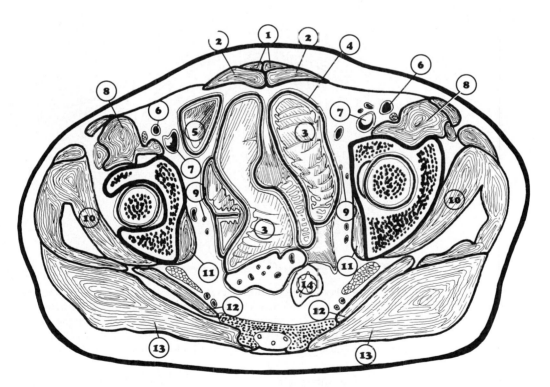

FIG. 8-24. Cross-section of the pelvis taken above the margins of the fifth anterior pair of sacral foramina and head of the femur. Pyramidalis muscle, *1;* rectus abdominis muscle, *2;* ileum, *3;* peritoneal cavity, *4;* cecum, *5;* external iliac artery, *6;* external iliac vein, *7;* iliopsoas muscle, *8;* ductus deferens, *9;* gluteus minimus muscle, *10;* obturator internus muscle, *11;* piriformis muscle, *12;* gluteus maximus muscle, *13;* rectum, *14.* (From Hagen-Ansert SL: The anatomy workbook, Philadelphia, 1986, JB Lippincott Co.)

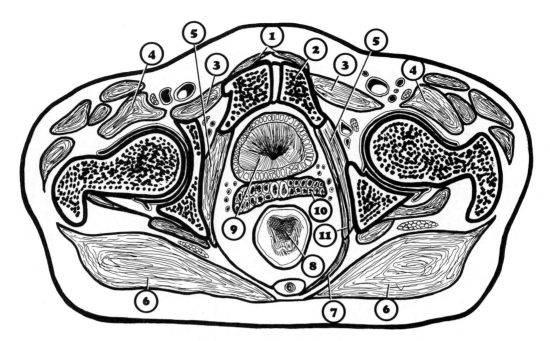

FIG. 8-25. Cross-section of the pelvis at the level of the coccyx, the spine of the ischium, the femur, and greater trochanter. Pyramidalis muscle, *1;* pubic os, *2;* pectineus muscle, *3;* iliopsoas muscle, *4;* obturator internus muscle, *5;* gluteus maximus muscle, *6;* coccygeus muscle, *7;* rectum, *8;* bladder, *9;* seminal vesicles, *10;* levator ani muscle, *11.* (From Hagen-Ansert SL: The anatomy workbook, Philadelphia, 1986, JB Lippincott Co.)

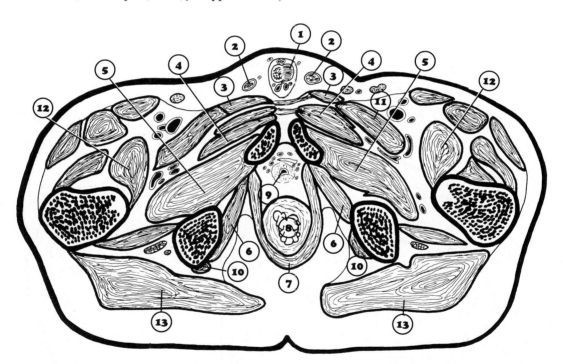

FIG. 8-26. Cross-section of the pelvis at the tip of the coccyx, the inferior ramus of the pubis, and the neck of the femur. Penile fascia, *1;* ductus deferens, *2;* adductor longus muscle, *3;* adductor brevis muscle, *4;* obturator externus muscle, *5;* obturator internus muscle, *6;* levator ani muscle, *7;* anus, *8;* rectum, *9;* ischiocavernous muscle, *10;* pectineus muscle, *11;* iliopsoas muscle, *12;* gluteus maximus muscle, *13.* (From Hagen-Ansert SL: The anatomy workbook, Philadelphia, 1986, JB Lippincott Co.)

margins of the obturator foramen. The gemellus inferior and superior, coccygeus, and levator ani muscles are shown. The rectum is seen in the midline. The trigone of the bladder and the urethral orifice are well shown, and the seminal vesicles and the ampulla of the vasa deferentia can be identified. The ejaculatory ducts enter the urethra in the lower portion of this section.

Fig. 8-26 passes below the tip of the coccyx, the upper portion of the tuberosity of the ischium and the inferior ramus of the pubis, the neck of the femur, and the lower portion of the greater trochanter. The rectum, prostate gland, penis, and corpus cavernosum are seen.

Fig. 8-27 passes through the femur, the scrotum, the upper portion of the left testicle, and the epididymis. The

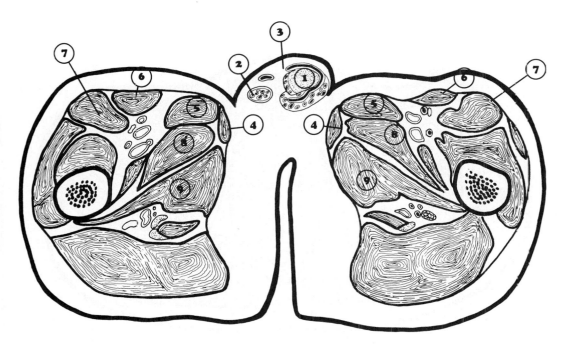

FIG. 8-27. Cross-section of the pelvis at the femur, scrotum, testicle, and epididymis. Testis, *1;* plexus pampiniformis, *2;* scrotum, *3;* gracilis muscle, *4;* adductor longus muscle. *5;* sartorius muscle, *6;* rectus femoris muscle, *7;* adductor brevis muscle, *8;* adductor minimus muscle, *9.* (From Hagen-Ansert SL: The anatomy workbook, Philadelphia, 1986, JB Lippincott Co.)

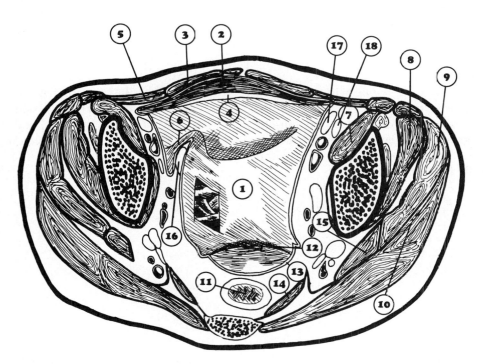

FIG. 8-28. Cross-section of the female pelvis just below the junction of the sacrum and coccyx. Uterus, *1;* pyramidalis muscle, *2;* rectus abdominis muscle, *3;* peritoneal cavity, *4;* obturator internus muscle, *5;* fallopian tube, *6;* iliopsoas muscle, *7;* gluteus minimus muscle, *8;* gluteus medius muscle, *9;* gluteus maximus muscle, *10;* rectum, *11;* pouch of Douglas, *12;* peritoneum, *13;* coccygeus muscle, *14;* piriformis muscle, *15;* ovary, *16;* external iliac vein, *17;* external iliac artery, *18.* (From Hagen-Ansert SL: The anatomy workbook, Philadelphia, 1986, JB Lippincott Co.)

lining, membrane, and tunica vaginalis of the scrotal cavity are seen, as are the vas deferens and the vascula plexus.

Fig. 8-28 is a section through the female pelvis just below the junction of the sacrum and coccyx, through the anterior inferior spine of the ilium and the great sciatic notch. The uterine artery and vein and the ureter are shown dissected beyond the uterine wall. The bladder is shown just anterior to the uterus, and the round ligament is shown. The ovaries are cut through their midsections on this level.

Fig. 8-29 is taken through the lower part of the coccyx and the spine of the ischium, the middle of the acetabulum, and the head of the femur. The superior gemellus

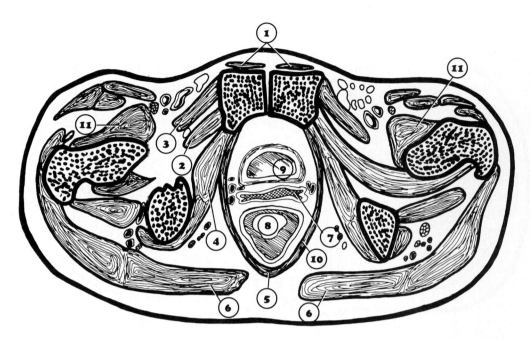

FIG. 8-29.   Cross-section of the female pelvis taken through the lower part of the coccyx and the spine of the ischium. Pyramidalis muscle, *1;* obturator externus muscle, *2;* pectineus muscle, *3;* obturator internus muscle, *4;* fascia of the pelvic diaphragm, *5;* gluteus maximus muscle, *6;* vagina, *7;* rectum, *8;* bladder, *9;* levator ani muscle, *10;* iliopsoas muscle, *11.* (From Hagen-Ansert SL: The anatomy workbook, Philadelphia, 1986, JB Lippincott Co.)

muscles and the pectineus muscle appear in this section, and the coccygeus muscle terminates here. The gluteus maximus, gluteus minimus, and gluteus medius muscles all begin their insertions in the lower part of this section. The external os of the cervix is shown. The ureters empty into the bladder at the base.

Fig. 8-30 to 8-41 are sagittal sections of the abdominal and pelvic viscera taken at 10 mm slices throughout the body. The muscular, vascular, and visceral relationships are essential to the sonographer's understanding of anatomy.

Text continued on p. 137.

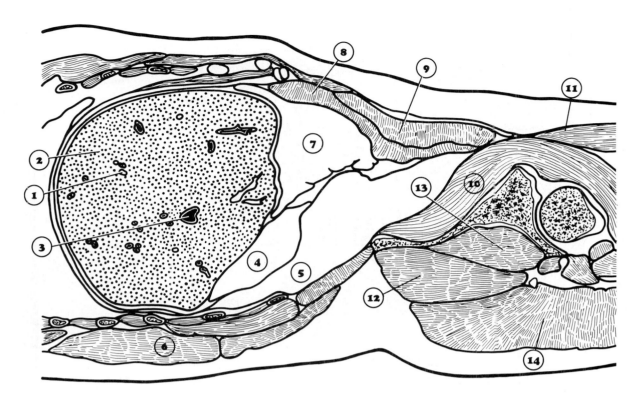

FIG. 8-30. Sagittal section of the abdomen taken along the right abdominal border. Portal vein, *1;* right lobe of the liver, *2;* hepatic vein, *3;* perirenal fat, *4;* retroperitoneal fat, *5;* latissimus dorsi muscle, *6;* omentum, *7;* internal oblique muscle, *8;* external oblique muscle, *9;* iliacus muscle, *10;* psoas major muscle, *11;* gluteus medius muscle, *12;* gluteus minimus muscle, *13;* gluteus maximus muscle, *14.* (From Hagen-Ansert SL: The anatomy workbook, Philadelphia, 1986, JB Lippincott Co.)

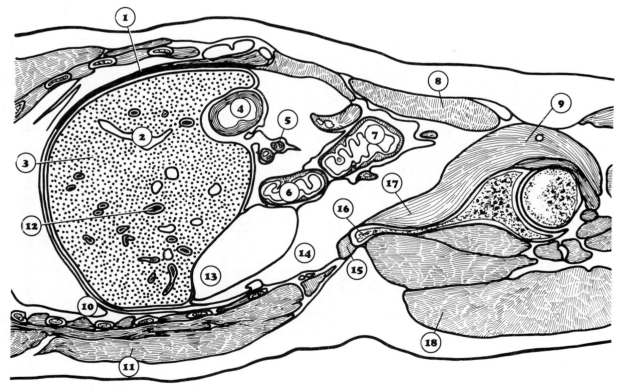

FIG. 8-31. Sagittal section of the abdomen 8 cm from the midline. Diaphragm, *1;* portal vein, *2;* liver, *3;* gallbladder, *4;* hepatic flexure, *5;* ascending colon, *6;* cecum, *7;* internal oblique muscle, *8;* psoas major muscle, *9;* costodiaphragmatic recess, *10;* latissimus dorsi muscle, *11;* hepatic vein, *12;* perirenal fat, *13;* retroperitoneal fat, *14;* quadratus lumborum muscle, *15;* ilium, *16;* iliacus muscle, *17;* gluteus maximus muscle, *18.* (From Hagen-Ansert SL: The anatomy workbook, Philadelphia, 1986, JB Lippincott Co.)

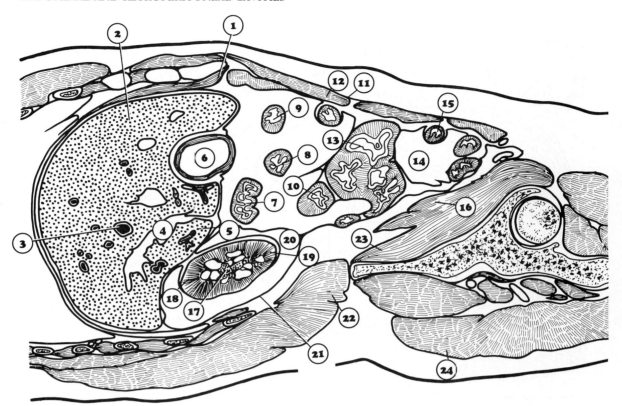

FIG. 8-32. Sagittal section of the abdomen 7 cm from the midline. Diaphragm, *1;* liver, *2;* hepatic vein, *3;* portal vein, *4;* caudate lobe of the liver, *5;* gallbladder, *6;* hepatic flexure, *7;* transverse colon, *8;* small bowel, *9;* ascending colon, *10;* rectus sheath, *11;* rectus abdominis muscle, *12;* cecum, *13;* mesentery, *14;* small bowel, *15;* psoas major muscle, *16;* renal medulla, *17;* right kidney, *18;* renal cortex, *19;* perirenal fat, *20;* perirenal fascia, *21;* quadratus lumborum muscle, *22;* iliacus muscle, *23;* gluteus maximus muscle, *24.* (From Hagen-Ansert SL: The anatomy workbook, Philadelphia, 1986, JB Lippincott Co.)

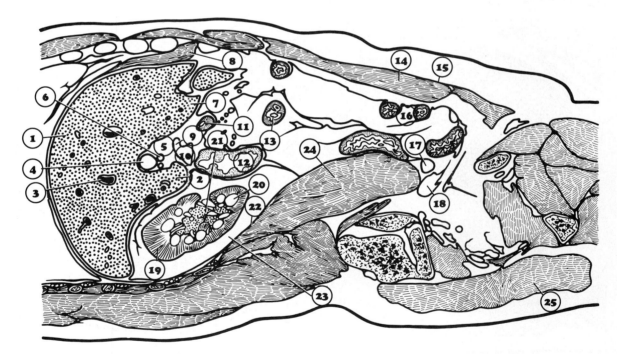

FIG. 8-33. Sagittal section of the abdomen 6 cm from the midline. Liver, *1;* caudate lobe, *2;* hepatic vein, *3;* portal vein, *4;* porta hepatis, *5;* hepatic artery, *6;* quadrate lobe of the liver, *7;* diaphragm, *8;* neck of the gallbladder, *9;* Hartmann's pouch, *10;* superior part of the duodenum, *11;* descending part of the duodenum, *12;* transverse colon, *13;* rectus abdominis muscle, *14;* anterior rectus sheath, *15;* mesentery, *16;* right external iliac artery, *17;* right external iliac vein, *18;* kidney, *19;* renal pyramid, *20;* renal sinus, *21;* perirenal fascia, *22;* perirenal fat, *23;* psoas major muscle, *24;* gluteus maximus muscle, *25.* (From Hagen-Ansert SL: The anatomy workbook, Philadelphia, 1986, JB Lippincott Co.)

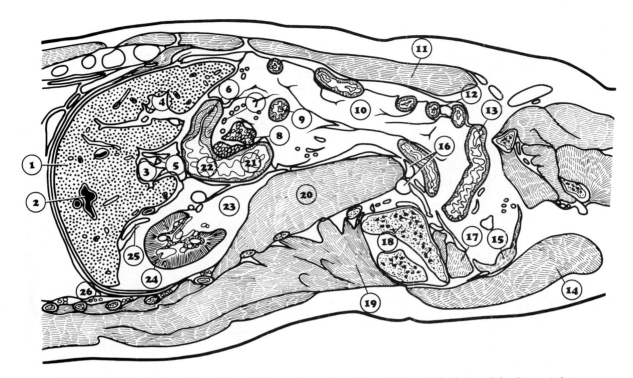

FIG. 8-34. Sagittal section of the abdomen 5 cm from the midline. Right lobe of the liver, *1;* hepatic vein, *2;* portal vein, *3;* left branch of the portal vein, *4;* cystic duct, *5;* pyloric sphincter, *6;* gastroduodenal artery, *7;* head of the pancreas, *8;* transverse colon, *9;* mesentery, *10;* rectus abdominis muscle, *11;* small bowel, *12;* ileum, *13;* gluteus maximus muscle, *14;* levator ani muscle, *15;* right external iliac artery, *16;* piriformis muscle, *17;* sacrum, *18;* erector spinae muscle, *19;* psoas major muscle, *20;* descending duodenum, *21;* superior duodenum, *22;* perirenal fat, *23;* right kidney, *24;* right suprarenal gland, *25;* costodiaphragmatic recess, *26.* (From Hagen-Ansert SL: The anatomy workbook, Philadelphia, 1986, JB Lippincott Co.)

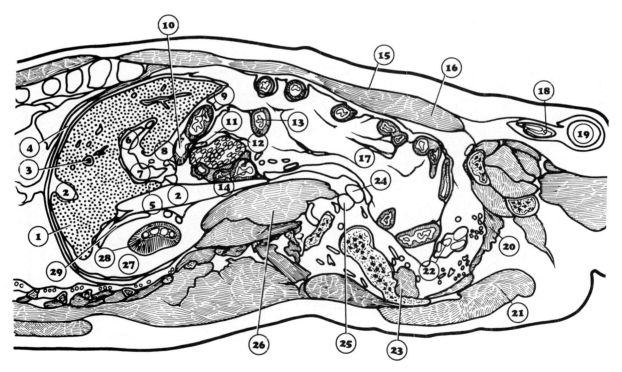

FIG. 8-35. Sagittal section of the abdomen 4 cm from the midline. Right lobe of the liver, *1;* inferior vena cava, *2;* hepatic vein, *3;* diaphragm, *4;* caudate lobe, *5;* left portal vein, *6;* hepatic artery, *7;* cystic duct, *8;* pylorus, *9;* descending part of the duodenum, *10;* gastroduodenal artery, *11;* head of pancreas, *12;* transverse colon, *13;* superior part of the duodenum, *14;* anterior rectus sheath, *15;* rectus abdominis muscle, *16;* mesenteric fat, *17;* spermatic cord, *18;* testis, *19;* levator ani muscle, *20;* gluteus maximus muscle, *21;* seminal vesicles, *22;* piriformis muscle, *23;* right common iliac artery, *24;* right common iliac vein, *25;* psoas major muscle, *26;* perirenal fat, *27;* right kidney, *28;* right suprarenal gland, *29.* (From Hagen-Ansert SL: The anatomy workbook, Philadelphia, 1986, JB Lippincott Co.)

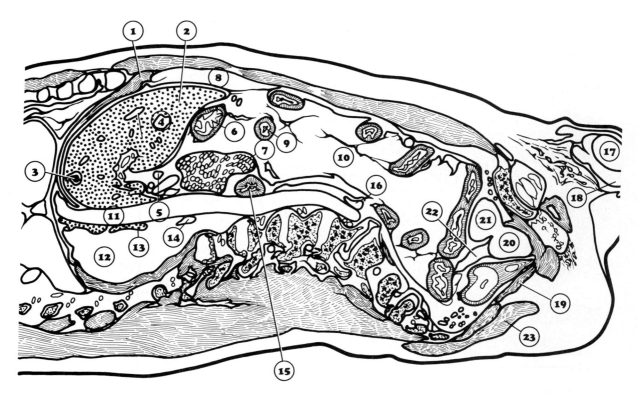

FIG. 8-36. Sagittal section of the abdomen 3 cm from the midline. Diaphragm, *1;* left lobe of the liver, *2;* hepatic vein, *3;* portal vein, *4;* hepatic artery, *5;* pyloric antrum, *6;* head of pancreas, *7;* falciform ligament, *8;* transverse colon, *9;* mesenteric fat, *10;* inferior vena cava, *11;* perirenal fat, *12;* right suprarenal gland, *13;* right renal artery, *14;* horizontal part of the duodenum, *15;* right common iliac artery, *16;* testis, *17;* scrotum, *18;* levator ani muscle, *19;* prostate, *20;* bladder, *21;* seminal vesicles, *22;* gluteus maximus muscle, *23.* (From Hagen-Ansert SL: The anatomy workbook, Philadelphia, 1986, JB Lippincott Co.)

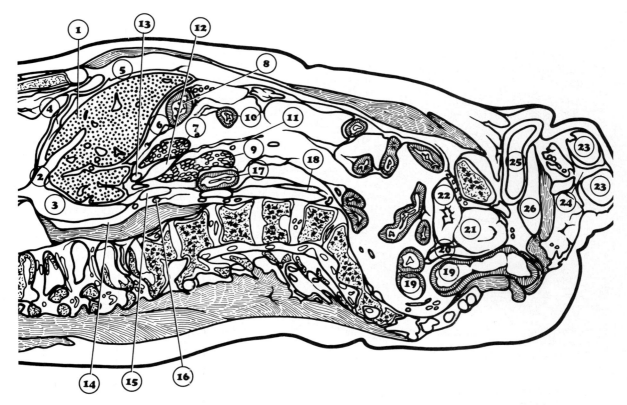

FIG. 8-37. Sagittal section of the abdomen 2 cm from the midline. Left lobe of the liver, *1;* hepatic vein, *2;* inferior vena cava, *3;* diaphragm, *4;* falciform ligament, *5;* lesser omentum, *6;* pancreas, *7;* pyloric antrum, *8;* uncinate process of pancreas, *9;* transverse colon, *10;* superior mesenteric vein, *11;* portal vein, *12;* hepatic artery, *13;* crus of diaphragm, *14;* left renal vein, *15;* right renal artery, *16;* horizontal part of the duodenum, *17;* right common iliac artery, *18;* rectum, *19;* seminal vesicles, *20;* prostate, *21;* bladder, *22;* testis, *23;* scrotum, *24;* corpus cavernosum penis, *25;* corpus spongiosum penis, *26.* (From Hagen-Ansert SL: The anatomy workbook, Philadelphia, 1986, JB Lippincott Co.)

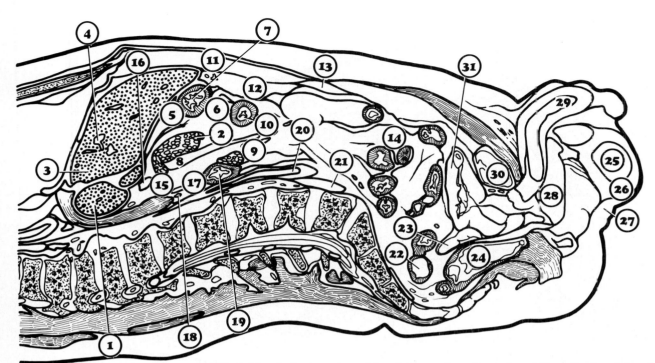

FIG. 8-38. Sagittal section of the abdomen 1 cm from the midline. Caudate lobe, *1;* body of pancreas, *2;* left lobe of liver, *3;* portal vein, *4;* lesser omentum, *5;* lesser sac, *6;* pyloric antrum, *7;* superior mesenteric vein, *8;* uncinate process of pancreas, *9;* transverse colon, *10;* falciform ligament, *11;* greater omentum, *12;* linea alba, *13;* mesenteric fat, *14;* crus of diaphragm, *15;* hepatic artery, *16;* left renal vein, *17;* right renal artery, *18;* horizontal part of the duodenum, *19;* aorta, *20;* left common iliac vein, *21;* rectum, *22;* seminal vesicles, *23;* rectum *24;* testis, *25;* epididymis, *26;* scrotum, *27;* corpus spongiosum penis, *28;* corpus cavernosum penis, *29;* symphysis pubis, *30;* bladder, *31.* (From Hagen-Ansert SL: The anatomy workbook, Philadelphia, 1986, JB Lippincott Co.)

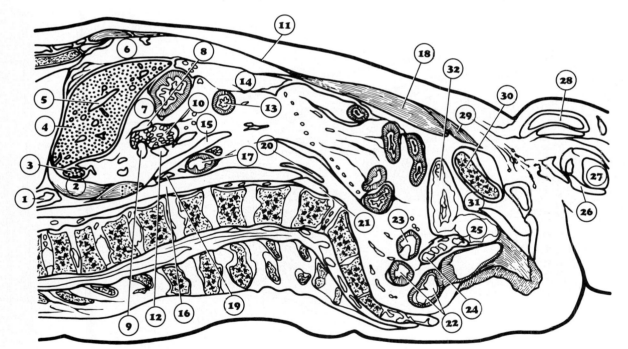

FIG. 8-39. Midline sagittal section of the abdomen. Esophagus, *1;* crus of the diaphragm, *2;* caudate lobe, *3;* left lobe of the liver, *4;* portal vein, *5;* falciform ligament, *6;* lesser omentum, *7;* lesser sac, *8;* splenic artery, *9;* pancreas, *10;* linea alba, *11;* splenic vein, *12;* transverse colon, *13;* greater omentum, *14;* superior mesenteric artery, *15;* aorta, *16;* horizontal part of duodenum, *17;* rectus abdominis muscle, *18;* left renal vein, *19;* inferior mesenteric artery, *20;* left common iliac vein, *21;* rectum, *22;* sigmoid colon, *23;* seminal vesicles, *24;* prostate, *25;* head of the epididymis, *26;* testis, *27;* corpus cavernosum penis, *28;* pyramidalis muscle, *29;* symphysis pubis, *30;* retropubic space, *31;* bladder, *32.* (From Hagen-Ansert SL: The anatomy workbook, Philadelphia, 1986, JB Lippincott Co.)

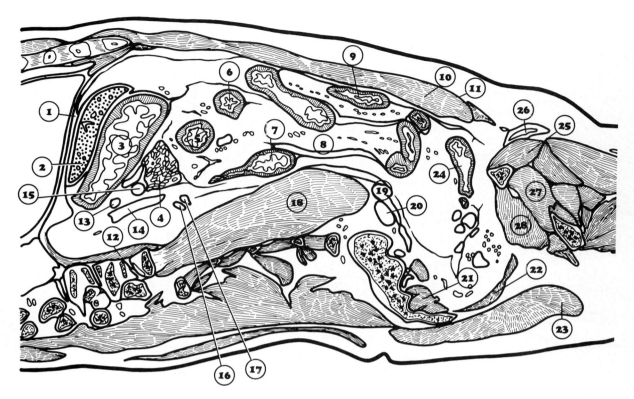

FIG. 8-40. Sagittal section of the abdomen 3 cm to the left of midline. Diaphragm, *1;* left lobe of the liver, *2;* body of the stomach, *3;* pancreas, *4;* ascending part of duodenum, *5;* transverse colon, *6;* jejunum, *7;* mesentery, *8;* small bowel, *9;* rectus abdominis muscle, *10;* rectus sheath, *11;* crus of the diaphragm, *12;* splenic artery, *13;* left suprarenal gland, *14;* splenic vein, *15;* left renal artery, *16;* left renal vein, *17;* psoas major muscle, *18;* left common iliac artery, *19;* left common iliac vein, *20;* piriformis muscle, *21;* levator ani muscle, *22;* gluteus maximus muscle, *23;* sigmoid colon, *24;* pectineus muscle, *25;* spermatic cord, *26;* obturator externus muscle, *27;* obturator internus muscle, *28.* (From Hagen-Ansert SL: The anatomy workbook, Philadelphia, 1986, JB Lippincott Co.)

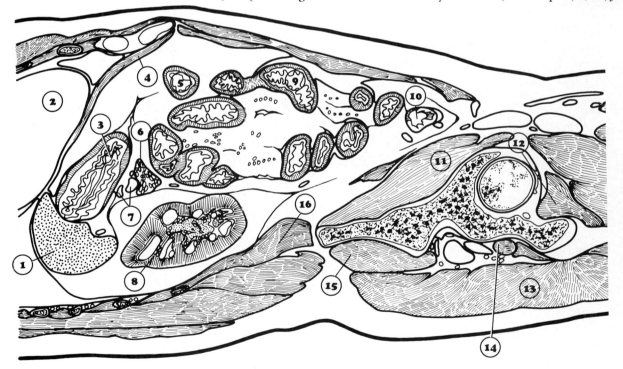

FIG. 8-41. Sagittal section of the abdomen along the left abdominal border. Spleen, *1;* heart, *2;* fundus of the stomach, *3;* diaphragm, *4;* transverse colon, *5;* pancreas, *6;* splenic artery and vein, *7;* left kidney, *8;* small bowel, *9;* sigmoid colon, *10;* iliacus muscle, *11;* obturator externus muscle, *12;* gluteus maximus muscle, *13;* obturator internus muscle, *14;* gluteus medius muscle, *15;* quadratus lumborum muscle, *16.* (From Hagen-Ansert SL: The anatomy workbook, Philadelphia, 1986, JB Lippincott Co.)

SUMMARY

1. The sonographer must have a thorough understanding of anatomy as it relates to the anterior-posterior relationships, superior-inferior relationships, oblique relationships, as well as understand the variations in normal anatomy.

2. The abdomen is divided into nine different regions. In addition, it consists of two horizontal planes and two vertical planes. It is also divided into four quadrants.

3. The anterior abdominal wall is composed of several layers of muscles, fibrous band, and fascia. The peritoneum is divided into two layers. The peritoneal cavity is the space between these two layers. The peritoneum lines the walls of the abdominal cavity. The mesentery and omentum are a double fold of peritoneum. The lesser sac is a completely enclosed recess of the peritoneal cavity that communicates with the rest of the peritoneal cavity behind the free edge of the lesser omentum at the upper border of the duodenum. There are ligaments, recesses, and gutters within the abdominal cavity.

4. The pelvis is divided into two parts, the true and the false pelvis.

9

Muscular System

SANDRA L. HAGEN-ANSERT

Muscles comprise most of the superficial bulk of the human body, and it is useful for the sonographer to have a general understanding of the various muscle groups encountered during the sonographic examination. A brief description of the muscle groups will be presented in this chapter.

An essential function of the human body is motion. This function is made possible by the development of the property of contractility in muscle tissue. Motion includes many movements, including body motion, breathing, heart contractility, gastrointestinal motility, as well as the rhythmic movement of the blood and lymph vessels.

TYPES OF MUSCLE

Three types of muscle can be identified by their function, structure, and location in the body: skeletal, smooth, and cardiac (Fig. 9-1).

Skeletal muscle

Skeletal muscle produces movements of the skeleton and is sometimes called voluntary muscle. This muscle is composed of striped muscle fibers and has two or more attachments.

There are four basic forms of dense connective tissue: tendons, ligaments, aponeuroses, and fasciae. The tendons attach muscle to bone; the ligaments connect the bones that form joints; aponeuroses are thin, tendinous sheets attached to flat muscles; and the fasciae are thin sheets of tissue that cover muscles and hold them in their place.

The individual fibers of a muscle are arranged either parallel or oblique to the long axis of the muscle. With contraction, the muscle shortens to one half or one third its resting length. Examples of such muscles are the rectus abdominis and the sternocleidomastoid.

Pennate muscles have fibers that run oblique to the line of pull, resembling a feather. A unipennate muscle is one in which the tendon lies along one side of the muscle and the muscle fibers pass oblique to it. A bipennate muscle has a tendon in the center, and the muscle fibers pass to it from two sides. The pectus femoris is a bipennate muscle. A multipennate muscle may have a series of bipennate muscles lying alongside one another, such as the deltoid, or it may have the tendon lying within its center and the fibers converging into it from all sides.

Smooth muscle

Smooth muscle is composed of long, spindle-shaped cells closely arranged in bundles or sheets. Its action is that of propelling material through vessels or the gastrointestinal tract and is known as peristalsis. In storage organs such as the bladder and uterus, the fibers are arranged irregularly and are interlaced with one another. In these organs, contraction is slower and more sustained to expel its contents.

Cardiac muscle

Cardiac muscle is only found in the myocardium of the heart and in the muscle layer of the base of the great blood vessels. These muscles consist of striated fibers that branch and unite with one another. The fibers tend to be arranged in spirals and have the ability to contract spontaneously and rhythmically. Specialized cardiac muscle fibers form the conducting system of the heart.

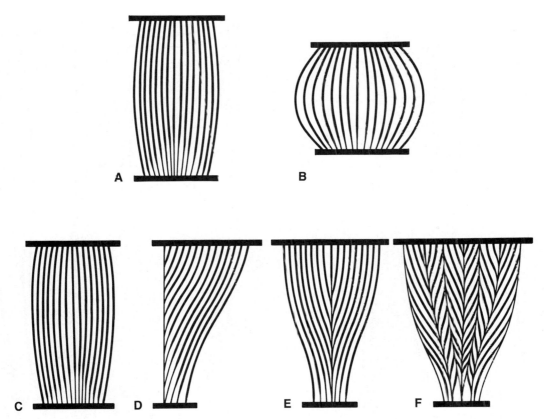

FIG. 9-1. Muscle groups. **A,** Resting muscle. **B,** Contracted muscle. **C to F,** Skeletal muscle. **C,** Parallel muscle. **D,** Unipennate muscle. **E,** Bipennate muscle. **F,** Multipennate muscle. (From Hagen-Ansert SL: The anatomy workbook, Philadelphia, 1986, JB Lippincott Co.)

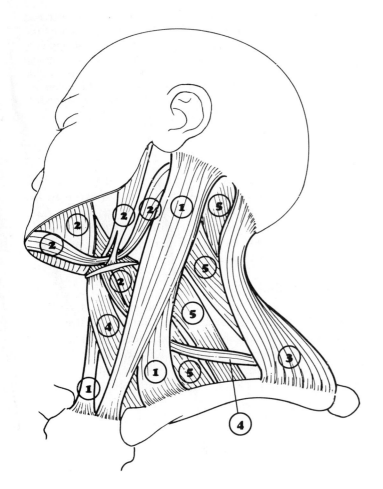

FIG. 9-2. Muscular system of the neck. *1,* Sternocleidomastoid muscles; *2,* suprahyoid muscles; *3,* trapezius muscles; *4,* infrahyoid muscles; *5,* posterior triangle of the neck. (From Hagen-Ansert SL: The anatomy workbook, Philadelphia, 1986, JB Lippincott Co.)

THE NECK

The larger muscle groups of the neck will be presented in this section as these will serve as landmarks for internal structures such as the thyroid and vascular structures found within the neck. The neck is divided into two triangles, anterior and posterior, by the sternocleidomastoid muscle. (Fig. 9-2).

The anterior triangle

The anterior triangle contains several important nerves and vessels and is bordered by the mandible above, the sternocleidomastoid muscle laterally, and the median plane of the neck. The infrahyoid muscle group consists of the sternohyoid, omohyoid, thyrohyoid, and sternothyroid muscles. These muscles arise from the sternum, the thyroid cartilage of the larynx, or the scapula and insert on the hyoid bone. Many vessels and nerves traverse this area.

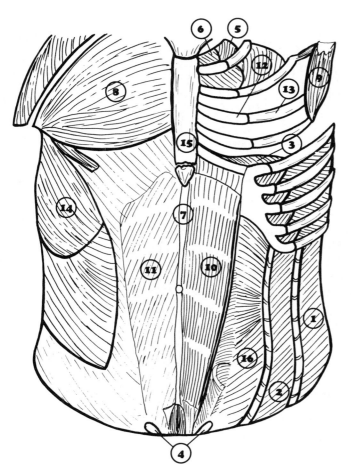

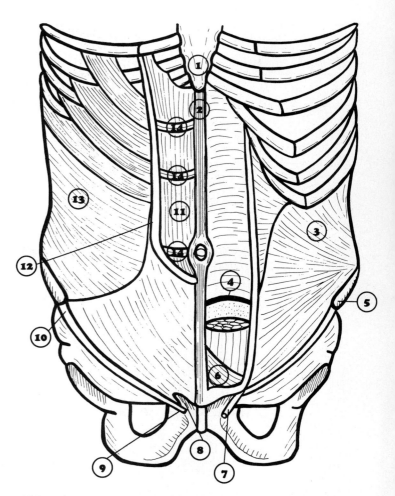

FIG. 9-3. Anterior view of the abdominal muscles. *1,* External oblique muscle; *2,* internal oblique muscle; *3,* diaphragm; *4,* external inguinal ring; *5,* external intercostal muscle; *6,* internal intercostal muscle; *7,* linea alba; *8,* pectoralis major muscle; *9,* pectoralis minor muscle; *10,* rectus abdominis muscle; *11,* rectus sheath; *12,* costal cartilage; *13,* rib; *14,* serratus anterior muscle; *15,* sternum; *16,* transversus abdominis muscle. (From Hagen-Ansert SL: The anatomy workbook, Philadelphia, 1986, JB Lippincott Co.)

FIG. 9-4. Anterior view of the rectus abdominus muscle and rectus sheath. *1,* Xyphoid process; *2,* linea alba; *3,* internal oblique muscle; *4,* arcuate line; *5,* anterior superior iliac spine; *6,* pyramidalis muscle; *7,* spermatic cord; *8,* superficial inguinal ring; *9,* pubic tubercle; *10,* inguinal ligament; *11,* rectus muscle; *12,* linea semilunaris; *13,* external oblique muscle; *14,* tendinous intersections. (From Hagen-Ansert SL: The anatomy workbook, Philadelphia, 1986, JB Lippincott Co.)

The posterior triangle

The posterior triangle is bounded anteriorly by the posterior border to the sternocleidomastoid, posteriorly by the anterior border of the trapezius, and inferiorly by the middle third of the clavicle. The muscles of this area arise from the head, the cervical vertebrae, the head of the ribs, the scapula, and the cervical and thoracic vertebral spines.

THE ABDOMEN
The anterior abdominal wall

The anterior abdominal wall is a muscular wall: the muscles are attached to the thoracic cage, to the lumbar spine, to the ilium, and to the pubis (Fig. 9-3). In some cases these attachments are indirect.

There are four muscles of the anterior abdominal wall. The central muscle is the rectus abdominis. The others are lateral to this muscle and are named, from the outside inwards: external oblique, internal oblique, and tranversus abdominis.

Linea alba

The linea alba is a fibrous band stretching from the xyphoid to the symphysis pubis. It is wider above than below and forms a central anterior attachment for the muscle layers of the abdomen. It is formed by the interlacing of the aponeuroses of the right and left oblique and transversus abdominis muscles.

Rectus sheath

The sheath of the rectus abdominis muscle is a sheath formed by the aponeuroses of the muscles of the lateral group (Fig. 9-4). The rectus muscle arises from the front of the symphysis pubis and from the pubic crest. It inserts into the fifth, sixth, and seventh costal cartilages and the xyphoid process. Upon contraction, the lateral margin forms a palpable curved surface, termed the linea semilunaris, that extends from the ninth costal cartilage to the pubic tubercle. The anterior surface of the rectus muscle is crossed by three tendinous intersections and are firmly attached to the anterior wall of the rectus sheath.

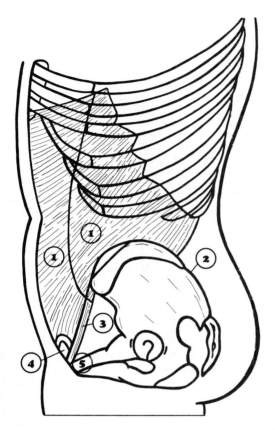

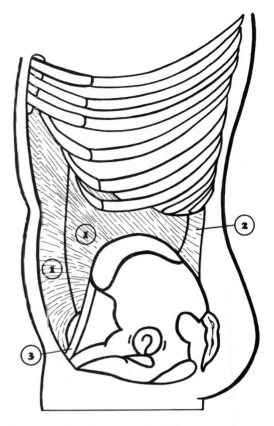

FIG. 9-5. External oblique muscle of the anterior and lateral abdominal wall. *1,* External oblique muscle; *2,* iliac crest; *3,* inguinal ligament; *4,* superficial inguinal ring; *5,* Pubic tubercle. (From Hagen-Ansert SL: The anatomy workbook, Philadelphia, 1986, JB Lippincott Co.)

FIG. 9-6. Internal oblique muscle of the anterior and lateral abdominal wall. *1,* Internal oblique muscle; *2,* lumbar fascia; *3,* inguinal ligament. (From Hagen-Ansert SL: The anatomy workbook, Philadelphia, 1986, JB Lippincott Co.)

External oblique muscle

The external oblique muscle arises from the lower eight ribs and fans out to be inserted into the xyphoid process, the linea alba, the pubic crest, the pubic tubercle, and the anterior half of the iliac crest (Fig. 9-5).

The superficial inguinal ring is a triangular opening in the external oblique aponeurosis and lies superior and medial to the pubic tubercle. (The spermatic cord or the round ligament of the uterus passes through this opening.)

The inguinal ligament is formed between the anterior superior iliac spine and the pubic tubercle, where the lower border of the aponeurosis is folded backward on itself.

The lateral part of the posterior edge of the inguinal ligament gives origin to part of the internal oblique and transverse abdominal muscles.

Internal oblique muscle

The internal oblique muscle lies very deep to the external oblique muscle (Fig. 9-6). The majority of its fibers are aligned at right angles to the external oblique muscle. It arises from the lumbar fascia, the anterior two thirds of the iliac crest, and the lateral two thirds of the inguinal ligament. It inserts into the lower borders of the ribs and their costal cartilages, the xyphoid process, the linea alba,

and the pubic symphysis. The internal oblique has a lower free border that arches over the spermatic cord or the round ligament of the uterus and then descends behind it to be attached to the pubic crest and the pectineal line. The lowest tendinous fibers are joined by similar fibers from the transversus abdominis to form the conjoint tendon.

Transversus muscle

This muscle lies deep to the internal oblique muscle, and its fibers run horizontally forward (Fig. 9-7). It arises from the deep surface of the lower six costal cartilages (interlacing with the diaphragm), the lumbar fascia, the anterior two thirds of the iliac crest, and the lateral third of the inguinal ligament. It inserts into the xyphoid process, the linea alba, and the pubic symphysis.

Diaphragm

The diaphragm is a dome-shaped muscular and tendinous septum that separates the thorax from the abdominal cavity (Fig. 9-8). Its muscular part arises from the margins of the thoracic outlet. The right crus arises from the sides of the bodies of the first three lumbar vertebrae; the left crus arises from the sides of the bodies of the first two lumbar vertebrae.

Lateral to the crura, the diaphragm arises from the me-

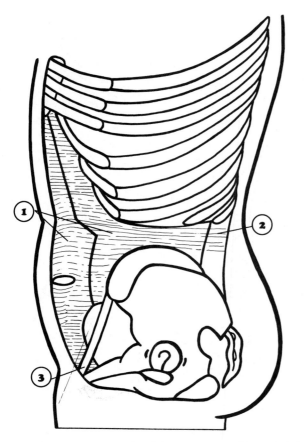

FIG. 9-7. Transversus muscle of the anterior and lateral abdominal wall. *1,* Transversus muscle; *2,* lumbar fascia; *3,* inguinal ligament. (From Hagen-Ansert SL: The anatomy workbook, Philadelphia, 1986, JB Lippincott Co.)

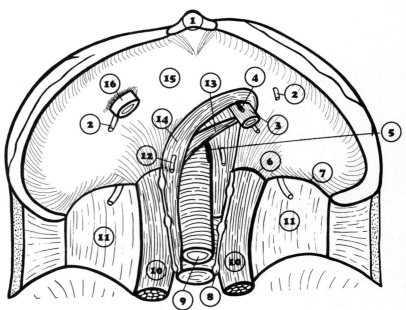

FIG. 9-8. Inferior view of the diaphragm. *1,* Xyphoid process; *2,* right and left phrenic nerves; *3,* esophagus; *4,* vagi; *5,* median arcuate ligament; *6,* medial arcuate ligament; *7,* lateral arcuate ligament; *8,* sympathetic trunk; *9,* aorta; *10,* psoas muscle; *11,* quadratus lumborum muscle; *12,* splanchnic nerves; *13,* left crus; *14,* right crus; *15,* central tendon; *16,* inferior vena cava. (From Hagen-Ansert SL: The anatomy workbook, Philadelphia, 1986, JB Lippincott Co.)

dial and lateral arcuate ligaments. The medial ligament is the thickened upper margin of the fascia covering the anterior surface of the psoas muscle. It extends from the side of the body or the second lumbar vertebra to the tip of the transverse process of the first lumbar vertebra. The lateral ligament is the thickened upper margin of the fascia covering the anterior surface of the quadratus lumborum muscle. It extends from the tip of the transverse process of the first lumbar vertebra to the lower border of the twelfth rib.

The median arcuate ligament connects the medial borders of the two crura as they cross anterior to the aorta.

The diaphragm inserts into a central tendon (Fig. 9-9). The superior surface of the tendon is partially fused with the inferior surface of the fibrous pericardium. Fibers of the right crus surround the esophagus to act as a sphincter to prevent regurgitation of the gastric contents into the thoracic part of the esophagus.

Back muscles of the body

The deep muscles of the back help to stablize the vertebral column (Fig. 9-10). They also have an influence on the posture and curvature of the spine. The muscles have the ability to extend, flex laterally, and rotate all or part of the vertebral column.

THE PELVIS

The pelvis is divided into two sections; the inferiormost section is the minor or "true" pelvis. The superior section is named the major or "false" pelvis.

True pelvis

The true pelvis is bounded posteriorly by the sacrum and coccyx (Fig. 9-11). The anterior and lateral margins are formed by the pubis, the ischium, and a small portion of the ilium. A muscular "sling" composed of the coccygeus and levator ani muscles forms the inferior boundary of the true pelvis and separates it from the perineum.

The true pelvis is divided into anterior and posterior compartments. The anterior compartments contain the bladder and reproductive organs. The posterior compartment contains the posterior cul-de-sac, the rectosigmoid muscle, perirectal fat, and the presacral space.

False pelvis

The false pelvis is defined by the iliac crests, the iliacus muscles, and the upper crest of the sacrum and is actually considered part of the abdominal cavity. The sacral promontory and the iliopectineal line form the boundary between the false pelvis and the true pelvis and delineate the boundary of the abdominal and pelvic cavities.

The uterus lies anterior to the rectum and posterior to the bladder and divides the pelvic peritoneal space into anterior and posterior pouches. The anterior pouch is termed the uterovesical space, and the posterior pouch is the rectouterine space or pouch of Douglas. The latter

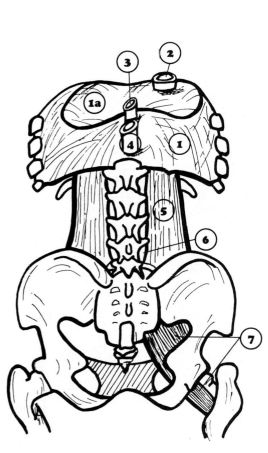

FIG. 9-9. Posterior view of the diaphragm. *1,* Diaphragm; *1a,* central tendon; *2,* inferior vena cava; *3,* esophagus; *4,* aorta; *5,* quadratus lumborum muscle; *6,* psoas major muscle; *7,* iliopsoas muscle. (From Hagen-Ansert SL: The anatomy workbook, Philadelphia, 1986, JB Lippincott Co.)

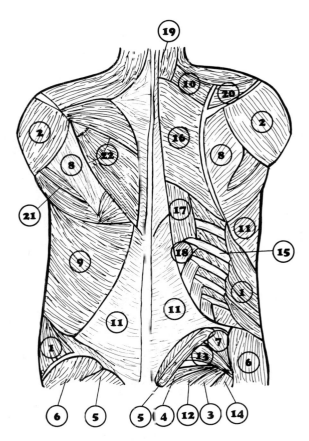

FIG. 9-10. Posterior view of the torso. *1,* External oblique muscle; *2,* deltoid muscle; *3,* gemellus inferior muscle; *4,* gemellus superior muscle; *5,* gluteus maximus muscle; *6,* gluteus medius muscle; *7,* gluteus minimus muscle; *8,* infraspinatus muscle; *9,* latissimus dorsi muscle; *10,* levator scapulae muscle; *11,* lumbodorsal fascia; *12,* obturator internus muscle; *13,* piriformis muscle; *14,* quadratus femoris muscle; *15,* ribs (7–12); *16,* rhomboid muscle; *17,* erector spinae muscle; *18,* serratus posterior inferior muscle; *19,* splenius capitis muscle; *20,* supraspinatus muscle; *21,* teres major muscle; *22,* trapezius muscle. (From Hagen-Ansert SL: The anatomy workbook, Philadelphia, 1986, JB Lippincott Co.)

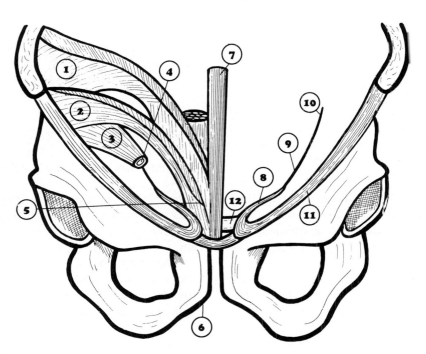

FIG. 9-11. Anterior view of the pelvis. *1,* Transversus muscle; *2,* Internal oblique muscle; *3,* cremaster muscle; *4,* spermatic cord; *5,* conjoint tendon; *6,* aponeurosis of the external oblique muscle; *7,* linea alba; *8,* pectineal ligament; *9,* pectineal line; *10,* iliopectineal line; *11,* inguinal ligament; *12,* pubic crest. (From Hagen-Ansert SL: The anatomy workbook, Philadelphia, 1986 JB Lippincott Co.)

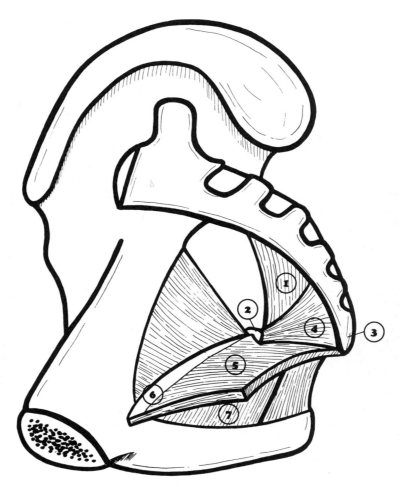

FIG. 9-12. Inferior wall of the pelvis. *1,* Sacrotuberous ligament; *2,* ischial spine; *3,* coccyx; *4,* coccygeus muscle; *5,* levator ani muscle; *6,* linear thickening of fascia covering the obturator internus muscle; *7,* obturator internus muscle. (From Hagen-Ansert SL: The anatomy workbook, Philadelphia, 1986, JB Lippincott Co.)

space is a common location in which fluids such as pus or blood may accumulate.

The fallopian tubes extend laterally from the fundus of the uterus and are enveloped by a fold of peritoneum known as the broad ligament. This ligament arises from the floor of the pelvis and contributes to the division of the peritoneal space into anterior and posterior pouches.

Pelvic muscles

The posterolateral surfaces of the true pelvis are lined by the obturator internus and pubococcygeus muscles (Fig. 9-12). The obturator internus muscles are symmetrically aligned along the lateral border of the pelvis with a concave medial border.

The pubococcygeus muscles are rounded, concave muscles that lie more posterior than the obturator internus muscles (Fig. 9-13). The psoas and iliopsoas muscles lie along the posterior and lateral margins of the pelvis major. The fan-shaped iliacus muscles line the iliac fossae in the false pelvis. The psoas and iliacus muscles merge in their inferior portions to form the iliopsoas complex. The posterior border of the iliopsoas lies along the iliopectineal line and may be used as a separation landmark of the true pelvis from the false pelvis.

Perineum

The true pelvis is subdivided by the pelvic diaphragm into the main pelvic cavity and the perineum (Fig. 9-14). The perineum has these surface relationships: anterior is the pubic symphysis; posterior is the tip of the coccyx; and lateral is the ischial tuberosities. The region is divided into two triangles by joining the ischial tuberosities by an imaginary line. The posterior triangle is the anal triangle, and the anterior triangle is the urogenital triangle.

The anal triangle has a posterior border of the coccyx, the ischial tuberosities, the sacral tuberous ligament, and the gluteus maximus muscle. The anus lies in the midline, with the ischiorectal fossa on each side.

The urogenital triangle is bounded anteriorly by the pubic arch and laterally by the ischial tuberosities. The superficial fascia is divided into the fatty layer, fascia of Camper, and the membranous layer, Colles' fascia.

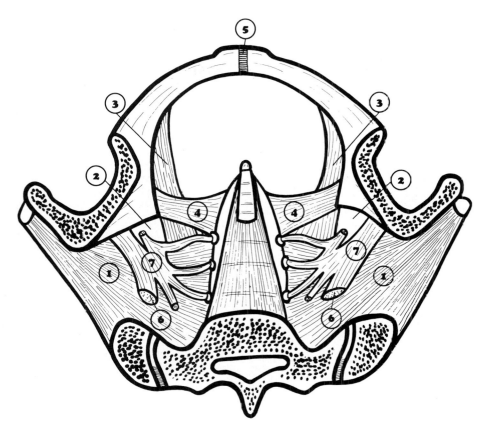

FIG. 9-13. Posterior wall of the pelvis. *1,* Piriformis muscle; *2,* greater sciatic foramen; *3,* sacro-tuberous ligament; *4,* sacrospinous ligament; *5,* pubic symphysis; *6,* lumbosacral trunk; *7,* sciatic nerve. (From Hagen-Ansert SL: The anatomy workbook, Philadelphia, 1986, JB Lippincott Co.)

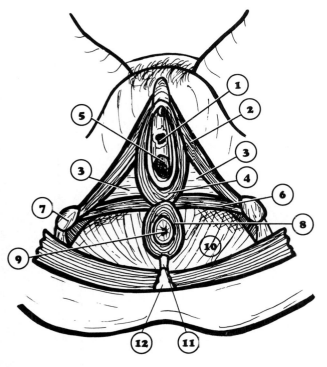

FIG. 9-14. Inferior view of the female pelvis. *1,* Urethra; *2,* ischiocavernosus muscle; *3,* urogenital diaphragm; *4,* bulbospongiosus muscle; *5,* vagina; *6,* transverse perineal muscle; *7,* ischial tuberosity; *8,* sphincter ani externus muscle; *9,* anus; *10,* levator ani muscle; *11,* anococcygeal ligament; *12,* Coccyx. (From Hagen-Ansert SL: The anatomy workbook, Philadelphia, 1986, JB Lippincott Co.)

SUMMARY

1. Because muscles comprise most of the superficial bulk of the body, it is very useful for the sonographer to have a general understanding of the various muscle groups that may be encountered during a sonographic examination.

2. Motion is an essential function of the human body. This function is made possible by the development of contractility in muscle tissue.

3. There are three types of muscle: skeletal, smooth, and cardiac.

4. There are four basic forms of dense connective tissue: tendons, ligaments, aponeuroses, and fasciae.

5. The neck is divided into the anterior and posterior triangle by the sternocleidomastoid muscle.

6. There are four muscles of the anterior abdominal wall: rectus abdominis, external oblique, internal oblique, and transversus abdominis.

7. The diaphragm separates the thoracic cavity from the abdominal cavity.

8. The back muscles of the body help to stabilize the vertebral column. They have the ability to extend, flex laterally, and rotate all or part of the vertebral column.

9. The pelvis is divided into two sections: the minor or "true" pelvis and the major or "false" pelvis. The

true pelvis is divided into anterior and posterior compartments. A muscular "sling" composed of the coccygeus and levator ani muscles forms the inferior boundary of the true pelvis and separates it from the perineum. The false pelvis is actually considered part of the abdominal cavity. An important landmark is the uterus as it lies anterior to the rectum and posterior to the bladder to divide the peritoneal space into anterior and posterior pouches: uterovesical space and rectouterine space (pouch of Douglas).

10. Multiple muscles align the walls of the true and false pelvis and should be recognized by the sonographer to determine normal anatomic relationships of pelvic organs.

10

Introduction to Scanning Techniques and Protocol

SANDRA L. HAGEN-ANSERT

The state of the art of ultrasound demands a high degree of manual dexterity and hand-eye coordination as well as a thorough understanding of anatomy, physiology, pathology, patient contours, equipment capabilities and limitations, and transducer characteristics. Ultrasound equipment today is so sophisticated that it demands a much greater understanding of the physical principles of sonography in order to produce quality images. The addition of Doppler techniques and color flow mapping has enhanced the understanding of physiology as it relates to blood flow dynamics.

Even though it is somewhat difficult to appreciate the actual scanning technique from a textbook, individual training in ultrasound is part of the sonographer's experience in producing high-quality scans. The sonographer must be aware of the special scanning techniques, artifacts encountered, and equipment malfunctions to be able to produce consistently high-quality scans. The specific applications of abdominal scanning will be discussed in this chapter.

SCANNING TECHNIQUES

Ultrasound has the capability of distinguishing interfaces among soft tissue structures of different acoustic densi-

ties. The strength of the echoes reflected depends on the acoustic interface and the angle at which the sound beam strikes the interface. Thus when performing a static scan, a compound sector-scanning motion is used to record a maximum number of interfaces. If too much sectoring is used, the scan will lose much of its detail; therefore the sonographer must judge during the performance of the scan when the scan has enough information for interpretation. This "overwrite" problem has really been eliminated with the development of high-quality real-time equipment.

ORIENTATION TO LABELING AND PATIENT POSITION
Labeling

An orderly procedure should be used to identify the anatomic position where the transverse and longitudinal scans have been taken. The illustrations in this book use the umbilicus or the symphysis pubis in the transverse supine position (Fig. 10-1); in the sagittal supine position the xyphoid and umbilicus are used (Fig. 10-2); for the prone position the iliac crest is used as a landmark.

All transverse supine scans are oriented with the liver on the left of the scan. Prone transverse scans orient the

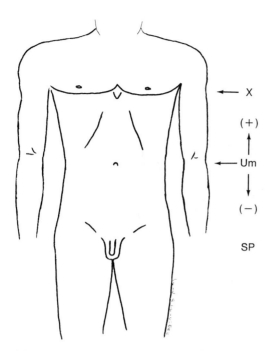

FIG. 10-1.   Orientation for transverse labeling. *Um,* umbilicus; *SP,* symphysis pubis; *X,* xyphoid.

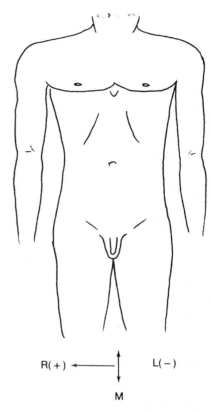

FIG. 10-2.   Orientation for sagittal labeling. *M,* midline; *R,* right of midline; *L,* left of midline.

liver to the right. Longitudinal scans present the patient's head to the left and feet to the right of the scan.

On a static scan, the umbilicus or iliac crest is usually considered the zero point for the upper abdomen. Scans cephalad from this point are labeled +, caudad are labeled −.

Longitudinal scans use the xyphoid, umbilicus, and symphysis to denote the midline of the scan. Right of the midline is designated +, and a − is used for the left. For example, a scan made 2 cm to the right is R + 2 cm; a scan made 1.5 cm to the left is 1 − 1.5 cm.

Real-time scans are generally labeled with a specific anatomic part in mind, such as the right upper quadrant (RUQ), gallbladder, pancreas, and so on.

All scans should be appropriately labeled for future reference. This includes the patient's name, date, and anatomic position.

Patient position
The position of the patient should be described in relation to the scanning table (i.e., a right decubitus would mean the right side down, a left decubitus the left side down). If the scanning plane is oblique, we merely state that is an oblique view without specifying the exact degree of obliquity.

CRITERIA FOR AN ADEQUATE SCAN WITH ARTICULATED ARM EQUIPMENT
There is a distinct difference in technique with articulated arm equipment as compared to a small real-time scanner. The images throughout the abdominal section will be a combination of both techniques. For teaching purposes, it is easier to understand the anatomic relationship of vari-

ous organs when the articulated arm is used, as a more global image is produced. When real time is used, it is sometimes more difficult to become oriented to all of the anatomic structures, as the sector or "pie" segment eliminates the surrounding anatomy.

Abdominal scans are probably the most difficult to produce with static ultrasound equipment because of the multiple interfaces and curved surfaces within the abdominal cavity. Some laboratories will require the complete abdominal contour on each scan. Precise scanning technique is required to be able to demonstrate the vessels in the midline with a single "pie" sweep (Fig. 10-3). Careful sector scanning along the lateral margin is necessary to outline the liver, the lateral and medial margins of both kidneys, and the spleen. Avoidance of the ribs is important to eliminate rib artifacts that may destroy necessary information. Quick sector scans over their borders usually work well to avoid these "ring-down" artifacts.

Transverse scans
1. The horseshoe-shaped contour of the vertebral column should be well delineated to ensure that the sound is penetrating through the abdomen without obstruction from gas interference (Fig. 10-4).

2. The prevertebral vessels should be well delineated anterior to the vertebral column (Fig. 10-5). These are best demonstrated with a single "pie" sweep technique.

3. The posterior surface of the liver edge should be seen as the transducer is arced across the anterior abdom-

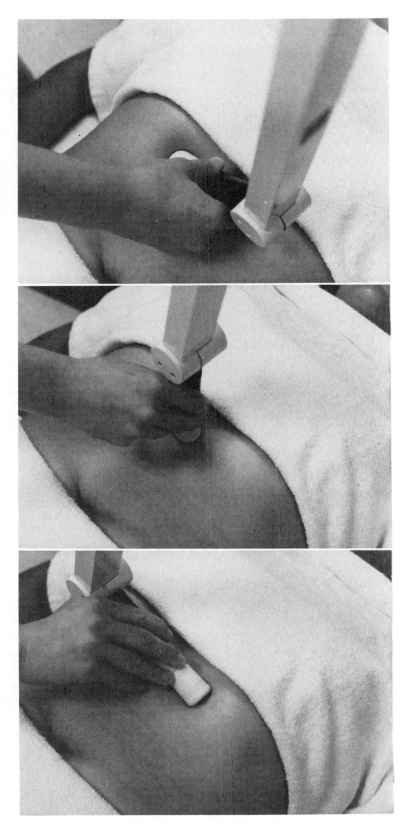

FIG. 10-3.   Articulated-arm single pie-sweep technique. The transducer face is angled sharply to the far right side of the abdomen and then slowly arced toward the far left side. The patient is in full inspiration throughout the single scan.

FIG. 10-4. The horseshoe-shaped contour of the vertebral column should be well delineated to ensure that the sound is penetrating through the abdomen without obstruction from gas interference.

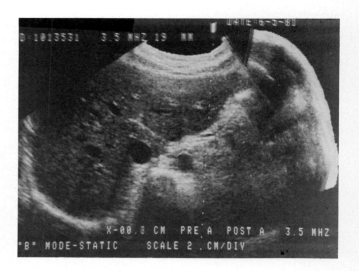

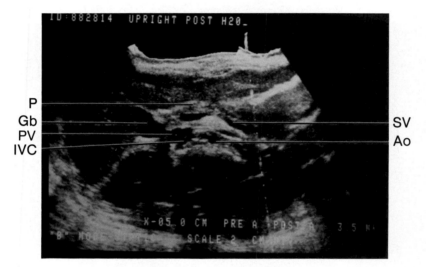

FIG. 10-5. The prevertebral vessels should be well delineated anterior to the vertebral column. These are best demonstrated with the single pie-sweep technique. *P*, pancreas; *Gb*, gallbladder; *PV*, portal vein; *IVC*, inferior vena cava; *SV,* splenic vein; *Ao,* aorta.

inal wall (Fig. 10-6). This ensures that the time gain compensation (TGC) is set correctly. If this posterior surface is not seen, the TGC may have to be broken earlier and the overall gain increased to allow adequate penetration. If there are too many echoes posterior to the liver, the overall gain should be decreased.

4. The individual organs should be well delineated with their specific echo patterns within their peripheral borders (Fig. 10-7).

Sagittal scans

Sagittal scans are somewhat easier to produce because usually a single "pie" sweep is used from under the diaphragm to below the umbilicus.

1. The diaphragmatic surface of the liver should be outlined to ascertain that the dome of the liver has been evaluated.

2. The posterior aspect of the liver should project the same fine echo pattern as the anterior surface. Gain ad-

justments should be made for overall penetration, or a lower frequency transducer could be used to increase penetration to the posterior surface (Fig. 10-8). For example, a 2.25 MHz large-diameter transducer could be substituted for a 3.5 MHz transducer to provide better penetration to the posterior structures.

3. The prevertebral vessels should be outlined with a single sweep technique (Figs. 10-9 and 10-10).

REAL-TIME PROTOCOL

Current real-time equipment has become so sophisticated that most ultrasound examinations are now being performed solely with such instrumentation. The small-diameter transducer is much easier to manipulate within the intercostal margins than the articulated arm transducer. There is greater flexibility with the real-time transducer, which means that anatomic landmarks are even more important to identify to completely survey the abdomen. Therefore a standard protocol is recommended.

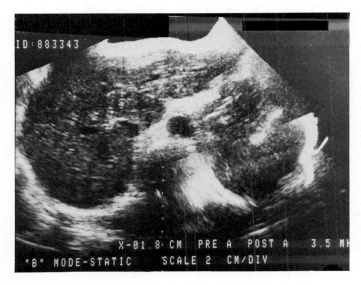

FIG. 10-6. The posterior surface of the liver edge should be seen as the transducer is arced across the anterior abdominal wall to ensure the time gain compensation is correctly set.

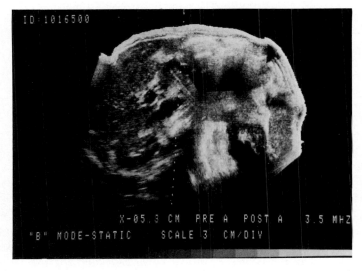

FIG. 10-7. The individual organs should be well delineated with their specific echo patterns within their peripheral borders. *L,* liver; *Gb,* gallbladder; *RK,* right kidney; *LK,* left kidney; *Sp,* spleen; *St,* stomach.

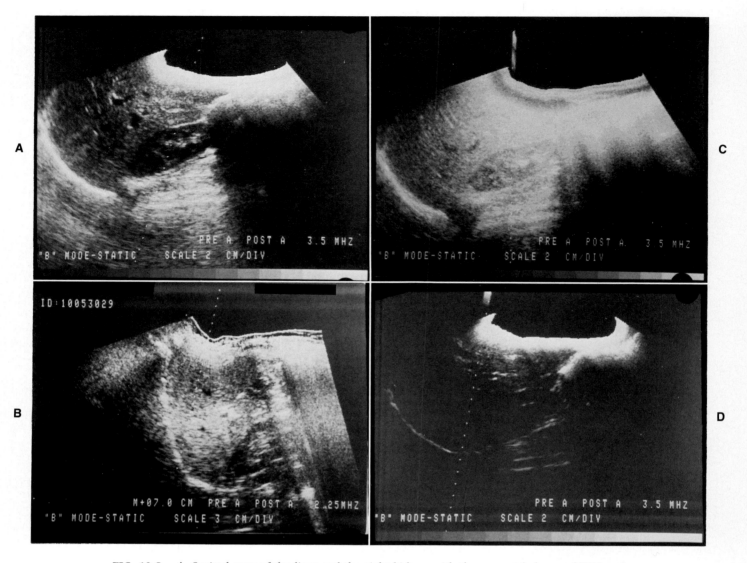

FIG. 10-8. **A,** Sagittal scan of the liver and the right kidney with the correct balance of TGC and sensitivity settings. **B,** Sagittal scan of the liver and right kidney with incorrect TGC settings. The near gain is too high and obliterates the anterior detail of the liver parenchyma. **C,** Sagittal scan of the liver and right kidney with the TGC set incorrectly. The white band of echoes in the middle of the liver indicates that the TGC is broken at this point; to balance the echoes, the TGC should be broken further back, closer to the posterior border of the liver. **D,** Sagittal scan of the liver with incorrect TGC and sensitivity settings. The sensitivity setting is too low and the TGC is set too steep.

The real-time protocol is as follows:
1. Transverse scans of (Figs. 10-11 to 10-20):
   a. Liver;
   b. Gallbladder;
   c. Right kidney;
   d. Special attention to left and right portal veins;
   e. Evaluate for ductal dilatation;
   f. Celiac axis;
   g. Tail of pancreas;

   h. Splenic-portal vein to include the body of the pancreas; look for the pancreatic duct;
   i. Superior mesenteric artery and vein to show uncinate process of pancreas and head of pancreas;
   j. If possible, the gastroduodenal artery and common bile duct for the lateral margin of the head of the pancreas; (water may be administered to separate the lateral margin from the duodenum);
   k. Aorta; look for an aneurysm or lymphadenopathy.

Text continued on p. 158.

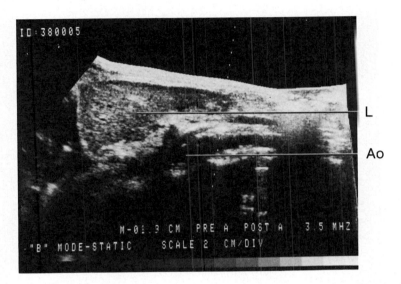

FIG. 10-9. The prevertebral vessels should be outlined in this sagittal scan with a single-sweep technique. *L,* liver; *Ao,* aorta.

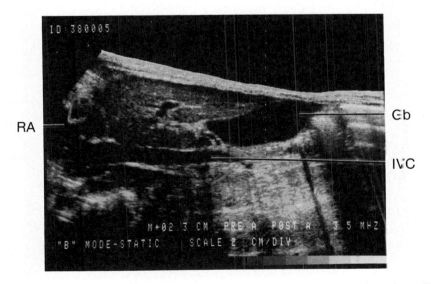

FIG. 10-10. The single-sweep technique is used in this sagittal plane to outline the gallbladder, *Gb,* and inferior vena cava, *IVC,* as it drains into the right atrium, *RA.*

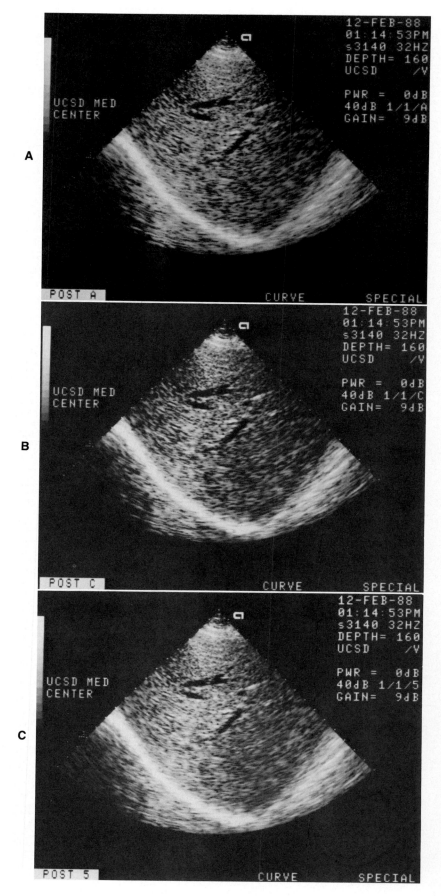

FIG. 10-11. For legend see opposite page.

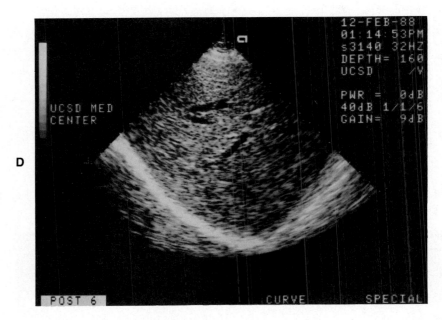

FIG. 10-11. A-D. Multiple scans over the right lobe of the liver with various post-processing curves allow the sonographer to reassign various gray levels within the liver parenchyma to produce a "softer" or more gray image, or to highlight the more reflective structures within the liver and thus produce a more contrast type of image. Some structures stand out better with changing these processing levels (i.e., some tumors, abscess collections, or hematomas may be more visible with this technique).

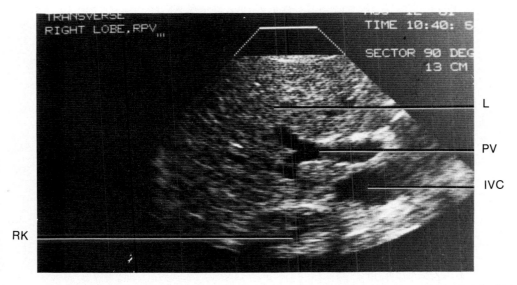

FIG. 10-12. Transverse scan of the liver, *L*, portal vein, *PV*, inferior vena cava, *IVC*, and right kidney, *RK*.

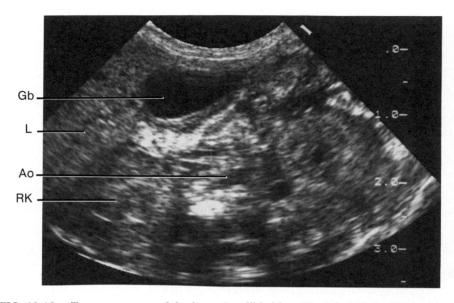

FIG. 10-13.   Transverse scan of the liver, *L,* gallbladder, *Gb,* right kidney, *RK,* and aorta, *Ao.*

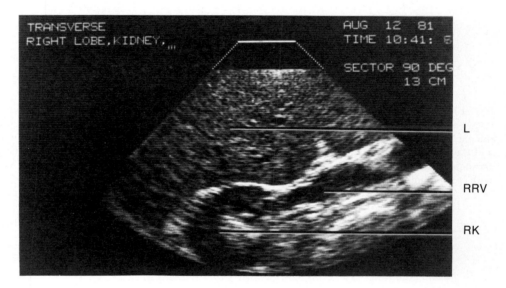

FIG. 10-14.   Transverse scan of the liver, *L,* right kidney, *RK,* and right renal vein, *RRV.*

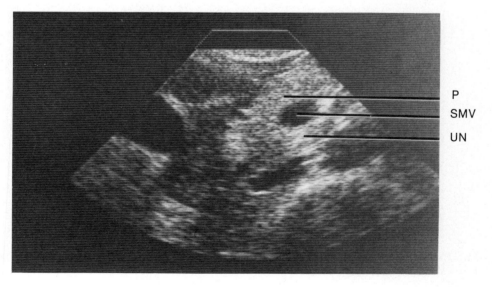

FIG. 10-15.   Transverse scan of the superior mesenteric vein, *SMV,* to show the uncinate process, *Un,* and head of the pancreas, *P.*

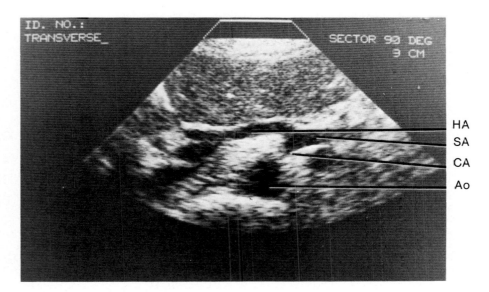

FIG. 10-16.   Transverse scan of the celiac axis, *CA,* splenic artery, *SA,* hepatic artery, *HA,* and aorta, *Ao.*

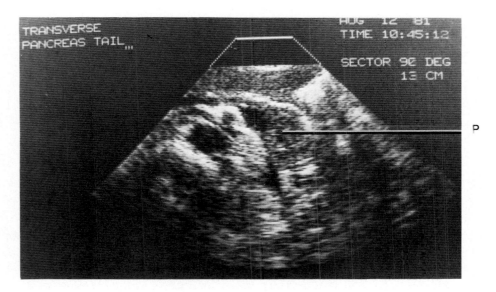

FIG. 10-17.   Transverse scan of the tail of the pancreas, *P.*

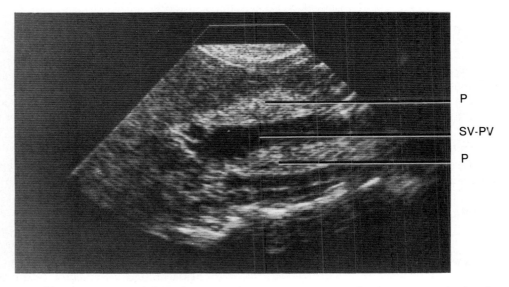

FIG. 10-18.   Transverse scan of the splenic-portal vein, *SV-PV,* as it marks the posterior body of the pancreas, *P.*

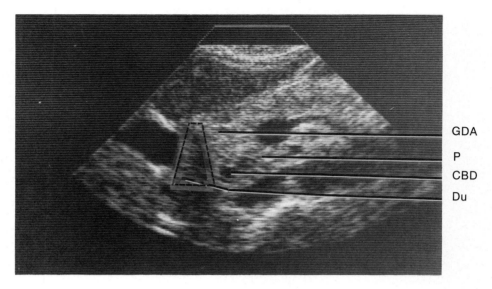

FIG. 10-19.   Transverse scan of the pancreas, *P,* gastroduodenal artery, *GDA,* common bile duct, *CBD,* and duodenum, *Du.*

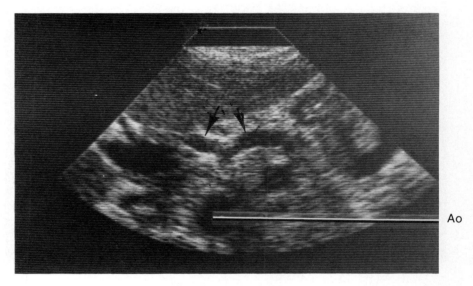

FIG. 10-20.   Transverse scan of the aorta, *Ao,* with the celiac axis arising from its anterior border *(arrow).*

2. Longitudinal scans to include (Figs. 10-21 to 10-27):
   a. Left lobe of liver;
   b. Tail of pancreas;
   c. Aorta, celiac axis, superior mesenteric artery, body of pancreas;
   d. Superior mesenteric vein, body and uncinate process of pancreas;
   e. Head of pancreas, gastroduodenal artery, common bile duct;
   f. Right lobe of the liver;
   g. Right kidney;
   h. Gallbladder.
3. Left decubitus views to include (Figs. 10-28 to 10-33):
   a. Gallbladder;
   b. Common bile duct;
   c. Head of pancreas;
   d. Right kidney;
   e. Right lobe of liver; this view is best for the part of the right lobe that is lateral or that is near the dome of the liver;
   f. Tail of the pancreas.
4. Right decubitus views to include (Figs. 10-34 and 10-35):
   a. Spleen;
   b. Tail of pancreas;
   c. Transverse and sagittal scans of the left kidney.

Unlike the articulated arm scans, which allow a panoramic view of the anatomic structures, real time provides a limited view sector of specific areas of the body. To make the scans easier to interpret, the area of interest

Text continued on p. 164.

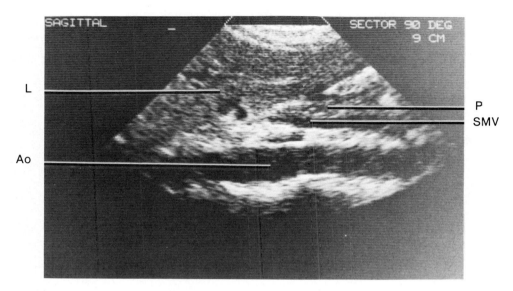

FIG. 10-21.   Sagittal scan of the superior mesenteric vein, *SMV,* pancreas, *P,* aorta, *Ao,* and liver, *L.*

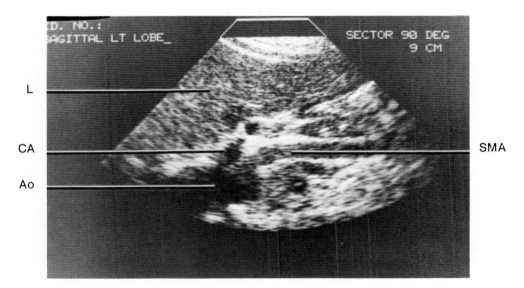

FIG. 10-22.   Sagittal scan of the left lobe of the liver, *L,* aorta, *Ao,* celiac axis, *CA,* and superior mesenteric artery, *SMA.*

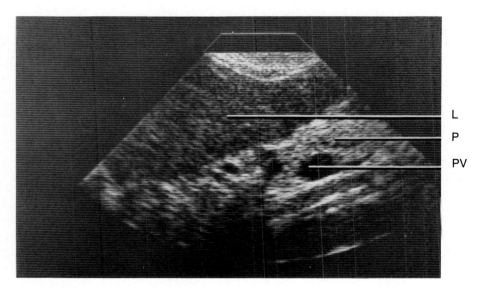

FIG. 10-23.   Sagittal scan of the tail of the pancreas, *P,* liver, *L,* and portal-splenic confluence, *PV.*

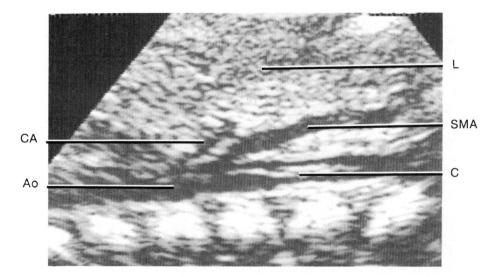

FIG. 10-24. Sagittal scan of the aorta, *Ao,* celiac axis, *CA,* superior mesenteric artery, *SMA,* and liver, *L,* on a neonate with an umbilical catheter in place, *C.*

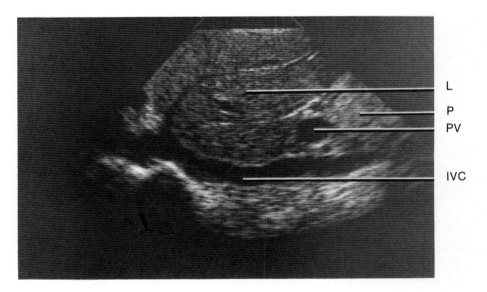

FIG. 10-25. Sagittal scan of the head of the pancreas, *P,* portal vein, *PV,* inferior vena cava, *IVC,* and liver, *L.*

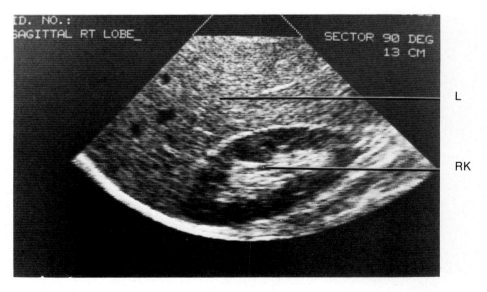

FIG. 10-26. Sagittal scan of the right lobe of the liver, *L,* and right kidney, *RK.*

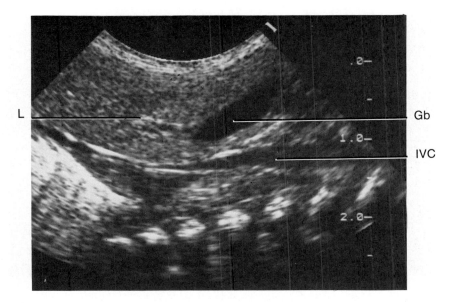

FIG. 10-27. Sagittal scan of the liver, *L*, gallbladder, *Gb*, and inferior vena cava, *IVC*.

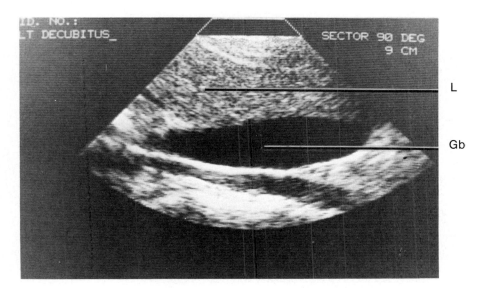

FIG. 10-28. Left decubitus scan of the liver, *L*, and gallbladder, *Gb*.

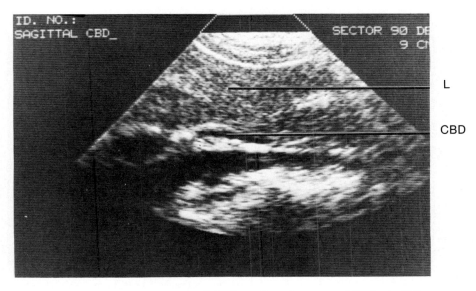

FIG. 10-29. Left decubitus scan of the liver, *L*, and common bile duct, *CBD*.

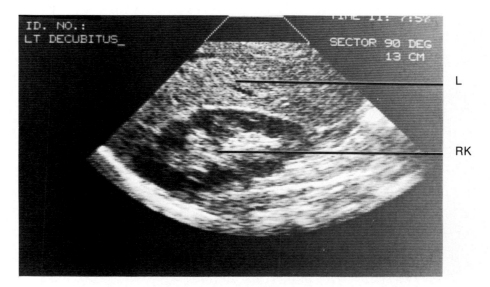

FIG. 10-30.   Left decubitus scan of the liver, *L,* and right kidney, *RK.*

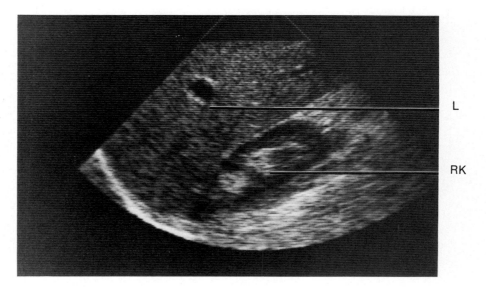

FIG. 10-31.   Left decubitus scan of the right lobe of the liver, *L,* and right kidney, *RK.*

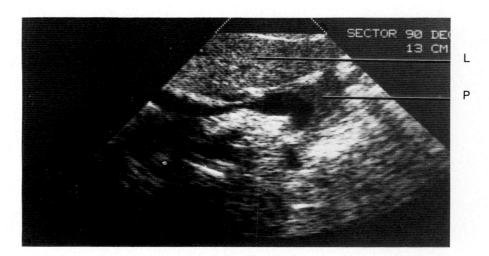

FIG. 10-32.   Right decubitus scan of the tail of the pancreas, *P,* as it drapes over the splenic portal vein. The liver, *L,* is seen anterior to the body of the gland.

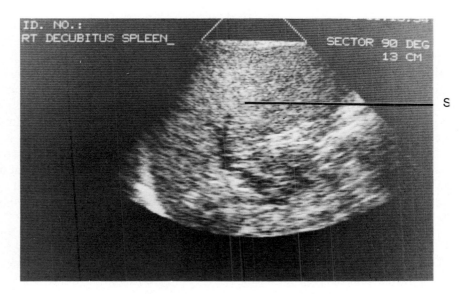

FIG. 10-33.   Sagittal right decubitus view of the spleen, *S.*

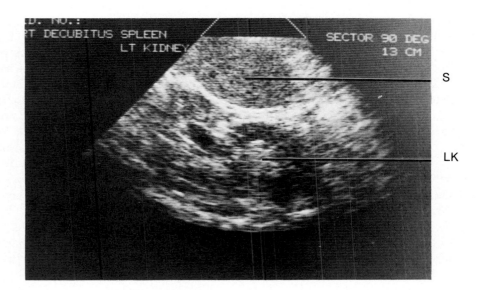

FIG. 10-34.   Transverse right decubitus view of the spleen, *S,* and left kidney, *LK.*

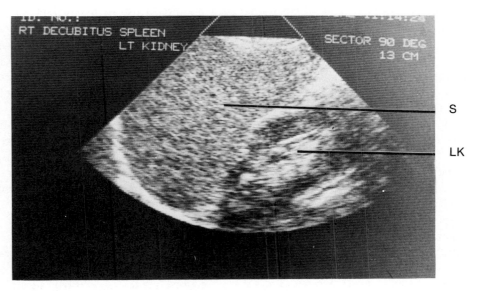

FIG. 10-35.   Sagittal right decubitus view of the spleen, *S,* and left kidney, *LK.*

on each scan is marked. For example, if the gallbladder and common bile duct are being examined, the scan would be marked Gb and CBD.

To avoid getting "carried away" with a particular piece of anatomy, it is important to adhere to a standard protocol when performing real time. Many times we have found, for example, the gallbladder to appear normal on the supine view only to contain stones when imaged with the decubitus or upright view.

It has been useful to administer fluid, either by mouth or by water enema if the pelvic area is in question, to follow the fluid pattern on real time and distinguish normal anatomy from fluid-filled loops of bowel.

GENERAL SCANNING PROTOCOL

Whenever a request arrives in the laboratory for an ultrasound examination, the diagnostic question is always the focal point of the examination. Therefore the patient's chart should be scanned by the sonographer to obtain the diagnostic problems to be solved, and the ultrasound examination should be tailored to solving the question.

The following protocol may be useful for either the articulated arm examination or the real-time examination. It may vary slightly according to the questions to be answered or the needs of the patient, but it is presented as an initial starting point for the sonographer. Specific illustrations of pathology are found in the individual chapters on the various organs.

Baseline upper abdomen

1. Transverse scan, 1 cm interval, from xyphoid to lower right lobe of the liver; pie sweep of pancreas and prevertebral vessels.
2. Longitudinal scan, 1 cm interval, to show:
   a. Aorta, superior mesenteric artery, celiac axis;
   b. Superior mesenteric vein;
   c. Inferior vena cava, portal-splenic vein;
   d. Common bile duct;
   e. Gallbladder (slight decubitus);
   f. Right kidney (slight decubitus).

Liver

1. Major area: liver.
2. Ancillary areas: gallbladder, diaphragm.
3. Essential scans:
   a. Survey longitudinal and transverse right upper quadrant at 1 cm intervals.
   b. Coronal scans of left decubitus views, if necessary.
   c. Patient supine, real-time initial survey of upper quadrant with patient in deep inspiration to demonstrate the uniform parenchymal texture of the liver.
   d. Left decubitus views of lateral portion of right lobe or subphrenic space as needed.

If the patient has jaundice, the sonographer should obtain information from the chart (laboratory values of bilirubin level, if there is a known primary lesion), as well as obtain information from other diagnostic examinations already performed. The decision should then be made whether the jaundice is obstructive or nonobstructive by scanning these areas:

1. Intrahepatic ducts:
   a. Look for ductal enlargement.
   b. Subcostal views of right upper quadrant every 2 cm.
   c. Longitudinal views important over area of right kidney because that is where the intrahepatic ducts are located.
2. Extrahepatic ducts:
   a. Longitudinal to see proximal duct anterior to portal vein.
   b. Look for distal duct draining into head of pancreas.
   c. If everything is normal in proximal duct and intrahepatic ducts, there probably is no obstruction.
      (1) Obstructive ducts: Look for dilated ducts, both intrahepatic and extrahepatic; if intrahepatic ducts are dilated and extrahepatic ducts are normal, then the obstruction is most likely from metastasis.
      (2) Nonobstructive ducts: If all ducts are normal, evaluate the liver closely for metastasis (primary tumor), cirrhosis, ascites.
      (3) Increased common bile duct or gallbladder: Look for cause of dilatation (stones, tumor, or stricture); whether patient is acutely or chronically ill (acute illness is most likely stones).
      (4) Distal duct posterior to head of pancreas; if patient is gassy, give water or scan upright or right side down; follow duct to see enlargement; look for stones on enlarged pancreas.

Gallbladder and biliary system

1. Major areas: gallbladder and biliary system.
2. Ancillary areas: right kidney, head of pancreas, liver, portal vein.
3. Essential scans:
   a. Real-time survey in both transverse and longitudinal views to visualize gallbladder and biliary system with the patient supine or in left decubitus or upright position.
   b. Longitudinal or oblique image of common bile duct.
   c. Transverse "Mickey Mouse" image of common bile duct, hepatic artery, and portal vein.
   d. Right upper quadrant survey to include liver and head of pancreas.

If there is a question of gallstones, first obtain pertinent information from the patient's chart (laboratory values, bilirubin level), previous radiographs, and previous surgery information (Was the gallbladder removed?). Then proceed with a real-time survey to demonstrate:

- Gallbladder and biliary system;
- Gallbladder wall thickness;
- Presence of echogenic bile;
- Presence of stones or polyps (change the position of the patient);
- Presence of "packed bag" (gallbladder full of stones).

Pancreas

1. Major areas: pancreas, abdominal vessels (aorta, inferior vena cava, superior mesenteric artery and vein, splenic-portal vein, left renal vein), and common bile duct.
2. Ancillary areas: liver, gallbladder, and intrahepatic ducts.
3. Essential scans:
   a. Longitudinal and transverse survey of right upper quadrant in supine position.
   b. Fluid-filled stomach views as needed to see tail of pancreas, or to separate pancreatic head from duodenum.
   c. Upright or decubitus scans to delineate pancreas from stomach, duodenum, and bowel.
   d. Longitudinal and transverse scan of common bile duct and pancreatic duct.

Aorta

1. Major areas: aorta, common iliacs.
2. Ancillary areas: superior mesenteric artery, celiac axis, kidneys, renal arteries.
3. Essential scans:
   a. Longitudinal and transverse at small intervals from the bifurcation to the xyphoid.
   b. Iliacs, longitudinal to each vessel and transverse to patient's body.
   c. Determine relationship of aneurysm when possible to superior mesenteric artery, celiac, and renal arteries.
   d. Visualize thrombus if aneurysm is present; look for dissection (flap).

Spleen

1. Major area: spleen.
2. Ancillary areas: left kidney, tail of pancreas, stomach diaphragm.
3. Essential scans:
   a. Patient supine: transverse scans of upper abdomen.
   b. Right decubitus, longitudinal and transverse (to spleen); prone or upright longitudinal and transverse scans to separate left upper pole of kidney, stomach, and tail of pancreas from the splenic border.

Kidneys

1. Major area: kidneys.
2. Ancillary areas: perirenal structures, renal pelvis, ureters (if enlarged), psoas muscle.
3. Essential scans:
   a. Decubitus, longitudinal and transverse scans to the kidneys.
   b. Supine of right kidney through the long axis of liver.
   c. Upright longitudinal if necessary to see left upper pole of kidney.
4. Renal transplant: A baseline study is acquired shortly after surgery to evaluate the transplant. The kidney and pelvic area is scanned to:
   a. Determine the axis of the kidney.
   b. Exclude abnormal fluid collections.
   c. Rule out ureteral obstruction.

Pelvis

1. Major areas: female—bladder uterus, ovaries, cervix; male—bladder, prostate, seminal vesicle.
2. Ancillary areas: female—iliopsoas, obturator internus, pubococcygeus, rectum male—iliopsoas, rectum.
3. Essential scans:
   a. Female—patient supine with a distended bladder, right or slight left decubitus to outline ovaries or adnexal area; water enema if adnexal mass is present.
   b. Male—patient supine with a distended bladder, longitudinal and transverse scans of bladder and prostate (if necessary, use steep angle of transducer to image prostate).

DOPPLER SCANNING TECHNIQUES IN VASCULAR ABDOMINAL STRUCTURES
General scanning techniques

The normal, routine sagittal transverse, coronal, and oblique scans of vascular structures are used to produce adequate images of vascular structures. Doppler techniques supplement the routine examination by permitting the detection and characterization of blood flow within those vessels. The Doppler principle has been previously explained in Chapter 5. Flow toward the transducer is positive, or above the baseline, while flow away from the transducer is negative, or below the baseline. Arterial flow pulsates with the cardiac cycle and shows its maximal peak during the systolic part of the cycle. Venous flow shows no pulsatility and has lower flow than arterial structures.

As seen in echocardiology, many of the abdominal vessels have characteristic waveforms. If the sample volume can be directed parallel to the flow, quantification of peak gradients can be estimated. However, in the tortuous course of most vascular structures, this is very difficult to attain.

The duplex Doppler equipment is the most common device used to evaluate abdominal flow patterns. This device uses a combined real time with pulsed or continuous-wave Doppler. The pulsed Doppler allows one to place the small sample volume within the vascular structure of interest by means of a trackball.

Aorta

The Doppler flow in the pulsatile aorta will demonstrate arterial signals in the patent lumen (Fig. 10-36). If the vessel were occluded, no arterial signals would be recorded.

Aortic dissection and pseudoaneurysms. Flow, often with two distinct patterns, can be seen in the true and false lumina by Doppler ultrasound.[1] The development of a pseudoaneurysm as a complication of an aortic graft procedure may be difficult to determine if pulsations are present or transmitted through the aortic wall. Doppler ultrasound may be useful to detect flow within the pseudoaneurysm.

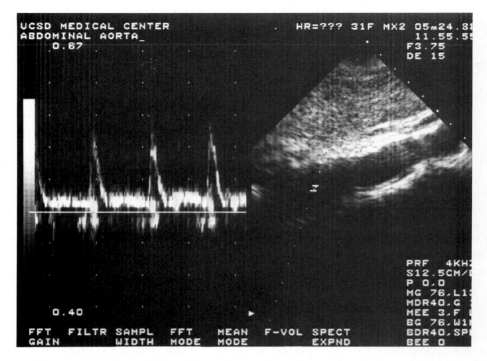

FIG. 10-36.   Doppler tracing of the abdominal aortic flow shows a prominent systolic wave with a smaller diastolic waveform corresponding to the cardiac cycle pulsations.

Hepatic artery

The identification of the hepatic artery from the common bile may be reliably assessed by pulsed Doppler techniques (Fig. 10-37). The sample volume may be placed directly in the pulsatile structures one assumes to be the hepatic artery, and arterial flow may be recorded. If this were the common bile duct, no flow would be recorded.

Aneurysms of gastrointestinal tract

Real-time imaging has the ability to detect small aneurysms of the hepatic, splenic, superior mesenteric, and gastroduodenal arteries (Figs. 10-38 to 10-40). However, with perianeurysmal fibrosis, the arterial pulsations may be reduced and thus pulsed Doppler may aid in making a specific diagnosis. If color flow is available, the low power mode may allow one to precisely outline the vascular structures, including the lumen and the aneurysm.

Renal arteries

The normal right renal artery (Fig. 10-41) arises anterolaterally from the aorta, passes anterior to the right crus of the diaphragm and posterior to the inferior vena cava. The left renal artery arises posterolaterally from the aorta. These points of origin are important in understanding the difficulties one encounters when performing a Doppler study of the renal arteries. It may be difficult to accurately record Doppler tracings from this vessel because of the somewhat tortuous nature of the artery. This is one of the reasons it is difficult to evaluate renal artery stenosis as the beam must be parallel to blood flow to accurately record maximum velocity flow patterns.

The evaluation of renal artery occlusion is quite accurate with Doppler. The arterial waveforms should always

be present from within the parenchyma of the kidneys. Their absence is diagnostic of arterial occlusion.[1]

Renal transplants

As will be discussed in Chapter 15, the transplanted kidney is subject to several vascular abnormalities, which include arterial and venous thrombosis, stenosis, and aneurysm formation.

If the renal artery is positioned so the blood flow is parallel to the Doppler beam, it may be possible to record arterial blood flow. If the vessel is stenotic, a high-velocity jet with distal turbulence may be recorded. As the beam is moved further downstream from the stenotic area, the flow will become more normal, but still slightly dampened.

Doppler analysis may be beneficial in demonstrating renal transplant rejection. Rejection causes decreased renal function as well as decreased renal blood flow, secondary to edema causing increased resistance in the capillary bed. The resistance is mirrored in the Doppler waveform by decreased flow during diastole.[1]

Inferior vena cava

The Doppler waveform recorded in the inferior vena cava shows a lower flow than is found in arterial structures (Fig. 10-42). The flow is increased in the presence of thrombus formation.

Portal venous system

Doppler flow patterns can be used to diagnose varices or collaterals in the portal venous system (Fig. 10-43). It is able to evaluate changes of flow patterns occurring in the course of portal hypertension. Bidirectional flow may also

Text continued on p. 171.

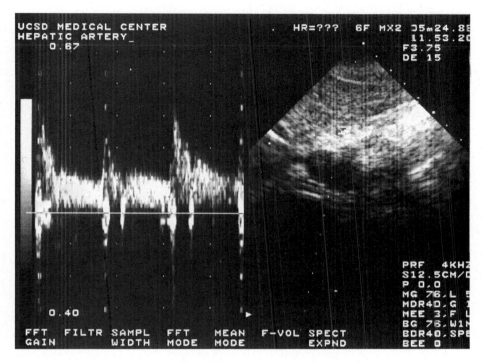

FIG. 10-37. Doppler waveform of the hepatic artery. The tracing is taken from the transverse plane. The artery is identified as a pulsatile vascular structure anterior to the aorta. If one were trying to separate the common bile duct from the hepatic artery, no pulsations or flow would be seen in the duct.

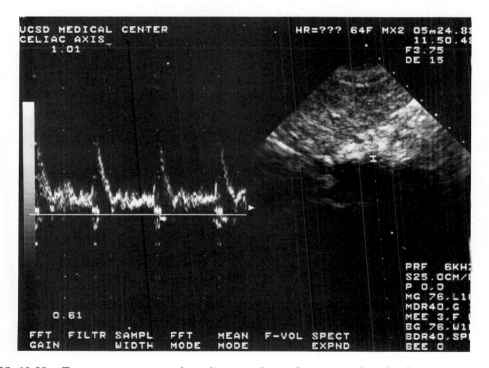

FIG. 10-38. Transverse scan over the celiac axis shows the positive Doppler flow pattern as the blood moves toward the transducer.

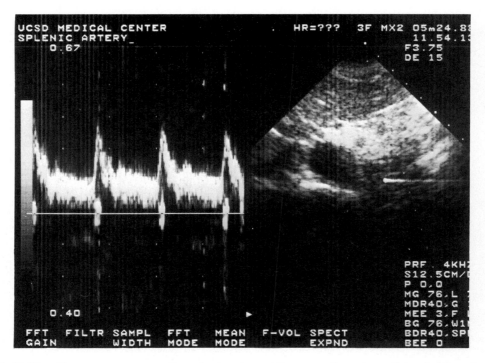

FIG. 10-39. Transverse scan over the splenic artery as it courses from the celiac axis. The arterial flow pattern is typical with increased flow during the systolic cycle.

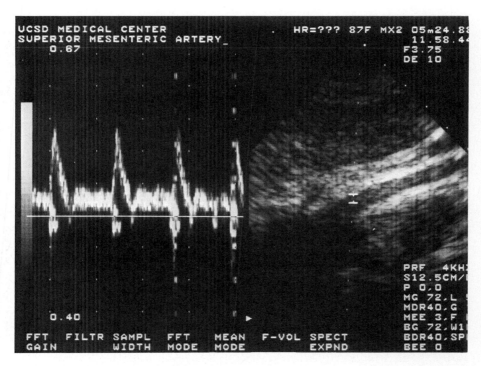

FIG. 10-40. Sagittal scan over the superior mesenteric artery demonstrates the normal Doppler arterial flow pattern.

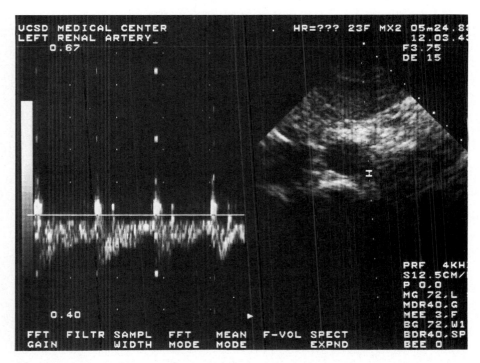

FIG. 10-41. Transverse scan at the level of the left renal artery shows the arterial Doppler flow with a negative deflection as the flow is moving away from the transducer into the kidney.

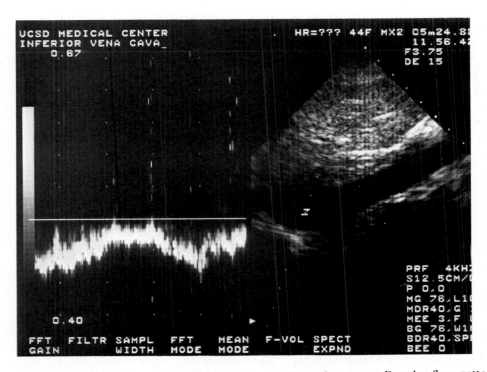

FIG. 10-42. Sagittal scan over the inferior vena cava shows the venous Doppler flow pattern. There is no sharp systolic segment as is seen in arterial flow patterns. The waveform is smoother and has less acceleration and amplitude. The Doppler flow is negative as the blood is moving into the right atrial cavity.

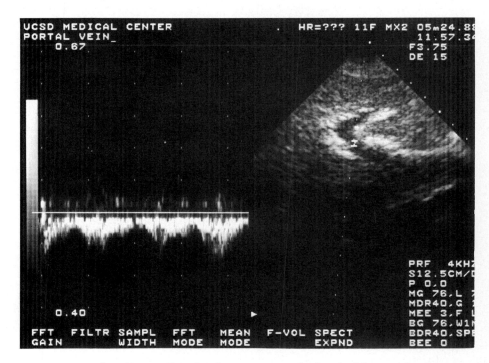

FIG. 10-43.   Venous Doppler flow pattern at the level of the portal vein.

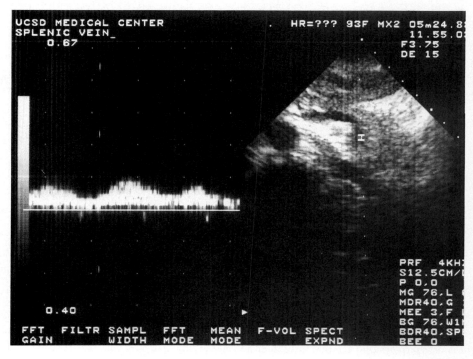

FIG. 10-44.   Venous Doppler flow pattern at the level of the splenic vein is very smooth, low profile, and small amplitude of flow in a positive direction as blood flows toward the transducer.

be seen. As liver function improves, normal hepatopetal flow is restored. If pressures worsen, there may be increased shunting away from the liver.

If a shunt is present in the porta hepatis, Doppler may be useful to determine the patency of the shunt.

Renal vein

Doppler ultrasound of renal vein thrombosis (Fig. 10-44) has been well described. If the occlusion is complete, no Doppler flow will be visualized. The entire vein should be evaluated so as to not miss a partial occlusion. The smaller veins within the kidney may also be evaluated. The absence of a flow signal from within the parenchyma may suggest venous thrombosis.

SUMMARY

1. State-of-the-art ultrasound demands a high degree of manual dexterity and hand-eye coordination as well as an understanding of anatomy, physiology, and pathology as it relates to specific sonographic findings.

2. Ultrasound has the capability of distinguishing interfaces among soft tissue structures of different acoustic densities. The strength of the echoes reflected depends on the acoustic interface and the angle at which the sound beam strikes the interface.

3. Labeling is used to identify the anatomic position where transverse and longitudinal scans have been taken.

4. The position of the patient should be described in relation to the scanning table.

5. It is important to adhere to a standard protocol when performing either articulated arm or real-time examination.

6. Doppler techniques supplement the routine examination by permitting the detection and characterization of blood flow within the vascular abdominal structures.

7. The duplex Doppler equipment is the most common device used to evaluate abdominal flow patterns. This device uses a combined real-time with pulsed or continuous-wave Doppler.

REFERENCES

1. Needleman L and Rifkin M: Vascular ultrasonography: abdominal applications, Rad Clin North Am 24(3), 1986.

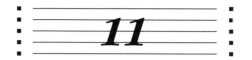

Vascular Structures

SANDRA L. HAGEN-ANSERT

The identification and recognition of vascular structures within the abdomen, retroperitoneum, and pelvis are extremely useful to the sonographer in identifying specific organ structures. It is important to understand the origin and anatomic variation of the major arterial and venous structures to identify the anatomy correctly on the sonographic image.

GENERAL COMPOSITION OF VESSELS

Blood is carried away from the heart by the arteries, and is returned from the tissues to the heart by the veins. Arteries divide into smaller and smaller branches, the smallest of which are the arterioles. These lead into the capillaries, which are minute-sized vessels that branch and form a network where the exchange of materials between blood and tissue fluid takes place. After the blood passes through the capillaries, it is collected in the small veins or venules. These small vessels unite to form larger vessels that eventually return the blood to the heart for recirculation.

A typical artery in cross-section consists of three layers (Fig. 11-1):
1. Tunica intima (inner layer), which itself consists of three layers: a layer of endothelial cells lining the arterial passage (lumen), a layer of delicate connective tissue, and an elastic layer made up of a network of elastic fibers.
2. Tunica media (middle layer), which consists of smooth muscle fibers with elastic and collagenous tissue.
3. Tunica adventitia (external layer), which is composed of loose connective tissue with bundles of smooth muscle fibers and elastic tissue.

Smaller arteries contain less elastic tissue and more smooth muscle than the larger arteries. The elasticity of the large arteries is important to the maintenance of a steady blood flow.

The veins have the same three layers as do the arteries, but they are different in their thinner tunica media layer. They appear collapsed because of little elastic tissue or muscle in their walls.

Veins have special valves within them that permit blood to flow only in one direction—toward the heart. They have a larger total diameter than do arteries, and the blood moves toward the heart slowly as compared to the arterial circulation.

MAIN SYSTEMIC VEINS
Inferior vena cava

The inferior vena cava (Fig. 11-2) is formed by the union of the common iliac veins behind the right common iliac artery. It ascends vertically through the retroperitoneal space on the right side of the aorta posterior to the liver, piercing the central tendon of the diaphragm at the level of the eighth thoracic vertebra to enter the right atrium of the heart. Its entrance into the lesser sac separates it from the portal vein.

The tributaries of the inferior vena cava are the hepatic veins, the right adrenal vein, the renal veins, the right testicular or ovarian vein, the inferior phrenic vein, the four lumbar veins, the two common iliac veins, and the median sacral vein.

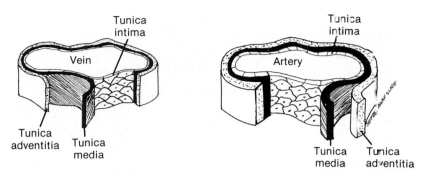

FIG. 11-1. Cross-section of an artery and vein showing the distinction between the three layers of each vessel: tunica intima (inner layer), tunica media (middle layer), and tunica adventitia (external layer).

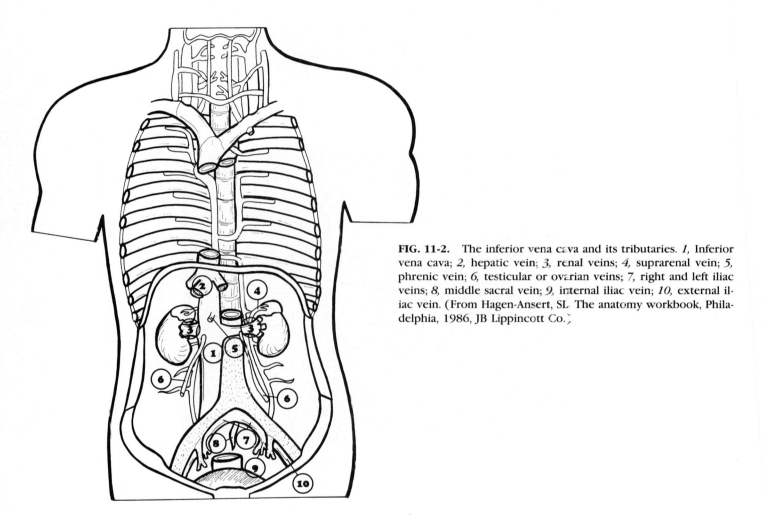

FIG. 11-2. The inferior vena cava and its tributaries. *1,* Inferior vena cava; *2,* hepatic vein; *3,* renal veins; *4,* suprarenal vein; *5,* phrenic vein; *6,* testicular or ovarian veins; *7,* right and left iliac veins; *8,* middle sacral vein; *9,* internal iliac vein; *10,* external iliac vein. (From Hagen-Ansert, SL The anatomy workbook, Philadelphia, 1986, JB Lippincott Co.)

Sonographic evaluation. On most sagittal sonograms, the inferior vena cava can be seen from the diaphragm to its bifurcation (Fig. 11-3). Differentiation from the aorta is easily made since the cava has a horizontal course with the proximal portion curving slightly anterior, whereas the aorta follows the curvature of the spine with the distal portion going more posterior. The proximal portion can often be seen to enter the right atrium on a sagittal scan.

The inferior vena cava serves as a landmark for many other structures in the abdomen and should be routinely visualized on all abdominal scans. On transverse scans (Fig. 11-4) its almond-shaped structure serves as a landmark for localization of the superior mesenteric vein, which is generally found anterior and slightly to the right of or just medial to the cava. On sagittal scans it serves as a landmark for the portal vein, which is located just anterior to and midway down the inferior vena cava (Fig. 11-5). It is also useful in locating the pancreas, which is found just inferior to the portal vein and anterior to the inferior vena cava, making a slight impression or indentation on the anterior wall of the cava.

Transverse scans should be made beginning at the xyphoid and moving toward the umbilicus at 1 cm incre-

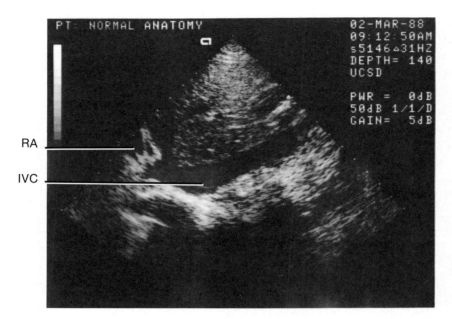

FIG. 11-3. Sagittal scan of the inferior vena cava, *IVC,* as it courses posterior to the liver to empty into the right atrial chamber, *RA.*

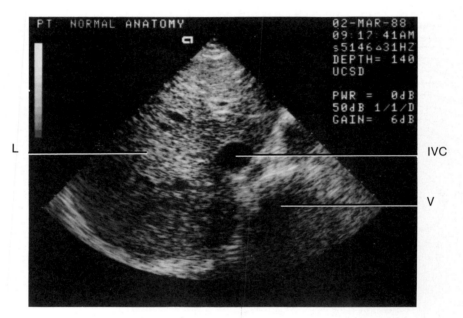

FIG. 11-4. Transverse scan of the inferior vena cava, *IVC,* liver, *L,* and vertebral column, *V.*

ments. Sagittal scans should begin at the midline and proceed in small intervals to the right until the entire vessel is visualized. Again a single sweep of the transducer should be used to image the vessels clearly. If patients are instructed to hold their breath, most likely they will perform a slight Valsalva maneuver toward the end of their breath holding. This maneuver allows normal veins to increase in size with expiration. The inferior vena cava may expand as much as 3 to 4 cm in diameter with this maneuver.

Real time will allow one to visualize the normal respiratory variation in the caliber of the inferior vena cava. It is not unusual for the cava to expand considerably in younger patients during a Valsalva maneuver.

Dilation of the inferior vena cava is noted in several pathologic conditions: right ventricular failure, congestive heart disease, constrictive pericarditis, tricuspid disease, and right atrial myxoma. Dilation of the cava is also seen in patients with hepatomegaly. The hepatic veins are dilated with increased pressure transmitted through the sinusoids, resulting in portal vein distention. If cirrhosis is present, the sinusoids may be unable to transmit pressure, and then the portal veins will not distend.

The presence of thrombus within the vessel should be evaluated especially in patients with a renal tumor. Other distortions of the inferior vena cava may be due to an extrinsic retroperitoneal mass, hepatic neoplasm, or pancreatic mass.

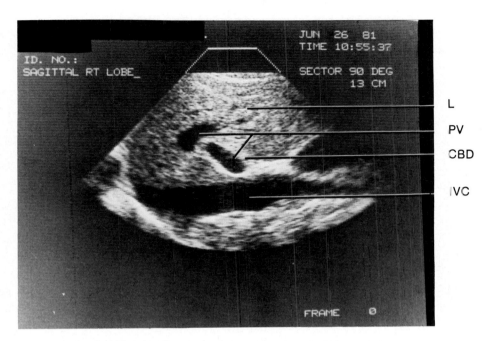

FIG. 11-5. The portal vein, *PV,* serves as a useful landmark on the sagittal scan for many abdominal structures. The pancreas is found just inferior to its margin and anterior to the inferior vena cava, *IVC.* The common bile duct, *CBD,* may be shown just anterior to the portal vein as it leaves the pancreas to enter the hilum of the liver, *L.*

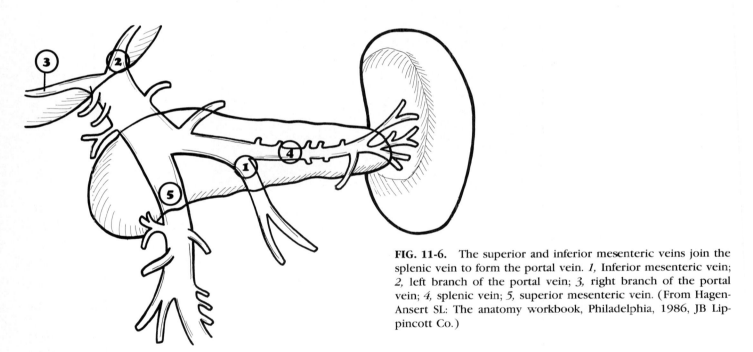

FIG. 11-6. The superior and inferior mesenteric veins join the splenic vein to form the portal vein. *1,* Inferior mesenteric vein; *2,* left branch of the portal vein; *3,* right branch of the portal vein; *4,* splenic vein; *5,* superior mesenteric vein. (From Hagen-Ansert SL: The anatomy workbook, Philadelphia, 1986, JB Lippincott Co.)

Portal vein

The portal vein is formed posterior to the pancreas by the union of the superior mesenteric and splenic veins (Fig. 11-6). Its trunk is 5 to 7 cm in length. It runs upward and to the right, posterior to the first part of the duodenum, and enters the lesser omentum. The portal vein then ascends in front of the opening into the lesser sac to the porta hepatis, where it divides into right and left terminal branches. It drains blood out of the gastrointestinal tract from the lower end of the esophagus to the upper end of the anal canal, from the pancreas, gallbladder, bile ducts,

and from the spleen. It has an important anastomosis with the esophageal veins, rectal venous plexus, and superficial abdominal veins. The portal venous blood traverses the liver and drains into the inferior vena cava via the hepatic veins.

Sonographic evaluation. The portal vein is clearly seen on both transverse and sagittal scans. On transverse scans it is a thin-walled circular structure, generally lateral and somewhat anterior to the inferior vena cava (Fig. 11-7). With the single-sweep technique, it is often possible to record the splenic vein crossing the midline of the

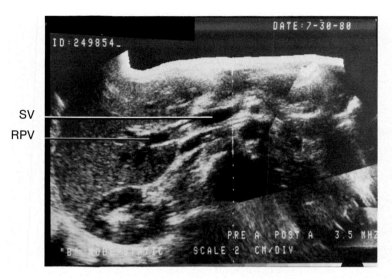

FIG. 11-7. Transverse scan of the portal vein and splenic vein. Right portal vein, *RPV,* splenic vein, *SV.*

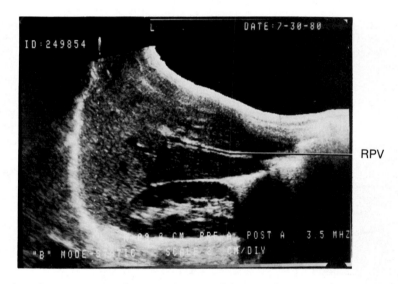

FIG. 11-8. With real-time imaging, the sagittal views of the portal vein can be systematically outlined as it bifurcates into the right and left portal veins to bring the blood supply to the liver parenchyma. Right portal vein, *RPV.*

abdomen to join the portal trunk. Thus a long section of the vein can be visualized. Often the right or left portal vein can be seen coming off the portal trunk and entering the hilum of the liver.

In the sagittal plane, slightly to the right of midline, the portal vein is situated between the inferior vena cava and the liver (Fig. 11-8). It is anterior to the inferior vena cava and posterior to the liver. A landmark for localizing the pancreas can be established with the demonstration of these vessels. The pancreas is anterior to the inferior vena cava and caudal to the portal vein.

Portal veins become smaller as they progress from the porta hepatis. Large radicles situated near or approaching the porta hepatis are portal veins, not hepatic veins (Fig. 11-9). They are characterized by high-amplitude acoustic reflections that presumably arise from the fibrous tissues surrounding the portal triad as it courses through the liver substance (Fig. 11-10).

The right and left portal veins course transversely through the liver. Thus transverse scans will display their longest extent. The right portal vein is most consistently demonstrated on the sonogram. Anatomically any intraparenchymal segment of the portal venous system lying to the right of the lateral aspect of the inferior vena cava is a branch of the right portal system. The left portal vein has a narrow-caliber trunk and may be seen coursing transversely through the left hepatic lobe from a posterior to an anterior position.

The caudate lobe of the liver lies just cranial to the bifurcation of the main portal vein and may separate the cava from the portal vein; however, it does not usually occur throughout the entire course of the vein (Fig. 11-11).

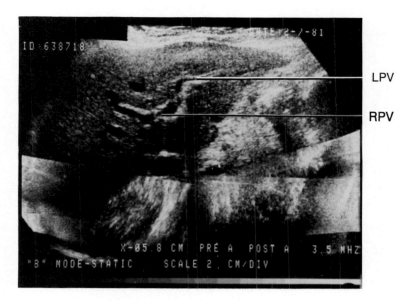

LPV

RPV

FIG. 11-9. Transverse scans of the bifurcation of the portal vein. Right portal vein, *RPV,* left portal vein, *LPV.*

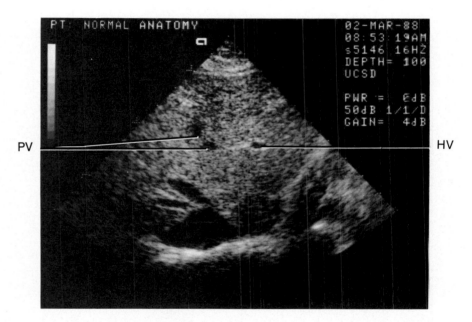

PV   HV

FIG. 11-10. Portal veins may be distinguished from the hepatic veins by their reflective properties as seen on the real-time image of the liver. The portal veins, *PV,* have a more reflective border than the thin-walled hepatic veins, *HV.* The hepatic veins drain into the inferior vena cava at the diaphragm, while the portal veins originate at the confluence of the splenic-portal junction. The main portal vein bifurcates into the right and left branches to fill the liver parenchyma.

This relationship is best seen on the longitudinal scan.

Since the portal radicle may have many different variations, it is important to become familiar with their patterns to be able to distinguish them from dilated biliary radicles.

Splenic vein

The splenic vein is a tributary of the portal circulation. It begins at the hilum of the spleen as the union of several veins and is then joined by the short gastric and left gastroepiploic veins. It passes to the right within the ileorenal ligament and runs posterior to the pancreas below the splenic artery. It then joins the superior mesenteric vein behind the neck of the pancreas to form the portal vein. It is joined by veins from the pancreas and the inferior mesenteric vein.

Sonographic evaluation. The splenic vein is best visualized in the transverse plane as it crosses the abdomen from the hilum of the spleen to join the portal vein slightly to the right of midline (Fig. 11-12). The splenic vein crosses anteriorly to the aorta and the inferior vena cava and generally relates to the medial and posterior borders of the pancreatic body and tail. Its course is variable, so small degrees of obliquity may be necessary. It is usu-

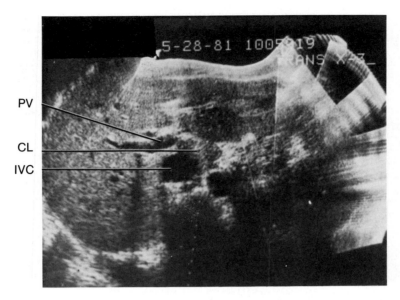

FIG. 11-11. The caudate lobe, *CL,* is the "tongue-like" projection of the liver lying between the portal vein, *PV,* and inferior vena cava, *IVC.* This may look very pronounced in some patients, depending on the angulation of the transducer.

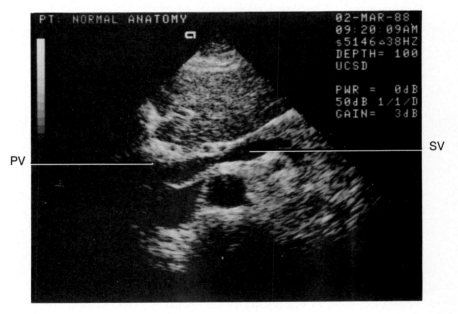

FIG. 11-12. Transverse scan of the splenic vein, *SV,* as it courses from the hilum of the spleen and flows posterior to the body of the pancreas to form the portal vein, *PV.*

ally smaller than the superior mesenteric vein and the main portal vein.

On sagittal scans the splenic vein can be visualized posterior to the left lobe of the liver and anterior to the major vascular structures. The pancreas may be seen inferior and slightly anterior to the vein (Fig. 11-13).

The larger diameter of the portal vein is the result of the influx of blood from the superior mesenteric vein. An obvious widening is demonstrated at the junction of the portal and splenic veins.

When splenomegaly is present, it is often possible to identify the origin of the splenic vein at the splenic hilum.

Superior mesenteric vein

The superior mesenteric vein is also a tributary as the portal circulation. It begins at the ileocolic junction and runs upward along the posterior abdominal wall within the root of the mesentery of the small intestine and on the right side of the superior mesenteric artery. It passes anterior to the third part of the duodenum and posterior to the neck of the pancreas, where it joins the splenic vein to form the portal vein. It also receives tributaries that correspond to the branches of the superior mesenteric artery, joined by the inferior pancreaticoduodenal vein to the right and the right gastroepiploic vein from

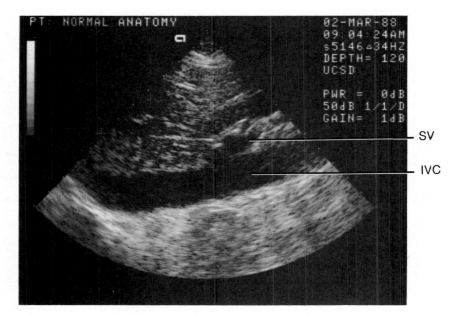

FIG. 11-13. Sagittal view of the splenic vein, *SV,* near the junction of the splenic-portal confluence. The inferior vena cava, *IVC,* is posterior.

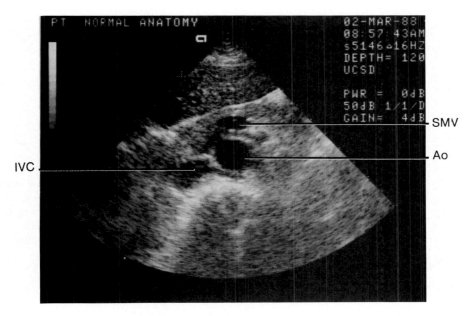

FIG. 11-14. The superior mesenteric vein, *SMV,* may serve as the posterior border of the body of the pancreas, the medial border of the head of the pancreas, or the anterior border of the uncinate process of the pancreas. *Ao,* aorta, *IVC,* inferior vena cava.

the right aspect of the greater curvature of the stomach.

Sonographic evaluation. The superior mesenteric vein is somewhat variable in its anatomic location. Generally it is related to the inferior vena cava in an anterior position. Often on ultrasound it is seen slightly to the right or to the left of the inferior vena cava and to the right of the superior mesenteric artery. Since the superior mesenteric vein drains into the portal vein (with the splenic vein), the sonographer should not be able to demonstrate these three structures together on a single transverse scan. Thus the superior mesenteric vein doubles as the posterior border of the neck of the pancreas and as

the anterior border of the pancreas where it crosses over the uncinate process of the pancreatic head (Fig. 11-14).

On sagittal scans, it is seen as a long tubular structure generally anterior to the inferior vena cava (Fig. 11-15). Often with correct oblique angulation of the transducer, one can follow the path of the superior mesenteric vein as it enters the portal system.

The following points help to distinguish the superior mesenteric artery from the vein:

1. The superior mesenteric vein is of larger caliber than the artery.
2. Respiratory variations are seen in the vein.

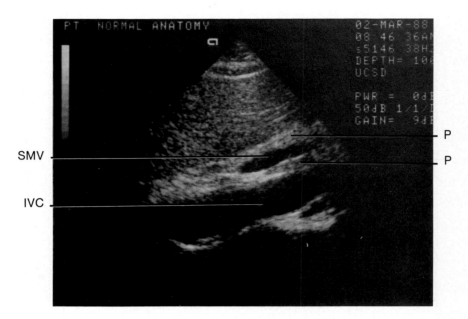

FIG. 11-15. Sagittal scan of the superior mesenteric vein, *SMV,* as it courses anterior to the unci-nate process of the pancreas, *P,* and posterior to the neck of the gland. *IVC,* inferior vena cava.

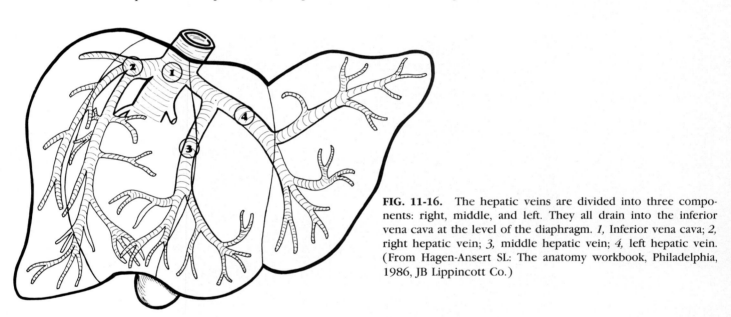

FIG. 11-16. The hepatic veins are divided into three compo-nents: right, middle, and left. They all drain into the inferior vena cava at the level of the diaphragm. *1,* Inferior vena cava; *2,* right hepatic vein; *3,* middle hepatic vein; *4,* left hepatic vein. (From Hagen-Ansert SL: The anatomy workbook, Philadelphia, 1986, JB Lippincott Co.)

3. On sagittal scans, the superior mesenteric artery angles away from the aorta whereas the vein tends to parallel the aorta or course anteriorly away from the aorta near the portal-splenic confluence.
4. Real-time identification of the confluence of superior mesenteric vein—portal vein or superior mesenteric artery is possible as the artery originates from the aorta.

Inferior mesenteric vein

The inferior mesenteric vein is a tributary of the portal circulation. It begins midway down the anal canal as the superior rectal vein. It runs up the posterior abdominal wall on the left side of the inferior mesenteric artery and duodenojejunal junction and joins the splenic vein behind the pancreas. It receives many tributaries along its way, including the left colic vein.

Sonographic evaluation. The inferior mesenteric vein is difficult to recognize on ultrasound because of its anatomic location and small diameter. It is generally cov-ered by small bowel tissue and has no major vascular structures posterior to it to aid in its recognition.

Hepatic veins

The hepatic veins are the largest visceral tributaries of the inferior vena cava. They originate in the liver and drain into the cava, returning blood from the liver that was brought to them by the hepatic artery and the portal vein. Their minor tributaries—the right hepatic vein in the right lobe, the middle hepatic vein in the caudate lobe, and the left hepatic vein in the left lobe—empty into the inferior vena cava at the level of the diaphragm (Fig. 11-16).

Sonographic evaluation. The hepatic veins are fre-

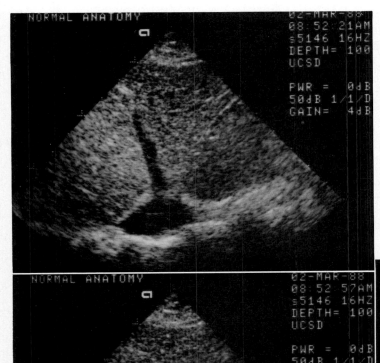

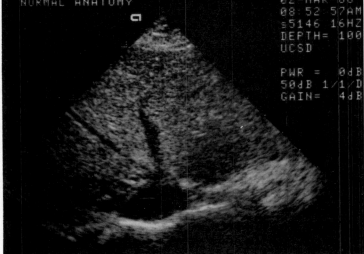

FIG. 11-17. Transverse scan with a cephalic angulation to show the hepatic veins draining into the inferior vena cava, A to C.

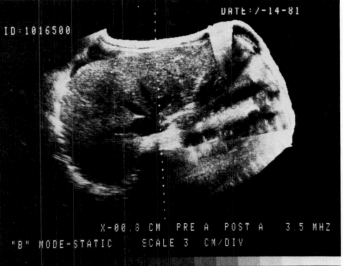

quently visualized on longitudinal scans of the liver. Transverse scans obtained with a cephalic tilt of the transducer at the level of the xyphoid often show at least two of the three veins draining into the inferior vena cava (Figs. 11-17 and 11-18). The two veins resemble the "playboy" bunny emblem on the sonogram.

The ability to distinguish hepatic veins from other vascular structures depends on recognition of their anatomic patterns. Hepatic veins drain cephalad toward the diaphragm and then dorsomedially toward the inferior vena cava. Hepatic veins increase in caliber as they approach the diaphragm. Unlike portal veins, they are not surrounded by bright acoustic reflections, although a slight amount of acoustic enhancement may be seen along their posterior border.

Renal veins

There are five to six veins that join to form the renal vein, which emerges from the hilum in front of the renal artery (Fig. 11-19). The renal vein drains into the inferior vena cava.

Sonographic evaluation. The right renal vein is seen best on the transverse sonogram as it flows directly from the renal sinus into the posterolateral aspect of the inferior vena cava (Fig. 11-20).

The left renal vein may not be seen so easily. However, when it is seen, it exits the renal sinus and takes a course anterior to the abdominal aorta and posterior to the superior mesenteric artery to enter the medial aspect of the inferior vena cava (Fig. 11-21).

Above the entry of the renal veins the inferior vena cava enlarges. The increased volume of blood returning from the kidneys to the cava accounts for this enlargement.

MAIN SYSTEMIC ARTERIES
Aorta

The systemic circulation leaves the left ventricle of the heart by way of the aorta. The aorta is the largest artery in the body (Fig. 11-22). After it arises a short distance from the left ventricle, it ascends behind the pulmonary artery. It then arches to the left and curves downward to form the descending or thoracic aorta. The descending aorta enters the abdomen through the aortic opening of the diaphragm in front of the twelfth thoracic vertebra in the retroperitoneal space. It descends anteriorly to the bodies

FIG. 11-18.   Sagittal view of the hepatic veins entering the inferior vena cava at the diaphragm.

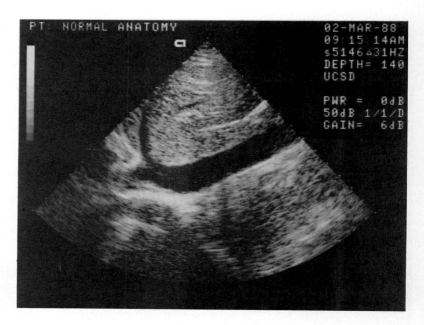

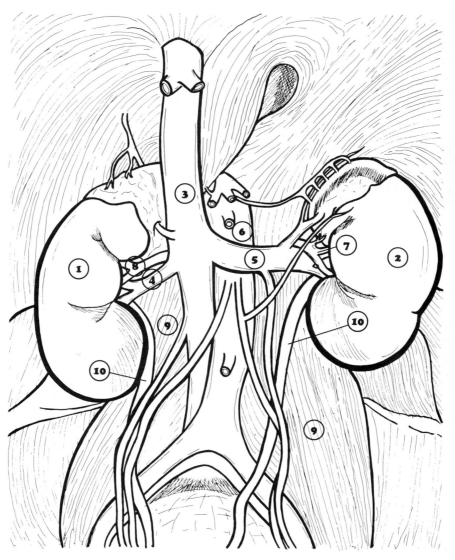

FIG. 11-19.   The kidneys and their vascular relationships. *1,* Right kidney; *2,* left kidney; *3,* inferior vena cava; *4,* right renal vein; *5,* left renal vein; *6,* aorta; *7,* left renal artery; *8,* right renal artery; *9,* psoas muscle; *10,* ureter. (From Hagen-Ansert SL: The anatomy workbook, Philadelphia, 1986, JB Lippincott Co.)

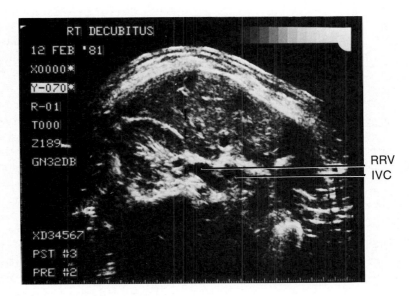

FIG. 11-20. Transverse scan of the right renal vein, *RRV*, as it enters the medial border of the inferior vena cava, *IVC*, directly from the right kidney.

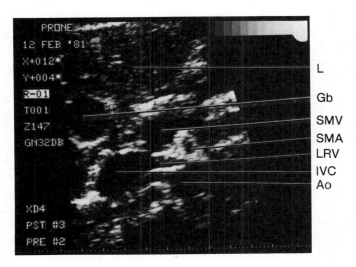

FIG. 11-21. The left renal vein leaves the renal hilus, travels anterior to the aorta and posterior to the superior mesenteric artery to enter the left border of the inferior vena cava. Liver, *L;* gallbladder, *Gb;* superior mesenteric vein. *SMV;* superior mesenteric artery, *SMA;* left renal vein, *LRV;* inferior vena cava, *IVC;* aorta, *Ao.*

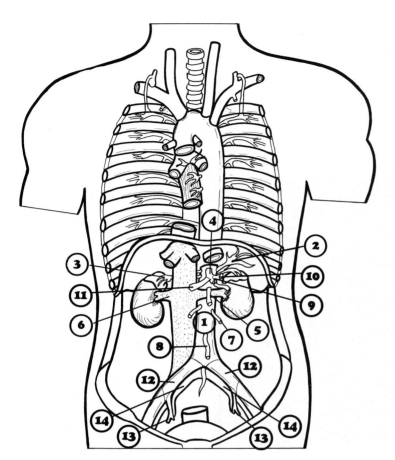

FIG. 11-22. The abdominal aorta and its tributaries. Abdominal aorta, *1;* inferior phrenic artery, *2;* suprarenal artery, *3;* celiac trunk, *4;* superior mesenteric artery, *5;* renal artery, *6;* testicular or ovarian artery, *7;* inferior mesenteric artery, *8;* left gastric artery, *9;* splenic artery, *10;* hepatic artery, *11;* common iliac arteries, *12;* internal iliac arteries, *13;* external iliac arteries, *14.* (From Hagen-Ansert SL: The anatomy workbook, Philadelphia, 1986, JB Lippincott Co.)

of the lumbar vertebrae. At the level of the fourth lumbar vertebra it divides into the two common iliac arteries.

The aorta is usually 2 to 4 cm in diameter. Although its diameter may vary slightly along the aortic contour as it branches to the visceral organs, the diameter is generally believed to be fairly uniform. The aorta has four main branches that supply other visceral organs and the mesentery: the celiac trunk, the superior and inferior mesenteric arteries, and the renal arteries.

The common iliac arteries arise at the bifurcation of the aorta and run downward and laterally along the medial border of the right and left psoas. At the level of the sacroiliac joint each iliac artery bifurcates into an external and an internal iliac artery.

The external iliac artery runs along the medial border of the psoas, following the pelvic brim. It gives off the inferior epigastric and deep circumflex iliac branches before passing under the inguinal ligament to become the femoral artery. The internal iliac artery enters the pelvis in front of the sacroiliac joint, at which point it is crossed anteriorly by the ureter. It also divides into anterior and posterior branches to supply the pelvic viscera, peritoneum, buttocks, and sacral canal.

Sonographic evaluation. The abdominal aorta is ordinarily one of the easiest abdominal structures to visualize by ultrasound because of the marked change in acoustic impedance between its elastic walls and its blood-filled lumen. Gray-scale sonography provides the diagnostic information needed to visualize the entire abdominal aorta, to assess its diameter, and to visualize the presence of thrombus, calcification, or dissection. Real time allows visualization of arterial pulsations, which may help to distinguish an artery from a vein.

The patient is routinely scanned in the supine position (Figs. 11-23 and 11-24). Gas-filled or barium-filled loops of bowel may prevent adequate visualization of the aorta, but this can be overcome by applying gentle pressure with the transducer to the area of interest or by changing the angle of the transducer or the patient. To outline the course of the vessel, initial scans should be made in the longitudinal plane. This scan should include the area from the xyphoid to well below the level of the bifurcation. In the normal individual the aorta shows a gradual tapering of its luminal dimension as it proceeds distally in the abdomen. A low to medium gain should be used to demonstrate the aorta without internal artifactual echoes.

Weak echoes may appear within the echo-free lumen. These are artifactual, due to reverberations and not to clot formation. Usually a clot will produce echoes of a greater intensity than reverberation echoes. By reduction of the sensitivity or adjustment of the time gain compensation, the electronic noise can be eliminated and thus a "cleaner" lumen obtained. Lateral resolution can also account for these spurious echoes. Poor lateral resolution results in echoes that are recorded at the same level as those from soft tissues that surround the vessel lumen. This is particularly true if the vessels are smaller in diameter than the transducer.

Since the aorta follows the anterior course of the vertebral column, it is important that the transducer also follow a perpendicular path along the entire curvature of the aorta. The anterior and posterior walls should be easily seen as a thin line for accuracy in measuring the diameter of the lumen. This facilitates measuring the anteroposterior diameter of the aorta, which in most institutions is done from the leading edge of the anterior wall to the leading edge of the posterior aortic wall.

In an effort to measure the anteroposterior width of the abdominal aorta, transverse scans are usually made every 1 to 2 cm from the xyphoid to the bifurcation (Fig. 11-25). The normal aorta is visualized as a circular structure anterior to the spine and slightly to the left of midline. In some cases the transverse diameter of the aorta differs from the longitudinal measurements; thus it is important to identify the vessel in two dimensions. If the patient has a very tortuous aorta, scans may be difficult to obtain in a single plane. As one scans in the longitudinal plane, the upper portion of the abdominal aorta may be well visualized but the lower portion may be out of the plane of view. In this case the examiner should obtain a complete scan of the upper segment and then concentrate fully on the lower segment. Transverse scans may

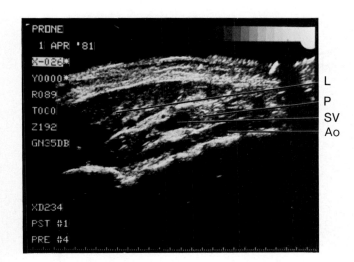

FIG. 11-23. Sagittal scan of the abdominal aorta. Liver, *L;* pancreas, *P;* splenic vein, *SV;* aorta, *Ao.*

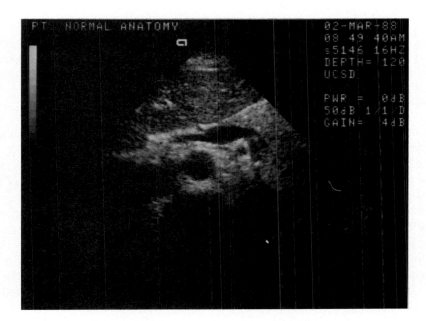

FIG. 11-24. Transverse scan of the abdominal aorta.

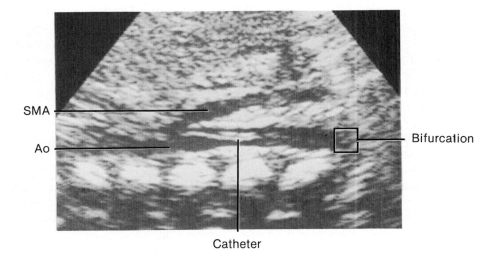

FIG. 11-25. Bifurcation of the abdominal aorta at the level of the umbilicus as seen in this neonatal abdomen. *SMA,* superior mesenteric artery, *Ao,* aorta.

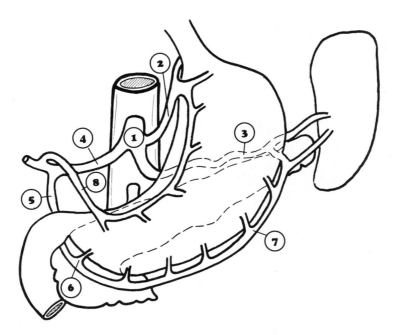

FIG. 11-26. Celiac artery and its branches. The celiac trunk originates within the first 2 cm of the abdominal aorta and immediately branches into the left gastric, splenic, and common hepatic arteries. Celiac artery, *1;* left gastric artery, *2;* splenic artery, *3;* common hepatic artery, *4;* gastroduodenal artery, *5;* right gastroepiploic artery, *6;* left gastroepiploic artery, *7;* right gastric artery, *8.* (From Hagen-Ansert SL: The anatomy workbook, Philadelphia, 1986, JB Lippincott Co.)

also be used to outline the tortuous aorta. In some patients, we have seen the aorta stretch from the far right of the abdomen to the far left.

To better visualize the aortic bifurcation, one may employ the lateral decubitus position. The patient should be examined in deep inspiration, which projects the liver and diaphragm into the abdominal cavity and serves as an acoustic window to visualize the vascular structures. If splenomegaly or a transonic left-sided mass is present, the right lateral decubitus position may be used. The patient should be rotated 5 to 10 degrees posteriorly from the true lateral position. Longitudinal scans along the axis of the abdominal aorta from the level of the xyphoid to the bifurcation should be made. Slight medial or lateral angulation may be needed to obtain the bifurcation. The inferior vena cava may be visualized anterior to the aorta in this plane.

Celiac trunk

The celiac trunk, originating within the first 2 cm of the abdominal aorta, is surrounded by the liver, spleen, inferior vena cava, and pancreas. It immediately branches into the splenic, common hepatic, and left gastric arteries (Fig. 11-26).

Splenic artery. The splenic artery is the largest of the three branches of the celiac trunk. From its origin, it takes a somewhat tortuous course horizontally to the left, usually along the upper margin of the pancreas. At a variable distance from the spleen it divides into two branches. One of these runs caudally into the greater omentum toward the right gastroepiploic artery. This branch is the left gastroepiploic artery. The other runs cephalically and divides into the short gastric artery, which supplies the

fundus of the stomach, and a number of splenic branches that supply the spleen.

Several small branches originate at the splenic artery as it runs along the upper border of the pancreas. The dorsal pancreatic, great pancreatic, and caudal pancreatic arteries are pertinent. The dorsal pancreatic (also known as the superior pancreatic) artery usually originates from the beginning of the splenic artery, but may also arise from the hepatic artery, celiac trunk, or aorta. It runs down behind and in the substance of the pancreas, dividing into right and left branches. The left branch comprises the transverse pancreatic artery. The right branch constitutes an anastomotic vessel to the anterior pancreatic arch and also a branch to the uncinate process. The great pancreatic artery originates from the splenic artery further to the left and passes downward, dividing into branches that anastomose with the transverse or inferior pancreatic artery. The caudal pancreatic artery supplies the tail of the pancreas and divides into branches that anastomose with terminal branches of the transverse pancreatic artery. The transverse pancreatic artery courses behind the body and tail of the pancreas close to the lower pancreatic border. It may originate from or communicate with the superior mesenteric artery.

Common hepatic artery. The common hepatic artery comes off the celiac trunk and courses to the right of the aorta at almost a 90-degree angle. It courses along the upper border of the head of the pancreas, behind the posterior layer of the peritoneal omental bursa, to the upper margin of the superior part of the duodenum, which forms the lower boundary of the epiploic foramen. It ascends into the liver with the hepatic duct, which lies to the right, and the portal vein, which is posterior. It then

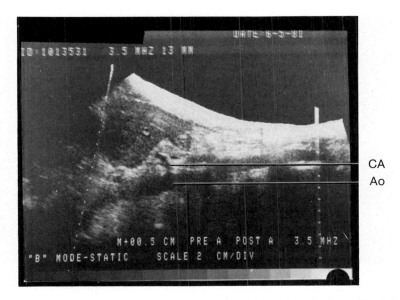

FIG. 11-27. Sagittal scan of the celiac artery, *CA,* as it arises from the anterior wall of the abdominal aorta, *Ao.*

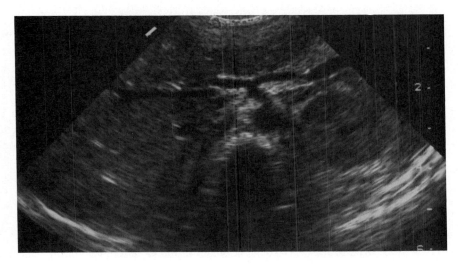

FIG. 11-28. Transverse scan over the upper abdomen shows the celiac trunk with its typical "seagull" appearance as it branches into the splenic and hepatic arteries.

divides into two major branches at the portal fissure that subdivide as they enter the liver to supply the right and left lobes:

1. The right hepatic branch, serving the gallbladder via the cystic artery.
2. The smaller left branch, serving both the caudate and the left lobes of the liver.

Within the liver parenchyma the hepatic arterial branches further divide repeatedly into progressively smaller vessels that eventually supply the portal triad.

The head of the pancreas, the duodenum, and parts of the stomach are supplied by the gastroduodenal artery, which arises from the common hepatic artery.

Left gastric artery. After the left gastric artery arises from the celiac trunk, it passes upward and to the left to reach the esophagus and then descends along the lesser curvature of the stomach. It supplies the lower third of the esophagus and the upper right part of the stomach.

Sonographic evaluation. The celiac trunk is best visualized sonographically on the longitudinal scan as the aorta pierces the diaphragm and extends into the abdominal cavity (Figs. 11-27 and 11-28). It is usually seen as a small vascular structure arising anteriorly from the abdominal aorta. Since it is only 1 to 2 cm long, it is sometimes difficult to record unless careful evaluation near the midline of the aorta is made. Sometimes the celiac trunk can be seen to extend in a cephalic rather than a caudal presentation. The superior mesenteric artery is usually just inferior to the origin of the celiac trunk and may be used as a landmark in locating the celiac trunk.

Transversely, one can differentiate the celiac trunk as the "wings of a seagull" arising directly anterior from the abdominal aorta.

The splenic artery may be seen to flow from the celiac trunk toward the spleen (Fig. 11-29). Since it is so tortuous, it is difficult to follow routinely on the transverse

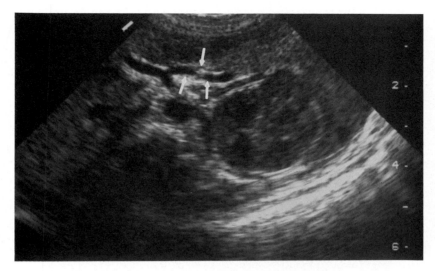

FIG. 11-29. Transverse scan of the splenic artery. This vessel may serve as the superior posterior border of the body and tail of the pancreas.

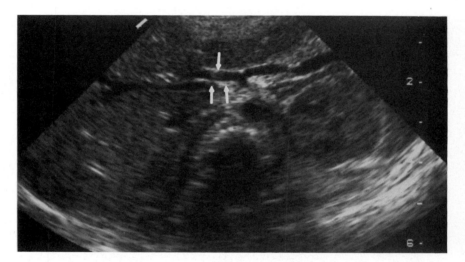

FIG. 11-30. The hepatic artery serves as the superior border of the head of the pancreas.

scan. Generally small pieces of the splenic artery are visible as the artery weaves in and out of the left upper quadrant.

The hepatic artery can be seen to flow anterior and to the right of the celiac trunk, where it then divides into the right and left hepatic arteries (Fig. 11-30).

The left gastric artery is of very small diameter and often is difficult to visualize by ultrasound (Figs. 11-31 and 11-32). It becomes difficult to separate from the splenic artery unless distinct structures are seen in the area of the celiac trunk branching to the left of the abdominal aorta.

Superior mesenteric artery

The superior mesenteric artery arises anteriorly from the abdominal aorta approximately 1 cm below the celiac trunk (Fig. 11-33). It runs posterior to the neck of the pancreas, passing over the uncinate process of the pancreatic head anterior to the third part of the duodenum,

where it enters the root of the mesentery and colon. It has five main branches: the inferior pancreatic, duodenal, colic, ileocolic, and intestinal arteries. These branch arteries to the small bowel themselves consist of 10 to 16 branches arising from the left side of the superior mesenteric trunk. They extend into the mesentery, where adjacent arteries unite with them to form loops or arcades. Their distribution is to the proximal half of the colon and small intestine.

Sonographic evaluation. The superior mesenteric artery is well seen on both transverse and longitudinal scans. As it arises from the anterior aortic wall it may follow a parallel course along the abdominal aorta or branch off at a slight angle to the anterior wall of the aorta and then follow a parallel course (Fig. 11-34). If the angle is severe, adenopathy should be considered.

Transversely the artery can be seen as a separate small circular structure anterior to the abdominal aorta and

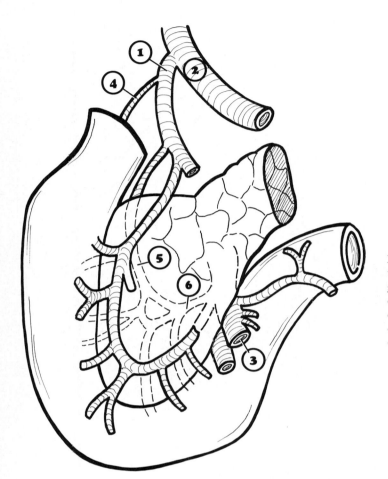

FIG. 11-31. The gastroduodenal artery is very useful in locating the head of the pancreas and serves as the lateral border of the gland. Gastroduodenal artery, *1;* hepatic artery, *2;* superior mesenteric artery, *3;* supraduodenal artery, *4;* anterior superior pancreaticoduodenal artery, *5;* posterior and anterior inferior pancreaticoduodenal artery, *6.* (From Hagen-Ansert SL: The anatomy workbook, Philadelphia, 1986, JB Lippincott Co.)

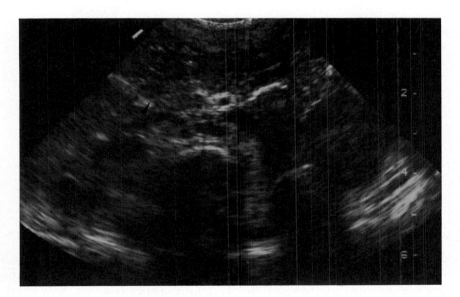

FIG. 11-32. Generally the transverse scan is the easiest view to localize the small circular gastroduodenal artery lateral to the head of the pancreas.

FIG. 11-33. The superior mesenteric artery arises anteriorly from the abdominal aorta approximately 1 cm below the celiac trunk. It supplies the proximal half of the colon and small intestine. Duodenojejunal flexure, *1;* superior mesenteric artery, *2;* inferior pancreaticoduodenal arteries, *3;* middle colic artery, *4;* right colic artery, *5;* ileocolic artery, *6;* ascending branch of ileocolic artery, *7;* intestinal arteries, *8;* cecal arteries, *9;* appendicular artery, *10;* ileal branches of the ileocolic artery, *11.* (From Hagen-Ansert SL: The anatomy workbook, Philadelphia, 1986, JB Lippincott Co.)

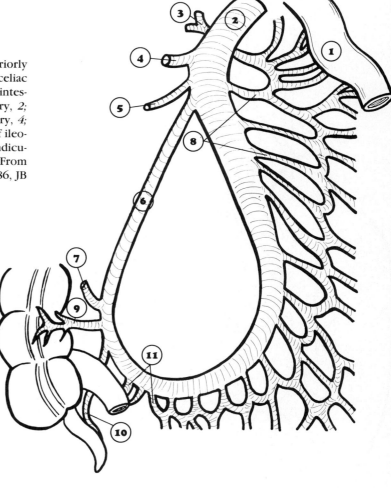

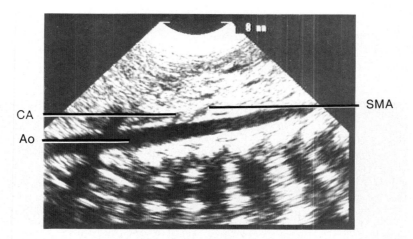

FIG. 11-34. Sagittal view of the superior mesenteric artery, *SMA,* as it arises from the anterior border of the abdominal aorta, *Ao,* inferior to the celiac axis, *CA.*

posterior to the pancreas (Fig. 11-35). Characteristically, it is surrounded by highly reflective echoes from the retroperitoneal fascia.

The origin of the superior mesenteric artery can be found by locating the left renal vein where it enters the inferior vena cava at the origin of the superior mesenteric artery.

Inferior mesenteric artery

The inferior mesenteric artery arises from the anterior abdominal aorta approximately at the level of the third or fourth lumbar vertebra. It proceeds to the left to distribute arterial blood to the descending colon, sigmoid colon, and rectum. It has three main branches: the left colic, sigmoid, and superior rectal arteries.

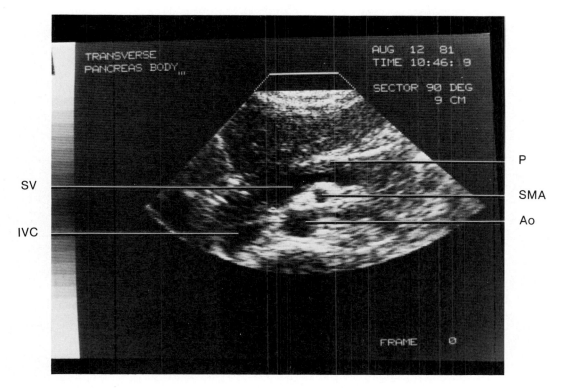

FIG. 11-35.   The transverse scan of the prevertebral vessels may show the small, reflective circular vessel of the superior mesenteric artery anterior to the abdominal aorta. The left renal vein may be seen to flow posterior to the vessel. Superior mesenteric artery, *SMA;* aorta, *Ao;* pancreas, *P;* splenic vein, *SV;* inferior vena cava, *IVC.*

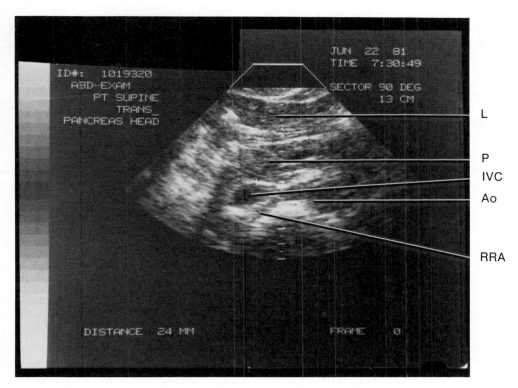

FIG. 11-36.   Transverse scan of the right renal artery as it flows from the medial wall of the aorta, posterior to the inferior vena cava, to enter the renal hilum. Right renal artery, *RRA;* portal vein, *P;* liver, *L;* inferior vena cava, *IVC,* aorta, *Ao.*

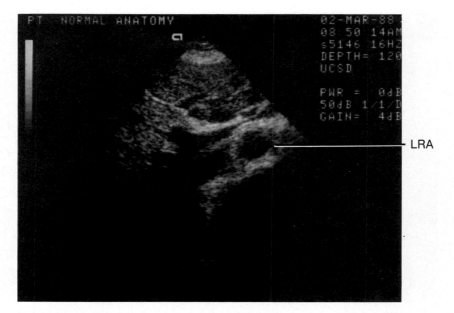

FIG. 11-37. Transverse scan of the left renal artery, *LRA,* as it leaves the lateral wall of the aorta to flow directly into the left renal hilum.

Sonographic evaluation. The inferior mesenteric artery is more difficult to visualize by ultrasound; but when it is seen, it generally is on a longitudinal scan. It is a small structure inferior to the superior mesenteric artery and celiac trunk. On transverse scans it is difficult to separate from small loops of bowel within the abdomen.

Renal arteries

The right and left renal arteries arise anterior to the first lumbar vertebra and inferior to the superior mesenteric artery from the posterolateral or lateral walls of the aorta. They divide into anterior and inferior suprarenal branches.

Sonographic evaluation. Both renal arteries are best seen on transverse sonograms (Figs 11-36 and 11-37). The right artery passes posterior to the inferior vena cava and anterior to the vertebral column in a posterior and slightly caudal direction. Occasionally on longitudinal scans a segment of the right renal artery is seen as a circular structure posterior to the inferior vena cava. The left renal artery has a direct course from the aorta anterior to the psoas and enters the renal sinus.

PATHOLOGY OF VASCULAR STRUCTURES
Aortic aneurysms

The greatest value of ultrasound in visualizing the abdominal aorta is the assessment of its luminal diameter for the purpose of ruling out an aneurysm (Fig. 11-38). These aneurysms usually are caused by atherosclerotic changes in the arterial wall. Less frequently they are due to mycotic or dissecting lesions.

The most common presentation of an atherosclerotic aneurysm is a fusiform dilation of the distal aorta at the level of the bifurcation (Fig. 11-39). Atherosclerosis will also cause decreased pulsations of the aortic walls with

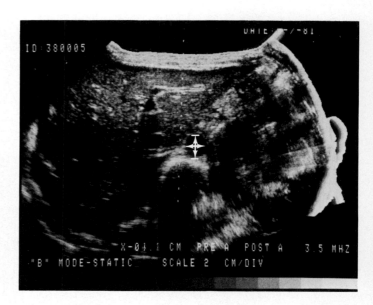

FIG. 11-38. The exact measurements of the aorta should be made on the ultrasound image to provide accurate follow-up for aneurysm development.

bright echoes reflecting the degree of thickening and calcification.

Saccular aneurysms that show only a small connection to the aorta have also been found by ultrasound. Often these are mistaken for a retroperitoneal mass or lymphadenopathy if the examiner does not carefully follow their extent and note their relationship to the aorta. Pulsations are usually diminished because of clot formation, or they may appear within the aneurysm because of transmission from the aorta.

Long-term clinical evaluation of patients with an aortic aneurysm has been conducted to determine whether the

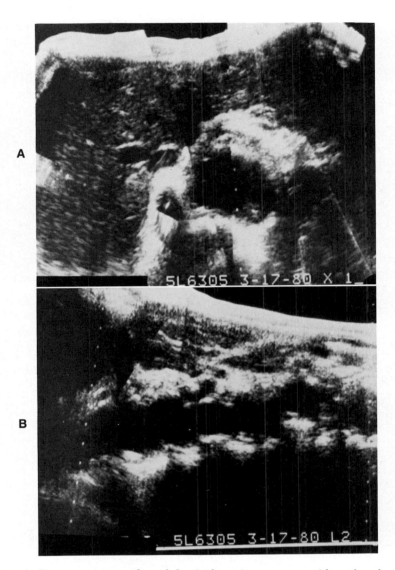

FIG. 11-39.   A, Transverse scan of an abdominal aortic aneurysm with a clot along its anterior wall. The aneurysm is larger in the transverse plane than in the anteroposterior plane. **B,** Sagittal scan of the aneurysm showing a fusiform dilation of the vessel.

size of an aneurysm changes (Fig. 11-40). Aneurysms of less than 5 cm maximum diameter (transverse, anteroposterior, width, and longitudinal measurements) rupture in 1% of cases, whereas those that exceed 6 cm show a 40% chance of rupture. Aneurysms that exceed 7 cm are more likely to rupture (60% to 80% of cases). The patient who presents with an aneurysm probably has a number of other medical problems as well. Thus it becomes important for the clinician to be able to evaluate the size of the aneurysm noninvasively and to follow it sequentially over a 3- to 6-month period by sonography. It is also important in these cases to mark on the films the exact location of the aneurysm, with the measurement given in the report so follow-up information will be accurate. It has been found that most aneurysms under 6 cm show little (less than 0.5 cm) or no change in growth over several years. Aneurysms over 6 cm may show dramatic increases in diameter (0.5 cm or more) over a 3- to 6-month interval.

Another important consideration is the relationship of the aneurysm to the renal arteries. Thus not only the diameter should be expressed, but also the longitudinal extent of the aneurysm as it relates to the origin of the renal vessels. Often bowel gas impairs adequate visualization of the renal arteries, and an indirect method must be used to locate the origin of the superior mesenteric artery. The renal arteries usually originate about the same level as the superior mesenteric artery.

If an aneurysm extends beyond the diaphragm into the thoracic aorta, it may be difficult to trace with ultrasound because of lung interference in the beam. Several attempts may be necessary to demonstrate this thoracic aneurysm. The transducer can be sharply angled from the xyphoid toward the sternal notch to visualize the lower extent of the aorta. In another technique the transducer may execute a longitudinal parasternal scan over the long axis of the heart. The thoracic aorta should be seen posterior to the cardiac structures. A third alternative is to scan

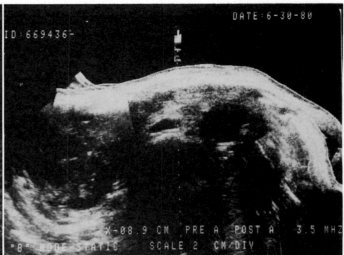

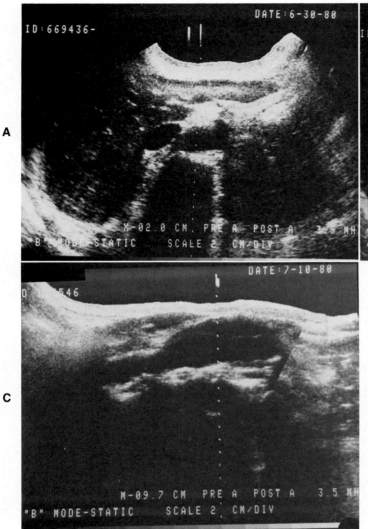

FIG. 11-40.   A, Transverse scan of a patient with an aneurysm. This scan was taken just below the xyphoid and shows a slight increase in aortic luminal size, especially in the transverse direction. **B,** This scan was taken 9 cm below the xyphoid and clearly shows the aneurysm near the level of the bifurcation. **C,** The sagittal scan shows the aneurysm at the level of the bifurcation with extension into the iliac vessel. Markers denote the relative position of the umbilicus and are useful in determining the superior or inferior extent of the aneurysm. The fine line denotes thrombus formation along the anterior border.

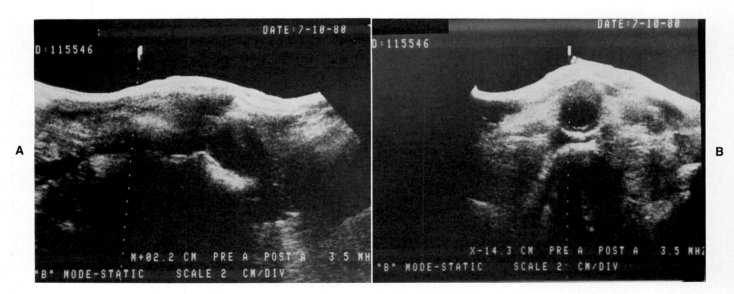

FIG. 11-41.   A, Sagittal scan of an iliac artery aneurysm. **B,** Transverse scan of the aneurysm with low-level thrombus along the anterolateral border.

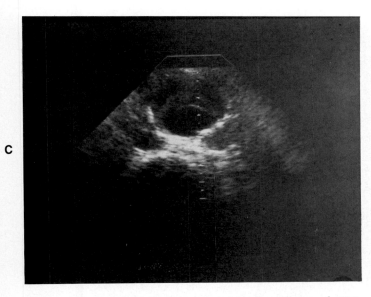

FIG. 11-41, cont'd.   C, Real-time imaging often allows a better appreciation of the amount and extent of thrombus material since the transducer is able to be more perpendicular to thrombus interfaces.

the patient's back with the patient upright or prone. The transducer should be angled slightly medial and placed in a sagittal plane along the left intercostal space. This is very effective if the thoracic aorta is deviated slightly to the left of the spine. Scalloped reverberations from the ribs will be recorded, with the luminal echoes directly posterior.

Thrombus within an aneurysm is shown ultrasonically as medium-to-low-level echoes (Figs. 11-41 and 11-42). Generally increased sensitivity is likely to highlight the thrombus echoes. The echoes should be seen in both planes on more than one scan to be separated from low-level reverberation echoes. Thrombus formation is usually more frequent along the anterior and lateral walls than along the posterior wall of the aorta.

An aneurysm that reaches the bifurcation may well extend into the iliac vessels. Real time allows the sonographer to rapidly assess the lumina of these vessels and to trace their course into the pelvic cavity.

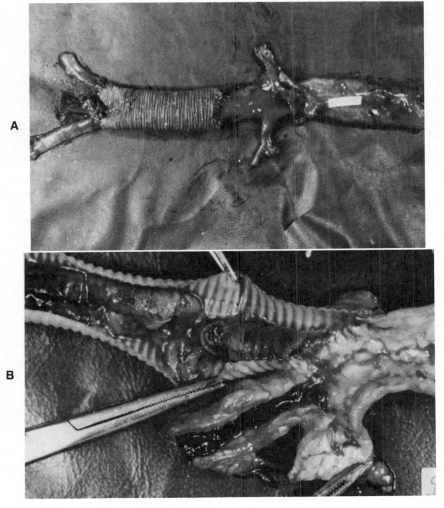

FIG. 11-42.   A, Gross specimen of the abdominal aorta with a graft attached below the renal arteries and above the iliac arteries. **B,** Thrombus and clot within the vessel at dissection.

A

B

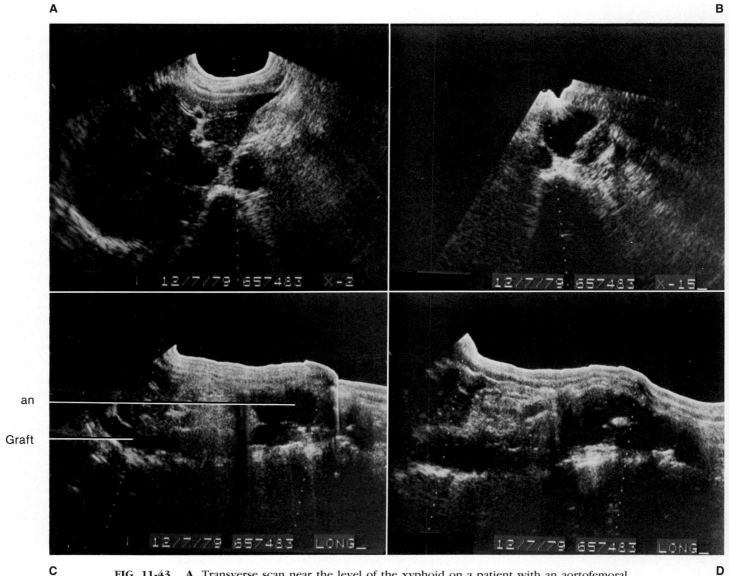

an

Graft

C

D

FIG. 11-43.   A, Transverse scan near the level of the xyphoid on a patient with an aortofemoral graft who presented with a 4 cm aneurysm. **B,** Transverse scan at the level of the bifurcation showing the aneurysm with echogenic clot along its lateral border. **C,** Sagittal scan of the aneurysm, *an,* and graft. **D,** Sagittal scan of the aneurysm as it extends into the iliac vessel. Echogenic thrombus is seen within the aneurysm.

Aortic grafts

An abdominal aortic aneurysm may be surgically repaired with a flexible graft material attached to the end of the remaining aorta. The synthetic material used for a graft produces bright echo reflections as compared with those from the normal aortic walls (Fig. 11-43) Postsurgically the attached walls may swell at the site of the attachment and form another aneurysm (pseudoaneurysm). Ultrasound is useful for postsurgical aneurysm studies as well as follow-up studies to visualize the graft and the normal aortic attachment.

Dissecting aneurysms

A dissecting aneurysm may be detected by ultrasound and usually displays one or more of the following characteristic signs:

1. Generally the patient is known to have an abdominal aneurysm, and sudden back pain may develop due to a dissection.
2. Since most aneurysms enlarge fairly symmetrically in the anteroposterior and lateral dimensions, an irregular enlargement with scattered internal echoes may represent an aneurysm with clot.
3. A double lumen may also represent a tear in the aortic wall. Real-time techniques are useful to detect the intimal flap or site of the dissection along the abdominal wall.

SUMMARY

1. Blood is carried away from the heart by the arteries and is returned from the tissues to the heart by the veins.

2. Arteries divide into smaller branches; the smallest are called arterioles. These lead into the capillaries.

3. The artery has three layers: tunica intima, tunica media, and tunica adventitia. The veins have the same three layers with the tunica media layer thinner than the arterial vessels.

4. The inferior vena cava is formed by the union of the common iliac veins behind the right common iliac artery. The tributaries of the inferior vena cava are the hepatic veins, right adrenal vein, renal veins, right testicular or ovarian vein, inferior phrenic vein, lumbar veins, common iliac veins, and the mean sacral vein.

5. The portal vein is formed posterior to the pancreas by the union of the superior mesenteric and splenic veins. The inferior mesenteric vein is a tributary of the portal circulation.

6. The aorta is the largest artery in the body. It leaves the left ventricle of the heart, ascends upward to its arch, then descends through the thoracic cavity into the abdominal cavity. At the fourth lumbar vertebra it divides into the two common iliac arteries. The abdominal aorta has four main branches that supply other visceral organs and the mesentery: celiac trunk, superior and inferior mesenteric arteries, and the renal arteries.

7. Ultrasound is very useful in measuring the luminal diameter of the aorta to rule out an aneurysm. It is also very useful to determine the presence of atherosclerosis and thrombus within the vessel.

12

Liver

SANDRA L. HAGEN-ANSERT AND WILLIAM J. ZWIEBEL

The liver is the largest organ in the body and is quite accessible to sonographic evaluation. The parenchyma of the normal liver is used to evaluate other organs and glands in the body (e.g., the kidneys are more echogenic than the liver, the spleen is about the same echogenicity, and the pancreas is about the same to slightly more echogenic than the liver). The size and shape of the liver determine the quality of the sonographic examination performed; that is, a prominent left lobe of the liver will facilitate visualization of the pancreas, which is situated just inferior to the border of the left lobe, whereas if the right lobe extends just below the costal margin, it may facilitate visualization of the gallbladder and right kidney.

ANATOMY

The liver occupies almost all of the right hypochondrium, the greater part of the epigastrium, and usually the left hypochondrium as far as the mammillary line. The contour and shape of the liver vary according to patient habitus and lie. Its shape is also influenced by the lateral segment of the left lobe and the length of the right lobe. The liver lies close to the diaphragm. The ribs cover the greater part of the right lobe (usually a small part of the right lobe is in contact with the abdominal wall). In the epigastric region the liver extends several centimeters below the xyphoid process. Most of the left lobe is covered by the rib cage.

Projections of the liver may be altered by some disease states. Downward displacement is often caused by tumor infiltration, cirrhosis, or a subphrenic abscess whereas ascites, excessive dilation of the colon, or abdominal tumors can elevate the liver. Retroperitoneal tumors may move the liver slightly forward.

Lobes

Right lobe. The right lobe is the largest of the four lobes of the liver (Fig. 12-1). It exceeds the left lobe by a ratio of 6:1. It occupies the right hypochondrium and is bordered on its upper surface by the falciform ligament, on its posterior by the left sagittal fossa, and in front by the umbilical notch. Its inferior and posterior surfaces are marked by three fossae: the porta hepatis, the gallbladder fossa, and the inferior vena cava fossa. A congenital anomaly, Riedel's lobe, can sometimes be seen as an anterior projection of the liver and may extend to the iliac crest.

Left lobe. This lobe lies in the epigastric and left hypochondriac regions (Fig. 12-2). Its upper surface is convex and molded onto the diaphragm. Its undersurface includes the gastric impression and omental tuberosity.

Caudate lobe. This small lobe is situated on the posterosuperior surface of the right lobe opposite the tenth and eleventh thoracic vertebrae (Fig. 12-3). It is bounded below by the porta hepatis, on the right by the fossa for the inferior vena cava, and on the left by the fossa for the venous duct.

Quadrate lobe. This lobe is oblong and situated on the posteroinferior surface of the right lobe (Fig. 12-4). In front it is bounded by the anterior margin of the liver, be-

A

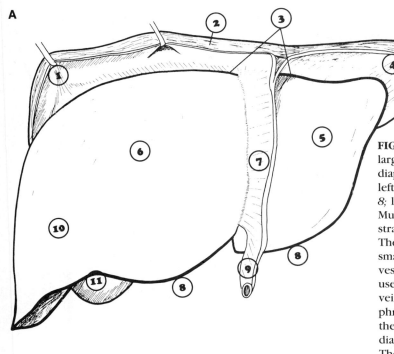

FIG. 12-1. A, Anterior view of the liver. The right lobe is the largest of the four lobes of the liver. Right triangular ligament, *1;* diaphragm, *2;* coronary ligament, *3;* left triangular ligament, *4;* left lobe, *5;* right lobe. *6;* falciform ligament, *7;* inferior margin, *8;* ligamentum teres, *9;* costal impression, *10;* gallbladder, *11.* **B,** Multiple sagittal scans over the right lobe of the liver demonstrate the fine stippled pattern throughout the liver parenchyma. The hepatic and portal vessels are seen throughout, usually as small circular structures as the image does not portray these vessels in their entire length on a routine survey unless care is used to follow the vessels back to their origin. (The hepatic veins drain into the inferior vena cava at the level of the diaphragm, while the portal veins originate in the porta hepatis at the junction of the splenic and superior mesenteric veins). The diaphragm should be demonstrated routinely on a sagittal scan. The upper pole of the right kidney shows that the scan is made along the far right margin of the abdomen, while views of the inferior vena cava and hepatic vein show the scan is more medial to the right kidney views. (**A** from Hagen-Ansert SL: The anatomy workbook, Philadelphia, 1986, JB Lippincott Co.)

B

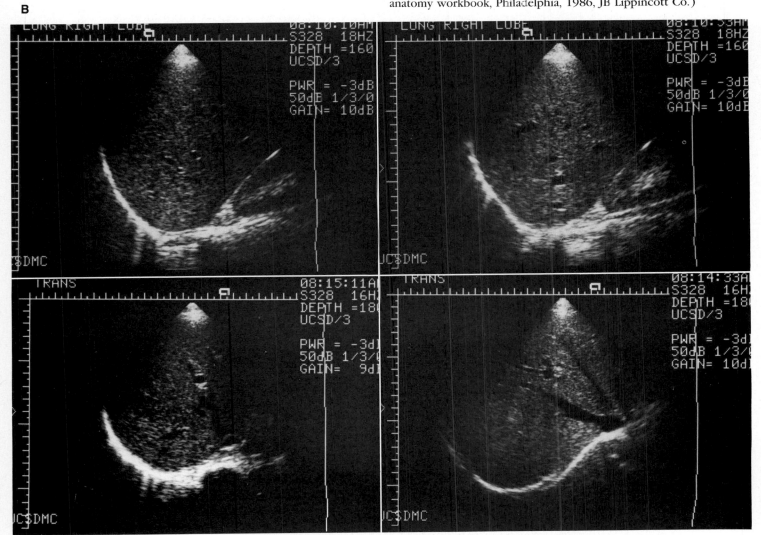

FIG. 12-2. Superior view of the liver. The left lobe of the liver lies in the epigastric and left hypochondriac regions. Fundus of the gallbladder, *1;* right lobe, *2;* diaphragmatic surface, *3;* coronary ligament, *4;* bare area, *5;* inferior vena cava, *6;* caudate lobe, *7;* left triangular ligament, *8;* diaphragmatic surface, *9;* left lobe, *10;* falciform ligament, *11.* (From Hagen-Ansert SL, The anatomy workbook, Philadelphia, 1986, JB Lippincott Co.)

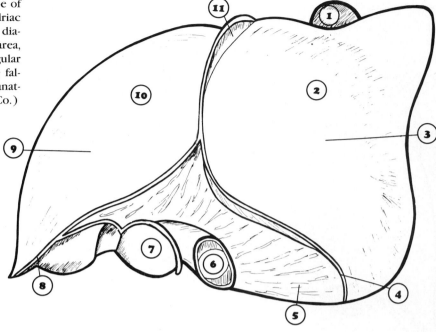

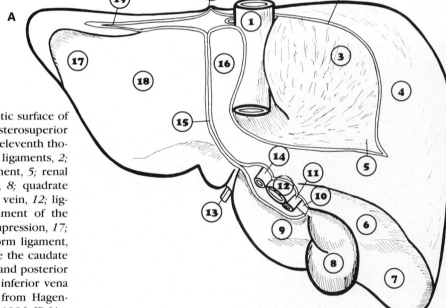

FIG. 12-3. **A,** Posterior view of the diaphragmatic surface of the liver. The caudate lobe is located on the posterosuperior surface of the right lobe, opposite the tenth and eleventh thoracic vertebrae. Inferior vena cava, *1;* coronary ligaments, *2;* bare area, *3;* right lobe, *4;* right triangular ligament, *5;* renal impression, *6;* colic impression, *7;* gallbladder, *8;* quadrate lobe, *9;* cystic duct, *10;* hepatic duct, *11;* portal vein, *12;* ligamentum teres, *13;* hepatic artery, *14;* attachment of the lesser omentum, *15;* caudate lobe, *16;* gastric impression, *17;* left lobe, *18;* left triangular ligament, *19;* falciform ligament, *20.* **B,** Transverse scans of the liver demonstrate the caudate lobe as it lies anterior to the inferior vena cava and posterior to the ligamentum venosum. Caudate lobe, *CL;* inferior vena cava, *IVC;* ligamentum venosum *(arrows).* (**A** from Hagen-Ansert SL: The anatomy workbook, Philadelphia, 1986, JB Lippincott Co.)

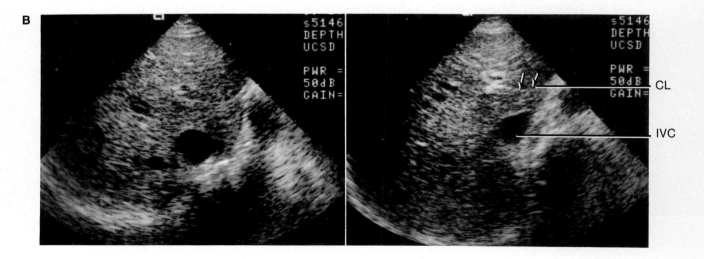

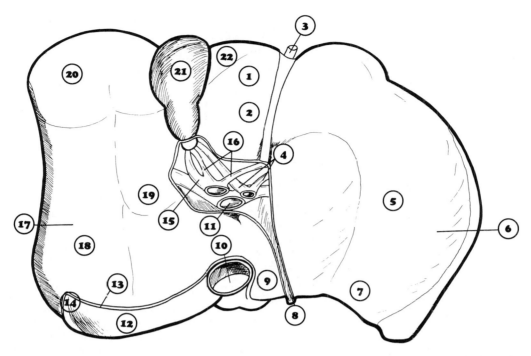

FIG. 12-4. Inferior view of the visceral surface of the liver. The quadrate lobe is located on the posteroinferior surface of the right lobe. Quadrate lobe, *1;* pyloric area, *2;* ligamentum teres, *3;* hepatic arteries, *4;* gastric impression, *5;* left lobe, *6;* esophageal impression, *7;* ligamentum venosum, *8;* caudate lobe, *9;* inferior vena cava, *10;* portal vein, *11;* bare area, *12;* coronary ligaments, *13;* right triangular ligament, *14;* cystic duct, *15;* hepatic duct, *16;* right lobe, *17;* renal impression, *18;* duodenal impression, *19;* colic impression, *20;* gallbladder. (From Hagen-Ansert SL: The anatomy workbook, Philadelphia, 1986, JB Lippincott Co.)

hind by the porta hepatis, on the right by the fossa for the gallbladder, and on the left by the fossa for the umbilical vein.

Portal and hepatic venous anatomy

As described by Marks et al.,[2] the portal venous system is a reliable indicator of various ultrasonic tomographic planes throughout the liver (Fig. 12-5).

Main portal vein. This vessel approaches the porta hepatis in a rightward, cephalic, and slightly posterior direction within the hepatoduodenal ligament. It comes in contact with the anterior surface of the inferior vena cava near the porta hepatis and serves to locate the liver hilum (Fig. 12-6). It then divides into two branches, the right and left portal veins.

RIGHT PORTAL VEIN. This branch is the larger of the two and requires a more posterior and more caudal approach (Fig. 12-7, *A* and *B*). It usually is possible to identify the anterior and posterior divisions of the right portal vein on sonography. The anterior division closely parallels the anterior abdominal wall.

LEFT PORTAL VEIN. This branch lies more anterior and cranial than the right portal vein. The main portal vein is seen to elongate at the origin of the left portal vein (Fig. 12-8). The vessel lies within a canal containing large amounts of connective tissue, which results in the visualization of an echogenic linear band coursing through the central portion of the lateral segment of the left lobe.

Hepatic veins. The hepatic veins are divided into three components: right, middle, and left (Fig. 12-9). The

right hepatic is the largest and enters the right lateral aspect of the inferior vena cava. The middle hepatic enters the anterior or right anterior surface of the IVC. The left hepatic, which is the smallest, enters the left anterior surface of the IVC.

Often it is possible to identify a long horizontal branch of the right hepatic vein coursing between the anterior and posterior divisions of the right portal vein.

Distinguishing characteristics of hepatic and portal veins. The best way to distinguish the hepatic from the portal vessels is to trace their points of origin. The hepatic vessels flow into the inferior vena cava whereas the portal system arises from the main portal vein. Real-time sector allows the sonographer to make this assessment within a few seconds.

Two other characteristics help distinguish the vessels:
1. Hepatic veins course between the hepatic lobes and segments; the major portal branches course within the lobar segments.
2. Hepatic veins drain toward the right atrium; the portal veins emanate from the porta hepatis (i.e., hepatic veins are larger near the diaphragm whereas portal veins are larger nearer the porta hepatis).

Segmental liver anatomy

The liver is divided essentially into two lobes, each of which has two segments. The right lobe is divided into anterior and posterior segments, and the left lobe into medial and lateral segments. The quadrate lobe is a portion of the medial segment. The caudate lobe is the poste-

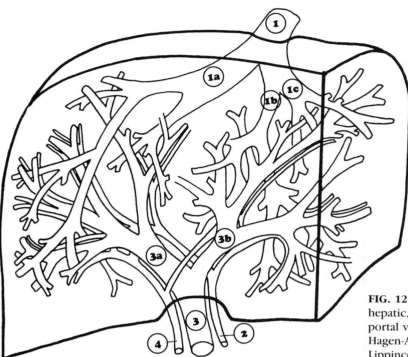

FIG. 12-5. Vascular system of the liver. Hepatic veins, *1;* right hepatic, *1a;* middle hepatic, *1b,* left hepatic, *1c;* hepatic artery, *2;* portal vein, *3;* right portal, *3a;* left portal, *3b;* bile duct, *4.* (From Hagen-Ansert SL: The anatomy workbook, Philadelphia, 1986, JB Lippincott Co.)

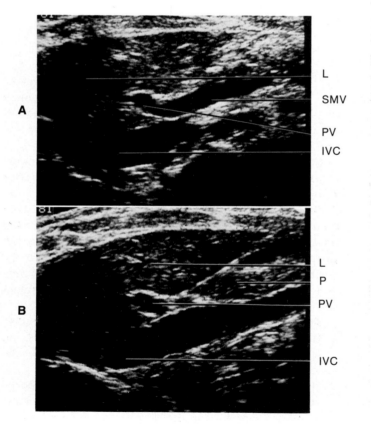

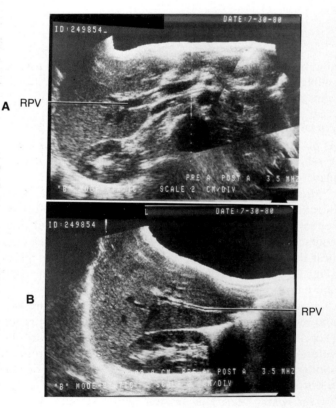

FIG. 12-6. A, Sagittal view of the main portal vein as it is formed by the union of the superior mesenteric vein and splenic vein. **B,** Sagittal view of the main portal vein as it lies anterior to the inferior vena cava. The pancreas may be identified as an echo-producing structure locating inferior to the portal vein and anterior to the inferior vena cava. Superior mesenteric vein, *SMV;* liver, *L;* main portal vein, *PV;* inferior vena cava, *IVC;* pancreas, *P.*

FIG. 12-7. A, Transverse view of the right portal vein. **B,** Sagittal view of the right portal vein, *RPV,* in the right lobe of the liver.

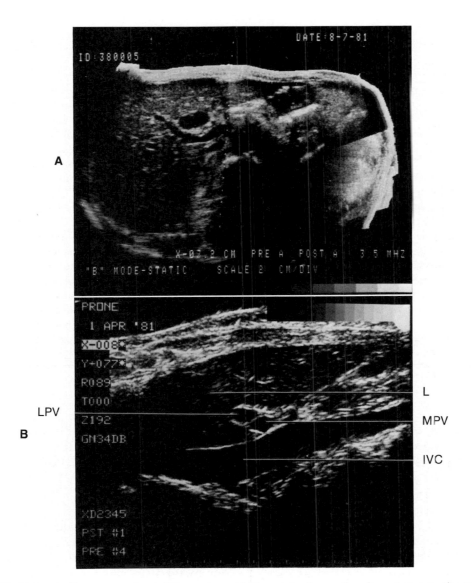

FIG. 12-8.   **A,** Transverse view of the main and left portal veins as they lie anterior to the inferior vena cava. **B,** Sagittal view of the main portal vein as it begins to bifurcate into the left portal vein. Liver, *L;* left portal vein, *LPV;* main portal vein, *MPV;* inferior vena cava, *IVC.*

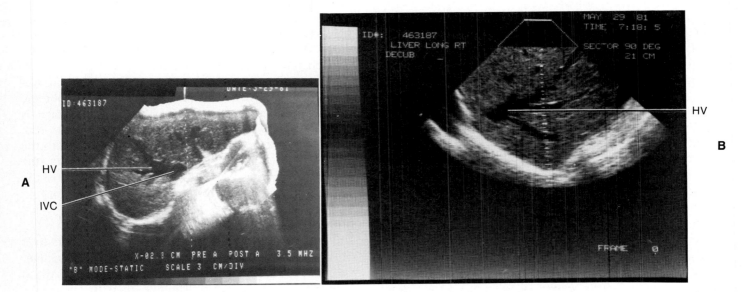

FIG. 12-9.   **A,** Transverse and, **B,** sagittal views of the hepatic veins as they drain into the inferior vena cava at the level of the diaphragm. Hepatic veins, *HV;* inferior vena cava, *IVC.*

Table 12-1   Anatomic Structures Useful for Dividing and Identifying the Hepatic Segments

Structure	Location	Usefulness
RHV	Right intersegmental fissure	Divides cephalic aspect of anterior and posterior segments of right hepatic lobe and courses between anterior and posterior branches of RPV
MHV	Main lobar fissure	Separates right and left lobes
LHV	Left intersegmental fissure	Divides cephalic aspects of medial and lateral segments of left lobe
RPV (anterior)	Intrasegmental in anterior segment of right hepatic lobe	Courses centrally in anterior segment of right hepatic lobe
RPV (posterior)	Intrasegmental in posterior segment of right hepatic lobe	Courses centrally in posterior segment of right hepatic lobe
LPV (initial)	Courses anterior to caudate lobe	Separates caudate lobe posteriorly from medial segment of left lobe anteriorly
LPV (ascending)	Turns anteriorly in left intersegmental fissure	Divides medial and lateral segments of left lobe
IVC fossa	Posterior aspect of main lobar fissure	Separates right and left hepatic lobes
Gb fossa	Main lobar fissure	Separates right and left hepatic lobes
Ligamentum teres	Left intersegmental fissure	Divides caudal aspect of left hepatic lobe into medial and lateral segments
Fissure of ligamentum venosum	Left anterior margin of caudate lobe	Separates caudate lobe from medial and lateral segments of left lobe

From Callen PW: J Clin Ultrasound 7(2):81, 1979.

rior portion of the liver lying between the fossa of the inferior vena cava and the fissure of the ligamentum venosum. The caudate lobe receives portal venous and hepatic arterial blood from both the right and the left systems. The anatomic features that assist in determining the positions of the various hepatic segments are listed in Table 12-1.

Functional division of the liver

The purpose of a functional division of the liver is to separate the liver into component parts according the blood supply and biliary drainage so one component can be removed in the event of tumor invasion or trauma. There are two functional divisions, a right and a left. The right functional lobe includes everything to the right of a plane through the gallbladder fossa and inferior vena cava (which corresponds to the anatomic right lobe) (Fig. 12-10). The left functional lobe includes everything to the left of the above plane (which corresponds to the left lobe, caudate lobe, and quadrate lobe).

Ligaments and fissures

There are three important ligaments and fissures to remember in the liver. The falciform ligament extends from the umbilicus to the diaphragm in a parasagittal plane, containing the ligamentum teres (Fig. 12-11, *A* and *B*). In the anteroposterior axis the ligament extends from the right rectus muscle to the bare area of the liver, where its reflections separate to contribute to the hepatic coronary ligament and attach to the undersurface of the diaphragm. The ligamentum teres appears as a bright echogenic focus on the sonogram and is seen as the rounded termination of the falciform ligament. Both the ligamentum falciform

and the ligamentum teres divide the medial segments of the left lobe of the liver. The fissure for the ligamentum venosum separates the left lobe from the caudate lobe (Fig. 12-12).

Relational anatomy

The fundus of the stomach lies posterior and lateral to the left lobe of the liver and may frequently be seen on transverse sonograms. The remainder of the stomach lies inferior to the liver and is best visualized on sagittal sonograms. The duodenum lies adjacent to the right and quadrate lobes of the liver. The pancreas is usually seen just inferior to the liver. The posterior border of the liver contains the right kidney, IVC, and aorta. The diaphragm covers the superior border of the liver. The liver is suspended from the diaphragm and anterior abdominal wall by the falciform ligament and from the diaphragm by the reflections of the peritoneum. Most of the liver is covered by peritoneum, but a large area rests directly on the diaphragm and this is called the bare area. The subphrenic space between the liver (or spleen) and the diaphragm is a common site for abscess formation. The lesser sac is an enclosed portion of the peritoneal space posterior to the liver and the stomach. This sac communicates with the rest of the peritoneal space at a point near the head of the pancreas. It also may be a site for abscess formation.

Intrahepatic vessels and ducts

The portal veins carry blood from the bowel to the liver whereas the hepatic veins drain the blood from the liver into the IVC. The hepatic arteries carry oxygenated blood from the aorta to the liver. The bile ducts transport bile, manufactured in the liver, to the duodenum.

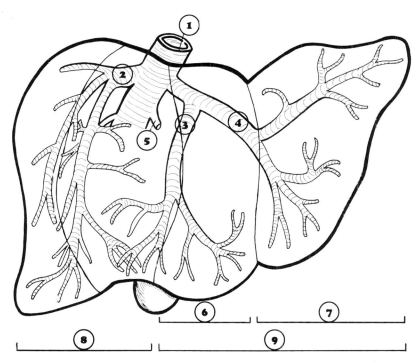

FIG. 12-10. Functional division of the liver. The purpose of a functional division is to separate the liver into component parts according to blood supply and biliary drainage so that one component can be removed in the event of tumor invasion or trauma. Inferior vena cava, *1;* right hepatic vein, *2;* middle hepatic vein, *3;* left hepatic vein, *4;* caudate lobe, *5;* medial segment, *6;* lateral segment, *7;* right lobe, *8;* left lobe, *9.*

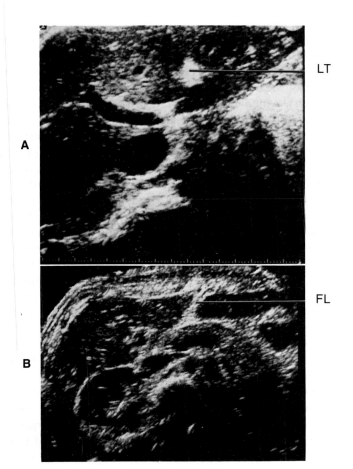

FIG. 12-11. A, The ligamentum teres, *LT,* appears as a very echogenic circular structure at the termination of the falciform ligament. Care should be taken not to confuse this with a mass in the liver. **B,** The falciform ligament, *FL,* is shown in this transverse scan; it divides the left lobe from the quadrate lobe of the liver.

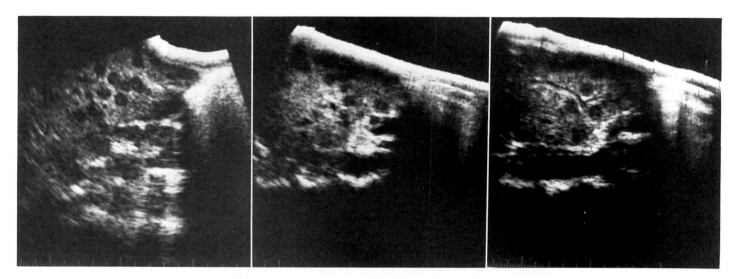

FIG. 12-32.   Sagittal scans made over the liver show multiple metastatic lesions within the liver. These are well demarcated with very low-lying echoes within.

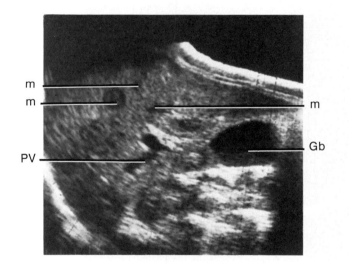

FIG. 12-33.   Sagittal scan over the right upper quadrant shows a distended gallbladder, portal structures, and small well-defined metastatic lesions within the liver. Mass *m;* gallbladder, *Gb;* portal vein, *PV.*

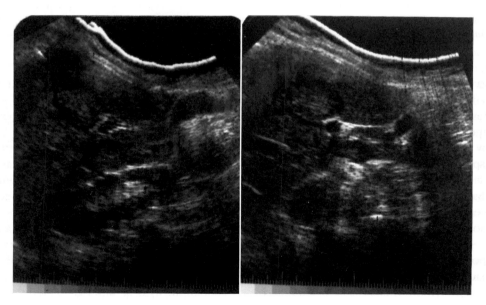

FIG. 12-34.   Sagittal scans show hepatomegaly and multiple filling defects within the liver representing metastatic disease. The defects are low echo producing with a "halo" type of echo pattern surrounding the lesion.

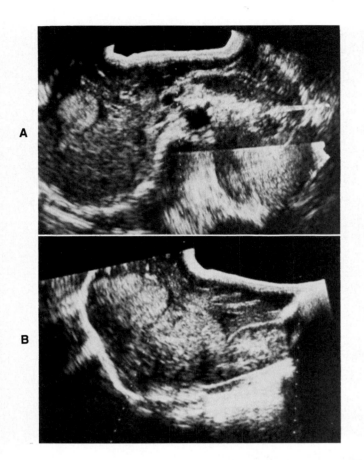

FIG. 12-35. **A,** Transverse and, **B,** sagittal scans of a 53-year-old man status post resection of distal colonic carcinoma. Extensive hyperechoic masses and para-aortic adenopathy were seen.

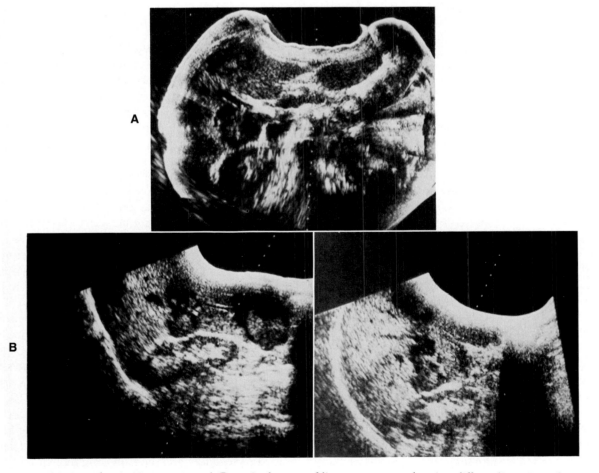

FIG. 12-36. **A,** Transverse and, **B,** sagittal scans of liver metastases showing diffuse distortion of the normal homogeneous parenchymal pattern.

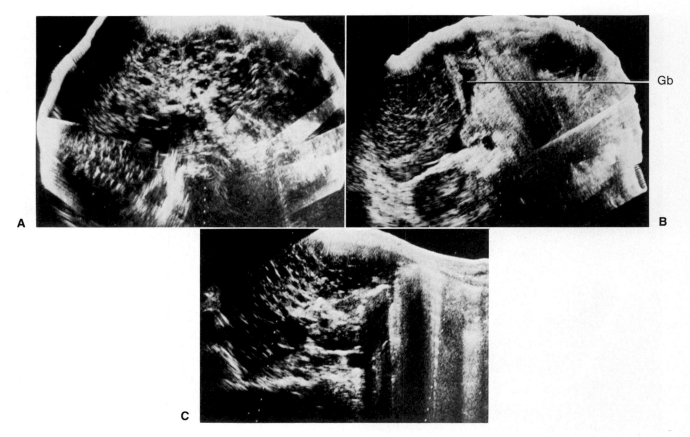

FIG. 12-37. **A** and **B**, Transverse and, **C**, sagittal scans of a patient with diffuse liver metastases. A thickened gallbladder, *Gb*, is also seen in **B**.

Lymphoma. Generally patients with lymphoma have hepatic involvement that shows sonographically as hepatomegaly with a normal liver pattern or a diffuse alteration of echo architecture with no evidence of a focal mass. Occasionally a focal echogenic or sonolucent mass is seen in a lymphoma patient. The presence of splenomegaly or retroperitoneal nodes may help to confirm the diagnosis of lymphadenopathy.

Diffuse abnormalities. Diffuse abnormalities of the liver may be seen sonographically as inhomogeneities within the liver parenchyma. Such abnormalities as biliary obstruction, hepatic metastases, common duct stones and stricture, extrahepatic masses, and passive hepatic congestion will be discussed as they present sonographically.

Biliary obstruction proximal to the cystic duct can be carcinoma of the common bile duct or hepatic metastases in the porta hepatis. In the former, jaundice and pruritus are the clinical signs. Laboratory data show an increase in direct bilirubin and alkaline phosphatase. The echo appearance of carcinoma of the common bile duct is tubular branching with fluid-filled structures (dilated hepatic ducts) that are best seen in the periphery of the liver on longitudinal scans. No mass is visualized. The gallbladder is of normal size, even after a fatty meal.

Hepatic metastases in the porta hepatis present the same clinical signs and laboratory data, except that there is abnormal hepatocellular function. The echo appearance is of an intrahepatic mass in the area of the porta hepatis that may be more or less echo producing than the normal parenchyma (Fig. 12-39). The dilated hepatic bile ducts are best seen on the longitudinal scans. Intrahepatic masses are usually associated with other hepatic metastases in other areas of the liver. The gallbladder is of normal size, even after a fatty meal.

Biliary obstruction distal to the cystic duct may be caused by common duct stones, extrahepatic masses in the porta hepatis, or common duct stricture.

1. Common duct stones cause right upper quadrant pain, jaundice, and pruritus as well as an increase in direct bilirubin and alkaline phosphatase. The echo appearance, best seen on sagittal scans, shows the dilated hepatic bile ducts in the periphery of the liver. The gallbladder size is variable, usually small. Gallstones are often present and appear as dense echoes along the bed of the gallbladder with an acoustic shadow posterior. The stones within the duct may be seen if they are large enough; a shadow may also be present.

2. Clinical signs of the extrahepatic masses at the porta hepatis include jaundice and symptoms referable to primary disease, and laboratory data are the same as for a stone in the common duct. The echo appearance shows an extrahepatic mass in the area of the porta hepatis, which could be lymph node enlargement, pancreatitis, a pseudocyst, or carcinoma in the head of the pancreas. The tubular branching and fluid-filled, dilated hepatic ducts are seen on longitudinal and transverse scans. The gallbladder is dilated, with no change in size after a fatty meal.

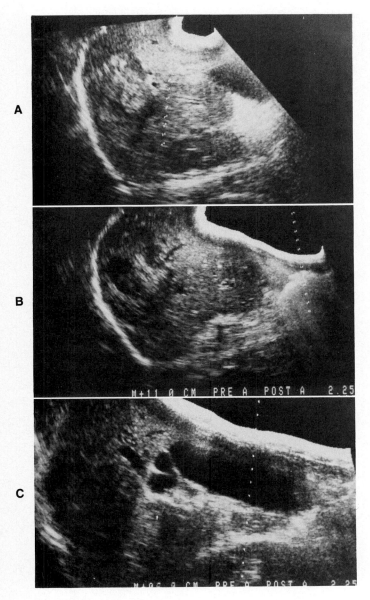

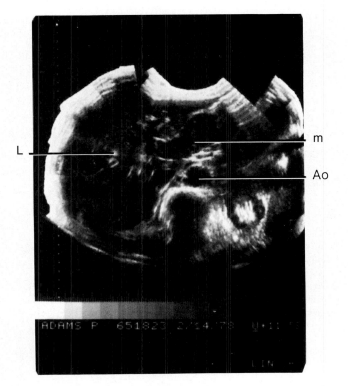

FIG. 12-39.   Transverse scan over the upper abdomen reveals a large, low-level echo-producing mass in the region of the porta hepatis. With further scanning one is able to demonstrate the mass as separate from the pancreas and retroperitoneal structures. Such a mass in the porta hepatis will also show dilated intrahepatic ducts. Liver, *L;* mass, *m;* aorta, *Ao.*

FIG. 12-38.   Sagittal scans of a young patient with oat cell carcinoma who now presents with jaundice, hepatomegaly, and anorexia. The scan showed a mass in the pancreatic head causing ductal obstruction and a distended gallbladder, **C,** and multiple liver metastases. The areas of inhomogeneity in the right lobe of the liver are evident in **A** and **B.**

3. Common duct stricture can be diagnosed by jaundice and past history of cholecystectomy. Direct bilirubin is increased, as is alkaline phosphatase. The echo appearance is dilated hepatic ducts with no porta hepatic mass.

Passive hepatic congestion is another diffuse hepatic abnormality. Generally it develops secondary to congestive heart failure, showing clinical signs of hepatomegaly. Laboratory data indicate normal or slightly abnormal hepatocellular function. The echo appearance shows dilated hepatic and portal veins that are more prominent centrally then peripherally. These structures are usually nonbranching (as the hepatic ducts are) and may decrease in size with expiration or increase with inspiration. The inferior vena cava is usually dilated, as are the superior mesenteric and splenic veins.

SUMMARY

1. The liver is the largest organ in the body and occupies almost all of the right hypochondrium, the greater part of the epigastrium, and the left hypochondrium as far as the mammillary line. The liver is divided into four lobes: right, left, caudate, and quadrate.

2. There are three important ligaments and fissures to remember in the liver: the falciform ligament, the ligamentum teres, and the ligamentum venosum.

3. The portal veins carry blood from the bowel to the liver. The hepatic veins drain the blood from the liver into the inferior vena cava. The hepatic arteries carry oxygenated blood from the aorta to the liver. The bile ducts transport bile manufactured in the liver to the duodenum.

4. The liver is a major center of metabolism and detoxification of the waste products of metabolism accumulated from other sources in the body and foreign chemicals that enter the body. These waste products are expelled through bile. The liver is a storage site for several compounds used in a variety of physiologic activities throughout the body.

5. Disease affecting the liver may be hepatocellular or obstructive.

6. The liver functions as a major site for conversion of dietary sugars into glucose. The liver is a principal site for metabolism of fats. The liver produces a wide variety of proteins. Enzymes are protein catalysts used throughout the body in all metabolic processes.

7. Bile is the excretory product of the liver. It is formed continuously by the hepatocytes, collects in the bile canaliculi adjacent to these cells, and is transported to the intestines via the bile ducts.

8. The majority of blood passing through the small and large bowel is collected in the portal venous system and transported to the liver.

9. The sonographic evaluation of the liver parenchyma includes assessment of its size, configuration, and contour. The hepatic parenchymal pattern changes with disease processes. Intrahepatic, extrahepatic, subhepatic, and subdiaphragmatic masses can be outlined and their internal composition recognized by specific echo patterns.

REFERENCES

1. Filly RA, Allen B, Menton M, et al: In vitro investigation of the origin of echoes within biliary sludge, J Clin Ultrasound 8:193, 1980.

2. Marks WM, Filly RA, and Callen PW: Ultrasonic anatomy of the liver: a review with new applications, J Clin Ultrasound 7:137, 1979.

13

Gallbladder and the Biliary System

SANDRA L. HAGEN-ANSERT

Ultrasonic evaluation of the gallbladder and biliary system has been very effective in the diagnosis of disease. Furthermore, real-time evaluation of the patient with gallbladder disease has proved to be an efficient method of diagnosing such diseases as cholelithiasis, cholecystitis, or duct dilation.

ANATOMY OF THE EXTRAHEPATIC BILIARY SYSTEM

The extrahepatic biliary apparatus consists of the right and left hepatic ducts, the common hepatic duct, the common bile duct, the gallbladder, and the cystic duct (Fig. 13-1).

Hepatic ducts

The right and left hepatic ducts emerge from the right lobe of the liver in the porta hepatis and unite to form the common hepatic duct, which then passes caudally and medially. The hepatic duct runs parallel with the portal vein. Each duct is formed by the union of bile canaliculi from the liver lobules.

The common hepatic duct is approximately 4 mm in diameter and descends within the edge of the lesser omentum. It is joined by the cystic duct to form the common bile duct.

Common bile duct

The normal common bile duct has a diameter of up to 6 mm. The first part of the duct lies in the right free edge of the lesser omentum (Fig. 13-2). In the second part the duct is situated posterior to the first part of the duodenum. The third part lies in a groove on the posterior surface of the head of the pancreas. It ends by piercing the medial wall of the second part of the duodenum about halfway down the duodenal length. There the common bile duct is joined by the main pancreatic duct, and together they open through a small ampulla (the ampulla of Vater) into the duodenal wall. The end parts of both ducts (common bile duct and main pancreatic duct) and the ampulla are surrounded by circular muscle fibers known as the sphincter of Oddi.

The proximal portion of the common bile duct is lateral to the hepatic artery and anterior to the portal vein. The duct moves more posterior after it descends behind the duodenal bulb and enters the pancreas. The distal duct lies parallel with the anterior wall of the vena cava.

Within the liver parenchyma the bile ducts follow the same course as the portal venous and hepatic arterial branches. The hepatic and bile ducts are encased in a common collagenous sheath forming the *portal triad.*

225

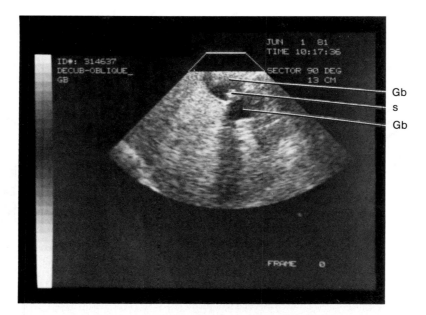

Gb
s
Gb

FIG. 13-5.   Oblique decubitus scan of a patient with a double gallbladder. A stone is in the more anterior sac. The acoustic shadow from the stone is seen posterior. Gallbladder, *Gb*; stone, *s*.

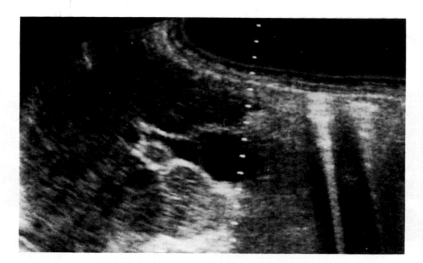

FIG. 13-6.   One anatomic variation of the normal gallbladder includes a folding of the fundus (Phrygian cap).

store bile for intermittent release in conjunction with eating.

To facilitate storage, the gallbladder mucosa concentrates bile by active transport of water; and as a result gallbladder bile may be twice as concentrated as hepatic bile. Filling of the gallbladder is passive and occurs during fasting, when the sphincter of Oddi (located at the junction of the common bile duct and the duodenum) is closed. The valves of Hyster in the neck of the gallbladder are not really valves and do not affect flow into or out of the gallbladder. Instead, they probably function to prevent kinking of the duct. Release of bile from the gallbladder appears to result from combined hormonal and neuronal activity, including simultaneous contraction of the gallbladder and relaxation of the sphincter of Oddi. The mechanism is not well established, however. Contraction of the gallbladder against a closed outlet is reported to

cause pressures of 100 to 200 mm of water, a factor no doubt accounting for the severe pain that occurs when a stone obstructs the cystic duct.

SONOGRAPHIC EVALUATION OF THE NORMAL GALLBLADDER AND BILIARY SYSTEM
Gallbladder

To ensure maximum dilation of the gallbladder, the patient should be given nothing to eat at least 8 to 12 hours prior to the ultrasound examination. The patient is initially examined in the supine position with a real-time sector scanner. Transverse, oblique, and sagittal scans are made over the upper abdomen to identify the gallbladder, biliary system, liver, right kidney, and head of the pancreas (Fig. 13-7). The patient should also be rolled into a steep decubitus or upright position in an attempt to sepa-

A   **B**

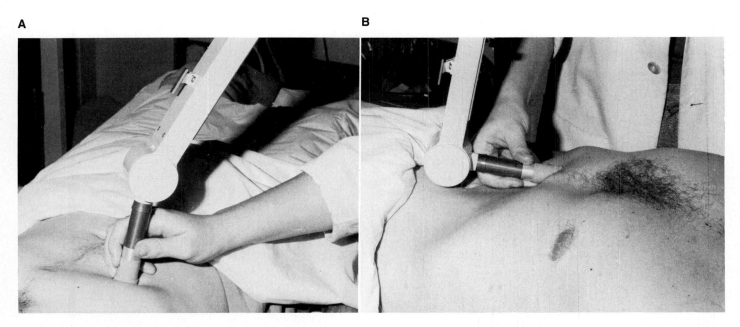

FIG. 13-7. **A,** Transverse oblique scan technique is used for better visualization of the gallbladder located under the costal margin. **B,** Sagittal oblique scans of the gallbladder area are performed with the patient in deep inspiration. The transducer is arced under the costal margin to record the interface of the gallbladder and liver.

rate small stones from the gallbladder wall or cystic duct (Fig. 13-8).

The gallbladder may be identified as a sonolucent oblong structure located anterior to the right kidney, lateral to the head of the pancreas and duodenum, indenting the inferior to medial aspect of the right lobe of the liver (Fig. 13-9). The sagittal scans show the right kidney posterior to the gallbladder. The fundus is generally oriented slightly more anterior, and on sagittal scans often reaches the anterior abdominal wall.

Carter et al.[2] have reported seeing on sagittal scans a bright linear echo within the liver connecting the gallbladder and the right or main portal vein in a high percentage of patients (Fig. 13-10). They stated that the neck of the gallbladder usually comes into contact with the main segment of the portal vein near the origin of the left portal vein. The gallbladder commonly resides in a fossa on the medial aspect of the liver. Because of fat or fibrous tissue within the main lobar fissure of the liver (which lies between the gallbladder and the right portal vein), this bright linear reflector was a reliable indicator of the location of the gallbladder. The gallbladder lies in the posterior and caudal aspect of the fissure. The caudal aspect of the linear echo "pointed" directly to or touched the gallbladder.

A small echogenic fold has been reported to occur along the posterior wall of the gallbladder at the junction of the body and infundibulum. It may be very small (3 to 5 mm) but may give rise to an acoustic shadow in the supine position. It is not duplicated in the oblique position (Fig. 13-11). The causes for such a junctional fold are the incisurae between the body and infundibulum or the Heister valves, which are spiral folds beginning in the neck of the gallbladder and lining the cystic duct.

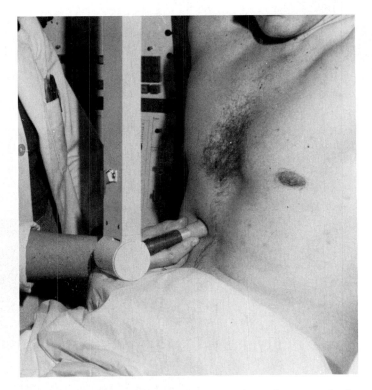

FIG. 13-8. Upright scan performed to evaluate the internal echoes within the gallbladder. Normally the bile should be sonolucent, but with disease low-level to bright-reflector echoes appear. A change in position should alter these echoes to prove that they are stones or real structures within the gallbladder parenchyma.

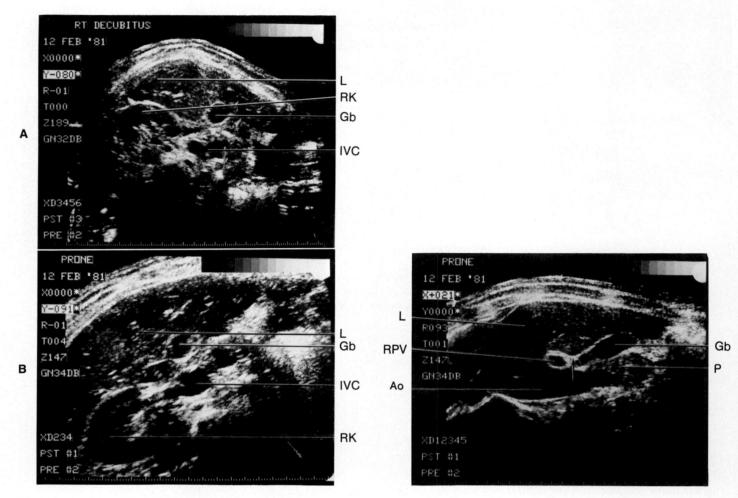

FIG. 13-9. **A,** Right decubitus and, **B,** transverse supine scans over the right upper quadrant show the gallbladder, *Gb,* as a sonolucent, rounded structure just anterior to the right kidney, *RK,* and inferior vena cava, *IVC,* and posterior to the liver, *L.*

FIG. 13-10. Sagittal scan of the gallbladder, *Gb,* right portal vein, *RPV,* and linear bright reflector of the main lobar fissure of the liver *(arrow).* Pancreas, *P;* liver, *L.*

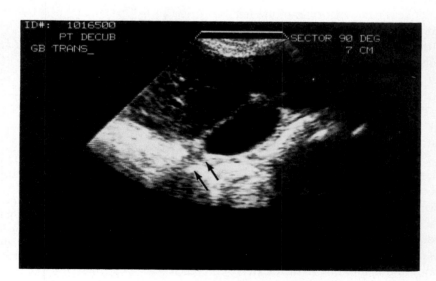

FIG. 13-11. The neck of the gallbladder may project soft shadowing due to the folds at the junction of the body and infundibulum *(arrows).*

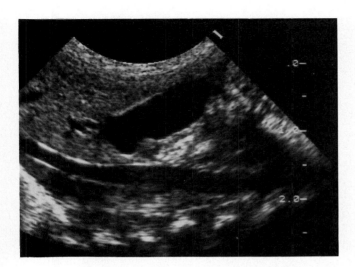

FIG. 13-12. Sagittal view of a distended gallbladder. The cystic duct is well seen. The inferior vena cava lies along the posterior border of the gallbladder.

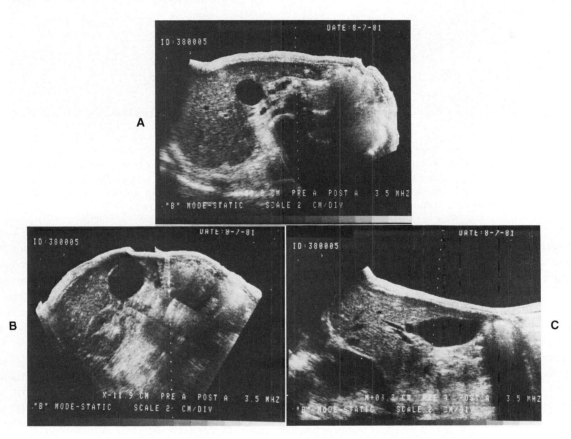

FIG. 13-13. **A** and **B,** Supine transverse scans of a prominent gallbladder. The AP diameter is 4.3 cm, slightly enlarged for a normal gallbladder. This patient should be given a fatty meal and rescanned in 40 minutes to see whether the gallbladder will contract. **C,** Sagittal scan of the gallbladder. The portal veins are shown superior to the neck of the gallbladder.

A prominent gallbladder may be normal in some individuals because of their fasting state (Figs. 13-12 and 13-13). A large gallbladder has been detected in patients with diabetes, patients who are bedridden with protracted illness or pancreatitis, and those who are taking anticholinergic drugs. Such a gallbladder may even fail to contract following a fatty meal, or intravenous cholecystokinin and other studies may be needed to make the diagnosis of obstruction.

If a gallbladder appears too large, a fatty meal may be administered and further sonographic evaluation made to detect whether the enlargement is abnormal or normal. If the gallbladder fails to contract during the examination, further investigation of the pancreatic area should be made. Courvoisier's sign indicates an extrahepatic mass compressing the common bile duct, which can produce an enlarged gallbladder (Fig. 13-14). In addition, the liver should be carefully examined for the presence of dilated bile ducts.

In a well-contracted gallbladder the wall changes from a single to a double concentric structure with three components recognized as reported by Marchal et al.[15]: (1) a

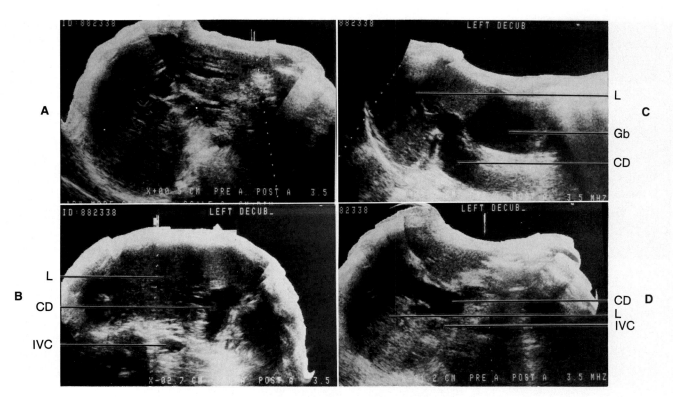

FIG. 13-14. This patient presented with jaundice and a palpable abdominal mass. Ultrasound was asked to rule out obstructive versus nonobstructive jaundice. A pancreatic mass was found with obstruction to the common duct. **A,** Transverse supine scan over the liver. **B,** Transverse left decubitus views over the dilated common duct. **C,** Sagittal left decubitus view over the dilated common duct and distended gallbladder. **D,** Left decubitus view showing the dilated common bile duct. *L,* liver; *CD,* common duct; *IVC,* inferior vena cava; *Gb,* gallbladder.

strongly reflective outer contour, (2) a poorly reflective inner contour, and (3) a sonolucent area between both reflecting structures.

Bile ducts

Sonographically the common duct lies anterior and to the right of the portal vein in the region of the porta hepatis and gastrohepatic ligament (Fig. 13-15). The hepatic artery lies anterior and to the left of the portal vein. On a transverse scan the common duct, hepatic artery, and portal vein have been referred to as the Mickey Mouse sign by Bartrum and Crow[1] (Fig. 13-16). The portal vein serves as Mickey's face, with the right ear the common duct and the left ear the hepatic artery. To obtain such a cross section, the transducer must be directed in a slightly oblique path from the left shoulder to the right hip.

On sagittal scans the right branch of the hepatic artery usually passes posterior to the common duct. The common duct is seen just anterior to the portal vein before it dips posteriorly to enter the head of the pancreas. The patient may be rotated into a slight (45-degree) or steep (90-degree) right anterior oblique position with the beam directed posteromedially to visualize the duct. This enables the examiner to avoid cumbersome bowel gas and to use the liver as an acoustic window.

When the right subcostal approach is used, the main portal vein may be seen as it bifurcates into the right and left branches. As the right branch continues into the right lobe of the liver, the right branch can be followed laterally in a longitudinal plane. The portal vein appears as an almond-shaped sonolucent structure anterior to the inferior vena cava. The common hepatic duct is seen as a tubular structure anterior to the portal vein. The right branch of the hepatic artery can be seen between the duct and the portal vein as a small circular structure.

The small cystic duct is generally not identified; and since this landmark is needed to distinguish the common hepatic from the common bile duct, a more general term of common duct is used to refer to these structures.

CLINICAL SYMPTOMS OF GALLBLADDER DISEASE

The most classic symptom of gallbladder disease is right upper quadrant abdominal pain, usually occurring after ingestion of greasy foods. Nausea and vomiting sometimes occurs and may indicate the presence of a stone in the common bile duct. A gallbladder attack may cause pain in the right shoulder, with inflammation of the gallbladder often causing referred pain in the right shoulder blade.

Gallstones

After a fatty meal the gallbladder contracts to release bile; and if the outflow tract is blocked by gallstones, pain results. As the bile is being stored in the gallbladder, small crystals of bile salts precipitate and may form gallstones

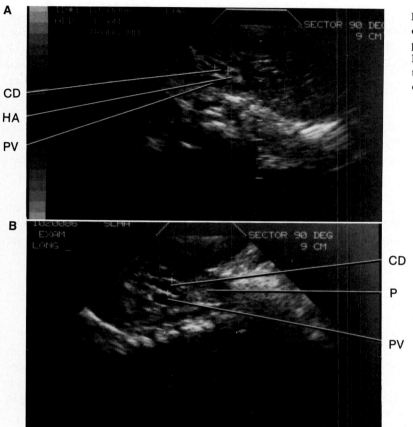

FIG. 13-15. **A,** Transverse scan of the portal vein, *PV,* common bile duct, *CD,* and hepatic artery, *HA.* The caliper markers measure the common bile duct at 7 mm. **B,** Sagittal scan of the common duct as it lies anterior to the portal vein, before dipping posteriorly into the pancreas, *P.*

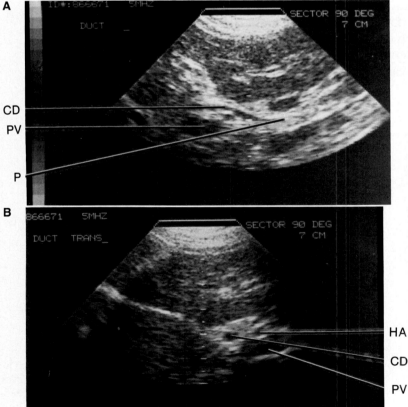

FIG. 13-16. **A,** Sagittal scan of the common bile duct as visualized anterior to the portal vein, *PV.* A 5 MHz transducer is used to image the very small vessel. **B,** Transverse view of the "Mickey Mouse" sign. The common bile duct, *CD,* is anterior and to the right of the portal vein, *PV,* while the hepatic artery, *HA,* lies anterior and to the left. *P,* pancreas.

varying from pinhead size to the size of the organ itself. There may be a single large gallstone or hundreds of tiny ones. The tiny stones are the most dangerous, since they can enter the bile ducts and obstruct the outflow of bile.

Jaundice

Jaundice is characterized by the presence of bile in the tissues with resulting yellow-green color of the skin. It may develop when a tiny gallstone blocks the bile ducts between the gallbladder and the intestines, producing pressure on the liver and forcing bile into the blood.

Cholecystitis

Inflammation of the gallbladder usually is a chronic illness punctuated by intermittent acute episodes, which occur when the cystic duct is obstructed by a calculus. Calculi (gallstones) are almost always associated with cholecystitis, although rare cases of "acalculus cholecystitis" are believed to occur. About 85% of gallstones are composed entirely of cholesterol; 10% are bile pigment stones, and 5% are a combination of bile pigments and cholesterol. Varying degrees of calcification may be superimposed, with the result that some stones are visible radiographically. Gallstones occur commonly in whites (more than 25% of persons over age 40) and occur with even higher incidence in specific populations such as Swedes and American Indians.

The relationship of gallstones to the pathogenesis of cholecystitis has long been a point of debate. Which comes first, the stone or the inflammation? The current tendency is to regard cholecystitis as a result of gallstone formation rather than a cause of it. This view is supported by the discovery of *lithogenic bile,* a form of bile supersaturated with cholesterol that is found in some individuals but not in others. *Lecithin* and bile salts keep cholesterol in *solution* in bile; hence the relative concentration of these elements may determine whether cholesterol precipitates and forms stones. In patients with lithogenic

bile the liver secretes too much cholesterol relative to the amount of lecithin and bile salts present. It is believed that precipitated cholesterol crystals in such patients aggregate and grow, forming stones. Gallstones may result in inflammation of the gallbladder mucosa through direct contact or by intermittent obstruction of the cystic duct. In the latter case, overdistension is believed to stretch the gallbladder wall excessively and produce ischemia. Obstruction also causes stasis, which promotes bacterial growth in the bile. Both ischemia and stasis are believed to account for the inflammation and scarring that occur in cholecystitis.

The gallbladder is not an essential organ. When the gallbladder is removed surgically, the common duct is believed to distend in some cases and take over the reservoir function.

PATHOLOGIC PATTERNS OF GALLBLADDER DISEASE
Gallbladder sludge

Occasionally a patient presents sonographically with a prominent gallbladder containing low-level internal echoes that may be attributed to thick or inspissated bile[3] (Fig. 13-17). Filly et al.[6] state that the source of echoes in biliary sludge is particulate matter (predominantly pig-

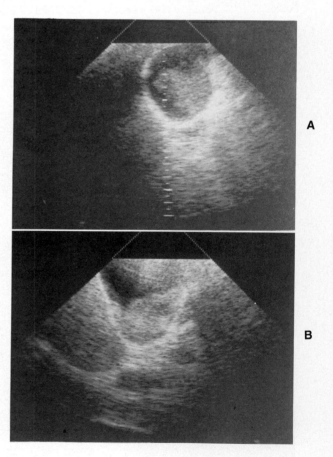

FIG. 13-18. A, Sagittal scan of a gallbladder with inspissated bile. **B,** Transverse scan with echogenic bile appearing very irregular and not layering out as would be expected. A tumor was questioned but ruled out because all the echoes were not reflective as one would expect tumor echoes to be.

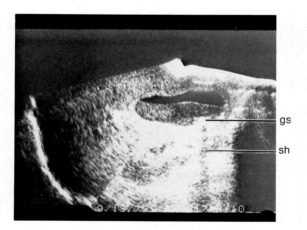

FIG. 13-17. Sagittal scan of a prominent gallbladder with echogenic bile layering along the posterior border. In addition, a bright reflector from a gallstone is seen along the posterior border with a shadow beyond. Gallstone, *gs;* shadow, *sh.*

ment granules with lesser amounts of cholesterol crystals). They report that the viscosity does not appear to be important in the generation of internal echoes in fluids. The particles can be very small and still produce perceptible echoes.

Some gallbladders may be so packed with inspissated bile that it becomes difficult to separate the gallbladder from the liver parenchyma (Fig. 13-18). Occasionally the thick bile is also found in the common duct due to obstruction.[4] Sludge is gravity dependent; thus with alterations in patient position, one may be able to separate sludge from occasional artifactual echoes found in the gallbladder. Filly et al.[6] state that sludge should be considered an abnormal finding, because either a functional or a pathologic abnormality exists when calcium bilirubin or cholesterol precipitates in bile (Fig. 13-19).

Wall thickness

The normal wall thickness of the gallbladder is 1 to 2 mm. Sonographically it may be underestimated when the wall has extensive fibrosis or is surrounded by fat.[8]

The sonographic appearance of acute cholecystitis has been identified as a gallbladder with an irregular outline of a thickened wall (Fig. 13-20). In addition, Marchal et al. [14,15] have found a sonolucent area within the thickened wall probably caused by edema. A study by Engel et al.[5] of wall thickness indicated that 98% of patients whose gallbladder walls were thick had disease whereas 50% with gallbladder disease had a wall thickness of less than 3 mm.

Sanders[17] states that the wall is not always thick in acute cholecystitis. Some walls will be thicker because of pericholecystic abscess. Occasionally a thickened gallbladder wall is seen in normal individuals. It seems to be related to the degree of contraction of a normal gallbladder. Sanders found the gallbladder wall thickened symmetrically with smooth outlines in patients with acute cholecystitis without abscess or ascites. If the thickened wall is localized and irregular, one should consider cholecystosis or carcinoma of the gallbladder.

Another condition wherein the gallbladder wall may be thickened is gangrenous cholecystitis. The wall is also edematous with focal areas of exudate, hemorrhage, and

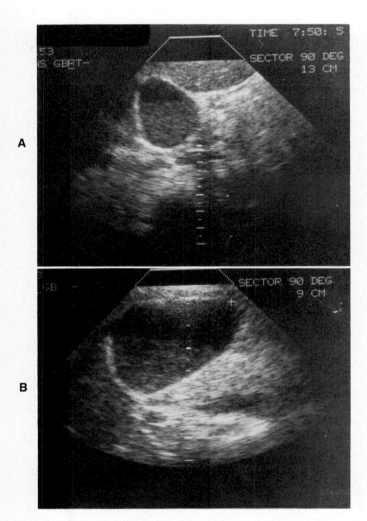

FIG. 13-19. **A,** Transverse and, **B,** sagittal scans of a prominent gallbladder with echogenic bile layering along the posterior border.

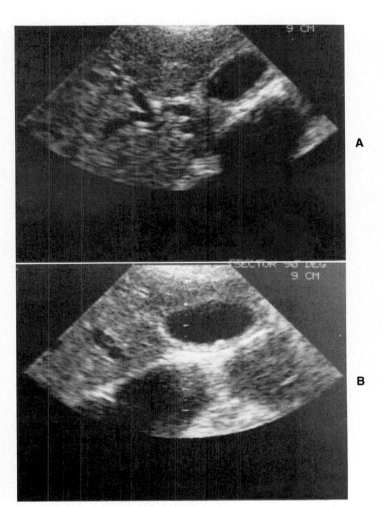

FIG. 13-20. This patient presented with jaundice and increased alkaline phosphatase values. **A,** Transverse view shows the thickened gallbladder walls with dilated ducts. **B,** Sagittal view demonstrates the gallbladder to be of normal size; however, the walls are thickened.

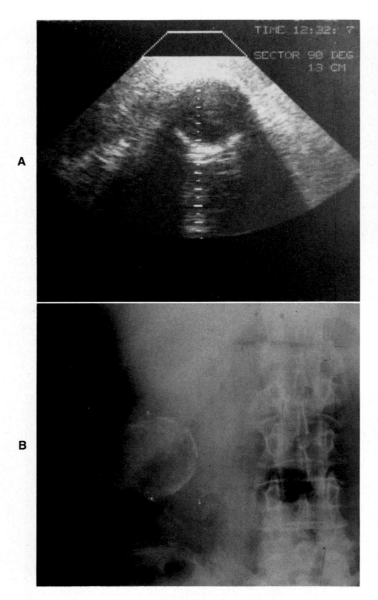

FIG. 13-21. **A,** If the gallbladder walls are calcified, wall thickness may be difficult to assess. These walls are very bright reflectors, and decreased through-transmission with shadowing is noted posteriorly. **B,** Radiography of the calcified "porcelain" gallbladder.

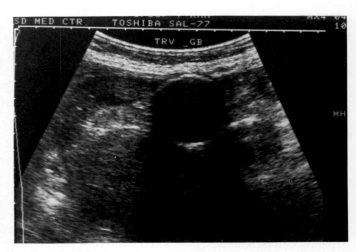

FIG. 13-22. Another patient who presents with a highly reflective gallbladder shows a distended gallbladder without wall thickness (as imaged with a 5 MHz transducer) and definite shadowing posterior to the "porcelain" gallbladder.

necrosis. In addition, there may be ulcerations and perforations resulting in pericholecystic abscesses or peritonitis. Gallstones or fine gravel occur in 80% to 95% of the patients. Kane[12] states that the common echo features of gangrene are the presence of diffuse medium to coarse echogenic densities filling the gallbladder lumen in the absence of bile duct obstruction. This echogenic material has three characteristics: (1) it does not cause shadowing, (2) it is not gravity dependent, and (3) it does not show a layering effect. The lack of layering is attributed to increased viscosity of the bile.

Fiski et al.[9] have stated that a thickened wall is a nonspecific sign and is not necessarily related to gallbladder disease. It may be found in the following conditions besides those previously discussed: hepatitis, adenomyomatosis, gallbladder tumor, or severe hypoalbuminemic states (Figs. 13-21 and 13-22).

Cholelithiasis

The evaluation of gallstones with real time has proven to be an extremely useful procedure in patients who present with symptoms of cholelithiasis. The gallbladder is evaluated for increased size, wall thickness, presence of internal reflections within the lumen, and posterior acoustic shadowing. Frequently patients with gallstones will have a dilated gallbladder. Stones that are less than 1 to 2 mm may be difficult to separate from one another by ultrasound evaluation and thus are reported as gallstones without comment on the specific number that may have been seen on the scan.

If an articulated arm scanner is used, care must be exercised in evaluating the gallbladder by use of a single-sweep technique and remaining perpendicular to the gallbladder and the stone. Slight sectoring will almost certainly fill in the shadow posterior to the stone and thus cause the stone to be overlooked (Fig. 13-23).

Regardless of the equipment used, the patient's position should be shifted during the procedure to demonstrate further the presence of the stones. Patients should be scanned in the right-side-up decubitus, right lateral, or upright position. The stones should shift to the most dependent area of the gallbladder. In some cases the bile has a thick consistency and the stones remain near the top of the gallbladder. Thus the density of the stones and the shadow posterior will be the sonographic evidence for stones (Figs. 13-24 to 13-28).

Gonzalez and MacIntyre[10] have evaluated the theory for acoustic shadowing formed from gallstones and discovered that scattered reflections do not affect shadowing as much as specular reflections do. The factors that produced a shadow were attributed to acoustic impedance of the gallstones; refraction through them or diffraction around them; their size, central or peripheral location, and position in relation to the focus of the beam; and the intensity of the beam.

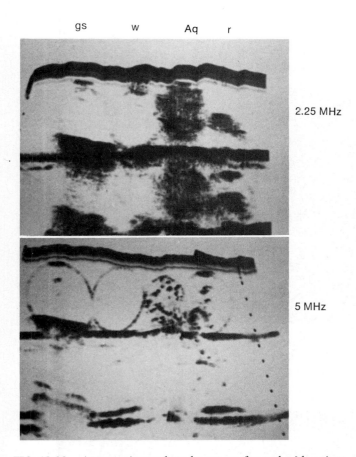

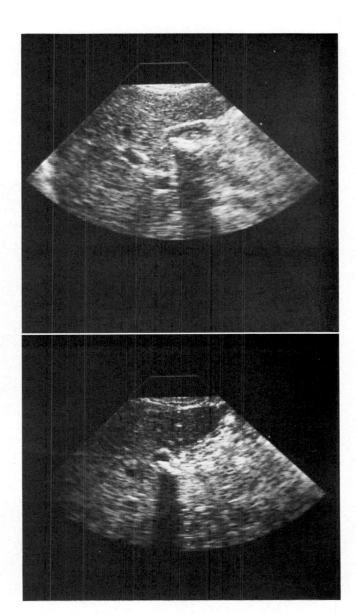

FIG. 13-23.   An experimental study was performed with a simulated gallbladder (a balloon) filled with sand to represent gallstones, *gs;* water to represent bile, *w;* aquasonic to represent thickened bile, *Aq;* and an actual gallstone, *r.* Scans were performed with a 2.25 and a 5.0 MHz transducer to evaluate resolution capabilities of the equipment. Low and high sensitivities were used to evaluate transmission quality.

FIG. 13-24.   Multiple echogenic foci (cholelithiasis) are identified in a gallbladder with posterior acoustic shadowing.

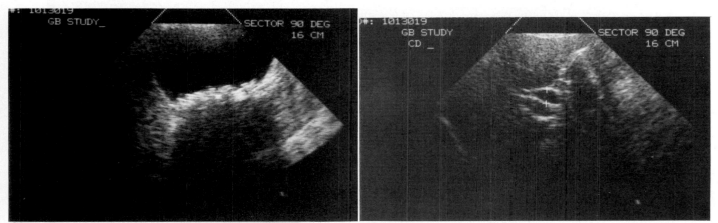

FIG. 13-25.   Nonviscous oral cholecystogram. **A,** Sagittal scan demonstrates a large gallbladder with multiple reflective stones along the posterior wall. An acoustic shadow is present. **B,** The common duct measures 12 mm and is considered to be enlarged.

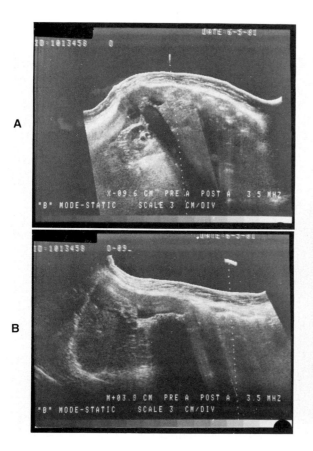

A

B

FIG. 13-26. This patient presented with liver metastases and a "packed bag." **A,** Transverse scan shows the anterior border of the gallbladder with a strong acoustic shadow posteriorly. **B,** Sagittal scan shows the sharply marginated shadow from the packed bag.

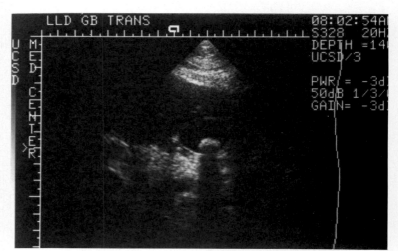

FIG. 13-27. Transverse scan over the gallbladder area shows a normal size gallbladder with a large single stone within. The shadow is well demarcated beyond the stone.

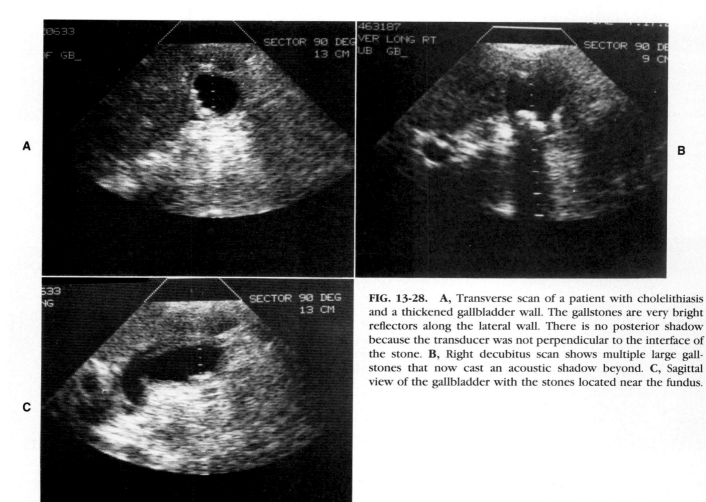

A

B

C

FIG. 13-28. **A,** Transverse scan of a patient with cholelithiasis and a thickened gallbladder wall. The gallstones are very bright reflectors along the lateral wall. There is no posterior shadow because the transducer was not perpendicular to the interface of the stone. **B,** Right decubitus scan shows multiple large gallstones that now cast an acoustic shadow beyond. **C,** Sagittal view of the gallbladder with the stones located near the fundus.

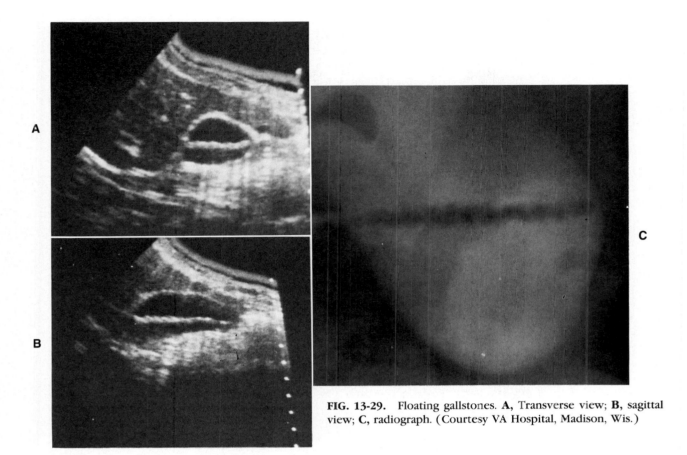

FIG. 13-29. Floating gallstones. **A,** Transverse view; **B,** sagittal view; **C,** radiograph. (Courtesy VA Hospital, Madison, Wis.)

Filly et al.[6,7] found in their in vitro phantom studies that all stones cast acoustic shadows regardless of the specific properties of the stones. The size of the stone was important, with stones greater than 3 mm always casting a shadow and those smaller than 3 mm sometimes not casting one. They found that any stone scanned two or more times with the same transducer and machine settings might or might not generate a shadow even though the scans were within seconds of each other. The shadow was highly dependent on the relationship between the stone and the acoustic beam. If the central beam was at or near the stone, a shadow would be seen. Thus some critical ratio between the stone diameter and the beam width must be achieved before shadowing is seen.

Floating gallstones

Some stones are seen to float when contrast material from an oral cholecystogram is present. This is because of the higher specific gravity of the contrast material than of the bile. The gallstones seek a level where their specific gravity equals that of the mixture of bile and contrast material[18] (Fig. 13-29).

Gas in the biliary tree shadow

Another cause for shadowing in the right upper quadrant is gas in the biliary tree. This is a spontaneous occurrence due to the formation of a biliary enteric fistula in chronic gallbladder disease.[8] The sonogram demonstrates the liver parenchyma to be disrupted by narrow bands of acoustic shadows lying behind well-defined discrete high-amplitude echoes deep within the liver parenchyma (Fig. 13-30).

Primary carcinoma of the gallbladder

Carcinoma of the gallbladder is very rare. A small tumor in the neck may not even be seen by sonography if secondary signs of obstruction and dilation are absent. The most frequent sonographic sign is a large, irregular, fungating mass that contains low-intensity echoes within the gallbladder. Sometimes the mass will completely fill the gallbladder, obscuring the gallbladder walls. There may be stones along with the tumor, causing posterior shadowing. The differential diagnosis of carcinoma, empyema, and xanthogranulomatous cholecystitis is virtually impossible by ultrasound, and surgical intervention may be the only recourse (Fig. 13-31).

Polyps in the gallbladder

A polyp appears sonographically as a low-level echo mass adjacent to the wall of the gallbladder. Generally it will not change in position or produce an acoustic shadow as will a gallstone. It is usually attached to the gallbladder wall by a short stalk (Fig. 13-32).

Dilated ducts

The common hepatic duct has an internal diameter of less than 4 mm (Figs. 13-33 and 13-34).[10,11] A duct diameter of 5 mm is borderline, and 6 mm requires further investi-

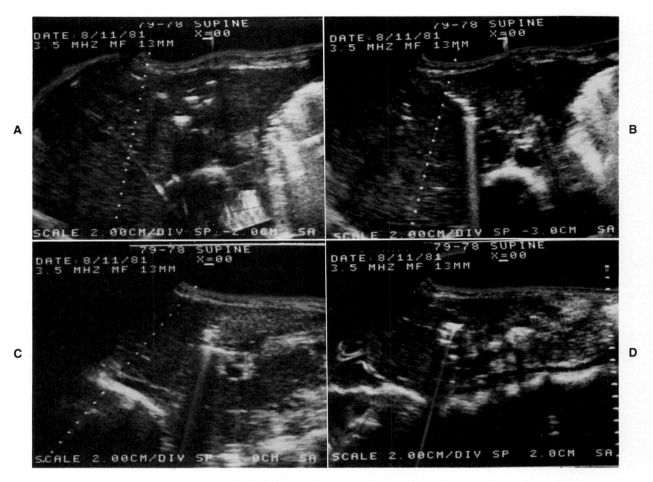

FIG. 13-30. Postoperative multiple bright reflectors within the hepatic parenchyma. There is an acoustic shadow beyond, which represented gas in the biliary tree. **A** and **B,** Transverse supine scans; **C** and **D,** sagittal scans. (Courtesy VA Hospital, Madison, Wis.)

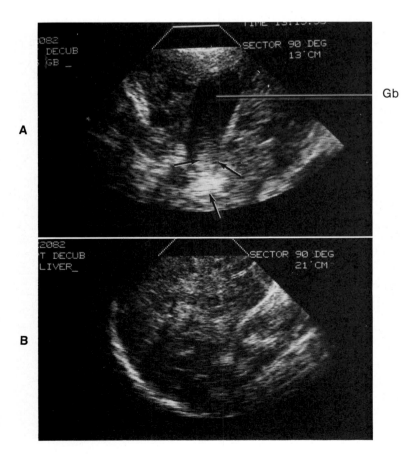

FIG. 13-31. This patient had liver metastases and a polypoid mass within the gallbladder, *Gb, (arrows).* **A,** Transverse and, **B,** sagittal scans of the liver with multiple focal defects.

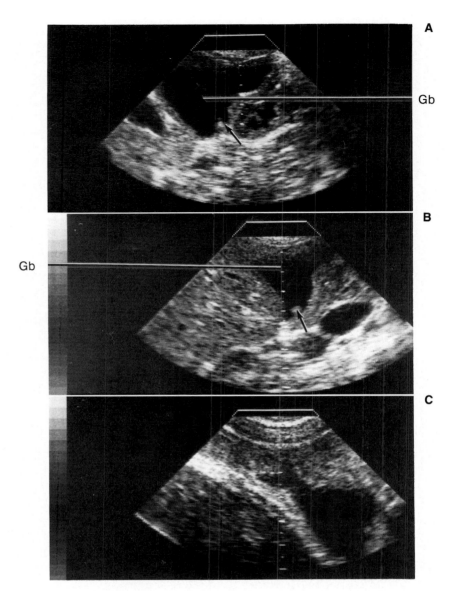

FIG. 13-32. **A** and **B,** Transverse scans of the distended gallbladder, *Gb,* with low-level irregularity attached to the wall *(arrow).* **C,** The small mass did not change position as the patient was rolled into a decubitus position.

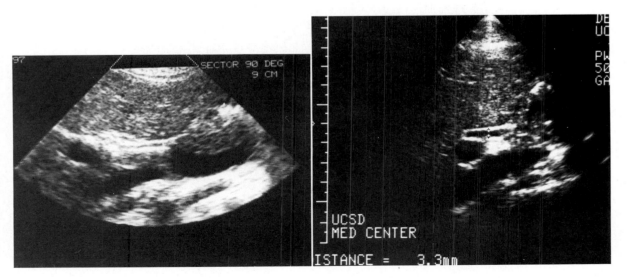

FIG. 13-33. Sagittal scans over the normal common bile duct. Under 5 mm is well within normal limits.

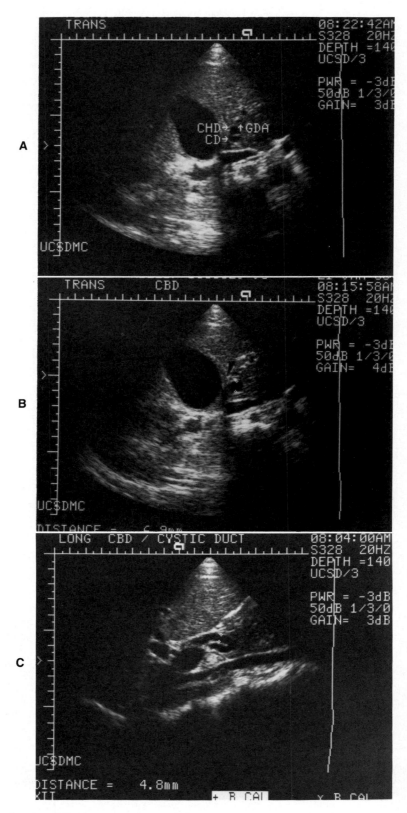

FIG. 13-34. **A** and **B,** Transverse scans of the prominent gallbladder, common hepatic duct, *CHD,* common duct, *CD,* and gastroduodenal artery, *GDA.* **C,** Sagittal scan of the common duct as it is draped anterior to the portal vein and inferior vena cava.

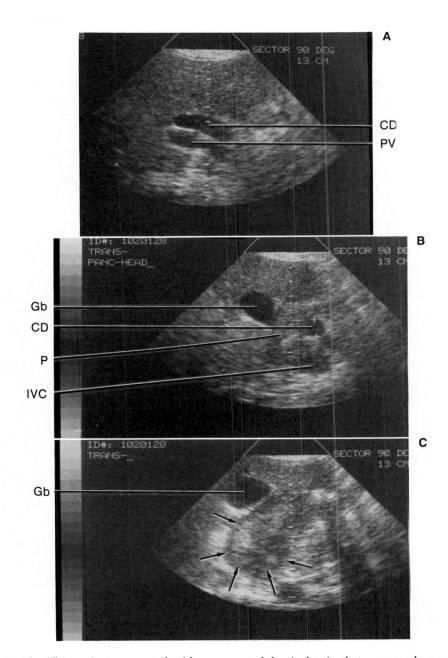

FIG. 13-35. This patient presented with recurrent abdominal pain that worsened upon eating. The sonogram showed a dilated common duct with a large irregular mass in the head of the pancreas. **A,** Sagittal scan of the common duct, *CD,* which measures 12 mm. **B,** Transverse of the common duct. Pancreas, *P;* gallbladder, *Gb;* inferior vena cava, *IVC.* **C,** Transverse of the gallbladder and pancreatic mass in the head of the gland *(arrows). PV,* portal vein.

gation. A patient may have a normal-sized hepatic duct and still have distal obstruction. The distal duct is often obscured by gas in the duodenal loop.

The common bile duct has an internal diameter slightly greater than that of the hepatic duct. Generally a duct over 6 mm is considered borderline, and over 10 mm is dilated (Fig. 13-34). Minimal dilation (7 to 11 mm) may be seen in nonjaundiced patients with gallstones or pancreatitis or in jaundiced patients with a common duct stone or tumor. However, a diameter of more than 11 mm suggests obstruction by stone or tumor of the duct or pancreas or some other source (Fig. 13-35). Parulekar[16] measured the common duct at 7.7 mm in nonjaundiced patients who had undergone cholecystectomy.

Dilated ducts may also be found in the absence of jaundice. The patient may have biliary obstruction involving one hepatic duct, an early obstruction secondary to carcinoma, or gallstones causing intermittent obstruction due to a ball-valve effect.

In an excellent study Laing, London, and Filly[13] give five characteristics that distinguish bile ducts from other intrahepatic structures (parasagittal scans provided the best visualization of the ducts):

1. Alteration in the anatomic pattern adjacent to the main (right) portal vein segment and the bifurcation. This was more pronounced in individuals who displayed greater degrees of dilation of the intrahepatic bile ducts.

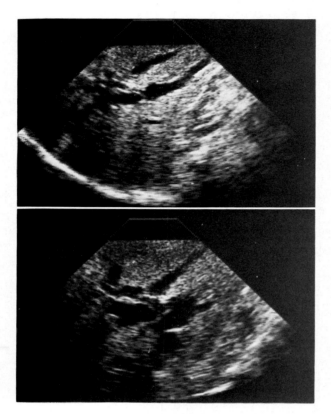

FIG. 13-36. Sagittal scans of the irregular walls of dilated bile ducts. As the ducts dilate, the course and caliber of the ducts become increasingly tortuous and irregular.

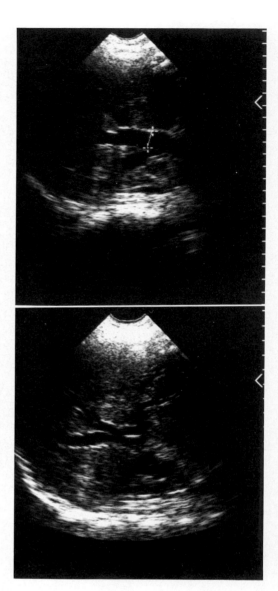

FIG. 13-37. The dilated ducts take on a stellate confluence within the right lobe of the liver.

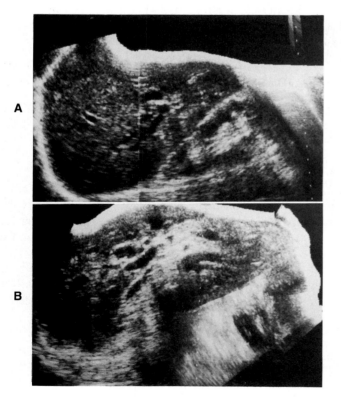

FIG. 13-38. **A,** This patient underwent cholecystectomy one year prior to the onset of jaundice and right upper quadrant tenderness. Pancreatic carcinoma with involvement to the lymph nodes caused intrahepatic duct dilation. **B,** Transverse scan of the dilated ducts within the liver.

2. Irregular walls of dilated bile ducts. As the intrahepatic biliary system dilates, the course and caliber of ducts become increasingly tortuous and irregular (Fig. 13-36).

3. Stellate confluence of dilated ducts. This was noted at the points where the ducts converge. Dilated ducts look like spokes of a wheel (Fig. 13-37).

4. Acoustic enhancement by dilated bile ducts. Both portal veins and ducts have high-amplitude reflections surrounding them.

5. Peripheral duct dilation. It is normally unusual to visualize hepatic ducts in the liver periphery whereas dilated bile ducts may be observed (Fig. 13-38).

SUMMARY

1. The extrahepatic biliary system consists of the right and left hepatic ducts, the common hepatic duct, the common bile duct, the gallbladder, and the cystic duct.

2. The gallbladder is divided into the fundus, body, and neck. It is located in the right upper quadrant closely related to the visceral surface of the liver.

3. The gallbladder functions to store bile for intermittent release in conjunction with eating.

4. The gallbladder resides in a fossa on the medial aspect of the liver. The neck of the gallbladder comes into contact with the main segment of the portal vein near the origin of the left portal vein.

5. The common duct lies anterior and to the right of the portal vein in the region of the porta hepatis and gastrohepatic ligament. The hepatic artery lies anterior and to the left of the portal vein. The common hepatic duct is a tubular structure anterior to the portal vein.

6. The most classic symptom of gallbladder disease is right upper quadrant pain, with extension to the right shoulder.

7. As the bile is stored in the gallbladder, small crystals of bile salts precipitate and may form gallstones varying from pinhead size to the size of the organ itself.

8. Jaundice is characterized by the presence of bile in the tissues with resulting yellow-green color of the skin. It may occur when small gallstones block the bile ducts between the gallbladder and the intestine.

9. Sometimes a large gallbladder may contain thick or inspissated bile.

10. The normal thickness of the gallbladder wall is 1 to 2 mm. The normal size of the common hepatic duct is less than 4 mm; while the common bile duct is less than 6 mm.

11. Five characteristics distinguish bile ducts from other intrahepatic structures: (1) alteration in the anatomic pattern adjacent to the main (right) portal vein segment and the bifurcation; (2) irregular walls of dilated bile ducts; (3) stellate confluence of dilated ducts; (4) acoustic enhancement by dilated bile ducts; and (5) peripheral duct dilation.

REFERENCES

1. Bartrum RJ and Crow HC: Inflammatory diseases of the biliary system, Semin Ultrasound 1(2), 1980.

2. Carter SJ, Rutledge J, Hirch JH, et al: Papillary adenoma of the gallbladder; ultrasonic demonstration, J Clin Ultrasound 6:433, 1978.

3. Conrad MR, James JO, and Dietchy J: Significance of low level echoes within the gallbladder, AJR 132:967, 1979.

4. Conrad MR, Landay MJ, and James JO: Sonographic parallel channel sign of biliary tree enlargement in mild to moderate obstructive jaundice, AJR 130:279, 1978.

5. Engel JM, Deitch EA, and Sikkema W: Gallbladder wall thickness: sonographic accuracy and relation to disease, AJR 134:907, 1980.

6. Filly RA, Allen B, Minton MJ, et al: In vitro investigation of the origin of echoes within biliary sludge, J Clin Ultrasound 8:193, 1980.

7. Filly RA, Moss AA, and Way LW: In vitro investigation of gallstone shadowing with ultrasound tomography, J Clin Ultrasound 7:255, 1979.

8. Finberg JJ and Birnholz JC: Ultrasound evaluation of the gallbladder wall, Radiology 133:693, 1979.

9. Fiski CE, Laing FC, and Brown TW: Ultrasonographic evidence of gallbladder wall thickening in association with hypoalbuminemia, Radiology 135:713, 1980.

10. Gonzalez L and MacIntyre WJ: Acoustic shadow formation by gallstones, Radiology 135:217, 1980.

11. Graham MF, Cooperberg PL, Cohen MM, et al: The size of the normal common hepatic duct following cholecystectomy; an ultrasonic study, Radiology 135:137, 1980.

12. Kane RA: Ultrasonographic diagnosis of gangrenous cholecystitis and empyema of the gallbladder, Radiology 134:191, 1980.

13. Laing FC, London LA, and Filly RA: Ultrasonographic identification of dilated intrahepatic bile ducts and their differentiation from portal venous structures, J Clin Ultrasound 6:73, 1978.

14. Marchal GJF, Casaer M, Baert AL, et al: Gallbladder wall sonolucency in acute cholecystitis, Radiology 133:429, 1979.

15. Marchal G, Van de Voorde P, Van Dooren W, et al: Ultrasonic appearance of the filled and contracted normal gallbladder, J Clin Ultrasound 8:439, 1980.

16. Parulekar SG: Ultrasound evaluation of common bile duct size, Radiology 133:703, 1979.

17. Sanders RC: The significance of sonographic gallbladder wall thickening, J Clin Ultrasound 8:143, 1980.

18. Scheske GA, Cooperberg PL, Cohen MM, et al: Floating gallstones; the role of contrast material, J Clin Ultrasound 8:227, 1980.

14

Pancreas

SANDRA L. HAGEN-ANSERT

With the advent of each new medical procedure, efforts to visualize the pancreas accurately have met with varying degrees of success. Prior to the relatively recent use of diagnostic ultrasound, computerized tomography, and magnetic resonance, other noninvasive procedures were unsuccessful in accurate visualization of the pancreas. The plain film of the abdomen is diagnostic of pancreatitis if calcification is visible in the pancreatic area; however, calcification does not occur in all cases. Localized ileus ("paralyzed gut," gas, and fluid accumulation near the area of inflammation) may be shown on the plain radiograph in patients with pancreatitis. The upper gastrointestinal test series provides indirect information about the pancreas when the widened duodenal loops is visualized. Other diagnostic methods such as hypotonic duodenography, isotope examination, arteriography, fiberoptic gastroscopy, and intravenous cholangiography all provide indirect information about the pancreas or prove limited in their diagnostic ability. Thus investigators have been striving to develop an examination that will be accurate, readily repeatable, and safe. Diagnostic ultrasound appears to be such an examination in many patients who are very slender in stature. The more obese patient images much better with computerized tomography.

The normal pancreas can be visualized in the majority of patients by using the neighboring organs and vascular landmarks as an aid in localization. The gland appears echographically as dense as or slightly denser than the hepatic parenchyma. Variations in patient positioning or utilization of contrast media through the stomach aids in visualizing the entire gland.

Difficulties encountered in making the proper diagnosis have been presented to give the sonographer a better understanding of the diagnostic signs of pancreatic disease.

At the present time there are still a few problems in pancreatic visualization with the ultrasonic technique. Familiar impediments are the reflections and absorptions caused by bone, gas, and air. If these occur over the area of interest, it becomes impossible to outline prevertebral vessels and thus visualization of the pancreas is limited. Obesity presents a problem in some cases. The far gain (or the overall gain) of the equipment may need adjustment for properly penetrating these patients. Normal organ movement makes exact repetition difficult in some cases, and several scans may have to be made before a confident analysis is possible. However, real time has overcome this problem, enabling the sonographer to follow the course of the prevertebral vessels accurately and delineate the borders of the pancreas with more precision.

For many reasons the pancreas may be a more difficult organ to visualize than the liver, gallbladder, spleen, or kidneys. Filly and Freimanis[3] have presented evidence that the normal pancreas is difficult to visualize by conventional bistable ultrasonic equipment since the gland produces many echoes at normal sensitivity due to multiple interfaces within it. With gray-scale ultrasound a nor-

246

Table 14-1   Ultrasound Correlations of Size (cm)

AP	Haber et al. (AJR 1976)	Weill et al. (Radiology, 1977)	Degraaff et al. (Radiology, 1978)	Arger et al. (J Clin Ultrasound, 1979)
Head	2.7 ± 0.7	3.0	2.01	2.5
Neck		2.1	1.00	
Body	2.2 ± 0.7	2.8	1.18	2.0
Tail	2.0 ± 0.4	2.8		2.0

mal pancreas can possess a degree of echogenicity greater than or equal to, but not less than, that of the liver.[4]

ANATOMY

The pancreas lies in the retroperitoneal cavity. It is usually 10 to 15 cm long, anterior to the first and second vertebral bodies. It is located deep in the epigastrium and left hypochondrium behind the lesser omental sac. Thus it is hidden from direct physical examination.

There is some variation in the size of the gland, for it has been described as sausage shaped, dumbbell shaped, or gradually tapering from its head to its tail. The gland is relatively larger (thicker) in children than in adults. It subsequently becomes smaller with advancing age. Several clinical studies have been made in efforts to determine the size of the normal gland (Table 14-1). Our own

experience corresponds with the measurements by Arger et al.[1]: head = 2.5 cm; body = 2 cm; and tail = 2 cm.

The pancreas is generally found in a horizontal oblique lie, extending from the concavity of the duodenum to the hilum of the spleen (Fig. 14-1). Other variations of the gland are transverse, horseshoe, sigmoid, L shaped, and inverted V.[11]

The gland is divided into four areas: head, neck, body, and tail. Each will be discussed as it relates to its surrounding anatomy (Fig. 14-2).

Head

The head of the pancreas is anterior to the inferior vena cava and left renal vein, inferior to the caudate lobe of the liver and the portal vein (Fig. 14-3), and lateral to the second portion of the duodenum. It lies in the "lap" of the

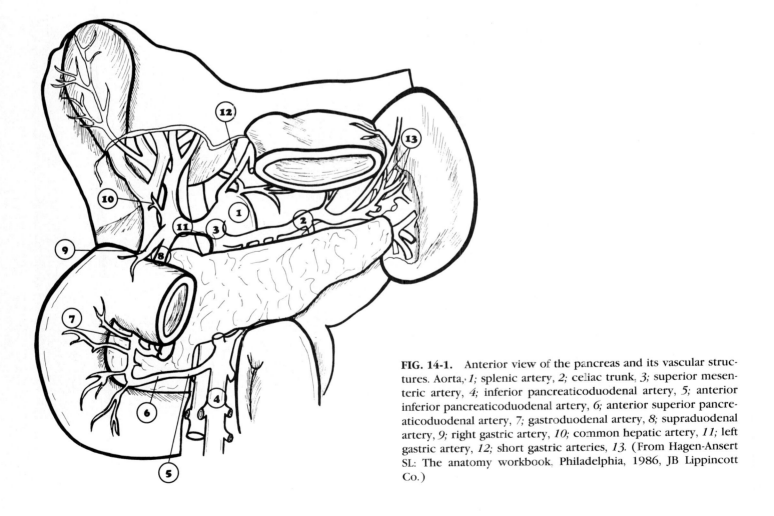

FIG. 14-1. Anterior view of the pancreas and its vascular structures. Aorta, *1;* splenic artery, *2;* celiac trunk, *3;* superior mesenteric artery, *4;* inferior pancreaticoduodenal artery, *5;* anterior inferior pancreaticoduodenal artery, *6;* anterior superior pancreaticoduodenal artery, *7;* gastroduodenal artery, *8;* supraduodenal artery, *9;* right gastric artery, *10;* common hepatic artery, *11;* left gastric artery, *12;* short gastric arteries, *13.* (From Hagen-Ansert SL: The anatomy workbook. Philadelphia, 1986, JB Lippincott Co.)

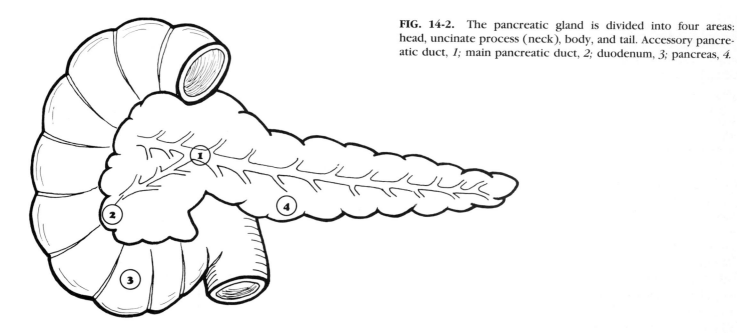

FIG. 14-2. The pancreatic gland is divided into four areas: head, uncinate process (neck), body, and tail. Accessory pancreatic duct, *1;* main pancreatic duct, *2;* duodenum, *3;* pancreas, *4.*

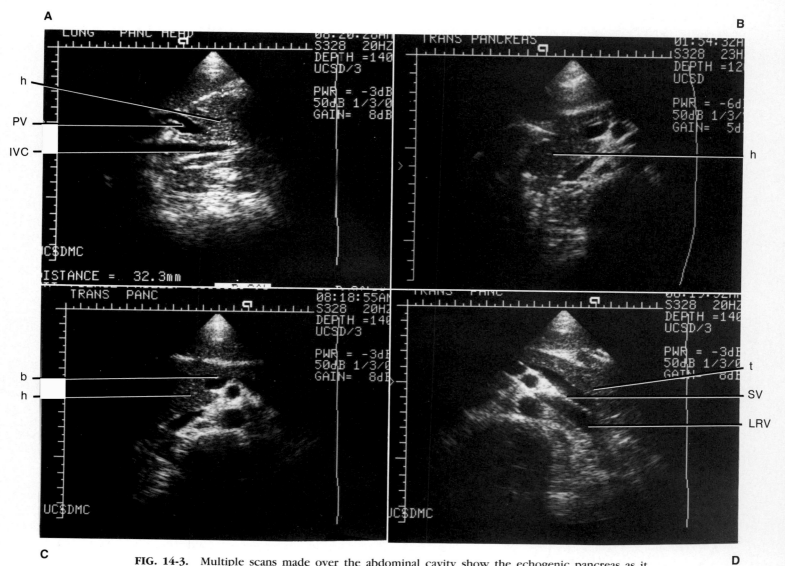

FIG. 14-3. Multiple scans made over the abdominal cavity show the echogenic pancreas as it drapes over the prevertebral vessels, inferior vena cava, and aorta. **A,** Sagittal scan of the portal vein, *PV,* pancreas, inferior vena cava, *IVC,* and head of pancreas, *h.* **B,** Transverse scan of the head of the pancreas, *h.* **C,** Transverse scan of the head and body, *b,* of the pancreas. **D,** Transverse scan of the tail of the pancreas, *t.* The splenic vein, *SV,* and left renal vein, *LRV,* are posterior to the gland.

duodenum. These structures pass posterior to the superior mesenteric vessels. It is also located posterior to the antrum of the stomach. The uncinate process is posterior to the superior mesenteric vessels. The common bile duct passes through a groove posterior to the pancreatic head, and the gastroduodenal artery serves as the anterolateral border.

Neck/body

The neck/body, the largest part of the gland, lies on an angle from caudal right to cephalic left posterior to the stomach and anterior to the origin of the portal vein. It rests posteriorly against the aorta, the origin of the superior mesenteric artery, the left renal vessels, the left adrenal gland, and the left kidney. The tortuous splenic artery is usually the superior border of the pancreas. The anterior surface is separated by the omental bursa from the posterior wall of the stomach. The inferior surface, below the attachment of the transverse mesocolon, is related to the duodenojejunal junction and the splenic flexure of the colon.

Tail

The tail of the pancreas lies in front of the left kidney close to the spleen and the left colic flexure. The splenic artery forms the anterior border, the splenic vein the posterior border, and the stomach the superoanterior border.

Pancreatic ducts

To aid in the transport of pancreatic fluid, the ducts have smooth muscle surrounding them. The *duct of Wirsung* is a primary duct extending the entire length of the gland (Fig. 14-4). It receives tributaries from lobules at right angles and enters the medial second part of the duodenum with the common bile duct at the *ampulla of Vater* (guarded by the *sphincter of Oddi*). The *duct of Santorini* is a secondary duct that drains the upper anterior head. It enters the duodenum at the minor papilla about 2 cm proximal to the ampulla of Vater.

Relational anatomy

The important structures related to the posterior surface of the pancreas include the inferior vena cava, the aorta, the superior mesenteric vessels, the splenic and portal veins, and the common bile duct. The splenic artery and stomach lie along the superior border of the pancreas, and the hilus of the spleen lies in contact with the tail of the gland. The anterior pancreatic surface is bounded by the stomach and the lesser peritoneal cavity whereas the inferior surface lies along the greater peritoneal cavity.

Because of the unyielding nature of the posterior abdominal wall, any enlargement of the gland will extend anteriorly.

PHYSIOLOGY

The pancreas is both an exocrine and an endocrine gland. Its exocrine function is to produce *pancreatic juice,* which enters the duodenum together with bile. The exocrine secretions of the pancreas and those of the liver,

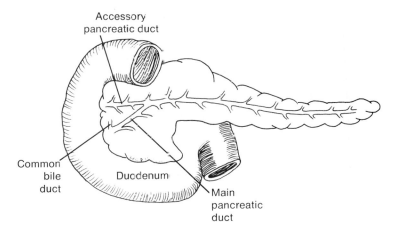

FIG. 14-4. The duct of Wirsung is the main pancreatic duct that extends the entire length of the gland. It receives tributaries from lobules at right angles and enters the medial second part of the duodenum with the common bile duct at the ampulla of Vater. The duct of Santorini is an accessory pancreatic duct that drains the upper anterior head of the gland.

which are delivered into the duodenum through duct systems, are essential for normal intestinal digestion and absorption of food. Pancreatic secretion is under the control of the vagus nerve and two hormonal agents, secretin and pancreozymin, that are released when food enters the duodenum. The endocrine function is to produce the hormone *insulin.* Failure of the pancreas to furnish sufficient insulin leads to diabetes mellitus.

The enzymes of the pancreatic juice are lipase, amylase, carboxypeptidase, trypsin, and chymotrypsin. The last three are secreted as inactive enzyme precursors to be activated when they have entered the duodenum. The pancreas contains acinar cells, exocrine secretory cells that are arranged in saclike clusters (acini) connected by small intercalated ducts to larger excretory ducts. The excretory ducts converge into one or two main ducts, which deliver the exocrine secretion of the pancreas into the duodenum.

Pancreatic juice is the most versatile and active of the digestive secretions. Its enzymes are capable of nearly completing the digestion of food in the absence of all other digestive secretions. Because the digestive enzymes that are secreted into the lumen of the small intestine require an almost neutral pH for best activity, the acidity of the contents entering the duodenum must be reduced. Thus the pancreatic juice contains a relatively high concentration of sodium bicarbonate, and this alkaline salt is largely responsible for the neutralization of gastric acid.

The nervous secretion of pancreatic juice is thick and rich in enzymes and proteins. The chemical secretion, resulting from pancreozymin activity, also is thick, watery, and rich in enzymes. Pancreatic juice is alkaline and becomes more so with increasing rates of secretion. This is because of a simultaneous increase in bicarbonates and decrease in chloride concentration.

The proteolytic enzyme trypsin may hydrolyze protein molecules to polypeptides. Chymotrypsinogen is activated by trypsin. Amylase causes hydrolysis of starch with the production of maltose, which is further hydrolyzed to glucose. Lipase is capable of hydrolyzing some fats to monoglycerides and some to glycerol and fatty acids. Although lipases are also secreted by the small intestine, what is secreted by the pancreas accounts for 80% of all fat digestion. Thus impaired fat digestion is an important indicator of pancreatic dysfunction.

LABORATORY TESTS

Amylase

In certain types of pancreatic disease the digestive enzymes of the pancreas escape into the surrounding tissue, producing necrosis with severe pain and inflammation. Under these circumstances there is an increase in serum amylase. A serum amylase level of twice normal usually indicates acute pancreatitis. Other conditions causing increased amylase are intestinal obstruction, mumps, and other disease of the salivary glands or ducts.

Glucose

The glucose tolerance test is performed to discover whether there is a disorder of glucose metabolism. An increased blood glucose level is found in severe diabetes, chronic liver disease, and overactivity of several of the endocrine glands. There may be a decreased blood sugar level in tumors of the *islets of Langerhans* in the pancreas.

Lipase

The lipase test is performed to assess damage to the pancreas. Lipase is secreted by the pancreas, and small amounts pass into the blood. The lipase level rises in acute pancreatitis and in carcinoma of the pancreas. (Both amylase and lipase rise at the same rate, but the elevation in lipase concentration persists for a longer period.)

SONOGRAPHIC TECHNIQUES OF THE NORMAL PANCREAS

Patient preparation

If the biliary system is to be evaluated along with the pancreas, the patient should eat nothing for 8 hours before performing the ultrasound examination. If just the pancreas is the main concern, however, I have found it helpful for the patient to be adequately hydrated. Often a full stomach serves as an advantage in outlining the more posterior pancreatic parenchyma. The patient may drink large quantities (16 to 32 ounces) of water, tomato, or orange juice prior to or following the initial examination in efforts to distend the stomach and fill the duodenal cap to outline the gland (Figs. 14-5 and 14-6).

Several investigators have used glucagon (1 mg) intravenously followed by 500 ml of water after 2 to 3 minutes.[14] The glucagon reduces the peristaltic action of the stomach and thus maintains a fluid-filled window for almost an hour. Simethicone and other "gas-eliminating" drugs have proved to be of little success. We have often found that they are more gas producing in the difficult "gassy" patients. Generally alterations in patient position

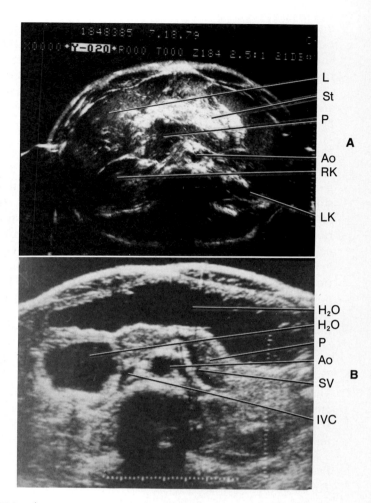

FIG. 14-5.   A, The stomach, *St,* can serve as an acoustic impediment or an acoustic enhancement if the patient is properly hydrated. This transverse scan shows the collapsed walls of a stomach that has just enough fluid within to permit adequate visualization of the posterior pancreas. **B,** This scan shows an extremely distended stomach, which helps to visualize the pancreas and prevertebral vessels posterior to its border. Water, H_2O; pancreas, *P*; aorta, *Ao*; inferior vena cava, *IVC*; splenic vein, *SV,* liver, *L;* left kidney, *LK;* right kidney, *RK*. (Courtesy John Deitz, Philadelphia, Pa.)

and ingestion of fluid are more conducive to obtaining an adequate examination.

Ultrasound should be performed prior to barium studies, for barium inhibits the transmission of sound.

Difficulties in visualization may be due to bowel gas, a transverse stomach obscuring the anatomy, or a small left lobe of the liver. A left lobe measuring 2 to 2.5 cm makes an excellent sonic window for pancreatic visualization. It can be used with a caudal tilt of the transducer (15 to 20 degrees) for better visualization of the gland. The distended gallbladder also can be used to bypass air in the duodenal cap for better visualizing the pancreatic head.

The patient is initially examined in the supine position. Subsequent RAO or LAO positions may be used to avoid bowel interference. A very effective alternative has been the erect position.[9] In this case air moves from the gastric antrum to the fundus. The upper viscera move downward from under the ribs. The liver moves caudad for an im-

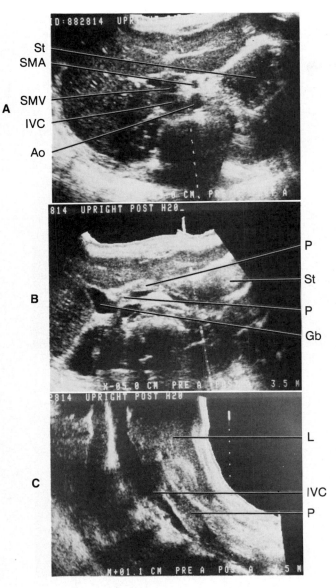

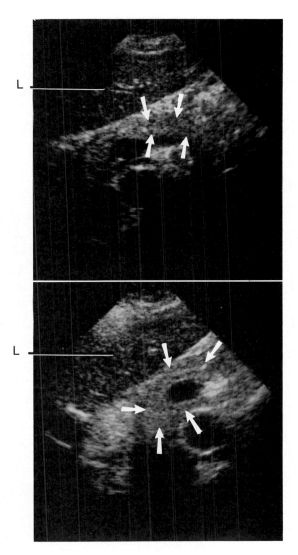

FIG. 14-7. The normal echo intensity of the pancreas is moderately greater than that of the liver (*arrows* demarcate pancreatic border). Liver, *L.*

FIG. 14-6. **A** and **B,** Transverse scans over the upper abdomen show the distended stomach, *St,* which is used to help identify the pancreas. The left lobe of the liver and prevertebral vessels are also very useful landmarks in demarcating the pancreatic borders. Often an upright scan, **C,** is useful to identify the distended inferior vena cava, *IVC,* as the posterior border of the pancreas, *P.* Superior mesenteric artery, *SMA;* superior mesenteric vein, *SMV;* aorta *Ao;* gallbladder, *Gb;* liver, *L.*

proved hepatic window. The erect position also results in distention of the venous structures, which aids in further localizing the pancreas.

Normal texture pattern

The echogenicity pattern of the pancreas is discussed in terms of how it relates to the liver's homogeneous "soft" echo pattern. Arger et al.[1] have stated that the normal pancreas has an echo pattern which is homogeneous and finer in texture than that of the surrounding retroperitoneum. The echo intensity is usually slightly less than that of the surrounding soft tissues. The echo intensity of the pancreas is moderately greater than that of the liver (Fig. 14-7).

Filly and London[4] have noted that retroperitoneal fat is strongly echogenic. Extensive fatty infiltrations of the pancreas are difficult to visualize by ultrasound. The pancreatic tissue blends with the surrounding retroperitoneal fat.

A lesser degree of fatty infiltration may not render the pancreas invisible but may raise the amplitude of returning *pancreatic* echoes, resulting in the clinical observation that the pancreas returns stronger echoes than the liver.[4]

Marks, Filly, and Callen[10] further investigated the echogenicity of the gland when they observed that a higher-amplitude pancreatic echogenicity is due to more than fat infiltration alone. Fibrous tissue may account for the portion of increased echogenicity not attributable to fat. Increased deposition of fat that has infiltrated along the pancreatic septa is a major determining factor of pancreatic echogenicity.

Sarti[12] and Sample et al.[11] have described a very effective technique for visualizing this echogenic organ. Pan-

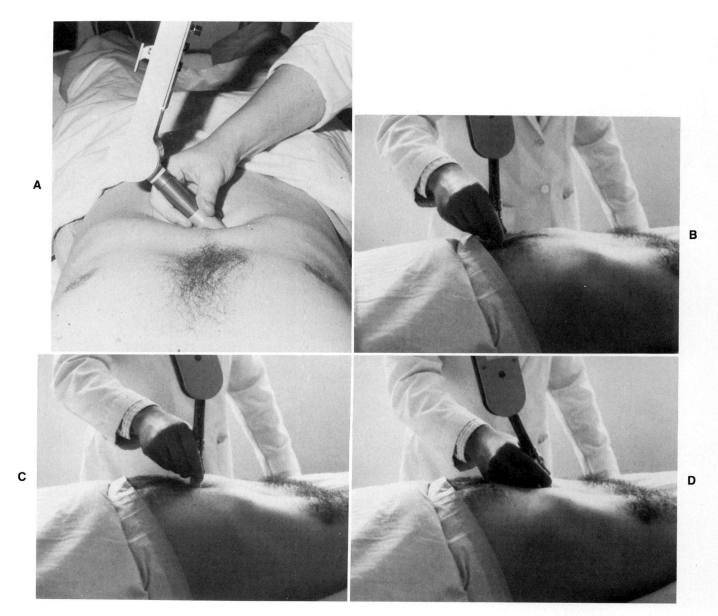

FIG. 14-8. Whether scans are made with an articulated arm scanner or real-time equipment, a similar protocol is used to evaluate the pancreas. **A,** Initial scans are made at the level of the xyphoid to search for the prevertebral vessels and pancreatic tissue. **B,** Single pie-sweep technique for better visualization of the midline structures such as the body of the pancreas, superior mesenteric vessels, and great vessels. **C,** The sagittal scan should be performed in full inspiration to outline the vessels to localize the pancreas. **D,** A slight arc motion of the transducer allows the beam to sweep under the xyphoid or costal margin.

creatic echoes will be in the highest shade (darkest) of gray when the liver echoes register in the higher shades. Thus the pancreatic echoes will be lost in the high-amplitude echoes of the surrounding fatty retroperitoneum. The gain settings should be adjusted so the liver echoes register in the middle to lighter shades. The pancreas will then register one to two shades darker than the liver but will not be viewed in the darkest shade.

Scanning techniques
Transverse scans

Transverse scans are used to make the initial visualization of the gland. The patient should be in full inspiration to distend the venous structures that act as landmarks in vi-

sualizing the pancreas. Generally we begin at the level of the xyphoid and proceed at 1 cm intervals until gas encumbers the examination. When the pancreas has been imaged, alterations in the angle of the transducer are made for more complete visualization. Alterations in patient positioning may be useful for fully visualizing the head or tail of the gland (Fig. 14-8).

The left lobe of the liver should be used as an ultrasonic window. The portal vein can be seen as an ovoid-circular structure anterior to the inferior vena cava (Fig. 14-9). Just anterior to the portal vein lie two small circular structures. The common duct is the more lateral, the hepatic artery the more medial (Fig. 14-10). This relationship has been termed by Bartrum and Crow the "Mickey

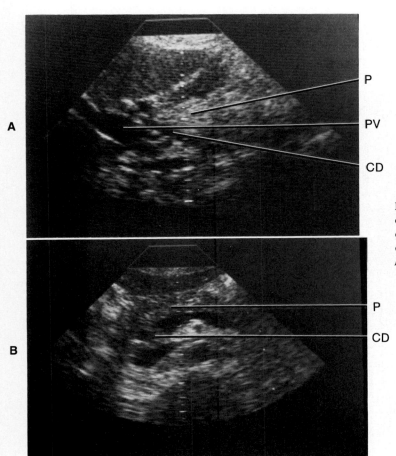

P

PV

CD

FIG. 14-9. A, Sagittal scan of the common bile duct as it lies directly anterior to the portal vein and posterior to the pancreas. **B,** On the transverse scan the common bile duct is the lateral margin of the head of the pancreas. Pancreas, *P;* portal vein, *PV;* common bile duct, *CD.*

P

CD

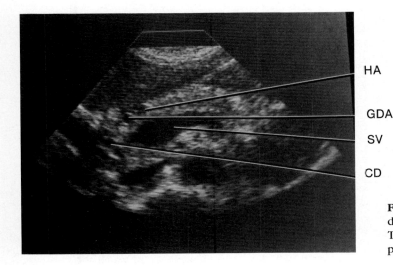

HA

GDA

SV

CD

FIG. 14-10. Transverse scan of the pancreas with the common duct, *CD,* hepatic artery, *HA,* and gastroduodenal artery, *GDA.* The splenic vein, *SV,* serves as the posteromedial border of the pancreas.

Mouse" sign—with the portal vein representing Mickey's face, the common duct his right ear, and the hepatic artery his left ear.

Often anterior to the common duct is the gastroduodenal artery or one of its branches. It is seen as a second circular structure lateral to the pancreatic head. Pancreatic reflections are usually seen at the junction of the splenic and portal veins. Another useful landmark for the pancreatic head and body is the junction of the superior mesenteric with the splenic/portal veins (Fig. 14-11). The SMV

and SMA both are posterior to the head and anterior to the uncinate process. The head is medial to the second and third parts of the duodenum. The fluid-filled duodenum can be a valuable landmark in identifying the pancreas (Fig. 14-12). It is especially useful to evaluate the peristaltic action of the duodenum in efforts to separate it from the lateral margin of the head. The collapsed duodenum appears ultrasonically as a dense central core with an echo-free periphery. It may be mistaken for part of the pancreas if not carefully evaluated.

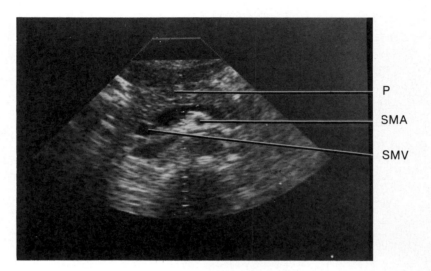

FIG. 14-11.   Transverse scan over the upper abdomen shows the inferior vena cava and aorta anterior to the spine. The superior mesenteric artery, *SMA,* is a small circular structure located anterior to the left renal vein and aorta and posterior to the body of the pancreas, *P.* The superior mesenteric vein, *SMV,* is shown as a circular structure on the transverse scan and is seen to join the splenic vein before forming the portal vein.

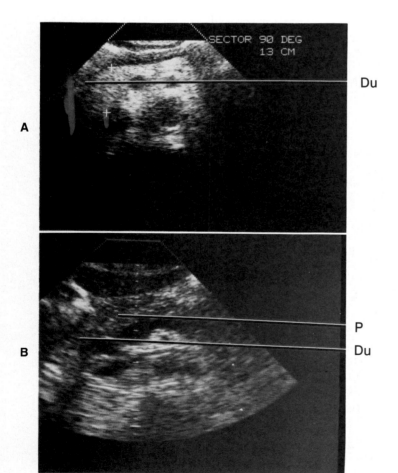

FIG. 14-12.   **A,** Transverse scan of the head of the pancreas as surrounded on the lateral border by the duodenum, *Du.* **B,** The duodenum often casts a shadow (due to air or gas within the duodenum). It may also be filled with fluid and thus serve as an excellent landmark for outlining the lateral margin of the pancreatic head. Variations in patient position will help the sonographer determine the motion of the duodenum. Also the real-time evaluation will allow the sonographer to watch the peristaltic action of the duodenum as it outlines the head of the gland. *P,* pancreas.

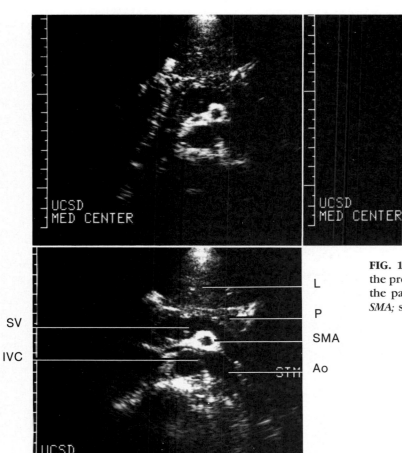

FIG. 14-13. Transverse scans over the upper abdomen show the prevertebral vessels as the posterior landmark of the body of the pancreas. Liver, *L;* pancreas, *P;* superior mesenteric artery, *SMA;* splenic vein, *SV;* inferior vena cava, *IVC;* aorta, *Ao.*

The body of the pancreas lies anterior to the SMV and SMA (Figs. 14-13 and 14-14). Shortly after the SMA originates, the curvilinear lucency of the left renal vein courses posterior to it and anterior to the aorta and can serve as a posterior landmark for the body of the gland.

Sagittal scans

Sagittal scans are begun at the midline and directed first to the patient's right at 1 cm intervals and then to the left at similar increments.

The portal vein is seen as a circular sonolucent structure anterior to the IVC and superior to the head of the pancreas. As one moves slightly toward midline, the common bile duct can be seen directly anterior to the portal vein as a small tubular structure posterior to the pancreatic head (Fig. 14-15). The gastroduodenal artery can sometimes be seen anterior and over the pancreatic head.

As the SMV flows cephalad to join the portal vein, it is seen as a long, tubular sonolucency posterior to the neck of the pancreas and anterior to the uncinate process.

The antrum of the stomach appears as a collapsed (Fig. 14-16) bull's-eye and is identified anterior and slightly caudal to the head/body. The splenic vein is a circular sonolucency posterior to the cephalic portion of the gland whereas the aorta, celiac axis, and SMA are posterior to the body of the gland. The left renal vein is a slitlike so-

nolucency between the aorta and the SMA and serves as a posterior border of the pancreas.

Pancreatic duct

The pancreatic duct can often be visualized on transverse scans as an echo-free tubular structure in the body of the gland (Fig. 14-17). Although the duct is largest in the head, its course is variable. Its smallest diameter is in the tail, and thus it is somewhat difficult to detect by ultrasound.

The normal caliber of the duct is generally considered to be 2 to 3 mm.[15] One should identify pancreatic tissue on both sides of the duct so as not to become confused by vascular structures that may overlie it (Fig. 14-18). However, the splenic vein is actually too posterior and the hepatic artery too anterior to be confused with the duct.

The duct appears as an echo-free area sharply marginated by two parallel echogenic lines. A thin strip of retroperitoneal fat may underlie the anterior aspect of the pancreas. This sonolucent linear pattern must not be mistaken for a duct structure.[2]

The posterior wall of the antrum can be seen on transverse scans as a relatively echo-free tubular structure overlying the anterior aspect of the pancreas. Again, one

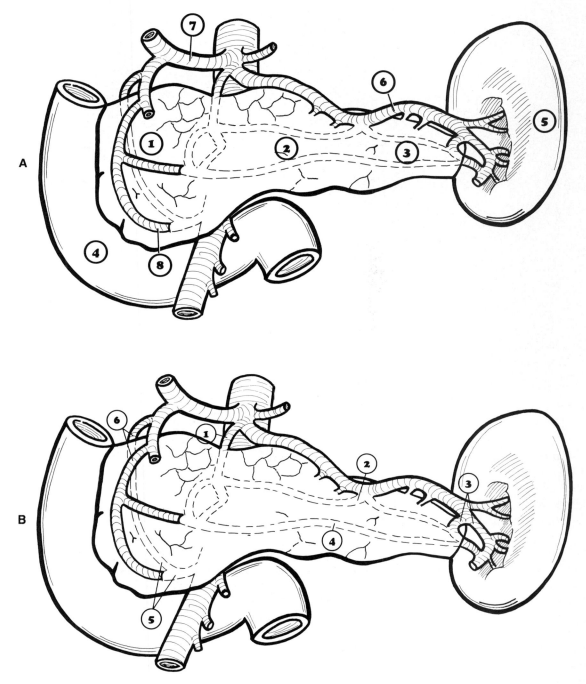

FIG. 14-14.   A, Arterial supply surrounding the pancreas. Head of the pancreas, *1;* body, *2;* tail, *3;* duodenum, *4;* spleen, *5;* splenic artery, *6;* hepatic artery, *7;* gastroduodenal artery, *8.* **B,** Pancreas and its main arterial supply. Dorsal pancreatic artery, *1;* great pancreatic artery, *2;* caudal pancreatic artery, *3;* inferior pancreatic artery, *4;* posterior and anterior inferior pancreaticoduodenal arteries, *5;* posterior and anterior superior pancreaticoduodenal arteries, *6.* (From Hagen-Ansert SL: The anatomy workbook, Philadelphia, 1986, JB Lippincott Co.)

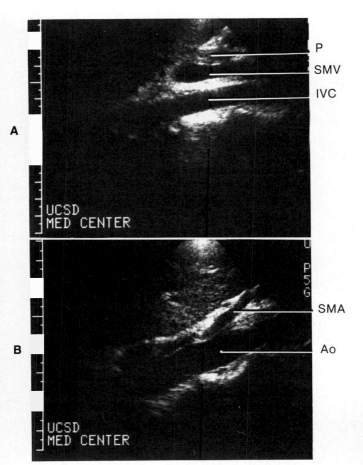

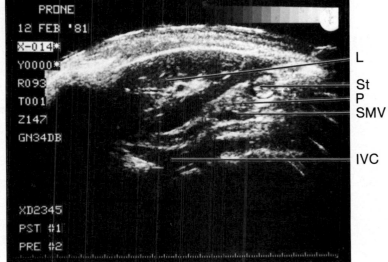

FIG. 14-15. A, Sagittal scans of the superior mesenteric vein, *SMV,* as it flows cephalad to join the portal vein. It is seen as a long tubular structure posterior to the neck of the pancreas, *P,* and anterior to the uncinate process. Inferior vena cava, *IVC.* **B,** Sagittal scan of the aorta, *Ao,* and superior mesenteric artery, *SMA.* The superior mesenteric artery is usually the posterior border of the body of the pancreas.

FIG. 14-16. The stomach may be seen as a collapsed bull's-eye anterior to the body of the pancreas on the sagittal scan. Liver, *L;* stomach, *St;* pancreas, *P;* superior mesenteric vein, *SMV;* inferior vena cava, *IVC.*

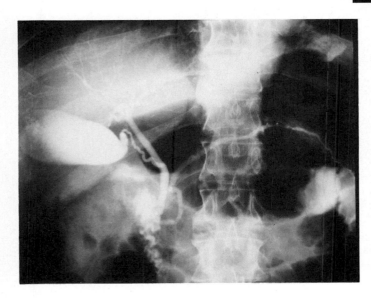

FIG. 14-17. Endoscopic retrograde pancreatogram demonstrating the pancreatic duct, common bile duct, and hepatic ducts.

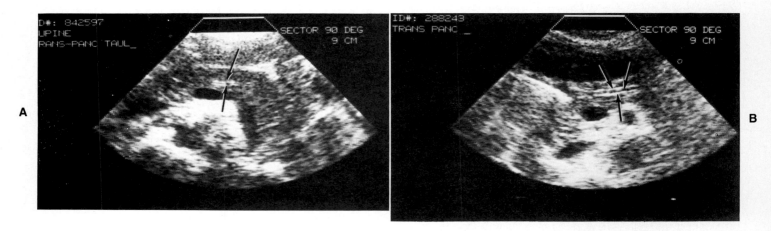

FIG. 14-18.   **A,** The pancreatic duct is very small when seen in the normal patient, appearing as a sonolucent area sharply marginated by two parallel echogenic lines *(arrows).* **B,** Pancreatic tissue must be identified on each side of the duct *(arrows)* so the duct can be distinguished from a collapsed antrum of the stomach or the splenic vein.

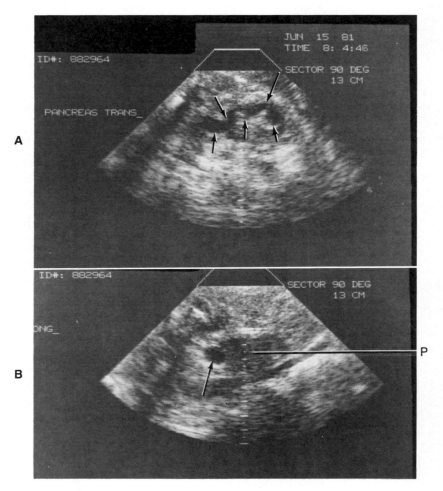

FIG. 14-19.   This patient presented with chronic pancreatitis and a dilated pancreatic duct. **A,** Transverse scan showing the dilated and tortuous pancreatic duct. Often such ducts will calcify and shadow. **B,** Sagittal scan of the prominent head of the pancreas and dilated pancreatic duct *(arrow).*

must not confuse this with a dilated duct. Confirmation can be made with the sagittal scan.[15]

Generally any degree of duct dilation is indicative of pancreatic disease (Fig. 14-19).

Pitfalls of pancreatic echography

Pancreatic echography can be obscured for any of the following reasons:

1. A small echo-free area medial to the liver may be fluid-containing duodenum that could be mistaken for the pancreas. Slight right anterior oblique decubitus scans should enable the sonographer to distinguish the duodenum from the pancreas. The patient may also be instructed to drink fluids to distend the stomach and fill the duodenum.
2. The pancreas may be difficult to visualize because of overlying structures such as stomach fat, muscles, and costal cartilage—in which case the position of the patient should be altered to avoid the interference.
3. Other solid masses in the retroperitoneal region, such as those of lymphadenopathy, may cause some confusion in the identification of the pancreatic region since the lymph nodes drape across the prevertebral vessels within the region where the pancreas may lie.

CLINICAL SIGNS AND PATHOLOGIC CONDITIONS OF THE PANCREAS
Congenital anomalies

Ectopic pancreatic tissue. This is the most common pancreatic anomaly, usually in the form of intramural nodules. The ectopic tissue may be found in various places in the gastrointestinal tract. Frequent sites are the stomach, duodenum, small bowel, and large bowel. On palpation these lesions may seem polypoid, and they characteristically have a central dimple. They are composed of elements of the pancreas, usually the acinar and ductal structures and less frequently the islets of Langerhans. They are generally small (0.5 to 2 cm), and acute pancreatitis or tumor may occur in them.

Annular pancreas. Annular pancreas is a rare anomaly in which the head of the pancreas surrounds the second portion of the duodenum. It is more common in males than in females, and all grades (from an overlapping of the posterior duodenal wall to a complete ring) may be found. It may be associated with complete or partial atresia of the duodenum and is susceptible to any of the diseases of the pancreas.

Fibrocystic disease of the pancreas. This hereditary disorder of the exocrine glands is seen frequently in children and young adults. The pancreas is usually firm and of normal size. Cysts are very small but may be present in the advanced stages. The acini and ducts are dilated. The acini are usually atrophic and may be totally replaced by fibrous tissue in many of the lobules. Nausea and vomiting may also occur, thus leading to malnourishment. The pancreatic secretion is gradually lost. With advancing pancreatic fibrosis, jaundice may develop from the common duct obstruction. A late manifestation is diabetes. Grossly the pancreas is found to be somewhat nodular and firm. There

may be edema and fat necrosis, but gradually fibrous replacement occurs in much of the parenchyma. Ducts may dilate and contain calculi. Calcification of the gland is seen radiographically in as many as 50% of the patients.

Pancreatitis

Causes. The most common cause of pancreatitis in the United States is biliary tract disease. Gallstone pancreatitis causes a relatively sudden onset of constant biliary pain. As the pancreatic parenchyma is further damaged, the pain becomes more severe and the abdomen becomes rigid and tender.

Alcohol abuse is the second most common cause of pancreatitis; and then comes trauma (surgical or blunt) to the abdomen, which may lead to ascites, the formation of a pancreatic pseudocyst, or pancreatitis.

Acute pancreatitis. The patient presents with moderate to severe tenderness in the epigastrium radiating to the back. The abdomen may be distended secondary to an ileus. Generally no jaundice is present. The pancreatitis may be either localized (associated with biliary disease or trauma) or generalized (associated with alcoholism).

SONOGRAPHIC FINDINGS. In the early stages of acute pancreatitis the gland becomes very swollen because of the increased prominence of lobulations and congested vessels. The early stage may clear completely only to recur with more severe symptoms and further damage to the pancreas.

By sonography the pancreas is normally as echogenic as or more echogenic than the liver. With pancreatitis the swollen gland becomes less echogenic than the liver parenchyma (Fig. 14-20). If localized enlargement is present, it may be difficult to separate from neoplastic involvement of the gland. Analysis of patient history and laboratory values should enable the clinician to make the distinction (Fig. 14-21). On longitudinal scans anterior compression of the inferior vena cava by the swollen head of the pancreas may be apparent.

The pancreatic duct may be obstructed in acute pancreatitis due to inflammation, spasm, edema, swelling of the papilla, or pseudocyst formation.[15]

Acute hemorrhagic pancreatitis. This disease is a rapid progression of acute pancreatitis. Patient symptoms may include intense and severe pain radiating to the back, shock, and ileus.

SONOGRAPHIC FINDINGS. In addition to the typical sonographic signs of pancreatitis, Sarti[12] states that one may find areas of necrosis of the parenchyma. Foci of freshly extravasated blood and fat necrosis are also seen. Necrosis of blood vessels results in the development of hemorrhagic areas referred to as Grey Turner's sign (discoloration of the flanks).

Chronic pancreatitis. Chronic pancreatitis results from recurrent attacks of acute pancreatitis and causes continuing destruction of the pancreatic parenchyma. It generally is associated with chronic alcoholism or biliary disease. Patient symptoms may include epigastric pain progressing with the disease, gastrointestinal problems, and jaundice secondary to common duct obstruction. The

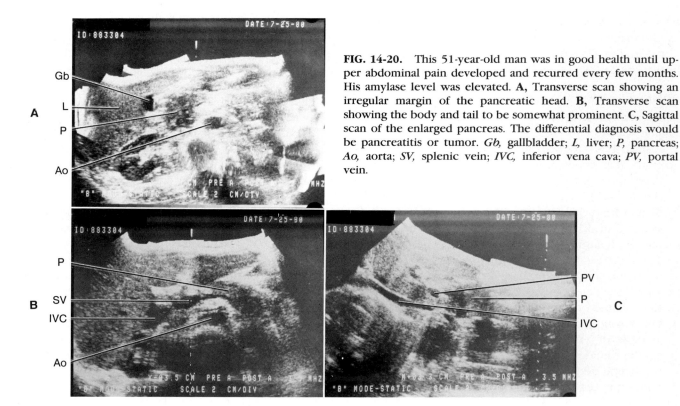

FIG. 14-20. This 51-year-old man was in good health until upper abdominal pain developed and recurred every few months. His amylase level was elevated. **A,** Transverse scan showing an irregular margin of the pancreatic head. **B,** Transverse scan showing the body and tail to be somewhat prominent. **C,** Sagittal scan of the enlarged pancreas. The differential diagnosis would be pancreatitis or tumor. *Gb,* gallbladder; *L,* liver; *P,* pancreas; *Ao,* aorta; *SV,* splenic vein; *IVC,* inferior vena cava; *PV,* portal vein.

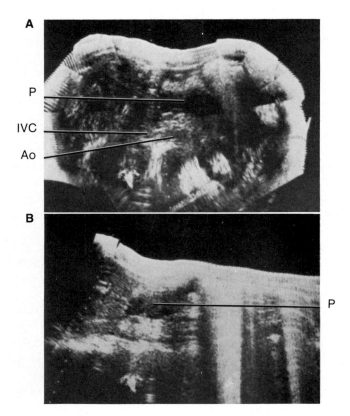

FIG. 14-21. This young woman was receiving chemotherapy for acute lymphocytic leukemia when epigastric pain developed and radiated to her back. The serum amylase level was elevated. The sonogram showed findings of acute pancreatitis. **A,** Transverse scan showing the sonolucent pancreatic tissue anterior to the great vessels. *P,* pancreas, *IVC,* inferior vena cava, and *Ao,* aorta. **B,** Sagittal scan of the inflamed pancreas. Subsequent follow-up scans 1 month later showed resolution of the drug-induced pancreatitis.

duct may dilate and contain calculi. There is calcification of the gland in 20% to 40% of the patients[15] (Fig. 14-22).

SONOGRAPHIC FINDINGS. Chronic pancreatitis may appear as a diffuse or localized involvement of the gland. The irregular borders of the gland are seen with an echogenic parenchyma if fibrosis or calcification is present. Shadowing will occur posterior to the calcification if the calculi are large enough.

The pancreatic duct may show strictures, stenosis, irregularities, and dilation (Fig. 14-23). The most common sites of obstruction are the papilla and the origin of the main pancreatic duct.[15]

Pancreatic abscess

An abscess may arise from a neighboring infection such as a perforated peptic ulcer, acute appendicitis, or acute cholecystitis. The sonographic appearance depends on the amount of debris present. The walls are thick, irregular, and highly echogenic. If air bubbles are present, an echogenic region with a shadow posterior will exist.

Pancreatic cysts

There are two types of pancreatic cysts—true cysts and pseudocysts. They may be either unilocular or multilocular.

True cysts. These microscopic sacs can be congenital or acquired. They arise from within the gland, usually in the head, then in the body, and then the tail. They have a lining epithelium (which may be lost with inflammation), and they contain pancreatic enzymes or are found to be continuous with a pancreatic duct.

Pseudocysts. In contrast, pancreatic pseudocysts are always acquired; they result from trauma to the gland or from acute or chronic pancreatitis. Approximately 11% to

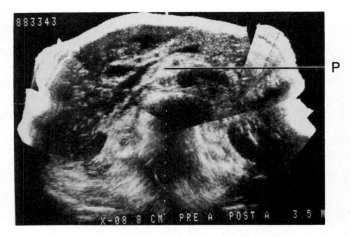

FIG. 14-22. Transverse scan of a patient with chronic pancreatitis. The gland is very dense. *P,* pancreas.

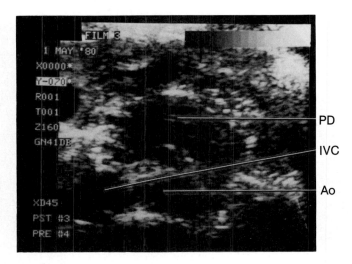

FIG. 14-23. Prominent pancreatic duct, *PD,* in a patient with acute pancreatitis. *IVC,* inferior vena cava, *Ao,* aorta.

18% of patients with acute pancreatitis develop pseudocysts. Encapsulated collections of pancreatic juice, blood, and debris form the pseudocyst. As Sarti[12] states, "the pancreatic enzymes that escape the ductal system cause enzymatic digestion of the surrounding tissue and pseudocyst development. The walls of the pseudocyst form in the various potential spaces in which the escaped pancreatic enzymes are found."[1] The pseudocyst usually presents few symptoms until it becomes large enough to cause pressure on surrounding organs.

Both pseudocysts and true cysts may protrude anteriorly in any direction, although the true cyst is generally associated directly with the pancreatic area. Pseudocysts usually develop through the lesser omentum, displacing the stomach or widening the duodenal loop.

A pseudocyst develops when pancreatic enzymes escape from the gland and break down tissue to form a sterile abscess somewhere in the abdomen. Its walls are not true cyst walls; hence the name *pseudo-* or false cyst. Pseudocysts may develop anywhere in the abdominal cavity and have been found as low as the groin and as high as the mediastinum. They generally take on the contour of the available space around them and therefore are not always spherical, as are normal cysts (Fig. 14-24). There may be more than one pseudocyst, so the sonographer should search for daughter collections when performing an echogram.

SONOGRAPHIC FINDINGS. Sonographically pseudocysts usually appear as well-defined masses with essentially sonolucent echo-free interiors. Because of debris, scattered echoes may be seen at the bottom of the cysts, and increased through-transmission is present (Fig. 14-25). The borders are very echogenic, and the cysts usually are thicker than other simple cysts. When a suspected pseudocyst is located near the stomach, the stomach should be drained so the cyst is not mistaken for a fluid-filled stomach. If the patient has been on continual drainage prior to the ultrasonic examination, this problem is eliminated.

UNUSUAL SONOGRAPHIC PATTERNS. Laing et al.[7] have reported a series of pseudocysts found to contain unusual

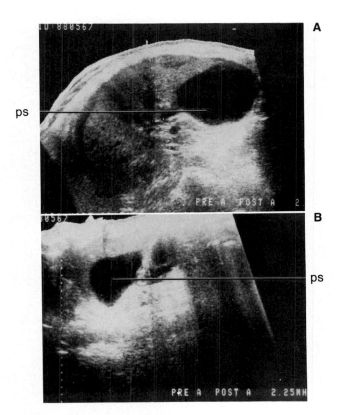

FIG. 14-24. Pancreatic pseudocysts present with a number of sonographic patterns. The most typical is fairly homogeneous with low-level debris, smooth borders, and good through-transmission; the sac assumes the available space in the retroperitoneum. **A,** Transverse scan of a pancreatic pseudocyst, *ps,* in the left upper quadrant. This must be separated from a liver cyst or a fluid-filled stomach. **B,** Sagittal scan showing the pseudocyst to occupy the available space in the retroperitoneum.

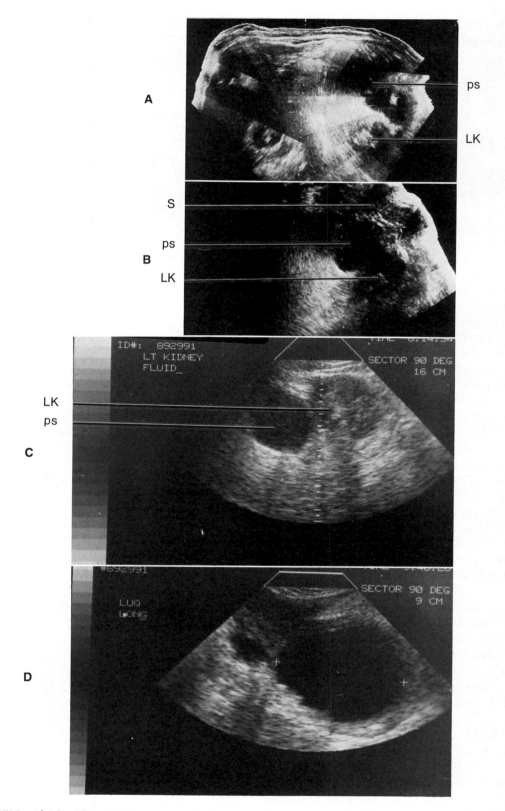

FIG. 14-25. This patient presented 11 days after surgery with left upper quadrant pain. A pseudocyst, *ps,* was found by ultrasound and was demonstrated to be separate from the left kidney, *LK,* and spleen, *S.* It was well encapsulated, which ruled out an abscess formation. **A,** Transverse and, **B,** transverse decubitus views of the spleen, *S,* left kidney, *LK,* and pseudocyst *ps.* **C,** Transverse and, **D,** sagittal scans of the pseudocyst as seen with real time.

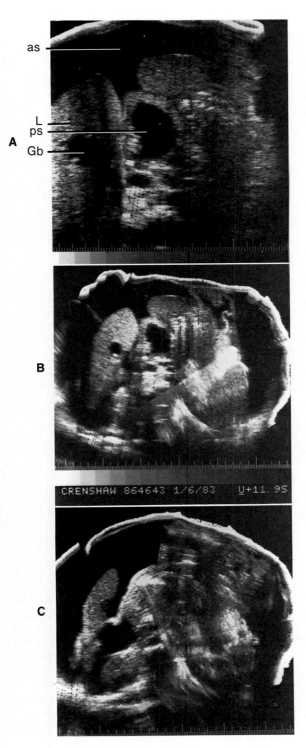

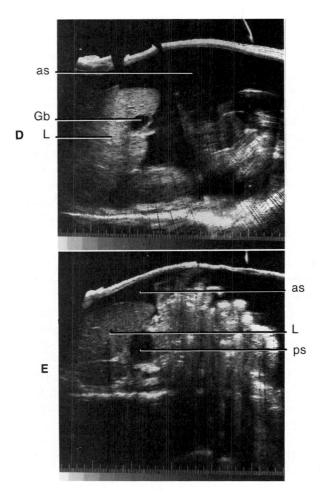

Fig 14-26, cont'd. **D** and **E** are sagittal scans demonstrating the ascitic fluid, *as,* cirrhotic liver, *L,* gallbladder, *Gb,* and pseudocyst *ps.*

FIG. 14-26. **A** to **C** show multiple transverse scans of a patient with cirrhosis, massive ascites, *as,* and a large pseudocyst, *ps,* located near the head of the pancreas.

internal echoes (Fig. 14-26). There were three classifications: (1) septated, which presented with multiple internal septations; (2) excessive internal echoes, caused by an associated inflammatory mass, hemorrhage, or clot formation; and (3) pseudocyst, with absence of posterior enhancement due to the rim of calcification.

SPONTANEOUS RUPTURE. Spontaneous rupture is the most common complication of a pancreatic pseudocyst, occurring in 5% of patients.[8]

In half of this 5% the drainage is directly into the peritoneal cavity. Clinical symptoms are sudden shock and peritonitis. The mortality rate is 50%. Ascites developing as a consequence of spontaneous rupture may be differentiated from that associated with cirrhosis in patients who have known rupture of a pseudocyst by analysis of the fluid for elevated amylase and protein content.[7]

In the other half of the 5% of patients the rupture is into the gastrointestinal tract. Such patients may present a confusing picture sonographically. The initial scan will show a typical pattern for a pseudocyst formation, but the patient may develop intense pain secondary to the rupture, and consequent examination will show the disappearance of the mass.

Benign tumors

Islet cell tumors. These are the most frequent benign tumor of the pancreas. Their size is small, diameter usually 1 to 2 cm, and they are well encapsulated with a good vascular supply. The tumors may be multiple and often are found in the tail of the gland. A large percentage occur in patients with hyperinsulinism and hypoglycemia.

Sonographically islet cell tumors are difficult to image

because of their small size. Greatest success is when they are located in the head of the gland.

Duct cell adenoma. This tumor may develop in the main pancreatic duct and cause obstruction. It has been responsible for the appearance of acute pancreatitis.[6]

Papilloma of the duct. These are found in the region of the ampulla and cause duct obstruction.

Cystadenoma. This lesion is a rare benign neoplasm arising from the pancreatic duct, most commonly in the tail of the pancreas. It occurs more commonly in women. Its size may range from 2 to 15 cm. The coarsely lobulated cystic tumors sometimes present sonographically with cyst walls thicker than the membranes between multilocular cysts.

Neoplasms of the pancreas

Adenocarcinoma. The most common primary neoplasm of the pancreas is adenocarcinoma, which usually occurs in the head. It is more commonly found in middle-aged men than in women. Symptoms usually appear late, the most common being pain radiating to the back or a dull, steadily aching mid-epigastrium pain. Weight loss, painless jaundice, nausea, vomiting, and changes in stools are also clinical symptoms. The painless jaundice usually appears first, followed by nausea and vomiting. The presence of a dilated gallbladder and a palpable mass is strongly suggestive of carcinoma (Courvoisier's law). A cyst or pancreatitis may occur behind the neoplastic obstruction of the duct. With obstruction of the pancreatic ducts, enzymes will be absent or present only in small amounts.

The sonographic appearance of adenocarcinoma is a general loss of the normal pancreatic parenchymal pattern. The gland becomes enlarged, with an irregular nodular border (Fig. 14-27). There may be secondary enlargement of the common duct due to enlargement of the pancreatic head (Fig. 14-28). A dilated pancreatic duct may be present.

Cystadenocarcinoma. Cystadenocarcinoma may be difficult to separate from carcinoma arising in a true cyst or cystic degeneration of a solid carcinoma. It is an irregular, lobulated cystic tumor with thick cellular walls. Metastases arise most commonly in the lymph nodes and liver. The course of this tumor may be slowly progressive with a tendency for the recurrent disease to remain localized.

Sonographic criteria for carcinoma. The detection of tumors less than 2 cm in diameter is difficult for the sonographer. Carcinoma of the pancreas often appears as an irregular mass with ill-defined borders and scattered internal echoes (Figs. 14-29 to 14-31). Arger et al.[1] state that their series of patients with a pancreatic neoplasm demonstrated these findings: (1) echo production less than in a normal pancreas; (2) unhomogeneous echoes, scattered larger echoes, and more intense echoes within the mass; (3) reduced sound transmission; and (4) areas of dense echogenicity in the large tumors. The detection of carcinoma of the pancreas can be difficult, especially if the tumor is infiltrating; therefore the examiner should be

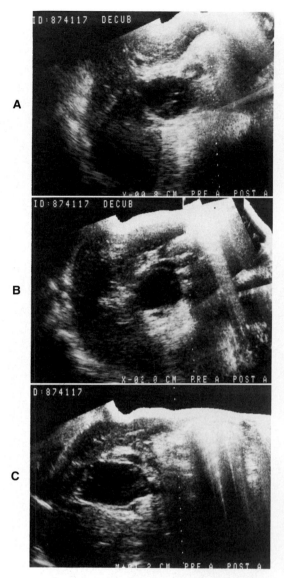

FIG. 14-27. An elderly woman presented with weight loss, gastrointestinal symptoms, and bowel obstruction. Ultrasound demonstrated the presence of a mass between the inferior vena cava and portal vein that was thought to be solid. It lay adjacent to the pancreatic head and most likely represented peripancreatic nodes. **A,** Transverse scan of the solid peripancreatic mass. **B,** The pancreas and vessels were displaced by the mass. **C,** Sagittal scan showing the mass in the area of the porta hepatis. This was found to be adenocarcinoma of the small intestine with invasion.

aware of other echographic findings. A large, noncontracting gallbladder may be tested with a fatty meal. After waiting 40 minutes from the administration of the fatty meal, rescan the patient to note full contraction of the gallbladder. Sokoloff et al.[13] state that typically large, unobstructed gallbladders are seen in fasting normal or vagotomized patients, in the presence of diabetes mellitus, or with contiguous inflammatory process. Weight loss following pancreatitis or with alcohol abuse in association with little pain is highly suggestive of pancreatic carcinoma if there is an ultrasonically detected enlargement of the pancreas. Other clinical signs are jaundice with a palpable mass, increased bilirubin, and increased alkaline

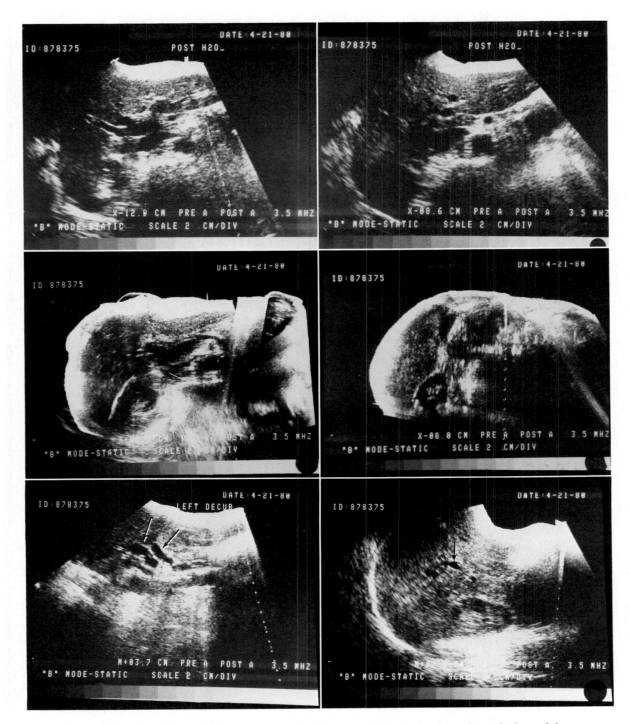

FIG. 14-28.   This 68-year-old man presented with severe abdominal pain and weight loss of three months' duration. A pancreatic carcinoma was found in the head of the gland. It had caused the biliary ducts to dilate *(arrows).*

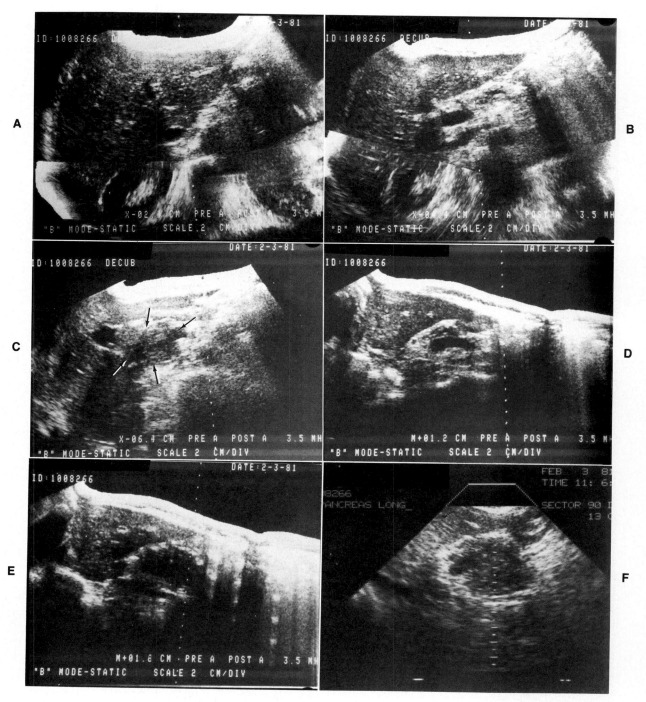

FIG. 14-29.   This 49-year-old man had a history of alcohol abuse, weight loss, and abdominal pain. An irregular mass was found in the head of the pancreas. **A,** Supine transverse scan of the upper abdomen. **B,** Area of the pancreas. The body appears to be of normal size and texture. **C,** Enlarged pancreatic head. **D,** Sagittal scan of the superior mesenteric vein as it bisects the body and uncinate process. **E,** Sagittal scan of the prominent pancreatic head. **F,** Real time of the pancreatic mass.

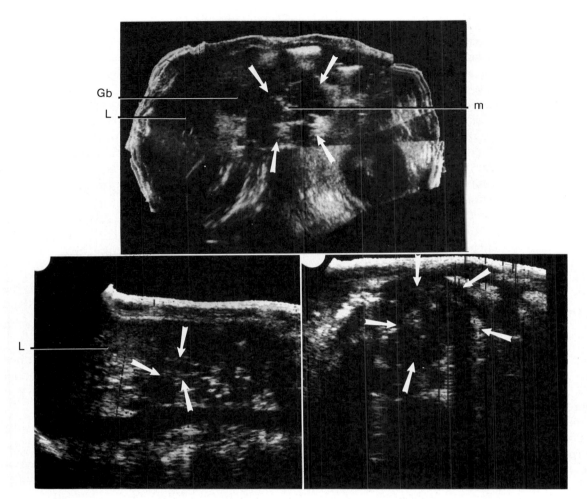

FIG. 14-30. This man presented with epigastric pain of three months' duration. On the sonogram there was a large, irregular, echo-producing mass in the region of the porta hepatis—head of the pancreas area *(arrows)*. This proved to be pancreatic carcinoma at the time of surgery. Liver, *L;* gallbladder, *Gb;* mass, *m.*

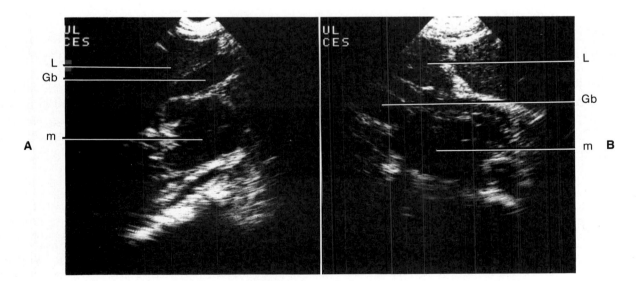

FIG. 14-31. **A,** Sagittal and, **B,** transverse scans of a patient with a large mass, *m,* in the body of the pancreas, which was proven surgically to be carcinoma. The mass is irregular in shape with low-lying internal echoes. The gallbladder was not distended, so the mass was not compressing the common bile duct.

phosphatase. The liver may be enlarged due to common duct obstruction, tumor, or metastatic disease.

Lymph node enlargement secondary to lymphoma or metastatic carcinoma may be confused with pancreatic carcinoma or pancreatitis. This diagnosis can be made by detecting splenic enlargement or the presence of nodes elsewhere in the abdomen. It is often difficult to differentiate carcinoma from pancreatitis. With pancreatitis the borders tend to be well defined whereas with carcinoma they are often poorly defined. If the pancreas is diffusely involved, this is highly suggestive of inflammatory disease. However, these findings in association with a mass in the region of the head of the pancreas do not exclude carcinoma, since pancreatitis and tumor can coexist. In these cases serial examinations may be very helpful in the evaluation of size changes in the gland.

Other "soft" signs for a pancreatic neoplasm by ultrasound include anterior indentation of the inferior vena cava due to enlargement of the pancreatic head, anterior displacement of the superior mesenteric vein due to enlargement of the head or uncinate process, and posterior displacement of the superior mesenteric vein due to enlargement of the head or body of the gland.[16]

Pancreatic duct in pancreatic carcinoma. The majority of pancreatic carcinomas arise from duct epithelium that causes duct dilation secondary to tumor. The pancreas may be poorly visualized if there is marked duct obstruction by tumor.[15]

When the lesion has so progressed that obstructive jaundice is apparent, the identification of a dilated pancreatic duct in conjunction with the dilated biliary tree helps pinpoint the distal site of the lesion. In patients in whom the lesion is small and has not obstructed the CBD, the presence of a periampullary lesion can be suggested by the dilated pancreatic duct.[5]

SUMMARY

1. The pancreas may be visualized ultrasonically in the majority of patients by using the neighboring organs and vascular landmarks to localize the gland.

2. The pancreas lies in the retroperitoneal cavity. It lies deep in the epigastrium and left hypochondrium behind the lesser omental sac.

3. The size and shape of the gland may vary in each patient. It is slightly larger in children than in adults.

4. The pancreas is divided into four sections: head, neck, body, and tail.

5. The head of the pancreas is anterior to the inferior vena cava and left renal vein, inferior to the caudate lobe of the liver and the portal vein and lateral to the second portion of the duodenum. The uncinate portion of the head of the pancreas is posterior to the superior mesenteric artery and vein. The common bile duct passes through a groove posterior to the pancreatic head, and the gastroduodenal artery serves as the anterolateral border.

6. The body of the gland lies on an angle from caudal right to cephalic left, posterior to the stomach and anterior to the origin of the portal vein. It is anterior to the aorta, superior mesenteric artery, left renal vein, left adrenal gland, and left kidney. The splenic artery is usually the superior border of the pancreatic body.

7. The tail of the pancreas lies anterior to the left kidney, close to the spleen and left colic flexure.

8. There are two ducts within the pancreas: the duct of Wirsung and the duct of Santorini.

9. The pancreas is both an exocrine and an endocrine gland. The exocrine function is to produce pancreatic juice. The endocrine function is to produce the hormone insulin.

10. The enzymes of the pancreatic juice are lipase, amylase, carboxypeptidase, trypsin, and chymotrypsin.

11. Failure to sonographically visualize the normal pancreas may be from: fluid-filled duodenum, overlying gas, or overlying solid masses in the retroperitoneum.

12. Congenital anomalies of the pancreas include ectopic pancreatic tissue, annular pancreas, and fibrocystic disease.

13. Pancreatitis may be caused from biliary tract disease or alcohol abuse. The disease may be acute or chronic. Pancreatic pseudocysts may develop with the onset of pancreatitis.

14. Benign tumors of the pancreas include islet cell tumors, duct cell adenoma, papilloma of the duct, and cystadenoma.

15. Neoplasms of the pancreas may include adenocarcinoma and cystadenocarcinoma. Small tumors of the pancreas may be very difficult to image well with ultrasound because of the overlying gas problems that may occur in the upper abdomen.

REFERENCES

1. Arger PH, Mulhern CB, Bonavita JA, et al: Analysis of pancreatic sonography in suspected pancreatic disease, J Clin Ultrasound 7:91, 1979.
2. Eisenscher A and Weill F: Ultrasonic visualization of Wirsung's duct: dream or reality? J Clin Ultrasound 7:41, 1979.
3. Filly RA and Freimanis AK: Echographic diagnosis of pancreatic lesions, Radiology 96:575, 1970.
4. Filly RA and London SS: The normal pancreas: acoustic characteristics and frequency of imaging, J Clin Ultrasound 7:121, 1979.
5. Gosink BB and Leopold GR: The dilated pancreatic duct: ultrasonic evaluation, Radiology 126:475, 1978.
6. Hassani SN, Smulewicz JJ, and Bard R: Pattern of pancreatic carcinoma by real time and gray scale ultrasonography, Appl Radiol, September-October 1977.
7. Laing FC, Gooding GAW, Brown T, and Leopold GR: Atypical pseudocysts of the pancreas: an ultrasonographic evaluation, J Clin Ultrasound 7:27, 1979.
8. Leopold GR, Berg RN, and Reinke RT: Echographic-radiological documentation of spontaneous rupture of a pancreatic pseudocyst into the duodenum, Radiology 120:699, 1972.
9. Macmahon H, Bowie JD, and Beezhold C:

Erect scanning of pancreas using a gastric window, AJR 132:587, 1979.

10. Marks WM, Filly RA, and Callen PW: Ultrasonic evaluation of normal pancreatic echogenicity and its relationship to fat deposition, Radiology 137:475, 1980.

11. Sample WF, Po JB, Gray RK, and Cahill PJ: Gray scale in ultrasonography techniques in pancreatic scanning, Appl Radiol, September-October, 1975.

12. Sarti DA: Rapid development and spontaneous regression of pancreatic pseudocysts documented by ultrasound, Radiology 125:789, 1977.

13. Sokoloff J et al: Pitfalls in the echographic evaluation of pancreatic disease, J Clin Ultrasound 2:321, 1974.

14. Weighall SL, Wolfman NT, and Watson N: The fluid-filled stomach: a new sonic window, J Clin Ultrasound 7:353, 1979.

15. Weinstein BJ, Weinstein DP, and Brodmerkel GJ: Ultrasonography of pancreatic lithiasis, Radiology 134:185, 1980.

16. Wright CH, Maklad F, and Rosenthal S: Grey scale in ultrasonic characteristics of carcinoma of the pancreas, Br J Radiol 52:281, 1979.

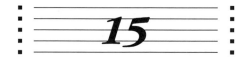

15

Kidneys and Adrenal Glands

SANDRA L. HAGEN-ANSERT AND BECKY LEVZOW

Kidneys

The evaluation of the kidneys with ultrasound is a noninvasive approach to diagnosing renal problems. Generally sonography is used after an *intravenous pyelogram* (IVP) has disclosed the need to investigate the acoustic properties of a mass (cystic or solid) or to further delineate an abnormal lie resulting from an extrarenal mass. In patients who cannot tolerate an IVP because of allergic reaction or other reason, sonography may be selected as the examination of choice to rule out renal disease.

In addition to delineating a renal mass, ultrasound can define perirenal fluid collections (e.g., hematoma or abscess), determine renal size and parenchymal detail, and detect enlarged ureters and hydronephrosis as well as congenital anomalies.

NORMAL ANATOMY

The kidneys lie in the retroperitoneal space under the cover of the costal margin (Fig. 15-1). The right kidney lies slightly lower than the left due to the right lobe of the liver. During inspiration both kidneys move downward by as much as 2.5 cm.

The normal adult kidney varies from 9 to 12 cm in length, 2.5 to 3 cm in thickness, and some 4 to 5 cm in width (Fig. 15-2). Generally both kidneys will attain approximately the same dimensions. A difference of more than 1.5 to 2 cm is significant.

The kidney is surrounded by a fibrous capsule, called the *true capsule,* that is closely applied to the renal cortex. Outside this capsule is a covering of perinephric fat. The perinephric fascia surrounds the perinephric fat and encloses the kidney and adrenal glands. The renal fascia (Geota's fascia) surrounds the true capsule and perinephric fat (Fig. 15-3).

The ureter is 25 cm long and resembles the esophagus in having three constrictions along its course: (1) where it joins the kidney, (2) where it is kinked as it crosses the pelvic brim, and (3) where it pierces the bladder wall. The pelvis of the ureter is funnel shaped in its expanded upper end. It lies within the hilum of the kidney and receives the major calyces. The ureter emerges from the hilum and runs downward along the psoas, which separates it from the tips of the transverse processes of the lumbar vertebrae. It enters the pelvis by crossing the bifurcation of the common iliac artery in front of the sacroiliac. It then runs along the lateral wall of the pelvis to the region of the ischial spine and turns forward to enter the lateral angle of the bladder.

On the medial border of each kidney is the rendhilum, which contains the renal vein, two branches of the renal

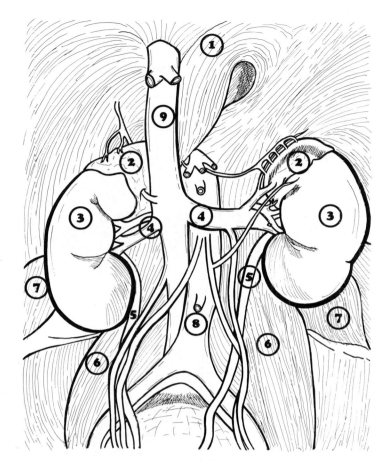

FIG. 15-1. Relationship of the kidneys, suprarenal glands (adrenal), and vascular structures to one another. Diaphragm, *1;* suprarenal gland, *2;* kidney, *3;* renal vein, *4;* ureter, *5;* psoas major muscle, *6;* quadratus lumborum muscle, *7;* aorta, *8;* inferior vena cava, *9.*

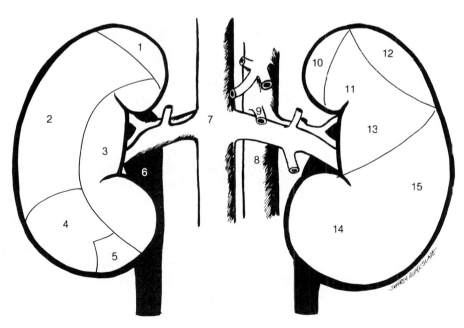

FIG. 15-2. Anatomic structures related to the anterior surfaces of the kidneys. Right adrenal gland, *1;* liver, *2;* duodenum, *3;* right colic flexure, *4;* small intestine, *5;* ureter, *6;* inferior vena cava, *7;* aorta, *8;* superior mesenteric artery, *9;* left adrenal gland, *10;* stomach, *11;* spleen, *12;* pancreas, *13;* jejunum, *14;* descending colon, *15.*

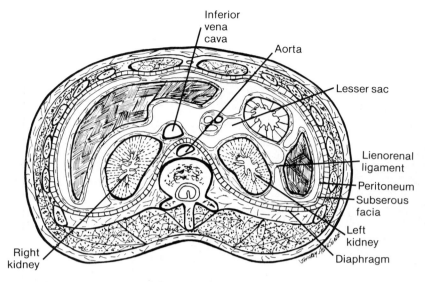

FIG. 15-3. Transverse section of the abdominal cavity through the epiploic foramen.

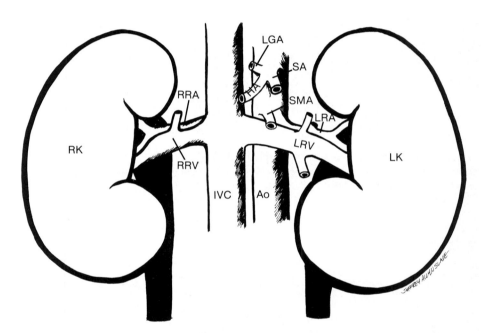

FIG. 15-4. Vascular relationship of the great vessels and their tributaries to the kidneys. Aorta, *Ao;* inferior vena cava, *IVC;* right renal vein, *RRV;* right renal artery, *RRA;* left renal vein, *LRV;* left renal artery, *LRA;* superior mesenteric artery, *SMA;* splenic artery, *SA;* hepatic artery, *HA;* left gastric artery, *LGA.*

artery, the ureter, and the third branch of the renal artery (Fig. 15-4).

The kidney is composed of an internal medullary portion and an external cortical substance (Fig. 15-5). The medullary substance consists of a series of striated conical masses, called the *renal pyramids,* that vary from 8 to 18 in number, and their bases are directed toward the outer circumference of the kidney. Their apices converge toward the renal sinus, where their prominent papillae project into the lumina of the minor calyces.

Within the kidney's upper expanded end (or pelvis) the ureter divides into two or three major calyces, each of which divides into two or three minor calyces. The 4 to 13 minor calyces are cup-shaped tubes that usually come into contact with at least one but occasionally two or

more of the renal papillae (forming the blunted apex of the renal pyramid). The minor calyces unite to form two or three short tubes, the major calyces; these, in turn, unite to form a funnel-shaped sac, the renal pelvis. Spirally arranged muscles surround the calyces and may exert a milking action on these tubes, aiding in the flow of urine into the renal pelvis. As the pelvis leaves the renal sinus, it rapidly becomes smaller and ultimately merges with the ureter.

The filtration-reabsorption system relies on a tubular excretory unit called the nephron, which is the structural and functional unit of the kidney. Each nephron contains a *capsula glomeruli* (Bowman's capsule), which consists of two layers of flat epithelial cells with a space between them and within which a cluster of nonanastomosing cap-

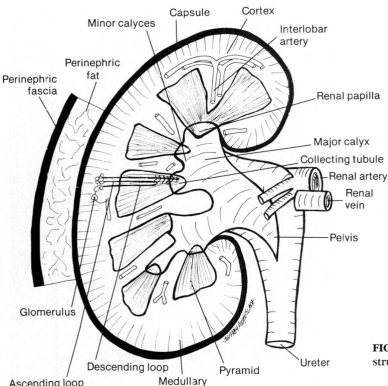

FIG. 15-5. The kidney cut longitudinally to show the internal structure.

illaries (the glomerulus) is enclosed. These two structures, the capsule and the glomerulus, together are named the renal corpuscle or malpighian body. Blood flows into each glomerulus via an afferent arteriole and out via an efferent arteriole. Extending from each Bowman's capsule is a renal tubule that contains several sections: the proximal tubule, descending limb (or loop of Henle), ascending limb, and distal convoluted tubule (which terminates in a straight or collecting tubule). These collecting tubules join larger tubules of one renal pyramid and converge to form a tube that opens at a renal papilla into one of the small calyces. Bowman's capsule and the convoluted tubules lie in the cortex of the kidney whereas the loops of Henle and the collecting tubules lie in the medulla.

The kidney is supplied with blood by the renal artery. Before entering the renal substance, branches of the renal artery vary in number and direction. In most cases the renal artery divides into two primary branches, a larger anterior and a smaller posterior. These arteries break down finally to minute arterioles and are called interlobar arteries. In the portion of the kidney between the cortex and medulla, these arteries are called arcuate arteries.

Likewise, veins of the kidney also break down into these categories. Five or six veins join to form the renal vein, which merges from the hilum anterior to the renal artery. The renal vein drains into the inferior vena cava. Further breakdown of the veins and arteries leads to the afferent and efferent glomerular vessels.

PHYSIOLOGY

The function of the kidney is to excrete urine. More than any other organ in the body, the kidneys adjust the amounts of water and electrolytes leaving the body so

that these equal the amounts of these substances entering the body.

The major function of the urinary system is to remove urea from the bloodstream so it does not accumulate in the body and become toxic. Urea is formed in the liver from ammonia, which in turn is derived from the simple proteins (amino acids) in body cells. The urea is carried in the bloodstream to the kidneys, where it is passed with water, salts, and acids out of the bloodstream and into the kidney tubules as urine.

The kidneys perform three functions to rid the body of unwanted material, which is excreted in the urine. The first is *filtration* of substances from the blood into Bowman's capsule. This occurs in the glomeruli. The second is *reabsorption* of most of the water and part of the solutes from the tubular filtrate into the blood. Most of the substances in the blood are needed by the body. Reabsorption is accomplished by the cells that compose the walls of the convoluted tubules, loop of Henle, and collecting tubules. The third process is *tubular secretion,* whereby acids and other substances that the body does not need are secreted into the distal renal tubules from the bloodstream. The distal renal tubules, carrying urine, merge to form the renal pelvis.

SONOGRAPHIC EVALUATION OF THE KIDNEYS
Normal texture and patterns

The kidneys are imaged by ultrasound as an organ with a smooth outer contour surrounded by reflected echoes of perirenal fat. The renal parenchyma surrounds the fatty central renal sinus, which contains the calyces, infundibula, pelvis, vessels, and lymphatics (Figs. 15-6 and 15-7). Because of the fat interface, the renal sinus is imaged as an

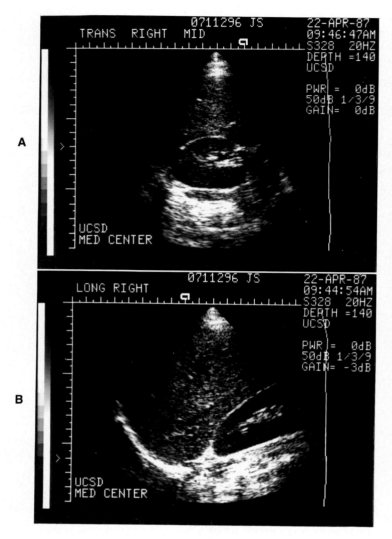

FIG. 15-6.   **A,** Transverse and, **B,** sagittal images of the right kidney as it lies posterior to the liver. Notice the subtle change in acoustic impedance as the sound penetrates the homogeneous liver parenchyma until it reaches the kidney parenchyma. The liver appears slightly more echogenic than the right kidney. The liver is extremely useful as a sonic window to visualize the renal area. As the patient takes a deep breath, the upper pole of the kidney is well visualized.

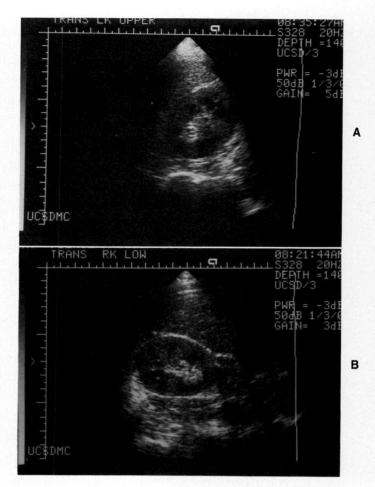

FIG. 15-7.   **A,** Transverse scan of the left kidney as it lies posterior to the spleen. The spleen is not as large as the liver and thus it is more difficult to image the left kidney as easily as the right. If one can avoid the air-filled stomach, the kidney may be imaged through the intercostal margins with the patient in deep inspiration. **B,** Transverse scan of the right kidney as it lies posterior to the liver.

area of intense echoes with variable contour. If two separate collections of renal sinus fat are identified, a double collecting system should be suspected.

Sinus fat and fibrous tissue, known as renal sinus fibrolipomatosis, may show ill-defined zones of low-level echoes within the renal sinus. It may be distinguished from hydronephrosis by its lack of well-defined borders but may be identical to a tumor within the renal sinus.[5]

Generally patients will be given nothing by mouth prior to their ultrasound or IVP examination. This state of dehydration causes the infundibula and renal pelvis to be collapsed and thus indistinguishable from the echo-dense renal sinus fat. If, on the other hand, the bladder is distended from rehydration, the intrarenal collecting system will also become distended.[3] An extrarenal pelvis may be seen as a fluid-filled structure medial to the kidney on transverse scans. Differentiation of the normal variant

from obstruction is made by noting the absence of a distended intrasinus portion of the renal pelvis and infundibula.[1] Dilation of the collecting system has also been noted in pregnant patients. The right kidney is generally involved with a mild degree of hydronephrosis. This distension returns to normal shortly after delivery.

Renal parenchyma

The parenchyma is the area from the renal sinus to the outer renal surface (Fig. 15-8). The arcuate and interlobar vessels are found within and are best demonstrated as intense specular echoes in cross section or oblique section at the corticomedullary junction.[4]

The cortex generally is echo producing (Fig. 15-9) (though its echoes are less intense than those from normal liver) whereas the medullary pyramids are echo free (Fig. 15-10). The two are separated from each other by bands of cortical tissue, called columns of Bertin, that extend inward to the renal sinus.

Rosenfield et al.[5] divided diseases of the renal paren-

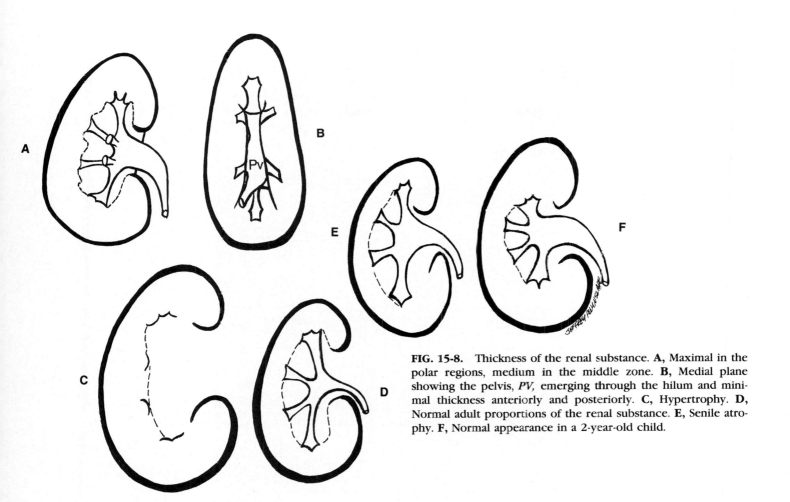

FIG. 15-8. Thickness of the renal substance. **A,** Maximal in the polar regions, medium in the middle zone. **B,** Medial plane showing the pelvis, *PV,* emerging through the hilum and minimal thickness anteriorly and posteriorly. **C,** Hypertrophy. **D,** Normal adult proportions of the renal substance. **E,** Senile atrophy. **F,** Normal appearance in a 2-year-old child.

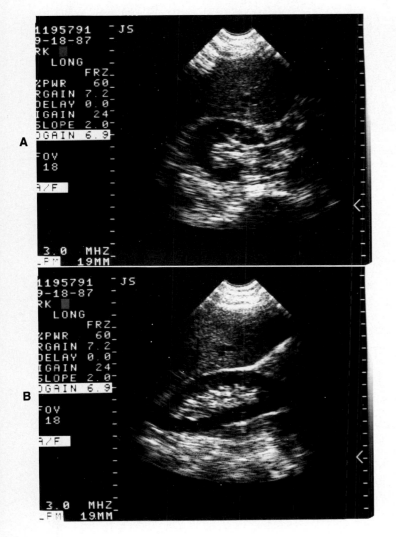

FIG. 15-9. **A** and **B,** Sagittal scans of the normal kidney. The cortex is the brightest of the echoes within the renal parenchyma. The medullary pyramids are echo free. The pyramids are separated from the cortex by bands of cortical tissue, the columns of Bertin, that extend inward to the renal sinus.

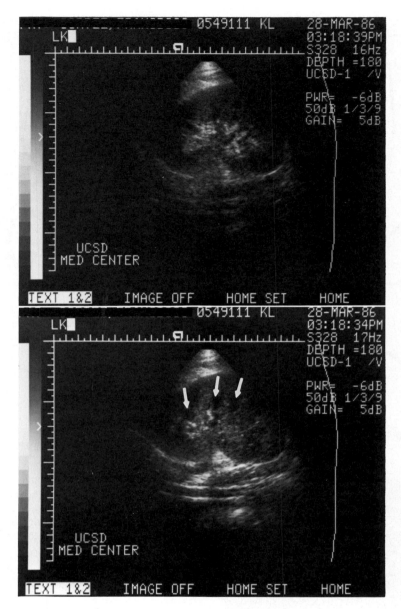

FIG. 15-10.   Transverse images of the left kidney demonstrating the echo-producing cortex and the small, echo-free renal pyramids (*arrows*).

chyma into those that accentuate cortical echoes but preserve or exaggerate the corticomedullary junction (Type I) and those that distort the normal anatomy, obliterating the corticomedullary differentiation in either a focal or diffuse manner (Type II).

The criteria for Type I changes were that (1) the echo intensity in the cortex be equal to or greater than that in the adjacent liver or spleen and (2) the echo intensity in the cortex equal that in the adjacent renal sinus. Minor signs would include the loss of identifiable arcuate vessels or the accentuation of corticomedullary definition.

Type II changes can be seen in a focal disruption of normal anatomy with any mass lesion, including cysts, tumors, abscesses, and hematomas..

Patient position and technique

The most efficient way to evaluate the kidneys is through the liver for the right kidney (Fig. 15-11) or through the

spleen for the left kidney (Fig. 15-12). The patient should be in a supine or decubitus position. The parenchymal echoes of the liver and spleen must be compared to the echo pattern of the renal parenchyma.

A proper adjustment of time gain compensation (TGC) with adequate sensitivity settings will allow a uniform acoustic pattern throughout the image. The renal cortical echo amplitude should be compared to the liver parenchymal echo amplitude at the same depth so the effect of an inappropriate TGC setting will be reduced.[1]

If the patient has a significant amount of perirenal fat, a high-frequency transducer may not penetrate the area properly and give the appearance as hypoechoic in the deeper areas of the kidney. Renal detail may also be obscured if the patient has hepatocellular disease, gallstones, or other abnormal mass collections between the liver and kidney.

Transverse, coronal, and longitudinal scans may be

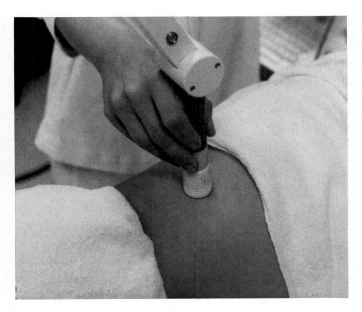

FIG. 15-11. The slight decubitus position is very effective for demonstrating the right kidney when the liver is used as an acoustic window.

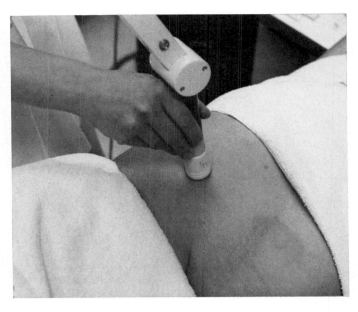

FIG. 15-12. The patient may be rolled into a right decubitus position to image the left kidney.

made through the intercostal margins to image the renal parenchyma. Relational anatomy should be identified to rule out possible metastases, abscess formation, or other incidental abnormality.

The upper pole of the left kidney may be difficult to image with the patient supine, and an upright prone or coronal approach through the spleen and left kidney may be more effective.

Real-time sector allows the rapid visualization of the lie of the kidney, which may be useful for accurate renal size determination.

Renal vascular structures

The renal vessels are best seen on transverse scans at the level of the hilum. Patency of the renal vein is a very important workup of renal carcinoma. Tumor extension into the renal vein or inferior vena cava may appear as low-level echoes within a dilated vascular structure.

The renal arteries flow posterior to the renal veins. On longitudinal scans the right renal artery is retrocaval and may be seen as a circular structure posterior to the IVC. The left renal vein (Fig. 15-13) may be seen as it passes anterior to the aorta and posterior to the SMA before flowing into the inferior vena cava.

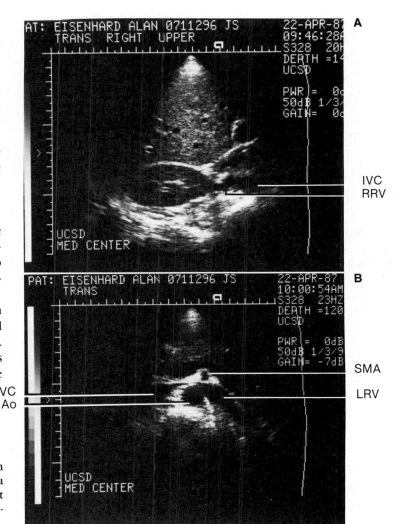

FIG. 15-13. **A,** Transverse scan of the right kidney, which shows the right renal vein, *RRV,* as it flows into the inferior vena cava, *IVC.* **B,** Transverse scan of the left renal vein, *LRV,* as it flows posterior to the superior mesenteric artery, *SMA,* and anterior to the aorta, *Ao.*

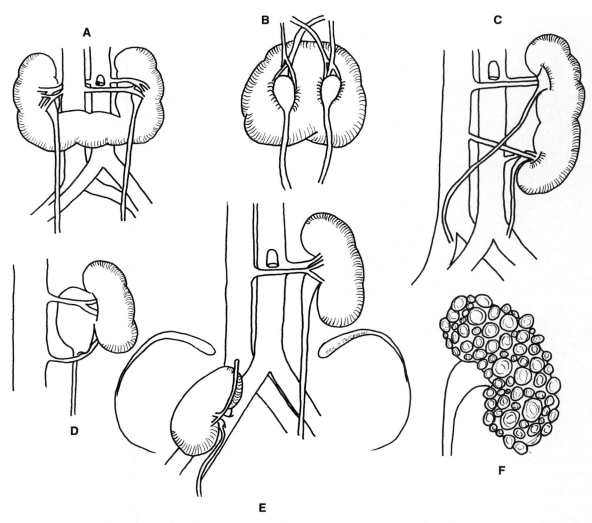

FIG. 15-14. Variations of renal anatomy, position within the retroperitoneal cavity, and pathology. **A,** Horseshoe kidney shown as two kidneys connected by an isthmus anterior to the great vessels and inferior to the inferior mesenteric artery. **B,** Cake kidney with a double collecting system. **C,** Double collecting system in a single kidney. **D,** Obstruction of the renal pelvis resulting in hydronephrosis. **E,** Pelvic kidneys with one kidney in the normal retroperitoneal position. **F,** Polycystic kidney.

Anatomic variations

A common renal variation is the dromedary hump, which is a localized bulge on the lateral border of the kidney. This hump will present the same echographic pattern as the rest of the renal parenchyma and thus will not be mistaken for a mass.

A double collecting system or elongated upper pole infundibulum may show a large column of Bertin in the midportion of the kidney. This has the appearance of a large and occasionally masslike zone of tissue, with echo characteristics much like cortex, insinuated between two separated portions of the echodense renal sinus.[2]

Other variations in renal anatomy are shown in Fig. 15-14.

CLINICAL SIGNS AND SYMPTOMS

Analysis of the patient's chart and medical history may disclose signs of renal disease such as a palpable flank mass, hematuria, polyuria, oliguria, pain, fever, urgency, or generalized edema. There may already be an acute onset of renal failure present.

Laboratory data that may indicate renal failure are an elevated blood urea nitrogen (BUN) and creatinine and an increased protein in the urine. Since the kidneys possess a significant reserve, loss of up to 60% of functioning renal parenchyma will not lead to elevation of either BUN or creatinine. Renal function is severely impaired when these levels are elevated.

PATHOLOGY AND SONOGRAPHIC PATTERNS
Congenital deformities

Agenesis. Congenital agenesis, absence of one kidney and ureter, may be difficult to assess clinically. Ultrasound can outline the normal kidney and tell with certainty whether one kidney is absent or pathologically afflicted.

Supernumerary kidney. Although rare, supernumerary kidney is a complete duplication of the renal system. It generally is found in the pelvis but occasionally will as-

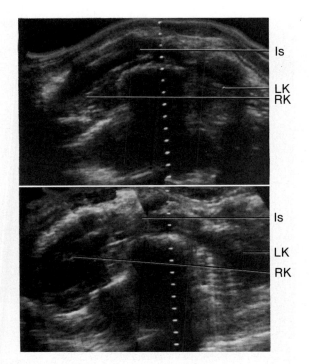

FIG. 15-15. Supine scans of the horseshoe kidney. The isthmus of the kidney drapes anterior to the prevertebral vessels, and careful scanning technique should be used to compress this part of the renal structure. Isthmus, *Is*; right kidney, *RK*; left kidney, *LK*.

cend with the other renal structures. Ultrasound may be able to outline two separate kidneys if they are within the normal renal area but may overlook the extra system if it is in the pelvis.

Horseshoe kidney. Horseshoe kidney occurs during fetal development, with fusion of the upper or lower poles. It does not ascend to its normal position in the retroperitoneal cavity. Generally the isthmus is found near the level of the iliac crest. It has separate ureters from either side of the kidney but is connected by tissue (the isthmus) draping across the midline.

Ultrasonically a horsehoe kidney should be evaluated from the supine position, since the kidneys generally appear lower in the abdomen and may be attenuated by the iliac crest in the prone position. The isthmus is best recorded with single-sweep technique and is seen as a sonolucent band draping over the great vessels. Lymphadenopathy is difficult to diagnose in a patient with a horseshoe kidney, since the isthmus may mimic the lymph nodes. Real-time equipment should allow visualization of the renal parenchyma with the isthmus connecting the two capsules and thus may aid in distinguishing other disease from the isthmus (Fig. 15-15).

Renal masses

Prior to the ultrasound examination for a renal mass, a complete review of the patient's chart and previous diagnostic examinations should be made. In most patients an IVP will already have been obtained; and these films should be used for assessing the size and shape of the kid-

neys, determining the location of the mass, detecting any distortion of the renal outline or pericalyceal system, and establishing the presence or absence of calcium or gas.

Renal masses are categorized as cystic, solid, or complex. A *cystic* mass will present sonographically with several characteristic features: smooth, well-defined circular borders, a sharp interface between the cyst and renal parenchyma, no internal echoes (aside from reverberations), and excellent through-transmission. On the other hand, a *solid* lesion will project as a nongeometric shape with irregular borders, a poorly defined interface between the mass and the kidney, low-level internal echoes, a poor posterior border due to the increased attenuation of the tumor, and very poor through-transmission. Areas of necrosis, hemorrhage, or calcification within the tumor may alter the above classification slightly and cause the mass to fall into the *complex* category.

In our experience the real-time sector scan allows a more complete evaluation of renal masses than does the articulated arm scan. If the mass is very small, respiration may cause it to move out of the field of view just enough to be missed on the articulated arm scan. The flexibility of the real-time sector enables the sonographer to do multiple rotations of the transducer and to view the kidney with the patient in normal respiration.

Simple cyst. These cysts may be located anywhere in the kidney and, if benign, are of no clinical significance unless they cause distortion of adjacent calyces to produce hydronephrosis or pain.

Peripelvic cysts are found within the region of the renal pelvis. Parapelvic cysts are outside the renal capsule but in the region of the pelvis.

Sonographic features include a smooth wall, a circular anechoic mass with good through-transmission, and the tadpole sign (Fig. 15-16) (i.e., narrow bands of acoustic shadowing posterior to the margins of the cyst at the borders of enhancement). A septum may occasionally be seen within the cyst as a well-defined linear line (Fig. 15-17). Sometimes small sacculations or infoldings of the cyst wall produce irregularity of the wall, and cyst puncture should be employed to ascertain that the mass is a cyst (Fig. 15-18).

Reverberation echoes may be seen along the anterior margin of the cyst. A change in transducer diameter and frequency may help to "clean up" the reverberation artifacts, especially in smaller cysts. Thus a higher-frequency smaller-diameter transducer would cause a small cyst to appear more sharply defined.

ULTRASONIC ASPIRATION TECHNIQUES. Once a renal mass has met the criteria for a cystic mass, a needle aspiration may be recommended to obtain fluid from the lesion for further evaluation of its internal composition.

The patient should be positioned with sandbags under the abdomen to help push the kidneys toward the posterior abdominal wall and provide a flat scanning surface. The cyst should be located in the transverse and longitudinal planes with scans performed at midinspiration. The depth of the mass should be noted from its anterior to

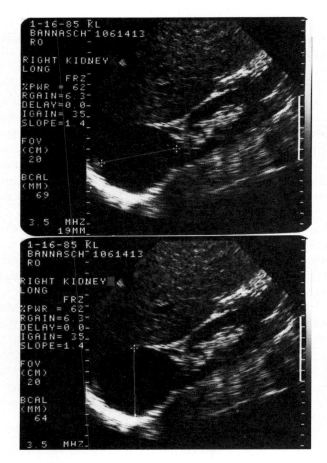

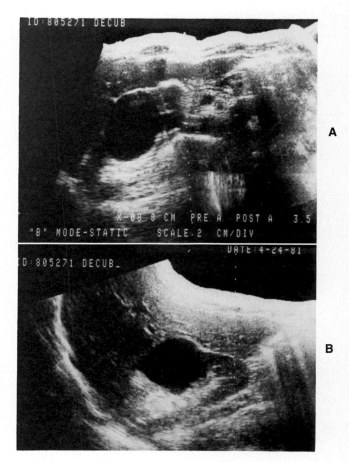

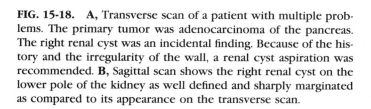

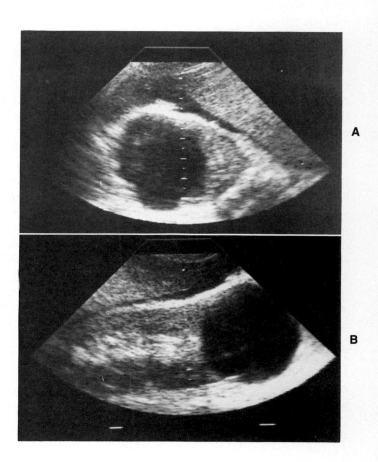

FIG. 15-16. Sagittal scans of a patient with a large right renal cyst in the upper pole. Measurements may be made in the long axis and AP axis of the kidney to aid in aspiration procedures, or in subsequent follow-up examinations.

FIG. 15-17. A, Supine transverse view of a right renal cyst. **B,** Sagittal supine view of the renal cyst as it compresses the calyceal echo pattern.

FIG. 15-18. A, Transverse scan of a patient with multiple problems. The primary tumor was adenocarcinoma of the pancreas. The right renal cyst was an incidental finding. Because of the history and the irregularity of the wall, a renal cyst aspiration was recommended. **B,** Sagittal scan shows the right renal cyst on the lower pole of the kidney as well defined and sharply marginated as compared to its appearance on the transverse scan.

posterior borders so the exact depth can be given to aid in placement of the needle.

A beveled needle will cause multiple echoes within the walls of the cyst. If the needle is slightly bent, many echoes will appear until the bent needle is completely out of the transducer's path. The larger the needle gauge, the stronger the reflection will be.

Sterile technique is used for aspiration and biopsy procedures. The transducer must be gas sterilized. Sterile lubricant is used to couple the transducer to the patient's skin.

When the area of aspiration is outlined on the patient's back, the distance is measured from the anterior surface to the middle of the cyst.

The volume of the cyst may be determined by measuring the radius of the mass and using the following formula:

$$V = \frac{4}{3} \pi r^3$$

The diameter of the mass can be applied to this formula:

$$V = d^3 \div 2$$

The patient's skin is painted with tincture of benzalkonium (Zephiran), and sterile drapes are applied. A local anesthetic is administered over the area of interest, and the sterile transducer is used to relocate the cyst. The needle is inserted into the central core of the cyst. The needle stop will help in making sure that the needle does not go through the cyst. The fluid is then withdrawn according to the volume calculations.

Inflammatory cyst. A simple renal cyst that becomes infected may present a complex echo pattern with thick walls, low-level echoes, and ill-defined borders.

Hemorrhagic cyst. This cyst may be difficult to define sonographically. Approximately 6% of simple cysts will hemorrhage, and the pattern may be hard to separate from that of a cystic neoplasm. Patterns range from one belonging to a simple cyst to one having irregular walls with low-level echoes and good through-transmission.

Calcified cyst. A cyst with calcified walls will present decreased through-transmission and echogenic walls. A cyst aspiration should be performed to rule out the presence of malignancy.

Cyst with milk of calcium.[1] These masses are calyceal diverticula that may or may not have lost their communication with the calyceal system. The condition presents no symptoms and generally is found incidentally at radiography. Within the cystic mass there is a layering, a linear band of strong echoes that are associated with an acoustic shadow.

Cystic mass with tumor.[1] The presence of a tumor mass in the cyst may signify a rapidly expanding cyst adjacent to a tumor. The tumor becomes incorporated into the expanding cyst. A cyst puncture should be made to define cellular contents.

Renal sinus lipomatosis. This is generally found by sonography to present as an area of low-level echoes

within the cystic area comparable to the pattern from the surrounding parenchyma.

Renal hematoma. Depending on the age of the hematoma, this process has a variety of sonographic findings. A fresh hematoma will present as a cystic structure without a smooth wall. As clot formation occurs, low-level echoes appear. Eventually the hematoma will liquefy or become organized, and its appearance will then become more cystic or complex.

Vascular cystic masses. Saccular aneurysms and arteriovenous malformations may appear as cystic multiloculations and cystic masses, respectively.

Hydronephrosis.[4] A cyst found at the upper pole of the kidney should elicit the question of a possible second dilated upper collecting system. If it is hydronephrotic, a tubular echo-free structure may be seen passing medial to the lower collecting system; this represents the dilated ureter. Septa may be seen if more than one calyx is involved.

General hydronephrosis presents as the loss of a pelvicalyceal system with cysts of similar size. Generally there is an absence of renal parenchyma (Figs. 15-19 to 15-21). This may be associated with a large extrarenal pelvis (one large medial cyst surrounded by and communicating with several laterally placed equal-sized smaller cysts). In another form of hydronephrosis a single cystic mass may be seen replacing the kidney. It may have a slightly lobulated border.

To separate a multicystic kidney from hydronephrosis, one must establish the presence or absence of a pelvicalyceal echo complex.

Multicystic kidney. This is a common cause of a mass in the neonatal abdomen. The kidneys have decreased or absent blood supply and are connected to an atretic ureter. Sonographically multiple cysts may be seen with no

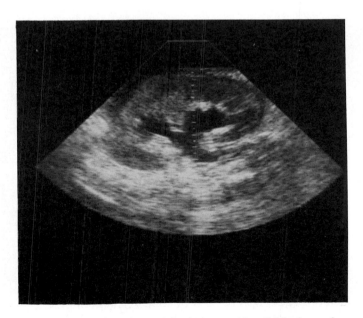

FIG. 15-19. Sagittal scan of the kidney with mild hydronephrosis of the pelvicalyceal system.

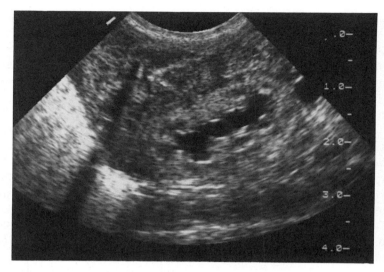

FIG. 15-20.   Sagittal scan of a neonate, which shows a mild form of hydronephrosis. It is not uncommon to see this pattern in the neonatal stage.

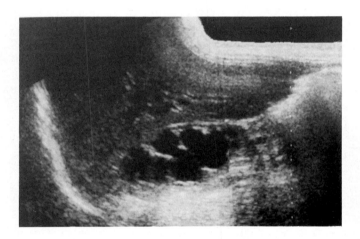

FIG. 15-21.   Sagittal scan of a patient with right hydronephrosis. There is loss of the pelvicalyceal system, with cysts of similar size representing the distended pelvis.

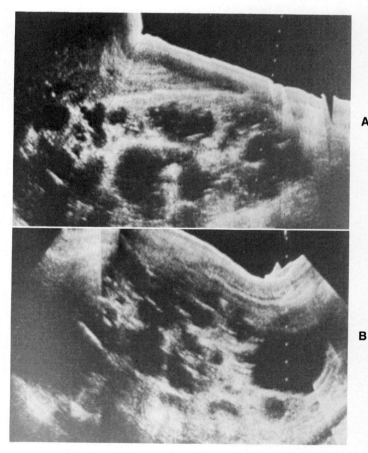

FIG. 15-22.   **A,** Adult polycystic disease is shown on these sagittal scans of the right kidney. **B,** Left kidney also shows polycystic disease. The renal parenchyma is completely filled with multiple cysts of varying sizes.

evidence of renal parenchyma or pelvicalyceal echo patterns.

Adult multicystic disease. Sonographically these patients will display calcified cysts with a small kidney and absent renal pelvis.

Adult polycystic disease. In this disease a cyst may arise from any portion of a collecting system (Fig. 15-22). Small cysts (under 1 cm) may not be readily detected although renal enlargement will be present. As the cysts grow, they become visible by sonography, with variable shapes and sizes and irregular walls. The pelvicalyceal echoes are seen, although they may be distorted by the cysts (Fig. 15-23).

Associated cysts in the liver (30% to 40%), pancreas (10%), and spleen (5%) have also been reported. Pitfalls in diagnosing them may arise if one becomes infected or hemorrhages. Severe hydronephrosis superimposed on chronic pyelonephritis may be distinguished from polycystic kidney disease by the communication of cysts with

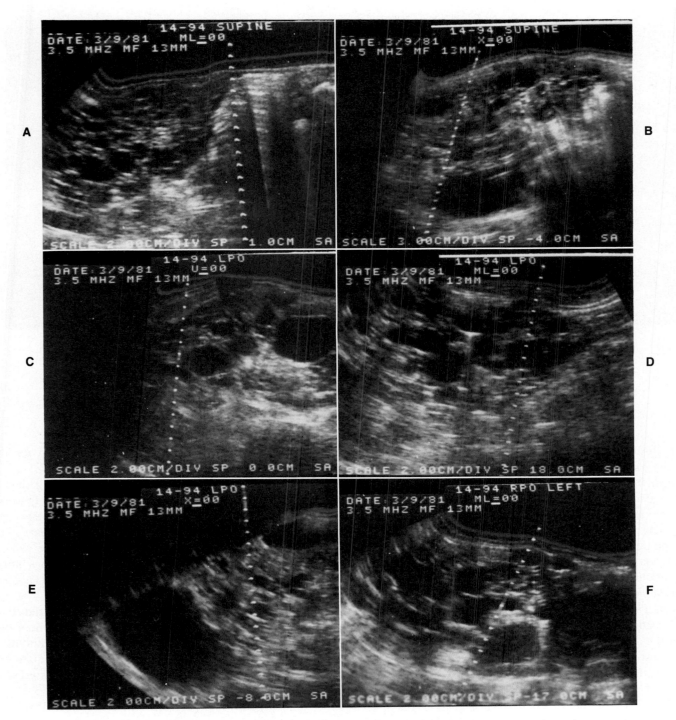

FIG. 15-23.   Patient with polycystic kidneys and liver disease. Multiple cysts are seen throughout the parenchyma of both organs. **A,** Supine transverse scan of the liver and kidney. There are so many cysts in both organs that it is difficult to separate one from the other. **B,** Supine transverse scan. **C** and **D,** Left posterior oblique scan of the right kidney. **E,** Left posterior oblique of a large cyst within the right kidney. **F,** Right posterior oblique view of the left kidney.

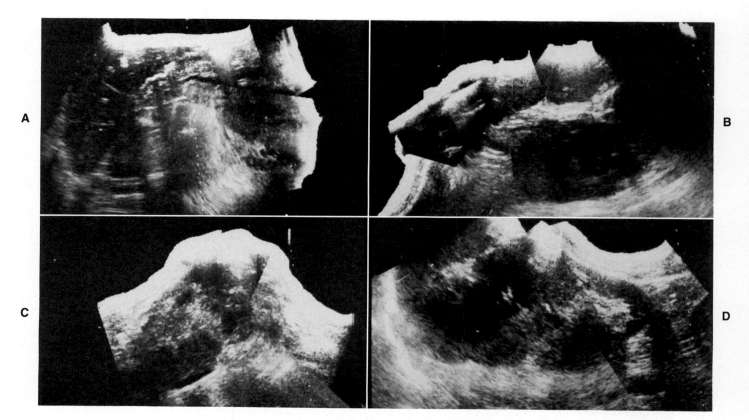

FIG. 15-24. Multiple scans of a large solid renal mass arising from the left kidney in a patient with a previous left renal carcinoma. **A,** Supine transverse scan showing the mass arising from the anterior border of the kidney. **B,** Coronal scan showing the left kidney displaced by the mass. **C,** Coronal transverse scans over the area of the solid mass. **D,** Coronal sagittal scan of the mass arising from the left upper pole of the kidney.

a longitudinal configuration. Polycystic cysts have a more circular lobulated appearance.

Infantile polycystic disease.[3] This form of tubular ectasia causes the tubules in the distal collecting systems to dilate and form small cystic structures. Sonographically they may appear as hepatic and portal fibrosis with renal enlargement with increased reflections throughout the parenchyma because of defined cystic masses in the cortex and medulla.

Hypernephroma[3] (renal adenocarcinoma). In contrast to a smoothly outlined cystic mass, hypernephromas are irregular in shape. The margins are well demarcated from the surrounding tissue, but the mass does not separate itself sonically from the renal parenchyma. Its edges are irregular, and low-level internal echoes are seen (Fig. 15-24). Usually these tumors will produce a "bump" on the IVP. The tumor may grow so large as to replace the renal volume. The smaller tumors, which do not distort the renal outline, are difficult to detect; one must look for subtle renal parenchymal widening or slight calyceal displacement (as seen on the IVP).

The amount of internal echo reflections may depend on the presence or absence of hemorrhage or necrosis within the tumor (Fig. 15-25).

If the mass appears to show evidence of a hypernephroma, attention should be directed to other structures and organs (e.g., the renal vein, inferior vena cava, liver) for possible metastases and to the retroperitoneum for the presence of enlarged nodes.

Transitional cell carcinoma. Symptoms generally range from incidental hematuria to grossly bloody urine. Most of these tumors are invasive without the presence of a bulky mass. When a bulky mass is found, it appears to be anechoic or to contain low-level echoes. These tumors become difficult to classify by sonographic findings alone, and thus a differential diagnosis must be given (Figs. 15-26 and 15-27).

Renal lymphoma. Patients with disseminated lymphomatous malignancies may have renal involvement that presents as nonspecific enlargement. If the lymphoma is focal in nature, a defined anechoic or low-level mass will be seen, and through-transmission will not be as great as seen with a simple cyst.

Angiomyolipoma (benign renal tumor). This mass presents as a homogeneous strongly echogenic area with significant acoustic impedance (Fig. 15-28). These characteristics are related to its high vascularity and increased fat content.

Inflammatory masses. Symptoms for inflammatory masses include fever, chills, and flank pain. Two acute inflammatory processes in the kidney can produce mass lesions capable of being mistaken for a renal tumor.[3] A *carbuncle or abscess* may present as a sonolucent mass with low-level echoes and shaggy margins. *Inflammatory cells*

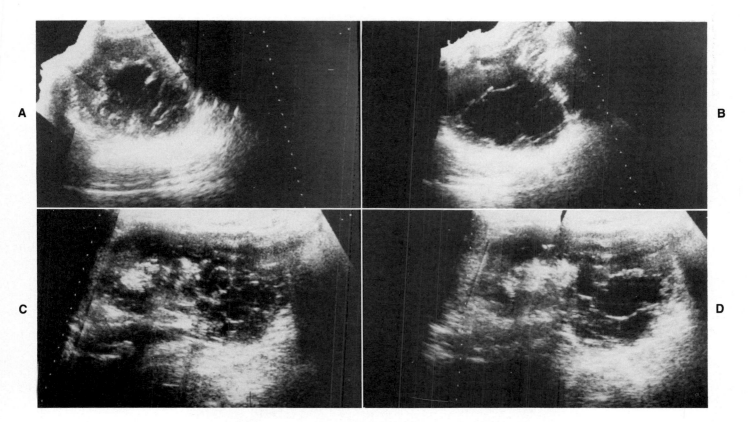

FIG. 15-25. This patient presented with a large complex renal tumor. **A,** Prone transverse scan over the area of the mass. **B,** On this scan, the mass appears somewhat homogeneous with good transmission, but the margins are very irregular. **C** and **D,** Sagittal prone scan showing the complex nature of the mass as it projects from the lower pole of the kidney.

may be seen in the renal parenchyma and can cause swelling and edema of the kidney with no discrete mass (Fig. 15-29).

A chronic renal abscess may produce a mass in the absence of clinical symptoms and present sonographically as a complex lesion.

Xanthogranulomatous pyelonephritis. Xanthogranulomatous pyelonephritis produces renal enlargement with multiple anechoic areas having central echogenic foci associated with acoustic shadowing.

Perinephric fluid collections. Fluid collections that lie adjacent to the kidney in the intraperitoneal or retroperitoneal space will show sonographically as a somewhat well-defined sonolucent area outside the kidney (Fig. 15-30). To separate this collection from an intrarenal mass requires that the renal outline be well defined. The patient should be scanned in the supine, prone, and decubitus positions so the collection can be visualized outside the kidney.

Renal failure

Hydronephrosis. Sonographic findings of moderate bilateral hydronephrosis were encountered by Morin and Baker[3] in a dehydrated patient undergoing rehydration. Renal sonography is most reliable in hydronephrosis if performed with the bladder empty and prior to initiation of rehydration.

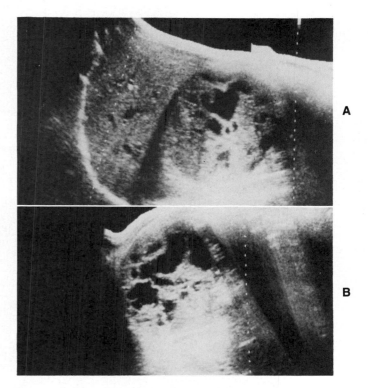

FIG. 15-26. This patient with a renal cell carcinoma presented at ultrasonography with a large solid mass that contained multiple necrotic areas arising from the right kidney. Since a clear margin was seen to separate the mass from the liver, its origin was thought to be renal or retroperitoneal. **A,** Sagittal supine scan. **B,** Transverse supine scan over the area of the complex tumor.

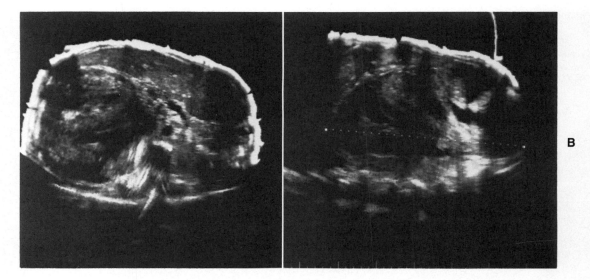

FIG. 15-27.   **A,** Transverse and, **B,** supine scans of a patient with a huge mass arising from the right kidney. The mass is very complex in nature. There is mild hydronephrosis of the pericalyceal system. This renal mass was further investigated.

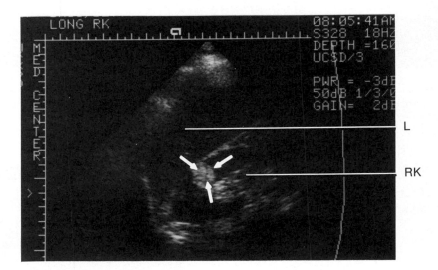

FIG. 15-28.   Sagittal scan of a patient with a small angiomyolipoma. This benign tumor is very echogenic and well defined. It may be separated as a discrete mass from the renal cortex. Liver, *L;* right kidney, *RK;* mass (*arrows*).

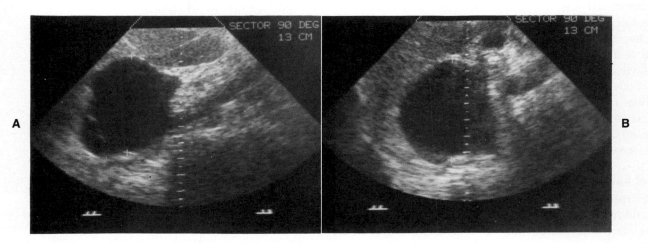

FIG. 15-29.   This patient presented with an elevated white blood count and spiking fever. **A,** The supine sagittal scan reveals a homogeneous, slightly irregular mass arising from the upper pole of the right kidney. **B,** Transverse scan of the renal abscess. Note the decreased through-transmission posterior to the abscess wall.

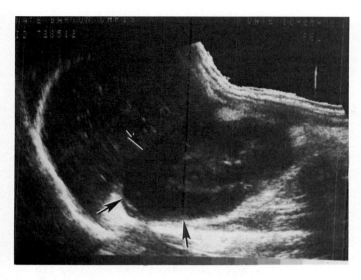

FIG. 15-30.   Sagittal scan over the right upper quadrant shows a large fluid collection between the liver and the right kidney. This represented a renal hematoma (*arrows*).

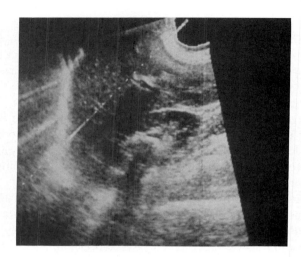

FIG. 15-31.   Sagittal scan of a staghorn calculus without obstruction to the pelvis.

Increased pressure in the kidney can affect the calyces or pelvis. A common pattern is calyceal distension without a prominent pelvis. By sonography this appears as a group of similar-sized cystic structures located in the central renal area. It may be distinguished from multicystic disease by the fact that the cysts are of similar size and there is an absence of echoes from the renal pelvic fat.

Resnick and Sanders[4] state that severe hydronephrosis may take on one of three patterns: a central septation, a blown-out (ovoid) sac, or the dumbbell or hourglass shape.

In patients with ureteropelvic junction obstruction the extrarenal pelvis is larger than the dilated infundibular component of the pelvicalyceal system. This type is the dumbbell pattern.

A rim of renal parenchyma surrounding the dilation may or may not be seen. The width of the remaining renal parenchyma may help in determining renal function and the prognosis of the disease.

Another pattern of hydronephrosis shows distended calyces with a medially located larger cystic structure representing the pelvis and upper ureter.[4] This has a sausage shape and may lead into the intrarenal component without a definite segmental narrowing. The cauliflower appearance of calyces flowing to the dilated pelvis may also be seen.

Besides cystic structures mimicking hydronephrosis, or vice versa, the presence of a staghorn calculus within a dilated collecting system may be a source of confusion. To distinguish this finding from another lesion, one should be able to see a prominent acoustic shadow posterior to the dense calculus (Fig. 15-31).

Pyonephrosis may be another variant of hydronephrosis. It will present as a dilated system with low-level echoes from the pus and may be difficult to distinguish from a tumor mass. Careful evaluation of the patient's chart and laboratory values may help make the diagnosis.

Small kidneys.   Small kidneys represent end-stage renal disease. In general, when compared to the liver, the renal parenchyma is more echogenic. Renal vascular disease may be another cause of small kidneys. If the infarct is focal, areas of decreased echoes will be seen. Within the infarcted small area, the kidneys will expand and contain fewer parenchymal echoes before shrinking to be echogenic.

Renal Transplant

BECKY LEVZOW

Renal transplantation and dialysis are currently used for the treatment of chronic renal failure or endstage renal disease. Ultrasound has emerged as an excellent tool in monitoring such transplant patients and may complement nuclear medicine and laboratory values in distinguishing the course of rejection. Since the sonogram does not rely on the function of the kidney, serial studies can be readily incorporated in determining the diagnosis and the treatment to be administered.

A number of complications may arise following transplantation: rejection, acute tubular necrosis (ATN), obstructive nephropathy, extraperitoneal fluid collections, hemorrhage or infarction, recurrent glomerulonephritis, graft rupture, and renal emphysema. Decreased renal function is commonly the main indication for ultrasonic evaluation.

THE PROCEDURE

Most renal transplant patients have had long-standing renal failure without obstructive nephropathy. Before the procedure, patient risk factors to be considered are age, primary diagnosis, secondary medical complications, and transplant source. It is found that recipients between 16 and 45 years of age with primary renal disease have the lowest risk for morbidity and mortality.

The major problem encountered with transplantation is graft rejection. The success of the transplant is directly related to the source of the donated kidney. There are two types of donors: living relatives and cadavers.

The surgical procedure begins with removal of the donor's left kidney, which is then rotated and placed in the recipient's right iliac fossa or groin region. The renal artery is attached by an end-to-end anastomosis with either the common or the external iliac artery (Fig. 15-32).

The ureter is inserted into the bladder above the normal ureteral orifice through a submucosal tunnel in the bladder wall. The tunnel creates a valve in the terminal ureter to prevent reflux of urine into the transplanted kidney.

Although the kidney is more vulnerable to trauma when it is placed in the iliopelvic region, this has rarely been a problem The advantage of such a location is its observation accessibility. There are complications that may arise following transplantation, however, and thus a variety of examinations may be incorporated to detect and follow the transplant. Useful information may be accumulated through laboratory tests, nuclear medicine, sonography, intravenous pyelography, and renal arteriography.

SONOGRAPHIC EVALUATION

As early as 48 hours after surgery a baseline sonographic examination is performed for the determination of renal size, calyceal pattern, and extrarenal fluid collections. Hydronephrosis can be easily recognized sonographically as the calyceal pattern dilates. Perirenal fluid collections (hematoma, abscess, lymphocele, or urinoma) can be diagnosed reliably and differentiated from acute rejection. Serial scans at 3- to 6-month intervals may be made to detect fluid collections at an early asymptomatic stage. The patient should be examined at the first sign of tenderness in the graft area or mass development.

Technique for sonographic examination

The patient is placed in the supine position. A full urinary bladder is required but should be monitored carefully since overdistension after surgery may result in urinary leakage at the neoureterocystostomy or cause pseudohydronephrosis (Fig. 15-33).

To locate the kidney precisely by ultrasound, transverse scans are made from the pubic symphysis to above the level of the graft. A mark is placed on the skin at the location of the superior and inferior poles, with an imaginary line drawn between the two points to determine the long axis of the kidney. If real time is available, rapid determination of the graft orientation may be obtained. Longitudinal and transverse scans at 1 cm intervals are then made parallel with and perpendicular to the long axis of the kidney (Fig. 15-34). From these scans accurate measurements of the renal length, width, and anteroposterior dimensions can be determined.

The normal transplant should appear as a smooth structure surrounding the homogeneous parenchymal pattern. A dense band of echoes in the midportion of the transplant represents the renal pelvis, calyces, blood vessels, and fatty fibrous tissues. The medullary pyramids are discrete sonolucent structures surrounded by the homogeneous grainy texture of the cortex (Fig. 15-35). The psoas

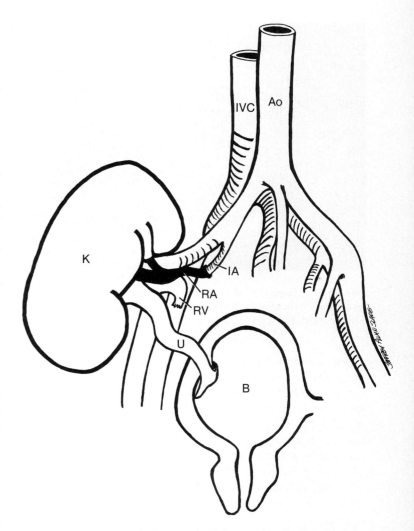

FIG. 15-32. Surgical placement of the renal transplant into the iliac fossa. Aorta, *Ao;* inferior vena cava, *IVC;* kidney, *K;* ureter, *U;* bladder, *B;* internal iliac artery, *IA;* renal artery, *RA;* renal vein, *RV.*

appears as parallel linear echoes posterior to the kidney transplant (Fig. 15-36).

A sonolucent appearance of the anterior portion of the kidney and, at times, an increased echogenic band across the anterior kidney occur on some scans due to inaccurate settings in the near field. Decreased amplification of the near gain in the first few centimeters of the slope will obliterate the decreased echoes of the near field and allow for better fill-in of the anterior portion of the kidney. This difference in anterior structure delineation is probably due to the attenuation of sound by subcutaneous fat, muscle thickness, skin texture, and scarring or to the fact that some patients transmit the sound frequency more readily than others.

The opposite is true for the problem of increased echoes in the near field. By decrease in the near gain, suppression of the echoes in the near field yields an image with uniform texture. Thus it is important to maintain proper penetration and delineation of internal structures with a good outline of adjacent musculature.

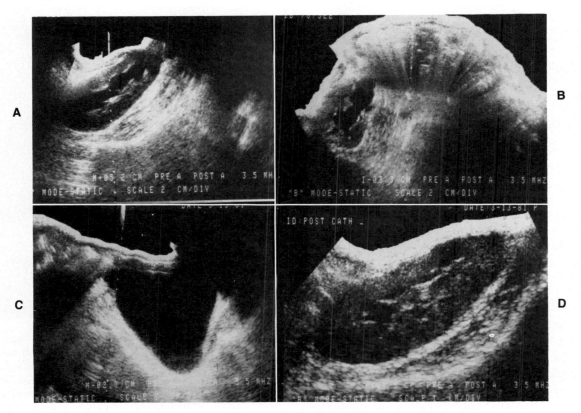

FIG. 15-33. A, Sagittal scan of a renal transplant patient showing distension of the calyceal system. **B,** Transverse scan of the hydronephrosis. **C,** The bladder was extremely overdistended and was the cause of the patient's "pseudohydronephrosis." **D,** Scan of the transplant after the patient voided; a normal compact calyceal system.

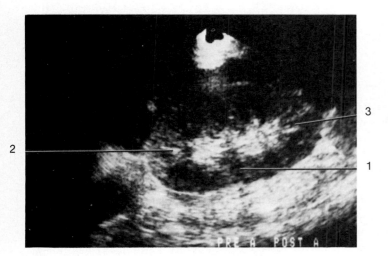

FIG. 15-34. When scanning the transplant, place the transducer over the midportion of the kidney, *1,* and gently arc to the superior pole, *2.* Now begin the scan and sweep the transducer to the inferior pole of the kidney, *3.*

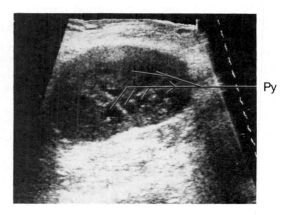

FIG. 15-35. The renal pyramids, *Py,* are discrete sonolucent structures.

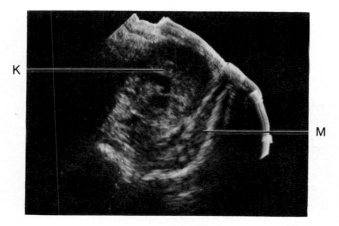

FIG. 15-36. The iliopsoas muscle, *M,* appears as a parallel linear group of echoes posterior to the kidney, *K.*

To record echoes from the parenchyma and distinguish the cortex from the medulla, the sonographer should scan the patient with low-gain and high-gain settings. The scans will include both kidneys as well as the pararenal area (i.e., iliac wing, iliacus iliopsoas).

RENAL TRANSPLANT REJECTION

Sonography can be useful in the diagnosis of rejection. Care must be taken to observe the size and shape; the appearance of the pyramids, cortex, and parenchyma; and the presence of any surrounding fluid collections. Maklad et al.[1] summarize the appearance of renal rejection by stating that there are five changes in the renal parenchymal echo pattern that have been observed during the process of rejection:

1. Enlargement and decreased echogenicity of the pyramids. This appearance is not at all uniform, and only a few pyramids may appear as such (Fig. 15-37).
2. Hyperechogenic cortex. The swollen sonolucent pyramids stand out against the background of increased echogenicity of the outer and interpyramidal cortex (Fig. 15-38).
3. A localized area of renal parenchyma, including both the cortex and the medulla presenting an anechoic appearance, is very difficult to fill in even when high sensitivity and TGC settings are used. This is usually seen in polar regions (Fig. 15-39).
4. Distortion of the renal outline due to localized areas of swelling involving both the cortex and the pyramids. The renal sinus echoes may appear compressed and displaced (Fig. 15-40).
5. Patchy sonolucent areas involving both cortex and medulla with coalescence on follow-up studies. These areas can become quite extensive, affecting a large portion of the renal parenchyma.

In long-standing rejection, Maklad et al.[1] state that two patterns have been observed: (1) a normal-sized renal transplant with very little differentiation between the parenchymal and renal sinus echoes and (2) a small kidney with irregular margins and an irregular parenchymal echo pattern.

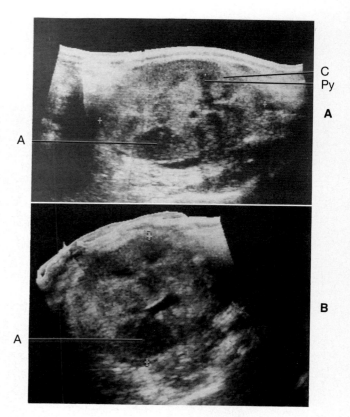

FIG. 15-37. **A,** Enlargement and decreased echogenicity of the pyramids, *Py,* due to edema and congestion with hemorrhage of the interstitial tissue. Ischemia and cellular infiltration (fibrosis) result in hyperechogenicity of the cortex, *C.* Anechoic, *A,* areas usually occur in the polar regions. **B,** Transverse scan of the same patient demonstrating the extent of the anechoic area.

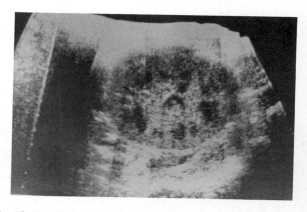

FIG. 15-38. Enlargement and decreased echogenic pyramids with a hyperechoic cortex.

These sonographic appearances correlate with the pathologic occurrences. When swelling with increased internal echoes within the cortex is present, rejection can be diagnosed. Edema, congestion, and hemorrhage of the interstitium produce swelling of the pyramids, which appears as decreased echogenicity (Fig. 15-41). Ischemia and cellular infiltration produce the increased echogenicity of the cortex. Increased areas of sonolucency may also occur in the cortex due to necrosis and infarction. These areas are usually seen in the polar regions of the trans-

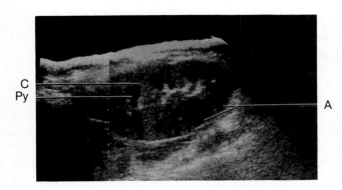

FIG. 15-39. This patient presented with enlargement and decreased echogenic pyramids, *Py*, hyperechogenic cortex, *C*, and a localized anechoic area of renal parenchyma, *A*. This correlated with pathology data of an edematous hemorrhagic cortex and medulla, with fibrin deposited throughout the kidney.

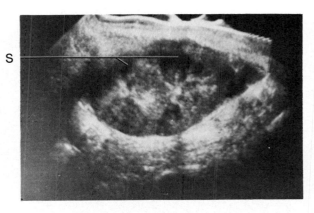

FIG. 15-40. The distortion of the renal outline is seen due to localized areas of swelling in the cortex and pyramids and patchy sonolucent, *S*, areas involving both the cortex and the medulla with coalescence on follow-up studies.

plant. If actual necrosis begins, the affected part appears as an area of decreased echogenicity, which suggests partial liquefaction. Irregular parenchymal echo patterns may result from parenchymal atrophy with fibrosis and shrinkage due to long-standing renal rejection.

Acute tubular necrosis

ATN is a common cause of acute posttransplant failure. Some degree occurs in almost every transplant patient, and it has been stated that as many as 50% of the recipients of cadaver kidneys experience ATN following transplantation. The incidence of ATN is usually higher in cadaver transplants than in donor-relative transplants or in kidneys that undergo warm ischemia or prolonged preservation, kidneys with multiple renal arteries, or kidneys obtained from elderly donors.

ATN usually resolves early in the postoperative period. Uncomplicated ATN is often reversible and can be treated by immediate use of diuretics and satisfactory hydration. It is important to recognize uncomplicated ATN and distinguish it from acute rejection, because the therapy for the two conditions is very different.

Clinically ATN may present a variety of different patterns. Urine volumes may be good initially, followed by oliguria or anuria, or there may be low urine output from the time of transplantation. The serum creatine level is always elevated. If urine output remains low and BUN and creatinine remain elevated, ATN may be difficult to distinguish from rejection. Other indications of rejection (e.g., hematuria, elevated eosinophile counts, or pain over the transplant) are helpful but may be late signs.

Sonographically there are usually no changes seen within the renal parenchyma. In the initial postoperative period the kidney may enlarge slightly due to secondary hypertrophy. This is believed to be a normal physiologic response of the newly transplanted kidney or is caused by swelling that often regresses within a week. However, if the swelling persists, then either ATN or rejection should be considered. With ATN the renal parenchymal pattern remains unchanged, in contrast to the earlier description of the parenchymal changes during rejection. If these

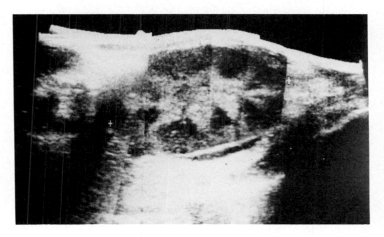

FIG. 15-41. Renal transplant rejection with prominent pyramids and echogenic renal cortex. A small amount of ascites is seen posterior to the transplant.

changes are lacking and the transplant fails to function, the cause is most likely ATN, provided the radionuclide evaluation has confirmed the patency of the vascular supply to the transplant.

Extraperitoneal fluid collections

There are numerous extraperitoneal fluid collections that may occur following transplantation: lymphoceles and lymph fistulas, urinary fistula and urinoma, perinephric abscess, and hematoma. These collections consist of lymph, blood, urine, pus, or a combination of the substances. A sign common to several of the complications is a decrease in renal function manifested by increased creatinine values. Sonographically the fluid collections may appear as round or oval structures with irregular and slightly thickened walls. Usually clinical or laboratory correlation will suggest the etiology of the fluid. Because the transplant is superficial, scans can easily be made and, if necessary, sonographic guidance can be rendered for aspiration of the contents for further analysis.

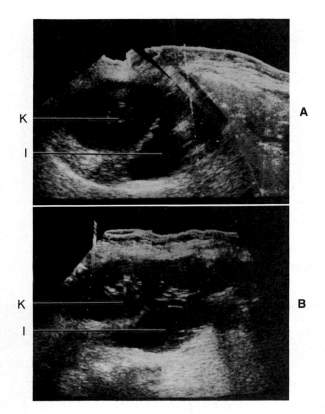

FIG. 15-42. **A,** Sagittal scan of a renal transplant, *K,* with a lymphocele, *l,* formation along the medial posterior border. **B,** Transverse scan of the transplant and lymphocele.

Lymphocele and lymph fistula. Lymphoceles are a common complication of transplantation, occurring in approximately 12% of all transplant patients. The source of the lymph collection is probably vessels severed during the preparation of recipient vessels, or it may be the kidney itself in the form of leakage from injured capsular and hilar lymphatics. The lymph drains into the peritoneal cavity, provoking a fibrous reaction and eventually walling itself off. Primary clinical signs are deterioration of renal function (usually within 2 weeks to 6 months of transplantation), development of painless fluctuant swelling over the transplant, ipsilateral leg edema, or wound drainage of lymph cells. If an IVP was performed, a mass indenting the bladder, ureteral deviation, ureteral obstruction, or kidney deviation will be seen.

Sonographically the lymphocele is a well-defined anechoic area, occasionally with numerous septations (Fig. 15-42). Urinomas may appear similar to lymphoceles, although usually they appear early whereas lymphoceles are more common chronically. If the mass is complex with solid components, hematoma or abscess must be considered.

Urinary fistula and urinoma. Abnormal collections of fluid surrounding the transplant may be readily detected by sonography.

Bladder leaks are derived from the anterior cystostomy or from the ureteroneocystostomy due to faulty surgical technique or bladder overdistension. Clinical signs include local tenderness, fever, sudden decrease in urine output, or urine leakage from the wound. Most fistulas become manifest in the first two postoperative weeks, but presentation may be delayed for over a month.

A collection of urine may be present within the pelvis as either a walled-off urinoma or free fluid. These collections are usually echo free. Differentiation of free urine from a loculated urinoma can easily be made by shifting the patient's position and repeating the examination in the same plane to show redistribution of the fluid.

Perinephric abscess. Perinephric infections can be very hazardous to the transplant patient undergoing immunosuppressive therapy. It is an uncommon complication reported as early as 12 days or many months after transplantation. If the patient presents with a fever of unknown origin, care must be taken to rule out an abscess formation. Sonographically an abscess may appear with septa in it. Edema and inflammation may be present around the mass, making the borders appear less distinct as compared to those found with lymphoceles and hematomas.

Hematoma. A hematoma may develop shortly after surgery. One of the major indications for an ultrasound scan may be a drop in the hematocrit value. Other clinical findings pertinent to hematomas include signs of bleeding, perinephric hemorrhage, a palpable mass, hypertension, and impaired renal function; or the hematoma may be an incidental finding during scanning. Hematomas appear as walled-off well-defined areas whose sonolucent echo production is dependent on the age or stage of the hematoma. It may appear sonolucent while the blood is fresh and be difficult to distinguish from a lymphocele or urinoma. As the clot becomes organized, the hematoma may tend to fragment and develop low-level internal echoes. The mass will then appear complex and eventually solid. After a time it may revert to a sonolucent mass and form a seroma.

Obstructive nephropathy

Early signs of obstruction are anuria or severe oliguria in a patient with satisfactory renal volumes. Numerous conditions may cause obstruction such as ureteral necrosis, abscess, lymphocele, fungus ball, retroperitoneal fibrosis, stricture at the ureterovesical junction, ureteral calculus, and hemorrhage into the collecting system with obstruction from clots. Sonographically obstruction appears as a splaying of the normally compact renal sinus echoes by echo-free spaces, which represent a dilated calyx and renal pelvis. If a renal calculus is the cause of obstruction, a dense echo with an acoustic shadow may be seen on the sonogram.

Graft rupture

Graft ruptures can occur in the first two postoperative weeks, presenting with an abrupt onset of pain and swelling over the graft, oliguria, and shock. Sonographically graft ruptures appear as a gross distortion of the graft contour and a perinephric or paranephric hematoma.

Adrenal Glands

The adrenal glands are small structures lying along the superomedial border of both kidneys. Ultrasound visualization of them may be a very tedious task in the normal patient. However, enlarged adrenal glands are imaged adequately with proper patient position, transducer selection, and time gain compensation settings.

ANATOMY

The adrenal glands are retroperitoneal organs that lie on the upper pole of each kidney (Fig. 15-43). At birth the ratio of their size to body weight is 20 times what it will be by adulthood, but by 1 year of age they are more proportional to body size. They are surrounded by perinephric fascia and are separated from the kidneys by the perinephric fat. Each gland has a cortex and a medulla.

The right adrenal gland is triangular or pyramidal and caps the upper pole of the right kidney. It lies posterior to the right lobe of the liver and extends medially behind the inferior vena cava. It rests posteriorly on the diaphragm.

The left adrenal gland is semilunar and extends along the medial border of the left kidney from the upper pole to the hilus. It lies posterior to the pancreas, the lesser sac, and the stomach. It also rests posteriorly on the diaphragm.

There are three arteries supplying each gland: (1) the suprarenal branch of the inferior phrenic artery, (2) the suprarenal branch of the aorta, and (3) the suprarenal branch of the renal artery. A single vein arises from the hilum of each gland and drains into the inferior vena cava on the right and into the renal vein on the left.

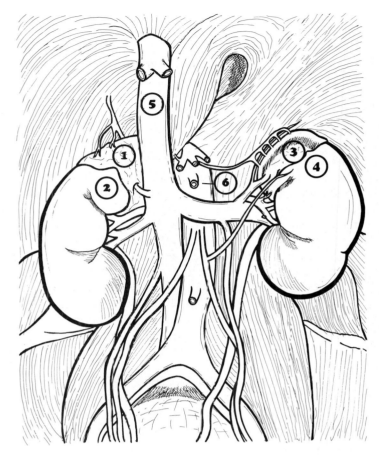

FIG. 15-43. The adrenal glands are retroperitoneal organs that lie on the upper pole of each kidney. Right adrenal gland, *1;* upper pole of right kidney, *2;* left adrenal gland, *3;* upper pole of left kidney, *4;* inferior vena cava, *5;* aorta, *6.* (From Hagen-Ansert SL: The anatomy workbook, Philadelphia, 1986, JB Lippincott Co.)

PHYSIOLOGY

Each adrenal gland is comprised of two endocrine glands. The cortex, or outer part, secretes a range of steroid hormones; the medulla, or core, secretes epinephrine and norepinephrine.

Cortex

The steroids secreted by the adrenal cortex fall into three main categories:

1. Mineralocorticoids—regulate electrolyte metabolism. Aldosterone is the principal mineralocorticoid. It has a regulatory effect on the relative concentrations of mineral ions in the body fluids and therefore on the water content of tissues. An insufficiency of this steroid leads to increased excretion of sodium and chloride ions and water into the urine. This is accompanied by a fall in sodium, chloride, and bicarbonate concentrations in the blood, resulting in a lowered pH or acidosis.
2. Glucocorticoids—play a principal role in carbohydrate metabolism. They promote deposition of liver glycogen from proteins and inhibit the utilization of glucose by the cells, thus increasing blood sugar level. Cortisone and hydrocortisone are the primary glucocorticoids. They diminish allergic response, especially the more serious inflammatory types (rheumatoid arthritis and rheumatic fever).
3. Sex hormones—androgens (male) and estrogens (female). The adrenal gland secretes both types of hormones regardless of the patient's sex. Normally these are secreted in minute quantities and have almost insignificant effects. With oversecretion, however, a marked effect is seen. Adrenal tumors in women can promote aggressive homosexuality and secondary masculine characteristics. Hypersecretion of the hormone in prepubertal boys accelerates adult masculine development and the growth of pubic hair. The adrenal cortex is controlled by ACTH (adrenocorticotropic hormone) from the pituitary. A diminished glucocorticoid blood concentration stimulates the secretion of ACTH. Consequent increase in adrenal cortex activity inhibits further ACTH secretion.

Hypofunction of the adrenal cortex in humans is called Addison's disease. Symptoms and signs include hypotension, general weakness, loss of appetite and weight, and a characteristic bronzing of the skin.

Oversecretion of the adrenal cortex may be caused by

an overproduction of ACTH due to a pituitary tumor or by a tumor in the cortex itself. Cushing's disease is one type of oversecretion disease of the adrenal cortex. Symptoms include increased sodium retension—which leads to tissue edema, increased plasma volume, and a mild alkalosis. Muscle and bone weakness is common. Secretion of androgens is increased and causes masculinizing effects in women.

Medulla[1]

The adrenal medulla makes up the core of the gland, in which groups of irregular cells are located amidst veins that collect blood from the sinusoids. This gland produces epinephrine and norepinephrine. Both of these hormones are amines, sometimes referred to as catecholamines. They elevate the blood pressure, the former working as an accelerator of the heart rate and the latter as a vasoconstrictor. The two hormones together promote glycogenolysis, the breakdown of liver glycogen to glucose, which causes an increase in blood sugar concentration.

The adrenal medulla is not essential for life and can be removed surgically without causing untreatable damage.

SONOGRAPHIC EVALUATION OF ADRENAL GLAND

Although sonography has proved useful in evaluating most soft tissue structures within the abdomen, visualization of the adrenal gland has been difficult because of its small size, medial location, and surrounding perinephric fat (Fig. 15-44).

If the adrenal gland is enlarged due to disease, it becomes an easy task to separate it from the renal parenchyma and thus determine whether the mass is cystic, solid, or somewhat calcified.

Normal texture and patterns

The right adrenal gland is located between the right lobe of the liver and the right crus of the diaphragm. The liver may serve as an acoustic window to visualize the echogenic adrenal gland. The gland is intimately related to the posterior aspect of the inferior vena cava and closely attached to Gerota's fascia.

Patient position and technique[5]

The right adrenal has a comma or triangular shape in the transaxial plane. Best visualization is obtained by a transverse scan with the patient in a left lateral decubitus position (Fig. 15-45). As the patient assumes this position, the inferior vena cava moves forward and the aorta rolls over the crus of the diaphragm, thus offering good visualization of the right kidney and adrenal area. The pie-sweep or single-sweep technique should be used with the patient in mid-inspiration (Fig. 15-46). If the patient is obese, it may be difficult to recognize the triangular or crescent-shaped adrenal gland. The adrenal should not appear rounded, for this would most likely represent some sort of abnormality.

On the longitudinal scan one may sector through the right lobe of the liver perpendicular to the right crus of

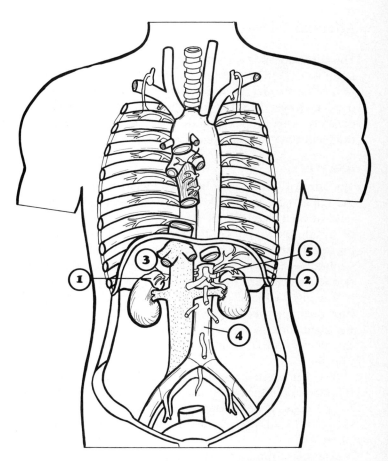

FIG. 15-44. The adrenal gland is very difficult to image with sonography due to its small size, medial location, and surrounding perinephric fat. Left adrenal gland, *1*; right adrenal gland, *2*; suprarenal arteries, *3*; abdominal aorta, *4*; inferior phrenic artery, *5*. (From Hagen-Ansert SL: The anatomy workbook, Philadelphia, 1986, JB Lippincott Co.)

the diaphragm. Care must be taken to separate the retroperitoneal fat reflections from reflections of the liver, crus, and normal adrenal tissue.

The left adrenal gland is closely related to the left crus of the diaphragm and the anterosuperomedial aspect of the left kidney (Fig. 15-47). It may be more difficult to image the left adrenal because of stomach interference. The patient should be placed in a right lateral decubitus position and transverse scans made in an attempt to align the left kidney and the aorta. The longitudinal plane has both a coronal and an oblique orientation.

The left adrenal is more triangular than the right. Variations in patient respiration may help to differentiate it from the superior pole of the left kidney.

Talmont[8] states that the exact coronal or longitudinal scanning plane may be determined by making transverse scans at the level of the lower, middle, and upper poles of the kidney. A mark is placed on the patient's abdominal side to show the relationship between the kidneys and great vessels. From these points the longitudinal oblique scan can be made to image the adrenal. A slightly anterior angulation of the transducer may be necessary to image the great vessels, diaphragmatic crus, and major organs adequately.

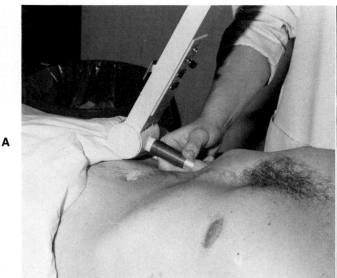

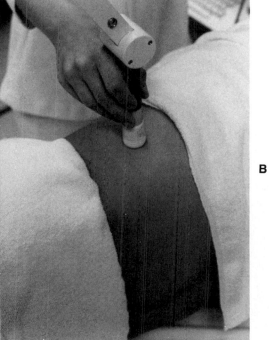

FIG. 15-45. **A,** Transverse and, **B,** decubitus views are the best for imaging the adrenal area.

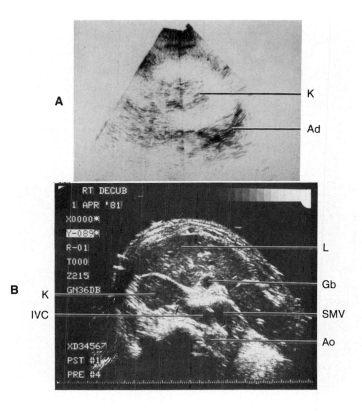

FIG. 15-46. **A,** Left decubitus position of the normal right adrenal gland, *Ad,* and kidney, *K.* **B,** *Arrow* indicates the area of the adrenal gland. Liver, *L;* kidney, *K;* gallbladder, *Gb;* inferior vena cava, *IVC;* superior mesenteric vein, *SMV;* aorta, *Ao.*

Ultrasound pitfalls[5]

1. Right crus of the diaphragm;
2. Second portion of the duodenum;
3. Esophagogastric junction (cephalad to the left adrenal gland)[2];
4. Medial lobulations of the spleen[7];
5. Splenic vasculature;
6. Body-tail region of the pancreas;
7. Fourth portion of the duodenum.

Sample[3] states the normal right adrenal gland can be visualized in over 90% of patients whereas the left is seen in 80% of patients.[4]

PATHOLOGY

Sonographically, adrenal cysts present a typical cystic pattern, as seen in other organs of the body having a strong back wall, no internal echoes, and good through-transmission. Adrenal cysts have the tendency to become calcified, which gives them the ultrasound appearance of a somewhat solid mass with no internal echoes (a sharp posterior border with poor through-transmission) (Fig. 15-48).

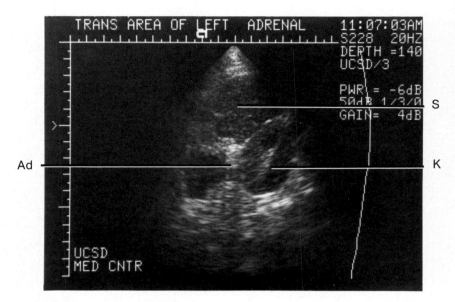

FIG. 15-47.   Transverse area of the left adrenal gland as it lies between the spleen *S* and left kidney *K*.

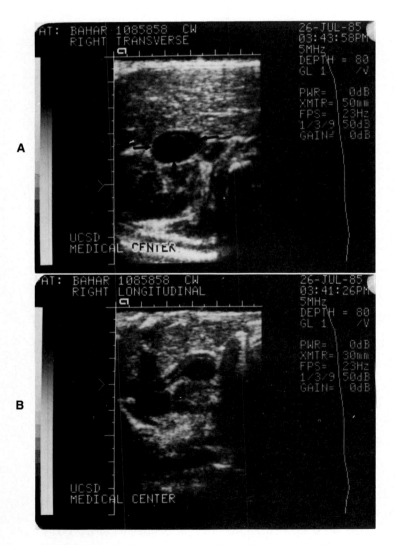

FIG. 15-48.   **A,** Transverse and, **B,** sagittal scans of a patient with a right adrenal cyst (*arrow*).

The cyst may have hemorrhaged, and then it appears as a complex mass with multiple internal echoes and good through-transmission.

Further pathology of the adrenal glands is related to the tumors arising within them and their hyposecretion or hypersecretion of hormones. Endocrine deficiencies may be produced when the glands are destroyed by hemorrhage, infarction, or tumor.[8] Pituitary dysfunction may also play a role in the function of the adrenals and their control of hormones.

There are several cortical syndromes that the sonographer may encounter while scanning for an adrenal mass[8]:

1. Addison's disease. This may be of adrenal or pituitary origin and is the chronic result of adrenal hypofunction. The deficiency may be due to a primary adrenal tumor or to metastases.
2. Adrenogenital syndrome. This is due to excessive secretion of the sex hormones.
3. Conn's syndrome. This is caused by excessive secretion of aldosterone, usually due to a cortical adenoma.
4. Cushing's syndrome. This is produced by excessive secretion of glucocorticoids due to hyperplasia, a benign tumor, or carcinoma. The syndrome can also be caused by an anterior pituitary tumor.
5. Waterhouse-Friderichsen syndrome. This is commonly due to bilateral hemorrhage into the adrenal glands.

The pheochromocytes of the adrenal medulla may produce a tumor called a pheochromocytoma that secretes epinephrine and norepinephrine in excessive quantities. These patients present with intermittent hypertension. The tumor has a homogeneous pattern that can be differentiated from a cyst by its weak posterior wall and poor through-transmission. Pheochromocytomas may be large bulky tumors with a variety of sonographic patterns

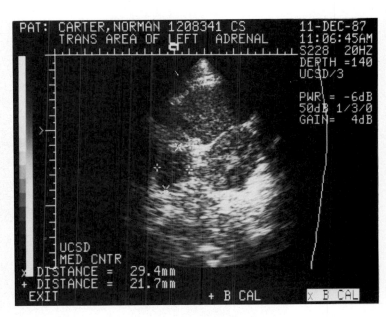

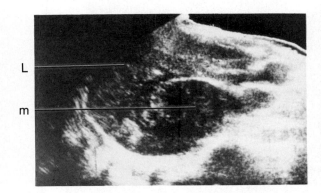

FIG. 15-49. Sagittal scan of a patient with a large pheochromocytoma in the right upper quadrant. Liver, *L;* mass, *m.* (Courtesy Marcia Lavery, Boston, Mass.)

FIG. 15-50. Transverse scan of a patient with a complex mass in the area of the left adrenal gland.

FIG. 15-51. Metastatic disease of the adrenal gland is shown in a 69-year-old man with a large-cell lung carcinoma and a nonhomogeneous defect. Liver, *L;* right kidney, *RK;* adrenal gland, *Ad.* **A,** Transverse scan showing the right adrenal mass just lateral to the vertebral column. **B** and **C,** Sagittal decubitus scans showing the adrenal mass separate from the liver and kidney. Low-level echoes are found within the mass to indicate the solid nature of the tumor.

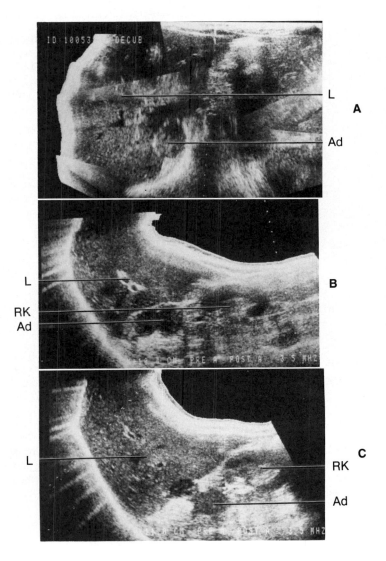

including cystic, solid, and calcified components[6] (Fig. 15-49).

Most adrenal carcinomas are not functional, but they may account for Cushing's syndrome or hyperaldosteronemia.[6] The origin of the tumor should be clearly defined. Metastases to the adrenals vary in size and echogenicity (Figs. 15-50 to 15-52). Often central necrosis will cause areas of sonolucency within the tumor.

The adrenal neuroblastoma is the most common malignancy of the adrenal glands in childhood and the most common tumor of infancy. Generally it arises within the adrenal medulla. Although children are usually asymptomatic, some do present with a palpable abdominal mass that must be differentiated from a neonatal hemorrhage and hydronephrosis.[6] Sonographically the tumor appears as an echogenic mass. It may be large, and evaluation of the surrounding retroperitoneum and liver should be made to rule out metastases (Fig. 15-53).

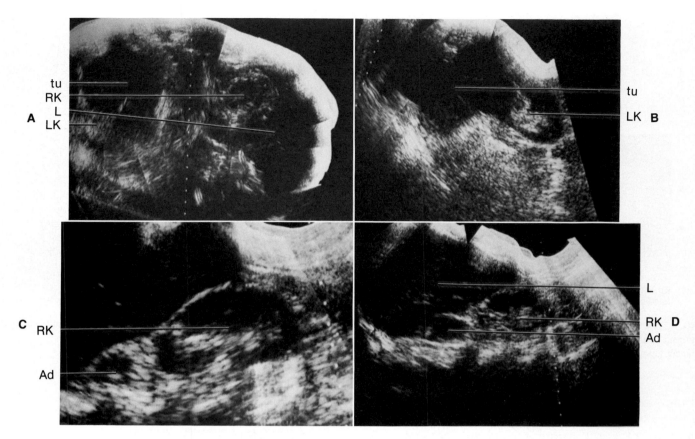

FIG. 15-52.   Metastatic disease of the adrenal gland in a patient with a large left renal tumor. **A,** Transverse prone scan. **B,** Sagittal prone scan. The tumor is growing off the upper pole of the left kidney. **C,** Supine sagittal scan of the right kidney and adrenal metastases. **D,** Supine sagittal scan through the liver, right kidney, and adrenal mass. The liver offers an excellent window to visualize the right kidney and adrenal gland. Left kidney, *LK;* tumor, *tu;* right kidney, *RK;* liver, *L;* adrenal gland, *Ad.*

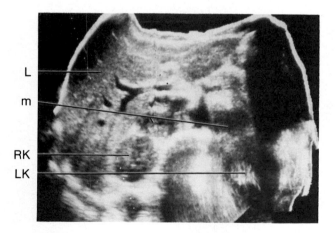

FIG. 15-53.   Transverse scan of a patient with bilateral adrenal metastases secondary to oat cell carcinoma. Liver, *L;* right kidney, *RK;* left kidney, *LK;* mass, *m.* (Courtesy Marcia Lavery, Boston, Mass.)

Summary

KIDNEYS

1. The kidneys lie in the retroperitoneal space. The right kidney is slightly lower than the left.

2. The kidney is surrounded by a fibrous capsule called the true capsule. Perinephric fat surrounds this capsule, with perinephric fascia surrounding the fat, called Geota's fascia.

3. The renal hilum is located on the medial border of each kidney and includes the renal vein, arterial branches, and the ureter.

4. The kidney is composed of an internal medullary portion and an external cortical substance. The medullary substance consists of a series of striated conical masses, called renal pyramids.

5. Within the kidney the ureter divides into two or three major calyces, each of which divides into two or three minor calyces. The major calyces unite to form the renal pelvis.

6. The filtration-reabsorption system relies on a tubular excretory unit called the nephron. Each nephron contains a capsula glomeruli. The capsule and glomerulus together are named the renal corpuscle.

7. The renal artery divides into two primary branches. These branches break down into interlobar arteries. In the portion of the kidney between the cortex and medulla, these arteries are called arcuate arteries.

8. Five or six smaller veins join to form the renal vein, which drains into the inferior vena cava. The renal vein merges from the hilum anterior to the renal artery.

9. The major function of the urinary system is to remove urea from the bloodstream so it does not accumulate in the body and become toxic.

10. The kidneys perform three functions to rid the body of unwanted material: filtration of substances from the blood into Bowman's capsule, reabsorption of most of the water and part of the solutes from the tubular filtrate into the blood, and tubular secretion whereby acids and other substances the body does not need are secreted into the distal renal tubules from the bloodstream.

11. Sonographically the renal parenchyma is slightly more echogenic than the liver parenchyma. The arcuate and interlobar vessels are found within and are demonstrated as intense specular echoes at the corticomedullary junction.

12. The cortex generally is echogenic whereas the medullary pyramids are echolucent. The two are separated from one another by bands of cortical tissue, called columns of Bertin, which extend into the renal sinus.

13. Congenital deformities of the kidney include agenesis, supernumerary kidney, or horseshoe kidney.

14. Renal masses may be classified as cystic, solid, or complex. Generally an intravenous pyelogram is performed first and sonography is used to further classify the nature of the mass.

15. Specific sonographic patterns for inflammatory, hemorrhagic, calcified, milk of calcium, cyst with tumor infiltration, lipomatosis, hematoma, hydronephrosis, multicystic, polycystic, hypernephroma, lymphoma, and carcinoma are included in this chapter.

RENAL TRANSPLANT

1. Renal transplantation and dialysis are currently used for the treatment of chronic renal failure or end-stage renal disease.

2. Complications following renal transplantation include rejection, acute tubular necrosis, obstructive nephropathy, extraperitoneal fluid collections, hemorrhage or infarction, recurrent glomerulonephritis, graft rupture, and renal emphysema.

ADRENAL GLANDS

1. The adrenal glands are small retroperitoneal structures that lie on the upper pole of each kidney. They are surrounded by perinephric fascia and are separated from the kidneys by the perinephric fat. Each gland has a cortex and a medulla.

2. Each adrenal gland is composed of two endocrine glands. The cortex secretes a range of steroid hormones; the medulla secretes epinephrine and norepinephrine.

3. Pitfalls in localizing the small normal adrenal gland include overlying right crus of diaphragm, second portion of duodenum, esophagogastric junction (to left adrenal), medial lobulations of the spleen, splenic vasculature, body-tail region of the pancreas, fourth portion of the duodenum.

4. Pathology of the adrenal gland that can be identified by sonography includes cysts, pheochromocytoma, and carcinoma.

REFERENCES
Kidneys

1. Elyaderani MK and Gabriele OF: Ultrasound of renal masses, Semin Ultrasound 11(1):21, 1981.
2. Finberg H: Renal ultrasound: anatomy and technique, Semin Ultrasound 11(1):7, 1981.
3. Morin ME and Baker DA: The influence of hydration and bladder distention on the sonographic diagnosis of hydronephrosis, J Clin Ultrasound 7:192, 1979.
4. Resnick MI and Sanders RC: Ultrasound in urology, Baltimore, 1979, The Williams & Wilkins Co.
5. Rosenfield AT, Taylor KJW, Crade M, and DeGraaf CS: Anatomy and pathology of the kidney by gray scale ultrasound, Radiology 128:737, 1978.

Renal Transplant

1. Maklad NF, Wright CH, and Rosenthal SJ: Gray scale ultrasonic appearances of renal transplant rejection, Radiology 131:711, 1979.

Adrenal Glands

1. Anderson PD: Clinical anatomy and physiology for allied health sciences, Philadelphia, 1976, W.B. Saunders Co.
2. Rao AKR and Silver TM: Normal pancreas and splenic variants simulating suprarenal and renal tumors, AJR 126:530, 1976.
3. Sample WF: A new technique for the evaluation of the adrenal gland with gray scale ultrasonography, Radiology 124:463, 1977.
4. Sample WF: Adrenal ultrasonography, Radiology 127:461, 1978.
5. Sample WF: Ultrasonography of the adrenal gland. In Resnick MI and Sanders RC, editors: Ultrasound in urology, Baltimore, 1979, The Williams & Wilkins Co.
6. Sample WF: Renal, adrenal, retroperitoneal, and scrotal ultrasonography. In Sarti DA and Sample WF, editors: Diagnostic ultrasound: text and cases, Boston, 1980, G.K. Hall & Co.
7. Sample WF and Sarti DA: Computed tomography and gray scale ultrasonography of the adrenal gland: a comparative study, Radiology 128:377, 1978.
8. Talmont CA: Adrenal glands. In Taylor KJW et al, editors: Manual of ultrasonography, New York, 1980, Churchill Livingstone, Inc.

16

Spleen and Retroperitoneum

SANDRA L. HAGEN-ANSERT

Spleen

ANATOMY
Normal anatomy

The spleen lies in the left hypochondrium, with its axis along the shaft of the tenth rib. Its lower pole extends forward as far as the midaxillary line. It is of variable size and shape but generally is considered to be ovoid with a convex superior and a concave inferior surface. The vessels that supply it enter at the hilum. The spleen is an intraperitoneal organ, being covered with peritoneum over its entire extent except for a small area at its hilum. Regardless of its shape, the ends of the spleen are called its posterior and anterior extremities; and its borders are superior and inferior. Accessory spleens occasionally are found near the hilum of the spleen.

The spleen is the largest single mass of lymphoid tissue in the body. It is active in blood formation during the initial part of fetal life. This function decreases so that by the fifth or sixth month of gestation the spleen assumes its adult character and discontinues its hematopoietic activity.

Relational anatomy

Anterior to the spleen lie; the stomach, tail of the pancreas, and left colic flexure (Fig. 16-1). The left kidney lies along its medial border. Posteriorly the diaphragm, left pleura, left lung, and ninth, tenth, and eleventh ribs are in contact with the spleen (Fig. 16-2).

Blood is supplied by the splenic artery, which travels along the superior border of the pancreas. Upon entering the spleen at the hilum, this artery immediately divides into about six branches.

The splenic vein leaves the hilum and joins the superior mesenteric vein to form the portal vein (Fig. 16-3). This vessel travels along the posterior medial aspect of the pancreas.

The lymph vessels emerging from the hilum pass through a few lymph nodes along the course of the splenic artery and drain into the celiac nodes. The nerves to the spleen accompany the splenic artery and are derived from the celiac plexus.

PHYSIOLOGY

The red pulp of the spleen is composed of two principal elements—the splenic *sinuses* alternating with splenic

300

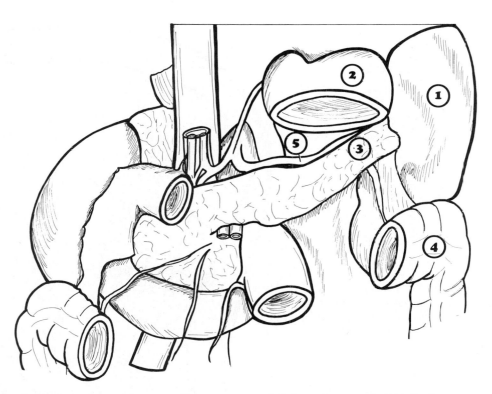

FIG. 16-1. The spleen and surrounding structures. *1,* Spleen; *2,* stomach; 3, tail of pancreas; *4,* descending colon; *5,* splenic artery. (From Hagen-Ansert SL: The anatomy workbook, Philadelphia, 1986, JB Lippincott Co.)

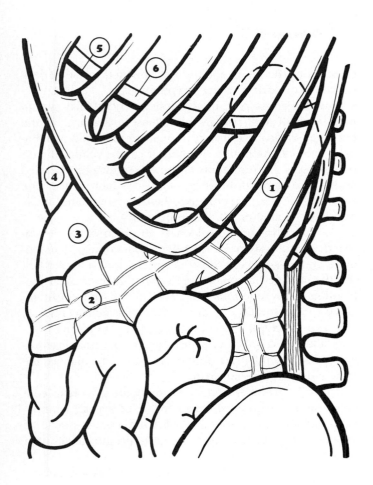

FIG. 16-2. Relationship of the spleen to adjacent structures as viewed from the left lateral position. *1,* Spleen; *2,* transverse colon; *3,* stomach; *4,* liver; *5,* diaphragm; *6,* costodiaphragmatic recess. (From Hagen-Ansert SL: The anatomy workbook, Philadelphia, 1986, JB Lippincott Co.)

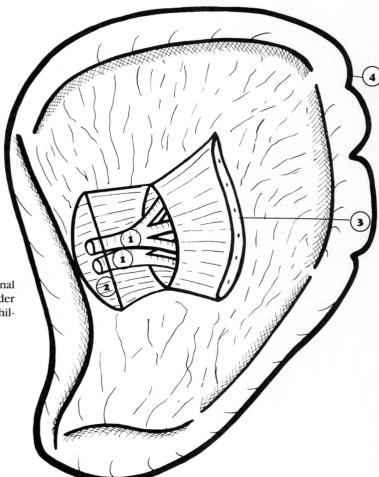

FIG. 16-3. Hilum of the spleen. *1,* Splenic vessels; *2,* lienorenal ligaments; *3,* gastrosplenic omentum; *4,* notched anterior border of spleen. (From Hagen-Ansert SL: The anatomy workbook, Philadelphia, 1986, JB Lippincott Co.)

cords. The sinuses are long irregular channels lined by endothelial cells or flattened reticular cells. A recent study indicated that there are pores or gaps between the lining cells, implying that the circulation is open and that blood cells can freely leave the sinuses to enter the intervening cords. The membrane shared by a cord and its adjacent sinuses is also perforated. Reticular cells with delicate processes sometimes bridge the cords. Thus these highly phagocytic cells create an open meshwork with the cords. The blood that leaves the splenic sinuses to enter the reticular cords passes through a complex filter.

The venous drainage of the sinuses and cords is not well defined, but it is assumed that tributaries of the splenic vein connect with the sinuses of the red pulp. From here the splenic vein follows the course of the artery, eventually joining the superior mesenteric vein to form the portal vein.

The white pulp of the spleen consists of the malpighian corpuscles, small nodular masses of lymphoid tissue attached to the smaller arterial branches. Extending from the splenic capsule inward are the trabeculae, containing blood vessels and lymphatics. The lymphoid tissue, or malpighian corpuscles, has the same structure as the follicles in the lymph nodes; but it differs in that the splenic follicles surround arteries, so that on cross section each contains a central artery. These follicles are scattered throughout the organ and are not confined to the peripheral layer or cortex, as are lymph nodes.

The spleen as part of the reticuloendothelial system plays an important role in the defense mechanism of the body and is also implicated in pigment and lipid metabolism. It is not essential to life, and it can be removed with no ill effects. The functions of the spleen may be classified under two general headings—those which reflect the functions of the reticuloendothelial system and those which are characteristic of the organ itself.

The functions of the spleen as an organ of the reticuloendothelial system are (1) the production of lymphocytes and plasma cells, (2) the production of antibodies, (3) the storage of iron, and (4) the storage of other metabolites. The functions characteristic of the organ include (1) maturation of the surface of erythrocytes, (2) reservoir function, (3) culling function, (4) pitting function, and (5) disposal of senescent or abnormal erythrocytes; also included are functions related to platelet life span and leukocyte life span.

The role of the spleen as an immunologic organ concerns the production of cells capable of making antibodies (lymphocytes and plasma cells); however, it should be understood that antibodies are also produced at other sites.

Phagocytosis of erythrocytes and the breakdown of the

hemoglobin occur throughout the entire reticuloendothe-lial system, but roughly half the catabolic activity is local-ized in the normal spleen. In splenomegaly the major por-tion of hemoglobin breakdown occurs in the spleen. The iron that is liberated is stored in the splenic phagocytes. In anomalies such as the hemolytic anemias, the splenic phagocytes become engorged with hemosiderin when erythrocyte destruction is accelerated.

In addition to storing iron, the spleen is subject to the storage diseases such as Gaucher's disease and Niemann-Pick disease. Abnormal lipid metabolites accumulate in all phagocytic reticuloendothelial cells but may also involve the phagocytes in the spleen, producing gross splenome-galy.

The functions of the spleen that are characteristic of the organ relate primarily to the circulation of erythro-cytes through it. In a normal individual the spleen con-tains only about 20 to 30 ml of erythrocytes. In splenom-egaly the reservoir function is greatly increased, and the abnormally enlarged spleen contains many times this vol-ume of red blood cells. The transit time is lengthened, and the erythrocytes are subject to destructive effects for a long time. In part, ptosis causes consumption of glucose, on which the erythrocyte is dependent for the mainte-nance of normal metabolism, and the erythrocyte is de-stroyed. Selective destruction of abnormal erythrocytes is also accelerated by the splenic pooling.

As erythrocytes pass through the spleen, the organ in-spects them for imperfections and destroys those it recog-nizes as abnormal or senescent. This is called the *culling* function. The *pitting* function is a process by which the spleen removes granular inclusions without destroying the erythrocytes. The normal function of the spleen keeps the number of circulating erythrocytes with inclusions at a minimum.

The spleen also pools platelets in large numbers. The entry of platelets into the splenic pool and their return to the circulation are extensive. In splenomegaly the splenic pool may be so large that it produces thrombocytopenia. Sequestration of leukocytes in the enlarged spleen may produce leukopenia.

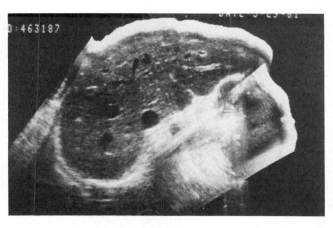

FIG. 16-4.   The normal texture of the spleen should be stippled with fine homogeneous echoes, as seen in the liver parenchyma.

SONOGRAPHIC EVALUATION OF THE SPLEEN
Normal texture and patterns

Sonographically the spleen should stipple in with fine ho-mogeneous low-level echoes as is seen within the liver parenchyma (Fig. 16-4). Cooperberg[1] states that the spleen has two components joined at the hilum. On trans-verse scans it has a crescentic appearance usually with a large medial component. As one moves inferiorly, only the lateral component is imaged. On longitudinal scans the superior component extends more medially than the inferior component. The irregularity of these components makes it difficult to assess mild splenomegaly accurately.

Patient position and technique

Real-time sector equipment is excellent for visualizing the left upper quadrant. The sonographer can successfully ma-nipulate the transducer between costal margins to image the left kidney, spleen, and diaphragm adequately (Table 16-1).

The patient may be scanned in the supine, prone, or right lateral decubitus position. The supine scan may have the problem of overlying air-filled stomach or bowel ante-rior to the spleen; thus the patient may be rotated into a

Table 16-1   Ultrasonic-pathologic classification of splenic disorders

Uniform splenic sonodensity		Focal defects		Perisplenic defects
Normal sonodensity	**Low sonodensity**	**Sonodense**	**Sonolucent**	
Erythropoiesis (in-cluding myelopro-liferative disorders)	Granulocytopoiesis (excluding myelodisorders)	Nonspecific (me-tastasis)	Nonspecific (benign primary neoplasm, cyst, abscess, ma-lignant neoplasm	Nonspecific (hematoma)
Reticuloendothelial hyperactivity	Lymphopoiesis		[lymphopoietic])	
Congestion	Other (multiple myeloma)			
	Congestion			

From Mittelstaedt CA and Partain CL: Radiology 134:697, 1980.

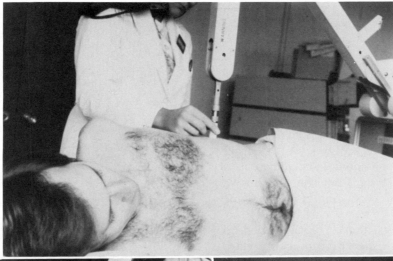

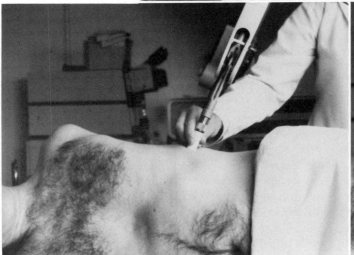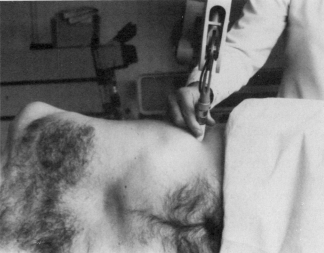

FIG. 16-5. The decubitus position permits the sonographer to scan between the ribs to record maximal information from the splenic parenchyma.

slight right decubitus position to permit better transducer contact without as much bowel interference (Fig. 16-5).

The prone scan is obtained with a slight cephalic angulation of the transducer head. Transverse scans are probably the easiest in which to orient the transducer (Fig. 16-6). When the left kidney is well seen, serial scans are made by moving the transducer gradually cephalad in 1 cm steps. As the scan moves superiorly from the calyceal area of the kidney, the spleen should be identified along the left lateral border. Single scans are probably the best for avoiding rib artifacts. This view may give additional information about the splenic parenchyma, but the best information is probably obtained from the right lateral decubitus position.

The decubitus, or axillary, position enables the sonographer to scan in an oblique fashion between the ribs (Fig. 16-7).

Various degrees of arcing the transducer through the costal margins may be necessary to demonstrate the fine homogeneous splenic parenchyma. Longitudinal decubitus scans can also be performed for an additional view.

One avoids the ribs by merely skipping over them as the scan is being made.

PATHOLOGIC CONDITIONS

As the largest unit of the reticuloendothelial system the spleen is involved in all systemic inflammations and generalized hematopoietic disorders, and many metabolic disturbances. It is rarely the primary site of disease. Whenever the spleen is involved in systemic disease, splenic enlargement usually develops; and therefore splenomegaly is a major manifestation of disorders of this organ (Table 16-2).[7]

Congenital anomalies

Complete absence of the spleen (asplenia or agenesis of the spleen) is rare and, by itself, causes no difficulties. Often, however, asplenia is associated with congenital heart disease (e.g., defects in or absence of the atrial or atrioventricular canal, pulmonary stenosis or atresia, transposition of the great vessels).

Accessory spleen is a more common congenital anom-

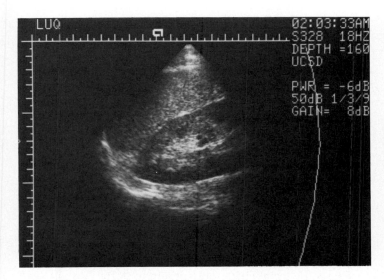

FIG. 16-6. Longitudinal scan of the left kidney and spleen. Note the finely stippled texture of the spleen as compared to the renal parenchyma.

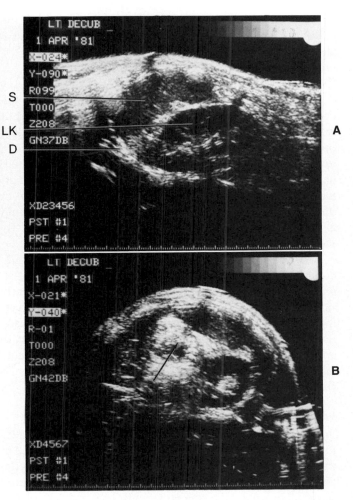

FIG. 16-7. A, Sagittal scan of the left upper quadrant with the patient in a decubitus position demonstrates the left kidney, *LK;* spleen, *S;* and diaphragm, *D.* **B,** Transverse view shows the stomach *(arrow)* anterior to the spleen and left kidney.

Table 16-2   Pathologic classification of splenic disorders

Hematopoietic	Reticuloendothelial hyperactivity (normal)
Granulocytopoiesis	Still's disease
Reactive hyperplasia to acute and chronic infection (low sonodensity)	Wilson's disease
Noncaseous granulomatous inflammation	Felty's syndrome
Myeloproliferative syndromes (normal)	Reticulum cell sarcoma
Chronic myelogenous leukemia	
Acute myelogenous leukemia	**Congestion (normal or low sonodensity)**
Lymphopoiesis (low sonodensity or focal sonolucent)	Hepatocellular disease
Chronic lymphocytic leukemia	
Lymphoma	**Nonspecific**
Hodgkin's disease	Neoplasm-metastasis (focal sonodense)
Erythropoiesis (normal)	Cyst (focal sonolucent)
Sickle cell disease	Abscess (focal sonolucent)
Hereditary spherocytosis	Malignant neoplasm (focal sonolucent)
Hemolytic anemia	Hodgkin's disease
Chronic anemia	Lymphoma
Myeloproliferative syndrome	Benign neoplasm (focal sonolucent)
Chronic myelogenous leukemia	Lymphangiomatosis
Acute myelogenous leukemia	Hematoma (perisplenic)
Other	
Multiple myeloma (low sonodensity)	

From Mittelstaedt CA and Partain CL: Radiology 134:697, 1980.

aly. One of every six accessory spleens is located in the tail of the pancreas. Lesions affecting the main spleen usually affect the accessory spleen as well.

Regressive changes

Amyloidosis. In systemic diseases leading to amyloidosis the spleen is the organ most frequently involved. It may be of normal size or decidedly enlarged, depending on the amount and distribution of amyloid. Two types of involvement are seen—modular and diffuse. In the modular type, amyloid is found in the walls of the sheathed arteries and within the follicles but not in the red pulp. In the diffuse type the follicles are not involved, the red pulp is prominently involved, and the spleen is usually greatly enlarged and firm.

Atrophy. Atrophy of the spleen (50 to 70 g) is not uncommon in normal individuals. It may also occur in wasting diseases. In chronic hemolytic anemias, particularly sickle cell anemia, there is excessive loss of pulp, increasing fibrosis, scarring from multiple infarcts, and incrustation with iron and calcium deposits. In the final stages of atrophy the spleen may be so small that it is hardly recognizable. Advanced atrophy is sometimes referred to as autosplenectomy.

Rupture

Rupture of the spleen is usually caused by a crushing injury or a severe blow. Much less often it is encountered in the apparent absence of trauma and is described as spontaneous rupture. Spontaneous rupture is encountered most often when the spleen is enlarged and soft in diseases such as infectious mononucleosis, leukemia, malaria, typhoid fever, and other types of acute splenitis.

Nonspecific acute splenitis

In nonspecific acute splenitis the spleen is enlarged by 200 to 400 g and is soft. The most common disease conditions producing acute splenitis are bacteremia, as in vegetative endocarditis; but any other severe systemic inflammatory disorder such as diphtheria, bacillary dysentery, or pneumonia may effect similar splenic changes. Acute splenitis may be induced by noninfectious disease and is encountered in any extensive tissue destruction of chemical or physical nature, presumably because the spleen is active in resorption of necrotic cell products.

Nonspecific subacute or chronic splenitis

The organ with nonspecific subacute or chronic splenitis is enlarged, but rarely as much as 1000 g, and is firm. This condition is seen most commonly in certain diseases that will be described later. The next most frequent cause is vegetative (bacterial) endocarditis.

Specific forms of splenitis

There are many infections that may affect the spleen. The more common infections will be discussed.

Syphilis. The spleen is often enlarged in congenital syphilis, but rarely more than twice its normal size. Sple-

nomegaly in the tertiary stage usually follows the congestive changes induced by luetic cirrhosis of the liver.

Sarcoid infectious mononucleosis. The spleen is enlarged in at least 50% of cases, usually two or three times its normal size. It is generally soft, fleshy, and hyperemic.

Vascular disease

Acute congestion. Active hyperemia accompanies the reaction in the spleen to acute systemic infections. The spleen is moderately enlarged, rarely over 250 g.

Chronic congestion. Chronic venous congestion may cause enlargement of the spleen, a condition referred to as congestive splenomegaly.

Long-standing congestive splenomegaly results in severe swelling of the spleen (1000 g or more).

The venous congestion may be of systemic origin, caused by intrahepatic obstruction to portal venous drainage or by obstructive venous disorders in the portal or splenic veins. Systemic venous congestion is found in cardiac decompensation involving the right side of the heart. It is particularly severe in tricuspid or pulmonary valvular disease and in chronic cor pulmonale.

The most common causes of striking congestive splenomegaly are the various forms of cirrhosis of the liver. It is also caused by obstruction to the extrahepatic portal or splenic vein (e.g., spontaneous portal vein thrombosis).

Hypersplenism. Hypersplenism is a symptom complex characterized by congestive splenomegaly, leukopenia, and anemia (McMichael, 1934). It was referred to as Bonti's disease and was considered a primary hematologic disorder with secondary involvement of the spleen. Currently splenic involvement is believed to be primary.

The hypersplenic syndrome has been divided into primary and secondary types. In primary hypersplenism there is increased splenic activity and size of unknown cause. Secondary hypersplenism may occur in patients whose splenomegaly has a known origin, such as leukemia or lymphoma. In both forms the spleen is almost always enlarged.

Infarcts. Splenic infarcts are comparatively common lesions caused by occlusion of the major splenic artery or any of its branches. They are almost always due to emboli that arise in the heart, produced either from mural thrombi, or from vegetations on the valves of the left side of the heart.

Disorders involving red cells

Hemolytic anemia. Hemolytic anemia is the general term applied to anemia referable to decreased life of the erythrocytes. When the rate of destruction is greater than can be compensated by the bone marrow, then anemia results.

Autoimmune hemolytic anemia. This type of anemia can occur in its primary form without underlying disease, or it may be seen as a secondary disorder in patients already suffering from some disorder of the reticuloendothelial or hematopoietic systems, such as lymphoma, leukemia, or infectious mononucleosis. In the secondary form the splenic changes are dominated by the underlying disease; in the primary form the spleen is variably enlarged.

Hereditary or congenital spherocytosis. In this disorder the spleen may be enlarged and sometimes weighs over 1000 g. An intrinsic abnormality of the red cells gives rise to erythrocytes that are small and spheroid rather than the normal, flattened, biconcave disks. The two results of this disease are the production by the bone marrow of spherocytic erythrocytes and the increased destruction of these cells in the spleen. The spleen destroys spherocytes selectively.

Sickle cell anemia. In the earlier stage of this disease, as seen in infants and children, the spleen is enlarged with marked congestion of the red pulp. Later the spleen undergoes progressive infarction and fibrosis and decreases in size until, in adults, only a small mass of fibrous tissue may be found, weighing less than 1 g (autosplenectomy). It is generally believed that these changes result when sickled cells plug the vasculature of the splenic substance, effectively producing ischemic destruction of the spleen.

Polycythemia vera. The spleen is variably enlarged, rather firm, and blue-red. It usually weighs about 350 g, and infarcts and thrombosis are common.

Thalassemia. The spleen is severely involved. This hemoglobinopathy differs from the others in that an abnormal molecular form of hemoglobin is not present. Instead, there is a suppression of synthesis of beta or alpha polypeptide chains, resulting in deficient synthesis of normal hemoglobin. The erythrocytes are not only deficient in normal hemoglobin but also abnormal in shape; many are target cells whereas others vary considerably in size and shape. Their life span is short because they are destroyed by the spleen in large numbers.

The disease ranges from mild to severe. The changes in the spleen are greatest in the severe form, called thalassemia major. The spleen is very large, often seeming to fill the entire abdominal cavity.

Disorders involving white cells

Leukemia. Chronic myelogenous leukemia may be responsible for more extreme splenomegaly than is any other disease. Depending on the duration of the disorder, the spleen may weigh anywhere from 1000 to 3000 g. Weights of 6000 to 8000 g are not rare. The organ is symmetrically enlarged and firm, and its capsule may be quite thickened.

Chronic lymphatic leukemia. This disorder produces less severe degrees of splenomegaly. The spleen rarely exceeds 2000 g.

Monocytic leukemia. This kind of leukemia causes mild splenomegaly, rarely producing a spleen over 500 g.

Reticuloendotheliosis

Gaucher's disease. All age groups can be affected by Gaucher's disease. About 50% of patients are under the age of 8 years and 17% under 1 year. Clinical features follow a chronic course, with changes in skin pigmentation and bone pain. Usually the first sign is splenomegaly, enlarging the spleen to as much as 8000 g.

Niemann-Pick disease. This rapidly fatal disease predominantly affects female infants. The clinical features consist of hepatomegaly, digestive disturbances, and lymphadenopathy.

Letterer-Siwe disease. This is sometimes called nonlipid reticuloendotheliosis, and there is proliferation of reticuloendothelial cells in all tissues but particularly in the spleen lymph nodes and bone marrow. Usually the spleen is only moderately enlarged, although the change may be more severe in affected older infants. This disease is generally found in children below the age of 2 years. Clinical features are hepatosplenomegaly, fever, and pulmonary involvement. It is rapidly fatal as well.

Hand-Schüller-Christian disease. This disorder is benign and chronic in spite of many features similar to those of Letterer-Siwe disease. It usually affects children over 2 years of age. The clinical features are a chronic course, diabetes, and moderate hepatosplenomegaly.

Primary tumors of the spleen

In general, primary tumors of the spleen (either benign or malignant) are rare.

Benign tumors. The cavernous hemangioma is the most common primary tumor of the spleen. Next in frequency is the lymphangioma. These may be very large, consisting of multicystic lesions. Other tumors that may arise in the spleen are fibromas, osteomas, and chondromas.

Malignant tumors. Any of the types of lymphomas or Hodgkin's disease found in the lymph nodes may be primary in the spleen, and they have the same characteristics as in the lymph nodes. Hemangiosarcomas with metastases, especially to the liver, are also known to occur.

The most common secondary tumors are sarcomas, principally the so-called malignant lymphoma group, and Hodgkin's disease.

Metastases of other types of tumors, especially carcinomas, are rare and usually occur only when generalized carcinomatosis has developed. An exception is widely disseminated melanocarcinoma that involves the spleen in about half the cases.

Sonographic patterns of pathology

Splenomegaly *(Figs. 16-8 to 16-11).* Although the spleen is sometimes difficult to visualize when the patient is supine, this position often allows a clearer insight into splenic enlargement. One can compare the size of the spleen with that of the liver. Usually the spleen is not well visualized until 9 to 11 cm above the umbilicus. Generally most of the liver is well visualized at the time of splenic visualization. In patients with splenomegaly the spleen may be seen as low as the umbilicus.

The determination of splenic enlargement is essential; once that has been established, the pathway to analyzing the cause for enlargement can be evaluated. It may be a general splenomegaly due to a blood disorder, alcoholic

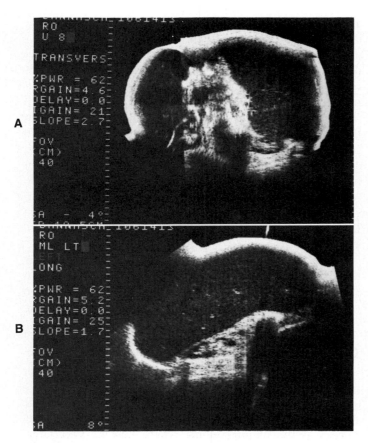

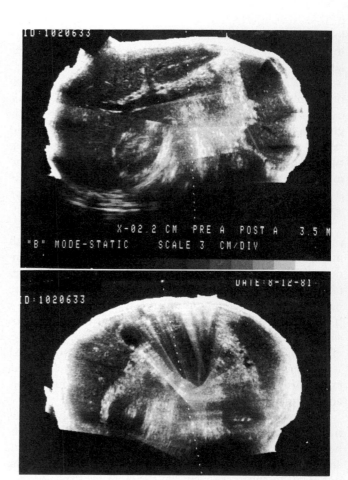

FIG. 16-8.   A, Transverse scan of a young patient with splenomegaly. The spleen is clearly much larger than the liver on this midabdominal view. **B,** Longitudinal scan over the enlarged spleen with a fine stippled pattern throughout.

FIG. 16-9.   Transverse scans of the left upper quadrant show the spleen to be mildly enlarged. Normally it does not exceed very far beyond the anterior border of the vertebral column.

cirrhosis, or other reasons; or it may be splenomegaly secondary to a hemorrhage, tumor, or cyst.

Splenic volume. Numerous authors have described a method for calculating splenic volume that correlates well with autopsy results. Koga's method[3] utilizes the decubitus long axis of the spleen. The splenic volume *(V)* in cubic centimeters is calculated as a function of the sectional area *(S)* in square centimeters by the following formula:

$$V = 7.53S - 77.56$$

Congenital anomalies. Splenic agenesis may be ruled out by the demonstration of a spleen. The sonographer should be alert not to confuse the bowel, which may lie in the same area, with the spleen. Evaluation of the left upper quadrant with real time should enable one to make the distinction.

An accessory spleen may be difficult to demonstrate by sonography if it is very small. When seen, it may appear as a low-level mass near the splenic hilum (Fig. 16-12).

Splenic trauma. If the patient has left upper quadrant pain secondary to trauma, a splenic hematoma or subcapsular hematoma should be considered (Fig. 16-13). The patient should be scanned in the supine position first; then scans should be made in the prone and decubitus

positions to define the hematoma. Increased gain settings can be used to define the extent of the hematoma. If the blood has organized, it may appear as an echo-free area within the spleen. If it has clotted, it may appear as a complex mass. A subcapsular hematoma generally will appear as a complex mass partially surrounding the splenic capsule. If the patient has a slightly enlarged spleen without signs of organized hematoma, serial scans performed 6 hours apart may be helpful in the clinical diagnosis. The serial scans are especially helpful for trauma patients who can afford to wait the 5 or 6 hours necessary between scans for a determination of enlargement to be made. A baseline scan is done as soon as the patient arrives, with follow-up serial scans over a 24-hour period.

Splenic cyst. Echographically a splenic cyst appears as an echo-free area with smooth well-defined borders and good enhancement posterior to its border (Fig. 16-14). Large cysts will be seen to cause splenomegaly and compression of normal splenic tissue whereas smaller cysts may be demonstrated within the outline of the spleen.[1]

It may be difficult to distinguish a splenic cyst from a renal cyst or pseudocyst. Careful evaluation of these other organ systems should define their normal contour and obviate the problem. Compression of normal structures sometimes is helpful in determining the origin of the

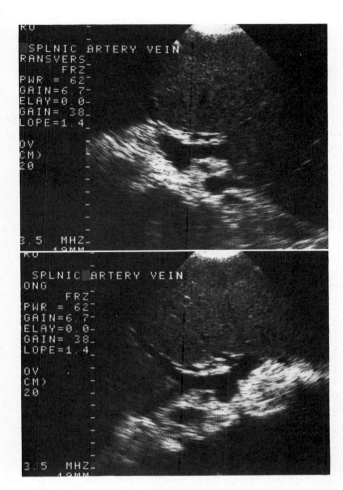

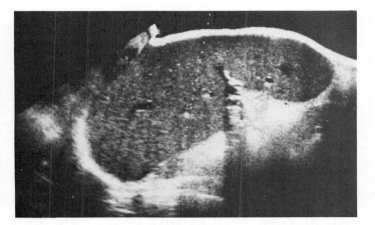

FIG. 16-11. Sagittal scan demonstrates the enlarged spleen, prominent hilus, and fine, uniform parenchymal pattern.

FIG. 16-10. Transverse scans of splenomegaly that also demonstrate congestion of the splenic hilus. The splenic artery and vein are very well seen.

mass. A splenic cyst may compress the renal parenchyma or even the tail of the pancreas. Of course, clinical evaluation of the patient is important in determining the differential diagnosis.

The sonographic appearance of a hemorrhagic splenic cyst has been described as a cystic mass with a gravity-dependent layering of two fluids each with distinctly different reflectivities. The difference in reflectivity is thought to be related to the amount of particulate matter within each fluid layer.[6]

Neoplasms. Splenic tumors are not seen as commonly as other tumors in the abdomen, and thus experience in their ultrasonic evaluation is limited.

Increased echogenicity of the spleen was reported by Siler et al.,[8] who stated that the spleen is often pathologically involved in patients with leukemia and lymphoma. In leukemia the spleen was grossly enlarged and firm and microscopically showed diffuse and focal infiltrates of leukemic cells. Numerous small infarcts could be seen throughout the parenchyma. Progression of the disease brought further disruption of architecture throughout the spleen. In non-Hodgkin's lymphoma, diffuse or nodular masses of cells were demonstrated. This underlying structural similarity between these diseases may be the reason for the increased echogenicity in infiltrating hematopoie-

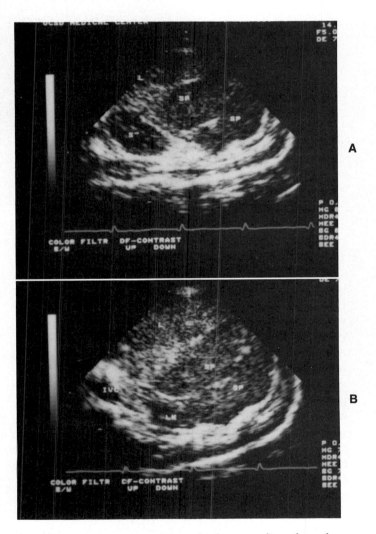

FIG. 16-12. In neonates with multiple anomalies, the spleen may be absent (asplenia) or multiple (polysplenia). **A,** Sagittal scan over the left upper quadrant shows two separate spleens, *SP.* The stomach is posterior. **B,** Sagittal scan of the liver, *L;* spleens, *SP;* left kidney, *LK;* and a piece of inferior vena cava, *IVC.*

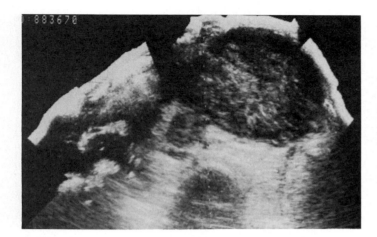

FIG. 16-13.   A young soccer player presented two days after suffering a severe blow to his left flank. A splenic hematoma was demonstrated on this decubitus view.

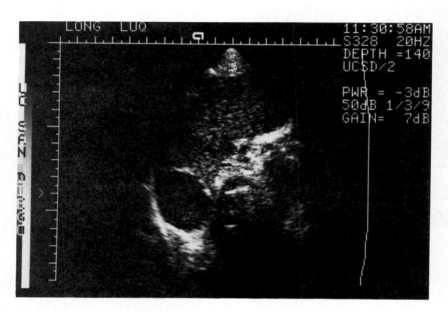

FIG. 16-14.   Sagittal scan over the left upper quadrant shows an echo-free area at the posterior aspect of the spleen that was consistent with a splenic cyst.

tic malignancies of the spleen. The particular stage at which the patient presents for a sonogram may also influence the echogenicity of the spleen.

In another study, by Murphy and Bernardino,[5] a limited number of patients with metastases to the spleen were studied by sonography. Hypoechoic lesions were seen in patients with histiocytic lymphoma, and both echogenic and hypoechoic lesions were seen in patients with melanoma. The dense echoes in patients with melanoma could be related to multiple microscopic metastases and a high tissue density. Although melanoma is one of the most frequent primary tumors to metastasize to the spleen, metastases from the breast, lung, or ovaries also may go to the spleen. Many of these patients are asymptomatic. Occasionally an enlarged spleen secondary to tumor may produce pain in the left upper quadrant or even cause a splenic rupture. A splenic infarction secondary to tumor emboli may also produce acute abdominal pain (Fig. 16-15). Thus splenomegaly may be found only incidentally at physical or sonographic evaluation.

The sonographic findings of lymphoma generally are low-level echoes emanating from splenomegaly.[9] The spleen may be of normal size and yet contain tumor in 33% of patients with Hodgkin's or non-Hodgkin's disease,[5] and another 33% with Hodgkin's disease may have splenomegaly with a pathologically normal spleen.

Cunningham[2] reports that both isolated lymphoma in the spleen and splenic abscess may give rise to ultrasonic images that show irregular zones of below-normal echo activity with unimpeded acoustic transmission. Since the clinical features of the two diseases are very similar, it may be difficult to separate the entities by sonographic evaluation.

Benign splenic tumors. Benign splenic tumors are occasionally seen by sonography. Generally splenomegaly will be the first indication of an abnormality. As the sensitivity is increased, the normal splenic parenchyma will fill in while the tumor will not.

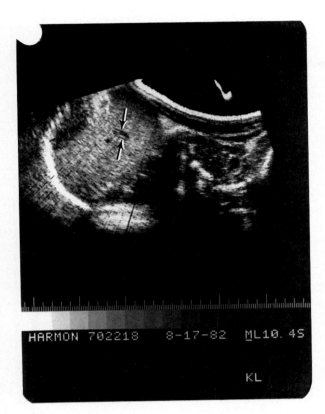

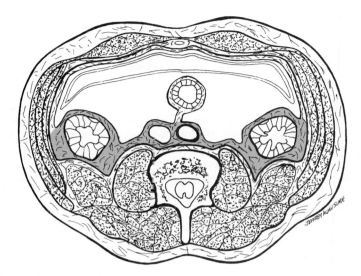

FIG. 16-16. Schematic transverse section of the abdominal cavity at the level of the fourth lumbar vertebrae. The retroperitoneal space is outlined in gray.

FIG. 16-15. Sagittal scan of the left upper quadrant shows a small collection within the spleen, which was representative of an infarct *(arrows)*.

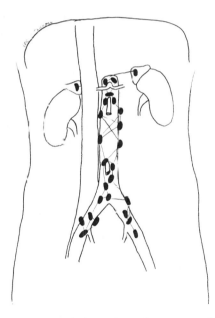

FIG. 16-17. Lymphatic chain along the aorta and iliac artery.

Retroperitoneum

ANATOMY

Retroperitoneal space

The retroperitoneal space is the area between the posterior portion of the parietal peritoneum and the posterior abdominal wall muscles. It extends from the diaphragm to the pelvis. Laterally the boundaries extend to the extraperitoneal fat planes within the confines of the transversalis fascia, and medially the space encloses the great vessels[1] (Fig. 16-16). It is subdivided into three categories: perinephric space or fascia of Gerota, anterior paranephric space, and posterior paranephric space. The perinephric space surrounds the kidney and perinephric fat, whereas the anterior paranephric space includes the extraperitoneal surfaces of the gut and pancreas. The iliopsoas, fat, and other soft tissues are within the posterior paranephric space.

Because it is protected by the spine, ribs, pelvis, and musculature, the retroperitoneum has been a difficult area to assess clinically; but ultrasound has become a useful diagnostic tool for detecting tumors and fluid collections (urinoma, abscess, hematoma, or ascites) located there.

Lymphatic system

There are two major node-bearing areas in the retroperitoneum: the iliac and hypogastric nodes within the pelvis

and the paraortic group in the upper retroperitoneum.

The lymphatic chain follows the course of the thoracic aorta, abdominal aorta, and iliac arteries (Fig. 16-17). Normal lymph nodes are smaller than the tip of a finger (less than 1 cm) and are not visualized by current ultrasound techniques. However, if these nodes enlarge because of infection or tumor, they become easier to visualize.

SONOGRAPHIC EVALUATION OF THE RETROPERITONEUM

Since the nodes lie along the lateral and anterior margins of the aorta, the best scanning is done with the patient in the supine position. It is important to examine the patient in two planes, since enlarged nodes seen in the longitudinal plane may mimic an abdominal aneurysm at lower gain settings. As the transverse scan is completed, the differential of an aneurysm versus lymphadenopathy can be made. The aneurysm will enlarge fairly symmetrically, whereas enlarged lymph nodes drape over the prevertebral vessels.

Longitudinal scans may be obtained first to outline the aorta and to search for enlarged lymph nodes. The aorta provides an excellent background for the somewhat sonolucent nodes. Longitudinal scans should begin at the midline and move both to the left and to the right at small increments. If an abnormality is noted on these sagittal scans, the area should be marked with a grease pencil for proper identification in the transverse plane.

Transverse scans are made from the xyphoid to the symphysis. Careful identification of the great vessels, organ structures, and muscle patterns is important. Patterns of a fluid-filled duodenum or bowel may make it difficult to outline the great vessels or may cause confusion in diagnosing lymphadenopathy.

Scans below the umbilicus are more difficult because of interference from the small bowel. Careful attention should be given to the psoas and iliacus within the pelvis, since the iliac arteries run along their medial border. Both muscles serve as a sonolucent marker in the pelvic sidewall. Enlarged lymph nodes can be identified anterior and medial to these margins. A smooth sharp border indicates no nodal involvement. The bladder should be filled to help push the small bowel out of the pelvis.

Splenomegaly should also be evaluated in patients with lymphadenopathy. As the sonographer moves caudal from the xyphoid, attention should be on the splenic size and great vessel area.

Lymph node evaluation

In our experience lymph nodes remain as consistent patterns whereas bowel and duodenum present changing patterns. As gentle pressure is applied with the transducer in an effort to displace the bowel, the lymph nodes remain constant. The echo pattern posterior to each structure is different. Lymph nodes are homogeneous and thus transmit sound easily; bowel presents a more complex pattern with dense central echoes from its mucosal pattern. Often the duodenum will have some air within its walls, causing a shadow posteriorly. Enlarged lymph nodes should be reproducible on ultrasound. After the abdomen is completely scanned, repeat sections over the enlarged nodes should demonstrate the same pattern as before.

The patient may be asked to return for a serial follow-up visit if there is uncertainty as to whether the pattern indicates enlarged lymph nodes or fluid-filled bowel.

Enlarged lymph nodes are more homogeneous than their surrounding organ structures, such as the pancreas, liver, kidneys, or spleen (Fig. 16-18). With increased sensitivity, diffuse low-level echoes may be seen within the nodes. Proper adjustment of the enhance control on most equipment is necessary for recording these fine echoes on the monitor. Their borders are generally smooth, but as

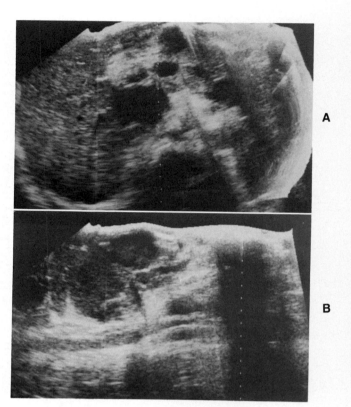

FIG. 16-18. A young man presented with ascites, edema, abdominal pain, and hypoproteinemia. His GI radiography showed displacement of the duodenum and stomach anteriorly with prominent proximal small bowel folds. Ultrasound showed a large lobuted retroperitoneal mass, ascites, and left hydronephrosis. **A,** Transverse scan showing splenomegaly and enlarged nodes anterior to the inferior vena cava. **B,** Sagittal scan of the enlarged nodes.

they enlarge they may take on a more irregular appearance (Figs. 16-19 to 16-23).

Asher and Freimanis (1969) stated that periaortic nodes are known to have specific characteristic patterns. They may drape or mantle the great vessels anteriorly. They may have a lobular, smooth, or scalloped appearance. As mesenteric involvement occurs, the adenopathy may fill most of the abdomen in an irregular complex pattern (Figs. 16-24 to 16-27).

The diagnosis of lymphadenopathy or a lymphomatous mass can be useful as a baseline study to the clinician. After treatment is administered, follow-up scans may be made to evaluate the shrinkage of the mass. If radiation therapy is used, it is helpful to mark the boundaries of the mass on the patient's skin for therapy planning.

PRIMARY RETROPERITONEAL TUMORS

A primary retroperitoneal tumor is one that originates independently within the retroperitoneal space. The tumor can arise anywhere, and most are malignant. As with other tumors, it may exhibit a variety of sonographic patterns

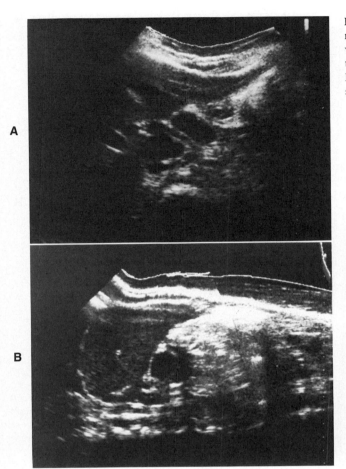

A

B

FIG. 16-19. Transverse, **A,** and sagittal, **B,** scans over the abdomen show a mass formation anterior to the aorta and inferior vena cava. Further investigation would require the sonographer to determine if this mass was part of the pancreas or an enlarged lymph node. The patient was found to have lymphoma and also showed an enlarged spleen on other scans.

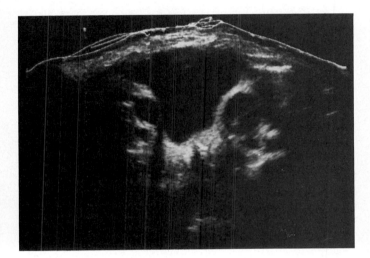

FIG. 16-20. The patient with lymphoma requires a complete abdominal and pelvic study to completely scan the nodal area. In this patient with a full bladder, enlarged nodes are seen bilaterally as they compress the lateral walls of the bladder.

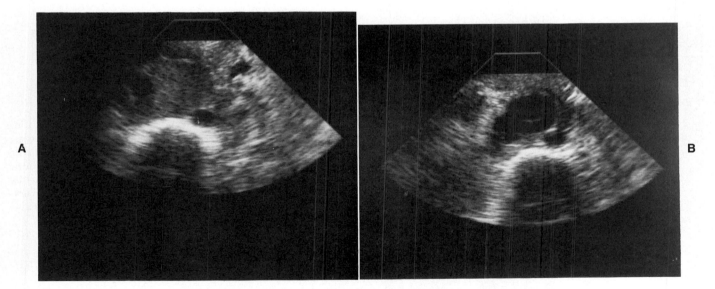

A

B

FIG. 16-21. This patient with a lymphoma had been receiving chemotherapy for a number of months. He now presented with fever, and the question of an abscess was raised. Because of his chemotherapy, the enlarged nodes were in various stages of regression, which can make them difficult to distinguish from abscess formation. The area in question was outlined by real-time examination for further needle aspiration and diagnosis. **A,** Transverse scan of a low-level node anterior to the great vessels. **B,** Transverse of a very homogeneous node anterior to the great vessels.

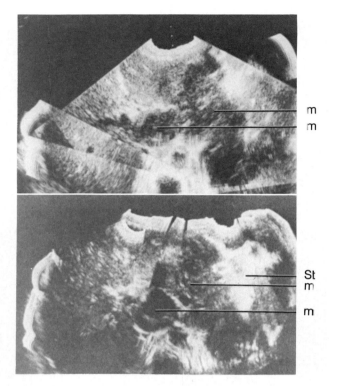

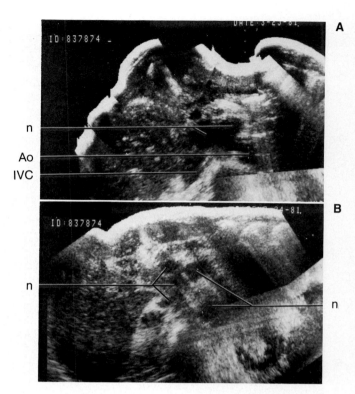

FIG. 16-22.   Transverse scans of a 44-year-old man with histocytic lymphoma of the upper abdomen. Ultrasound shows the lymphomatous mass, *m*, surrounding the stomach. The mass extends across the midline into the area of the head of the pancreas.

FIG. 16-23.   This patient presented with para-aortic node enlargement, an enlarged common bile duct, and right hydronephrosis. **A,** Transverse scan of the enlarged nodes, *n*. **B,** Several small nodes anterior to the great vessels are dilated. *Ao,* aorta; *IVC,* inferior vena cava.

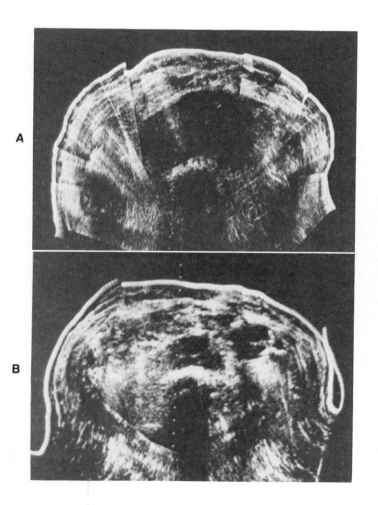

FIG. 16-24.   Ultrasound is a very effective tool for monitoring patients with lymphoma. This patient shows a dramatic decrease in the size of the para-aortic mass after treatment. **A,** Initial scan showing the homogeneous lymph mass to encircle the aorta completely. As sensitivity is increased, the aortic border may be seen better. **B,** Comparable transverse scan 15 months later. Note the regression in size of the mass surrounding the aorta.

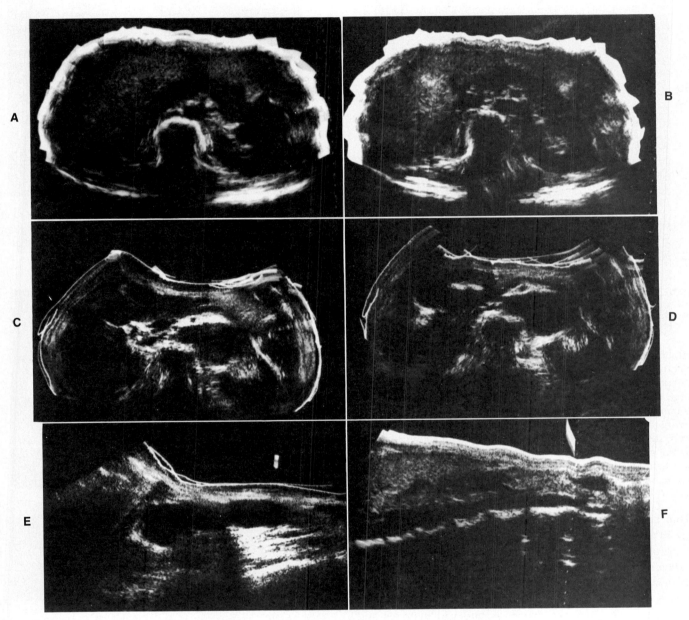

FIG. 16-25.   A to **D,** Multiple transverse scans over the upper abdomen in a patient with Hodgkin's disease. The dilated lymph nodes are seen in every scan as they hug the border of the great vessels. **E** and **F,** Sagittal scan showing the dilated lymph node in **E** and anterior to the aorta in **F.**

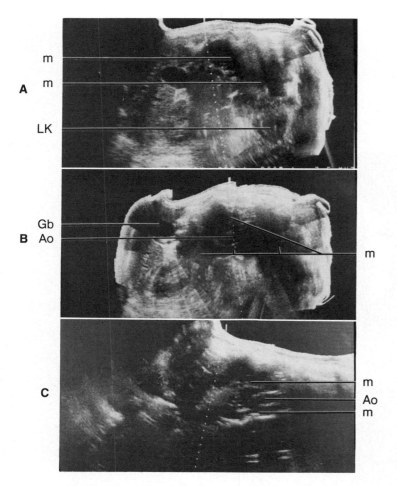

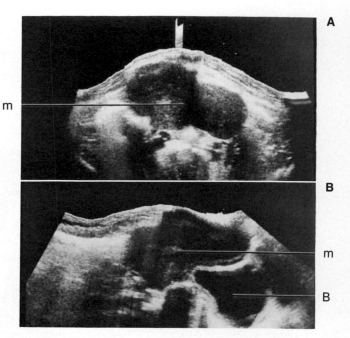

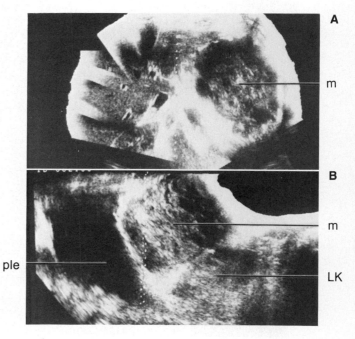

FIG. 16-26.   This 56-year-old patient with known laryngeal carcinoma complained of abdominal pain, jaundice, and malaise. Lymphoma was found at biopsy. Ultrasound demonstrated a large solid mass at the level of the porta hepatis obstructing the common bile duct and causing intrahepatic duct dilation and an enlarged gallbladder. Both the inferior vena cava and the aorta were distorted by the mass. **A,** Transverse scan shows mild left hydronephrosis. The mass is seen anterior to the great vessels and kidney. **B,** Transverse scan of the dilated gallbladder, *Gb,* and mass, *m.* **C,** Sagittal scan of the mass encircling the aorta, *Ao.*

FIG. 16-27.   Transverse, **A,** and sagittal, **B,** scans of a 12-year-old boy treated seven years earlier for Burkitt's lymphoma. He now presented with a scar associated with a fibroma that was enlarging. Bladder, *B;* mass, *m.*

FIG. 16-28.   Transverse **A,** and sagittal, **B,** scans of a patient with a large, solid retroperitoneal mass, *m,* separated from the left kidney, *LK.* A large pleural effusion, *ple,* is also seen above the diaphragm.

from homogeneous to complex to solid (Figs. 16-28 and 16-29).

Neurogenic tumors are usually encountered in the paravertebral region, where they arise from nerve roots or sympathetic chain ganglia. Sonographically their pattern is quite variable.

Leiomyosarcomas are prone to undergo necrosis and cystic degeneration. Their sonographic pattern is complex. Liposarcomas produce a highly reflective sonographic pattern due to their fat interface.

Fibrosarcomas and rhabdomyosarcomas may be quite invasive and may infiltrate widely into muscles and adjoining soft tissues. They often present with extension across the midline and appear very similar to lymphomas. Sonographically they are highly reflective tumors.

Teratomatous tumors may arise within the upper retroperitoneum and the pelvis. They may contain calcified echoes from bones, cartilage, and teeth as well as soft tissue elements.

Tumors of uniform cell type generally have a homogeneous appearance unless there is hemorrhage or necrosis. Often the presence of necrosis depends on the size and growth of the mass (Fig. 16-30).

SECONDARY RETROPERITONEAL TUMORS

Secondary retroperitoneal tumors are primarily recurrences from previously resected tumors. Recurrent

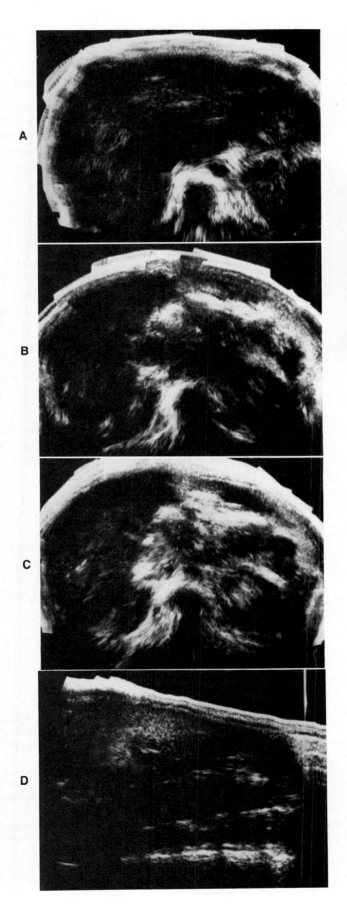

A

B

C

D

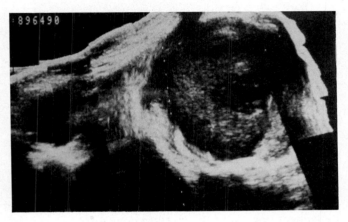

FIG. 16-29. **A** to **C,** Multiple transverse scans over the upper abdomen show a large retroperitoneal mass that extends from the area of the porta hepatis to the level of the umbilicus. The mass appears separate from the aorta and liver. **D,** Sagittal scan showing the extension of the mass from the umbilicus to well into the mid portion of the liver.

FIG. 16-30. A large retroperitoneal tumor exhibiting central necrosis is surrounded by low-level echoes.

masses from previous renal carcinoma are frequent. Ascitic fluid along with a retroperitoneal tumor usually indicates seeding or invasion of the peritoneal surface. Evaluation of the paraaortic region should be made for extension to the lymph nodes. The liver should also be evaluated for metastatic involvement.

RETROPERITONEAL FLUID COLLECTIONS

Urinoma. A urinoma is a walled-off collection of extravasated urine that develops spontaneously after trauma, surgery, or a subacute or chronic urinary obstruction. Urinomas usually collect about the kidney or upper ureter in the perinephric space. Occasionally urinomas dissect into the pelvis and compress the bladder. Generally their sonographic pattern is sonolucent unless they become infected.

Hemorrhage. A retroperitoneal hemorrhage may occur in a variety of conditions, including trauma, vasculitis, bleeding diathesis, leaking aortic aneurysm, or bleeding neoplasm. Sonographically it may be well localized and produce displacement of other organs, or it may present as a poorly defined infiltrative process.

Fresh hematomas present as sonolucent areas whereas organized thrombus and clot formation show echo densities within the mass. Calcification may be seen in longstanding hematomas.

Abscess. Abscess formation may result from surgery, trauma, or perforations of the bowel or duodenum. Sonographically the abscess usually has a more complex pattern with debris. Gas within the abscess will be reflective

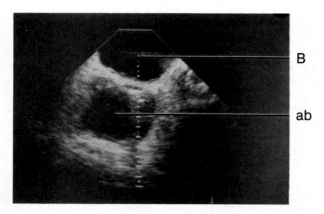

FIG. 16-31. A young man who had been stabbed in the left flank presented with pain, hematuria, urgency, and fever. A large abscess, *ab*, was found anterior to the rectum and posterior to the bladder, *B*.

and cast an acoustic shadow (Fig. 16-31). One should be careful not to miss a gas-containing abscess for "bowel" patterns. The radiograph should be evaluated in this case. The abscess frequently extends along or within the muscle planes, is of an irregular shape, and lies in the most dependent portion of the retroperitoneal space.

RETROPERITONEAL FIBROSIS

Retroperitoneal fibrosis is a disease of unknown etiology characterized by thick sheets of fibrous tissue in the retroperitoneal space. The disease may occur in association with abdominal aortic aneurysms. It may encase and obstruct the ureters and vena cava, with resultant hydronephrosis. A discrete mass of abnormal tissue lying anterior and lateral to the great vessels has been described by Sanders et al.[2] It may mimic lymphoma and thus must be further delineated for benignity or malignancy.

SUMMARY
Spleen

1. The spleen is the largest single mass of lymphoid tissue in the body. It lies in the left hypochondrium. Important neighboring organs include the stomach, pancreas, and left kidney.

2. The functions of the spleen may be classified under two general headings: those that reflect the functions of the reticuloendothelial system and those characteristic of the organ itself.

3. Sonographically the normal spleen should have the same texture as the homogeneous liver parenchyma.

4. The spleen is involved in all systemic inflammations and generalized hematopoietic disorders, and many metabolic disturbances. It is rarely the primary site of disease. Whenever the spleen is involved in systemic disease, splenic enlargement usually develops; and therefore splenomegaly is a major manifestation of disorders of this organ.

Retroperitoneum

5. The retroperitoneal space is the area between the posterior portion of the parietal peritoneum and the posterior abdominal wall muscles. It extends from the diaphragm to the pelvis. It is subdivided into three categories: perinephric space (fascia of Gerota), anterior paranephric space, and posterior paranephric space.

6. There are two major node-bearing areas in the retroperitoneum: the iliac and hypogastric nodes within the pelvic and the paraaortic group in the upper retroperitoneum.

7. A primary retroperitoneal tumor is one that originates independently within the retroperitoneal space. The tumor can arise anywhere and most are malignant.

8. Secondary retroperitoneal tumors are primarily recurrences from previously resected tumors. The presence of ascites may also occur.

9. Other masses within the retroperitoneal space include urinoma, hemorrhage, and abscess formation.

REFERENCES
Spleen

1. Cooperberg PL: Ultrasonography of the spleen. In Sarti DA and Sample WF, editors: Diagnostic ultrasound: text and cases, Boston, 1980, GK Hall & Co.

2. Cunningham J: Ultrasonic findings in isolated lymphoma of the spleen simulating splenic abscess, J Clin Ultrasound 6:412, 1978.

3. Koga T: Correlation between sectional area of the spleen by ultrasonic tomography and actual volume of the removed spleen, J Clin Ultrasound 7:119, 1979.

4. Mittelstaedt CA and Partain CL: Ultrasonic-pathologic classification of splenic abnor-

malities: gray scale patterns, Radiology 134:697, 1980.

5. Murphy JF and Bernardino ME: The sonographic findings of splenic metastases, J Clin Ultrasound 7:195, 1979.

6. Propper RA, Weinstein BJ, Skolnick L, et al: Ultrasonography of hemorrhagic splenic cysts, J Clin Ultrasound 7:18, 1979.

7. Robbins SL and Cotran RS: Pathologic basis of disease, Philadelphia, 1979, WB Saunders, Co.

8. Siler J, Hunter TB, Weiss J, and Haber K: Increased echogenicity of the spleen in benign and malignant disease, AJR 134:1011, 1980.

9. Taylor KJW and Moulton D: The spleen. In Taylor KJW, editor: Atlas of gray scale ultrasonography, New York, 1978, Churchill Livingstone, Inc.

Retroperitoneum

1. Goldberg BB, Pollack HM, and Bancks NH: Retroperitoneum. In Resnick MI and Sanders RC, editors: Ultrasound in urology, Baltimore, 1979, The Williams & Wilkins Co.

2. Sanders RC, Duffy T, McLaughlin MG, et al: Sonography in the diagnosis of retroperitoneal fibrosis, J Urol 118:944, 1977.

Part Three

SUPERFICIAL STRUCTURES

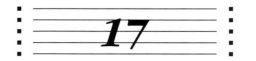

High-Resolution Ultrasonography of Superficial Structures

LAURA SCHORZMAN

The recent development of high-resolution ultrasound instruments provides a means of effectively evaluating superficial organs and structures. A number of systems have been designed that utilize frequencies in the 7 to 10 MHz range and incorporate water or oil path delays. High-resolution imaging and optimal use of the focal zone are satisfied by such instrumentation. The appellation "small-parts scanning" has been applied to this technology.

The material for this chapter was obtained by a system utilizing a 10 MHz 13 mm diameter transducer. The transducer is focused at a depth of approximately 2.2 cm from the skin surface and provides an axial resolution of 0.4 mm and a lateral resolution of 1 or 2 mm. The transducer is housed in a water bath and mechanically driven back and forth in a linear fashion. This produces a 3×4 cm rectangular image format. Update of the information at 30 frames per second provides the real-time capability of the system. A thin, pliable membrane covering the water bath housing is placed in contact with the skin.

The real-time feature of small-parts scanners provides ease and flexibility for rapid and thorough evaluation of structures.

THYROID GLAND
Anatomy

The thyroid gland consists of a right and a left lobe connected in the midline by an isthmus. Each lobe is lateral to the trachea and is bounded posterolaterally by the carotid artery and internal jugular vein (Figs. 17-1 and 17-2). The conical upper pole partly covers the lower portion of the thyroid cartilage, and the rounded lower poles partially cover the third and fourth tracheal rings. The sternocleidomastoid and strap muscles (sternothyroid, sternohyoid, and omohyoid) are situated anterolateral to the thyroid (Fig. 17-2).

The two lobes of the gland are of similar size and shape in most persons, although the right lobe is often slightly larger. The isthmus, which lies anterior to the trachea, is variable in size. A triangular cephalad extension of the isthmus, the pyramidal lobe, is present in 15% to 30% of thyroid glands. When present, it too is of varying size and is more frequently located on the left. A fibrous capsule encloses the gland and gives it a smooth contour.

Blood is supplied to the thyroid via four arteries. Two superior thyroid arteries arise from the external carotids and descend to the upper poles. Two inferior thyroid ar-

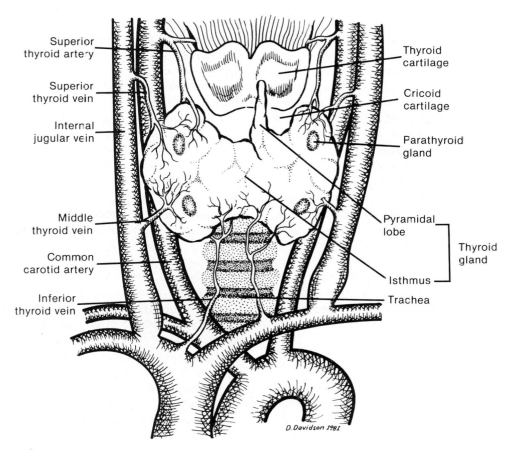

FIG. 17-1. Anterior view of the thyroid and parathyroid regions. (Modified from Forsham PH: Endocrine system and selected metabolic diseases, ed, 3, Summit, NJ, 1974, Ciba Parmaceutical Co.)

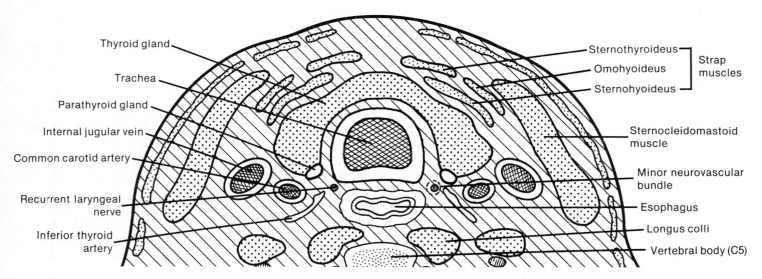

FIG. 17-2. Cross-section of the thyroid region showing organ, vessel, and muscle relationships. (Modified from Forsham PH: Endocrine system and selected metabolic diseases, ed, 3, Summit, NJ, 1974, Ciba Pharmaceutical Co.)

teries arise from the thyrocervical trunk of the subclavian artery and ascend to the lower poles. Corresponding veins drain into the internal jugular vein (Fig. 17-1).

Physiology

The role of the thyroid, an endocrine gland, is to maintain normal body metabolism, growth, and development by the synthesis, storage, and secretion of thyroid hormones.

The mechanism for production of thyroid hormones is iodine metabolism. The thyroid gland traps iodine from the blood and, through a series of chemical reactions, produces the thyroid hormones triiodothyronine (T3) and thyroxine (T4). These are stored in the colloid of the gland. When thyroid hormone is needed, release into the bloodstream is accomplished by the action of thyrotropin or thyroid-stimulating hormone (TSH), produced by the pituitary gland. The secretion of TSH is regulated by thyrotropin-releasing factor, which is produced by the hypothalamus. The level of thyrotropin-releasing factor is controlled by the basal metabolic rate. A decrease in the BMR, which is a result of a low concentration of thyroid hormones, causes an increase in thyrotropin-releasing factor. This causes increased secretion of TSH and a subsequent increase in the release of thyroid hormones. When the blood level of hormones is returned to normal, the BMR returns to normal and TSH secretion stops.

Pathology

Enlargement of the thyroid gland is termed *goiter*. This can be diffuse and symmetric or irregular and nodular (focal). It may be a result of hyperplasia or neoplasia, inflammatory processes, or colloid distension of the follicles. A goiter can be associated with normal thyroid function, hyperfunction, or hypofunction.

Hyperthyroidism is a hypermetabolic state in which increased amounts of thryoid hormones are produced as a result of pituitary-thyroid regulatory system failure. The hormonal increase may be caused by an adenoma that independently secretes the thyroid hormone or by an increase in TSH. Manifestations of this condition are weight loss, nervousness, and increased heart rate; exophthalmos may develop when the condition is severe. Hyperthyroidism associated with diffuse goiter is Graves' disease.

Hypothyroidism is a hypometabolic state resulting from inadequate secretion of thyroid hormones. It is usually caused by an abnormality of the gland that restricts production of the hormones. Lethargy, sluggish reactions, and a deep husky voice are manifestations. Congenital hypothyroidism is cretinism.

Benign lesions

CYST. About 20% of solitary thyroid nodules are cysts. Many are thought to represent cystic degeneration of a follicular adenoma. Blood or debris may be present within them. Cysts are almost uniformly benign.

ADENOMA. Adenomas, more common in females, account for approximately 70% of true solitary thyroid nodules. They have a well-developed fibrous capsule encasing distinct internal architecture and are more firm than surrounding thyroid tissue. These solitary discrete lesions, ranging in size from 3 to 10 cm, are typically slow growing but may grow suddenly due to internal hemorrhage.

DIFFUSE NONTOXIC GOITER (COLLOID GOITER). This compensatory enlargement of the thyroid gland is due to thyroid hormone deficiency. The gland becomes diffusely and uniformly enlarged and is firm but not hard. In the first stage hyperplasia occurs; in the second stage, colloid involution. Progression of this process leads to asymmetric and multinodular glands.

ADENOMATOUS HYPERPLASIA (MULTINODULAR GOITER). This goiter is one of the most common forms of thyroid disease. Nodularity of the gland can be the end stage of diffuse nontoxic goiter, which can be followed by focal scarring, by focal areas of ischemia and necrosis and cyst formation, or by fibrosis or calcification. Some of the nodules are poorly circumscribed; others appear to be encapsulated. Enlargement can involve one lobe to a greater extent that the other and sometimes causes difficulty in breathing and swallowing.

THYROIDITIS. Thyroiditis can be a result of infections or autoimmune causes. The disease may be chronic (lymphocytic and Hashimoto's disease), which presents as mild swelling of the gland, or subacute (De Quervain's), which presents with pain and fever.

Malignant lesions.

Thyroid carcinoma is relatively rare and is not a frequent cause of death (approximately 1100 persons die annually versus 100,000 for lung cancer). Evidence suggests an increased risk of thyroid cancer in adults with a childhood history of face, neck, or upper mediastinal radiation. A 7% to 9% prevalence has been cited in these persons.

Any nodule newly discovered or that exhibits a rapid increase in size is suspect for malignancy. In addition, stony hard nodules fixed to surrounding structures and/or palpable cervical lymph nodes are suspect. Primary cancers of the thyroid can be categorized into four types: papillary, follicular, medullary, and anaplastic. Malignant lymphoma and metastatic tumors also occur.

PAPILLARY CARCINOMA. Papillary carcinoma is the most common thyroid gland malignancy (60% to 70%). The incidence is greatest among young adults (less than 40 years of age), but the lesion also occurs in the older population or in young children. This particular type of thyroid cancer is seen more frequently in females. It is one of the least aggressive and least malignant of human cancers, but in rare instances it can cause death.

The lesions may be tiny or may range up to 10 cm. They grow slowly, tend to infiltrate locally, and spread to cervical lymph nodes.

The clinical presentation is usually the incidental discovery of a nonpainful asymptomatic neck lump. Since metastases to regional cervical and mediastinal nodes are frequent, it is not uncommon for an enlarged lymph node to be detected prior to detection of the primary thyroid nodule.

Papillary carcinomas may be pure or mixed papillary and follicular; however, the long–term behavior is that of pure papillary carcinoma. Whether or not cervical node metastases are present, papillary carcinoma seems to be curable by hemithyroidectomy followed by thyroid hormone therapy.

FOLLICULAR CARCINOMA. This form of thyroid cancer accounts for about 15% to 20% of thyroid cancers. Its frequency increases with advancing age, and again females are more often affected.

An irregular, firm, nodular enlargement or a solitary, seemingly encapsulated, enlarging nodule is characteristic. Enlargement of the lesion is slow but somewhat more rapid than that of papillary carcinoma.

Metastases travel through the blood to lungs and bone. Lymph node involvement is uncommon. This type of thyroid cancer is more aggressive than papillary cancer; however, the prognosis is good, especially if diagnosed and treated before tissue invasion and before the age of 40 years.

MEDULLARY CARCINOMA. This form accounts for 5% to 10% of thyroid cancers. It presents as a hard bulky mass that may cause enlargement of a portion of a lobe or involve large areas of the entire gland.

Multiple endocrine neoplasia syndromes (e.g., Sipple's syndrome) have medullary carcinoma associated with pheochromocytoma and parathyroid adenoma. Medullary carcinoma is one type of thyroid carcinoma that may be familial.

Sharply circumscribed but unencapsulated medullary carcinomas frequently invade surrounding structures. They metastasize to cervical lymph nodes and other distant sites. Although their course is rather slow, the 5-year survival rate is 40% to 50%.

ANAPLASTIC (UNDIFFERENTIATED) CARCINOMA. About 10% to 15% of thyroid cancers are of this form. It usually occurs after 50 years of age, with no predilection for either sex. It is one of the most malignant and deadly of all carcinomas occurring in humans.

The lesion presents as a hard fixed mass with rapid growth and produces pressure symptoms, possibly tenderness. Its growth is locally invasive into surrounding neck structures, and it usually causes death by compression and asphyxiation due to invasion of the trachea. Since there is no effective treatment, most patients die within a year after diagnosis has been established.

LYMPHOMA. Primary lymphomas of the thyroid arise in the 60 to 70 year-old patient population, with the incidence somewhat greater in females. Although uncommon, they usually occur in a patient with a huge goiter of recent development. The prognosis is generally poor.

METASTATIC TUMORS TO THE THYROID. Cancers from various organs of the body can metastasize to the thyroid gland. Breast cancer is the most common thyroid metastatic lesion; but metastases also come from the lung, kidney, and colon.

Ultrasound evaluation

Management, whether surgical or medical, of thyroid nodules is handled on the basis of the nodule's being benign or malignant. The date of origin, physical findings, and various laboratory tests are used as aids in differentiation. It is frequently impossible to distinguish a single nodule from multiple nodularity by physical examination. A multinodular gland is less likely to be malignant than one with a solitary lesion, excluding patients who have received prior head and neck irradiation; however, benign lesions and carcinomas can coexist.

Although it has resolution limitations (nodules smaller than 1 cm are not demonstrable) and differentiation of cystic from solid lesions is not possible, the radioisotope scan is commonly used in the management of thyroid nodules. After intravenous injection of a radioisotope,[131] I or technetium-99^m pertechnetate, a rectilinear scanner or gamma camera is used to detect the concentration of the radioisotope in the nodule and in the remaining gland. The nodules are then classified as cold or hot depending upon how they concentrate the isotope.

Cold nodules concentrate less isotope than the surrounding thyroid tissue. Approximately 20% of cold thyroid nodules are malignant and about 20% are cystic. Most of the remainder are benign adenomas.

Hot nodules represent increased thyroid activity or are nodules that concentrate more radionuclide than the remaining thyroid. They are almost never malignant if hot by ^{131}I scan.

The role of ultrasound is to detect and characterize thyroid nodules. Size and location can be accurately assessed for initial evaluation and for follow-up study. Masses as small as 3 mm can be demonstrated, and differentiation of cystic versus solid nodules easily made, by ultrasound. Sonographic characterization of solid nodules as to benignity or malignancy is a desirable feature that has yet to be clearly established.

Ultrasound is instrumental also in needle aspiration procedures of cystic and solid lesions. Since areas of hemorrhage and necrosis have a poor cytologic yield, they should be avoided. Sonography can provide guidance for accurate needle placement to obtain optimal diagnostic aspirate material.

Scanning technique. When a patient is referred for ultrasound evaluation of a thyroid or neck mass, the isotope examination should be obtained for correlation.

The sonographic examination is begun with the patient lying supine. A sponge or pillow is placed under the neck to hyperextend it. This moves the mandible out of the field of interest and permits better transducer access. The head is turned slightly away from the side being examined, further optimizing transducer access (Fig. 17-3). This position is important for visualization, but one must also consider patient comfort. A comfortable and cooperative patient is instrumental in obtaining a diagnostic examination.

Because of the limited field of view of high-resolution scanners, it is not possible to image the entire thyroid gland in each scan. The lobes must be evaluated independently. In addition, because of the limited view that is ultimately documented, it is prudent for the interpreter of the examination to observe the study being performed.

A methodical routine for thorough investigation of the

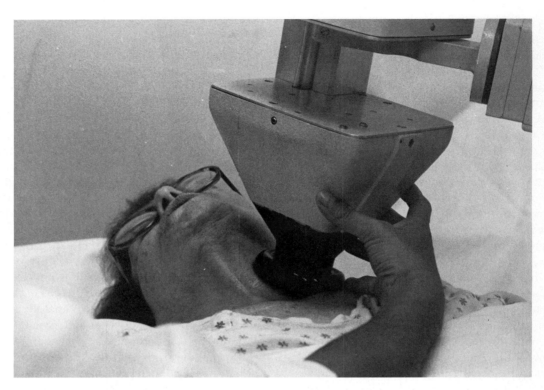

FIG. 17-3. Patient and transducer positions for longitudinal scanning of the thyroid gland.

gland should always be followed. Transverse scanning begins at the lower pole of one lobe and continues up through the entire gland. The transducer is glided over the neck perpendicular to the skin. Because of variations in neck anatomy, experimentation with scanning head angulations may be necessary to achieve maximum transducer-to-skin contact. The carotid artery and jugular vein are used as lateral landmarks, and the trachea as a medial reference. If the preliminary survey reveals a normal gland, representative images should be recorded at the lower, middle, and upper poles, care being taken to document the medial and lateral extents of the gland. If an abnormality is encountered, all characteristics of the anomaly (cystic areas, calcifications, halo, etc.) should be demonstrated. It is not uncommon for sonography to demonstrate multiple nodules in a gland previously suspected of having only a solitary lesion.

Longitudinal scans are then performed from the medial aspect of the gland to the lateral surface through the lower, middle, and upper poles. Again, imaging should represent each pole of the thyroid in the normal situation. An abnormality is imaged as in transverse scanning. One lobe is explored in both transverse and longitudinal planes before the opposite lobe is.

After each lobe is evaluated, the isthmus must be scanned. Transverse sections are usually more satisfactory for visualizing this area. The examination is complete when normal and pathologic relationships have been understood and documented.

Ultrasound appearances

NORMAL. The normal thyroid gland has a smooth homogeneous texture of medium-level echoes. Lateral to the gland the carotid artery and internal jugular vein are identified in the transverse plane (Fig. 17-4, A). The vein, which is usually partly collapsed, is lateral and slightly superficial to the artery. A Valsalva maneuver by the patient will cause jugular vein distension. Thyroid vessels are occasionally seen anterior to the gland or coursing within the parenchyma. The strap muscles are anterolateral to the gland and the longus colli can often be identified posteriorly. The trachea is in the midline, posterior to the isthmus.

On longitudinal section the strap muscles and longus colli border the gland anteriorly and posteriorly, respectively (Fig. 17-4, B). The upper and lower poles appear as conical projections. During swallowing the normal gland glides along the musculature in a cephalocaudad direction.

CYST. Simple cysts as small as 1 mm can be identified with high-resolution scanners. As in cysts elsewhere, well-demarcated smooth margins and lack of internal echoes are present (Fig. 17-5). Many cysts, however, have internal architecture that may be the result of hemorrhage. Recent hemorrhage can have an echolucent appearance or a fine smooth diffuse echographic pattern. Dense echoes or septations, which represent organization of blood, may be seen within cysts of longer duration. Many clinicians currently postulate that thyroid cysts are simply the result of degeneration of adenomas.

ADENOMA. Adenomas, which comprise the majority of "cold" nodules (60%), have a broad spectrum of ultrasound appearances. They range from predominantly echolucent to completely echodense and commonly have a peripheral halo (Fig. 17-6). The echolucent areas are a result of cystic degeneration (probably from hemorrhage)

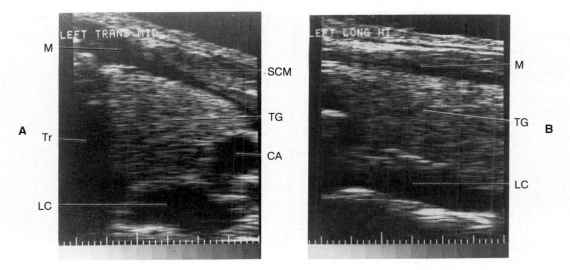

FIG. 17-4.   A, Transverse scan of the left lobe of the normal thyroid gland, *TG,* demonstrating the relationships of the carotid artery, *CA,* trachea, *Tr,* and muscles. Note the homogeneous texture of the gland. **B,** Longitudinal scan of the upper pole of the normal thyroid, *TG.* Strap muscles, *M,* border the gland anteriorly and the longus colli, *LC,* borders posteriorly. *SCM,* sternocleidomastoid muscle.

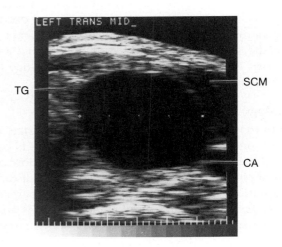

FIG. 17-5.   A 2 cm thyroid cyst occupies most of the left lobe on this transverse scan. TG, thyroid gland, isthmus; CA, carotid artery; SCM, sternocleidomastoid muscle.

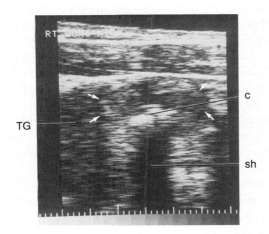

FIG. 17-6.   Longitudinal scan of a thyroid adenoma demonstrating a halo *(arrows)* and a large central calcification, *c,* with shadow, *sh. TG,* thyroid gland.

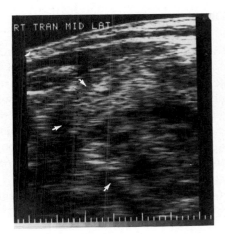

FIG. 17-7.   Areas of cystic degeneration and a poorly defined halo *(arrowheads)* can be identified on this transverse scan of a multinodular goiter. Discrete nodule margins are difficult to perceive.

and usually lack a well-rounded margin. This lack of a discrete cystic margin is helpful in differentiation from a simple cyst. Calcification, characteristically rimlike, can also be associated with adenomas. Its acoustic shadow may preclude visualization posteriorly (Fig. 17-6). The halo or thin echolucent rim surrounding the lesion may represent edema of the compressed normal thyroid tissue or the capsule of the adenoma. In a few instances it may be blood around the lesion. Although the halo is a relatively consistent finding in adenomas, additional statistical information is necessary to establish its specificity.

MULTINODULAR GOITER. Individual lesions in multinodular goiter have many of the features of true adenomas. The multiple nodules of adenomatous hyperplasia may demonstrate halos and may or may not have discrete margins (Fig. 17-7). The echo texture of the solid portion of the

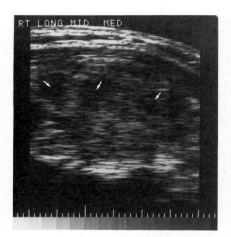

FIG. 17-8. Longitudinal scan of subacute thyroiditis showing diffuse enlargement of the thyroid gland with multiple nodular masses *(arrows)*.

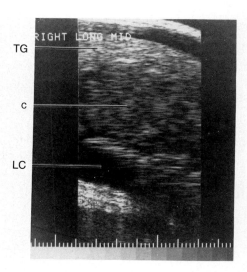

FIG. 17-9. Longitudinal section revealing the 3 cm thyroid carcinoma, *c,* to be less echogenic than the normal thyroid, *TG.* Longus colli, *LC.*

lesion is typically similar to that of normal thyroid. Various degrees of cystic degeneration as well as calcification may be present within the nodules.

THYROIDITIS. Thyroiditis usually appears as an enlarged gland with a generalized lower-amplitude echogenicity than normal thyroid parenchyma. Chronically inflamed glands are inhomogeneous and have disordered parenchymal echoes. Areas of relative sonolucency and/or high reflectivity may be seen as well as discrete solid nodules (Fig. 17-8).

In acute thyroiditis the resultant diffuse edema of the disease produces a homogeneous diminished echo pattern when compared to normal thyroid. The affected lobe or lobes are enlarged.

CARCINOMA. Cancers of the thyroid produce areas of lower-amplitude echoes than does normal thyroid parenchyma (Fig. 17-9). The interfaces of the lesion are often poorly defined and a halo is rarely present. Cystic degeneration, if present, is minimal. Specks of calcium, although not common, may also be noted but are seldom peripheral as with adenomas.

PARATHYROID GLANDS
Anatomy
The parathyroid glands are usually closely attached to or embedded in the sheath of the posteromedial surface of the capsule of the thyroid gland (Figs. 17-1 and 17-2). Their numbers and locations are variable. Usually there are two pairs, a superior and an inferior, which lie behind the middle third and lower third of the thyroid. It is the inferior pair that tends to be more variable in position and may be anterior to the thyroid or may be retrosternal in the mediastinum.

The glands are typically somewhat flattened oval structures of approximately 3 × 4 mm in the adult.

Physiology
The parathyroid glands are the calcium-sensing organs in the body. They produce parathormone (PTH) and monitor the serum calcium feedback mechanism.

The stimulus PTH secretion is a decrease in the level of blood calcium. When the serum calcium level decreases, the parathyroid glands are stimulated to release PTH. When the serum calcium level rises, parathyroid activity decreases. PTH acts on bone, kidney, and intestine to enhance calcium absorption.

Pathology
Primary hyperparathyroidism. This is a state of increased function of the parathyroid glands and is characterized by hypercalcemia, hypercalciuria, and low serum levels of phosphate. Kidney damage and bone disease are manifestations of this situation. Primary hyperparathyroidism occurs when increased amounts of PTH are produced by an adenoma, primary hyperplasia, or rarely carcinoma.

ADENOMA. By far the most common cause of primary hyperparathyroidism is an adenoma. A single hyperfunctioning lesion is responsible for 80% of cases. This benign tumor is usually very small (rarely larger than 3 cm) and often is not palpable. It is well encapsulated and is most common in the inferior parathyroid glands. Differentiation between adenomas and hyperplasia is difficult on histologic and morphologic grounds.

PRIMARY HYPERPLASIA. Primary hyperplasia is hyperfunction of all parathyroid glands with no apparent cause. Only one gland may significantly enlarge and the remaining glands be only mildly affected, or all glands may be enlarged. In any case, they rarely reach greater than 1 cm in size.

CARCINOMA. Histologic differentiation between adenoma and carcinoma is very difficult. Metastases to regional nodes or distant organs, capsular invasion, or local recurrence must be present for the diagnosis of cancer to be made.

Most cancers of the parathyroid glands are small, irregular, and rather firm masses. They sometimes adhere to surrounding structures. If death results, it is more likely to

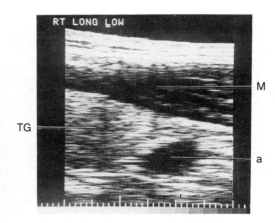

FIG. 17-10. Parathyroid adenoma, *a,* posterior to the lower pole of the thyroid gland, *TG,* on this longitudinal scan. Strap muscles, *M.*

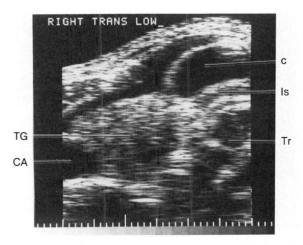

FIG. 17-11. Transverse scan at the level of the thyroid gland, *TG,* demonstrating a thyroglossal duct cyst, *c,* in the midline anterior to the trachea, *Tr.* Carotid artery, *CA;* isthmus of thyroid gland, *Is.*

be due to hyperparathyroid complications than to the malignancy itself.

Secondary hyperparathyroidism. A chronic hypocalcemia, caused by renal failure, vitamin D deficiency (rickets), or malabsorption syndromes, induces PTH secretion and leads to secondary hyperparathyroidism. The hyperfunction of the parathyroids is apparently a compensatory reaction; renal insufficiency and intestinal malabsorption cause hypocalcemia, which leads to stimulation of PTH. All four glands are usually affected.

Ultrasound evaluation

Patients with unexplained hypercalcemia detected on routine blood chemistry screening are the most common referrals for parathyroid echography. Symptomatic renal stones, ulcers, and bone pain are other indications.

Scanning technique. The sonographic examination is carried out much like the thyroid examination but with emphasis placed on the anticipated locations of the parathyroid glands (Fig. 17-3).

Transversely the evaluation should begin at the most caudal level possible (sternal notch) and extend as far cephalad as possible (mandible). If no pathology is identified, representative scans should be recorded at the lower, middle, and upper areas of the thyroid gland, which is a major reference organ. Landmarks such as thyroid, trachea, carotid artery, and longus colli should be demonstrated.

Longitudinally the cephalocaudal extent on each side of the neck should be examined from medial to lateral. The trachea represents the medial limit, and the carotid artery the lateral extent. Representative scans of the medial and lateral aspects of the lower, middle, and upper thyroid should be recorded.

Ultrasound appearances

NORMAL. Theoretically one would expect high-resolution scanners to be capable of resolving the parathyroid glands; however, to date this has not been true. The anatomic relationships (i.e., closely attached to or embedded in the thyroid gland and the apparent lack of acoustic differences between the thyroid and parathyroid glands) are probable explanations.

Since in many cases a prominent longus colli appears as a discrete area posterior to the thyroid, it is important not to confuse this normal anatomy with a mass. Longitudinal sections can usually solve the problem. A linear appearance of the muscle is evident in this plane (Fig. 17-4, *B*). The minor neurovascular bundle, composed of the inferior thyroid artery and recurrent laryngeal nerve, may also be a source of confusion (Fig. 17-2). Again, longitudinal scans can usually eliminate this confusion by identification of its tubular appearance.

ADENOMA. Parathyroid adenomas are homogeneous, well-circumscribed, and less echogenic than normal thyroid tissue (Fig. 17-10). A dense sharp outer margin may be present around the lesion and is helpful in determining its extrathyroidal nature.

HYPERPLASIA. Since hyperplastic parathyroid glands and parathyroid adenomas both appear as relatively sonolucent masses, they cannot be sonographically discriminated. Hyperplasia involves all parathyroid glands to some extent; however, all glands may not be sufficiently enlarged to be seen by sonography.

MISCELLANEOUS NECK MASSES

The role of ultrasound in evaluation of palpable neck masses is to determine site of origin and assess lesion texture.

Developmental cysts

Thyroglossal duct cyst. Thyroglossal duct cysts are congenital anomalies that present in the midline of the neck anterior to the trachea (Fig. 17-11). They are fusiform or spherical masses and are rarely larger than 2 or 3 cm.

A remnant of the tubular development of the thyroid gland may persist between the base of the tongue and the

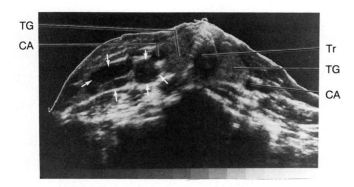

FIG. 17-12. Multiple lucencies *(arrows)* lateral to the right lobe of the thyroid gland, *TG,* on this transverse scan from a contact static B-scanner. These represent enlarged lymph nodes of Hodgkin's disease. *CA,* carotid artery; *Tr,* trachea.

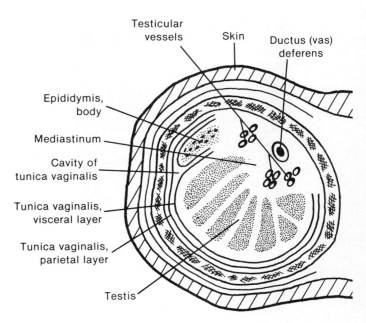

FIG. 17-13. Cross-section through the midpoint of the scrotum and right testis. (Redrawn from Anson BJ: Morris' human anatomy, ed 12, New York, 1966, McGraw-Hill Book Co.)

hyoid bone. This narrow hollow tract, which connects the thyroid lobes to the floor of the pharynx, normally atrophies in the adult. Failure to atrophy creates the potential for cystic masses to form anywhere along it.

Branchial cleft cyst. Branchial cleft cysts are cystic formations that are usually located laterally. During embryonic development the branchial cleft is a slender tract extending from the pharyngeal cavity to an opening near the auricle or into the neck. A diverticulum may extend either laterally from the pharynx or medially from the neck.

Although primarily cystic in appearance, these lesions may present with solid components, usually of low-level echogenicity, particularly if they have become infected.

Cystic hygroma. Cystic hygromas of the neck result from congenital modification of the lymphatics. They present from the posterior occiput and are most frequently seen as large cystic masses on the lateral aspect of the neck. They can be multiseptated and multilocular.

Abscesses

Abscesses can arise in any location in the neck. Their sonographic appearance ranges from primarily fluid filled to completely echogenic. Most commonly they are masses of low-level echogenicity with rather irregular walls. Chronic abscesses may be particularly difficult to demonstrate since their indistinct margins blend with surrounding tissue.

The role of ultrasound in evaluation of abscesses is localization for percutaneous needle aspiration and follow-up examination during and after treatment.

Adenopathy

Low-level echogenicity of well-circumscribed masses is the classical sonographic appearance of enlarged lymph nodes. However, in some cases they appear echo free. Inflammatory processes may also exhibit a cystic nature.

Differentiation of inflammatory from neoplastic processes is not always possible by sonographic criteria alone. In some instances, because of the limited field of view of small-parts scanners and the magnitude of the pa-

thology, alternative examinations are necessary. A contact static image B-scanner may be required to display the anatomy and pathology of the questionable area adequately (Fig. 17-12).

SCROTUM AND TESTES
Anatomy

Scrotum. The scrotum is a pendant sac that is divided by a septum into two compartments. Each compartment contains a testis, an epididymis, and a portion of spermatic cord and ductus deferens. The left side commonly extends farther caudad than the right.

The innermost investment of the scrotum is formed by the tunica vaginalis. It is a double sac with a parietal or outer layer and a visceral or inner layer (Fig. 17-13). The space between the parietal and visceral layers normally contains a small amount of fluid.

Testes. The two testes, the male organs of reproduction, are ovoid and slightly flattened from side to side. The upper pole is normally a little more anterior than the lower. The average dimensions are 4 to 5 cm long and 2.5 to 3 cm wide. Posteriorly, at the superior and inferior borders of the testes, the head and tail of the epididymis are attached. The spermatic cord is also attached posteriorly. Support of the testes is provided mainly by the spermatic cord and the scrotum.

The visceral layer of the tunica vaginalis covers the testicular surface, except at the epididymis and spermatic cord attachments. Just under the tunica vaginalis is the tunica albuginea, a fibrous capsule encasing the testis (Fig. 17-14). From the fibrous capsule, septa pass into the interior of the testis and form compartments or lobules. These lobules contain the seminiferous tubules, whose lining creates spermatozoa. The union of the septula,

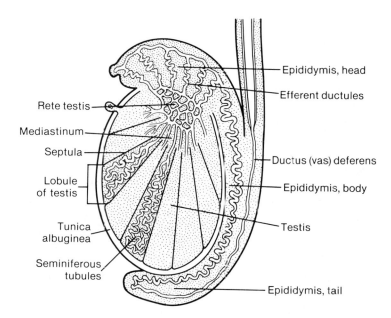

Epididymis, head

Efferent ductules

Rete testis

Mediastinum

Septula

Lobule
of testis

Ductus (vas) deferens

Epididymis, body

Testis

Tunica
albuginea

Seminiferous
tubules

Epididymis, tail

FIG. 17-14. Longitudinal section of the testis and epididymis. (The size of the seminiferous tubules is exaggerated). (Redrawn from Anson, BJ: Morris' human anatomy, ed 12, New York, 1966, McGraw-Hill Book Co.)

ducts, nerves, and vessels is the mediastinum testis. In the mediastinum the tubules join to form the rete testis, from which the efferent ductules open into the epididymis.

Testicular development occurs in the retroperitoneum near the kidneys. Since the testes are attached to the peritoneum, their descent through the future inguinal canal into the scrotum drags the peritoneum with them. The peritoneum then lines each half of the scrotum, covers most of the testes, and is the tunica vaginalis. The passage between the scrotal peritoneum (tunica vaginalis) and the abdominal peritoneum, which was formed during descent of the testicle, is usually obliterated by fusion of the walls. If the connection persists, a congenital hernia results.

Epididymis. The epididymis, which lies along the posterolateral border of the testis, is the first portion of the duct of the testis and is its excretory system. The head (globus major) is at the superior pole of the testis and the tail (globus minor) is attached inferiorly (Fig. 17-14). Laterally and posteriorly the epididymis is covered by the visceral layer of the tunica vaginalis.

The spermatic cord, which ascends from the testis cephalad through the inguinal canal, is formed by the ductus (vas) deferens and testicular vessels and nerves.

Physiology

The testes, which produce spermatozoa, are considered exocrine glands. However, since they also produce male sex hormones, they also can be considered endocrine glands. Testosterone is the hormone responsible for spermatogenesis and the development of male sexual organs and characteristics.

Pathology
Scrotum

EDEMA. Edema of the scrotum is due to vascular or lymphatic disturbance or stasis. It can be a result of inflamma-

tion, allergic states, chronic cardiac insufficiency, enlarged inguinal lymph nodes, or parasitic obstruction of the lymphatics (elephantiasis). Prolonged stasis of the lymphatics causes the scrotal walls to become thickened by connective tissue. Epididymoorchitis frequently has associated scrotal edema.

HYDROCELE. A hydrocele is scrotal sac enlargement caused by serous fluid accumulation between the layers of visceral and parietal tunica vaginalis. As much as 300 ml of fluid can be present, but most hydroceles contain 50 to 100 ml. The usual anterior location of a hydrocele causes posterior displacement of the testis within the scrotum.

Acute hydroceles are a result of trauma, infection of the testis or epididymis, or tumor. Chronic hydroceles are frequently idiopathic but can mask an underlying testicular malignancy. Most hydroceles are asymptomatic and are a manifestation of other disease processes.

HERNIA. An inguinal hernia occurs when a loop of bowel protrudes into a patent vaginalis-peritoneal communication. When the bowel contains air or fluid, hernia can be confusing since it can have sonographic features similar to those of other scrotal masses.

Testes

ORCHITIS AND EPIDIDYMITIS. Infections limited to the testes are rare. They occur more frequently in the epididymis, with secondary involvement of the testis. Epididymitis is the most common of the intrascrotal inflammations. Organisms from infected urine, the prostate, or the seminal vesicles travel to the epididymis via the vas deferens. Infection can also be lymphatic or blood borne. An acute hydrocele often coexists with intrascrotal infections.

Orchitis and epididymitis can be classified as specific (gonorrhea, syphilis, mumps, tuberculosis), nonspecific, and traumatic. Gonorrhea and tuberculosis affect the epididymis first; syphilis and mumps involve the testis. If the disease is not adequately treated, abscesses can develop.

Nonspecific epididymitis with subsequent orchitis is usually the result of a urinary tract infection.

Traumatic epididymitis can result from strenuous exercise in which infected prostatic secretions or urine are forced into the epididymis.

Testicular abscess is usually a complication of preexisting acute epididymitis. Pain, fever, redness, and edema are the presenting features. It is frequently difficult to assess the epididymal versus testicular nature of this infection because of difficulty on palpation.

NEOPLASMS. Testicular malignancy is primarily a disease of young men (20 to 40 years of age). It is the second leading cause of cancer death in this age group. There is a higher incidence of malignancy in undescended testes; however, surgical correction before the age of 6 virtually eliminates the risk. Approximately 95% of testicular neoplasms arise from germ (sex) cells of the testes.

Seminoma is the most common type of testicular tumor. For unknown reasons it is more frequent in the right testis than in the left. It is a lobulated homogeneous tumor devoid of hemorrhage or necrosis and is well circumscribed but not encapsulated. Frequently the entire testis is replaced by tumor. Elevated serum titers of follicle-stimulating hormone (FSH) are sometimes present in patients with this tumor.

Being the least malignant of germ cell tumors in its pure form and being highly sensitive to radiation, seminoma has a reasonably good prognosis. With orchiectomy followed by radiation of abdominal and thoracic nodes, the 2-year survival is 92%.

Embryonal carcinoma represents 19% to 25% of malignant testicular tumors. Because of its multiple histology, it is one of the most confusing. Areas of hemorrhage and necrosis are seen within these firm tumors, which typically have poorly demarcated borders. The tumor can partially or completely replace the testis. Elevated serum levels of α-fetoprotein (AFP) and/or human chorionic gonadotropin (hCG) can be found in patients with any nonseminomatous tumor.

The 5-year survival with this aggressive and lethal tumor is only 30% to 35%. It is generally not responsive to radiation and is treated with chemotherapy.

Choriocarcinoma is a highly malignant form of testicular tumor. It is rarely a pure tumor, usually mixed with other cell types. Typically it is small and does not cause testicular enlargement. Elevated serum or urine levels of hCG are usually detected in patients with choriocarcinoma.

Pure testicular choriocarcinoma is fatal. As a result of widespread metastases, almost all patients die within a year of diagnosis.

Teratoma, a tumor consisting of a heterogeneous mixture of tissues, accounts for approximately 7% to 10% of testicular tumors. Three basic types of testicular teratomas (dermoid, differentiated, and undifferentiated) have been classified and are of varying degrees of malignancy.

Because of the possibility of small foci of cancer, many authorities believe that all solid teratomas in adults should be managed as malignant. Abnormal serum levels of hCG and AFP are present in some patients with malignant teratoma.

Orchiectomy with surgical removal of any metastases (usually lymph nodes) is the treatment. The grade of malignancy of teratoma is between those of seminoma and embryonal carcinoma.

Testicular tumors are frequently composed of more than one of the previously discussed cell types (i.e., *mixed tumors*). Approximately 40% are of this nature, with the teratoma-embryonal carcinoma mixture the most common. Teratocarcinomas are those teratomas that have other neoplastic elements.

Ultrasound evaluation

Since it is often difficult to assess the intratesticular versus extratesticular nature of a scrotal mass by physical examination alone, ultrasound evaluation has become an important clinical tool to assist in differentiation.

Scanning technique. For sonographic evaluation the patient is placed in the supine "semifrogleg" position. The scrotum is supported with one hand of the operator while the transducer head is manipulated with the other. Again, because of the limited field of view, each hemiscrotum must be evaluated separately. Examination is made by gentle placement of the water path on the hemiscrotum. The testis and epididymis can be manipulated against the membrane from lateral to medial as scanning is performed.

Longitudinal views are easier to interpret; therefore it is suggested that they be performed first. A survey through the entire hemiscrotum should be made prior to image recording. The recording sequence begins at the lower pole of the testis with lateral to medial scanning. Static images should document the relationship of the testis to the epididymis, the presence or absence of fluid, and the texture of the testis and epididymis. The midportion and upper pole of the testis are evaluated in a similar fashion. Evaluation of the upper pole should include the epididymis and its texture. The area cephalad to the head of the epididymis is also evaluated and documented. If a pathologic process is identified, characteristics of the abnormality and anatomic relationships should be clearly documented.

Transverse scans are performed in a similar manner. Beginning at the lower pole, the testis is manipulated so the lateral to medial examination can be accomplished. The midportion and upper pole and the epididymis are similarly examined, with the same emphasis on pathosis as described for longitudinal scanning. The opposite hemiscrotum is always scanned for comparison.

Ultrasound appearances

TESTES. The *normal* testis exhibits a granular homogeneous medium-level echogenicity (Fig. 17-15). A small amount of fluid is present between the layers of the tunica vaginalis and can be identified in most cases.

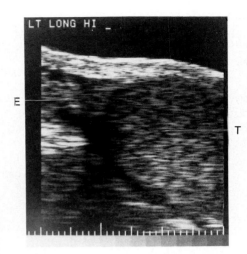

FIG. 17-15. Longitudinal scan showing the homogeneous texture with medium-level echogenicity of the normal testis, *T*, and the slightly more echogenic epididymis, *E*. A normal amount of fluid is present around the epididymis and testis.

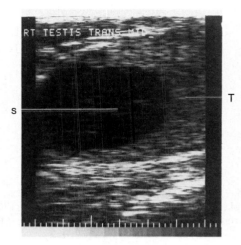

FIG. 17-16. Transverse scan of a testicular seminoma, *s*, showing less echogenicity than in the normal testicle, *T*.

Inflammation of the testis can be diffuse orchitis or a focal abscess. In orchitis the testicle becomes enlarged and exhibits a lower echogenic pattern than the normal testicle. An abscess appears as a localized area of inhomogeneity within the testis and often has cystic areas.

Testicular *tumors* tend to be of lower echogenicity than normal testicular tissue (Fig. 17-16). They can exhibit rather well-circumscribed borders or may appear to invade the testicular tissue. Although this is the typical pattern for tumor, it is not specific since chronic abscess, hematoma, and granuloma may appear similar. There are no characteristic sonographic patterns for malignant versus benign disease. Reactive hydroceles often coexist with both malignant and benign conditions of the testis.

EPIDIDYMIS. The epididymis is usually distinguishable because it has a coarser ultrasonic texture than the normal testis (Fig. 17-15). The epididymal head can nearly always be identified and appears to cap the testicular upper pole. The body of the epididymis is more difficult to identify and the tail is not frequently seen.

The most common intrascrotal inflammation is epididymitis. It appears sonographically as uniform enlargement of the epididymis and is most evident in the globus major. Compared to normal, the texture is less echodense. In chronic epididymitis the epididymis is very echodense and can contain calcium and shadowing. Focal abscesses may appear as sonolucent areas within the epididymis.

EXTRATESTICULAR COLLECTIONS. These can be idiopathic or associated with a known disorder.

HYDROCELES. As previously mentioned, can be associated with infectious processes or tumors. They appear as a fluid collection surrounding the testis (Fig. 17-17). Depending on their volume, they may surround the testis or be visualized at only the upper or the lower pole

A *spermatocele* is cystic dilation of the spermatic cord. Since it does not invaginate the tunica vaginalis, it appears

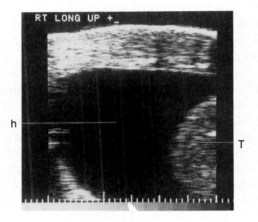

FIG. 17-17. A large hydrocele, h, surrounds the upper pole of the testis, *T*, on this longitudinal scan.

cephalad to the testis as a loculated fluid collection often containing low-level echoes.

Hematoceles are uncommon and can be primarily cystic or contain echoes from organization of clotted blood. They also are located cephalad to the testes.

Hydrocele of the cord is the encasement of fluid in a sac of peritoneum within the spermatic cord. It also presents as a cystic mass cephalad to the testis. In contrast to hematoceles and spermatoceles, hydroceles of the cord are almost always entirely echo free.

A *varicocele* is cystic varicose enlargement of the veins of the spermatic cord. The cystic enlargement, cephalad to the testis, is usually of a tortuous nature resembling a bag of worms.

VASCULAR ACCESS FOR HEMODIALYSIS

Approximately 40,000 patients in the United States are undergoing chronic hemodialysis for end-stage renal disease. These are patients whose severely damaged kidneys are not capable of removing toxic products from the blood. Dialysis removes these substances and maintains

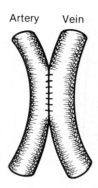

Artery   Vein

FIG. 17-18. Typical side-to-side arrangement for an arteriovenous fistula. (Redrawn from Massry S and Sellers A: Clinical aspects of uremia and dialysis, Springfield, Ill, 1976, Charles C Thomas, Publisher.)

electrolyte hemostasis by passing the patient's blood through a dialyzing solution.

Anatomy and physiology

Circulatory access for hemodialysis is dependent on creation of an easily accessible high-flow vascular system. This is accomplished by some form of surgical connection between an artery and vein. After anastomosis the veins frequently enlarge due to increased flow of arterialized blood through them. Needles can then be inserted into the arterialized veins to provide adequate flow for dialysis.

Creation of a successful arteriovenous (AV) anastomosis requires a situation in which adequate arteries and veins can be joined without stress and without jeopardy to circulation of the extremity involved. The forearm and thigh are usual locations, with common hookups being radial artery to cephalic vein, brachial artery to antecubital vein, and femoral artery to saphenous vein. The anastomosis can be of the side-to-side, end-to-end, or end-to-side design. This description refers to the respective arterial-venous or graft-venous relationship.

Vascular access systems are of two types. One is a direct AV fistula using the patient's own vessels; the other involves the use of tubes, either heterologous (usually bovine) or synthetic materials.

Arteriovenous fistula. The AV fistula proved to be a major advance over the previously used external Silastic (Scribner) shunts in terms of complications and failures. It is usually the arrangement of choice for initial vascular access.

A side-to-side anastomosis between an artery and the largest available adjacent vein is made (Fig. 17-18). Increased blood flow created by fistula formation causes the subcutaneous veins to become progressively dilated, thereby providing sufficient blood flow for hemodialysis.

Bovine heterograft. Bovine heterografts made from processed carotid arteries of cows are usually reserved for patients whose vessels will not permit establishment of an AV fistula or whose fistula has failed.

The anastomosis is frequently the end-to-side type (Fig. 17-19). A loop fistula between the radial or ulnar artery and the antecubital or a deep vein in the forearm is also common. The thigh is usually reserved as a last resort be-

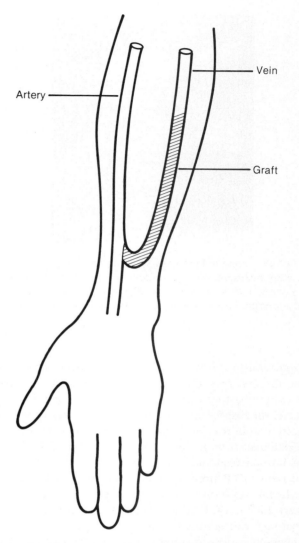

Artery —

Vein

Graft

FIG. 17-19. Schema of a bovine heterograft. (Courtesy Christine Skram, RDMS, University of California Medical Center, San Diego.)

cause of an increased incidence of graft complications in this location.

Synthetic graft. Polytetrafluoroethylene (Gore-Tex) has become a popular material for use in vascular access. Grafts of synthetic material are easier to handle and easier to reoperate on, and they have a better rate of patency than do bovine heterografts.

Straight or U-shaped anastomoses are used with preference for the proximal radial artery and a medial vein at or above the elbow joint (Fig. 17-20).

Pathology

A number of complications can lead to failure of the access. AV fistulas and bovine heterografts have higher complication rates in patients with proved arterial disease. The most likely cause is low blood flow.

Thrombosis. The most common complication to cause access failure is thrombosis. It develops due to low blood flow, which is a result of inadequate arterial inflow or high venous resistance (outflow obstruction). Com-

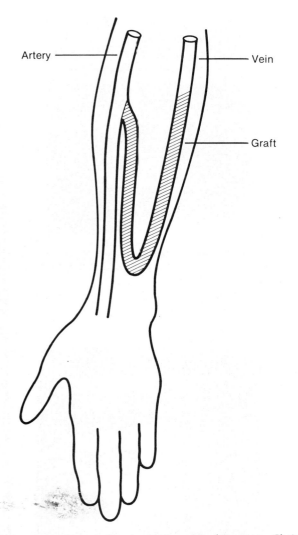

Artery

Vein

Graft

FIG. 17-20. Schema of a synthetic graft. (Courtesy Christine Skram, RDMS, University of California Medical Center, San Diego.)

mon sites of thrombosis are anastomotic and puncture sites. Occlusion can develop as a result of thrombus accumulation. Thrombectomy or reconstruction can be performed in an attempt to salvage the access.

Infection. Early detection of infection is crucial in vascular accesses since graft replacement is often required in inadequately treated cases. Infection can result from repeated venipunctures or after operation. Bovine heterografts are especially susceptible to infection, but it is not a significant problem with radiocephalic AV fistulas. Treatment with systemic and/or topical antibiotics is effective. Localized abscesses can be drained; but if they are grossly infected, the graft must be removed.

Aneurysm. An aneurysm is the result of weakness of the venous wall due to high venous pressure or repeated dialysis trauma. Thrombus can develop within the aneurysm. More ominously, graft degeneration with hemorrhage or infection may occur.

Pseudoaneurysm. A false aneurysm, which probably results from extravasation, may develop as a result of trauma or infection. It is usually found at the site of anastomosis (usually arterial) or at a needle puncture tear.

Ultrasound evaluation

Scanning technique. For evaluation of arm fistulas the patient is placed recumbent, primarily for purposes of stability and support of the arm. The arm of interest is closest to the operator and is extended (hand up) and supported on the bed beside the patient. If the arm cannot be positioned as described, a firm flat device for support from shoulder to hand may be used. The patient's arm is abducted approximately 45 degrees with the support device positioned under it and the shoulder. If necessary, the examination may be performed with the patient in a wheel-chair. Support of the extended arm can be obtained with the device stabilized on the arm of the wheelchair.

For evaluation of leg fistulas the patient is supine on a bed with the leg of interest closest to the operator. A slight frogleg position facilitates transducer access.

A preliminary review of the patient's surgical anatomy (and pathosis if present) should be undertaken prior to image recording.

Since the vein is usually of larger caliber and easier to identify, it is located first and the survey is begun longitudinally near the elbow. With an AV fistula the vein is traced toward the wrist to the anastomosis. After examination of the anastomosis the artery is then traced back to the elbow. A graft is evaluated similarly: scanning is performed toward the wrist through the vein, venous anastomosis, and graft. The arterial anastomosis and artery are then identified, and the sonographer continues to scan back toward the elbow.

After preliminary exploration, scanning is repeated with image documentation of the vein, venous anastomosis, graft, arterial anastomosis, artery, and any pathologic condition that may be present. Transverse scanning is performed using this routine. The flexibility of real time allows the vasculature to be delineated with relative ease.

Ultrasound appearances

ARTERIOVENOUS FISTULA. Since existing vasculature is used in creation of an AV fistula, the artery and vein are seen as anechoic tubular channels. With survey through the vessels the anastomosis, usually side-to-side, can be identified where the vein becomes contiguous with the artery (Fig. 17-21). The vascular thrill detected on palpation is helpful in localizing the anastomosis.

BOVINE HETEROGRAFT. The appearance of a normal bovine heterograft is of an anechoic tubular channel whose walls are smooth and regular. It has essentially the same echographic appearance as a patient's normal blood vessels. The anastomoses can be difficult to identify because of the echographic similarity of the heterograft and the native vessel; however, a slight wall irregularity is often evident at the suture site. The end-to-side arterial anastomosis can be identified by tracing the heterograft to its insertion into the side of the artery.

SYNTHETIC GRAFT. The synthetic graft appears as a very discrete anechoic channel (Fig. 17-22). Because of its acoustic properties, synthetic graft material demonstrates a greater beam attenuation than do native vessels. The anastomosis can be clearly identified by the sharp differ-

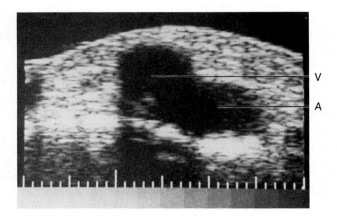

FIG. 17-21. Transverse section through arterial, *A*, to venous, *V*, anastomosis of a normal arteriovenous fistula.

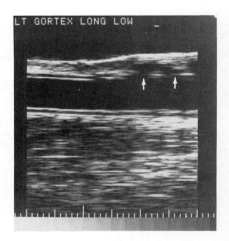

FIG. 17-22. Longitudinal sonogram of a synthetic graft. Note the smooth walls of the graft interrupted at the needle puncture sites *(arrows)*.

ence in echo attenuation between the graft and the host vessel (Fig. 17-23).

COMPLICATIONS. A number of complications have been reported.

Thrombosis of a vascular access appears as an irregular echo reflection within the otherwise anechoic lumen of the vessel and may create an acoustic shadow. The amount and extent of resultant stenosis can be demonstrated. Special note should be made of wall irregularities from needle puncture, since they may be sites of thrombus deposition.

On rare occasions, soft or early thrombus may not create sufficient acoustic impedance to be sonographically evident. Doppler sonography may be useful in these instances.

Infection can appear as a sonolucent or complex mass around the graft or as vegetations within the graft appearing as echoes projecting from the wall of the lumen. Vegetations may flap with pulsations that can be documented by real time. Special attention should be paid to repeated venipuncture sites since they are potential abscess formation sites.

A palpable mass of vascular grafts is frequently an *aneurysm*. A localized increase in the normal caliber of the vein is characteristic. Thrombus may occur within the aneurysm, which is an area of relative stasis.

A *pseudoaneurysm* occurs most commonly at the anastomotic site or at a needle puncture site. A thrombus may totally fill the pseudoaneurysm (Fig. 17-24).

NEONATAL APPLICATIONS

The newborn infant is especially suited for small-parts scanning since many organ systems in these children are within the depth limits (4 to 5 cm) of the transducer. The real-time capability is useful for rapidly surveying areas of interest and diminishing the problem of patient motion.

Technique of neonatal sonography

Examination of the neonate requires a few special considerations. Prior to examination the transducer assembly, especially the water path, must be cleaned with a disinfec-

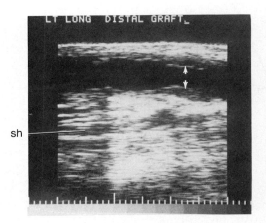

FIG. 17-23. Scan of synthetic graft anastomosis. The junction between the graft and the host vein can be identified by the shadowing, *sh*, deep to the graft. Minimal stenosis *(between arrowheads)* is also present within the vein.

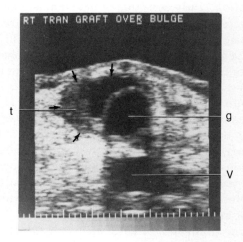

FIG. 17-24. Transverse scan of a synthetic graft, *g*, demonstrating a pseudoaneurysm *(arrows)* partially filled with thrombus, *t*. Native vessel, *V*.

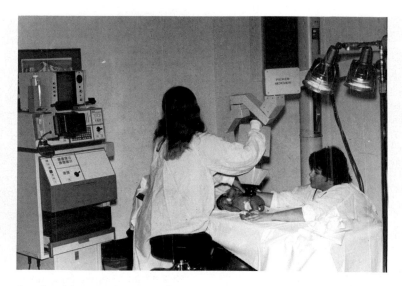

FIG. 17-25. Overhead heating lamps, a clean environment, and a member of the neonatal ward team are necessary for examination of the neonate. (From Canty T et al: Ultrasonography of pediatric surgical disorders, New York, 1981, Grune & Stratton, Inc.)

tant. The operator's hands should be washed and a clean gown should be worn.

Control of the ambient temperature is crucial since premature infants are very sensitive to temperature changes. Overhead heating lamps or an insulated heating pad under the infant can be used (Fig. 17-25). The acoustic coupling agent and the water path membrane must also be warmed.

Coordination of the examination between the ultrasound department and the neonatal ward team is especially important. Because of the critical status of many premature infants, unneccessary detainment in the ultrasound department should be avoided. Scheduling must be arranged for equipment availability upon the infant's arrival in the department.

The infant should be recently fed (unless otherwise indicated). A happy child is more likely to be still.

A member of the neonatal ward team should accompany the infant. The sonographer cannot be expected to provide the specialized monitoring sometimes necessary for these infants.

Clinical applications
Abdomen

URINARY TRACT. A palpable abdominal mass in neonates is usually of renal origin. Ureteropelvic junction obstruction, multicystic dysplastic kidney, and renal vein thrombosis are the most frequent abnormalities.

The ultrasound examination can be performed with the infant in the supine, decubitus, or prone position. If the supine or decubitus position is used, examination is performed in the midaxillary line; if prone, examination is from the posterior. Longitudinal scanning of the kidney from medial to lateral is performed followed by transverse scanning cephalad to caudad. Recorded images should be representative of the corticomedullary areas and the renal pelvis.

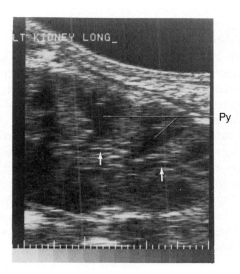

FIG. 17-26. The medullary portions, pyramids, *Py,* of the neonatal kidney, are clearly seen on this prone longitudinal scan. A normal amount of urine within the renal collecting system *(arrows)* is also identified.

In the *normal* neonatal kidney the medullary portions (pyramids) are clearly visible as areas of lower echogenicity than the surrounding cortex (Fig. 17-26). An irregular renal outline, called fetal lobulation, can often be identified. The normal renal pelvis contains a small amount of urine. Since renal sinus fat is minimal or absent in the neonate, the renal sinus does not appear as dense as in the adult.

In *congenital ureteropelvic junction* (UPJ) *obstruction* the renal pelvis becomes dilated and variable degrees of calyectasis occur (Fig. 17-27). Some normal parenchyma can usually be seen. With other causes of hydronephrosis, expecially reflux, the renal pelvis becomes dilated to a lesser degree and more uniformly than with UPJ obstruction.

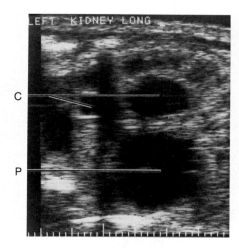

FIG. 17-27. Prone longitudinal scan of a ureteropelvic junction obstruction in a neonate. The renal pelvis, *P,* and calyces, *C,* are grossly dilated.

In *multicystic dysplastic kidney* the contour is quite irregular and the parenchyma disorganized. Multiple cysts of varying size can usually be identified in these nonfunctioning kidneys.

Infants of diabetic mothers and very sick dehydrated babies are at risk for *renal vein thrombosis.* Enlargement of the affected kidney, absence of urine in the renal pelvis, and swollen pyramids are characteristic of this disorder.

HEPATOBILIARY SYSTEM. Excellent resolution of the premature infant's liver is possible with small-parts scanners (Fig. 17-28). Depth limitations, however, may preclude complete evaluation of the liver in full-term infants.

In an infant who has not recently been fed, the gallbladder can usually be identified. Sludge, whose significance is unknown at this age, has been seen on occasion; and cholelithiasis, although unusual in newborns, may be demonstrated.

A choledochal cyst, dilation of a segment of the extrahepatic biliary system, may be suspected in an infant who presents with a palpable abdominal mass and jaundice. The sonographic feature is a right upper quadrant cystic mass in the porta hepatis that is separable from the gallbladder. The intrahepatic bile ducts may be dilated or of normal caliber.

IDIOPATHIC HYPERTROPHIC PYLORIC STENOSIS. Infants who present with vomiting and are suspected of having pyloric stenosis are candidates for sonography. The ultrasonic appearance of pyloric stenosis is a thick (at least 4 mm) circular hypoechoic ring that represents the muscular thickening (Fig. 17-29).

Miscellaneous

SPINAL CORD. Infants who present with cutaneous defects overlying the sacrum such as a sacral dimple, hairy patch, or hemangioma are at risk for tethering of the cord. A tethered cord is anomalous insertion lower than normal and relatively fixed. Early diagnosis is crucial since it can cause irreversible nerve deficits if not surgically corrected.

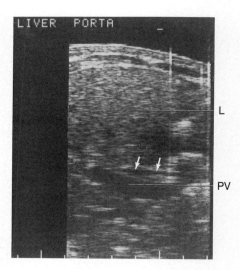

FIG. 17-28. Supine longitudinal scan demonstrating the liver, *L,* and the common bile duct *(arrows)* in this neonate. *PV,* portal vein.

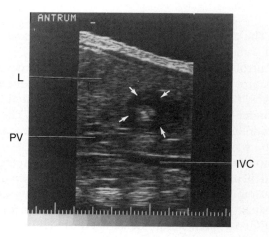

FIG. 17-29. This supine longitudinal scan of the epigastrium shows the thick muscular ring *(arrows)* of pyloric stenosis. *L,* liver; *PV,* portal vein; *IVC,* inferior vena cava.

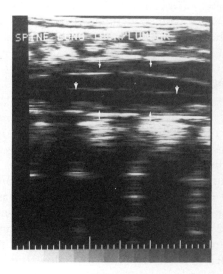

FIG. 17-30. Lumbar spinal cord within the subarachnoid space *(arrows)* on a prone longitudinal scan. The linear echo within the spinal cord is the central canal *(arrowheads).*

Longitudinal imaging is begun in the posterior midline at the midthoracic level. The spinal cord, central canal of the cord, and fluid in the subarachnoid space can be seen (Fig. 17-30). As scanning progresses caudally, the cauda equina and filum terminale can be viewed.

Normally the cord moves freely within the spinal canal. The most striking sonographic features of a tethered cord are the lack of cord motion and thickening of the filum. The cord exhibits a rigid appearance within the spinal canal.

For documentation of dynamic events, the videotape format is necessary. Static photography, however, can be used for anatomic representation.

SUMMARY

1. The recent development of high-resolution ultrasound instruments provides a means of effectively evaluating superficial organs and structures.

2. Although it has resolution limitations and differentiation of cystic from solid lesions is not possible, the radioisotope scan is commonly used in the management of thyroid nodules.

3. Patients with unexplained hypercalcemia detected on routine blood chemistry screening are the most common referrals for parathyroid echography.

4. The role of ultrasound in evaluation of palpable neck masses is to determine site of origin and assess lesion texture.

5. Since it is often difficult to assess the intratesticular versus extratesticular nature of a scrotal mass by physical examination alone, ultrasound evaluation has become an important clinical tool to assist in differentiation.

6. The newborn infant is especially suited for small-parts scanning since many organ systems in these children are within the depth limits (4 to 5 cm) of the high-frequency transducer.

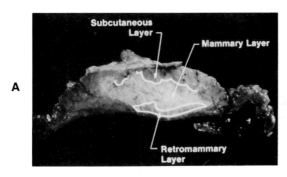
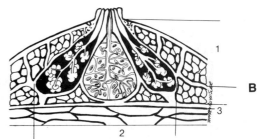

FIG. 18-3.   Three layers of breast tissue. **A,** Anatomic section. **B,** Diagram. *1,* Subcutaneous fatty layer; *2,* mammary layer; *3,* retromammary layer. (Modified from Townsend CM: Clin Symp 32[2]:1, 1980.)

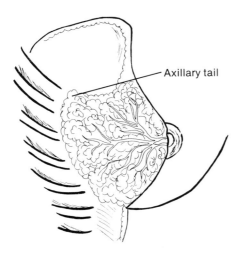

FIG. 18-4.   A projection of tissue, called the axillary tail or tail of Spence, usually extends from the upper outer quadrant into the axilla.

retromammary layer consists of fat lobules that are separated anteriorly from the mammary layer by the deep connective tissue plane and posteriorly by the fascia over the pectoralis major.

During pregnancy the ducts and parenchymal elements of the breast expand to such a degree that the mammary layer takes up the entire breast. The subcutaneous fat layer and the retromammary layer are so squeezed that they appear very narrow on the sonogram. The interfaces in the pregnant breast will be less echogenic.

The major portion of the breast contained within the superficial fascia of the anterior thoracic wall is situated between the second or third rib superiorly, the sixth or seventh costal cartilage inferiorly, the anterior axillary line laterally, and the sternal border medially.[9] The greatest amount of glandular tissue is located in the upper outer quadrant of the breast, which explains why tumors are more frequently found here.

The major pectoral muscle lies posterior to the retromammary layer. The minor pectoral muscle lies superolaterally posterior to it. The pectoralis minor courses from its rib cage origin to the point where it inserts into the coracoid process. The lower border of the pectoralis ma-

jor forms the anterior border of the axilla. Breast tissue can extend into this region and is referred to as the axillary tail or tail of Spence (Fig. 18-4).

Vascular supply and lymph drainage

The principal blood supply to the breast is from branches of the internal mammary and the lateral thoracic arteries. The intercostal artery plays a subordinant role. Venous drainage is through superficial and deep veins. The superficial veins are usually arranged in a transverse or longitudinal pattern and can be seen on the sonogram. The deep veins are not visible. In the axilla the axillary vein is sonographically visible, with the axillary artery located superior and a bit posterior to it.

The lymphatics of the breast originate in the lymph capillaries of the mammary connective tissue grid. The lymph capillaries are similar to blood capillaries and are abundant in the breast tissue. They have valves to assure flow in the direction of the venous system (away from the tissues). The lymph vessels empty into lymph nodes; thus when cancer cells invade the lymphatic system, they reach the lymph nodes, which act as a filter and retain the malignant cells. These then grow at the expense of the node and gradually destroy it.

The axillary lymph nodes are closely related to the axillary vein. The majority of the lymph drainage passes to this group of nodes. Other drainage pathways are along the inferior margin of the pectoralis major. Flow may also be directed to groups of lymph nodes around the third, fourth, and fifth prongs of the serratus anterior as well as toward the intercostal and mediastinal node group. Lymph drainage is also routed to the subdiaphragmatic lymph nodes. Medial lymph drainage eventually reaches the peristernal and anterior mediastinal lymph nodes. In addition, there are abundant lymphatic connections to the opposite breast.

Variations in parenchymal patterns

The first pattern, and the one most difficult to image by sonography, is the fatty breast. Fatty replacement of the parenchymal elements of the breast occurs with each pregnancy. With the onset of menopause there is atrophy of the ducts. As a result, all three layers appear fatty. Gen-

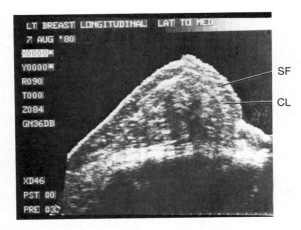

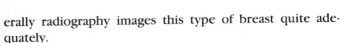

FIG. 18-5. Central shadow in a fatty replaced breast. *SF,* subcutaneous fat; *CL,* Cooper's ligaments.

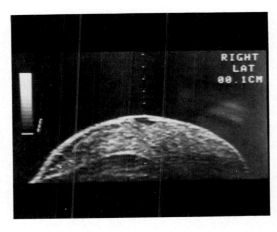

FIG. 18-6. Sagittal scan of a young dense breast in compression.

erally radiography images this type of breast quite adequately.

The second pattern is still largely fat. Histologically there is some periductal connective tissue, which sonographically presents as bright reflectors. The breast basically appears fatty.

The next pattern is complex. It consists of progressing degrees of fibrosis. Sonographically degrees of coalescence of the dense connective tissue and a scalloped effect of the superficial connective tissue plane can often be seen. There is still some residual fat present in this pattern.

The last pattern shows no residual fat in the mammary layer. The fat is replaced by dense connective tissue. If this breast is examined with a water path scanner with the patient prone and the breast in a free-hanging position, an area of no information occurs in the central portion (Fig. 18-5). The extent of the shadow will depend on the beam width, depth of placement of the focus, frequency of the transducer, and tissue structure of the nipple. If multiple transducers are used, a compound scan may help to elminate this shadow. However, a more effective technique is compression. The use of compression allows the breast tissue to be flattened, thus compressing the dense tissue and allowing the acoustic beam to be perpendicular to more interfaces (Fig. 18-6).

PHYSIOLOGY

The breast is an endocrine gland and is affected in its physical and microscopic state by the changing hormonal levels. The growth of the breast begins before the onset of menstruation. At puberty the combined influences of the hypothalamus and anterior pituitary, and later the ovaries, cause growth of the breast. Although these are the primary endocrine sources responsible for breast growth, complete development also requires normal levels of insulin and thyroid hormone secretions.[4]

During the first year or two of menstruation, ovulation does not occur and there is an increased output of estrogen. This causes the mammary ducts to elongate. Their epithelial lining reduplicates and proliferates as the ends of the mammary tubules form sprouts of future lobules. Estrogen stimulates the vascularity of the breast tissue, increases the volume and elasticity of the connective tissues, and induces fat deposition in the breast.

With the onset of maturity (i.e., when ovulation occurs and the progesterone-secreting corpora lutea are formed) the second stage of mammary development occurs.[8] This is the formation of the lobules and acinar structures and gives the mammary gland the characteristic lobular structure found during childbearing years. Further acinar development continues in proportion to the intensity of the hormonal stimuli during each menstrual cycle.

During pregnancy, changes occur that make milk production possible. In addition to estrogen and progesterone, hormones such as placental lactogen, prolactin, and chorionic gonadotropin are required for complete gestational development of the breast.[11] At delivery there is a loss of estrogen and progesterone. Prolactin then predominates and the alveolar cells actively synthesize and secrete milk. During the three months following cessation of lactation, involution of the breast occurs. The breast remains larger due to the fatty tissue replacement. Post-lactation involution is a decrease in the size of the lobular-alveolar components as compared to their enlargement during pregnancy.

EVALUATION OF THE PATIENT WITH A BREAST MASS
Medical history

A complete medical history is very important in assessing the patient with a breast mass. Several pertinent questions may aid the clinician in the final diagnosis:

- Age (the greater the age the higher the risk, especially over 35)
- Previous cancer of the breast (up to 16% will develop cancer in the other breast)
- Family history (40% chance of developing cancer if mother had cancer)
- Late first pregnancy (28 or over)

- Nulliparous women
- Late menopause (54 or older)
- Previous biopsy for benign disease
- Exposure to radiation at an early age
- Mammographic appearance of a prominent duct pattern or marked dysplasia
- Obesity
- Suppression of emotions (especially anger)

The age of the patient is important since malignancy is rarely found in women under 25 and the incidence steadily increases with age. If the patient or the clinician detects a breast mass, symptoms such as pain, tenderness, or nipple discharge should be noted. The patient is questioned whether these symptoms occur cyclicly, during pregnancy, or in relation to trauma or previous breast disease. Patients with a previous biopsy-proved breast lesion or who have had breast cancer are at an increased risk for cancer. The incidence of cancer is greater in a patient whose mother or sister has had breast cancer. Early menarche and late menopause have also been associated with an increased risk of breast cancer.[8]

Diagnostic techniques

A complete physical examination of the patient's breasts should be performed after the medical history has been taken. It is essential that the size, location, consistency, and mobility of the mass be noted, as well as the site of biopsy scars, asymmetry between the breasts, skin changes or discoloration, and the presence of skin dimpling.

One of the most reliable methods for detecting breast masses is palpation, which may be done by either the physician or the patient. Premenopausal women should examine their breasts at the same time of the month, preferably 5 to 7 days after cessation of menses, so subtle changes can be detected.

Most breast lumps are benign, with only 20% to 25% of those surgically removed revealing malignancy. More than 90% of the lumps are found by breast self-examination.

Mammography

The most accurate noninvasive method for the detection of breast lesions is mammography. With dedicated mammographic equipment, either film-screen radiography or xeroradiography, the diagnosis of cancer can be made if the examination is optimally performed and interpreted.

The mammographic diagnosis of breast cancer depends on the demonstration of a mass having poorly defined stellate or knobby margins or a cluster of tiny rod-shaped calcifications. The benign lesions are known to have sharply defined margins and smooth contours. If calcifications are present in the benign lesion, they are round or oval shape. To better visualize these small areas of calcification, fine detail is critical. The development of mammographic magnification offers improved detail and sharpness for the interpreter to determine if the lesion is benign or malignant.

The American Cancer Society recommends that all women between the ages of 35 and 40 have a baseline mammogram performed, followed by an annual or biennial mammogram screening until the age of 50. Women beyond 50 years should have a mammogram yearly. With the development of high resolution and low radiation techniques, this recommendation is actively being promoted across the nation in an effort to reduce the mortality figures from breast cancer.

Technologic advances in combining mammography with ultrasound have produced an even higher diagnostic accuracy. While mammography is the most sensitive technique for detecting cancer in the fatty breast tissue, ultrasound is more useful in women under 35 years and in women with dense, fibrous, glandular breasts. Ultrasound also gives information about tissue characteristics that mammography does not provide.

Ultrasound

Ultrasound has been found clinically useful in the following conditions: patients with radiographic dense breasts (any age), younger patients, those patients with an equivocal mammographic finding, symptomatic patients who are pregnant or lactating, and patients with breast prostheses. It is also of great value in distinguishing a cystic from a solid lesion in a patient with a known breast mass.

REAL-TIME TECHNIQUE. Patients who present with a palpable breast lesion may be examined with high-resolution real-time ultrasound.

The patient may be examined in a supine-oblique position, as she is rolled about 35 degrees toward the side opposite the breast to be examined. A sponge or folded towel is placed under her hips and shoulders to support her position. Her arm (on the side of the breast to be examined) is placed behind her head to help provide a stable scanning surface.

A high-frequency, 5.0 or 7.5 MHz, small-diameter transducer is used to image the breast parenchyma. The time gain compensation is adjusted to balance the skin echo, subcutaneous fat, dense breast core or mammary layer, retromammary layer, and pectoral muscles. The sensitivity of the equipment is adjusted to visualize the low-level subcutaneous layer, the echogenic mammary layer, and bright reflection from the retromammary layer, and the medium-level reflection from the pectoral muscles.

The mass is localized and its boundaries noted with a marking pen. The area surrounding the mass in a 3 cm square is then marked off with the marking pen. Scans are made in the transverse direction beginning at the inferior margin and moving cephalad by the smallest intervals possible. Subsequent scans are made in the sagittal direction beginning at the medial border of the square and moving laterally by small intervals. Extreme care should be taken to scan very lightly over the breast area so as not to distort the architecture. If the mass is very mobile, you may need to isolate it between two fingers. This will secure the lesion so it will not slip from under the transducer as you are scanning. The characteristics of the mass should be noted: shape, size, definition of borders, amount of transmission or attenuation, presence or absence of internal echoes, and degree of reflection from the anterior or posterior wall. Because the mass must be evaluated so carefully, it is important to assess these characteristics when the beam is directly over the major part of the lesion. Small lesions, under 1 cm, may not be easily visualized by this technique to the wide beam width, which fails to visualize a mass smaller than the transducer diameter.

The limitation of the real-time system is that it deforms the skin and underlying tissues by the direct transducer contact. Generally there is a poor portrayal of skin and subcutaneous detail. In addition, it is very difficult to scan adequately near the nipple area.

Another problem arises in examining the patient with a multicentric process such as fibrocystic disease. Then the entire breast should be evaluated, and it becomes very cumbersome to scan the whole breast accurately in small intervals since the breast is such a mobile flaccid structure in the supine position. Thus a dedicated breast water path unit was developed for a complete evaluation of the breast.

DEDICATED WATER PATH BREAST INSTRUMENTATION. The commercially available water path systems allow the patient to either lie prone on a special examining bed with the breast suspended in a large water tank or supine with a water bag suspended over the breast (Fig. 18-7).

In one available system, the transducer or transducers are mounted within the tank. The diameter of the transducer is much larger than found in the conventional hand-held transducer to allow the beam to be focused more precisely in the breast tissue. The focal length is dependent on the amount of water present between the breast and the transducer.

The patient lies in the prone swimmer's position with the arm (by the breast to be examined) placed at her side (Fig. 18-8). This allows the tail of the breast to be coupled with water.

Scans may be performed by small, 1 to 2 mm intervals in the transverse, sagittal, coronal, or rotational mode (depending on the particular instrumentation used). A mass lesion should be visualized in two axes and its characteristic pattern noted with a single transducer.

There are several approaches to visualizing the breast with the water path system. The multiple transducer ap-

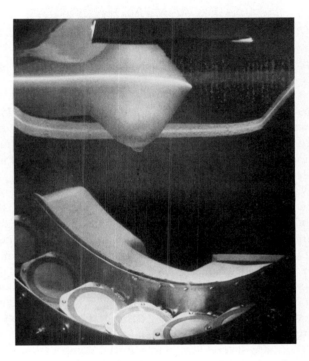

FIG. 18-7. Commercially available water path system that uses several large-aperture transducers to examine the breast.

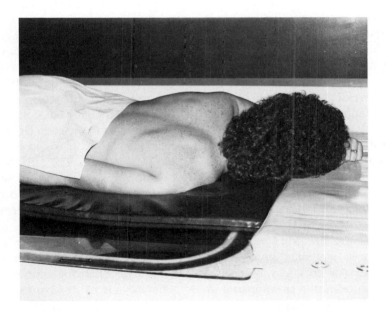

FIG. 18-8. It is necessary that the patient be placed in an oblique position so water contact and perpendicularity of the beam with the breast and the tail of Spence will be maintained.

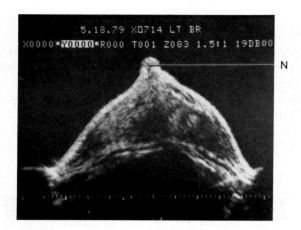

FIG. 18-9. Transverse scan of a noncompressed breast. *N,* nipple.

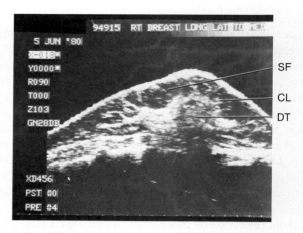

FIG. 18-10. Subcutaneous fat, *SF,* displays areas of low reflectivity interspersed with bright reflectors from Cooper's ligament, *CL. DT,* dense tissue.

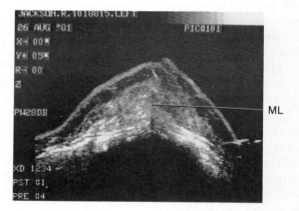

FIG. 18-11. Transverse scan of the mammary layer of the breast, *ML.*

proach provides an image with little or no nipple shadow; however, the multiple transducer *overwrite* may eliminate the attenuation or transmission characteristics of a lesion that might be clearly shown with a single transducer.

Various areas of the breast that cannot be seen on one view may be well shown on another. For example, the blind area on the transverse scan is near the inferomedial margin of the breast whereas on the sagittal scan it is near the inferior margin. Thus a mass may be better shown in one view than another.

COMPRESSION TECHNIQUES. A flexible nonattenuating material may be draped under the breasts or wrapped around the chest to enable the breast tissue to be compressed or flattened.

There are several advantages to the compression technique. Generally if the nipple shadow was present, it will disappear with compression to allow a better view of the subareolar area. Kelly-Fry[5] further states two additional advantages to the compression technique: (1) it decreases the length of the tissue path that the sound field must traverse and allows transducers with higher frequencies to be used; and (2) the problem of the loss of sound at a sharp angle of entrance to the breast is eliminated by the flattening of the tissues and thus delineation of the lesion is improved.

The disadvantages of compression are that it distorts the anatomy and sometimes eliminates the skin line information.

ULTRASONIC DESCRIPTION OF THE NORMAL BREAST. There are many variations in the normal breast, and these must be fully appreciated for interpretation of the sonographic image and differentiation of normal patterns from pathologic processes. The breast of a premenopausal patient will be discussed in detail.

The boundaries of the breast are the skin line, nipple, and retromammary layer. These generally give strong bright echo reflections. The areolar area may be recognized by the slightly lower echo reflection as compared to the nipple and skin. The internal nipple may show low to bright reflections and is quite variable (Fig. 18-9).

Subcutaneous fat displays areas of generally low reflectivity intermixed with bright reflectors from Cooper's ligaments and other connective tissue (Fig. 18-10). The Cooper ligaments will be seen if the beam strikes them at a perpendicular angle. Often compression of the breast will allow even more ligaments to be visualized.

The mammary layer, often referred to as the breast core or active glandular breast tissue, is generally displayed as a somewhat cone-shaped or triangular area beneath the subcutaneous fat layer and anterior to the retromammary layer. It is shown to converge toward the nipple (Fig. 18-11). The fatty tissue interdispersed throughout the mammary layer will dictate the amount of intensity reflected from the breast parenchyma. If little fat is present, there is a uniform architecture with a strong echogenic pattern (due to collagen and fibrotic tissue) throughout the mammary layer. When fatty tissue is present, areas of low-level echoes become intertwined with areas of strong echoes from the active breast tissue. The analysis of this pattern becomes critical to the final diagnosis, and one must be able to separate lobules of fat from a marginated lesion.

The use of compression may help to determine

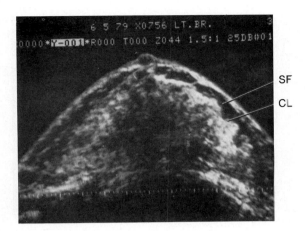

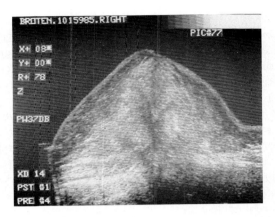

FIG. 18-13. Fatty replaced breast.

FIG. 18-12. Dense breast. *SF,* subcutaneous fat; *CL,* Cooper's ligament.

whether a suspected lesion maintains its shape or loses it, as fatty tissue does when compressed. Some instruments allow one to rotate around a point; thus fatty tissue will be very irregular and merge into the breast parenchyma whereas a lesion will be marginated from the parenchyma.

The retromammary layer is similar in texture to the subcutaneous layer, although the boundary echoes resemble skin reflections. The pectoral muscles are shown as low-level echo areas posterior to the retromammary layer. Ribs and intercostal margins are seen as bright and anechoic areas posterior to the pectoral muscles.

The echo appearance of the breast does change with age: the younger the patient, the greater the volume of the mammary layer, the denser the breast, and the more effective sonography is over mammography (Fig. 18-12). The older patient has more fatty tissue, and it is more difficult to distinguish disruptions in architecture than in the younger denser breast (Fig. 18-13).

Many breast lesions occur diffusely within the breast parenchyma (i.e., fibrous infiltration and fibrocystic disease). The recognition of these processes involves assessing the magnitude, texture, and distribution of echoes throughout the breast core.

Changes associated with a diffuse breast lesion may be characterized by
1. Increase in fibrotic tissue (more echogenic)
2. Increase in amplitude of echoes
3. Increase in fatty tissue (less echogenic)
Usually fatty infiltrations are not well circumscribed. Diffuse conditions lack the uniformity and texture seen in normal breast tissue.

Localized lesions may exhibit cystic or solid appearances depending on their particular characteristics. Observation of the lesions should be made using the following criteria:
1. Boundary echoes
2. Attenuation or transmission characteristics
3. Shape and position of the lesion
4. Disruption of normal architecture
5. Nature of surrounding tissues

6. Homogeneity
7. Presence of calcifications
8. Skin changes

Each of these changes will be discussed in the next section as they relate to cystic versus solid lesions and the distinction between benign and malignant breast lesions.

PATHOLOGY OF BREAST MASSES

The most common pathologic lesions of the female breast are, in order of decreasing frequency, fibrocystic disease, carcinoma, fibroadenoma, intraductal papilloma, and duct ectasia.[11] Benign lesions are the most common breast lesions, occurring in 70% of proved lesions biopsied or removed. Several parameters must be considered when a dominant mass has been palpated: patient's age, physical characteristics of the mass, and previous medical history. Lesions more common to younger women are fibrocystic disease and fibroadenomas. Older or postmenopausal women are more likely to have intraductal papillomas, duct ectasia, and cancer.

The benign and malignant masses will be discussed with their clinical findings and symptoms, mammographic findings,[3] and ultrasound findings.

Characteristic signs of breast masses[9]

Contour or margin	Anterior and/or posterior
Smooth	Strong
Irregular	Weak
Spiculated	Absent
Shape	Attenuation effects
Round	Acoustic enhancement
Oval	Acoustic shadowing
Tubular	Central
Lobulated	Bilateral
	Unilateral
Internal echo pattern	
Anechoic (homogeneous)	Distal echoes
Strong	Strong
Intermediate	Intermediate
Weak	Weak
Mixed	Absent
Boundary echoes	Disruption of architecture

Benign disease

Fibrocystic disease. This breast syndrome has histologic changes that occur on the terminal ducts and lobules of the breast in both the epithelial and the connective tissue and is usually accompanied by pain in the breast.

Its etiology is thought to be a disturbance in the estrogen-progesterone balance since it does not occur during puberty. It is a cyclic dysplasia, with signs and symptoms that vary according to the menstrual cycle. (Other diseases such as mammary dysplasia, fibroadenoma, cystosarcoma phylloides, and papillomas do not change with the menstrual cycle.)

The changes in fibrocystic disease occur in the breast parenchyma according to the patient's age. General symptoms are pain, nodularity, a dominant mass, cysts, and occasional nipple discharge.

There are three distinct stages:
1. Mastodynia or mazoplasia
2. Adenosis
3. Cystic disease

Stage 1, *mazoplasia,* is characterized by an increased proliferation of the stroma and by the small number of lobules or acini.[10] Stage 2, *adenosis,* is hyperplasia and proliferation of the epithelial component of the ducts.[10] Stage 3, *cystic disease,* is the involution of the lobules and hyperplasia of the surrounding stroma, leading to the formation of cysts.[10]

Another facet of fibrocystic disease is the dilation of the ducts, known as *comedomastitis.* This is seen in middle-aged women and is characterized by the dilation of ducts filled with a secretion produced by desquamated cells from the duct wall. The secretion will be manifested clinically by a multicolored and sticky nipple discharge. It often is accompanied by a retroareolar or periareolar redness and burning pain and itching. If untreated, the terminal ducts dilate and thicken. If the process is chronic, the ducts become tortuous (varicocele of Bloodgood) and may cause nipple retraction that simulates cancer.

Fibrocystic disease is a benign condition although a patient with duct hyperplasia and atypia is subject to a five-times greater risk of developing breast cancer.[10]

Apocrine metaplasia with atypia carries a similar but slightly decreased risk factor and has been termed *precancerous mastopathy* by Haagensen.[2]

Gross cystic disease and breast cancer occur in the same age group of patients, 40 to 50 years. Thus the method for diagnosis and treatment must be specific, to rule out a benign process versus a malignant one.

In the stage of mastodynia or mazoplasia the breasts are very painful, especially in the premenstrual period. The upper outer quadrants seem to be the most sensitive. This process is commonly seen in young women. Since it is a benign condition, it may subside spontaneously with time, medication, or pregnancy.

Stage 2 or adenosis is commonly seen in women 25 to 40 years of age. The pain is premenstrual and less severe. The patient may also have nipple discharge. (To be clinically significant, the discharge must be spontaneous and

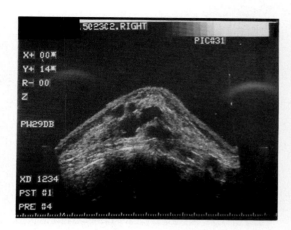

FIG. 18-14. Transverse noncompression scan of a patient with fibrocystic disease showing multiple characteristic cystic structures throughout the breast.

unprovoked.) The breast parenchyma is more pronounced and irregular due to nodularity. The nodules are usually of small size; they are considered more dominant as they reach 1 cm.

If the hyperplasia is surrounded by an intense proliferation of fibrous tissue, these areas may form a dominant mass that may be mistaken clinically for cancer. It is helpful to distinguish a tumor, which will have three dimensions (height, width, and depth) and occupy space, whereas a mass will have only two dimensions (height and width) and represents thickening.

MAMMOGRAPHIC FINDINGS
1. Scattered fine, coarse, round, or lobulated densities and masses in combination with proliferation of parenchyma and linear strands of fibrous (stromal) tissue

ULTRASOUND FINDINGS (FIG. 18-14)
1. Average amount of subcutaneous fat
2. Areas of fibrous stroma that appear brighter than the parenchyma
3. Small cysts scattered throughout the breast (cystic stage)
4. Large cysts that may also be present (Fig. 18-15)

Cystic disease. This disease is commonly seen in women 35 to 55 years of age. Symptoms include history of a changing menstrual cycle, pain (especially when the cyst is growing rapidly), recent lump, and tenderness. The disease may be microcystic or macrocystic. The small cyst may regress incompletely during the premenstrual phase. In the microcystic form, the cysts are multiple with some pain and tenderness of the breast. The macrocystic form has three-dimensional lesions, well delineated and slightly mobile (Fig. 18-16). These cysts may be aspirated for analysis of the fluid.

MAMMOGRAPHIC FINDINGS
1. Usually smooth walled with sharp borders
2. Hard to differentiate between a cyst and a noncalcified fibroadenoma
3. Lucent rim of fat around cyst

ULTRASOUND FINDINGS[4]
1. Smooth, sharp, well-defined borders (Fig. 18-17)

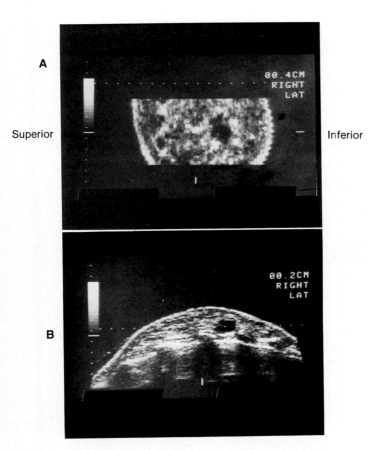

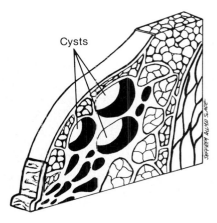

FIG. 18-16. Schema of multiple cysts in a breast. (Modified from Townsend CM: Clin Symp 32[2]:1, 1980.)

FIG. 18-15. A, The C-scan coronal slice of this cystic mass is taken parallel with the chest wall. It demonstrates the medial to lateral extent of the mass at this particular mass. **B,** Sagittal compression scan of the cystic mass with a septation. (Courtesy University of California, San Francisco.)

2. Lateral edge shadowing (arises from the low energy loss as the beam passes normally through the distal cyst wall, leaving sufficient energy to cause multireflections between the distal cyst wall and the chest wall[6])
3. Anechoic
4. Posterior enhancement

Fibroadenoma. This is one of the most common benign breast tumors, *the* most common in childhood, and occurs primarily in young adult women. It may be found in one breast only or bilaterally.

The growth of the fibroadenoma is stimulated by the administration of estrogen. Under normal circumstances hormonal influences on the breast (estrogen) result in the proliferation of epithelial cells in lactiferous ducts and in stromal tissue during the first half of the menstrual cycle. During the second half this condition regresses, allowing breast tissue to return to its normal resting state. In certain disturbances of this hormonal mechanism the regression fails to occur and results in the development of fibrous and epithelial nodules that become fibroadenomas, fibromas, or adenomas, depending on the predominant cell type. They may also be related to pregnancy and lactation.

Clinically the fibroadenoma is firm, rubbery, freely mobile, and clearly delineated from the surrounding breast tissue (Fig. 18-18). It is round or ovoid, smooth or lobu-

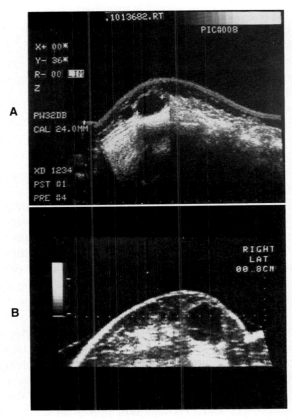

FIG. 18-17. A, Transverse scan of a cystic anechoic mass. **B,** Postoperative sagittal scan of a complex hemorrhagic mass with layering (Courtesy MD Anderson Medical Center, Houston.)

lated, and usually does not cause loss of contour of the breast unless it develops to a large size. It rarely causes mastodynia, and it does not change size during the menstrual cycle. It grows very slowly. A sudden increase in size with acute pain may be due to hemorrhage within the tumor. Calcification may follow hemorrhage or infarction, and thus the tumor may mimick a carcinoma.

MAMMOGRAPHIC FINDINGS

1. Smooth contour

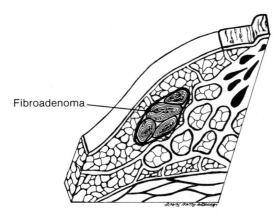

FIG. 18-18. Schema of a fibroadenoma. The lesion is palpated as a solitary, smooth, firm, well-demarcated nodule. (Modified from Townsend CM: Clin Symp 32[2]:1, 1980.)

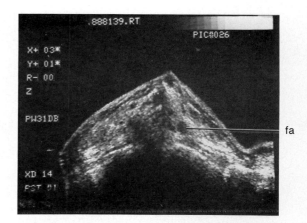

FIG. 18-19. Transverse scan of a small fibroadenoma, *fa*, displaying low-level internal echoes.

2. Difficult to differentiate from a cyst (except when lobulated)
3. May contain calcium deposits, which make differential diagnosis easier; as degeneration of tumor progresses, size and number of deposits increase

ULTRASOUND FINDINGS[1]
1. Smooth or lobulated borders (Fig. 18-19)
2. Strong anterior wall
3. Intermediate posterior enhancement
4. Low-level homogeneous internal echoes (sometimes strong)

Cystosarcoma phyllodes. This disease is an uncommon breast neoplasia, yet it is the most frequent sarcoma of the breast. It is more commonly found in women in their 50s and usually is unilateral. It may arise from a fibroadenoma as well as de novo. Many patients may notice a small breast mass that has been present for a long time suddenly begin to grow rapidly. At least 27% of these tumors are malignant; 12% will metastasize.

When the tumor is small, it is well delineated, firm, and mobile, much like a fibroadenoma. As it enlarges, the surface may become irregular and lobulated. Skin changes can develop due to increasing pressure. Edema may produce a skin change. As pressure increases, it causes trophic changes and eventual skin ulcerations. Infection and abscess formation may be a secondary complication. The tumor never adheres to the adjacent soft tissue or underlying pectoral muscle, and therefore dimpling of the skin or fixation of the tumor is not observed.[10]

MAMMOGRAPHIC FINDINGS
1. May be solitary and extremely large or a conglomerate of several masses
2. Borders smooth and sharp
3. Calcifications not usually seen as with fibroadenomas
4. Overlying skin thickened and stretched
5. More difficult to recognize in the young dense breast, where tumor occupies most of the breast

ULTRASOUND FINDINGS (FIG. 18-20)
1. Borders somewhat irregular
2. Anechoic or low level
3. Usually very large

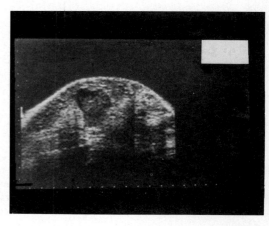

FIG. 18-20. Sagittal scan showing a lobulated complex mass in the breast of a 48-year-old woman. Cystosarcoma phyllodes. (Courtesy Thomas Jefferson University Hospital, Philadelphia.)

4. Weak posterior margin
5. Architectural disruption

Lipoma. A pure lipoma is entirely composed of fatty tissue. Other forms of lipoma consist of fat with fibrous and glandular elements interspersed (fibroadenolipoma). The lipoma may assume a large size before it is clinically detected. It is usually found in middle-aged or menopausal women.

Clinically on palpation a large, soft, poorly demarcated mass is felt that cannot be clearly separated from the surrounding parenchyma. There is no thinning or fixation of the overlying skin.

MAMMOGRAPHIC FINDINGS
1. Sharply defined capsule
2. Radiolucent (fat cells)
3. No calcification; appears benign and homogeneous
4. May extend to beneath the skin and displace the subcutaneous fat

ULTRASOUND FINDINGS
1. Difficult or impossible to detect in the fatty breast
2. Internal low-level echo content similar to that of fat
3. Posterior enhancement
4. Smooth walls

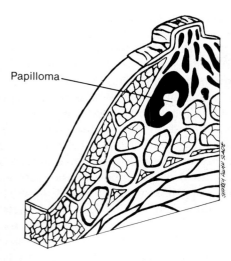

FIG. 18-21. Solitary intraductal papilloma. (Modified from Townsend CM: Clin Symp 32[2]:1, 1980.)

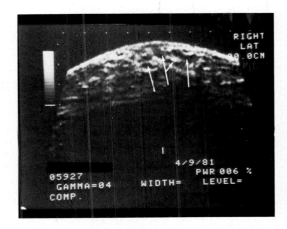

FIG. 18-22. Young breast with dilated milk-filled ducts (Courtesy MD Anderson Medical Center, Houston.)

Intraductal papilloma. This disease occurs most frequently in women 40 to 50 years of age. The predominant symptom is spontaneous nipple discharge arising from a single duct. When the discharge is copious, it is usually preceded by a sensation of fullness or pain in the areola or nipple area and is relieved as the fluid is expelled.

Papillomas are usually small, multiple, and multicentric. They consist of simple proliferations of duct epithelium projecting outward into a dilated lumen from one or more focal points (Fig. 18-21) each supported by a vascular stalk from which it receives the blood supply. Trauma may rupture the stalk, filling the duct with blood or serum. Papillomas may also grow to a large size and thus become palpable lesions. They are somewhat linear, resembling the terminal duct, and are usually benign.

Fat necrosis. Fat necrosis may be caused by trauma to the breast or plasma cell mastitis; or it may be related to an involutional process or other disease present in the breast, such as cancer. It is more frequently found in older women.

Clinical palpation reveals a spherical nodule that is generally superficial under a layer of calcified necrosis. A deep-lying focus of necrosis may cause scarring with skin retraction and thus mimic carcinoma.

MAMMOGRAPHIC FINDINGS

1. Area of nodular fibrosis or typical linear cystlike calcifications

ULTRASOUND FINDINGS

1. Irregular complex mass with low-level echoes
2. May mimic a malignant lesion
3. May appear as fat but is separate and different from the rest of the breast parenchyma

Acute mastitis. This process may be due to infection, trauma, mechanical obstruction in the breast ducts, or other reasons. It often occurs during a lactation, beginning in the lactiferous ducts and spreading via the lymphatics or blood (Fig. 18-22). Acute mastitis is often confined to one area of the breast.

Diffuse mastitis results from the infection's being car-

ried via the blood or breast lymphatics and thus affecting the entire breast.

MAMMOGRAPHIC FINDINGS

1. Increased density, ill defined
2. Difficult to diagnose in the dense lactating breast unless sufficient fat is interspersed to provide differences in density
3. Skin thickening due to edema

Chronic mastitis. An inflammation of the glandular tissue is considered to be chronic mastitis. It is very difficult to differentiate by ultrasound; the echo pattern will be mixed and diffuse with sound absorption. It usually is found in elderly women. There is a thickening of the connective tissue that results in narrowing of the lumina of the milk ducts. The cause is inspissated intraductal secretions, which are forced into the periductal connective tissue.

Clinically the patient usually has a nipple discharge, and frequently the nipple has retracted over a period of years. Palpation reveals some subareolar thickening but no dominant mass.

MAMMOGRAPHIC FINDINGS

1. Coarse road-type calcifications
2. Skin thickening
3. Nipple retraction (may or may not be present)

Abscess. This complication may be single or multiple. Acute abscesses have a poorly defined border, whereas mature abscesses are well encapsulated with sharp borders. A definite diagnosis cannot be made from the mammogram alone. Aspiration is needed.

Clinical findings will show pain, swelling, and reddening of the overlying skin. The patient may be febrile, and swollen painful axillary nodes may be present.

ULTRASOUND FINDINGS

1. Diffuse mottled appearance of the breast
2. Dense breast
3. Irregular borders (some may be smooth)
4. Posterior enhancement
5. May have low-level internal echoes

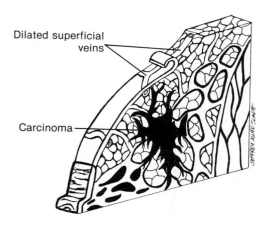

FIG. 18-23. Vascular signs of malignant disease (Modified from Townsend CM: Clin Symp 32[2]:1, 1980.)

Differential diagnosis of breast masses

Symptoms of breast masses include pain, a palpable mass, spontaneous or induced nipple discharge, skin dimpling, ulceration, or nipple retraction. The benign process is usually associated with pain, tumor, and nipple discharge. Skin dimpling or ulceration and nipple retraction are nearly always due to cancer. *Solid tumors* are rubbery, mobile, and well delineated (as seen in a fibroadenoma) or stone hard and irregular (as in a carcinoma). Soft tumors usually represent a lipoma (fat tissue). *Cystic masses* are like a balloon of water, well delineated but not as mobile as fibroadenomas because they form part of the breast parenchyma whereas a fibroadenoma has a capsule.

Malignant disease generally develops over a long period. It is not unusual for several years to pass from the first appearance of atypical hyperplasia to the final diagnosis of in situ cancer. This becomes the critical time for detection and treatment.

Malignant cells will grow along a line of least resistance, such as in fatty tissue. In fibrotic tissue most cancer growth occurs along the borders. Lymphatics and blood vessels are frequently used as pathways for new tumor development (Fig. 18-23). If the tumor is encapsulated, it will continue to grow in one area, compressing and distorting the surrounding architecture. When the carcinoma is contained and has not invaded the basal membrane structure, it is considered *in situ.* Most cancer will originate in the ducts whereas a smaller percentage will originate in the glandular tissue.

Cancer of the breast is of two types: sarcoma and carcinoma. *Sarcoma* refers to breast tumors that arise from the supportive or connective tissues. Sarcoma is the usual type, growing rapidly and invading fibrous tissue. *Carcinoma* refers to breast tumors that arise from the epithelium, in the ductal and glandular tissue, and usually has tentacles. Other malignant diseases affecting the breast are a result of systemic neoplasms such as leukemia or lymphoma.

Cancer is further classified as infiltrating and noninfiltrating. *Infiltrating* carcinoma has infiltrated the tissue beyond the basement membrane and into adjacent tissue.

Chances of metastases are enhanced with the time and type of growth present. Infiltrating carcinomas are histologically designated into several types. Some produce more fibrosis and therefore are categorized as infiltrating ductal carcinoma with productive fibrosis. Others, such as medullary carcinoma, have little associated fibrosis. Colloid carcinoma is a type of cancer in which mucin production occurs and the fibrotic reaction may be variable. Over 80% of carcinomas fall into the category of infiltrating ductal carcinoma with productive fibrosis. *Noninfiltrating* carcinoma is carcinoma of the lactiferous ducts that has not infiltrated the basement membrane but is proliferating within the confines of the ducts and its branches. There is no danger of metastases under these circumstances. This also may be referred to as carcinoma in situ. Most in situ lesions develop from longstanding epithelial hyperplasia of ducts and lobules.

The more favorable cancers, which remain localized to the breast longer and have a 75% survival after 10 years, represent only 10% to 12% of all breast cancer.[12] This group includes medullary, intracystic papillary, papillary, colloid, adenoid cystic, and tubular carcinoma.

Malignant cystosarcoma phyllodes and stromal sarcomas rarely metastasize to regional nodes and have a better than average prognosis after treatment. Occasional spread to distant areas of the body has been reported with these tumors.

The exact type of tumor can be determined only by a histologic diagnosis, not by other noninvasive means. It is the role of mammography and ultrasound to clarify whether a mass is present and whether it has cystic or solid characteristics; then a differential can be made as to its benign or malignant probabilities.

The characteristics most often seen by ultrasound in a malignant mass are as follows:
1. Irregular spiculated contour or margin
2. Round or lobulated
3. Weak nonuniform internal echoes
4. Intermediate anterior and absent or weak posterior boundary echoes
5. Great attenuation effects

The exception to this list of criteria is medullary carcinoma. Due to its cellularity and occasional encapsulation, it may present more like a fibroadenoma. Its characteristics are smooth borders and round uniform to absent internal echoes.

Intraductal solid carcinoma (comedocarcinoma). Macroscopically the lactiferous ducts are filled with a yellow pastelike material that looks like small plugs (comedones) when sectioned. Histologically the ducts are filled with plugs of epithelial tumor that have a central necrosis, giving rise to the pastelike material. Both invasive and noninvasive forms exist.

The clinical picture depends on the stage of the disease. Noninvasive forms may lack any clinical or palpatory findings. If there is a nipple discharge, it is more frequently clear than bloody (unlike papillary carcinoma, in which bloody discharge is typical). The patient may complain of pain or the sensation of insects crawling on the

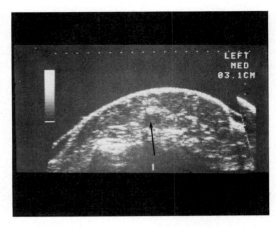

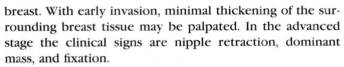

FIG. 18-24. Sagittal scan of the breast of a 57-year-old woman with an infiltrating duct carcinoma *(arrow)*. The mass had irregular borders with increased fibrosis surrounding it. (Courtesy Massachusetts General Hospital, Boston.)

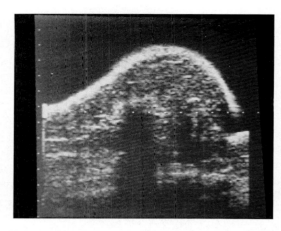

FIG. 18-25. Sagittal scan of an infiltrating duct carcinoma with acute attenuation of the sound. (Courtesy Thomas Jefferson University Hospital, Philadelphia.)

breast. With early invasion, minimal thickening of the surrounding breast tissue may be palpated. In the advanced stage the clinical signs are nipple retraction, dominant mass, and fixation.

MAMMOGRAPHIC FINDINGS

1. Microcalcifications

ULTRASOUND FINDINGS

1. Irregular border (Fig. 18-24)
2. Diffuse internal echo pattern
3. Attenuation with shadowing (Fig. 18-25)

Juvenile breast cancer. This disease is similar to the intraductal carcinoma and infiltrating ductal carcinoma found in adults. Generally it occurs in young females, between 8 and 15 years of age, and has a good prognosis when treated.

Papillary carcinoma. This tumor initially arises as an intraductal mass. It may also take the form of an intracystic tumor, but that is rare.

The early stage of papillary carcinoma is noninfiltrating. The tumor occasionally arises from a benign ductal papilloma. It is associated with little fibrotic reaction.

Both intraductal and intracystic forms exist, and these represent 1% to 2% of all breast carcinomas. The earliest clinical sign of *intraductal* papillary carcinoma is bloody nipple discharge. Occasionally a mass can be palpated as a small, firm, well-circumscribed area; this may be mistaken for a fibroadenoma. There may be nodules of blue or red discoloration under the skin with central ulceration. A diffusely nodular appearance overlying the skin is a special variant of multiple intraductal papillary carcinoma. *Intracystic* papillary carcinoma is clinically indistinguishable in its early stages from a cyst or fibroadenoma. When the tumor has invaded through the cyst wall, it is palpable as a poorly circumscribed mass.

MAMMOGRAPHIC FINDINGS

1. Intraductal—not often diagnosed in early stages
2. Intracystic—recognized when invasion beyond the wall of the cyst occurs; the sharp contours of the cyst are lost because of surrounding edema and infiltration

ULTRASOUND FINDINGS

1. Irregular borders
2. Heterogeneous internal echo pattern
3. Attenuation with acoustic shadowing

Paget's disease. Paget's disease arises in the superficial subareolar or deeper lactiferous ducts and grows in the direction of the nipple, spreading into the intraepidermal region of the nipple and areola. It may be confused with a melanoma.

The disease induces changes of the nipple and areola. Any ulceration, enlargement, or deformity of the nipple and areola should suggest Paget's disease. This is a relatively rare tumor, accounting for 2.5% of all breast cancers. It occurs in older women, over 50 years of age. Differential diagnosis includes benign inflammatory eczematous condition of the nipple, since palpatory findings are frequently not present. The primary duct cancer may be quite deep or embedded in fibrotic tissue.

MAMMOGRAPHIC FINDINGS

1. Thickened areolar tissue due to eczema or tumor infiltration
2. Solid tumor mass occasionally
3. Microcalcifications (if seen in either a punctate or a linear display, strongly suggestive of duct carcinoma)

ULTRASOUND FINDINGS

1. Irregular borders
2. Heterogeneous internal echoes
3. Attenuation with posterior shadow
4. Subareolar solid mass
5. Skin echo thin and deformed, suggesting infiltration

Scirrhous carcinoma. This tumor is a type of duct carcinoma with extensive fibrous tissue proliferation (productive fibrosis). There may also be focal calcification present. Histologically the cells are found in narrow files or strands, clusters, or columns and may form lumina with varying frequency.

Scirrhous is the most common form of breast cancer. The classical clinical signs are a firm, nodular, frequently nonmovable mass often with fixation as well as flattening

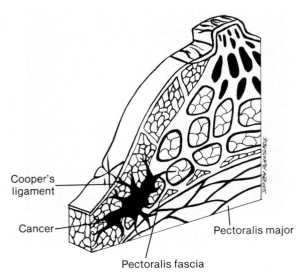

FIG. 18-26.   Skin dimpling. (Modified from Townsend CM: Clin Symp 32[2]:1, 1980.)

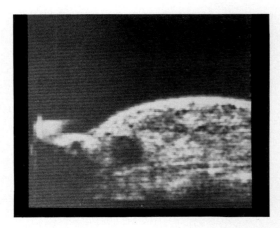

FIG. 18-27.   This benign-appearing solid mass was pathologically proved to be a medullary carcinoma. (Courtesy Thomas Jefferson University Hospital, Philadelphia.)

of overlying skin and nipple retraction. The retraction is a result of an infiltrative shortening of Cooper's ligaments due to productive fibrosis (Fig. 18-26). Fixation and retraction of the nipple may be the result of a subareolar carcinoma but may also be caused by benign fibrosis of the breast. It is important to note that some patients normally have inverted nipples. The size of the cancer may vary from a few millimeters to involvement of nearly the entire breast. The deep-lying scirrhous carcinoma may grow into and become fixed to the thoracic wall. A sanguineous discharge is rare in this tumor.

MAMMOGRAPHIC FINDINGS
1. Central mass with lobular and ill-defined contour from which numerous fibrous strands extend into surrounding breast tissue
2. Diagnosis easier in the fatty breast than in the dense breast
3. Microcalcification present in 35%

ULTRASOUND FINDINGS
1. Irregular mass with ill-defined borders
2. Attenuation with posterior shadow
3. Disruption of architecture

Medullary carcinoma. This type of duct carcinoma is a densely cellular tumor containing large, round, or oval tumor cells. It usually is a well-circumscribed mass whose center is frequently necrotic as well as hemorrhagic and cystic.

Medullary carcinoma is relatively rare, comprising less than 5% of breast cancers. The age of occurrence is slightly lower than for the average breast cancer. The skin fixation over the mass is an infrequent finding. It will occasionally reach large proportions and may have a diameter up to 10 cm. Discoloration of the overlying skin is often seen. Bilateral occurrence is more frequent than in other cancers.

MAMMOGRAPHIC FINDINGS
1. Round, oval, or lobulated mass

2. Margins appear to be smooth, but with nonuniformity and adjacent edema
3. Connective tissue strands occasionally
4. In larger tumors, secondary signs of subcutaneous fatty tissue infiltration, skin thickening, and increased vascularity

ULTRASOUND FINDINGS
1. May resemble fibroadenoma (Fig. 18-27)
2. Well-defined border
3. Homogeneous internal echoes
4. Posterior enhancement

Colloid carcinoma (mucinous). This is also a type of duct carcinoma. The cells of the tumor produce secretions that fill lactiferous ducts or the stromal tissues that the tumor cells are invading.

Clinically it presents as a smooth not particularly firm mass at palpation. Due to its smooth, nonfibrosing nature, one does not see plateauing or fixation, as with scirrhous carcinoma.

MAMMOGRAPHIC FINDINGS
1. Smoothly contoured mass resembling a benign tumor

ULTRASOUND FINDINGS
1. Similar to a fibroadenoma
2. Well-defined borders
3. Posterior enhancement

Lobular carcinoma. This disease originates in the ductules of the lobules. When the basement membrane is not invaded and there are no signs of infiltration, the disease is called lobular carcinoma in situ. Secondary involvement of adjacent terminal ductules and neighboring lobules may occur. Multiple foci of lobular carcinoma throughout the breast are not rare.

It most commonly is found in women between the ages of 40 and 50. Frequently it is found in the upper outer quadrants, perhaps because in the involuted breast the residual breast tissue remains in the upper outer quadrants whereas the other areas are replaced by fat. There are no typical clinical symptoms that indicate lobular carcinoma in situ. The indication for biopsy depends on abnormal palpatory findings. It commonly occurs bilat-

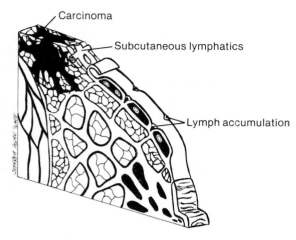

FIG. 18-28. Skin edema (Modified from Townsend CM: Clin Symp 32[2]:1, 1980.)

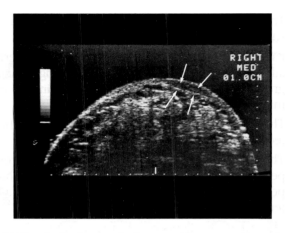

FIG. 18-29. Sagittal scan of a breast with metastatic carcinoma. The area of skin thickening shows decreased echogenicity due to the collection of lymphatic fluid. (Courtesy Massachusetts General Hospital, Boston.)

erally; thus prophylactic biopsy and mammography of the opposite breast are recommended.

MAMMOGRAPHIC FINDINGS

1. Microcalcifications (Some clinicians believe that the tumor is adjacent to the calcifications. However, it is not certain whether the calcifications occur as a result of the lobular carcinoma itself or whether the two processes have an increased tendency to occur together.)

ULTRASOUND FINDINGS

1. Weak internal echo pattern, irregular distribution
2. Intermediate anterior and lateral wall echoes
3. Absent posterior wall
4. Irregular central shadow present
5. Tumor surrounded by bright punctate echoes of breast stroma, especially in the mammary layer

Diffuse carcinoma (inflammatory carcinoma). This tumor presents with all infiltrative types of breast carcinoma (scirrhous, medullary, colloid, etc.). Characteristically there is a diffuse spread of disease throughout the breast due to capillary invasion and involvement of lymphatics of the skin (Fig. 18-28).

It usually is found in middle-aged to older women. The breast is often very large, the progression of inflammatory carcinoma very rapid, and the course very short. The skin shows an erythematous blotchy pattern, and the nipple may be retracted. There is diffuse skin thickening.

MAMMOGRAPHIC FINDINGS

1. Generalized skin thickening
2. Parenchyma not as cloudy as with inflammatory mastitis, but proliferation of abnormal tissue of increased density
3. Occasionally a dominant mass from which the carcinoma originates
4. Sometimes malignant calcifications in linear or intraductal forms

ULTRASOUND FINDINGS

1. If dominant mass present, borders irregular with high attenuation by shadow (Fig. 18-29)
2. Skin thickening in comparison with the normal breast

BIOPSY TECHNIQUES FOR BREAST TUMORS

Three events have occurred that affect the number and type of invasive diagnostic procedures used on women with breast masses.

First, women are becoming more informed about their diagnostic choices. They are asking their physicians to order an ultrasound examination to determine whether the mass is cystic or solid before subjecting themselves to an excisional biopsy.

Second, as physicians have the availability of ultrasound, they are being more confident in its use and are more willing to perform a needle aspiration of a cystic area rather than the more invasive excisional biopsy. This judgment depends on the physical characteristics of the breast mass, the age of the patient, and the associated risk factors determined from the patient's history.

Third, needle biopsy is more acceptable to both patients and physicians. Although it is not as accurate as the open biopsy, it has become a useful diagnostic tool in breast lesions suspected of being carcinomatous. The advantages of the technique are that it is an office procedure, it is cost effective, it is simple to perform, and it is relatively atraumatic. Needle biopsy or excisional biopsy is the only reliable method for determining the exact malignancy of a breast mass.

SUMMARY

1. One out of eleven American women will develop breast cancer.
2. The clinical diagnosis of breast cancer may fall under several categories depending on the age of the patient, whether the lesion is palpable, the risk factors of the patient, and previous medical history.
3. The self-examination technique is an important issue in the detection of early lesions or subtle changes in the breast parenchyma that one may notice only from a routine examination.
4. The function of the female breast is to secrete milk during lactation.

19

Neonatal Echoencephalography

RAUL BEJAR
GUSTAVO VIGLIOCCO
HECTOR GRAMAJO
MARY ALLARE

Brain damage is a common event in the immature infant. Intraventricular-subependymal hemorrhages (IVHs/SEHs) occur in 40% to 70% of premature neonates less than 34 weeks of gestation. Multifocal necrosis of the white matter (WMN) or periventricular leukomalacia (PVL) can develop in 12% to 20% of infants weighing less than 2000 g. These lesions are associated with increased mortality and abnormal neurologic outcome.*

The understanding of intracranial lesions in newborn infants has increased considerably with the advancements in ultrasonography and computerized tomography during the last ten years.† Echoencephalography (ECHO) continues to be the technique of choice to visualize the neonatal brain. This technique is a nonionizing, noninvasive bedside procedure very well tolerated by even the smallest and sickest infants. It allows very early and frequent studies of the population at risk. Furthermore, ECHO diagnosis correlates well with examinations obtained by computed tomography (CT) and autopsy studies.[5,32,53,58,59]

This chapter describes the echoencephalography technique to study the newborn infant's brain through the fontanelles and the sutures as well as the sonographic characteristics of the most frequent pathologic conditions found in newborn infants.

TECHNIQUE

Mechanical or phased array sector scanners are the equipment of choice to perform echoencephalography studies rather than linear array transducers. The small transducer makes it possible to obtain excellent contact with the skull through the fontanelles and sutures and to avoid the curvature of the calvarium (as would be found with a linear array transducer). Consequently, good visualization of the brain is achieved even in infants with small fontanelles.[4,9,10,12,58] With modern scanners most of the studies in small premature infants should be performed with a 7.5 MHz transducer. In larger babies the studies can be obtained with a 7.5 MHz transducer for structures located close to the fontanelles and a 5 MHz transducer for visualization of the anatomy in areas situated farther away from the transducer.

Different planes and views are used to study the supratentorial and infratentorial compartments.[9,10,12] Supratentorial studies show both cerebral hemispheres, the basal ganglia, the lateral and third ventricles, the interhemispheric fissure, and the subarachnoid space surrounding the hemispheres. Infratentorial studies visualize the cere-

---

*References 1, 11, 23, 31, 37, 38, 54, 55, 70.
†References 1, 4, 5, 9-12, 23, 31, 32, 37, 38, 53-55, 58, 59, 63, 70.

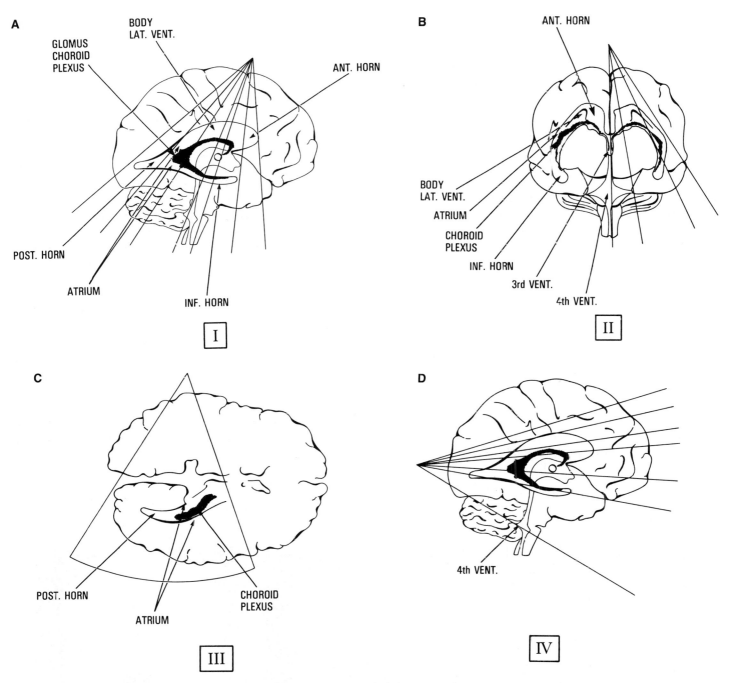

FIG. 19-1. Schema of the different views used to study the supratentorial compartment. **A,** Coronal studies. **B,** Sagittal and parasagittal studies. **C,** Axial studies through the mastoid fontanelle. **D,** Axial studies through the posterior fontanelle. Note the distance of the structures of the brain from the transducer in the different views.

bellum, the brain stem, the fourth ventricle, and the basal cisterns.

Supratentorial compartment

The supratentorial compartment is imaged from the anterior fontanelle in the coronal, modified coronal, sagittal, and parasagittal planes and in the axial plane from the mastoid fonticullus and the posterior fontanelle. (Fig. 19-1).

Coronal and modified coronal studies. To perform these studies the transducer is placed on the anterior fon-

tanelle with the scanning plane following the coronal suture. The middle of the crystal must be centered in the coronal suture to reduce bone interference and to procure the most extensive image of the brain. Symmetrical images must be obtained. This is accomplished using the skull bones and the middle cerebral arteries at the Sylvian fissure as landmarks (Fig. 19-2). The skull bones and the arteries should have the same size bilaterally. After a symmetric view is obtained, the transducer is angled anteriorly and posteriorly to enable complete visualization of the lateral and third ventricles, the deep subcorti-

NORMAL RTE OF PRETERM INFANTS

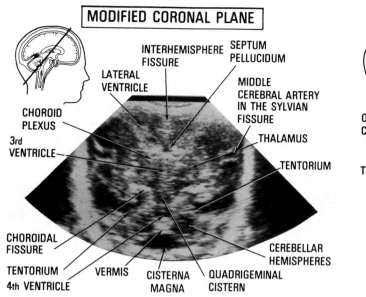

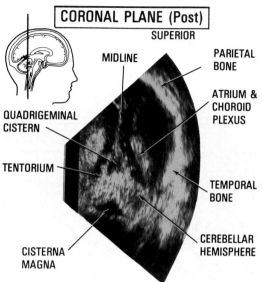

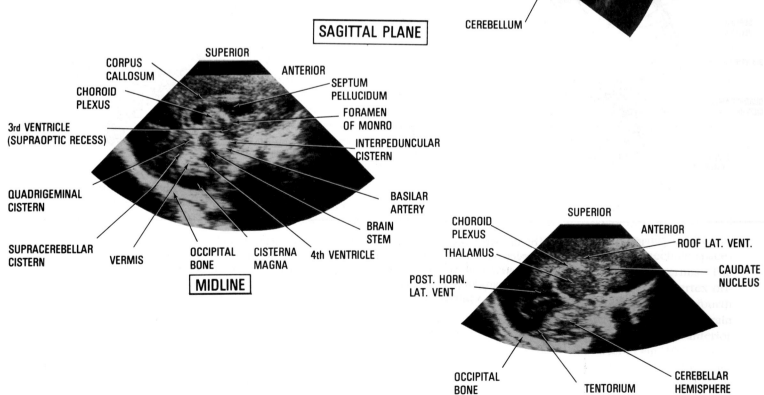

FIG. 19-7. Normal ultrasound studies focused in the infratentorial compartment. In the parasagittal study, note the normal ultrasonographic characteristics of the cerebellar hemispheres. See text for more descriptions.

the parasagittal plane. The cerebellar hemispheres appear as round, low echogenic formations with moderately hyperechoic surfaces (Fig. 19-7).

Modified coronal studies. The modified coronal plane demonstrates the body of the lateral ventricles, the third ventricle, and the posterior fossa. To obtain this view the transducer is positioned over the anterior fontanelle with an angle of approximately 30 to 40 degrees between the scanning plane and the surface of the fontanelle. In this view the tentorium, the cerebellar vermis, the fourth ventricle, the cerebellar hemispheres, and the cisterna magna can be seen in the infratentorial compartment. The vermis is a very echogenic structure in the midline. The fourth ventricle appears in the midline as a small anechoic space approximately 2 to 3 mm wide, located anteriorly to the vermis. The cerebellar hemispheres have low echogenicity and are contiguous with the echogenic vermis. The cisterna magna corresponds to a nonechogenic space between the vermis, the cerebellar hemispheres, and the occipital bone (Fig. 19-7).

Coronal studies. A "straight" coronal view of the posterior fossa is obtained by placing the transducer on the mastoid fontanelle or the occipitotemporal suture, immediately behind the ear. The scanning plane should be kept perpendicular to the canthomeatal line. The tentorium, the cerebellar hemispheres, the cisterna magna, and the supracerebellar cistern are visualized (Fig. 19-7). Angling the transducer anteriorly brings the fourth ventricle and the brain stem into view. The fourth ventricle appears as a triangle inside the cerebellum, and the most ventral aspect of the supracerebellar cistern is also seen (Fig. 19-7).

Studies from the cervical spinal column. Pathology in the posterior fossa and in the spinal cord can be studied through the neck using a high-definition short-focused transducer. The transducer is placed at the posterior part of the neck just below the occipital bone, with the scanning plane in the same direction as the spinal cord (sagittal plane) (Fig. 19-8, *A*). Then the transducer is rotated up to visualize the medulla and the cervical spinal cord surrounded by the anechoic subarachnoid space. At the top of this view the cisterna magna and the inferior part of the vermis can easily be identified (Fig. 19-8, *B*). Since the structures of the posterior fossa are distant from the transducer when they are scanned from the anterior fontanelle, studying the posterior fossa in the coronal plane from the mastoid fonticullus and in the sagittal plane through the neck enables more precise identification of subarachnoid and intracerebral hemorrhages.

ECHOENCEPHALOGRAPHIC DIAGNOSIS OF NEONATAL BRAIN LESIONS

Real-time echoencephalography is ideal for timing the onset and sequentially following the evolution of a large number of brain lesions in newborn infants.

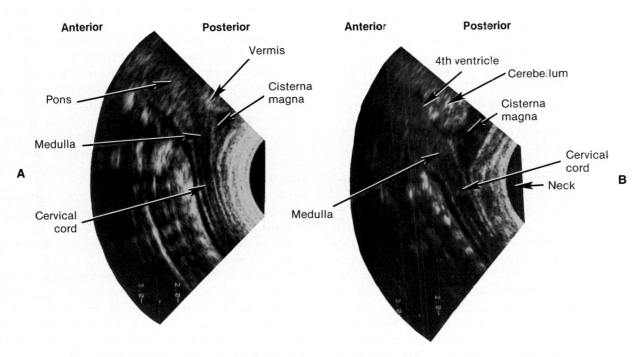

FIG. 19-8. Sagittal visualization of the posterior fossa from the cervical column (nuchal view). To obtain a view similar to **A**, the transducer should be applied in the middle of the cervical column with the scanning plane oriented in the sagittal plane. The cervical cord, the brain stem, the cisterna magna, and the inferior part of the cerebellum may be seen. After obtaining view **A**, the transducer should be oriented upward to visualize the cisterna magna, the cerebellum, and the brain stem in more detail, **B.** Note the normal echogenicity of the spinal cord compared with the subarachnoid space and the vermis of the cerebellum.

Hemorrhagic pathology

Subependymal-intraventricular hemorrhages (SEH-IVH). Subependymal-intraventricular hemorrhages (SEHs-IVHs) are the most common hemorrhagic lesions in preterm newborn infants. These lesions affect 30% to 50% of infants less than 34 weeks of gestation.* SEHs-IVHs are a developmental disease since they originate in the subependymal germinal matrix.[31,54] The germinal matrix is the tissue where neurons and glial cells develop before migrating from the subventricular (subependymal) region to the cortex. The germinal matrix is highly cellular, has poor connective supporting tissue, and is richly vascularized with very thin capillaries. This increased capillary fragility may explain the high frequency of these hemorrhages in tiny infants. Furthermore, the germinal matrix has a high fibrinolytic activity that may be important for the extension of the capillary hemorrhages that originate in this tissue.[25,31,54,67] By 24 weeks of gestation most of the neuronal and glial migration has occurred. However, pockets of germinal matrix remain until 40 weeks of gestation in the subependymal area at the head of the caudate nuclei. This may explain why subependymal hemorrhages are less frequent in term infants and why the majority of the intraventricular hemorrhages in these infants originate in the choroid plexus.[37,54,70]

Subependymal hemorrhages (SEHs) are caused by capillary bleeding in the germinal matrix. The most frequent location is at the thalamic-caudate groove. If bleeding continues, the hemorrhage enlarges, pushing the ependyma into the ventricular cavity, which can then become completely occluded by the subependymal hemorrhage. Eventually a large SEH will rupture through the ependyma into the ventricular cavity, forming an intraventricular hemorrhage (IVH).

IVHs and SEHs are easily detected with real-time echoencephalography as very echodense structures, since fluid and clotted blood have higher acoustic impedance than the brain parenchyma and the cerebrospinal fluid (CSF). Overall, ECHO is more sensitive for detecting IVHs-SEHs than computerized tomography (CT). Hemoglobin concentrations greater than 5 to 6 mg/dl are required to detect blood in the ventricular cavities with CT, while ECHO can visualize blood when the concentration of red blood cells in the CSF is only 1 to 2 mg/dl (Fig. 19-9).[10,12]

SEHs-IVHs can be studied in the coronal, modified coronal, sagittal, parasagittal, and axial planes. A subependymal hemorrhage is usually seen at the thalamic-caudate notch as a very echodense lesion pushing up the floor and external wall of the lateral ventricle with partial obliteration of the ventricular cavity. The SEH can extend by continuous bleeding and perforate the ventricular wall with partial or total flooding of the ventricular system (intraventricular hemorrhage, IVH). IVHs appear as echodense structures inside the anechoic ventricular cavities. Depending on the amount of blood, the ventricle can become full and dilated. Subsequently the SEH may obstruct the circulation and absorption of the cerebrospi-

nal fluid, causing the ventricles to dilate further with CSF and ultimately resulting in posthemorrhagic hydrocephalus (Fig. 19-9).

Fig. 19-9 depicts SEHs-IVHs as they are seen in the different views. In Fig. 19-10 the corresponding pathologic specimen is demonstrated, showing that ECHO can visualize very small SEHs (3 mm in diameter or less). Fig. 19-11 and 19-12 show the evolution of SEHs-IVHs at different stages. Fig. 19-13 shows a large SEH-IVH with subsequent posthemorrhagic hydrocephalus, before and after placement of a ventriculoperitoneal shunt. Fig. 19-14 illustrates a large intraventricular hemorrhage with a changing fluid meniscus, depending on the infant's head position. This is quite different from the typical clot and a most unusual event illustrating that ECHO can detect unclotted blood in the cerebral ventricular system.

Studies from the anterior fontanelle may not detect small IVHs, since intraventricular blood tends to "settle out" in the posterior horns. These small IVHs can be diagnosed when the occipital horns are visualized in the axial plane from the mastoid or from the posterior fontanelles. Since these fontanelles are closer to the occipital horns than the anterior fontanelle, the occipital horns are within the focal range of the transducer, and a greater amount of ultrasonic energy can reach the sedimented red blood cells.

IVHs-SEHs are not a sudden event: they usually expand slowly (Figs. 19-11 and 19-12). This phenomenon is probably secondary to the high fibrinolytic activity of the germinal matrix. However, in some infants the IVHs-SEHs may extend very fast; sudden flooding and distension of the ventricles by hemorrhage is associated with the clinical symptoms of shock, seizures, hypoxemia, and a sudden decrease in the hematocrit. Typically, when a small IVH-SEH progresses to a large IVH-SEH (usually during the first four postpartum days), the IVHs/SEHs are asymptomatic. Since approximately 70% of hemorrhages are asymptomatic, it is necessary to have a technique, such as ECHO, to routinely scan all the infants at risk for these lesions.

Classification of SEH-IVH hemorrhage is based on the extension of the hemorrhage and the resultant changes in the ventricular size:

- Grade I: SEH or IVH without ventricular enlargement
- Grade II: SEH or IVH with minimal ventricular enlargement
- Grade III: SEH or IVH with moderate or large ventricular enlargement
- Grade IV: SEH or IVH with intraparenchymal hemorrhage

Only ventricular enlargement produced by the intraventricular hemorrhage should be considered. Small SEHs-IVHs may occlude the foramen of Monro or the aqueduct of Sylvius and thereby produce moderate to large dilatation of the lateral ventricles by CSF.

The ventricular size is measured in the sagittal plane (height of the body of the ventricles at the midthalamus) and in the axial plane (width of the atrium at the level of the choroid plexus). Based on these measurements, ventricular dilatation may be classified as follows:

- Mild dilatation: Ventricular size measuring 8 to 10 mm

---

*References 1, 23, 39, 54, 55, 70.

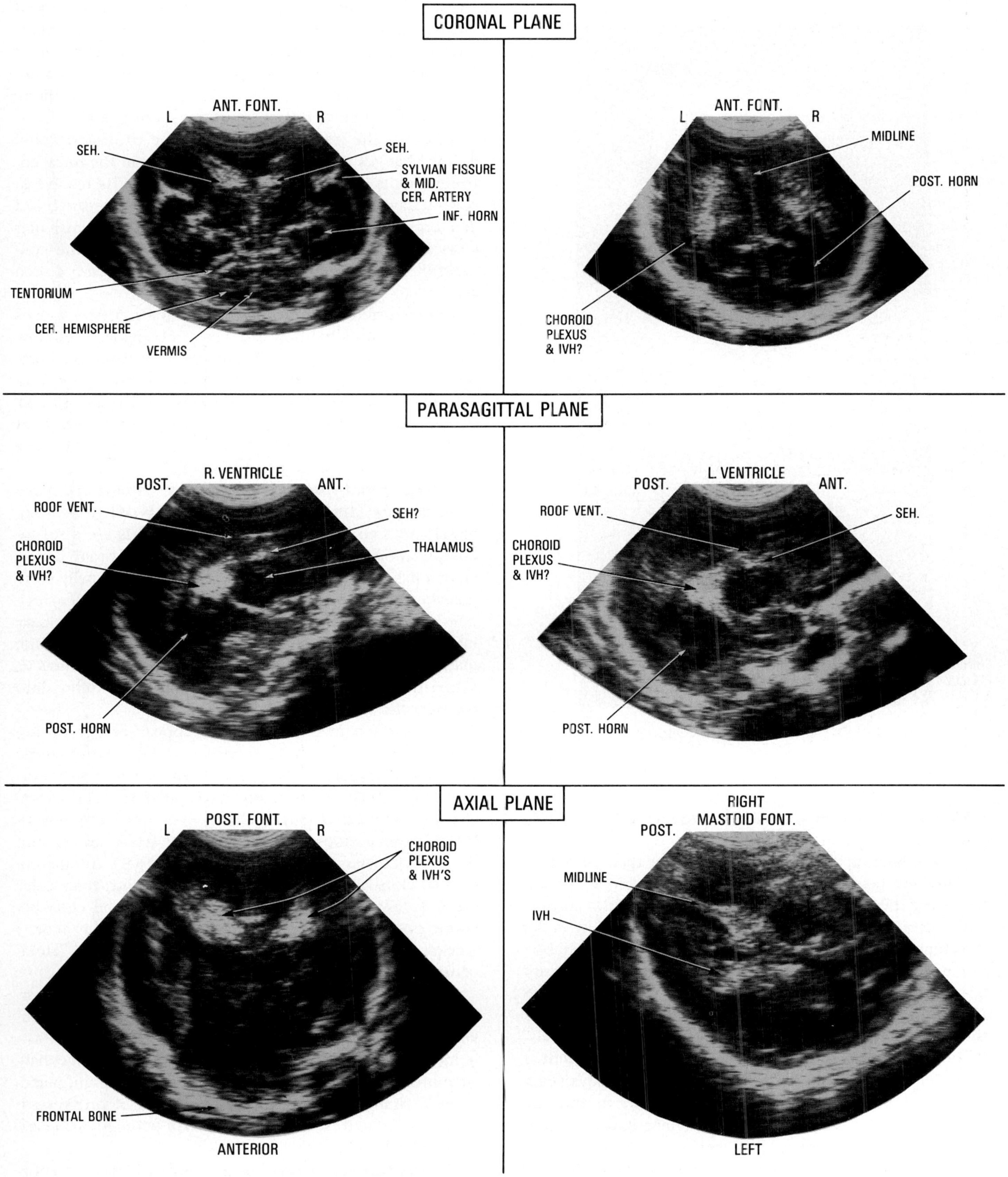

FIG. 19-9. Postmortem ultrasound and pathologic studies in a premature infant with small SEHs-IVHs. The ventricular cavities are partially obstructed by SEHs. The small SEH (2 mm) in the right caudate nucleus is seen in the coronal and sagittal planes. The studies of the axial plane through the posterior and mastoid fontanelle showed IVHs. These hemorrhages were not clearly visualized in the modified coronal and sagittal studies from the anterior fontanelle.

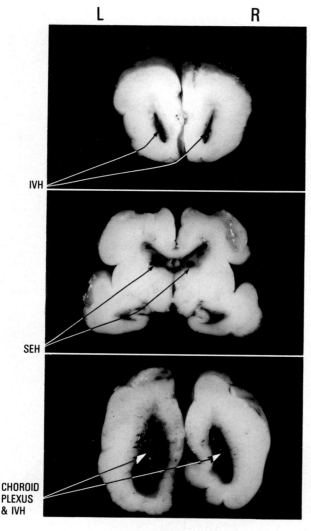

FIG. 19-10. See legend for Fig. 19-9.

- Moderate dilatation: Ventricular size measuring 11 to 14 mm
- Large dilatation: Ventricular size greater than 14 mm

After the hemorrhage has occurred, the blood spreads following the CSF pathways, reaching the fourth ventricle and eventually the cisterns in the posterior fossa, with the development of subarachnoid hemorrhages (SAH). Subsequently, obstruction of the CSF pathways and obliterans arachnoiditis occurs, causing imbalance between production and reabsorption of CSF. Posthemorrhagic ventricular dilatation develops as a consequence of this imbalance.[70] If the ventricular dilatation is progressive, the patient is considered to have posthemorrhagic hydrocephalus (Figs. 19-12 and 19-13). This complication occurs in approximately 35% of infants with large hemorrhages. Usually mild to moderate ventricular dilatation resolves spontaneously. However, placement of a ventriculoperitoneal shunt may be necessary for severely dilated ventricles.

Posthemorrhagic hydrocephalus may be silent, since the white matter of newborn infants is very compliant and easily compressed as the ventricles widen.[70] This factor explains why initial ventricular dilatation occurs without changes in the head circumference. The head circumference starts to enlarge only after significant compression of the white matter has developed.[70] Sequential studies are required in infants with SEHs-IVHs to diagnose posthemorrhagic ventricular dilatation in the silent phase.

ECHO is the most reliable technique to diagnose and follow changes in the ventricular size and in the intraventricular clots (Figs. 19-11 to 19-13). IVHs-SEHs resolve in several days or weeks, depending on the size of the bleed and on the individual patient. Although intraventricular clots are easily detected by CT, as they resolve the concentration of hemoglobin decreases and they are not seen after 10 to 14 days in CT studies.[4,32,58,59]

Intraventricular clots undergo characteristic changes with time. Initially they are very echogenic, then low echogenic areas appear. Eventually they become completely cystic with visualization of the choroid plexus inside the cystic ventricular cast (Figs. 19-12 and 19-13). Large cystic intraventricular clots may cause persistent ventricular dilatation despite drainage of the CSF by a ventriculoperitoneal shunt (Fig. 19-13).

Intraparenchymal hemorrhages. Intraparenchymal hemorrhages (IPHs) complicate SEHs-IVHs in approximately 15% to 25% of the infants.[46,70] IPHs are a severe complication since they indicate that the brain parenchyma has been destroyed. Although IPHs originally were considered to be an extension of SEHs-IVHs, recent evidence suggests that this lesion may actually be a primary infarction of the periventricular and subcortical white matter with destruction of the lateral wall of the ventricle. When the necrotic tissue liquefies, the IVH extends into the necrotic areas.[69]

Intraparenchymal hemorrhages appear as very echogenic zones in the white matter adjacent to the lateral ventricles. Echogenic areas in the white matter may correspond to IPHs or to hemorrhagic infarctions or extensive periventricular leukomalacia. In the classic grade IV IPH there is a clot extending from the white matter into the ventricular cavity (Figs. 19-15 to 19-18). Intraparenchymal clots follow the same evolution as intraventricular clots. A few days after the acute bleeding the clots become cystic and are reabsorbed completely in 3 or 4 weeks, leaving a cavity communicating with the lateral ventricle (porencephalic cyst) (Figs. 19-15 to 19-18).

When SEHs-IVHs associated with IPH evolve to posthemorrhagic hydrocephalus, the increased intraventricular pressure is transmitted to the porencephalic cyst. Posthemorrhagic hydrocephalus associated with porencephaly is an indication for early ventriculoperitoneal shunt placement to minimize the deleterious effects of progressive compression and ischemia of the brain parenchyma (Figs. 19-15 and 19-16).

Subarachnoid hemorrhages. Subarachnoid hemorrhages (SAHs) may be isolated or secondary to IVHs-SEHs. The etiology of isolated SAH is not clearly understood. Birth trauma and hypoxia/asphyxia have been considered the most probable causes.[70] In the case of IVHs-SEHs,

Text continued on p. 376.

CORONAL PLANE

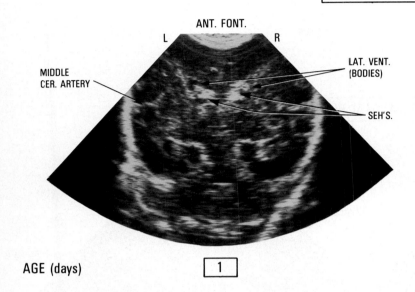

ANT. FONT.

L R

MIDDLE CER. ARTERY

LAT. VENT. (BODIES)

SEH'S.

AGE (days) 1

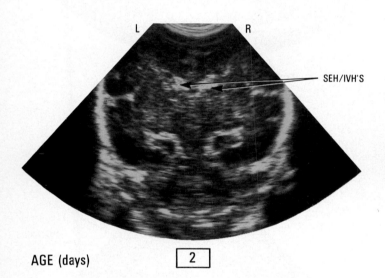

L R

SEH/IVH'S

AGE (days) 2

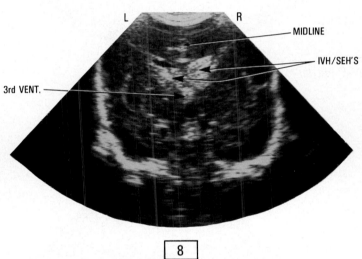

L R

MIDLINE

IVH/SEH'S

3rd VENT.

8

FIG. 19-11. Sequential studies showing the slow extension of a small SEH-IVH. The infant had small SEHs-IVHs bilaterally, which progressed to large SEHs-IVHs. Note the dilatation of the ventricles by the intraventricular clots, the cystic transformation of the intraventricular casts with the choroid plexus inside, and the initiation of posthemorrhagic ventricular enlargement by CSF.

L R

MIDLINE

SEH

IVH

3rd VENT.

INF. HORN

19

PARASAGITTAL PLANE

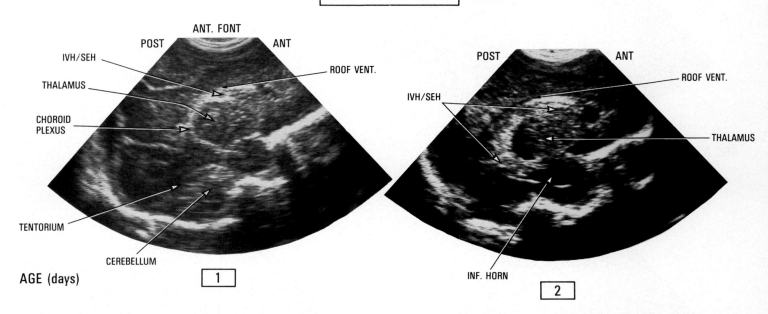

AGE (days) ☐1☐

☐2☐

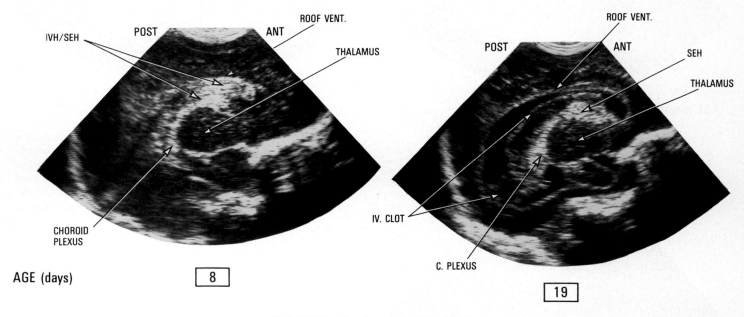

AGE (days) ☐8☐

☐19☐

FIG. 19-12. See legend for Fig. 19-11.

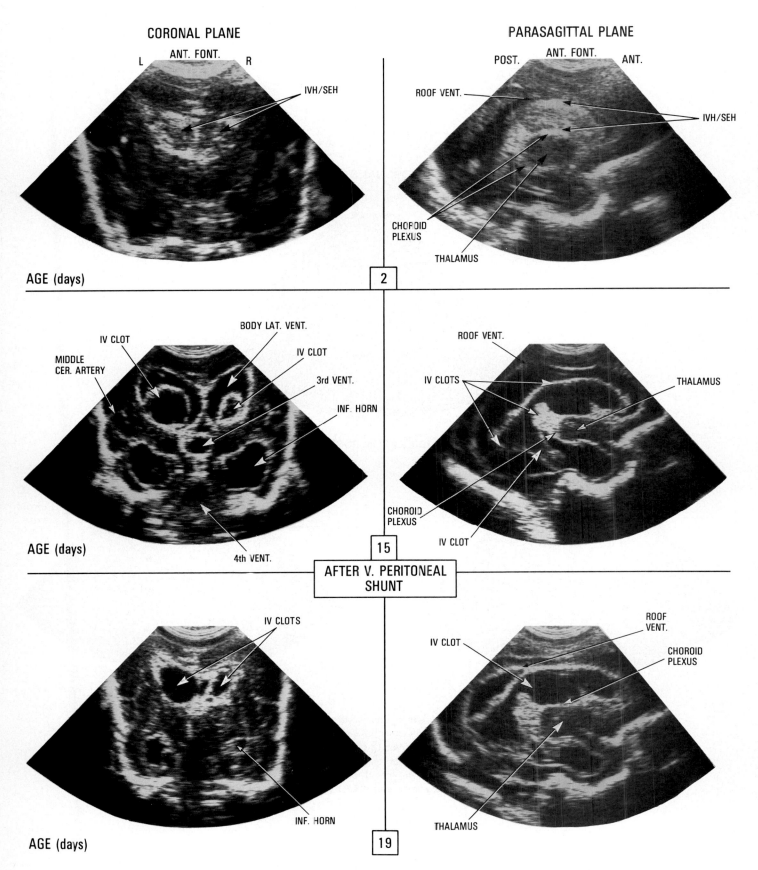

FIG. 19-13. Large IVH/SEH, posthemorrhagic hydrocephalus, and changes in the size of the ventricles produced by a ventriculoperitoneal shunt (VPS). The ventricles are filled with very echogenic material (blood) and distended by cerebral spinal fluid. Note that the ventricular cast appears "anchored" to the choroid plexus and the caudate nucleus. A VPS reduced significantly the size of the ventricular cavities draining practically all the CSF; however, the ventricles remained dilated by the intraventricular clots.

CORONAL STUDY

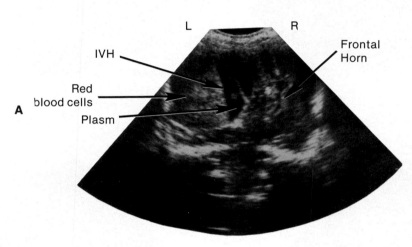

AXIAL STUDIES FROM POST FONTANELLE

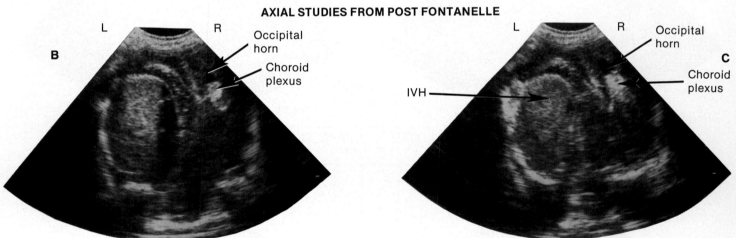

Head lying on left side

After turning to the right side

FIG. 19-14.   Very large acute IVH. The coronal and axial images show a very large IVH in the left side. The intraventricular blood is liquid because of a sedimentation of the red blood cells. In images **A** and **B,** the infant's head was lying over the left side. Image **C** was obtained immediately after turning the head to the right side. In this image the separation between red blood cells and plasma is lost because of the mixing of the red blood cells and plasma. These images are clear evidence that real-time echoencephalography can detect unclotted blood in the cerebral ventricular system.

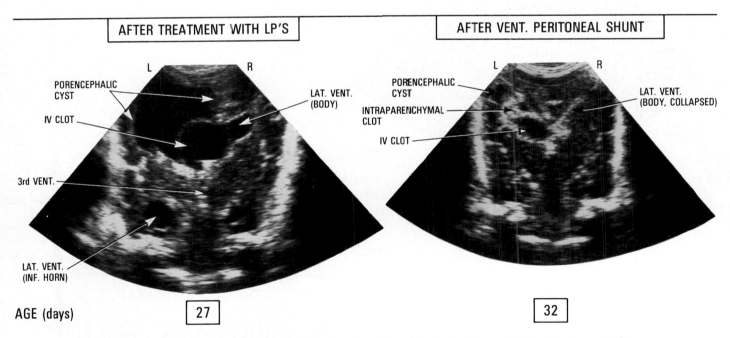

FIG. 19-15. Coronal, sagittal, parasagittal, and axial studies in a preterm infant with large IVH/ SEH, extensive IPH, posthemorrhagic hydrocephalus, and porencephaly. Note the unique clot extending from the ventricle into the brain parenchyma and the changes in the intraparenchymal clot with the development of a large porencephalic cyst. The cyst communicates with the body of the left lateral ventricle. The parasagittal studies through the lateral wall of the ventricle and the axial views were useful to define precisely the extension of the IPH and the porencephalic cyst. A VPS produced significant reduction of the ventricular size and the porencephalic cyst.

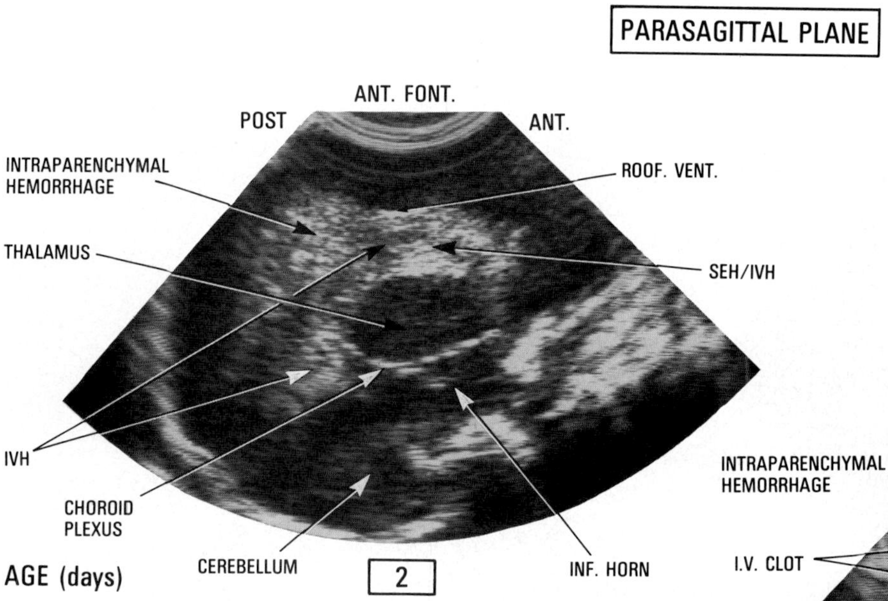

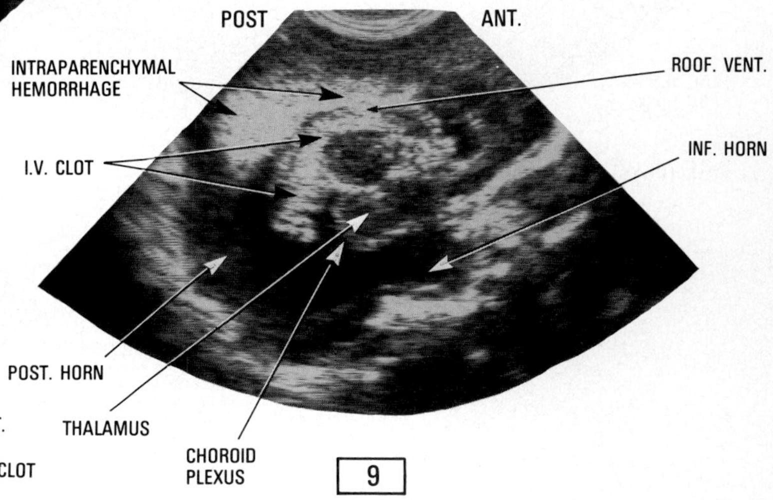

PARASAGITTAL PLANE

ANT. FONT.

POST   ANT.

INTRAPARENCHYMAL
HEMORRHAGE   ROOF. VENT.

THALAMUS   SEH/IVH

IVH

CHOROID
PLEXUS

AGE (days)   CEREBELLUM   2   INF. HORN

POST   ANT.

INTRAPARENCHYMAL
HEMORRHAGE   ROOF. VENT.

I.V. CLOT   INF. HORN

POST. HORN

THALAMUS

CHOROID
PLEXUS   9

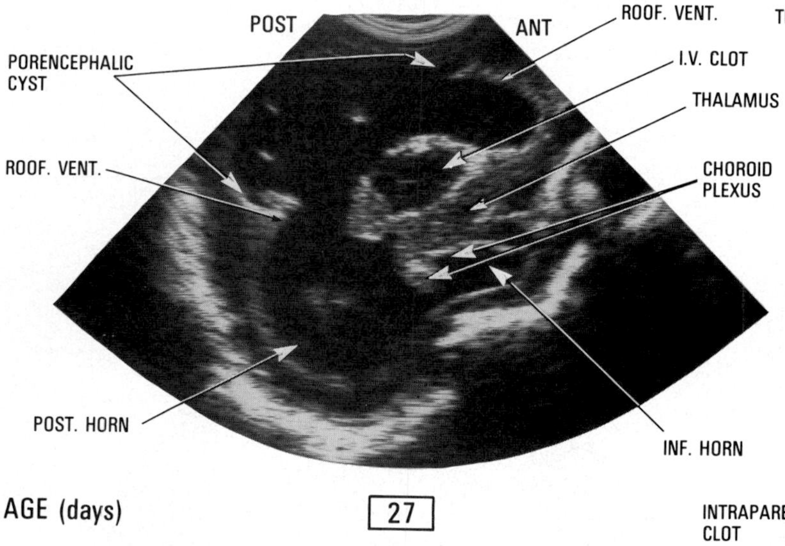

POST   ANT.   ROOF. VENT.

PORENCEPHALIC
CYST   I.V. CLOT

                                                THALAMUS

ROOF. VENT.   CHOROID
                                                PLEXUS

POST. HORN

AGE (days)   27   INF. HORN

FIG. 19-16. See legend for Fig. 19-15.

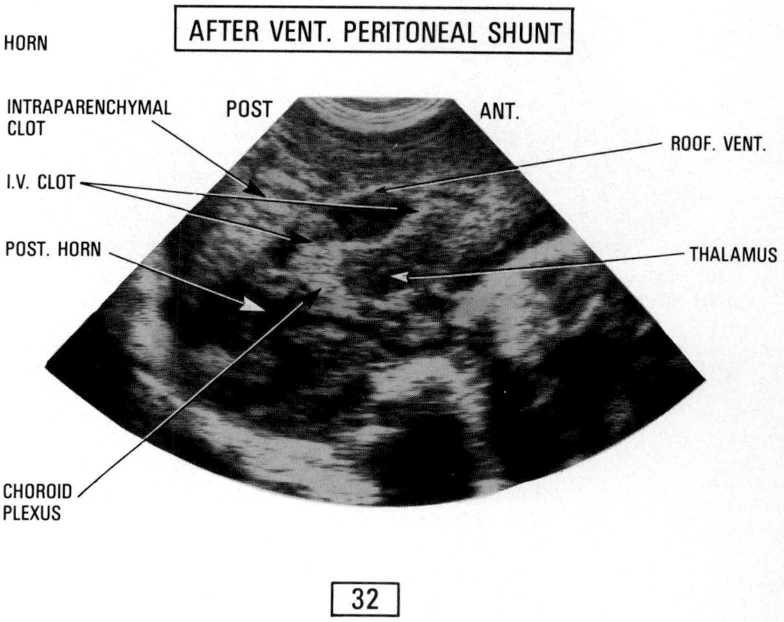

AFTER VENT. PERITONEAL SHUNT

INTRAPARENCHYMAL
CLOT   POST   ANT.

I.V. CLOT   ROOF. VENT.

POST. HORN   THALAMUS

CHOROID
PLEXUS   32

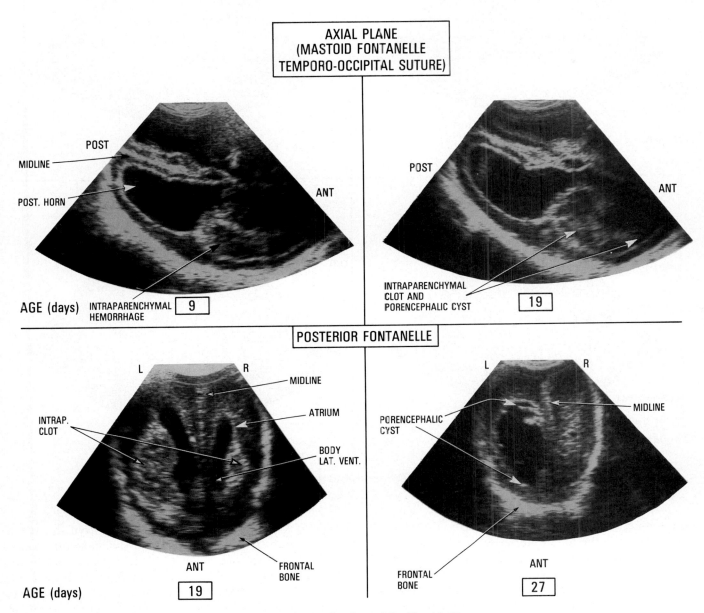

FIG. 19-17.   See legend for Fig. 19-15.

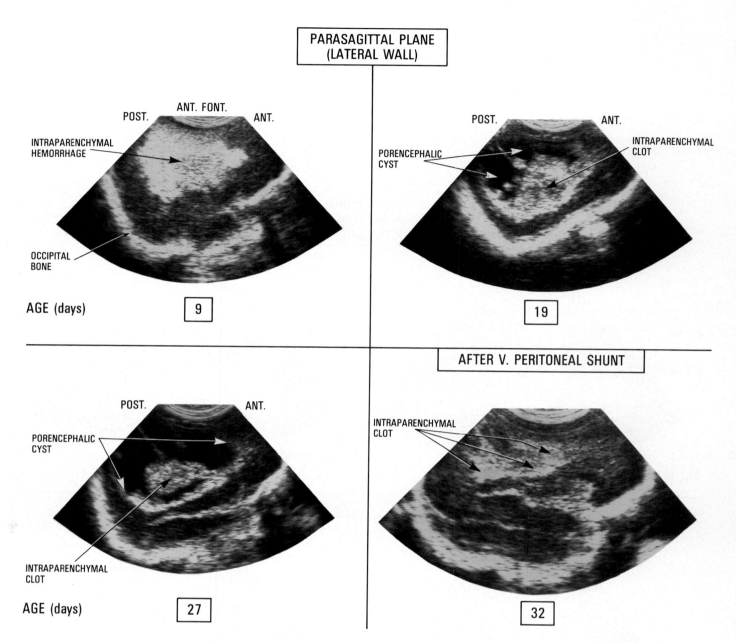

FIG. 19-18. See legend for Fig. 19-15.

blood coming from the germinal matrix or the choroid plexus collects in the infratentorial subarachnoid cisterns (cisterna magna and supracerebellar cistern). The blood may extend to the subarachnoid space surrounding the convexity of the cerebral hemispheres. The diagnosis of SAHs is important, inasmuch as obstruction of the CSF pathways may occur with subsequent development of hydrocephalus or transitory ventricular dilatation.

Subarachnoid hemorrhages are characterized by strong echoes in the anechoic subarachnoid space.[9,28] Increased echogenicity in the Sylvian fissure has been considered diagnostic of SAH. However, this criterion is associated with high incidence of false negative and false positive diagnoses. SAHs can be diagnosed easily if the cisterns in the posterior fossa are studied. Scanning the posterior fossa in the coronal, modified coronal, and sagittal planes, and from the neck enables unequivocal diagnosis of SAHs

(Figs. 19-19 and 19-20). Blood coming from the ventricles may obstruct the aqueduct of Sylvium and the foramina of Luschka and Magendie. Bicompartmental hydrocephalus may develop, since the fourth ventricle has choroid plexus. This process may lead to gigantic dilatation of the fourth ventricle with displacement and compression of the brain stem (Fig. 19-20).

Intracerebellar hemorrhages. Four categories of intracerebellar hemorrhage have been described:
- Primary intracerebellar hemorrhage
- Venous infarction
- Traumatic laceration due to occipital diastasis
- Extension to the cerebellum of a large SEH-IVH

In premature neonates there are areas of germinal matrix located around the fourth ventricle in the cerebellar hemispheres. The cerebellar germinal matrix has the same vulnerability to hemorrhage as the telencephalic germinal

LARGE SAH IN THE CISTERNA MAGNA

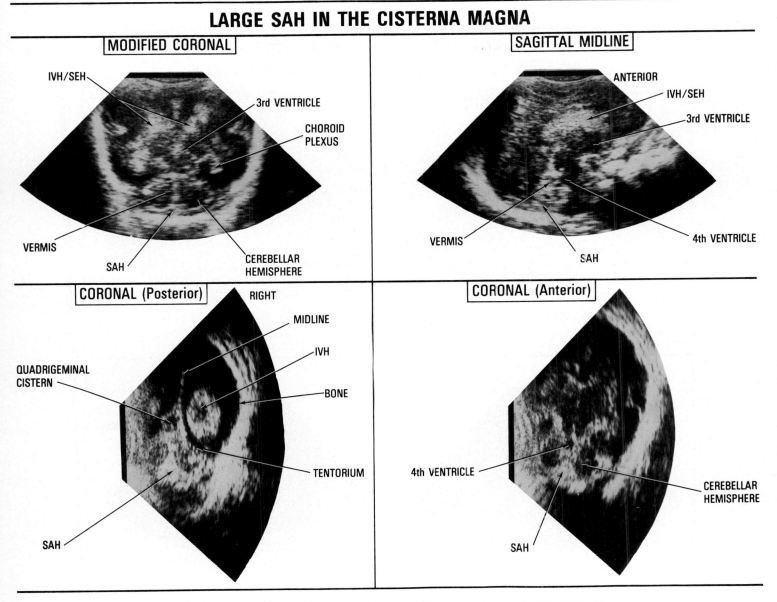

FIG. 19-19.   Large SAHs in the posterior fossa in two premature infants with IVHs-SEHs. The coronal studies of the posterior fossa through the mastoid fontanelle were useful to diagnose SAH in the first patient. Note the increased echogenicity in the cisterna magna and in the supracerebellar cistern. In the second patient the fourth ventricle enlarged acutely. Lumbar punctures decompressed transiently the fourth ventricle without significant change in the size of the lateral ventricles. By 19 days the fourth ventricle was gigantic, displacing the brain stem anteriorly. A ventriculoperitoneal shunt corrected the hydrocephalus but failed to reduce the size of the fourth ventricle, indicating bicompartmental hydrocephalus.

matrix. Intracerebellar hemorrhages have been reported in approximately 5% to 10% of postmortem studies of neonatal populations.[70] The incidence in live infants is significantly lower. This discrepancy is probably a result of the difficulties in diagnosing these hemorrhages.

Using modified coronal, sagittal, and parasagittal views of the posterior fossa (infratentorial compartment), it is possible to diagnose unequivocally intracerebellar hemorrhages.[9] These hemorrhages appear as very echogenic structures inside the less echogenic cerebellar paren-

chyma. Coronal views through the mastoid fontanelle may be essential to differentiate intracerebellar hemorrhages from large SAHs in the cisterna magna and/or in the supracerebellar cistern. Intracerebellar hemorrhages become cystic with time, leaving cavitary lesions in the cerebellar hemispheres. These characteristic sequential changes are useful in making a positive diagnosis of intracerebellar hemorrhages (Figs. 19-21 and 19-22).

Epidural hemorrhages and subdural collections. Epidural hemorrhages and subdural fluid collections are

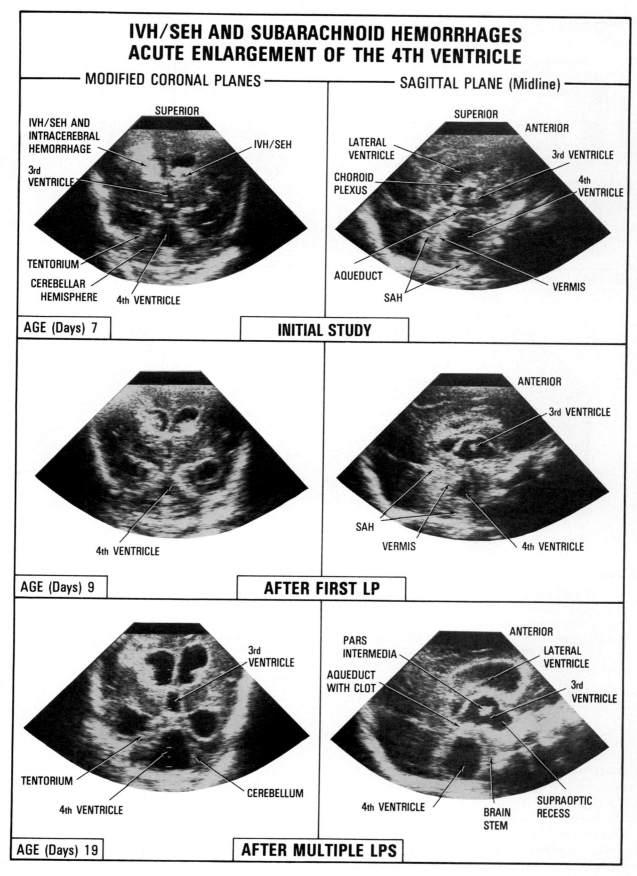

FIG. 19-20.   See legend for Fig. 19-19.

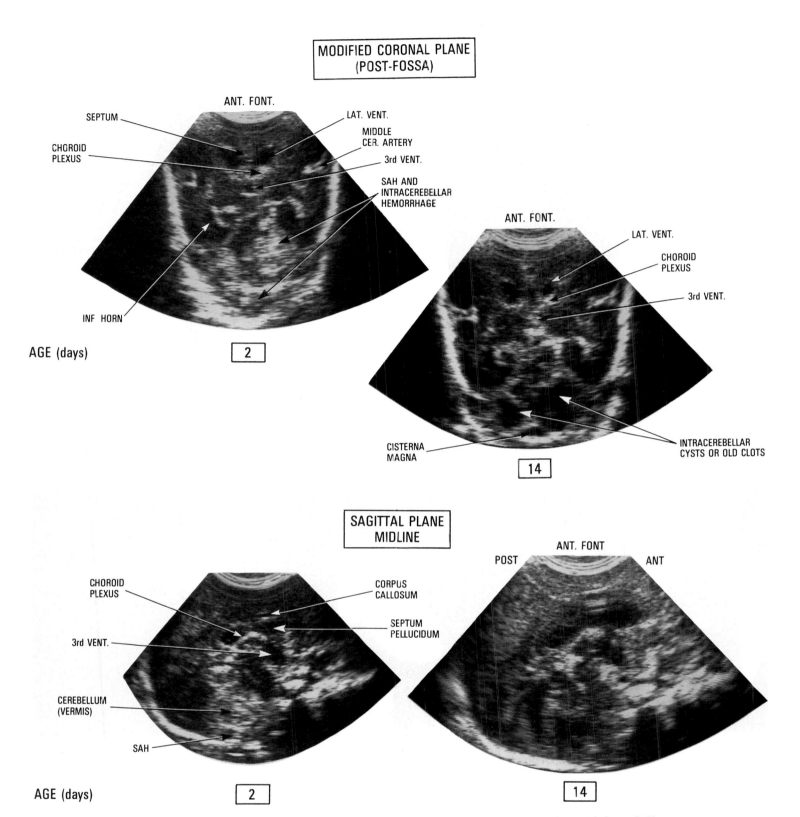

FIG. 19-21. Postmortem ultrasound and pathologic studies in a premature infant with large SAH in the posterior fossa and extensive intracerebellar hemorrhages (hemorrhagic infarctions). The modified coronal and sagittal studies found an enlarged posterior fossa occupied by very echogenic material. Simultaneous studies in the coronal plane from the mastoid fontanelle through the cerebellar hemispheres found intracerebellar hemorrhages. Note the changes in the echogenicity of the intracerebellar hemorrhages with time. *Continued.*

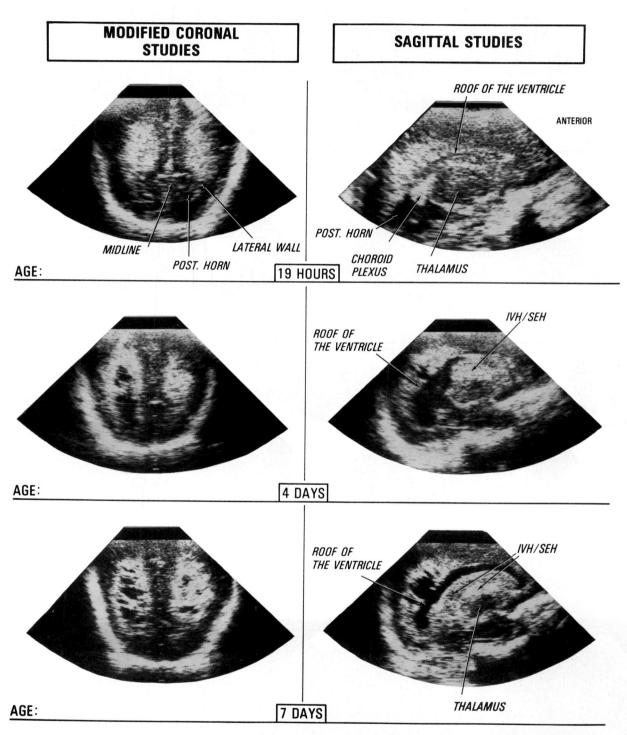

FIG. 19-28. Antenatal multifocal white matter necrosis. Cavitary lesions appear in the very echogenic white matter by the fourth day after delivery, indicating that the brain was damaged prenatally.

CORONAL PLANE

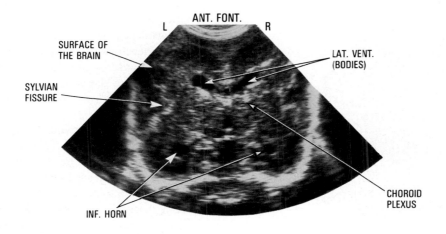

MODIFIED CORONAL PLANE

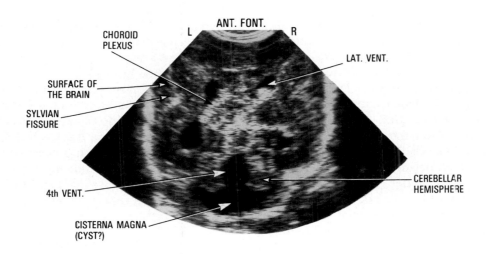

SAGITTAL PLANE (MIDLINE)   **PARASAGITTAL PLANE**

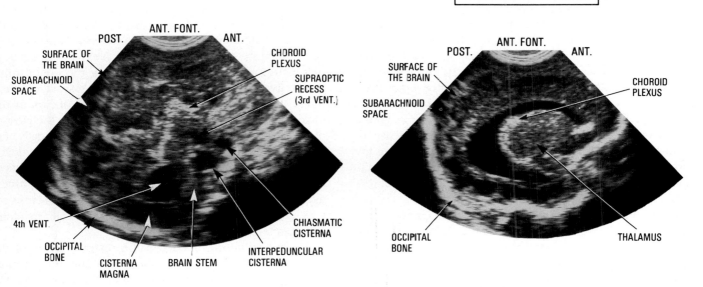

FIG. 19-29. Brain atrophy. Note the enlargement of the subarachnoid space, the widening of the Sylvian fissure, and the cisterns associated with moderate dilatation of the lateral ventricles. This patient had cerebellar infarctions imitating a Dandy-Walker malformation.   *Continued.*

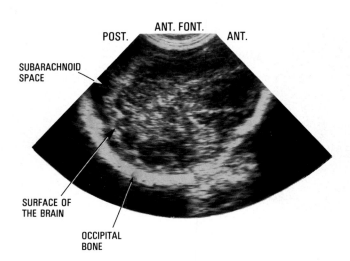

PARASAGITTAL PLANE (EXTERIOR)

ANT. FONT.

POST. ANT.

SUBARACHNOID SPACE

SURFACE OF THE BRAIN

OCCIPITAL BONE

FIG. 19-29, cont'd. Brain atrophy.

The chronic stage of WMN is identified with ultrasound when echolucencies develop in the echogenic white matter (Figs. 19-24 to 19-28). Pathologic studies have confirmed that echolucent lesions correspond to cavitary lesions in the white matter.[11,51] The presence of echolucencies is prima facie evidence that necrotic injury exists in the cerebral white matter. Echodensities alone suggest, but do not prove, that the echodense white matter is necrotic. The absence of cystic lesions in the echoencephalogram precludes definitive diagnosis of WMN. Since very echogenic white matter can be simply congestion without coagulation, and in fact not necessarily white matter necrosis at all, careful sequential observations must be performed to identify cavitary lesions developing in the echodense white matter. Cystic lesions in WMN may be microscopic or smaller than the resolution of the ultrasound scanners. Consequently WMN may exist in the absence of cavitary lesions in the sonograms.

Both neuropathologic and echoencephalographic studies have shown that a period of 1 to 6 weeks ensues between the acute stage of WMN and the development of cystic lesions. Echogenic areas and cysts decrease in size and eventually disappear 2 to 5 months after the diagnosis of acute necrosis. If the necrosis was extensive, brain atrophy may be the only indication that WMN occurred during the perinatal period. ECHO is also useful to diagnose the atrophic phase of the chronic stage. This phase is identified by an enlarged subarachnoid space, widened interhemispheric fissure, and persistent ventricular dilatation in an infant with a normal or small head circumference (Fig. 19-29).

Using cavitary lesions as the criteria to diagnose white matter necrosis, Bejar et al.[13] found that WMN is present in 17% of premature infants less than 34 weeks gestation. Approximately half of the patients had cavitary lesions at birth or during the first four postpartum days, indicating that the onset of these lesions occurred antenatally (Figs. 19-29 and 19-30). The remainder of the infants had echogenic areas in the white matter during the first postpartum week, and cavitary lesions developed between 10 and 27 days after delivery. Since the cavities appeared after the first postpartum week, the white matter necrosis was considered to have a postnatal onset (Figs. 19-24 to 19-27). Therefore WMN can be classified as either antenatal white matter necrosis, when the cavities appear at birth or prior to day four, or as postnatal white matter necrosis when cavities develop after the fourth postpartum day.

Focal brain necrosis. These necrotic lesions occur within the distribution of large arteries. This complication is present in term and preterm infants, but it is infrequent under 30 weeks gestational age.[7,70] Vascular maldevelopment, asphyxia/hypoxia, embolism from the placenta, infectious diseases, thromboembolism secondary to disseminated intravascular coagulation, and polycythemia have been implicated as etiologic factors in this condition.[62,70] These insults may occur prenatally or early in postnatal life, leading subsequently to the dissolution of the cerebral tissues and formation of cavitary lesions. The term porencephaly is used to describe a single cavity, multicystic encephalomalacia for multiple cavities, and hydranencephaly for a large single cavity with entire disappearance of the cerebral hemispheres.[62,70]

The images observed with ECHO in these injuries are very echogenic localized lesions within the distribution of the major vessel. The echodense lesions are considered to correspond to cerebral infarctions (Figs. 19-30 to 19-33). After several days echolucencies will appear within the echogenic areas. Subsequently the infarcted regions will be replaced by cavities that may or may not communicate with the ventricle (Fig. 19-32).

DISORDERS OF BRAIN DEVELOPMENT

Major events occur during the development of the brain.[70,71] Dorsal induction refers to the changes occurring in the dorsal aspect of the embryo by which the brain and the spinal cord are formed. The first step in the formation of the neural plate on the dorsum of the embryo is the differentiation of the ectoderm. This occurs at approximately 18 days of gestation. Next the margins of this plate invaginate and close, forming the neural tube. Distinctive portions of the neural tube fuse at different times. The first fusion of the neural folds occurs in the lower medulla at approximately 22 days. Then the closure of the neural tube progresses rostrally and caudally, finishing at 24 to 26 days. The cellular differentiation develops from 28 to 32 days, forming the definitive segments of the medulla. Disruption of this developmental process may result in malformations such as craniorachischisis totalis, anencephaly, myeloschisis, encephalocele, myelomeningocele, and Arnold-Chiari.[70,71]

Ventral induction occurs in the rostral portion of the embryo at 5 to 6 weeks gestation, resulting in the formation of the face and forebrain. After the closure of the neural tube there is segmentation of the forebrain with subsequent development of two lateral extensions: the

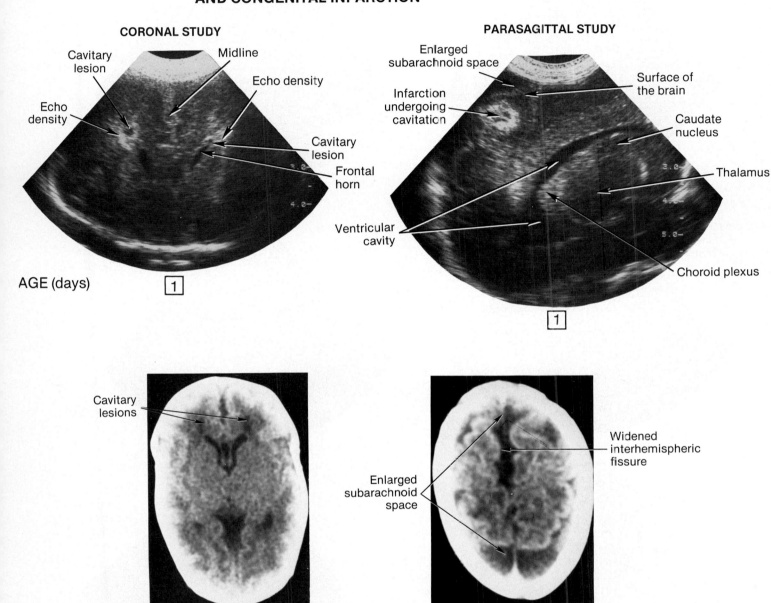

FIG. 19-30.   Antenatal infarction in the subcortical white matter of the left parietal lobe in a premature infant born with antenatal white matter necrosis and brain atrophy. Echodense areas in the periventricular white matter associated with cavitary lesions were detected in the first echoencephalogram on day 1. Sagittal studies on the same day showed an area of increased echogenicity with echolucencies in the subcortical white matter of the left parietal lobe. Note the enlargement of the subarachnoid space. CT studies showed cavitary lesions in the frontal lobes and extensive enlargement of the subarachnoid space, indicating brain atrophy.

LARGE INFARCTION IN THE FRONTAL LOBE

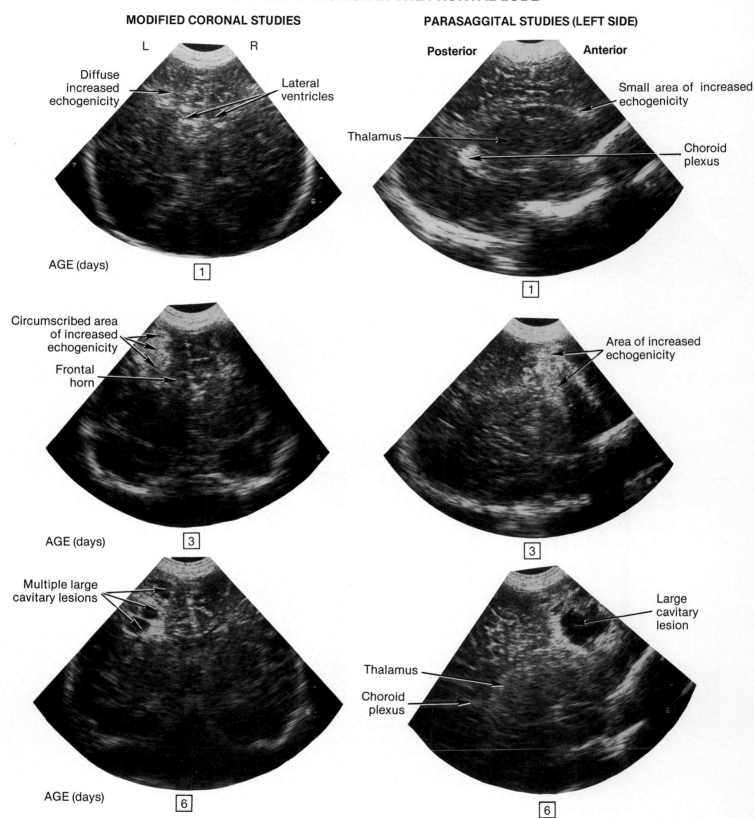

MODIFIED CORONAL STUDIES

PARASAGGITAL STUDIES (LEFT SIDE)

FIG. 19-31. Large infarction in the frontal lobe. Echoencephalogram on day one shows diffuse increased echogenicity in the frontal lobes without clear visualization of the lateral ventricles, which appear collapsed. Two days later the subcortical and deep white matter in the left frontal lobe is more echogenic. A circumscribed area of increased echogenicity is clearly seen. By day 6 large cavitary lesions had developed in the echogenic white matter. Since large cavitary lesions were present on day 6, it is quite possible that the initial insult to the brain occurred antenatally.

CORONAL STUDIES

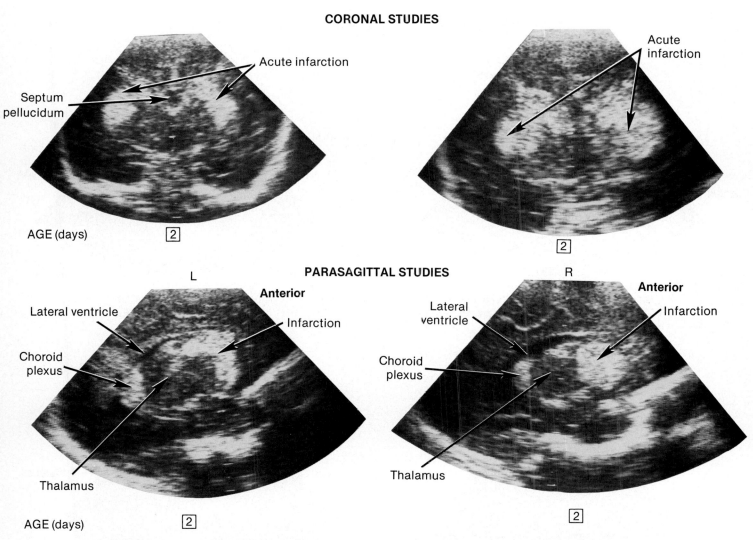

FIG. 19-32. Necrosis in the internal capsule and basal ganglia. Note the location and "commalike" shape of the echogenic areas. Compare the location and shape of these echodensities with the echogenic areas shown in patients with multifocal white matter necrosis. Parasagittal studies are useful to identify the location of the necrotic zones, which in this patient includes the caudate nuclei, the internal capsule, the anterior nuclei of the thalami, and quite possibly the globus pallidus.

telencephalon and an interior structure, the diencephalon. Diverticulation of these extensions will form the cerebral hemispheres from the telencephalon, and the basal ganglia and third ventricle from the diencephalon. Disturbance of this process may cause holoprosencephaly, holotelencephaly, and faciotelencephalic malformations.[70,71]

ECHO has been found useful in the diagnosis of the following malformations.

Arnold-Chiari malformation

Arnold-Chiari malformation is characterized by the following:

- Displacement of the fourth ventricle and upper medulla into the cervical canal
- Displacement of the inferior part of the cerebellum through the foramen magnum
- Defects in the calvarium and spinal column

Arnold-Chiari malformation is frequently associated with myelomeningocele, hydrocephalus, dilatation of the third ventricle, and absence of the septum pellucidum. Eighty-five percent to ninety percent of infants with myelomeningocele have Arnold-Chiari malformations. Hydrocephalus is usually caused by obstruction of the CSF pathway at the fourth ventricle or in the posterior fossa, or secondary to aqueductal stenosis, which is present in 40% to 75% of infants with Arnold-Chiari malformations.*

Arnold-Chiari malformation can be correctly diagnosed with ECHO. Sagittal studies from the anterior fontanelle show a small cerebellum, absence of the cisterna magna, low position of the fourth ventricle, and displacement of the cerebellum through the foramen magnum associated with hydrocephalus, absence of the septum pellucidum, and widening of the third ventricle (Fig. 19-33).

---

*References 8, 34, 49, 56, 70, 71.

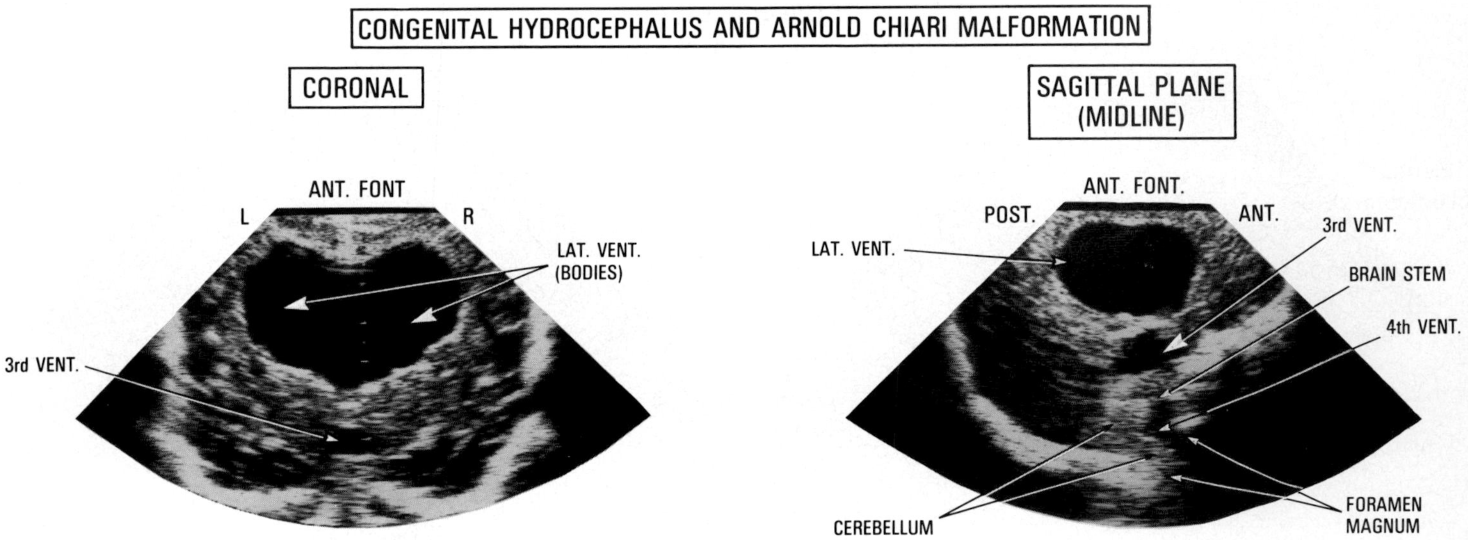

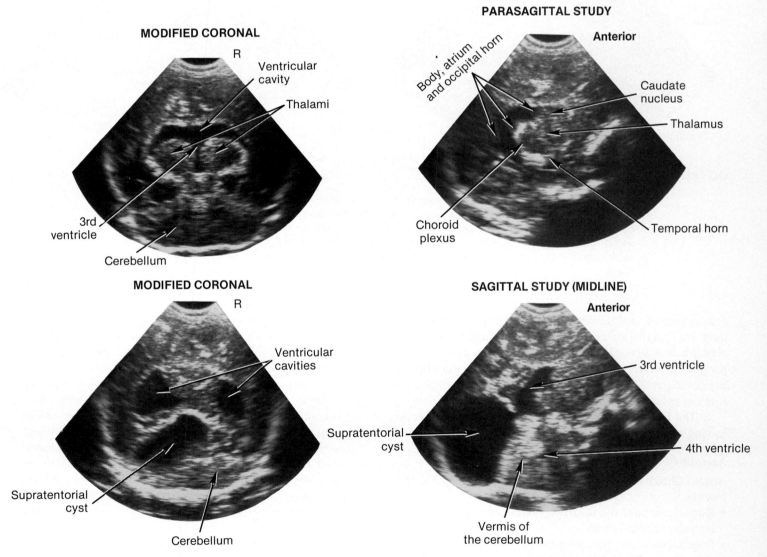

FIG. 19-33. Arnold-Chiari malformation. Note the low position of the fourth ventricle, the absence of the cisterna magna, and the extension of the inferior part of the cerebellum into the foramen magnum.

FIG. 19-34. Holoprosencephaly. Note the crescent shape of the central cavity extending into the third ventricle, the absence of corpus callosum, septum pellucidum, and frontal horns (parasagittal studies), and the large supratentorial cyst protruding from the third ventricle.

Holoprosencephaly

Holoprosencephaly is caused by disturbances in the process of ventral induction very early in life. The neuropathologic features include a single cerebrum with single ventricular cavity, absence of the corpus callosum and frontal horns and a thin membrane arising from the roof of the third ventricle which may extend posteriorly forming a supratentorial cyst* (Fig. 19-34).

After the ventral induction has occurred, ischemic lesions in the midline may induce malformations of the telencephalon similar to holoprosencephaly. As in holoprosencephaly, there is a single ventricular cavitary and absence of the corpus callosum. However, the presence of two frontal horns helps in differentiating these malformations caused by ischemic lesions from true holoprosencephaly. When holoprosencephaly is suspected, it is important to obtain modified coronal studies of the whole frontal lobes to determine whether two frontal horns are present (Figs. 19-35 and 19-36).

Dandy-Walker malformation

The typical Dandy-Walker malformation is characterized by absence of the cerebellar vermis, cystic changes in the fourth ventricle with the development of a large cyst in the posterior fossa (Dandy-Walker cyst), and hydrocephalus. The hydrocephalus is caused by the atresia of the foramina of Luschka and Magendie (congenital obstructive hydrocephalus). When the vermis is absent, the fourth ventricle communicates directly with the cyst[34,44,59] (Fig. 19-37). A Dandy-Walker variant is present when there is an enlarged cisterna magna communicating with the fourth ventricle in the presence of a normal or hypoplastic cerebellar vermis (Fig. 19-38).

Agenesis of the corpus callosum

The corpus callosum is the great commissure connecting the brain hemispheres. Hypoplasia or agenesis of the corpus callosum may occur during the processes of ventral induction or cellular migration. Agenesis of the corpus callosum is often combined with migrational disorders such as heterotopias and polymicrogyria.[24,35,70,71] Absence of the corpus callosum may also be induced by ischemic lesions in the midline or by intrauterine encephalomalacia (Fig. 19-36). Other defects associated with this defect are porencephaly, hydrocephalus, microgyria, and fusion of the hemispheres.

Complete absence of the corpus callosum is distinguished by narrow frontal horns as well as marked separation of the anterior horns and bodies of the lateral ventricles associated with widening of the occipital horns and the third ventricle. The ventricular cavities acquire the distinctive appearance of "vampire wings." These characteristics are easily identified by ECHO (Figs. 19-39 and 19-40).

---

*References 8, 24, 34, 49, 56, 70, 71.

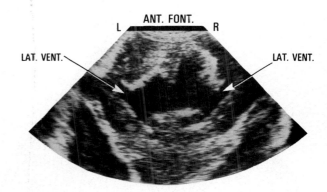

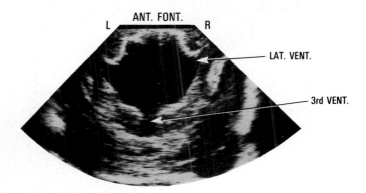

FIG. 19-35. Absence of the corpus callosum caused by a large midline infarction. Note the areas of increased echogenicity in the frontal lobes close to the midline. These echodense zones are associated with destruction of the corpus callosum and a large porencephalic cavity communicating with the lateral ventricles.

Congenital hydrocephalus

Hydrocephalus refers to any condition in which enlargement of the ventricular system is caused by an imbalance between production and reabsorption of CSF. When this instability ensues in the fetus, the widening of the ventricular system is present at birth. Infants born with ventricular enlargement are considered to have congenital hydrocephalus. Hydrocephalus is infrequently caused by overproduction of fluid. Excessive fluid production may occur in infants with papilloma of the choroid plexus, a tumor that actively secretes CSF.[45,47,71]

Two anatomic types of hydrocephalus are distinguished.

Obstructive hydrocephalus. This type of hydrocephalus is characterized by interference in the circulation of CSF within the ventricular system itself, causing subsequent enlargement of the ventricular cavities proximal to the obstruction.[70,71]

Communicant hydrocephalus. In this variety the CSF pathways are open within the ventricular system but there is decreased absorption of CSF. Absorption of CSF can be impeded by occlusion of the subarachnoid cisterns in the posterior fossa or the obliteration of the subarach-

Text continued on p. 399.

MULTIPLE INFARCTION CAUSING "FALSE" HOLOPROSENCEPHALY MALFORMATION

CORONAL STUDIES

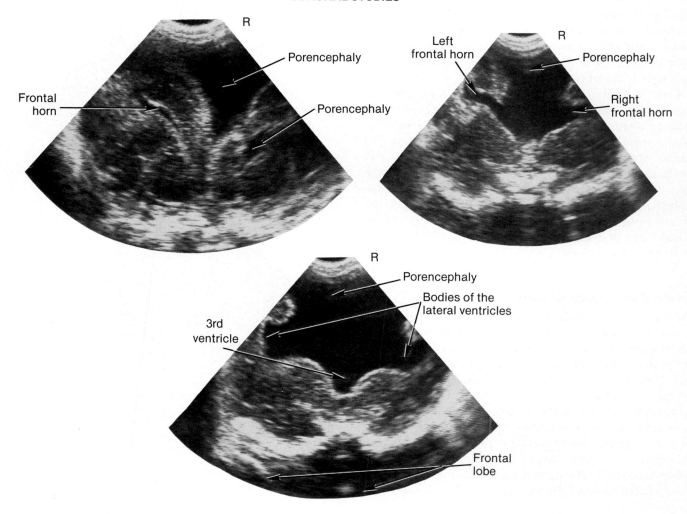

MODIFIED CORONAL STUDIES

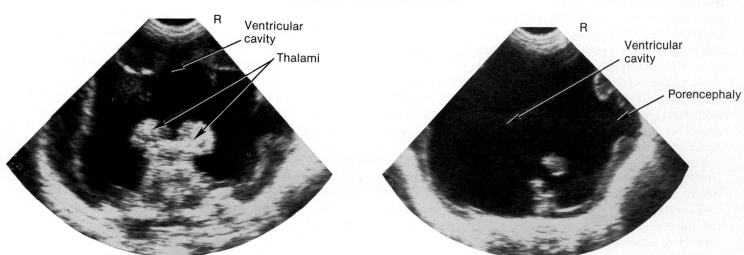

FIG. 19-36. Absence of the corpus callosum and holoprosencephaly-like brain caused by multiple infarctions. This patient has a more advanced stage of the necrotic process than the patient in Fig. 19-35. The difference between this patient and the patient in Fig. 19-34 (real holoprosencephaly) is that the brain in this illustration has remanents of midline structures and two frontal horns.

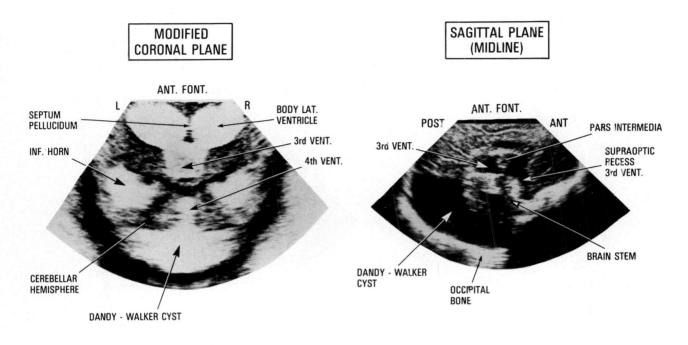

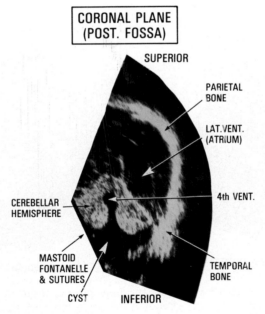

FIG. 19-37. Echoencephalograms in Dandy-Walker malformation. Note the posterior fossa cyst in the modified coronal and sagittal planes. The coronal studies show that the vermis was absent and that there was an open communication between the fourth ventricle and the cyst.

LARGE CISTERNA MAGNA

MODIFIED CORONAL STUDIES

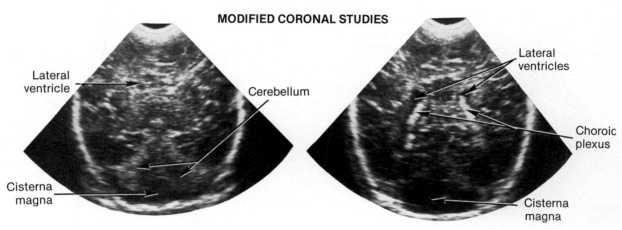

SAGITTAL STUDY (MIDLINE)   PARASAGITTAL STUDY

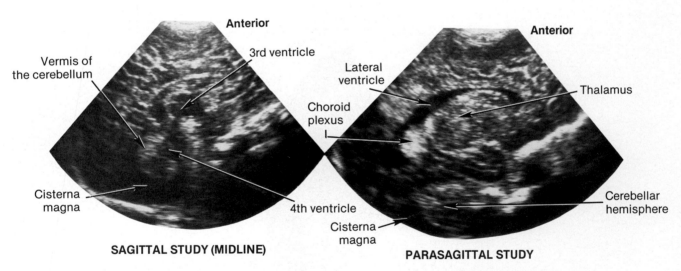

FIG. 19-38.   Redundant cisterna magna. Note the large cisterna magna in the posterior fossa. The enlarged cistern may be confused with a Dandy-Walker cyst. However, this patient has normal vermis and fourth ventricle, indicating that this is not a Dandy-Walker malformation.

AGENESIS OF THE CORPUS CALLOSUM

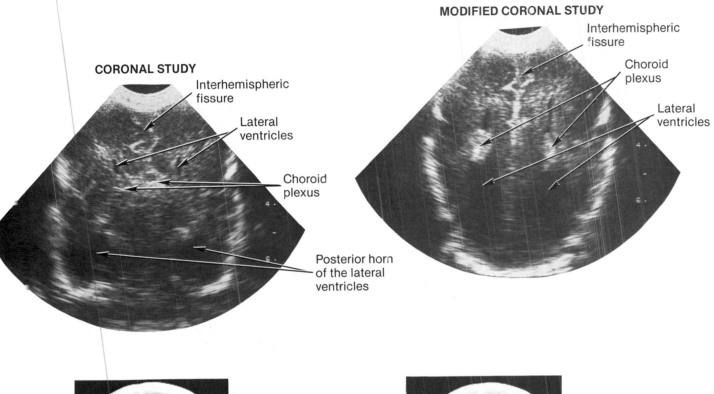

MODIFIED CORONAL STUDY

Interhemispheric fissure

Choroid plexus

Lateral ventricles

CORONAL STUDY

Interhemispheric fissure

Lateral ventricles

Choroid plexus

Posterior horn of the lateral ventricles

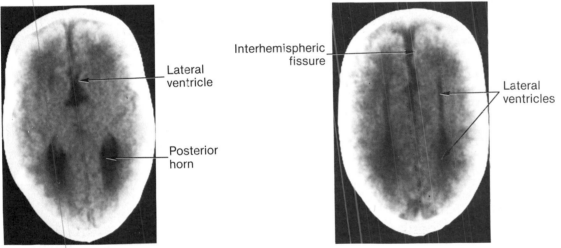

Lateral ventricle

Posterior horn

Interhemispheric fissure

Lateral ventricles

FIG. 19-39. Agenesis of the corpus callosum. Note the location and shape of the lateral ventricles. The ventricles are parallel to the midline. The interhemispheric fissure is widened, suggesting brain atrophy. The CT studies confirm the ultrasound diagnosis and show the enlarged third ventricle displaced upward and posteriorly.

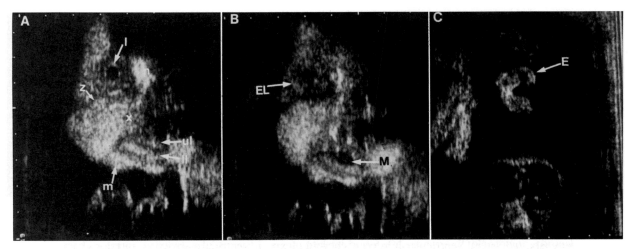

FIG. 20-17. **A,** Coronal view demonstrating facial features, *l,* lens; *z,* zygomatic bone; *x,* maxilla; *ul,* upper lip; *ll,* lower lip; *m,* mandible; *n,* nasal bones. **B,** Coronal view in same fetus obtained in a more anteriorly placed scan demonstrating the eyelid, *EL,* and mouth, *m.* **C,** Tangential view of the fetal ear, *E.*

lies the cisterna magna within the posterior fossa space (Fig. 20-15). Recognition of a normal posterior fossa aids in the detection of space-occupying masses and in the early detection of ventriculomegaly. Below this level the orbital rings and nasal bones are appreciated (Fig. 20-16).

Lower in the fetal head the anterior, middle, and posterior cranial fossae are observed within the base of the skull. The sphenoid bones create a V-shaped appearance as they divide the anterior fossa from the middle fossae with the petrous ridges further separating the middle fossae from the posterior fossa. At the junction of the sphenoid wings and petrous ridges, the area of the sella turcica (site of pituitary gland) can be identified.[25]

The face. Superior real-time imaging has allowed operators to explore facial anatomy in recent years. In addition to delineating minute details of facial architecture, ultrasound investigators have been exposed to an exciting new arena of facial imaging and behaviors. Facial expressions and movements (rapid eye movements, yawning) provide for an enlightening scanning session and may ultimately prove helpful in detecting abnormal behavioral states of the fetus.

Images of the face can be viewed as early as the late first trimester of pregnancy. Facial morphology becomes more apparent as the fetus develops. Remarkable clarity of facial features can be seen by the nineteenth to twenty-second weeks of pregnancy. The bony skeletal structures and soft tissue architecture of the face are visible during most obstetrical examinations.

ANATOMIC LANDMARKS OF THE FACIAL PROFILE. Images of the fetal forehead are achieved by viewing the facial profile. In this view the contour of the frontal bone, the nose, the upper and lower lips, and the chin are observed. Profile views of the fetal face are useful in determining the relationship of the nose to the lips and in the exclusion of forehead malformations (i.e., anterior cephaloceles) (see Fig. 23-15). Prominence of the forehead may be associated with certain forms of skeletal dysplasia (see Chapter 23).

ANATOMIC LANDMARKS OF THE CORONAL FACIAL VIEW. By placement of the transducer in a coronal scanning plane, sectioning through the face will reveal both orbital rings, the parietal bones, ethmoid bones, nasal septum, zygomatic bone, maxillae, and mandible (Fig. 20-17). Scans obtained in an anterior plane over the orbits will demonstrate the eyelids and, when directed posterior to this plane, the orbital lens (Fig. 20-17). The eyeglobes, hyaloid artery, and vitreous matter have been sonographically identified.[4]

The oral cavity and tongue are frequently outlined during fetal swallowing (Fig. 20-17). Tangential views of the face aid in differentiating the nostrils, nares, nasal septum, maxillae, and mandible (see Fig. 23-15). This view is helpful in the diagnosis of craniofacial anomalies such as cleft lip (see Chapter 23).

The fetal ears may be defined in the second trimester as lateral protuberances emerging from the parietal bones. Later in pregnancy the components of the external ear (pinna) may be seen[25] (Fig. 20-17). The semicircular canals and internal auditory meatus have been sonographically recognized.[25,39]

Fetal hair is often observed along the periphery of the skull.

The vertebral column. The anatomy of the vertebral column should be assessed in all fetuses referred for obstetrical evaluation. A gross anatomic survey of the spine should be attempted to exclude major spinal malformations (i.e., meningomyelocele) (see Chapter 23).

The fetal spine is studied in either sagittal or transverse scanning planes. In a sagittal section the spine will appear as two curvilinear lines extending from the cervical spine to the sacrum. The normal fetal spine tapers near the sacrum and widens near the base of the skull (Fig. 20-18). This double line appearance of the spine is referred to as the "railway" sign and is generated by echoes from the posterior and anterior laminae and spinal cord.[33]

When the scanning plane cross-sects both laminae and equal amounts of tissue are noted on either side of the spinal echoes, the transverse processes and vertebral bod-

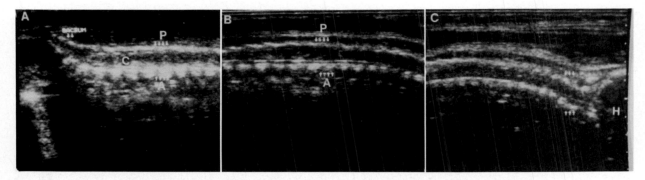

FIG. 20-18. Sagittal sections of the lumbosacral, **A**, thoracic, **B**, and cervical, **C**, spine in a 37-week fetus displaying the "railway" sign produced by the anterior, *A*, and posterior, *P*, laminae. Note the tapering of the spine at the sacrum and the widening at the entrance into the base of the skull, *H.* Between the laminae lies the spinal canal, *C.* Frequently the spinal cord is outlined as a linear echo coursing through the center of the canal.

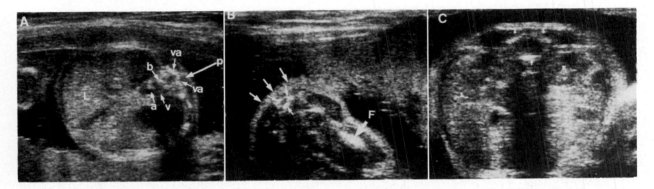

FIG. 20-19. Transverse scans of the vertebral column demonstrating the echogenic ring produced by the vertebral body and laminae. **A**, Thoracic vertebrae with typical landmarks. *L*, liver; *a,* aorta; *v,* vertebral body; *va*-vertebral arch; *p,* posterior vertebral muscles. **B**, Sacral vertebra outlined *(small arrows)*. Note the intact posterior wall found in the normal fetus *(large arrows)*. *F.* femur. **C**, Transverse view through the spine at the level of the kidney, *K,* demonstrating the closed circle appearance *(arrows)* of the spine created by the intact vertebral arch. *L*, liver.

ies are delineated.[33] This is the appropriate plane in which to screen for spinal defects.[33]

In a transverse plane the spinal column will appear as an echogenic closed circle. The circle of echoes represents the center of the vertebral body, the pedicles, and the posterior ossification center[19] (Fig. 20-19). These elements should be identified in the normal fetus while the pedicles will appear splayed in a V-, C- or U-shaped configuration and the posterior ossification echo (vertebral arch) will be absent in a fetus with a spinal defect (see Chapter 23).

When evaluating the spine, it is imperative for the sonographer to align the transducer in a perpendicular axis to the spinal elements. Incorrect angles may falsely indicate an abnormality. The spinal muscles and posterior skin border can be viewed posterior to the circular ring of the ossification centers (Fig. 20-19). It is important to note the integrity of the skin surface as this membrane will be absent in fetuses with open spina bifida. Inspection of the spine is often technically difficult when the fetus is lying with the spine down. The optimal viewing of the spine occurs when the fetus is lying on its side in a transverse direction.

The thorax. Although the respiratory system of the fetus is nonfunctional inutero, the fetal lungs are important landmarks to routinely visualize within the thoracic cavity. The lungs serve as lateral borders for the heart and therefore are useful landmarks in assessing the relationship and position of the heart with the chest. Identification of fetal lung location is beneficial in observing fetal breathing movements that are centered over the diaphragm and chest. In addition, like many fetal organs, the lungs are subject to abnormal development. Lung size, texture, and location should be assessed routinely to exclude a lung mass.

The fluid-filled fetal lungs are observed as solid homogeneous masses of tissue bordered medially by the heart, inferiorly by the diaphragm, and laterally by the rib cage (Fig. 20-20). As the heart occupies a midline position within the chest, displacement of the heart warrants further study to exclude a possible mass of the lung that may deviate the position of the heart (see Chapter 23).

In sagittal views of the thorax, lung tissue is present superior to the diaphragm and lateral to the heart (Fig. 20-20). Investigators have attempted to define textural variations of the lung in comparison to the liver.[2] Fetal

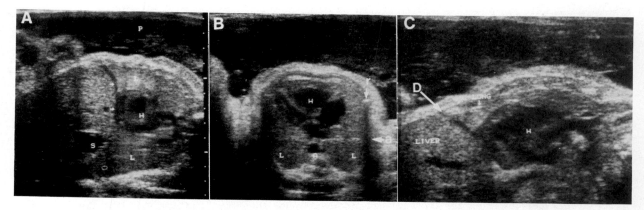

FIG. 20-20. **A,** Sagittal scan depicting the homogeneous lungs located lateral to the heart, *H,* and superior to the diaphragm *(arrows).* Note the normal placement of the stomach, *S,* inferior to the diaphragm. *P,* placenta. **B,** Transverse section, in same fetus, demonstrating the position of the lungs, *L,* in relation to the heart, *H.* Note the apex of the heart to the left side of the chest. The base of the heart is in the midline and anterior to the aorta, *A.* Displacement of the heart should alert the investigator to search for a mass of the lung, heart, or diaphragm. Note the rib, *r,* and corresponding acoustic shadow, *a.* **C,** In the late third trimester of pregnancy the lung tissue can be seen and compared to the liver texture, which is located inferior to the diaphragm, *D. H,* heart.

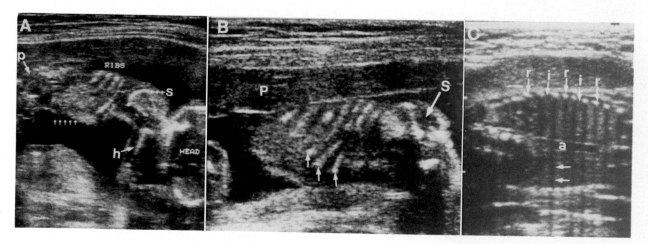

FIG. 20-21. **A,** Sagittal view demonstrating the ribcage, scapula, *S,* anterior abdominal wall *(arrows),* and humerus, *h,* in a fetus in a back-up position. *p,* pelvis. **B,** Tangential view depicting the length of the ribs *(arrows). P,* placenta; *S,* shoulder. **C,** Sagittal representation of the ribcage. Note that the sound waves will not pass through the bony rib; therefore a "dropout" of sound *(arrows)* occurs posterior to the rib. Sound will pass through the intercostal space, *i. a,* aorta.

lung tissue will appear more dense than the liver as pregnancy progresses.

The ribs, scapulae, and clavicles are bony landmarks of the chest cavity. As these structures are composed of bone, acoustic shadowing occurs posterior to these landmarks. The entire rib cage may be identified when sections are obtained through the posterior aspects of the spine and rib cage (Fig. 20-21). Oblique sectioning of the ribs will reveal the total length of the ribs as well as the floating ribs. On sagittal planes the echogenic rib interspersed with obthe intercostal space creates the typical "washboard" appearance of the rib cage (Fig. 20-21). Sound waves strike the rib and are reflected upward, leaving the characteristic void of echoes posterior to the bony

element, while sound waves will pass through the intercostal space.

On a transverse cross-section through the chest and upper abdomen, the curved rib can be appreciated immediately anterior to the skin. It is important to differentiate this structure from the skin wall, especially when attempting to measure the abdominal circumference (see Chapter 21). Although the entire rib cage may be impractical to routinely examine, in fetuses at risk for congenital rib anomalies, study of the ribs is warranted (i.e., rib fractures found in osteogenesis imperfecta).

The clavicles are most easily observed in transverse sections through the upper thorax (Fig. 20-22). The clavicle can be viewed in its length and measured to deter-

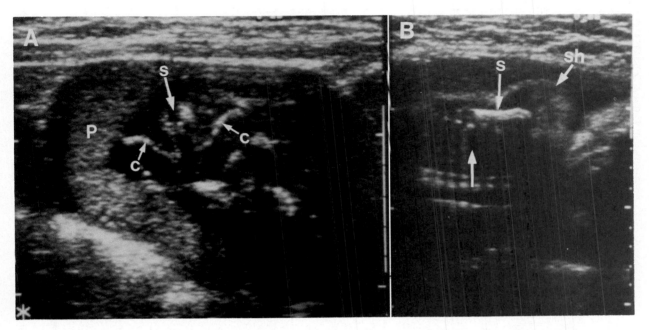

FIG. 20-22.   A, Coronal section of upper thoracic cavity revealing the clavicles, *c,* and spine, *s. P,* placenta. **B,** Sagittal section demonstrating the scapula, *s,* in relation to the shoulder, *sh,* and ribs *(arrow).*

mine gestational age.[73] In this same view the spinal elements, esophagus, and carotid arteries may be seen. The clavicles may also be demonstrated as small echogenic dots superior to the ribs. Measurements of the clavicles may be useful in predicting those fetuses with shoulder dystocia (large shoulders, which may obstruct delivery of the macrosomic fetus; see Chapter 22) or those with congenital clavicular anomalies.

The scapula can easily be recognized in the upper chest. On sagittal sections the scapula appears as a dense linear echo adjacent to the rib shadows, whereas on transverse sections it is viewed medial to the humeral head (Fig. 20-22). Oblique views will demonstrate the entire configuration of the scapula. The sternum may be seen in axial sections as a bony sequence of echoes beneath the anterior chest wall.

The heart. The anatomy of the fetal heart will be addressed in Chapter 36.

The diaphragm and thoracic vessels. The diaphragm represents the division between the thorax and abdomen and is most easily viewed in the longitudinal plane. The diaphragm lies inferior to the heart and lungs and superior to the liver, stomach, and spleen (Fig. 20-23). The diaphragm is difficult to study on transverse sections through the chest.

Sonographically the diaphragm can be identified as a thin curvilinear interface between the lung and liver. The diaphragm is more easily seen on the right side because of the strong liver interface.

The diaphragm is an important landmark in the exclusion of congenital diaphragmatic hernia (see Chapter 23). Therefore when the diaphragm is noted, it is helpful to identify the contour of the diaphragm from one chest wall

to the opposite chest wall. In addition, the stomach should be demonstrated inferior to the diaphragm.

Several vascular structures may be observed within the thoracic cavity and neck. Vessels emanating from the heart are visible within the fetal neck. The carotid arteries (lateral to the esophagus) and the jugular veins (lateral to the carotid arteries) are frequently noted when the fetal neck is extended. The subclavian artery has been identified by Jeanty and associates.[38]

The trachea can often be identified as a midline structure seen in both sagittal and transverse planes. The esophagus is a landmark that aids in determining the location of the carotid arteries and is outlined when amniotic fluid is swallowed by the fetus.

Large thoracic vessels such as the aorta, inferior vena cava, and superior vena cava are routinely observed. The aorta is recognized on sagittal planes as it exits the left ventricle and forms the aortic arch (Fig. 20-23). As the vessels course posteriorly the thoracic aorta and descending aorta with the bifurcation of the iliac arteries are apparent. The sonographer should check for arterial pulsations to confirm the aorta. Further division of the aortic vasculature can be seen within the fetal pelvis as the common iliac vessel, internal iliac vessels, and umbilical arteries (coursing around the bladder) are seen. In addition, the external iliac arteries may be seen entering the femoral arteries.[29]

The inferior vena cava is identifiable to the right of the aorta and will parallel the course of the aorta throughout the thorax, abdomen, and into the pelvis. On transverse cross-sections the inferior vena cava appears to lie to the right of the aorta. The sonographer should note that the inferior vena cava appears anterior to the aorta within the

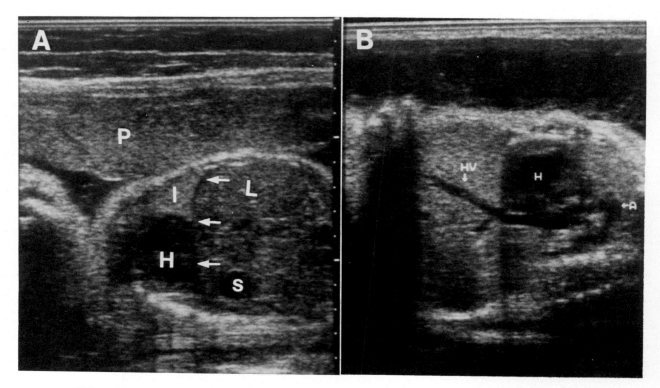

FIG. 20-23.   A, Sagittal scan demonstrating the diaphragm *(arrows)* separating the thoracic and abdominal cavities. *P,* placenta; *H,* heart; *L,* liver; *s,* stomach; *l,* lung. **B,** Sagittal view showing a hepatic vessel coursing through the liver before joining the inferior vena cava as it passes through the diaphragm and empties into the right atrium. Note the aortic arch, *A,* exiting the heart superiorly.

chest. This is caused by the anterior entrance of the vena cava at the junction of the right atrium.[29]

Divisions of the inferior vena cava may be observed (renal veins, hepatic veins, and iliac veins).[29] The superior vena cava can be outlined entering the right atrium from above the heart. By following the superior vena cava into the neck, the jugular veins may be observed.

The upper quadrant. The fetal hepatobiliary system includes the liver, portal venous system, the hepatic veins and arteries, the gallbladder, and bile ducts. Currently the liver, gallbladder, portal, and hepatic vessels can be appreciated by antenatal ultrasonography of the right upper quadrant.

The circulation of blood between the placenta and hepatobiliary system warrants discussion as this event is unique to intrauterine life.

Physiologically the liver is nonfunctional in utero, although it serves the important function of shunting blood to the heart. Oxygenated blood flows from the placenta through the umbilical vein, within the cord, to the umbilicus on the fetal anterior abdominal wall (see Fig. 20-33). The umbilical vein enters the fetal abdomen and courses superiorly along the falciform ligament and joins the portal vein as it runs transversely into the liver tissue[34] (Fig. 20-24). At this transverse junction the vessel is called the umbilical portion of the left portal vein (LPV).[34] The LPV then courses caphalad with further branching into the ductus venosus, right anterior, and posterior portal veins. This is the level at which the abdominal circumference is

measured to determine estimated fetal weight. This is the area in which growth abnormalities may be first detected as the fetal liver is sensitive to accelerations in growth (macrosomia) or lagging fetal growth (growth retardation). In this same cross-section the fetal stomach, aorta and IVC, and spine are noted.

The hepatic veins can be imaged in sagittal planes or in cephalad-directed transverse planes (Fig. 20-23). The right, left, and sagittal hepatic vessels are often delineated and followed as they drain into the inferior vena cava.[34]

Differentiation between a hepatic or portal vessel may be accomplished by evaluating the thickness of the vessel wall. In general, the walls of the portal vessels are more echogenic than the hepatic vessels.

The borders of the liver are delineated between the diaphragm and bowel. The dense texture of the liver may be used to compare the texture of the bowel. The right lobe of the liver is easily viewed on transverse sections. The fetal gallbladder is identified on transverse scans as a cone-shaped cystic structure (inverted teardrop) located on the right side of the abdomen at the level of the liver (Fig. 20-24). The gallbladder should not be misinterpreted as the left portal vein. Remember that the LPV is a midline structure appearing more tubular than the gallbladder. In addition, the LPV can be traced to the umbilical cord and portal venous system.[34]

The fetal pancreas can be identified posterior to the stomach and anterior to the splenic vein when the fetus is lying with the spine down.[34,41]

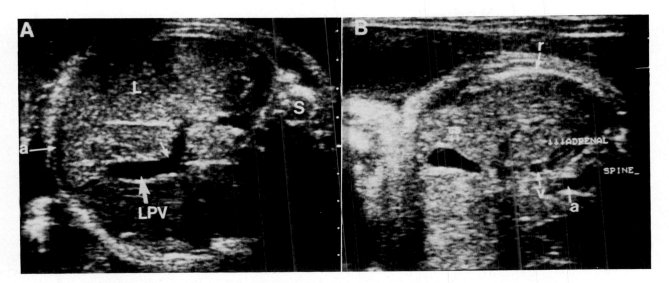

FIG. 20-24. **A,** Transverse section through the liver demonstrating liver tissue, *L,* and the umbilical portion of the left portal vein, *LPV,* as it courses transversely within the liver and branches medially *(arrow)* into the portal sinus. *S,* spine; *a,* abdominal wall musculature. **B,** Section of upper quadrant revealing the gallbladder, *GB,* adrenal gland *(arrows),* inferior vena cava, *v,* aorta, *a,* and spine. *r,* rib.

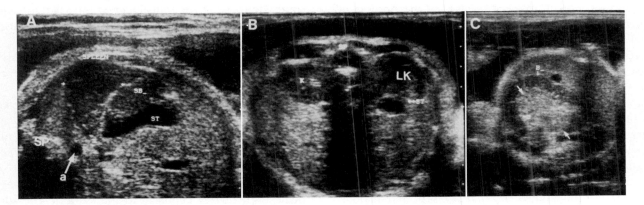

FIG. 20-25. **A,** Transverse scan identifying the spleen *(arrows),* small bowel, *SB,* and fluid-filled stomach, *ST.* SP, spine shadow; *a,* aorta. **B,** Transverse section of right kidney, *K,* and stomach, *ST,* anterior to the left kidney, *LK,* in a fetus in a spine-up position, *SP.* **C,** Transverse scan of the transverse colon, *B,* and small bowel *(arrows)* with the fetus in a spine-down position.

The left-sided fetal spleen can be viewed as a soft-tissue mass on sagittal or transverse scans of the left upper abdomen (Fig. 20-25). When the stomach is full, the spleen can be appreciated lateral and posterior to the stomach. Recognition of the spleen is beneficial in Rh-sensitized fetuses as splenomegaly may be identified.[68]

The gastrointestinal system. The fetal gastrointestinal tract is composed of the esophagus, stomach, small bowel, and colon.

The fluid-filled esophagus may be seen when the fetus has swallowed amniotic fluid.

The fetal stomach appears as a cystic organ within the left upper abdomen (Fig. 20-25). Because of the swallowing of amniotic fluid, the stomach appears full of fluid and therefore appears cystic. The stomach is seen by the second trimester of pregnancy and should be routinely identified in all fetuses. Failure to observe the stomach may occur because of recent fetal regurgitation or emptying of the stomach contents into the small bowel prior to the study. By repeating the scan within approximately one-half hour, the stomach is almost always identified. Enlargement of the stomach may not represent an abnormality, as a fetus may ingest greater quantities of amniotic fluid in pregnancies complicated by excessive amounts of amniotic fluid. The stomach may appear enlarged when the first portion of the duodenum is viewed; however, this usually represents a normal anatomic variant.

The fetal bowel is viewed as tubular echogenic structures located in the abdomen and pelvis (Fig. 20-25). The different bowel segments (duodenum, jejunum, ileum, and colon) have been described. The ascending, transverse, and descending colon are distinguishable. In addition, the hepatic and splenic flexures are recognizable.[5]

The bowel loops may be distinguished from the liver

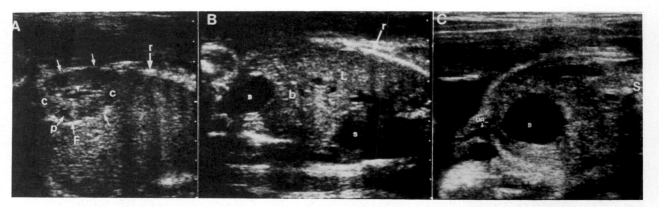

FIG. 20-26. **A,** Longitudinal representation of the kidney at 37 weeks of gestation revealing the renal cortex, *c*, pelvis *(arrowhead)*, and pyramids, *p*. The kidney is marginated by the capsule of the kidney *(arrows)*, which is sonographically enhanced due to perirenal fat, *F. r*, rib. **B,** Sagittal view of fluid-filled bladder, *B*, in the pelvis. Note the more cephalic location of the stomach, *s*, in the upper abdomen. *L*, liver; *b*, bowel; *r*, rib. **C,** Transverse view of the bladder, *B*, with demonstration of the umbilical arteries, *UA*, as they course around the bladder after exiting the umbilical cord. *S*, spine.

by noting the dense borders of the liver and its nonhomogenicity. In addition, intestinal peristalsis will aid in identifying the bowel. In early pregnancy the borders of the liver and bowel may be indistinguishable.

Small bowel commonly appears as a cluster of rings bordered by the large bowel and may be clearly seen by the late second trimester of pregnancy. Nyberg and associates state that the colon will appear prominent and commonly contain meconium particles in the late third trimester.[57] This represents a normal finding while cystic dilatation of the bowel may indicate an obstructive process (see Chapter 23). The bowel may measure up to 18 mm at term.[57]

The urinary system. The urinary system of the fetus is composed of the kidneys, adrenals, ureters, and bladder.

The kidneys are located on either side of the spine in the posterior abdomen and are apparent as early as the fifteenth week of pregnancy.[5] The appearance of the developing kidney changes with advancing gestational age. In the second trimester of pregnancy the kidneys appear as ovoid retroperitoneal structures that lack distinctive borders. The pelvocaliceal center may be difficult to define in early pregnancy while, with continued maturation of the kidneys, the borders become more defined and the renal pelvis becomes more distinct[5] (Fig. 20-26). The renal pelvis appears as an echo-free area in the center of the kidney. The normal renal pelvis will frequently appear minimally dilated (1 to 3 mm in diameter),[23] and this is currently believed to be of no clinical significance.

In the third trimester the renal borders are highly demarcated with identification of the renal pyramids, calyces, and cortex. This is thought to occur because of the increasing presence of perirenal and sinus fat within the kidney.[5] The renal parenchyma or medulla can also be outlined in most instances. The kidneys may be evaluated in either sagittal or transverse scanning planes. The investigator usually begins by studying the fetus in a transverse cross-section (Fig. 20-27). When the fetus is lying on its side, the upper kidney is readily apparent adjacent to the spine, although the distal kidney is shadowed by the spine. By rotating the transducer to the sagittal plane, the long axis of the shadowed kidney is seen and anatomy then evaluated (Fig. 20-26).

When the fetal spine is directed anterior or posterior, both kidneys should be apparent on either side of the spine (Fig. 20-27).

The length, width, thickness, and volume of the kidney have been determined for different gestational ages.[27] This information is extremely useful when a renal malformation is suspected or one is being serially followed (see Chapter 23).

The fetal adrenal glands are observed in a transverse plane immediately cephalad to the kidneys. The adrenals are seen as early as the 20th week of pregnancy and, by 23 weeks, they assume a "rice-grain" appearance[26] (Fig. 20-24). The center of the adrenal gland appears as a central echogenic line surrounded by tissue that is less dense. The central midline interface will widen after the 35th week of gestation.[35] The transverse aorta can be used to locate the left adrenal because of the close proximity of the anterior surface of the gland. Likewise, the inferior vena cava is helpful in isolating the right adrenal. Occasionally the adrenal glands may be identified in sagittal planes, although rib shadowing may interfere with this evaluation.

It is important to note that adrenal glands may appear large in utero and therefore should not be confused with the kidneys. Nomograms for normal adrenal size are available.[26]

The normal fetal ureter cannot be visualized using current sonographic imaging. Dilated or obstructed ureters are readily apparent and have been described elsewhere (see Chapter 23).

Urinary bladder identification in the fetus can be achieved in either transverse or sagittal sections through the anterior lower pelvis (see Fig. 20-26). The bladder is

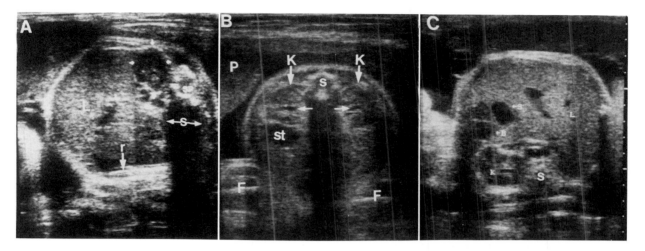

FIG. 20-27. **A,** When the fetus is lying on its side, the upper kidney *(arrows)* is visualized adjacent to the spine, *SP.* The kidney on the downside is shadowed by the acoustic shadow, *s,* from the spine. *L,* liver; *r,* rib. **B,** Kidneys, *K,* visualized in a spine-up position, *s.* Note the renal pelvices *(arrows),* which are filled with urine—a normal pregnancy finding. The stomach, *st,* is noted anterior to the left kidney. Note the spinal shadow emanating from the bony spine. *F,* femurs; *P,* placenta. **C,** When the fetus is lying with the spine-down, *S,* the kidneys are seen. The left kidney, *K,* is viewed posterior to the bowel, *B,* and the stomach, *s.* The liver, *L,* is observed, although the right kidney is not seen at this level.

located in the midline and appears as a round fluid-filled cavity. The size of the bladder varies, depending on the amount of the urine contained within the bladder cavity. As the fetus generally voids once an hour, failure to see the bladder initially should prompt the investigator to recheck for bladder filling at the end of the exam. The bladder should be visualized in all normal fetuses. If one repeatedly fails to identify the urinary bladder in the presence of oligohydramnios (severe lack of amniotic fluid), one should suspect a renal abnormality (see Chapter 23).

The fetal bladder size may appear increased in pregnancies complicated by hydramnios (large quantities of amniotic fluid). The fetal bladder is an important indicator of renal function. When the bladder and normal amounts of amniotic fluid are noted, one can assume that at least one kidney is functioning.

The genitalia. Identification of the male and female genitalia is possible provided the fetal legs are abducted and sufficient quantities of amniotic fluid are present. Providing information regarding sex identification is clinically important when a fetus is at risk for a sex-linked disorder (i.e., aqueductal stenosis, hemophilia). Relaying information about the sex of the fetus may have significant emotional impact; therefore, guidelines should be established within each department as to whether this information should be given to the patient. Only those investigators with proven sex detection skills should attempt to exchange this information.

When attempting to localize the genitalia, the scanner should follow the long axis of the fetal lie caudally toward the hips. The bladder is a helpful landmark within the pelvis in which to identify the anteriorly located genital organs. Tangential scanning planes directed between the thighs are also useful in defining the genitalia. The sex of the fetus can be appreciated as early as 14 to 16 weeks

gestation, although clear delineation can be achieved by the 20th to 22nd weeks in the cooperative fetus. When the fetus is in a breech lie, it is often difficult to distinguish the gender.

The female genitalia can be noted in several scanning planes. In a transverse plane the thighs and labia are identified ventral to the bladder, while in tangential projections, the entire labial folds, and often the labia minora, are demonstrated (Fig. 20-28). In scans of the perineum obtained parallel to the femurs, the shape of the genitalia will appear rhomboid.[35] Keep in mind that the labia may appear edematous and swollen. This normal finding should not be confused with the scrotum.

The scrotum and penis are fairly easy to recognize in either scanning plane (Fig. 20-28). The male genitalia can generally be differentiated as early as the 15th and 16th weeks of pregnancy. The scrotal sac is seen as a mass of soft tissue between the hips with the frequent identification of the scrotal septum and testicles. Fluid around the testicles (hydrocele) is a common normal finding during intrauterine life.

The upper and lower extremities. The fetal limbs are accessible to an anatomic and biometric surveillance. Bones of the upper and lower appendicular skeleton have been described extensively along with the generation of numerous nomograms detailing the normal growth patterns for each limb.[35]

Fetal long-bone measurements aid in the assessment of fetal age and growth and further allow the detection of skeletal dysplasias and various congenital limb malformations. The sonographer must attempt to not only measure fetal limb bones, but to also survey the anatomic configurations of the individual bones whenever possible.

The upper extremity consists of the humerus, elbow, radius, ulna, wrist, metacarpals, and phalanges.

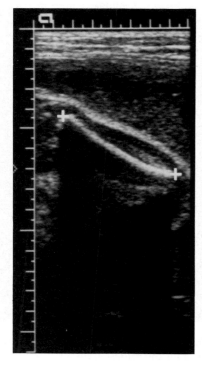

FIG. 21-4. Longitudinal section of the femur demonstrating a correct measurement *(between crosses)*. The femoral head is not included. The acoustic shadow is clearly defined.

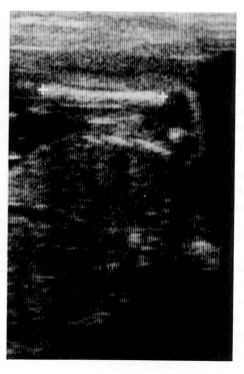

FIG. 21-5. Longitudinal section through the humerus. The length is determined by the crosses.

tinct, and an acoustic shadow should be cast due to the absorption of the sound waves into the bone (Fig. 21-4). All authors have measured the femur from the major trochanter to the external condyle. The femoral head is not taken into account even when it is visible.[25] Yeh et al.[45] claim that the fetal femur can predict gestational age between 25 and 35 weeks with less than 5 days accuracy, and within 6 days at 40 weeks.

Overestimation of the length of the femur by high gain settings or by including the femoral head or distal epiphysis in the measurement is possible. Underestimation can be obtained by using incorrect plane orientation and not obtaining the full length of the bone.

The humerus is sometimes more difficult to measure than the femur. It is almost always found very close to the anterior fetal abdomen. This falls in the near field zone where detail is not always focused, and the acoustic shadow is less clear cut (Fig. 21-5).[25]

Other bone lengths are sometimes valuable in the assessment of gestational age. The ulna can be recognized by following the humerus down until two parallel bones are visualized and then rotating the transducer slightly until the full length of the bones are identified. The forearms are very commonly found by the fetal face. The ulna can be distinguished from the radius because it penetrates much deeper into the elbow. The tibia-fibula measurement can be obtained by the same technique by following the femur. The tibia can be identified because the tibial plateau is larger rather than fine and tapering as in the fibula.

Orbits

Another parameter useful in predicting gestational age are fetal orbit measurements. The ocular distance (OD), binocular distance (BD), and interocular distance (ID) can be measured. Gestational age can best be predicted from the BD.[25] This measurement is more strongly related to BPD and gestational age than are the other orbital parameters.[33] The fetal orbit should be measured in a plane slightly more caudal than the BPD. The orbits are accessible in every head position except the occipitoanterior position (i.e., face looking down). All measurements should be taken from outer border to outer border (Fig. 21-6). The ocular distances measure the single fetal orbit itself. The binocular distance includes both of the fetal orbits at the same time, whereas the interocular diameter measures the distance between the two orbits. Jeanty and Romero[25] state that (1) both eyes should have the same diameter, (2) the largest diameter of the eyes should be used, and (3) the image should be symmetrical. Care should be taken not to underestimate the measurement when there is oblique shadowing from the ethmoid bone. This parameter is especially useful when other fetal growth parameters are affected as in hydrocephaly or skeletal dysplasia. With careful sonographic examinations, the fetus with hypotelorism, hypertelorism, anophthalmos, or microphthalmos can be diagnosed.

Abdominal circumference

In 1975, Campbell and Wilken[4] first described the use of the fetal abdominal circumference (AC) for use in the prediction of fetal weight.

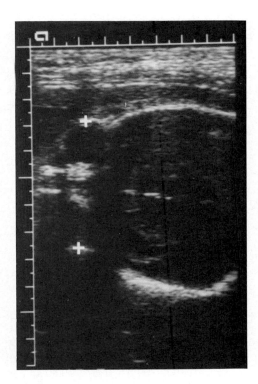

FIG. 21-6. Transverse section of the fetal head demonstrating the orbits. The markers outline the binocular distance.

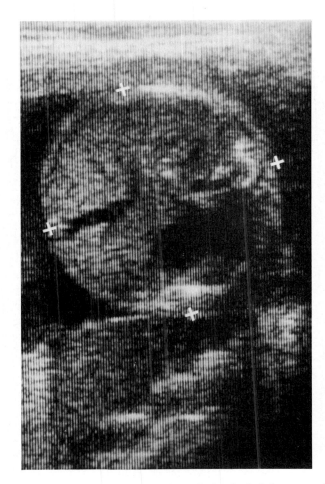

FIG. 21-7. Transverse section through the fetal abdomen at the level of the fetal stomach and umbilical vein as it branches into the left portal sinus.

The abdominal circumference is very useful in monitoring normal fetal growth and in detecting intrauterine growth retardation, macrosomia, and isoimmunization. It is more useful as a growth parameter than it is in predicting gestational age.

The fetal abdomen should be measured at the level where the umbilical vein branches into the left portal sinus. The stomach bubble can often be seen at this level (Fig 21-7).[22] The abdomen should be more circular than oval, as an oval shape can lead to an oblique cut and a false estimation in size.

The abdominal circumference can be measured with the same instruments used to measure head circumference. The calipers should be placed along the external perimeter of the fetal abdomen to include subcutaneous soft tissue. The following formula can be used to calculate the AC:

$$AC = \frac{D_1 + D_2}{2} \times \pi$$

where D_1 = diameter from fetal spine to anterior abdominal wall and D_2 = transverse diameter perpendicular to D_1. There is no consistent relationship noted between the AP and transverse diameters as recognized in the fetal head.[24]

Using multiple fetal growth parameters

No single fetal parameter is perfect in the prediction of gestational age. Hadlock et al[19] have suggested that there

is a significant improvement in estimating fetal age when two or more parameters are used (Table 21-1). Use of multiple parameters in the estimation of fetal age is appropriate only when the fetus is growing normally. Congenital anomalies of the head, abdomen, and skeleton as well as functional disturbances must be taken into consideration before using multiple parameters.

Hohler[24] used a technique to average together the BPD, HC, AC, and FL. The value of using multiple parameters is that while it is possible that any of the measurements may be technically incorrect, it is very unlikely that all of the measurements will be overestimated or underestimated.

Other parameters

There have been numerous other nomograms correlating almost any aspect of fetal anatomy with gestational age. Among the most interesting of these are the cerebellum, epiphyseal ossification, and the fetal intestines.

McLeary and co-workers[34] found the fetal cerebellum to be a more accurate reflection of gestational age than the BPD in cases of oligohydramnios, dolicocephaly, breech, twins, or in the presence of a uterine anomaly. They claim this is true since the posterior fossa is not af-

Table 21-1   Predicted Normal Values for Measurements of the Fetus in Utero

Menstrual age (weeks)	Head circumference (HC)			Abdominal circumference (AC)			Femur length			HC/AC ratio			Estimated weight percentiles		
	-2SD (cm)	Mean (cm)	+2SD (cm)	-2SD (cm)	Mean (cm)	+2SD (cm)	-2SD (cm)	Mean (cm)	+2SD (cm)	-2SD	Mean	+2SD	10th (kg)	50th (kg)	90th (kg)
12	5.1	7.0	8.9	3.1	5.6	8.1	0.2	0.8	1.4	1.12	1.22	1.31			
13	6.5	8.9	10.3	4.4	6.9	9.4	0.5	1.1	1.7	1.11	1.21	1.30			
14	7.9	9.8	11.7	5.6	8.1	10.6	0.9	1.5	2.1	1.11	1.20	1.30			
15	9.2	11.1	13.0	6.8	9.3	11.8	1.2	1.8	2.4	1.10	1.19	1.29			
16	10.5	12.4	14.3	8.0	10.5	13.0	1.5	2.1	2.7	1.09	1.18	1.28			
17	11.8	13.7	15.6	9.2	11.7	14.2	1.8	2.4	3.0	1.08	1.18	1.27			
18	13.1	15.0	16.9	10.4	12.9	15.4	2.1	2.7	3.3	1.07	1.17	1.26			
19	14.4	16.3	18.2	11.6	14.1	16.6	2.3	3.0	3.6	1.06	1.16	1.25			
20	15.6	17.5	19.4	12.7	15.2	17.7	2.7	3.3	3.9	1.06	1.15	1.24			
21	16.8	18.7	20.6	13.9	16.4	18.9	3.0	3.6	4.2	1.05	1.14	1.24	0.28	0.41	0.86
22	18.0	19.9	21.8	15.0	17.5	20.0	3.3	3.9	4.5	1.04	1.13	1.23	0.32	0.48	0.92
23	19.1	21.0	22.9	16.1	18.6	21.1	3.6	4.2	4.8	1.03	1.12	1.22	0.37	0.55	0.99
24	20.2	22.1	24.0	17.2	19.7	22.0	3.8	4.4	5.0	1.02	1.12	1.21	0.42	0.64	1.08
25	21.3	23.2	25.1	18.3	20.8	23.3	4.1	4.7	5.3	1.01	1.11	1.20	0.49	0.74	1.18
26	22.3	24.2	26.1	19.4	21.9	24.4	4.3	4.9	5.5	1.00	1.10	1.19	0.57	0.86	1.32
27	23.3	25.2	27.1	20.4	22.9	25.4	4.6	5.2	5.8	1.00	1.09	1.18	0.66	0.99	1.47
28	24.3	26.2	28.1	21.5	24.0	26.5	4.8	5.4	6.0	0.99	1.08	1.18	0.77	1.15	1.66
29	25.2	27.1	29.0	22.5	25.0	27.5	5.0	5.6	6.2	0.98	1.07	1.17	0.89	1.31	1.89
30	26.1	28.0	29.9	23.5	26.0	28.5	5.2	5.8	6.4	0.97	1.07	1.16	1.03	1.46	2.10
31	27.0	28.9	30.8	24.5	27.0	29.5	5.5	6.1	6.7	0.96	1.06	1.15	1.18	1.63	2.29
32	27.8	29.7	31.6	25.5	28.0	30.5	5.7	6.3	6.9	0.95	1.05	1.14	1.31	1.81	2.50
33	28.5	30.4	32.3	26.5	29.0	31.5	5.9	6.5	7.1	0.95	1.04	1.13	1.48	2.01	2.69
34	29.3	31.2	33.1	27.5	30.0	32.5	6.0	6.6	7.2	0.94	1.03	1.13	1.67	2.22	2.88
35	29.9	31.8	33.7	28.4	30.9	33.4	6.2	6.8	7.4	0.93	1.02	1.12	1.87	2.43	3.09
36	30.6	32.5	34.4	29.3	31.8	34.3	6.4	7.0	7.6	0.92	1.01	1.11	2.19	2.65	3.29
37	31.1	33.0	34.9	30.2	32.7	35.2	6.6	7.2	7.8	0.91	1.01	1.10	2.31	2.87	3.47
38	31.9	33.6	35.5	31.1	33.6	36.1	6.7	7.3	7.9	0.90	1.00	1.09	2.51	3.03	3.61
39	32.2	34.1	36.0	32.0	34.5	37.0	6.9	7.5	8.1	0.89	0.99	1.08	2.68	3.17	3.75
40	32.6	34.5	36.4	32.9	35.4	37.9	7.0	7.6	8.2	0.89	0.98	1.08	2.75	3.28	3.87

From Hadlock FP, Deter RL, and Harrist RB: Sonographic detection of fetal intrauterine growth retardation, Appl Radiol 12:28, 1983.

fected by any of these conditions. The measurement can be taken approximately 30 degrees from Reid's base line, which should demonstrate the contents of the posterior fossa. The widest diameter of the cerebellum should be measured (Fig. 21-8).

Chinn et al.[8] have correlated the distal femoral epiphyseal ossification (DFE) and the proximal tibial epiphyseal ossification (PTE) with advanced gestational age. The DFE and PTE appear as a high amplitude echo that is separate but adjacent to the femur or tibia. They found the DFE can be identified in gestations greater than 33 weeks, and the PTE is identified greater than 35 weeks. It is not necessary to measure these ossifications; they are either there or absent. They also stated that the importance of their finding is that in their neonatal unit, greater than 33-week gestation neonates have a 95% survival rate. This can be helpful when other growth parameters are compromised due to a congenital anomaly or in the differentiation of an immature fetus from one with intrauterine growth retardation.

Zilianti and Fernandez[46] have found that the changes in the fetal bowel correlate to gestational age. They state the changes appear to be related to the increase in meconium content and its gradual displacement to the colon by a progressively more efficient peristalsis.

They have graded these changes as follows[46]:

1. The intestine has a uniform gray appearance.
2. The colon can be identified by small echo-free areas close to the kidneys and bladder.
3. These areas become larger and delineate large segments of the colon. (The small bowel can also be seen represented by clusters of numerous transsonic areas that continuously change their shape.)
4. The colon becomes redundant, haustra appear, and echo-free areas of small bowel are larger and show an active peristalsis.

Their results are as follows:

- At 26 to 30 weeks gestation, 84% of fetuses are in stage 1
- At 31 to 35 weeks gestation, 54% of fetuses are in stage 2
- At 36 to 37 weeks gestation, 48% of fetuses are in stage 3
- At 38+ weeks gestation, 84% of fetuses are in stage 4

Although this method is not perfect, it has value during a third trimester-pregnancy.

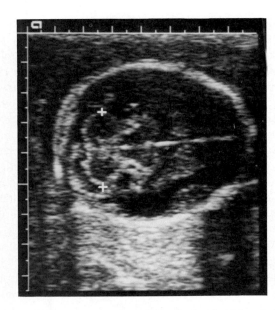

FIG. 21-8. Transverse section through the fetal head demonstrating the cerebellum and transverse cerebellar distance outlined by crosses. The thalami and the cavum septum can also be identified at this level.

INTRAUTERINE GROWTH RETARDATION

Intrauterine growth retardation (IUGR) is a decreased rate of fetal growth and is difficult to define. The most common definition is a fetal weight below the 10th percentile for a given gestational age.[18] Birth weight standards, however, cannot differentiate between an infant who is constitutionally small and one who is IUGR. The ponderal index may be useful to help distinguish between these two types of infants.

There are two types of IUGR: symmetrical and asymmetrical. A symmetrically growth retarded infant is small in all parameters. Typical causes of this type are low genetic growth potential, intrauterine infection, severe maternal malnutrition, chromosomal aberration, and severe congenital anomalies.[39] When IUGR is diagnosed before the third trimester, a level II sonogram and amniocentesis is indicated to rule out a major fetal anomaly. Asymmetrical IUGR is more common and usually is the result of placental insufficiency. This form of IUGR usually begins in late second or early third trimester with relative sparing of head size.

An early diagnosis of IUGR and monitoring of fetal well-being will be of significant help in the management of the pregnancy. Ultrasound is an easy and noninvasive method of following fetal growth and well-being.

Biparietal diameter

Because of the head sparing, a single biparietal diameter (BPD) measurement is not reliable in detecting IUGR. Campbell and Dewhurst[2] have described two patterns of head growth with serial cephalometry. The "low profile" pattern of head growth is constantly low but continues throughout gestation and is associated with fetal factors. The "late flattening" pattern slows or stops during the third trimester and is associated with maternal factors. In diagnosing IUGR, the BPD has more value when it is used in conjunction with other parameters.

Abdominal circumference

The abdominal circumference (AC) is a poor predictor of gestational age but is valuable in assessment of fetal growth.[7] This measurement is affected early in the process as the fetal liver is one of the most severely affected body organs.[9]

Head circumference/abdominal circumference

Campbell and Thoms[3] developed the head circumference to abdominal circumference ratio (H:A ratio) to detect IUGR in cases of uteroplacental insufficiency.

The ratio should decrease as the gestational age increases. With the loss of fat and subcutaneous tissue, the ratio will increase. The H:A ratio can also be used to distinguish between symmetrical and asymmetrical IUGR.[7] Crane and Kopta[9] found the H:A ratio to be a highly sensitive predictor of IUGR.

Total intrauterine volume

Total intrauterine volume (TIUV) was described as a useful screening tool for IUGR by Gohari et al.[15] in 1977. The rationale behind TIUV was that along with fetal volume, the placental volume and amniotic volume are decreased. Because this measurement requires the use of a static scanner and is affected by technique and degree of bladder filling,[18] this method is of limited usefulness today.

Estimated fetal weight (EFW)

With modern sonographic technology, fetal weight can be estimated with reasonable accuracy. This estimation is based on the premise that volume can be derived from measurements of the fetus, and fetal volume is related to fetal weight. This relationship is justified as volume is equal to the product of mass and density; and the overall fetal density is close to unity throughout gestation. Several authors have used multiple parameters, including BPD, OFD, head circumference, abdominal circumference, thoracic measurements, head and abdomen volume measurements, CRL, limb lengths, and the total fetal volume based on three-dimensional sonographic reconstruction, to derive equations for the prediction of fetal weight.[7] Perhaps the most widely used equation is the Shepard et al.[43] equation (see Appendix E). This equation uses the BPD and AC to derive the fetal weight and has an accuracy of ±10%. Ott et al.,[37] using the 10th percentile as the cut-off for IUGR fetuses, found normal ultrasonic weight curves to be sensitive in picking up small-for-gestational-age (SGA) fetuses.

EFW has recently been described in the prediction of IUGR. Chervenak et al.[7] have defined three zones of estimated fetal weight. Each zone has a different prevalence of IUGR. In zone 1 the EFW is above the lower 20% confidence limit and IUGR is ruled out. For zone 3 the EFW is below the lower 0.5% confidence limit and has an 82% prevalence of IUGR. Patients in this zone should be delivered as soon as lung maturity can be proven. If the EFW is between zone 1 and zone 3, it falls into zone 2, which has a 24% prevalence of IUGR. Patients in this zone should have serial sonograms and fetal heart rate monitoring.[7]

Femur length/abdominal circumference

Previously discussed fetal parameters have been dependent on gestational age. If the gestational age is unknown, the diagnosis of IUGR can be difficult to make. Hadlock et al.[20] proposed the femur length to abdominal circumference ratio as a gestational age–independent variable. They found the ratio expressed as FL:AC x 100 did not change after 20 weeks gestation. The normal value for the ratio is 22 ± 2. Any value over 24 indicates IUGR. The FL:AC ratio is not valuable in the detection of symmetrical IUGR.

Abdominal circumference growth

Divon et al.[12] reported another gestational age–independent variable to detect IUGR. Since the growth of the abdominal circumference appears to be linear from 15 weeks onward, the rate of AC growth can be an indication of the SGA fetus. The rate of growth of the fetal abdominal circumference is expressed as millimeters per 14 days and is calculated from two serial ACs taken 14 days apart with the following equation: rAC = final AC - previous AC x 14 (number of days between exam). Divon et al.[12] have found that a rate of growth of less than or equal to 10 mm/14 days is suggestive of a small-for-gestational-age fetus.

Decreased amniotic fluid

The association between oligohydramnios and intrauterine growth retardation is well recognized. It has been speculated that one of the mechanisms leading to oligohydramnios in gestations with intrauterine growth retardation is related to uteroplacental insufficiency with fetal hypoxia, which results in diminished renal plasma flow. The decreased renal flow leads to diminished glomerular filtration and, subsequently, diminished fetal urine and amniotic fluid product.[23] Manning et al.[31] proposed a method of qualitatively evaluating the amniotic fluid volume. They proposed the "1 cm rule." When the greatest pocket of amniotic fluid measured less than 1 cm, oligohydramnios was present. Hoddick et al.,[23] in a retrospective study of 125 SGA infants, found the 1 cm rule correctly determined only 4% of the cases and was falsely negative in 96% of the cases. Hill et al.[21] tested the 1 cm rule and found that this degree of oligohydramnios was associated with severe IUGR or a congenital anomaly. They found using a subjective decrease of amniotic fluid as a marker for SGA fetuses was more sensitive as a screening tool.

Placental grade

Placentas of newborn infants who were SGA have been found to have increased ischemic lesions, infarction, fibrin, and calcium deposits. Grannum and associates[16] proposed a grading system for placental maturity starting with grade 0 in early pregnancy to grade III in late pregnancy—a grade III placenta being one with extensive calcification with the placental substance divided into compartments.

Kazzi et al.[27] found that a small fetus with a grade III placenta was associated with a fourfold increased risk of SGA birth when compared to pregnancies with a less than grade III placenta. When Kazzi et al.[26] studied the placental grading and sonographic biometry, they found that the presence of a grade III placenta and a BPD of 87 mm or less suggested a patient at increased risk for IUGR. Patterson et al.[38] examined early placental maturation and perinatal outcome. They found that the mean birth weight of patients in the early maturation group were significantly less than those patients in the matched control group.

Functional fetal assessment

An early diagnosis and an estimation of fetal well-being are the main problems in the management of IUGR. Functional fetal assessment is useful in determining when fetal growth has slowed or stopped. Fetal breathing motions and fetal urine production were the first fetal functions to be assessed. Fetal urine production rate was described by Campbell et al.[5] The fetal bladder was measured in three dimensions and the volume calculated. Serial bladder volume measurements were taken and the hourly increase was measured. This method was too cumbersome for widespread use.

Marsal[32] noted that the incidence of fetal breathing movements was lower in growth retarded fetuses. Decreased fetal movements and breathing motions have been reported in SGA fetuses. Manning et al.[31] developed the biophysical profile, which consists of five fetal biologic variables: (1) fetal breathing movement, (2) fetal motion, (3) amniotic fluid volume, (4) fetal tone, and (5) the nonstress test. A score of two is given for each variable that was normal and a score of zero for an abnormal variable. If a fetus had a score of less than six, there was a marked increase in perinatal mortality.[39] Based on this, the biophysical profile can be used to assess fetal well-being and is helpful in planning delivery of the growth retarded fetus.

Doppler ultrasound

Fetal Doppler ultrasound is one of the newest techniques to detect IUGR. There have been many reports on fetal Doppler. Continuous-wave (CW) Doppler uses a transmitting crystal and a receiver crystal. A CW probe cannot discriminate between different signals along the beam path. The CW transducer samples along the whole beam. Pulsed-wave (PW) Doppler is depth selective and uses the same crystal to send and receive signals. Two-dimensional imaging is necessary with PW Doppler so that the proper depth can be selected along the beam path.[17]

Umbilical artery, uterine artery, and fetal aorta are the most common vessels studied by fetal Doppler. Each vessel has its own wave form that can be easily identified. The ratio of systolic peak to end diastole is measured from these wave forms. Campbell and colleagues[6] reported a reduction in the S:D ratio from 6.5 at 16 weeks to about 2.5 at term.[17,29] in normal fetuses. The S:D ratio appears to reflect the umbilical vascular resistance. As the resistance increases, the S:D ratio increases. Preliminary studies have shown that fetuses with increased S:D ratios are at risk for IUGR or poor perinatal outcome.[42]

MACROSOMIA

Macrosomia has classically been defined as a birth weight of 4000 g or greater. With respect to delivery, however, any fetus that is too large for the pelvis through which it must pass is "macrosomic."[11] Early identification of the fetus that is at risk for unusually large size is essential to obstetrical management. Macrosomia has been shown to be 1.5 to 2 times more frequent than the normal in women who are multiparous and 35 or over, prepregnancy weights of greater than 70 kg, a ponderal index in the upper 10th percentile, weight gains of 20 kg (44 lb), or post-term.[1,28] The macrosomic fetus has an increased incidence of morbidity and mortality as the result of head and shoulder injuries and of cord compression. A recent study[1] showed that 30% to 43% of cases of meconium aspiration, brachial palsy, and clavicular fracture occurred in the 10% of infants weighing over 4000 g.

Timing and mode of delivery of the potential macrosomic fetus is of great concern to the obstetrician. Boyd et al.[1] demonstrated in their study that the incidence of macrosomia increased from 1.7% at 36 weeks to 21% at 42 weeks. They further suggested the prevention of macrosomia could be curbed by selective induction, avoiding an increase in the already high percentage of cesarean sections.

Clinical considerations of macrosomia should include the genetic constitution (e.g., growth regulators set unusually high) and the environmental factors (e.g., maternal diabetes or prolonged gestation).[11] Deter and Hadlock[11] have introduced two new terms relating to macrosomic fetuses: mechanical and metabolic macrosomia. They identified three different types of mechanical macrosomia: fetuses that are (1) generally large, (2) generally large but with especially large shoulders, and (3) those that have a normal trunk but a large head. The first type can occur as a result of genetic factors, prolonged gestation, or multiparity. The second is found in the diabetic pregnancy, and the third type can be caused by genetic constitution or pathologic processes such as hydrocephalus. Only one type of metabolic macrosomia was identified by these authors, and that was the group of large-for-gestational-age (LGA) fetuses based on a standard weight curve appropriate for the population being studied and a normal range extending to 2 SD above the mean.

Biparietal diameter

Accurate sonographic predictors of macrosomia would be invaluable to the obstetrical management of macrosomia. Crane et al.[10] first described the detection of fetal macrosomia by BPD. All fetuses in their study with BPD values within the normal range were AGA at birth while 25 of 26 fetuses with two or more BPD values above the normal range (97.5th percentile) were LGA.[10] Most investigators believe, however, that BPD alone is not the optimal method to predict macrosomia.

Abdominal circumference

The abdominal circumference measurements described by Campbell and Wilkin[4] added yet another parameter to the assessment of fetal size. Indeed, the abdominal circumference is probably the single most valuable biometric parameter in the assessment of fetal growth. Ogata et al.[36] evaluated fetal growth in fetuses of the diabetic mother with serial measurements of the BPD and AC. In fetuses with birth weights less than 4000 g, both the BPD and AC were within the range determined for normal fetuses. In those fetuses with birth weights greater than 4000 g, normal BPD values were found but the AC values were greater than 2 SD after 28 to 32 weeks.

Estimated fetal weight

Using the sonographic estimation of fetal weight to determine macrosomia is of some value. A significant number of false positives or false negatives can be expected unless the actual weight is either less than 3600 g or greater than 4500 g.[11] This might be due to the lack of parameters reflecting the amount of muscle and adipose tissue present (e.g., thigh circumference).

An evaluation of two equations for the predicting of fetal weight using BPD and AC was presented by Shepard et al.[43] Weight estimates above the 95th percentile were used to classify fetuses as macrosomic.

Femur length/abdominal circumference

Hadlock et al.[20] described another approach in the detection of macrosomia: the femur lengths/abdominal circumference ratio (FL:AC), a time-dependent body proportionality ratio. Fetuses in this study with FL:AC values less than the 10th percentile and newborns with birth weights above the 90th percentile were classified as macrosomic, both prenatally and postnatally. It was suggested that these parameters might better be applied in diabetic pregnancies where asymmetric macrosomia is more likely.[35]

Chest area

Waldimeroff et al.[44] have described that chest area may be useful in ultrasonic detection of the LGA fetus. Measurement of the chest area has been reported to result in an 80% detection rate in relation to the 90th percentile, and in 47% in relation to the 95th percentile. The authors concluded the measurement of the chest area is a method of choice in the detection of the large-for-gestational-age infant. Serial measurements of the chest area should be carried out in cases of positive discrepancy in fundal heights and in cases of maternal diabetes.

Macrosomia index

Elliott et al.[13] calculated a macrosomia index by subtracting the biparietal diameter (BPD) from the chest diameter. In this study group, 87% of the infants weighing greater than 4000 g had a chest/biparietal diameter of 1.4 cm or greater. Fetal weight less than 4000 g was predicted accurately in 92% of those infants having chest/biparietal diameters of 1.3 or less. This positive correlation holds true for weights above and below 4000 g.

Other methods

In addition to the numerous biometric parameters previously discussed as useful in diagnosis of macrosomia, other ultrasound observations could at least suggest macrosomia. Diabetics may accumulate more amniotic fluid (polyhydramnios) than nondiabetics. The presence of an excessive amount of amniotic fluid in a nondiabetic patient could alert the physician to the presence of glucose intolerance in the undiagnosed gestational diabetic. True polyhydramnios that can occur in the diabetic should alert the physician to the possibility of fetal anomaly,[22] especially those of the neural tube, known to be higher in this patient population as well as macrosomia.

The placentas of macrosomic fetuses can become significantly enlarged as they are not immune to the growth-enhancing effects of fetal insulin. Enlarged placentas should be suspected when the thickness is more than 5 cm in sections obtained at right angles to its long axis.[22]

In conclusion, early documentation of gestational age in both the symmetric and asymmetric macrosomic groups would be useful in the clinical management of the LGA fetus, thus avoiding early delivery of the LGA fetus with potentially immature lungs.

SUMMARY

1. The gestational sac is the first structure to be identified on an early obstetrical ultrasound examination. It first appears at 4 weeks of menstrual age as a complete circle of echoes in the fundus or midportion of the uterine cavity.

2. The crown-rump length (CRL) is the most accurate sonographic technique that can be used to establish gestational age in the first trimester. In early pregnancy there is an excellent correlation between fetal length and age as pathologic disorders will minimally affect the growth of the fetus during this time.

3. The biparietal diameter (BPD) is the most widely accepted means of measuring the fetal head and estimating the gestational age in the second trimester. When measuring BPD, it is important to accurately determine the landmarks.

4. Femur length is almost as accurate as BPD in the determination of gestational age. Other bone lengths are valuable in the assessment of gestational age. Orbital distances and the transverse cerebellar diameter are useful adjuncts for fetal age determination.

5. Intrauterine growth retardation, a decreased rate of fetal growth, needs to be diagnosed early and the fetus monitored closely. Abdominal circumference, head circumference/abdominal circumference ratio, estimated fetal weight, oligohydramnios, functional fetal assessment, and Doppler ultrasound are important ways of monitoring fetal growth.

REFERENCES

1. Boyd ME, Usher RH, and McLean FH: Fetal macrosomia: prediction, risks, proposed management, Obstet Gynecol 61:715, 1983.
2. Campbell S, Dewhurst CJ: Diagnosis of the small-for-dates foetus by serial ultrasonic cephalometry, Lancet 2:1002, 1971.
3. Campbell S, Thoms A: Ultrasound measurement of the fetal head to abdomen circumference ratio in the assessment of growth retardation, Br J Obstet Gynaecol 84:165, 1977.
4. Campbell S and Wilken D: Ultrasonic measurement of fetal abdominal circumference in the estimation of fetal weight, Br J Obstet Gynaecol 82:689, 1975.
5. Campbell S, Wladimiroff JW, Dewhurst CJ: The antenatal measurement of fetal urine production, J. Obstet Gynaecol. Br Commonw 80:680, Aug 1973.
6. Campbell S, Griffin DR, Pearce JM, et al: New Doppler technique for assessing uteroplacental blood flow. Lancet 1:675, 1983.
7. Chervenak FA, Jeanty P, and Hobbins JC: Current status of fetal age and growth assessment, Clin Obstet Gynecol Pec 10:424, 1983.
8. Chinn D, Bolding D, Callen P, et al: Ultrasonic identification of fetal lower extremity epiphyseal ossification centers, Radiology 147:815, 1983.
9. Crane JP and Kopta MM: Prediction of in-

trauterine growth retardation via ultrasonically measured head/abdominal circumference ratios, Obstet Gynecol 54:597, 1979.
10. Crane JP, Kopta MM, Welt SI, et al: Abnormal fetal growth patterns: ultrasonic diagnosis and management, Obstet Gynecol 50:205, 1977.
11. Deter RL and Hadlock FP: Use of ultrasound in the detection of macrosomia: a review, J Clin Ultrasound 13:519, 1985.
12. Divon MY, Chamberlain PF, Sipos L, et al: Identification of the small-for-gestational-age fetus with the use of gestational age—independent indices of fetal growth, Am J Obstet Gynecol 155:1197, 1986.
13. Elliott JP, Garite FJ, Freemany KK, et al: Ultrasound prediction of fetal macrosomia in diabetic patients, Obstet Gynecol 60:159, 1982.
14. Ford K and McGahan J: Cephalic index: its possible use as a predictor of impending fetal demise, Radiology 143:517, 1982.
15. Gohari P, Berkowitz RL, and Hobbins JC: Predictions of intrauterine growth retardation by determination of total intrauterine volume, Am J Obstet Gynecol 127(3):255, 1977.
16. Grannum PA, Berkowitz RL, Hobbins JC: The ultrasonic changes in the maturing placenta, Am J Obstet Gynecol 133(8):915, 1979.
17. Griffin D, Cohen-Overbeck T, and Campbell S: Fetal and uteroplacental blood flow, Clin Obstet Gynecol 10:565, 1983.

18. Hadlock FP, Deter RL, and Harrist RB: Sonographic detection of abnormal fetal growth patterns, Clin Obstet Gynecol 27:342, 1984.
19. Hadlock F, Deter R, Harrist R, and Park S: Computer assisted analysis of multiple fetal growth parameters, Radiology 152:497, 1984.
20. Hadlock FP, Harrist RB, Fearneyhough TC, et al: Use of femur length/abdominal circumference ratio in detecting the macrosomic fetus, Radiology 154:503, 1985.
21. Hill LM, Breckle R, Wolfgrom KR, and O'Brien PC: Oligohydramnios: ultrasonically detected incidence and subsequent fetal outcome, Am J Obstet Gynecol 147:497, 1983.
22. Hobbins JC, Winsberg F, and Berkowitz R: Ultrasonography in OB/GYN, Baltimore, 1983, Williams & Wilkins Co.
23. Hoddick WK, Cullen PW, Filly RA, and Creasy RK: Ultrasonographic determination of qualitative amniotic fluid volume in intrauterine growth retardation: reassessment of the 1 cm rule, Am J Obstet Gynecol 149:758, 1984.
24. Hohler CW: Ultrasound estimation of gestational age, Clin Obstet Gynecol 27:2, 1984.
25. Jeanty P and Romero R: Obstetrical ultrasound, New York, 1984, McGraw-Hill Book Co.
26. Kazzi GM, Gross TL, and Sokol RJ: Fetal bi-

parietal diameter and placental grade: predictors of intrauterine growth retardation, Obstet Gynecol 62:755, 1983.

27. Kazzi GM, Gross TL, Sokol RJ, and Kazzi NJ: Detection of intrauterine growth retardation: a new use for sonographic placental grading, Am J Obstet Gynecol 145:733, 1983.

28. Klebanoff MA, Mills JL, and Berendes H: Mother's birth weight as a predictor of macrosomia, Am J Obstet Gynecol 153:253, 1985.

29. Kurjak A, Kirkinen P, and Fatin V: Biometric and dynamic ultrasound assessment of small-for-dates infants: report of 260 cases, Obstet Gynecol 56:281, 1980.

30. London L: Obstetric ultrasound. In Hagen-Ansert S, editor: Textbook of diagnostic ultrasonography, St. Louis, 1983, The CV Mosby Co.

31. Manning FA, Platt LP, and Sypus L: Antepartum fetal evaluation: development of a biophysical profile, Am J Obstet Gynecol 136:787, 1980.

32. Marsal K: Ultrasonic assessment of fetal activity, Clin Obstet Gynecol 10:541, 1983.

33. Mayden K, Tortora M, Berkowitz R, et al: Orbital diameters: a new parameter for prenatal diagnosis and dating, Am J Obstet Gynecol 144:289, 1982.

34. McLeary R, Kuhns L, and Barr M: Ultrasonography of the fetal cerebellum, Radiology 151:441, 1984.

35. Modanlou HD, Komatsu G, Dorchester W, et al: Large-for-gestational-age neonates: anthropometric reasons for shoulder dystocia, Obstet Gynecol 60:417, 1982.

36. Ogata ES, Sabbagha RE, Metzger BE, et al: Serial ultrasonography to assess evolving fetal macrosomia, JAMA 243:2405, 1980.

37. Ott WJ and Doyle S: Ultrasonic diagnosis of altered fetal growth by use of a normal ultrasonic fetal weight curve, Obstet Gynecol 63(2):201, 1984.

38. Patterson RM, Hayashi RH, and Cavazos D: Ultrasonographically observed placental maturation and perinatal outcome, Am J Obstet Gynecol 147:773, 1983.

39. Sabbagha RE: Intrauterine growth retardation avenues of future research in diagnosis and management by ultrasound, Sem Perinatol 8:31, 1984.

40. Sabbagha R, Hughey M, and Depp R: Growth-adjusted sonographic age (GASA): a simplified method, Obstet Gynecol 51:383, 1978.

41. Sabbagha RE, Tamura RK, and Dal Campo S: Fetal dating by ultrasound, Sem roentgenol 17(3):July 1982.

42. Schulman H, Fleischer A, Stein W, et al: Umbilical velocity wave ratio in human pregnancy, Am J Obstet Gynecol 148:985, 1984.

43. Shepard MJ, Richards VA, Berkowitz RL, et al: An evaluation of two equations for predicting fetal weight by ultrasound, Am J Obstet Gynecol 142:47, 1982.

44. Waldimeroff JW, Bloemsma CA, and Wallenberg HCS: Ultrasonic diagnosis of the large-for-dates infant, Obstet Gynecol 52:285, 1978.

45. Yeh M, Bracero L, Reilly K, et al: Ultrasonic measurement of the female length as an index of fetal gestational age, Am J Obstet Gynecol 144:519, 1982.

46. Zilianti M and Fernandez S: Correlation of ultrasonic images of fetal intestine with gestational age and fetal maturity, Obstet Gynecol 62:5, 1983.

22

Ultrasound and High-risk Pregnancy

LAURA J. ZUIDEMA

KARA L. MAYDEN ARGO

Ultrasound has come to play an important role in the management of obstetric patients. It can provide a "window" through which the physician can "see" inside the uterus and look at the fetus. The information that ultrasound can provide regarding pregnancy is extensive. For example, when a mother presents with vaginal bleeding, a common obstetric complication, placental location can easily be determined. Gestational age can be determined and fetal growth can be monitored to assess whether the fetus is growing appropriately. Twins and triplets can be diagnosed early in pregnancy—information that the physician will use in providing prenatal care.

Ultrasound has also improved patient care. With ultrasound guidance, amniocentesis no longer needs to be done blindly. The physician can see that the tip of the needle is in the pocket of amniotic fluid and not in the fetus. Ultrasound has changed the method of intrauterine transfusions in Rh disease. Whereas intrauterine transfusion was formerly performed using fluoroscopic guidance, it can now be done using ultrasound guidance with less radiation to the fetus and mother.

There are many more examples of the way in which ultrasound can influence obstetric management of the pregnant patient. This chapter deals with the interaction between high-risk obstetrics and ultrasound.

MULTIPLE PREGNANCY

The mother who has just been told that she is pregnant with twins is usually very excited. Having twins is an unusual event. The physician providing medical care for the patient, however, now views her not as routine but as a high-risk patient. The mother is at increased risk for obstetric complications such as preeclampsia, third-trimester bleeding, and prolapsed cord.[26] The twins are at increased risk for premature delivery and congenital anomalies.[13,24] As a result, a twin has a five times greater chance of perinatal death than a singleton fetus.[9] The physician may periodically order ultrasound scans for this patient.

Before ultrasound was used routinely, as many as 60% of twins were not diagnosed before delivery.[13] With routine use of ultrasound, most twins are diagnosed before the onset of labor. During the first trimester, multiple pregnancy can be identified by visualizing more than one gestational sac within the uterus (Fig. 22-1). A firm diagnosis should not be made unless a fetal pole can be seen within each sac, regardless of the number of sacs that are

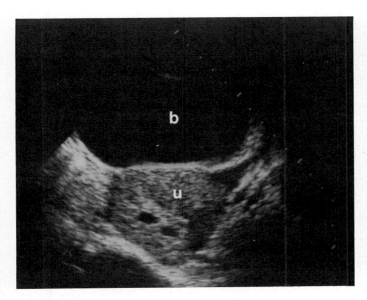

FIG. 22-1. Early twin pregnancy manifested by two echolucent gestational sacs. Fetal poles are not yet seen. *B,* bladder; *u,* uterus.

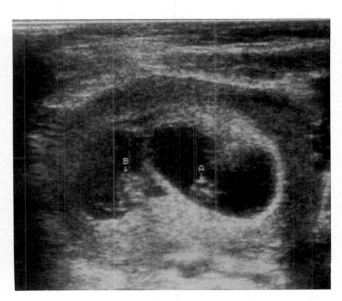

FIG. 22-2. Early twin pregnancy demonstrating two fetal poles, *A* and *B.*

seen (Fig. 22-2). In the second and third trimesters, several clinical findings may prompt an ultrasound examination. The patient's uterus may be larger on exam than expected for dates. Maternal serum α-fetoprotein (MSAFP) screening is being performed routinely now for detection of neural tube defects. Twin pregnancies, by virtue of having two fetuses rather than one, are associated with elevations of maternal serum α-fetoprotein. Therefore a patient with elevated MSAFP may present for a scan to rule out neural tube defects and be found to be carrying twins. The physician may detect two fetal heart beats or palpate two heads, prompting an ultrasound examination. Finally, the twins may be unsuspected and found serendipitously (Fig. 22-3).

Once a twin gestation has been identified, a detailed ultrasound examination should be performed specifically looking for fetal anomalies since twins are at increased risk for anomalies. To understand why this is so, the etiology of twinning must be reviewed.

There are two types of twins, monozygotic (identical) or dizygotic (fraternal). Dizygotic twins arise from two separately fertilized ova. Each ovum will implant separately in the uterus, will develop its own placenta, chorion, and amniotic sac (diamniotic, dichorionic). The placentas may implant in different parts of the uterus and be distinctly separate, or may implant adjacent to each other and fuse. While the placentas are fused, their blood circulations remain distinct and separate from each other.

Monozygotic twins (identical) arise from a single fertilized egg which then divides, resulting in two genetically identical fetuses. Depending on whether the fertilized egg divides early or late, there will be one or two placentas, chorions, and amniotic sacs. If the division occurs early, 1 to 3 days postconception, there will be two amnions and two chorions (diamniotic dichorionic). If the division occurs at 4 to 8 days, there will be one chorion and two am-

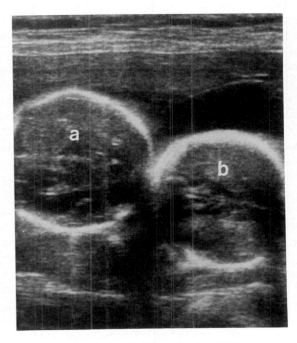

FIG. 22-3. Twin heads, *A* and *B.*

niotic sacs (diamniotic, monochorionic). If the division occurs after 8 days, two fetuses will be present but only one amniotic sac and one chorion (monoamniotic, monochorionic). If the division occurs after 13 days, the division may be incomplete and conjoined twins may result. The twins may be joined at a variety of sites, including head, thorax, abdomen, and pelvis (Fig. 22-4).

Monozygotic twins present a very high-risk situation. Besides being associated with an increased incidence of fetal anomalies, if there is only one amniotic sac, the twins may entangle their umbilical cords, cutting off their blood supply. Since monozygotic twins may share a placenta,

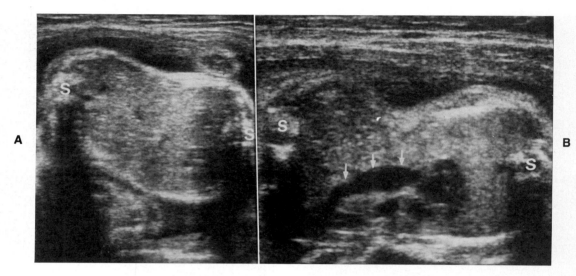

FIG. 22-4. **A,** Conjoined twins, seen through cross-sections of abdomen. **B,** Conjoined twins on cross-section with loop of bowel *(arrows)* seen crossing from one to other. *s,* spine.

they are at increased risk for a syndrome known as twin-to-twin transfusion. This exists when there is an arterio-venous shunt within the placenta. The arterial blood of one twin is pumped into the venous system of the other twin. As a result, the donor twin becomes anemic and growth retarded while the recipient twin is normal size or hydropic. The donor twin may be so growth retarded that it will eventually die in utero. In the event that twin-to-twin transfusion exists, the growth of the twins will be discordant, the donor twin falling off the growth curve. Oligohydramnios may also be present in the amniotic sac of the donor twin (if there are two sacs).

One twin may die in utero while the other one continues to grow. One ultrasound study showed that 70% of pregnancies that began with twins terminate as singletons.[18] Many of these losses occur very early and are never detected. Others are detected early when the patient presents with vaginal bleeding in the second trimester and two sacs are visualized, one with a healthy fetus and one with a demise (Fig. 22-5). If the demise occurs very early, complete resorption of both embryo and gestational sac or early placenta may occur. If the fetus dies after reaching a size too large for resorption, the fetus will be markedly flattened due to loss of fluid and most of the soft tissue. This is termed fetus papyraceous.

When scanning twin pregnancies, the sonographer should always attempt to determine whether there are one or two amniotic sacs by locating the membrane that separates the sacs (Figs. 22-6 and 22-7). If two sacs are seen, the pregnancy is known to be diamniotic, but the sonographer will not be able to determine whether the twins are identical. As mentioned before, both monozygous and dizygous twins may have two amniotic sacs.

The location of the placenta should be determined. An attempt should also be made to determine the number of placentas. Occasionally, clearly separate placentas may be identified (Fig. 22-8). If two placentas are implanted immediately adjacent to each other and fuse, it may be diffi-

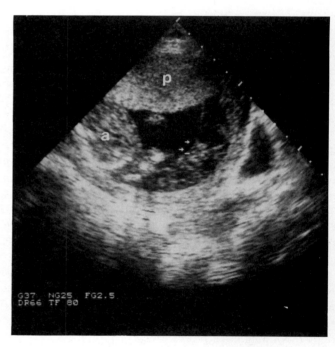

FIG. 22-5. Early twin pregnancy with intrauterine demise of twin B in sac to right *(arrows)*. *p,* placenta; *a,* surviving fetus.

cult to determine whether there are one or two placentas. The placenta will appear to be one large placenta. The body of the placenta should be scanned to determine whether a line of separation can be seen (Figs. 22-9 to 22-11).

The twins should each then be scanned for corroboration of dates and size, measuring parameters that include biparietal diameter (BPD) and head circumference (HC), abdominal circumference (AC), and femur length (FL). Currently, growth parameters for twins are usually determined from singleton growth charts. These charts have been determined for the single fetus in an uncomplicated

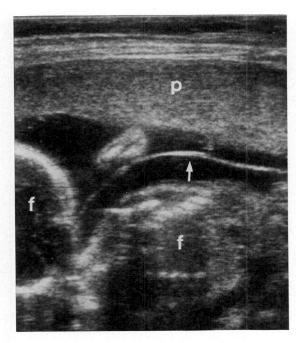

FIG. 22-6. Twin pregnancy with membrane separating the two sacs. *p,* placenta; *f,* fetus.

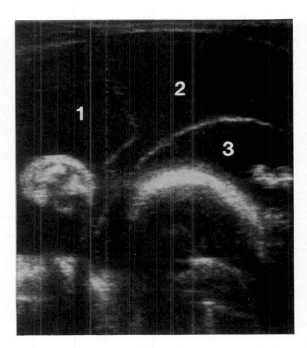

FIG. 22-7. Triplet pregnancy with identification of three separate sacs.

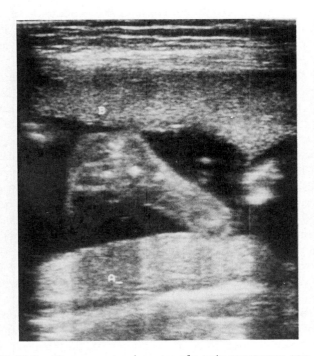

FIG. 22-8. Two separate placentas of a twin pregnancy: one, *B,* anterior and the other, *A,* posterior.

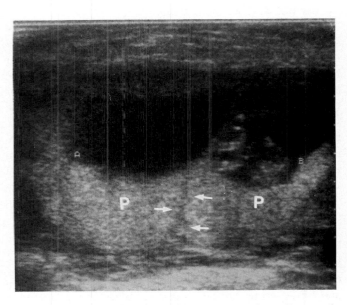

FIG. 22-9. Twin pregnancy with two separate but adjacent placentas. *Arrows* show line of demarcation. *p,* placenta.

pregnancy. Similar growth charts have not been uniformly established for twins.

There is a difference of opinion as to whether the growth of the BPD for twins is the same as that of singletons. Crane et al.[5] demonstrated that the growth of the BPD in normal twins was similar to that of a singleton. Other authors showed a decrease in the growth of BPD for twin gestations after approximately 30 weeks.[17,27] The BPD should not be used alone as an index of fetal growth.

Dolichocephaly can be common in twin pregnancies due to crowding. In dolichocephaly the BPD is shortened and the occipitofrontal diameter (OFD) is lengthened due to compression. Hence the BPD will underestimate gestational age with dolichocephaly. The sonographer should always determine the cephalic index (cephalic index = BPD/OFD × 100). A cephalic index (CI) of less than 75% suggests dolichocephaly. The normal CI is 75% to 85%.

The association between BPD and AC has been exam-

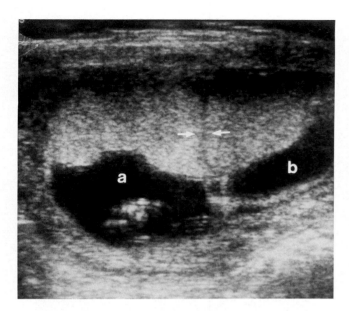

FIG. 22-10. Twin pregnancy showing two sacs, *a* and *b,* and two immediately adjacent placentas. *Arrows* point to the separating line between the two placentas.

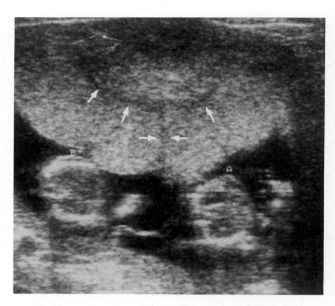

FIG. 22-11. Early twin pregnancy showing separation between the two placentas *(horizontal arrows)* and also a small uterine contraction *(vertical arrows).*

ined. Socol et al.[31] showed a slowing of growth for BPD and AC in twins was noted by 32 and 34 weeks, respectively. When the twins were examined at birth, however, AC but not BPD was found lagging.

It is known that twins are smaller in size at birth than singleton fetuses of comparable gestational age. Of concern is the ability to detect growth retardation in one or both fetuses. In trying to detect whether both fetuses are growth retarded, the singleton growth charts are used for estimated fetal weights. When attempting to determine whether only one twin is growth retarded, differences between the measurements of the two twins must be examined. A difference in estimated fetal weight of more than 20%, a difference in BPD of 6 mm, a difference in AC of 20 mm, and a difference in femur length of 5 mm have been reported as predictors of discordancy of growth between twins.[34]

IMMUNE AND NONIMMUNE HYDROPS
Immune hydrops

Erythroblastosis fetalis, whether due to ABO, Rh, or irregular blood group antigen incompatibility, is a problem of which the sonographer must be aware. Isoimmunization due to blood group incompatibility results when fetal red blood cells obtain entry into the maternal blood system. The fetal red cells possess antigens to which the mother, lacking that antigen, mounts an immune response. The resulting antibody can cross the placenta because of its small size. It attaches to the fetal red blood cell and destroys the fetal red blood cell (hemolysis). This hemolysis then results in fetal anemia, and the fetal bone marrow must then replace the destroyed red blood cells. If the bone marrow cannot keep up with the destruction, extramedullary sites of red blood cell production such as the liver and spleen are recruited into erythropoiesis

(production of red blood cells). If the production of red blood cells cannot keep up with the destruction, the anemia can become severe and congestive heart failure and edema of fetal tissues may occur.

An isoimmunized fetus can be very sick. If the severely anemic fetus does not receive a blood transfusion, it may die in utero. If a transfusion is not performed in utero and the fetus is delivered prematurely, complications due to prematurity, such as respiratory distress syndrome and intracranial hemorrhage, may threaten the life of the infant.

The perinatal death rate for Rh-sensitized pregnancies was 25% to 35% before intrauterine transfusions were performed.[28] With the institution of aggressive treatment and modern intensive neonatal care, the perinatal death rate has decreased significantly. The death rate depends on the severity of the hydrops. The more severe the disease, the greater the chance of fetal death. In 45% to 50% of cases of Rh sensitization, the disease will be mild, while 25% of the time the disease will be severe.[28]

Blood group isoimmunization is diagnosed by maternal ABO and Rh determination and antibody screening during pregnancy. Once an antibody known to cause hydrops fetalis has been identified, the antibody titer must be determined. If the antibody titer is less than 1:16, experience at most centers shows that intrauterine death is unlikely. If the antibody titer is greater than 1:16, then the pregnancy must be monitored with serial amniocentesis.

Since hemolysis results in breakdown of red blood cells, and the by-products, namely bilirubin, will stain the amniotic fluid, a spectrophotometric analysis of the fluid can give a measure of the degree of hemolysis. The gestational age at which the first amniocentesis is performed depends on past obstetric history. For example, if the current pregnancy is the first sensitized pregnancy, the first amniocentesis is performed at 26 to 28 weeks gestation. If

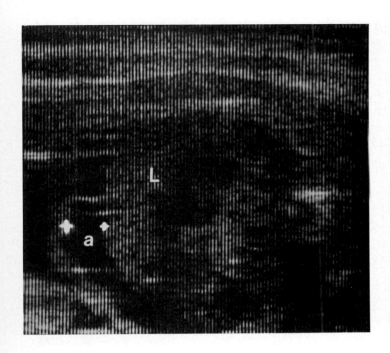

FIG. 22-12. Cross-section of fetal abdomen showing ascites. *L,* liver; *a,* ascites.

the mother has had prior affected infants or fetuses requiring intrauterine transfusions, the physician may need to perform the first amniocentesis earlier than 26 to 28 weeks.

Once the amniocentesis is performed, the amniotic fluid is sent for spectrophotometric analysis. Specifically, a measure of change in the optical density at 450 nm wavelength is measured (Δ OD450). The Δ OD450 is then plotted on a Liley curve.[19] The value will fall into one of three zones:

1. Low zone: Rh negative and mildly affected fetuses are found here. They should be followed expectantly and delivered at term.
2. Mid-zone: A downward trend within the mid-zone indicates the fetus is probably affected but will survive, and delivery should occur at 38 weeks gestation. A horizontal or rising trend indicates that the fetus is in danger of intrauterine or neonatal death and that preterm delivery or intrauterine transfusion and preterm delivery are indicated.
3. High zone: Fetal death zone. The fetus in the high zone will require immediate treatment or will die.

The ultrasound team plays an important role in the management of the isoimmunized pregnancy. Early in pregnancy, ultrasound confirmation of dates is important in aiding the clinician to decide when the first amniocentesis will be performed. During the pregnancy the fetus can be monitored for signs of hydrops up until delivery regardless of whether the pregnancy is being monitored solely by amniocentesis or whether the fetus is undergoing intrauterine transfusion.

In examining a fetus for signs of hydrops, the sonographer is looking for signs of edema. Scalp edema may be present. The fetus may have ascites (Figs. 22-12 and 22-13), pleural effusions, or pericardial effusion. Polyhydram-

nios is generally present if the fetus is hydropic. The placenta will be large and thick (Fig. 22-14). There may be an increase in umbilical vein diameter[23] (Fig. 22-15). Because the liver and spleen are involved in production of red blood cells, they will be large in size. The size of the liver has been measured in isoimmunized fetuses to see whether the severity of the disease can be predicted.[35]

Ultrasound also plays a key role in transfusion of the fetus. Before ultrasound was available for use in transfusion, intrauterine transfusion was performed using fluoroscopic guidance. Now transfusions are done exclusively using ultrasound guidance.

There are two methods of transfusing a fetus. The first, intraperitoneal, is the original method. Using ultrasound guidance, a catheter is placed in the peritoneal cavity of the fetus. The blood is then transfused into the peritoneal space through the catheter. The fetus will slowly absorb the red blood cells from the peritoneal cavity. The second method is that of direct intravascular transfusion via the umbilical vein (percutaneous umbilical blood sampling, PUBS).[6] Using ultrasound guidance, a fine needle is directed through the maternal abdomen toward the umbilical vein where it enters the placenta (Fig. 22-16). The red blood cells are transfused directly into the umbilical vein. This method is preferred since a specimen of fetal blood can be obtained pretransfusion to confirm that the fetus is isoimmunized and that it is indeed anemic, requiring transfusion. A specimen can be obtained posttransfusion to document that the fetal hematocrit is adequate.

Nonimmune hydrops

Nonimmune hydrops (NIH) is a term used to describe a group of conditions in which hydrops is present in the fetus but is not due to fetomaternal blood group incompatibility. Numerous fetal, maternal, and placental disorders

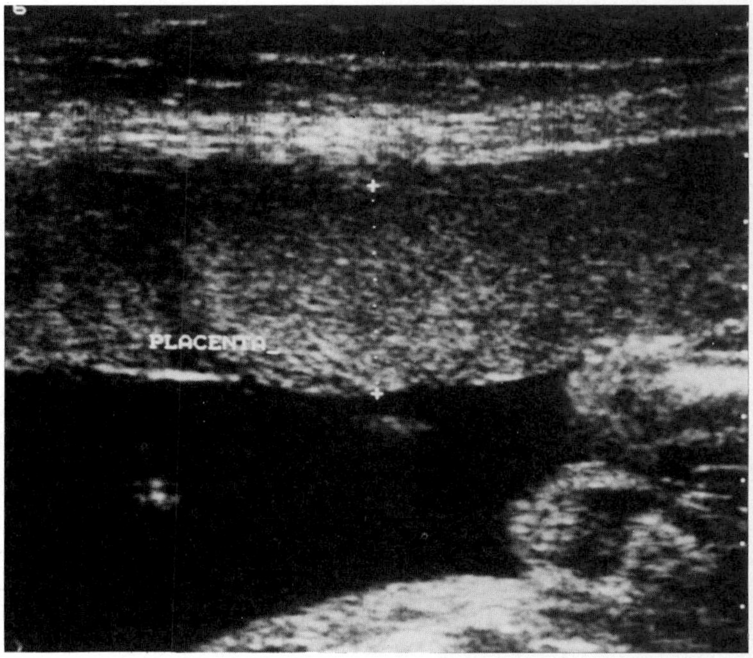

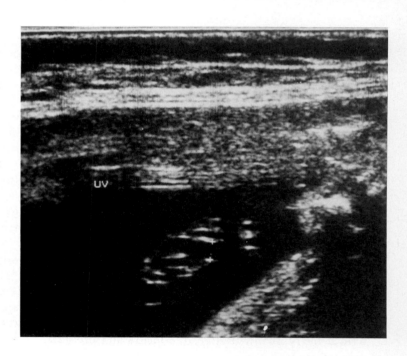

FIG. 22-13.   Measurement of thickness of placenta in an Rh-sensitized pregnancy.

FIG. 22-14.   Measurement of a cross-section of umbilical vein.

are known to cause or be associated with nonimmune hydrops, including cardiovascular, chromosomal, hematologic, urinary, and pulmonary problems as well as twin pregnancies, malformation syndromes, and infectious diseases[14] (see boxed material).

The incidence of nonimmune hydrops is approximately 1 in 2500 to 1 in 3500 pregnancies, but nonimmune hydrops accounts for about 3% of fetal mortality.[20,21] In the past, 46% to 80% of hydrops fetalis cases were due to rhesus isoimmunization. With the widespread use of Rh immune globulin, the incidence of hydrops fetalis due to Rh isoimmunization has steadily declined to the point where the ratio of nonimmunologic to immunologic cases of hydrops fetalis is rising.

The exact mechanism of why nonimmune hydrops occurs is uncertain. A variety of maternal, fetal, and placental problems are known to cause or have been found in association with NIH, some of which are listed in the boxed material. While the causes of NIH are varied, certainly the same processes described for the hydrops associated with Rh sensitization may apply to NIH.

Cardiovascular lesions are often the most frequent causes of NIH.[14] Congestive heart failure may result from functional cardiac problems such as dysrhythmias, tachy-

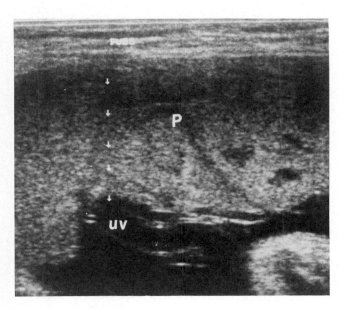

FIG. 22-15. Identification of insertion of umbilical cord into placenta. This is the site at which percutaneous umbilical blood sampling would be performed. *P,* placenta; *uv,* umbilical vein.

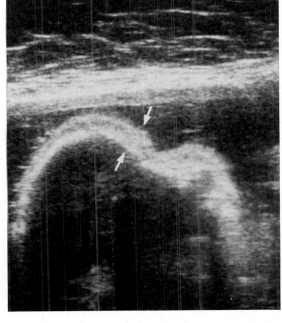

FIG. 22-16. Fetus of a diabetic mother showing increased subcutaneous fat on body. *Arrows* point to adipose tissue.

Disorders Associated with Nonimmune Hydrops

Cardiovascular problems	Respiratory problems
Tachyarrhythmia	Diaphragmatic hernia
Complex dysrhythmia	Cystic adenomatoid
Congenital heart block	malformation of the
Anatomic defects	lung
Cardiomyopathy	Tumors of the lung
Myocarditis	Gastrointestinal problems
Intracardial tumors	Jejunal atresia
Chromosomal problems	Midget volvulus
Trisomy 21	Meconium peritonitis
Turner's syndrome	Liver problems
Other trisomies	Hepatic vascular
XX/XY mosaicism	malformations
Triploidy	Biliary atresia
Twin pregnancy	Infectious problems
Twin-to-twin transfusion	CMV
Hematologic problems	Syphilis
α-Thalassemia	Herpes simplex, type I
Arteriovenous shunts	Rubella
In utero closed-space	Toxoplasmosis
hemorrhage	Placenta/umbilical cord
Glucose-6-phosphate	problems
deficiency	Chorioangioma
Urinary problems	Fetomaternal transfusion
Obstructive uropathies	Placental and umbilical
Congenital nephrosis	vein thrombosis
Prune belly syndrome	Umbilical cord anoma-
Ureterocele	lies

cardias, and myocarditis as well as from structural anomalies such as hypoplastic left heart and other types of congenital heart disease. Obstructive vascular problems occurring outside of the heart such as umbilical vein thrombosis and pulmonary diseases such as diaphragmatic hernia can cause nonimmune hydrops. Large vascular tumors functioning as arterial venous shunts can also result in NIH.

Severe anemia of the fetus is another well-recognized etiology for NIH.[14] Although the anemia is not a result of isoimmunization, the result is the same. Severe anemia in the donor twin of a twin-to-twin transfusion syndrome will cause hydrops as well as anemia due to α-thalassemia and significant fetomaternal hemorrhage.

To make the diagnosis of nonimmune hydrops, Rh or irregular blood group antibody (such as Kell or Duffy) isoimmunization is ruled out with an antibody screen. Ultrasonically the fetus may appear very similar to a sensitized baby. Scalp edema as well as pleural and pericardial effusions may be present along with ascites. Other findings may be present in addition, indicating the cause of the hydrops. If the hydrops is a result of a cardiac tachyarrhythmia, a heart rate in the range of 200 to 240 is common. If a diaphragmatic hernia is present, bowel will be visible in the chest cavity. If twin-to-twin transfusion is causing hydrops of one twin, there should be a discordancy in the size of the two twins. The twin supplying the blood should be growth retarded whereas the recipient will be normal or large for gestational age. A thorough examination of the fetus along with fetal echocardiography must be carried out since, as is evident from the boxed material, abnormalities of almost every organ system have been described with nonimmune hydrops. In addition to the ultrasound examination, genetic amniocentesis for karyotype is indicated as chromosomal abnormalities have been described as etiologies for nonimmune hydrops.

Many times an etiology for nonimmune hydrops cannot be determined. If an etiology is found, treatment depends on the cause. As an example, if the hydrops is due to a tachycardia, medicine can be given to the mother in an attempt to slow the fetal heart rate. Ultrasound can be useful in monitoring the progress of the fetus. Resolution of ascites and gross edema has been documented after the fetal heart was converted to a normal rhythm. If the fetus is anemic due to twin-to-twin transfusion, intrauterine transfusion will not be successful in solving the anemia problem since most of its blood is being shunted away. Ultrasound can assist the clinician in assessing how sick the fetus is by the severity of the hydrops and by biophysical profile (discussed later). The clinician can then make an informed choice as to when he or she should deliver the fetus.

MATERNAL DISEASE OF PREGNANCY
Diabetes

The ultrasound team is often called on to perform multiple examinations of pregnant diabetics. Diabetic pregnancies are high risk. There is an increased risk for unexplained stillbirth and congenital anomalies among insulin-dependent pregnant diabetics.[25,32] Diabetic pregnancies may be complicated by frequent hospitalizations for glucose control, serious infections such as pyelonephritis, and problems at the time of delivery.

Glucose is the primary fuel for fetal growth. If glucose levels are very high and uncontrolled (as happens in diabetes resulting from an inability to produce enough insulin), the fetus may have many possible problems. The fetus may become macrosomic. A macrosomic infant may become too large to fit through the mother's pelvis, making cesarean section necessary. If delivery is accomplished vaginally, however, the physician may have difficulty delivering the shoulders of the baby after the head has delivered. This is termed shoulder dystocia. Brachial plexus nerve injuries may occur due to the traction placed on the head and neck in attempts to get the remainder of the baby delivered. Once delivered, an infant of a diabetic mother may have many problems, including glucose control in the nursery necessitating intravenous glucose administration. If the maternal glucose control is good, these problems can be avoided. This is why glucose control in a diabetic pregnant patient is so important.

There are two types of diabetics, insulin-dependent (IDD) and noninsulin-dependant or diet-controlled (NIDD). A diabetic pregnant patient may have diabetes antedating her pregnancy. Some pregnant diabetics, however, may manifest signs of diabetes only during pregnancy and have normal glucose levels when they are not pregnant (i.e., gestational diabetics). Gestational diabetics may be diet controlled or require insulin.

Pregnancy dates should be confirmed with ultrasound. Because of unexplained stillbirth and pregnancy compli-

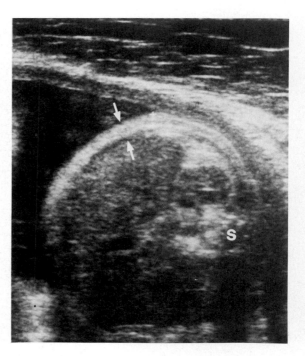

FIG. 22-17. Fetus of diabetic mother with increased subcutaneous fat. *Arrows* point to subcutaneous adipose tissue. *s*, Spine on cross-section of abdomen.

cations, the physician may elect to deliver the diabetic at 38 to 40 weeks or when fetal lung maturity is demonstrated. Correct dating is very important. A diabetic baby delivered preterm may end up in the high-risk nursery with respiratory distress syndrome.

Scans may give the clinician information about glucose control in the diabetic. Polyhydramnios is associated with poor glucose control. A fetus measuring large for gestational age will also raise concerns about diabetic compliance. Increased adipose tissue may be seen on the fetus in utero (Fig. 22-17). If the estimated fetal weight is greater than 4000 g at term, the clinician will be alert to the problems of dystocia with a vaginal delivery and may prefer cesarean delivery.

Ultrasound plays a very important role in scanning for fetal anomalies. Caudal regression syndrome (lack of development of lower limbs) is seen almost exclusively in diabetics.[25] Congenital defects of the heart and neural tube defects are anomalies commonly seen if defects are present.[25,32] Finally, ultrasound assists the clinician with amniocentesis for lung maturity studies. When the fetal lung profile (tests that indicate maturity of fetal lungs: lecithin sphingo) myelin [4s] ratio and phosphatidyl glycerol [PG]) is mature, the fetus can safely be delivered.

Hypertension

Hypertension is a medical complication of pregnancy that occurs frequently in high-risk populations. Hypertension places both mother and fetus at risk. Hypertensive pregnancies may be associated with small placentas because of the effect of the hypertension on the blood vessels. If the placenta develops poorly, the blood supply to the fetus may be restricted and growth retardation may result.

Growth-retarded fetuses are at increased risk of fetal distress and death in utero.

There are various forms of hypertensive disease during pregnancy. In the past, toxemia has been used to describe hypertensive disorders. It was believed that a "toxin" in the mother's bloodstream caused the hypertension. Currently, hypertension is considered to be caused by prostaglandin abnormalities.

The terminology currently used in clinical practice to describe hypertensive states during pregnancy includes (1) pregnancy-induced hypertension (which includes preeclampsia, severe preeclampsia, and eclampsia) and (2) chronic hypertension, which was present before the woman was pregnant. Preeclampsia is a pregnancy condition in which high blood pressure develops with proteinuria (protein in the urine) or edema (swelling). If the hypertension is neglected, the patient may develop seizures that can be life threatening to both mother and fetus. Severe preeclampsia may develop in some cases and refers to the severity of hypertension and proteinuria. Severe preeclampsia generally indicates the patient must be delivered immediately. Eclampsia represents the occurence of seizures or coma in a preeclamptic patient. Chronic hypertension is diagnosed in patients in whom high blood pressure is found prior to 20 weeks' gestation. Chronic hypertension can result from primary essential hypertension or from secondary hypertension (renal, endocrine, or neurologic causes).

The ultrasound team may be called on to perform serial scans for fetal growth and to monitor for the adequacy of amniotic fluid. If fetal growth is falling off the normal growth curve or oligohydramnios occurs, theobstetrician may intervene and deliver the fetus, fearing that intrauterine fetal demise is imminent. Hypertensive pregnancies are also associated with abruptio placenta.

Other maternal disease

Ultrasound can be useful in the workup of vomiting in the pregnant woman. Nausea and vomiting are common symptoms associated with pregnancy. Hyperemesis gravidarum exists when a pregnant woman vomits so much that she develops dehydration and electrolyte imbalance. When this occurs, hospitalization with intravenous fluid administration is usually necessary. The physician must ensure that the vomiting is due strictly to pregnancy and not to other disease such as gallstones, peptic ulcers, or trophoblastic disease. Trophoblastic disease can easily be ruled out by demonstrating a viable intrauterine pregnancy. Gallstones can be ruled out by careful sonographic examination of the gallbladder.

Ultrasound can also be useful in the workup of urinary tract disease. Approximately 4% to 6% of pregnant women have asymptomatic bacteriuria. If the bacteriuria is not treated, 25% of these women may develop pyelonephritis.[15] While pyelonephritis usually presents with flank pain, fever, and white blood cells in the urine, hydronephrosis is another condition that presents with flank pain. Pregnancy is normally associated with mild hydronephro-

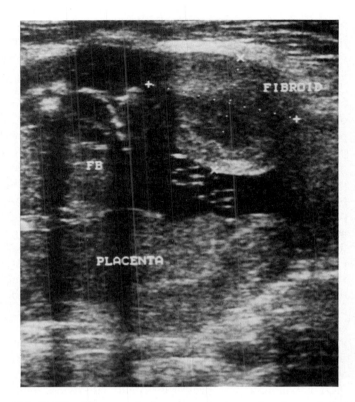

FIG. 22-18. Ultrasound of a pregnant uterus showing a uterine fibroid.

sis.[8] The hydronephrosis may be due to a combination of effects. First, progesterone has a dilatory effect on the smooth muscle of the ureter.[8] Second, the enlarging uterus also compresses the ureters at the pelvic brim, causing a hydronephrosis of obstruction.[12] If a woman presents with more than one episode of pyelonephritis or has continued flank pain, ultrasound examination may provide information as to the etiology.

Physiologic ovarian cysts may be associated with early pregnancy. These cysts may be large, ranging from 8 to 10 cm. The cyst should shrink as the pregnancy progresses. If the cyst does not resolve, surgical exploration may be necessary to rule out ovarian cancer. Periodic ultrasound examinations will be necessary for follow-up of the cyst.

Finally, pregnant women may periodically present with problems related to uterine fibroids. Fibroids are actually benign tumors of uterine smooth muscle that may be stimulated to excessive growth by the hormones of pregnancy, specifically estrogen. If the growth is very rapid, the fibroid may outgrow its blood supply and undergo necrosis. This in turn may cause pain and premature labor. Ultrasound examination of the uterus in a pregnant woman may detect uterine fibroids. This is important information for the clinician (Fig. 22-18).

PLACENTAL ABNORMALITIES
Placental abruption

Placental abruption is where the placenta separates from its site of implantation in the uterus before the delivery of the fetus. In cases where the majority of the placenta separates from the uterus, fetal death will follow if the fetus is not delivered immediately since its source of oxygen has been disrupted. The incidence of abruption severe enough to cause fetal death is estimated at 1 in 500 deliveries.[36]

There are many causes or associations of abruption, including abdominal trauma, short umbilical cord, sudden decompression of the uterus, and pregnancy-induced hypertension.[36] Abruption is a diagnosis made clinically. The patient may present with a number of signs, including preterm labor, vaginal bleeding, abdominal pain, fetal distress or a dead fetus, and uterine irritability. Often when a patient is "abrupting" the uterus will be "rock-hard" to palpation (i.e., the uterus will be continuously contracting and not relax between contractions). If the patient is undergoing a major abruption, no time can be lost in delivering the patient. In this case, treatment of the patient should not be delayed to obtain an ultrasound examination. However, there are instances in which ultrasound examination is helpful.

Not every abruption is a complete abruption, and not every patient with abruption will have pain. Traditionally, the difference between placenta previa and placental abruption is that although they both present as third-trimester bleeding, the previa is usually associated with painless bleeding and the abruption is associated with pain. There are exceptions, of course. A patient with placenta previa can have a placental abruption. A posterior placenta that is abrupting may not clinically be associated with abdominal pain. Abruption may occur acutely and proceed rapidly or may proceed more slowly. Patients may present with unclear signs and the diagnosis may be difficult.

When abruption occurs, the bleeding will be retroplacental (behind the placenta) and may either remain localized as a hemotoma or dissect retroplacentally and extend to beneath the chorioamnion to gain access to the cervix (Fig. 22-19). If the blood remains retroplacental, the patient will have no visible bleeding. This bleeding may be very significant. On ultrasound examination, a cystic area will be seen retroplacentally. If the abruption does not extend but the process quiesces, the hematoma will no longer remain clearly cystic but will develop echoes inside. In early pregnancy one may see elevation of the membranes. This is not necessarily a sign of abruption. Pregnancy with this finding can progress uneventfully.

Placenta previa

The placenta normally implants in the body of the uterus. In roughly 1 out of every 200 pregnancies,[36] however, the placenta implants over or near to the internal os of the cervix. This is termed placenta previa.

The placenta may be considered (1) a complete or total previa, (2) a partial previa, (3) a marginal previa, or (4) low-lying (Fig. 22-20). With complete previa the cervical internal os is completely covered by placental tissue. A partial previa only partially covers the internal os. A marginal previa does not cover the os but its edge comes to the margin of the os. While a low-lying placenta is im-

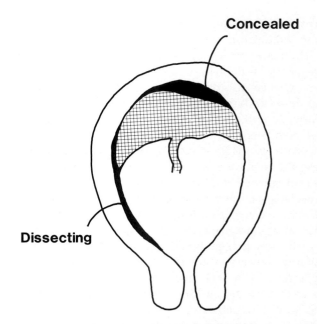

FIG. 22-19. Types of placental abruption.

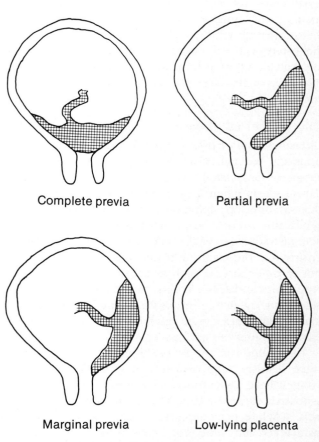

Complete previa   Partial previa

Marginal previa   Low-lying placenta

FIG. 22-20. Types of placenta previa.

planted in the lower uterine segment, its edge does not reach the internal os.

A pregnancy complicated by placenta previa is high risk because of the threat of life-threatening hemorrhage. As the pregnancy progresses into the third trimester, two very important changes occur. First, the lower uterine segment is "developing," that is, thinning and elongating in preparation for labor. As the lower uterine segment develops, the placental attachment to the lower uterine wall may be disrupted, resulting in bleeding. Second, the cervix softens and some dilatation can occur before the onset of labor. Cervical dilatation may also disrupt the attachment of a placenta located over or near the cervical os.

Classically a patient with placenta previa will present with painless bleeding in the third trimester of pregnancy. The bleeding can be impressive. When a pregnant patient presents with third-trimester bleeding, diagnosis is imperative since the treatment will be different based on the clinical diagnosis. If the clinical diagnosis is placental abruption, the obstetrician will deliver the fetus or it may die. If the diagnosis is placenta previa, the fetus is preterm, and the mother is not bleeding heavily, the clinical management may be conservative with transfusion and close observation until the point where the fetus is mature or the pregnancy must be terminated because of bleeding.

When the time for delivery arrives, if the placenta completely covers the os, the fetus will have to be delivered by cesarean section. If the placenta only partially covers the os, it is possible that the fetus may deliver vaginally. The pressure of the fetus as it passes through the cervix and birth canal may compress the part of the placenta that has been disrupted and stop the bleeding.

Ultrasound plays an important role in localization of the placenta. Historically the diagnosis of placenta previa could be made radiologically only by injecting a radio contrast dye into the amniotic cavity to demonstrate the position of the placenta or by angiography. When a patient presented with third-trimester bleeding and needed to be delivered and previa was suspected clinically, it could be confirmed by "double set-up" examination. The patient was taken to the operating room and examined vaginally with an operating room team on standby. If placenta previa was confirmed with digital examination, the patient was delivered operatively. Otherwise vaginal delivery was allowed. Ultrasound has changed the management of the pregnant patient with previa because the clinician can be relatively sure that a previa exists.

While ultrasound allows easy localization of the placenta, the diagnosis of previa is difficult at times. Early in pregnancy, while the uterus is small, the relative endometrial surface covered by placenta is large.[16] As the pregnancy progresses, however, the amount of endometrial surface the placenta covers decreases. Therefore, placentas can appear as previas early in pregnancy and many can be marginal. As the lower uterine segment develops, however, and the placenta decreases relative to the uterus in size, there may be an increase in distance between the lower edge of the placenta and the internal os. The relationship of the placenta will change as pregnancy progresses, and a large number of low-lying placentas will become fundal placentas by term.[30]

The concept that the placenta changes its position within the uterine cavity has been termed "migration,"[16] implying that the placenta actually moves and relocates. It may be that the placenta actually does not move but that the position appears changed because of the physiologic changes occurring around it (i.e., enlargement of the uterus and development of the lower uterine segment).

While the majority of placentas that are considered previas in the second trimester convert to fundal or low-lying placentas by the third trimester, there are exceptions. If the placenta is a complete previa in the second trimester, it is unlikely to change its position drastically. In all likelihood when the third trimester arrives, it will remain a complete previa.[10]

In performing a routine obstetrical ultrasound, the sonographer should always describe the position of the placenta. The placenta should be scanned longitudinally to see whether it extends into the lower segment. If it does, a transverse scan should be obtained to determine whether the placenta is located centrally or whether it lies to one side of the cervix (Figs. 22-21 and 22-22). Oblique scans may be necessary to visualize the relationship of the placenta to the cervix.

To see the internal os of the cervix, the patient should have a full bladder. In this way the relationship of the placenta to the internal os can be visualized. In theory this works well. In practice, having a full bladder and visualizing the internal os is not always easy. If a patient is actively bleeding or laboring, the sonographer may not have time to wait for the patient to fill her bladder. If the fetal head is low in the pelvis, diagnosis of a posterior placenta previa may be difficult as the fetal skull bones will block transmission of the ultrasound at a critical point. If the physician can elevate the fetal head out of the pelvis, it may be possible to distinguish between a posterior low-lying and a posterior previa.

An overfilled bladder may push the internal os up, making it appear higher than it actually is. This may give the false impression of a previa. Emptying the bladder will reduce the pressure on the lower uterine segment and allow the cervix to assume a more normal position. The placenta may not be a previa at all.

Describing the location of the placenta has clinical importance. A previa noted on scan will alert the obstetrician that no pelvic examination should be performed on the patient. A finger inadvertently pushed through an unknown previa can result in a frightening amount of bleeding not only for the patient, but also the physician. If a placenta is noted to be low-lying early in pregnancy, the placenta location can be followed with consecutive scans to see whether this location persists.

Ultrasound now plays a major role in diagnosis and management of placenta previa. It is safe and accurate and

5. Anterior abdominal wall: exclude omphalocele/gastroschisis
6. Fetal spine: survey for large defects
7. Fetal limbs: count and assess integrity of limbs

Further sonographic evaluation prior to selecting a sample site should address the placenta and amniotic fluid. While a posterior placenta may afford an easier access to the amniotic fluid, an anterior placenta may be penetrated provided the obstetrician is directed through the thinnest portion of the placenta and away from the insertion site of the umbilical cord. A 20 to 22-gauge needle is preferred in patients with anterior placentas. The pregnancy loss rate in pregnancies in which the placenta was traversed as compared to nonplacental taps was similar when ultrasound was used throughout the procedure.[39] It is desirable to avoid the placenta in patients who are Rh-negative. In all Rh-negative patients, RhoGAM is administered within 72 hours of the procedure.

The evaluation of the amount of amniotic fluid is crucial to the successful performance of amniocentesis. Decreased amounts of amniotic fluid or inaccessible amniotic fluid pockets may prohibit successful amniocentesis procedures. A relationship must be established between the position of the fetus and the desired amniotic fluid pocket. In many instances, manipulation of the fetus by the obstetrician, ambulation of the mother, or changes of fetal position are necessary to achieve an adequate sampling site. Bladder filling or emptying may also aid in the redistribution of amniotic fluid. Frequently, because of reduced amounts of amniotic fluid for unexplained reasons or the inability to find a "safe" pocket to tap, the patient is rescheduled to return in 1 week for an additional attempt. In the majority of cases, upon a repeat study, fetal position and the amniotic fluid amount are usually favorable for tapping. Amniotic fluid is continuously produced, and therefore increases as gestation advances.

Second, the sonographer should assist in determining the amniotic tap site. The optimal place to collect amniotic fluid is: (1) away from the fetus, (2) devoid of placental tissue when possible, (3) away from the umbilical cord, and (4) close to the maternal midline (lateral needle insertions should not be attempted because of the laterally positioned uterine vessels).

Technique of genetic amniocentesis

Ultrasound-guided amniocentesis has been described using static B-scanners and real-time imaging.[61] Using this method, ultrasound is used to determine an amniotic fluid pocket, and the skin is marked to denote the amniocentesis site. The transducer is removed, the skin prepped and anesthetized, and the needle inserted for aspiration. This technique has allowed the successful retrieval of amniotic fluid; however, it is limited as operators are unaware of the intrauterine events between site selection and insertion of the needle. The fetus is continuously moving and may potentially move into the presumed empty pocket of amniotic fluid. In 1983, Jeanty et al.[80] proposed ultrasound-monitored amniocentesis or simultaneous needle insertion under continuous real-time observation. With

this technique, the amniocentesis area is determined, but a specific site is not chosen until immediately before the needle insertion. Instead, the quadrant of the uterus involved is aseptically prepared to encompass a large surface area. The transducer is placed in a sterile glove or plastic bag (gas sterilized) to enable ultrasound monitoring on the sterile field during the procedure. Sterile coupling gel is applied to the maternal skin in the area of the proposed amniocentesis site. The amniocentesis site is rescanned to confirm the amniotic fluid pocket, and then the exact site and pathway for the introduction of the needle is determined. The distance to the amniotic fluid can be measured using the electronic calipers, which is extremely useful in obese patients, as a longer needle is frequently used to obtain amniotic fluid. In many instances, a new site is chosen as a result of fetal movements or myometrial contractions in the proposed amniocentesis site. In the event a new site is chosen, the transducer is moved to the new site as the majority of the uterus is prepped. Upon successful identification of the amniocentesis site, a finger is placed between the transducer and the patient's skin, which produces an acoustic shadow due to the air interface. The needle is then inserted, under continuous observation, parallel to the transducer (Fig. 23-2). As the needle is inserted perpendicular to the transducer, it will be visualized at the uterine wall (2 to 3 cm into the abdomen). The needle tip echo will be evident once it has entered the uterine cavity and will appear as a bright echo as it penetrates the amniotic fluid (Fig. 23-3). With this technique, the exact location of the needle tip can be appreciated, and if incorrectly placed, it can be redirected immediately. It is critical that the transducer and needle are positioned in a perpendicular fashion. If the needle is angled, it will not be evident within the ultrasound beam. Several investigators prefer to scan away from the sterile field and employ an "angle" technique. In skilled hands, this method has proven to be reliable.[4] There appears to be a significant decrease in bloody and dry taps, along with a decrease in the number of insertions required to obtain amniotic fluid using the sonographically monitored amniocentesis technique.[126] This is the method used in intrauterine transfusions (see Chapter 22) and fetal surgery.

The amniotic fluid is then aspirated through a syringe connected to the needle hub. Frequently the first few millimeters of fluid are discarded to avoid contamination. It is typical to extract 20 to 30 ml of amniotic fluid for chromosomal analysis and α-fetoprotein evaluation. Frequently in advanced pregnancies (20 to 21 weeks), additional amounts of amniotic fluid are required (30 to 40 ml). In the event that amniocentesis is performed because of fetal anomalies, additional amniotic fluid is necessary for the study of acetylcholinesterase and viral studies (TORCH titers). After aspiration, the stylet is placed in the needle and removed under sonographic guidance from the uterus.

Immediately following amniocentesis, fetal cardiac activity should be identified and documented. The use of videotaping allows the continuous recording of the prescan, the amniocentesis, and postamniocentesis events.

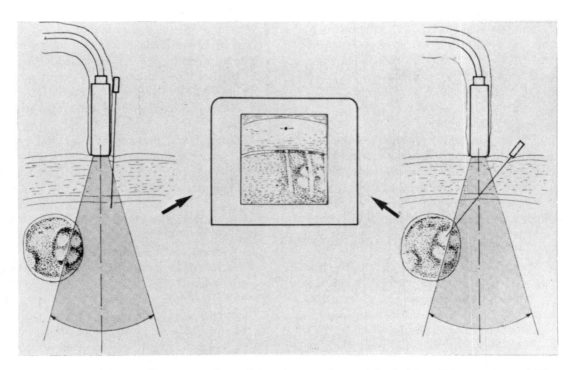

Fig. 23-2. If the needle is inserted parallel to the transducer, only the tip will be represented. If the needle is inserted at an angle with the transducer, the beam will intersect the needle, but it will not demonstrate its tip, which could be in a harmful position. Notice that in both cases the image on the screen will be the same. Angling the needle is a dangerous procedure that should be avoided. (From Jeanty P, Rodesch F, Romero R, et al: Am J Obstet Gynecol 146:593, 1983.)

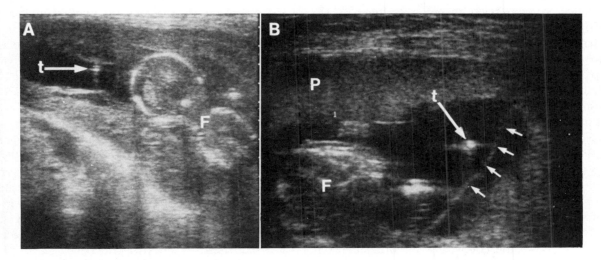

Fig. 23-3. **A,** Genetic amniocentesis at 15.6 weeks using direct visualization method. The needle tip, *t,* is identified within the amniotic cavity. *F,* Fetus. **B,** Genetic amniocentesis at 16 weeks of gestation in a twin pregnancy. The needle tip, *t,* is identified within the sac above the dividing amniotic membrane *(arrows). P,* Placenta; *F,* fetus.

Documentation of the amniocentesis procedure is important. A description of the amniocentesis site, the amount of amniotic fluid obtained, the color and quality of the fluid (clear, blood-tinged, etc.), and any procedure-related complications should be detailed. If the placenta is penetrated, a search for placental hemorrhage should be attempted. In the majority of cases, the bleeding ceases within a short period of time.

The continuous-monitoring amniocentesis technique is invaluable in cases of oligohydramnios, anterior placentas, and in patients with rupture of the membranes because only small pockets of fluid are usually available. This method allows the precise identification of small amniotic fluid pockets and enables the guidance of the needle into small amniotic fluid pockets.

Genetic amniocentesis and multiple gestations

Amniocentesis in multiple gestations warrants special consideration. Preliminary sonographic studies, as described for singleton fetuses, should be performed. For each fetus in a multiple pregnancy, it is imperative to study fetal anatomy and perform individual growth profiles for each fetus. The identification of the dividing amniotic membrane is important (see Chapter 22). Amniotic fluid should be evaluated, and when a membrane can be sonographically defined, a study of the amniotic fluid within each sac should be attempted.

The amniocentesis technique for multiple gestations is similar to the singleton method, except each individual sac is entered (Fig. 23-3,B). The first sac is identified, fluid is aspirated, and indigo carmen dye (0.5 ml from a separate syringe) is injected into the sac. The second amniocentesis site is then chosen in the opposite fetal sac (by recognition of membrane) and the needle is inserted. If clear amniotic fluid is obtained, the second sac has been entered; however, if dye-stained fluid is visible, the first sac has been repenetrated. Triplet pregnancies have also been successfully tapped. Documentation of each amniocentesis and meticulous labeling of fluid samples is essential in multiple amniocenteses procedures.

COMPREHENSIVE ULTRASOUND AND PRENATAL DIAGNOSIS

High-resolution ultrasound has had a dramatic effect on the detection of congenital defects of the fetus before birth. Reports of ultrasound-detected congenital abnormalities inundate the obstetrical and radiologic literature. The knowledge that has been gained over the past 15 years has opened the door to more aggressive searches for fetal lesions, has markedly changed the obstetrical management of these pregnancies, and has inspired others to develop and perform fetal surgery in an attempt to correct anatomic malformations of the fetus.

As a result of this increasing volume of information, a new sophistication has arisen in the detection of fetal disease. Ultrasound equipment has become more exacting with superior resolution capabilities, a new approach has evolved to systematically evaluate the fetus at risk or with a known birth defect, and there has been an increasing demand for sonographers to become more aware of genetic disorders. It is important for the sonographer to understand the intricacies of prenatal diagnosis. Many specialists are involved in the counseling, performance, and interpretation of ultrasound studies. The prenatal diagnostic team includes radiologists, obstetricians, sonographers, perinatologists, pediatricians, neonatologists, pediatric surgeons, neurosurgeons, geneticists, genetic counselors, and perinatal social workers.

In this chapter, comprehensive ultrasound examinations will pertain to specialized scans of the fetus that are performed in women with a high risk for a fetal anomaly. In contrast to the antepartum obstetrical scan, this examination isolates particular fetal organs that may be involved in particular congenital diseases. This scan is commonly referred to as a genetic scan or a level II scan. The name level II scan may be an inappropriate title since it refers to the second-stage scan performed after amniotic fluid α-fetoprotein elevations. This term has carried over

into general obstetrical scanning; however, it appears to be inappropriate for fetal anomaly detection. Therefore, in this text, the comprehensive ultrasound examination will refer to specialized scans to (1) detect or confirm a fetal anomaly, (2) evaluate the fetus at risk for an anomaly, and (3) follow the fetus with a known anomaly throughout gestation.

Following are indications for comprehensive ultrasound examinations:
1. Patients who have previously delivered a child with a congenital anomaly that could be detected by ultrasound
2. Fetuses with suspected or known fetal anomalies
3. A history of chromosomal anomalies with associated structural malformations of the fetus
4. Any screening ultrasound examination suggestive of a fetal anomaly
5. Any screening ultrasound examination that demonstrates severe hydramnios or oligohydramnios
6. Elevations of amniotic fluid α-fetoprotein
7. Patients in whom pregnancies are confounded by conditions that may cause fetal anomalies
8. Insulin-dependent diabetic pregnancies
9. Fetal hydrops (see Chapter 22)
10. Teratogenic agent exposure (severe radiation exposure, drug ingestion, etc.)

Comprehensive ultrasound examinations require an average of 45 minutes to 1 hour to perform to study the at-risk lesion and to correlate sonographic findings with pertinent genetic and clinical indices.

The causes of congenital birth defects are extensive. Major congenital abnormalities requiring surgical treatment occur in 2% to 4% of newborns. Minor congenital anomalies are present in an additional 10% to 12% of children.[107]

Sixty-five to seventy percent of congenital anomalies have unknown causes. Twenty percent of congenital malformations are genetically transmitted and 10% result from chromosomal defects. Environmental factors (drugs, radiation, maternal metabolic disease, and infections) can explain the presence of congenital anomalies in approximately 10% of pregnancies.[107] Maternal infections (cytomegalovirus, rubella, and toxoplasmosis) account for approximately 4% of birth defects.

The risk of congenital anomalies is increased in women who are insulin dependent (8% to 9% increase).[87,107] This increased incidence was found in women who were diabetic prior to conception. Cardiovascular, central nervous system defects (anencephaly and spina bifida), sacral abnormalities (caudal regression syndrome), and limb abnormalities have been noted to be prevalent in this high-risk group.[119]

The sonographer should be knowledgable about the effects of certain teratogens (drugs or agents that give rise to abnormalities in fetal development) on the fetus. Many agents are known to cause specific anatomic aberrations whereas others are considered to be possible teratogens. For this reason patients are referred for comprehensive ultrasound studies to exclude specific anomalies that may

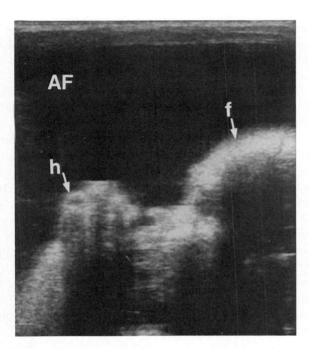

Fig. 23-4. Polyhydramnios in a fetus with a diaphragmatic hernia. Excessive amounts of amniotic fluid are found because of the lack of normal swallowing. Fetal features are enhanced as amniotic fluid surrounds the fetus and improves visualization of anatomic structures. *AF,* Amniotic fluid; *F,* forehead; *h,* hand.

Fetal Conditions Associated with Polyhydramnios and Oligohydramnios

POLYHYDRAMNIOS

Nonanomalous conditions
Diabetes mellitus
Rh isoimmunization
Multiple gestation
Fetal anomalous conditions
Anencephaly
Encephalocele
Hydrocephaly
Microcephaly
Cardiac failure
Cystic hygromas
Lung masses
Ectopic cordis
Diaphragmatic hernia
Esophageal duodenal atresia
Omphalocele/gastroschisis
Bowel obstruction
Mesenteric/ovarian cyst
Ureteropelvic junction obstruction
Placental abnormalities
Fetal teratomas

OLIGOHYDRAMNIOS

Nonanomalous conditions
Intrauterine growth retardation
Premature rupture of membranes
Postdates pregnancy (42 weeks)
Fetal anomalous conditions[82]
Infantile polycystic kidney disease
Renal agenesis
Posterior urethral valve syndrome
Dysplastic kidneys
Chromosomal abnormalities

Modified from Seeds JW and Cefalo RC: Anomalies with hydramnios—diagnostic role of ultrasound, Contemp Ob/Gyn 23:32, 1984.

have formed because of exposure to a teratogenic medication or agent.

When a fetal anomaly is found, investigators should search for other malformations, since isolated fetal malformations are uncommon.

AMNIOTIC FLUID

An important parameter to evaluate in pregnancies at risk for anomalies is the amount of amniotic fluid. The exact amount of amniotic fluid is difficult to measure; however, a subjective impression of an abnormal volume (increased or decreased) may infer an underlying congenital malformation.

Polyhydramnios (excessive amounts of amniotic fluid) may be associated with congenital malformations (Fig. 23-4). For example, impairment of fetal swallowing can result in polyhydramnios (diaphragmatic hernia, gastrointestinal defects). Many anomalies are associated with polyhydramnios; therefore comprehensive ultrasound studies should be performed to search for associated fetal defects (see boxed material). Assessment of the amount of amniotic fluid remains largely a subjective observation that relies on the expertise of the investigator. Considerable operator experience is necessary to differentiate between normal and abnormal amniotic fluid states. Varying degrees of excessive amounts of amniotic fluid can be present. Sonographic characteristics suggestive of severe polyhydramnios are (1) the appearance of a freely floating fetal body and limbs within the amniotic cavity, (2) accentuated fetal anatomy, and (3) a freely moving fetus. When polyhydram-

nios is discovered, nonanomalous fetal conditions should also be considered (diabetes mellitus, Rh disease).

Oligohydramnios (significantly reduced amounts of amniotic fluid) can result from severe renal disease (e.g., posterior urethral valve syndrome [see Fig. 23-34], renal agenesis and infantile polycystic kidney disease [see Fig. 23-32]) or from nonanomalous fetal conditions (see boxed material). In addition, there can be diminished amounts of amniotic fluid (oligohydramnios) due to inadequate urinary function (intrauterine growth retardation) or to an obstruction that causes a blockage to normal excretion.[82] On recognition of oligohydramnios, a careful search for normal-appearing fetal kidneys and bladder should ensue. In all obstetrical cases it is imperative to identify the fetal bladder and a normal amniotic fluid volume, which signifies at least unilateral renal function. In cases of normal amniotic fluid and nonvisualization of the fetal bladder, fetal voiding may have occurred prior to the examination. After prolonged observation periods, the bladder should be noted. In all cases of equivocal or proven oligohydramnios, fetal renal abnormalities should be considered. If severe oligohydramnios is noted prior to the 28th week of gestation, renal anomalies must be suspected. Rupture of the membranes may occur in the second trimester of pregnancy. Therefore correlation with the obstetrical history is imperative in evaluation of the fetus with oligohydramnios. Nonanomalous conditions yielding decreased amounts of fluid are well known. Intrauterine growth retardation and premature rupture of the membranes should be considered after 28 weeks of gestation. Postdates-related oligohydramnios should be considered in every pregnancy evaluated after 40 weeks of gestation (see Chapter 22).

The ultrasound criteria for oligohydramnios are nonspecific, yet relate to the appearance of fetal crowding and scanty amounts of amniotic fluid throughout the amniotic cavity. Amniotic fluid, kidney architecture, and bladder function must be evaluated conjunctively to diagnose renal disease.

In pregnancies with oligohydramnios, sonographic resolution is poor because of lack of an acoustic interface (amniotic fluid), and at times examinations may be limited.

Oligohydramnios may cause various fetal malformations such as clubbing of the hands or feet, pulmonary hypoplasia, and hip displacement.[82]

ABNORMALITIES ALTERING CONTOUR OF THE CRANIUM

The fetal calvarium is sonographically echogenic and, therefore, easily recognized on ultrasound (see Chapter 20). The contour of the fetal skull is smooth and should appear as an intact structure. Several cranial malformations alter the normal-appearing contour of the fetal cranium.

Anencephaly

Anencephaly represents the most common defect of the neural tube. The incidence of anencephaly is 1 per 1500 births in North America,[70] with a higher incidence in the United Kingdom.

Anencephaly is a defect characterized by the absence of the fetal skull. The defect usually involves the frontal and parietal bones, but the occipital bones and orbits are commonly present. Neural tissue, the brain stem, and the midbrain are present, and the cerebral hemispheres are missing.

Anencephaly occurs from failure of the fetal neural tube to fuse at the cephalic portion of the fetal cranium between the second and third weeks of embryonic development. As a result, there is an abnormality in the formation of the forebrain.

Anencephaly is a lethal disorder; therefore early diagnosis of this lesion is desirable in the second trimester of pregnancy. Many cases of anencephaly can be diagnosed by ultrasound following an abnormally elevated maternal serum α-fetoprotein value. In anencephaly there is an open defect (thick membrane) between the neural tissue and the amniotic fluid, and α-fetoprotein leaks into the fluid and maternal circulation.

The cause of anencephaly is unknown. Recent investigators are studying the correlation of vitamin deficiencies with the occurrence of neural tube defects.[141]

The primary diagnostic tool for the confirmation of anencephaly is ultrasound, since the fetal cranium can be identified as early as the twelfth week of gestation. Although the diagnosis of anencephaly can be suspected as early as the twelfth to thirteenth weeks of gestation, a final diagnosis should not be attempted until 14 to 15 weeks of gestation. Campbell et al.[14] first reported the antenatal diagnosis of anencephaly at 17 weeks of gestation by sonography in 1972. The inability to visualize the cranium at any gestational age should lead to the consideration of anencephaly.

Sonographically, the anencephalic fetus will demonstrate several characteristics:
1. Absence of bony fetal cranium, typically above the level of the fetal orbits (Fig. 23-5, A)
2. Fetal brain tissue can be seen extending from the defect (cerebrovasculosa)
3. Fetal orbits may appear to be protruding because of absent frontal bone
4. Polyhydramnios is present in 40% to 50% of pregnancies (may result from impaired swallowing due to a malformed brain stem);
5. Associated spinal lesions may be identified
6. Other associated lesions: cleft palate, umbilical hernia, club feet

In anencephalic fetuses, cranial measurements (biparietal diameter, head circumference) will not be obtainable. In cases when the fetal cranium is low in the maternal pelvis, a full bladder is beneficial to elevate the fetal head out of the pelvis.

Fetal acrania, a variant of anencephaly, can present with complete but abnormal brain development with an associated cranial defect in the skull.[115]

It is important to differentiate anencephaly from fetal microcephalus. Fetal microcephalus represents a condition marked by an abnormally small fetal calvarium; therefore this can potentially be misinterpreted as anencephalus. Amniotic band syndrome may be considered when there are large defects in the fetal skull.

The majority of anencephalics will be detected by maternal serum α-fetoprotein screening, by ultrasound in patients at risk for anencephaly, and by serendipitous recognition of anencephaly during routine obstetrical ultrasound examinations. To detect anencephaly during the antepartum period, an effort should be made to elucidate the cranium on all fetuses undergoing ultrasound.

A common technical problem sonographers will encounter is the evaluation of the fetal cranium when it is positioned low in the maternal pelvis. This is frequently observed in the patient in labor. Cranial measurements in many cases are unobtainable because of a deep fetal head position (engaged in the pelvis). Aside from this limita-

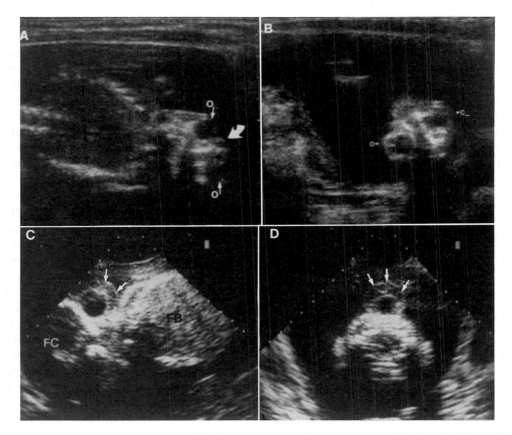

Fig. 23-5. A, Sagittal scan demonstrating an absence of the cranium above the level of the orbits *(arrow)* in a fetus with anencephaly at 22 weeks of gestation. Note the protuberant appearance of the orbits, *o;* **B,** In same patient, the orbits and nasal structures are noted in a transverse scan. Cranial structures were unidentifiable above the orbital level. *o,* Orbit. **C,** Transverse section of an occipital cephalocele *(arrows).* Protruding brain tissue could not be visualized within the cephalocele. *FC,* Fetal cranium; *FB,* fetal body. **D,** Transverse scan of cephalocele *(arrows)* with occiput of head projected anteriorly.

tion, the contour and echogenicity of the cranium should be identified.

Cephaloceles

Cephaloceles are neural tube defects involving the protrusion of meninges and, in many cases, fetal brain tissue through a defect in the fetal cranium. Cephaloceles occur in 1 per 2000 births.[25] These lesions result from a failure of the neural tube to close in the cephalic portion of the fetal skull.

Cephaloceles are most frequently found in the occipital region of the cranium in the cranial midline. Cephaloceles may involve the parietal, nasopharyngeal, or frontal bones.[25] Various forms of cephaloceles are possible. An encephalocele (protrusion of brain tissue) or meningocele (protrusion of meninges only) must be sonographically distinguished.

Although large cephaloceles are easily seen, small cephaloceles may be missed. Sonographic criteria for evaluation of a cephalocele include:

1. Herniation of a cranial saclike structure (Fig. 23-5, *C*)
2. Recognition of a bony defect in fetal cranium (small defects may be difficult to visualize)
3. Presence or absence of brain tissue within the cephalo-

cele (prognosis may vary based on presence or absence of brain tissue) (Fig. 23-5, *C*)
4. Location of the cephalocele should be determined (midline, occipital, parietal, nasopharyngeal, frontal); compare location of cephalocele to interhemispheric fissure and facial structures[25]

If a cephalocele has been identified on ultrasound, further evaluation of the fetus is necessary to search for coexisting fetal anomalies. Following are additional fetal organs that should be evaluated:

1. Fetal cranium: determine cranial size and normalcy of ventricles (macrocephaly—enlarged fetal head can be identified in fetuses with associated fetal hydrocephalus; microcephaly—small fetal head due to herniation of brain tissue into cephalocele)
2. Fetal spine: spina bifida can occur in conjunction with the existing neural tube defect of the cranium
3. Fetal kidneys: Meckel's syndrome—cephalocele, polycystic kidneys, polydactyly—is an autosomal recessive disease with the cephalocele as a marker for the syndrome
4. Specific fetal organs according to genetic syndrome (cephaloceles can occur with skeletal dysplasias and chromosomal anomalies)

The width of the lateral ventricle is represented as the distance from the interhemispheric fissure (falx) to the distal border of the lateral ventricle. The width of the cerebral hemisphere (HW) is calculated from the interhemispheric fissure (falx) to the first echo of the inner skull table. Both measurements should be obtained in the same perpendicular axis and within the distal hemisphere. To avoid interference by artifacts within the proximal (upper) cranial hemisphere, the distal ratio is most frequently determined. The sonographer must avoid measuring in an oblique plane or incorrectly determining the LVW/HW ratio at the level of the BPD. The insular echo located at the level of the BPD should not be confused with the lateral border of the ventricle. The insula is positioned lower in the head and can be recognized by identifying the pulsations of the middle cerebral artery (see Chapter 20).

Intracranial landmarks helpful in identifying the correct level to measure the LVW/HW ratio include (1) the temporal horns of the lateral ventricles lie above the biparietal diameter landmarks (thalamus, third ventricle, insula), (2) the lateral border of the ventricle courses in parallel with the interhemispheric fissure (falx), and (3) the cerebral hemispheres should be noted to be symmetric. Measurements of the LVW/HW ratio should be obtained in the same location and level on repeated studies.

The LVW/HW ratio is considered abnormal when it exceeds 95% for the given gestational age (Table 23-1). In general, after the twenty-second week of gestation the LVW/HW ratio should not exceed 50%, or in other words, the lateral border of the temporal ventricle should be less than halfway between the falx and outer skull table. It is important to remember that a borderline ratio does not conclusively indicate ventriculomegaly. A small percentage of normal fetuses will have larger-than-average-sized ventricles, and this abnormal LVW/HW ratio merely represents a normal variant.[18] Follow-up ultrasound studies are recommended to isolate those fetuses with pathologically dilated ventricles. In the second trimester (less than 24 weeks), ventricular enlargement may be difficult to diagnose by the LVW/HW ratio. Pretorius and associates[118] have suggested further criteria for determining ventriculomegaly in the second trimester. The LVH/HW ratio should be compared to normal ratios at each gestational age, the lateral ventricle width should measure less than 1.1 cm and the choroid plexus should appear to fill the ventricular body and atria. Progressive ventriculomegaly can be suspected when the LVW/HW ratio fails to decrease in size and remains constant during the second trimester.

Management decisions (options for intrauterine shunting, early delivery, or cephalocentesis) are based on the progression of cerebral ventricle dilatation and clinical factors.[19,47,108] Increases in the LVW/HW ratio may be indicative of worsening ventriculomegaly and may prompt the need for fetal surgery or delivery.

Ultrasound examination of the fetus at risk for ventriculomegaly, as indicated by family history, should include the following:

1. Antepartum obstetrical ultrasound examination (see Chapter 20)
2. Evaluation of the occipital, temporal, and frontal horns of the ventricular system
3. Evaluation of the integrity of the interhemispheric fissure (falx cerebri)
4. Evaluation of the posterior fossae (Dandy-Walker and Arnold-Chiari malformations originate in this space)
5. Calculation of the LVW/HW ratio and standard cranial measurements

Several sonographic studies are often necessary to diagnose fetal ventriculomegaly. As the natural history of ventriculomegaly is unknown in the majority of cases, it is difficult to predict the time of development of ventriculomegaly in at-risk fetuses. For example, if a fetus at risk for ventriculomegaly is found to have normal ventricles at 19 weeks of gestation, this does not guarantee the fetus will not manifest dilated ventricles later in pregnancy. Therefore serial ultrasound evaluations of these fetuses are performed throughout the course of gestation. Typically the fetus at risk for hydrocephaly is evaluated beginning at the 17th to 18th week of gestation, with follow-up studies at 19 to 20 and 22 to 24 weeks to allow the option for termination of pregnancy in the affected fetus. In addition, early scanning and recognition of ventriculomegaly will allow for the consideration of fetal surgical shunting techniques.

After ventriculomegaly has been documented by ultrasound, the patient is commonly scanned weekly to follow the progression of ventricular dilatation. Fetuses who exhibit an increasing expansion of the ventricles may be candidates for fetal surgery or early delivery.

The following sonographic criteria are diagnostic for fetal ventriculomegaly:

1. Dilatation of the occipital and temporal horns of the ventricles, which exceeds the ranges of normal for the given gestational age (based on LVW/HW ratio and sonographic observations) (Fig. 23-6, A)
2. Massive dilatation of the cerebral ventricles (LVW/HW ratio commonly unobtainable)
3. Enlargement of the third and/or fourth ventricle found in conjunction with dilatation of the temporal and occipital ventricles (Fig. 23-6, B)
4. Diminished amounts of cortical mantle that appear displaced toward the lateral aspects of the fetal skull by dilated ventricles as determined by LVW/HW ratio (Fig. 23-6)
5. Ability to clearly reproduce evidence of ventriculomegaly

When the sonographic diagnosis of ventriculomegaly has been made, a comprehensive survey of the fetus is performed to detect coexisting malformations (Table 23-2). Evaluation of the intracranial and extracranial contents is important in the evaluation of the fetus with ventriculomegaly. Most fetuses with ventriculomegaly have additional fetal anomalies.

The contour of the skull should be inspected for cephaloceles or irregularities in the contour of the calvarium. Clover-leaf skull deformities have been found in association with ventriculomegaly.[20]

Table 23-2   Fetal Anatomy Evaluation in Fetuses with Ventriculomegaly

Region	Anatomical site	To evaluate for
Cranium	Contour of skull	Cephalocele, clover-leaf skull
	Cranial size	Normocephaly, macrocephaly, microcephaly
	Interhemispheric fissure	Holoprosencephaly, arachnoid cyst, porencephaly, space-occupying lesion
	Texture of brain tissue	Calcifications associated with intrauterine infection (CMV, toxoplasmosis)
	Extent of ventriculomegaly	Dilatation of temporal, occipital, frontal horns of lateral ventricles, third and fourth ventricles
	Intracranial anatomy	Additional structural anomalies (cerebellar agenesis, agenesis of corpus callosum)
	Posterior cranial fossa	Dandy-Walker or Arnold-Chiari malformation
	Cortical mantle	Hydranencephaly, severe ventriculomegaly
Face	Orbits	Hypotelorism, hypertelorism, cyclopia
	Nose	Single or absent nostrils
	Lips, palate	Cleft lip, cleft palate
Thorax	Heart	Structural cardiac anomalies (fetal echocardiography)
Abdomen	Liver	Ascites, cysts
	Stomach, bowel	Gastrointestinal anomalies
	Kidneys, bladder	Polycystic kidneys (Meckel's), renal agenesis (bilateral), unilateral renal agenesis
		Dysplastic kidneys
	Genitalia	Sex determination for sex-linked disorders (aqueductal stenosis)
Vertebral column	Spine	Spinal defects
Skeleton	Limbs	Skeletal dysplasias
	Hands, feet	Structural deformities
Biometric profile	BPD, HC, OFD	Cranial growth
	Orbital distances	Orbital distance anomalies
	Abdominal circumference	Estimation of fetal weight
	Limb lengths	Fetal gestational age and growth
	H/A ratio	Head to abdomen disproportion
	LVW/HW ratio	Degree of ventriculomegaly

The size of the fetal cranium is significant in the prognosis, management, and delivery of the fetus with dilated ventricles. In many cases fetal cranial size is normal, even in the presence of ventriculomegaly. Ventriculomegaly can be appreciated in most fetuses prior to any enlargement of the fetal calvarium. Enlargement of the fetal cranium may occur secondary to fetal ventriculomegaly as the fetal sutures are distensible and will expand from increased pressure and enlargement of the ventricles. Macrocephaly is used to refer to the fetal cranium, which is large for the gestational age secondary to fetal ventriculomegaly. In contrast, the fetal cranium may be abnormally small in fetuses with ventriculomegaly (Fig. 23-7). Isolated microcephaly can present with the typical features of a small calvarium and dilatation of the ventricles. The presence of microcephaly in conjunction with fetal ventriculomegaly may signify an underlying syndrome or defect. For instance, fetuses with holoprosencephaly may manifest with microcephaly, hydrocephaly, and varying orbital and facial anomalies.[105] The accurate estimation of cranial biometry is therefore essential in differentiating various types of cranial malformations.

The interhemispheric fissure (falx cerebri) is an important landmark to identify in the fetus with ventriculomegaly. Absence of this fissure may suggest hydranencephaly

or alobar holoprosencephaly[26] (Fig. 23-8). Arachnoid cysts have been noted to obscure the normal course of the interhemispheric fissure. A shift of the midline echo complex may be indicative of a porencephalic cyst or other space-occupying lesion that may cause marked deviations of the normal cranial structures.[18]

The texture of the brain tissue should be inspected for calcifications, which may suggest intrauterine infection as the cause for enlarged ventricles (e.g., cytomegalic inclusion virus [CMV], toxoplasmosis). Identification of calcifications within the fetal brain should prompt the sonographer to evaluate the fetal abdomen for ascites, which has been noted in conjunction with maternal infection during pregnancy.

All ventricular chambers should be evaluated in the fetus with enlarged ventricles. The extent of dilatation should be assessed in the frontal, temporal, occipital, and third and fourth ventricles.

Intracranial anatomy, in addition to ventricular evaluation, needs to be studied. Recognition of normal-appearing intracranial structures is extremely beneficial in the diagnosis and counseling of patients. Cerebral agenesis and agenesis of the corpus callosum may be sonographically appreciated.[35]

The posterior cranial fossa should be routinely evalu-

increased pressure within the fetal cranium resulting from dilated ventricles by the percutaneous insertion of a shunt directed into the fetal brain under ultrasound guidance. Fetal surgery was designed to arrest hydrocephalus to prevent further brain damage as a result of enlarging ventricles. Severe compression of the developing fetal brain may invoke irreversible brain damage, which may not be amenable to correction after birth.[58] The intent of an intrauterine shunt, therefore, was to drain fluid from the dilated ventricle via the intracranial shunt and into the amniotic cavity. This allowed a temporary decrease in intracranial pressure and, in many cases, stabilization of the ventriculomegaly. With the arrest of ventriculomegaly, it was hoped that developing brain tissue would continue to proliferate, thereby preserving brain tissue until delivery and neonatal correction could be achieved.

Early attempts at intrauterine treatment for fetal hydrocephalus were performed by Osathanondh and Birnholz.[9,114] A needle was introduced into the cranium under ultrasound guidance to decompress the fetal head to permit delivery. Although this technique was encouraging because it proved successful in decompressing the fetal cranium, it failed to prevent the reaccumulation of ventricular fluid.

Clewell and associates in 1982[34] devised a procedure that decompressed the ventricular system by inserting an indwelling shunt into the ventricle, thereby relieving intraventricular pressure and decompressing the dilated ventricular system. The technique incorporates a temporary shunt that, when functioning, prevents further compression of the fetal brain, thus allowing the pregnancy to advance to delivery and neonatal correction.

The intrauterine surgical shunting technique entails the following: (1) under local anesthesia and maternal/fetal sedation, a needle is sonographically guided into the parietal bone of the fetal skull; (2) the shunt is then passed through the center of the needle and into the dilated ventricle and the needle is withdrawn; (3) one end of the shunt is secured within the ventricle and the opposite end is left within the amniotic cavity in order to allow the cerebrospinal fluid to drain into the amniotic fluid.[47]

Ultrasound is used to monitor the procedure in the placement of the shunt and in the observation of fetal cardiac activity and movements. The LVW/HW ratio is performed prior to shunt placement and following fetal surgery. Decreases in the LVW/HW ratio may be indicative of a functioning intrauterine shunt whereas a rapid accumulation of ventricular fluid may indicate failure of the shunt or dislodgement.[47] Localization of the shunt within the fetal calvarium should be documented on serial sonographic studies.

Candidates for fetal surgery have been defined by the Society of Fetal Medicine[35,108]:

1. Fetuses with isolated ventriculomegaly (no evidence of sonographic, chromosomal, or other associated fetal abnormalities)
2. Fetuses with isolated ventriculomegaly less than 30 weeks of gestation (after 30 weeks and pulmonic maturity, delivery is preferred)
3. Progressive ventriculomegaly with diminution of cortical mantle as identified by ultrasound
4. Singleton fetuses
5. Patients receiving informed consent concerning experimental nature of the procedure (known benefits and risks)
6. Patients willing to undergo neonatal follow-up and study of child who received intrauterine shunt

The majority of fetuses with ventriculomegaly are not candidates for intrauterine fetal treatment due to associated fetal malformations or advanced gestational age. The crucial role of ultrasound is to determine which fetuses have isolated ventriculomegaly. It is important to realize that many abnormalities that may coexist with ventriculomegaly may be undetectable by ultrasound. The sonographic team must diligently scrutinize the fetus for sonographically detectable defects once ventriculomegaly has been identified by evaluating all major organ systems to identify those fetuses with single or multiple lesions.

The fetal surgical team includes an obstetrician skilled in surgical procedures and intrauterine transfusions, pediatric neurosurgeons, neonatologists, and pediatric surgeons for treatment following delivery. In addition, experienced sonographers/sonologists skilled in the detection of fetal malformations, geneticists, and anesthesiologists complete the team.[35,108]

Forty-four fetuses have undergone intrauterine shunting procedures.[108] The conclusions of the International Fetal Surgery Registry[104,108] have summarized that the current technique of indwelling catheter placement in hydrocephalic fetuses is generally poor and experimental. Factors leading to this conclusion stem from the lack of information regarding the natural history of ventriculomegaly, the limitations of ultrasound techniques to clearly elucidate fetal malformations, suboptimal results in maintaining a functioning shunt, and blockage and dislodgement of the shunt resulting in additional shunting procedures.

Intrauterine treatment for fetal ventriculomegaly has not proven to be clearly beneficial and is burdened by the risks of fetal death, chorioamnionitis, and premature labor. Consequently, this has discouraged fetal surgeons in the current treatment of the hydrocephalic fetus.[108] Recent animal studies have shown that indwelling shunts may stop fetal ventriculomegaly and has shown the potential for growth of cortical tissue.[108] Further animal investigations and long-term follow-up of human fetuses who were shunted in the antenatal period are necessary to determine the efficacy of therapy for the fetus with ventriculomegaly.

Hydranencephaly

Hydranencephaly is a condition characterized by the failure of the cerebral hemispheres to develop. Hydranencephaly occurs as a result of an obstruction to the internal carotid vessels, which prohibits the formation of the cerebral hemispheres. Consequently, there is impairment to the absorption of cerebrospinal fluid, which results in the accumulation of fluid within the fetal cranium. Because of this cerebral defect, the cerebral hemispheres (which would normally develop above the carotid vessels) fail to form. The portion of the fetal brain that is vascularly supplied by the basilar artery, however, will develop. Therefore the midbrain, basal ganglia, and cerebellum—and occasionally the occipital lobes of the brain—will be present.[45,60]

During sonographic evaluation the fetal cranium will appear to be filled with large quantities of fluid surrounding the midbrain structures. As a consequence of this process, fetal brain tissue is damaged and replaced by cerebrospinal fluid.

The prognosis for hydranencephaly is dismal, and therefore recognition of this defect in the antenatal period is desirable.

Sonographic evaluation of all fetuses with ventriculomegaly should attempt to scrutinize intracranial contents and cerebral mantle to detect fetuses with this condition. The sonographic diagnosis of hydranencephaly may be difficult to distinguish from severe ventriculomegaly as the cerebral mantle may be thinned in the latter, although brain tissue can usually be recognized within the frontal and occipital lobe regions.[60]

Several sonographic signs are suggestive of hydranencephaly[18,45,60,115]:

1. Grossly enlarged fluid-filled cavity within fetal cranium
2. Inability to define the interhemispheric fissure (absent in this condition)
3. Sonographic demonstration of the midbrain, basal ganglia, and cerebellum surrounded by large quantities of fluid
4. Absence of cortical mantle tissue (may be found in occipital region)
5. Polyhydramnios may occur in conjunction with hydranencephaly

Extreme caution should be exerted in the consideration of fetal hydranencephaly as severe forms of ventriculomegaly and holoprosencephaly may mimic this cranial defect.[18,60] In the event that the specific fetal malformation cannot be defined by antenatal ultrasound, it is important to remember that the prognoses for hydranencephaly, alobar holoprosencephaly, and severe ventriculomegaly are equally poor.[18] In many instances neonatal sonography and computerized axial tomography are necessary to differentiate between these lesions.

Holoprosencephaly

Holoprosencephaly represents an intracranial abnormality characterized by a common dilated ventricular cavity. It is important to recognize the fetus with this condition as the management and prognosis differs from ventriculomegaly. Holoprosencephaly encompasses a spectrum of cerebral malformations that result from the faulty sagittal cleavage of the forebrain (prosencephalon). This defect is commonly found with varying facial anomalies that occur along the midline facial plane of the fetus. Holoprosencephalic defects range from the severe alobar type to the less severe semilobar and lobar forms.[26,60]

Embryologically the prechordal mesoderm is responsible for the cleavage of the prosencephalon and development of the nasofrontal areas. The ethmoid, nasal bones

and septum, premaxilla, and vomer bone represent these processes. When these structures fail to form, facial malformations develop that can affect the orbits, nose, lips, and palate. Facial defects vary in severity, ranging from fused or single orbits to hypotelorism (decreased distance between the orbits). Nasal anomalies range from the absence of the nostrils/nasal structures to single nostrils, although in all forms the nasal bones may appear normal. Often midline clefts involve the lip and soft palate.[26,60]

In the most severe form of holoprosencephaly (alobar), there is a failure of the cerebral hemispheres to divide, and consequently the falx cerebri and interhemispheric fissure are absent. A common ventricular chamber and fused thalamus are seen. The single ventricle occupies the parietal, occipital, and frontal regions of the fetal skull and has a C-shape configuration (Fig. 23-8). Although difficult to diagnose antenatally, there is often absence of the corpus callosum and olfactory bulbs (arhinencephaly). Facial anomalies that have been identified in alobar holoprosencephaly range from cyclopia (single bony orbit with a proboscis—fleshy piece of tissue found above the orbit), ethmocephaly (proboscis located between separate orbits) (Fig. 23-9), cebocephaly (hypotelorism with a single-nostril nose),[105] and clefts of the lip and/or palate. Facial malformations are frequently observed in alobar holoprosencephaly; however, this is not a universal finding. When facial anomalies are sonographically detected in conjunction with a common ventricle, fused thalami, and absent interhemispheric fissure, alobar holoprosencephaly should be suspected. The differential diagnosis of alobar holoprosencephaly includes severe ventriculomegaly, hydranencephaly, massive Dandy-Walker cysts, porencephalic cysts, and arachnoid cysts.[45]

The size of the fetal cranium may vary in fetuses with alobar holoprosencephaly. Microcephaly is most commonly found because of a reduced amount of brain tissue; however, an enlarged fetal cranium (macrocephaly) may be found when ventriculomegaly is associated. A normal cranial head size may be found with this condition and is more common with the milder forms of holoprosencephaly.[26]

The prognosis for alobar holoprosencephaly is extremely poor with survival unlikely; therefore differentiation of this cranial disorder from other cystic lesions is needed for proper counseling and obstetric management.[26,115] Intrauterine shunting procedures are contraindicated in these cases, and often the mode of delivery will vary, depending on the ultrasound findings.[26]

Semilobar holoprosencephaly represents an intermediate form of holoprosencephaly and is manifested by a partial separation of the cerebral hemispheres.[26]

In lobar holoprosencephaly the cerebral hemispheres are present and usually completely divided, although fusion may occur in the frontal portion of the fetal brain. In this form the brain is usually normal and the septum pellucidum absent.[45] Identification of the septum pellucidum negates the possibility of lobar holoprosencephaly.

Facial abnormalities may be absent in both types, although hypotelorism may be recognized. The sonographic diagnosis of semilobar and lobar holoprenceph-

OTHER CRANIAL ANOMALIES

A number of rare intracranial malformations can be visualized with sonography. Many of these disorders may be difficult to categorize by antenatal ultrasound and most often are differentiated based on family history and newborn evaluation.

Porencephalic cysts are fluid-filled structures that are produced secondary to fetal intracerebral hemorrhage. [60,115] These cysts can vary in size and location and may distort normal cranial landmarks. Porencephalic cysts may produce a shift of the midline echo structures. The prognosis for porencephaly may be extremely poor; therefore recognition of this type of lesion is important.

Fetal intracranial hemorrhages have been sonographically diagnosed. When the hemorrhage is within the ventricle, the ventricular cavity will appear highly echogenic, and in some cases ventriculomegaly will be present.

Evaluation of the posterior fossa and cerebellum is necessary in the comprehensive examination of the fetal cranium. The cerebellum and posterior fossae can be studied in a transverse section through the fetal head at a level caudad to the biparietal diameter plane. The cerebellar hemispheres and cisterna magna are identifiable at this level (see Chapter 20). Intracranial lesions of the posterior fossae can be identified by comparing the size of each cerebellar hemisphere[115] and by evaluation of the cisterna magna.[37]

Anomalies of the posterior fossae may involve total or partial absence of the cerebellum. Normal dimensions of the cerebellum[94] and the cisterna magna have been reported.[37,100] Enlargement of the cisterna magna may indicate hypoplasia of the cerebellum or may be associated with hydrocephalus or represent a normal variant.[37] In Dandy-Walker malformations an obstruction of the foramen of Magendie results in the formation of a cyst of the fourth ventricle; consequently, a cystic mass lies within the posterior fossae. In Joubert syndrome there is a congenital absence of the cerebellum, therefore evaluation of the posterior fossae is necessary in the evaluation of patients at risk for this lesion.[115] Cerebellar agenesis may be found in association with chromosomal trisomies, ventriculomegaly, microcephaly, and spina bifida.[37,115]

Arteriovenous malformations may be diagnosed by sonography and present as cystic masses of the fetal brain, which may cause dilatation of the ventricles. Doppler techniques (see Chapter 21) may be useful in isolating an arteriovenous anomaly.

ABNORMALITIES OF THE FACE

Remarkable enhancements in sonographic imaging have generated a tremendous interest in imaging the facial structures of the fetus. These advancements in the identification of facial morphology have been exemplified previously (see Chapter 20). A knowledge of normal anatomic facial structures is imperative to appreciate subtle malformations of facial architecture.

Craniofacial malformations are common birth defects with an incidence of 1 per 600 births.[33,139] Facial defects discovered during comprehensive sonographic studies represent significant findings, as coexisting fetal anomalies usually exist. Many fetuses with facial defects have chromosomal abnormalities. Therefore a careful investigation of the fetal face should be pursued during all studies for fetal anomalies.

Although sophisticated equipment promises to allow investigators to identify even more subtle facial details, it is unrealistic to hope that superior facial detail will be identifiable in all fetuses at risk for anomalies. Conditions that may interfere with comprehensive facial studies include unfavorable fetal lie, oligohydramnios, maternal obesity, and unsophisticated ultrasound equipment. In most cases the fetal face will be accessible for examination. Frequently, subtle manipulation of the fetus and operator patience is necessary to obtain optimal and interpretable views of the face.

Fetal facial structures are most easily recognized after the 22nd week of gestation; however, the antenatal diagnosis of congenital lesions is desirable prior to that time; therefore conclusive studies of the face remain a challenge for even the most experienced scanners. In lieu of the above-mentioned limitations, dedicated studies of the face need to continue. Certainly several facial anomalies are recognizable during the second trimester of pregnancy.

As discussed earlier, deformities of the fetal face may often identify the type of cranial abnormality. For example, recognition of a single orbit and a proboscis is highly indicative of alobar holoprosencephaly.

Abnormalities of the forehead

Views of the fetal forehead can best be appreciated by evaluation of the fetal profile. This can be achieved by a series of midsagittal scans through the fetal face.[116] The fetal forehead (frontal bone) in this view should appear as a curvilinear surface with differentiation of the forehead, nose, lips, and chin. This view will allow the diagnosis of anterior cephaloceles, which can arise in the frontal region of the skull. The characteristics of anterior cephaloceles are typical of cephaloceles in other locations. Anterior cephaloceles may cause abnormally wide-spaced orbits (hypertelorism).[129]

Clover-leaf skull deformities present with prominence of the forehead, which may be identifiable by ultrasound techniques. Clover-leaf skull deformities have been associated with skeletal dysplasias (dwarfism) and ventriculomegaly.[20,129] Any irregularities in the contour of the forehead should prompt the investigator to search for additional fetal malformations. Profile views of the fetal skull are also helpful in the study of fetuses at risk for thantophoric dysplasia, achondroplasia, and osteopetrosis in which a prominent forehead is characteristic.[63]

Abnormalities of the orbits

Orbital architecture has become increasingly important in the evaluation of craniofacial anomalies. The anatomy of the orbits (see Chapter 20), their use in gestational age assessment (see Chapter 21),[78] and their role in detecting ocular abnormalities[105] have been investigated. Orbital

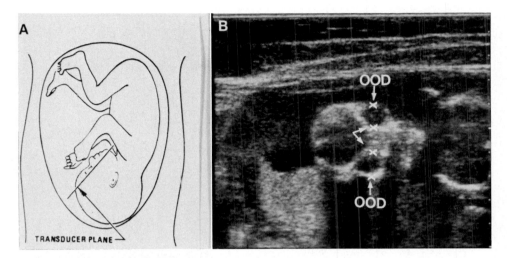

Fig. 23-11.   A, Frontal view demonstrating a fetus in a vertex presentation with the fetal cranium in an occipitotransverse position. The transducer is placed along the coronal plane (approximately 2 cm posterior to the glabella-alveolar line). **B,** Coronal sonographic plane demonstrating outer orbital distance, *OOD,* and inner orbital distance, *IOD (angled arrows).* The IOD is measured from the medial border of the orbit to the opposite medial border *(angled arrows).* The OOD is measured from the outermost lateral border of the orbit to the opposite lateral border.(**A** from Mayden KL, Tortora M, Berkowitz RL, et al: Am J Obstet Gynecol 144:289, 1982.)

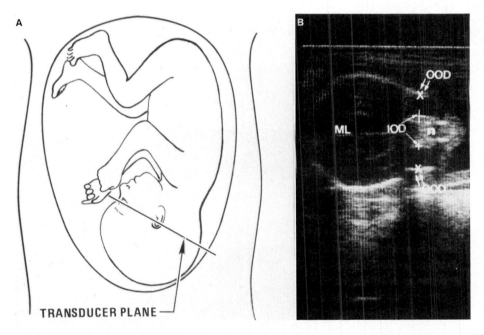

Fig. 23-12.   A, Frontal view demonstrating the fetal cranium in an occipitotransverse position. The transducer is placed along the orbitomeatal line (approximately 2 to 3 cm below the level of the biparietal diameter). **B,** Sonogram through the fetal cranium in this position demonstrating midline, *ML,* nasal process, *n,* outer orbital distance (OOD—*double small arrows*), and inner orbital distance (IOD—*white bars*). (From Mayden KL, Tortora M, Berkowitz RL, et al: Am J Obstet Gynecol 144:289, 1982.)

distance measurements are beneficial in the diagnosis of fetal conditions in which hypotelorism or hypertelorism is a feature. Both of these conditions are frequently associated with other fetal anomalies, and often the orbital problem will elucidate the type of cranial anomaly or genetic syndrome. Therefore both an anatomic and biometric evaluation of the fetal orbits should be attempted in fetuses at risk for orbital malformations.

The fetal orbits can be measured reliably in two planes when the fetal head is in an occipitotransverse position (fetal cranium on the side): (1) a coronal scan posterior to the glabelloalveolar line (Fig. 23-11) and (2) a transverse scan at a level below the biparietal diameter (along the orbitomeatal line) (Fig. 23-12). In these views the individual orbital rings, nasal structures, and maxillary processes can be identified. When the fetus is in an occipito-

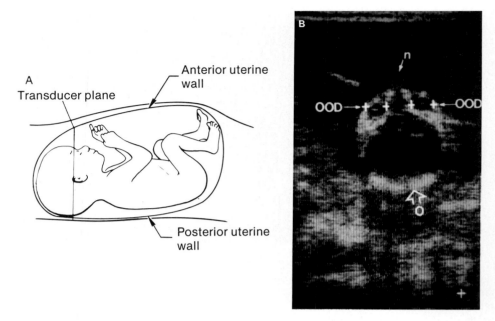

Fig. 23-13. **A,** Side view demonstrating the fetus in an occipitoposterior position. The transducer is placed in a plane that transects the occiput, orbits, and nasal process. **B,** Sonogram through the fetal cranium in an occipitoposterior position. *Open arrow*, occiput; IOD—crosses, inner orbital distance; OOD, outer orbital distance; *arrow* = nasal process. Note the linear echo within each orbit representing the lenses of the eyes. (**A** From Mayden KL, Tortora M, Berkowitz RL, et al: Am J Obstet Gynecol 144:289, 1982. **B** From Mayden KL: J Med Ultrasound 8:117, 1984.)

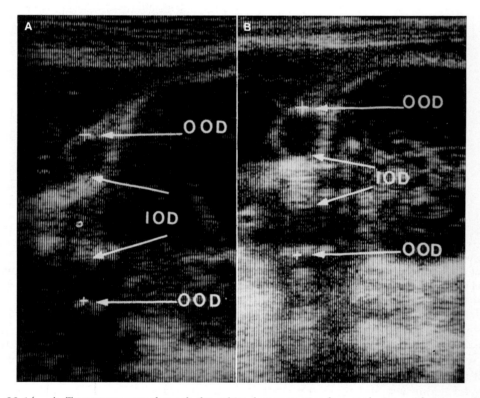

Fig. 23-14. **A,** Transverse scan through the orbits demonstrating hypertelorism with inner orbital distance, *IOD*, and outer orbital distance, *OOD*, that are increased for the gestational age of 31 weeks. **B,** Transverse scan through the orbits of a normal fetus at 31 weeks of gestation demonstrating normal IOD and OOD. (From Chervenak FA, Tortora M, Mayden KL, et al: Am J Obstet Gynecol 149:94, 1984.)

Table 23-3 Predicted BPD and Weeks Gestation from the Inner and Outer Orbital Distances

BPD (cm)	Gestation (wk)	IOD (cm)	BPD (cm)	OOD (cm)	Gestation (wk)	IOD (cm)	OOD (cm)
1.9	11.6	0.5	1.3	5.8	24.3	1.6	4.1
2.0	11.6	0.5	1.4	5.9	24.3	1.6	4.2
2.1	12.1	0.6	1.5	6.0	24.7	1.6	4.3
2.2	12.6	0.6	1.6	6.1	25.2	1.6	4.3
2.3	12.6	0.6	1.7	6.2	25.2	1.6	4.4
2.4	13.1	0.7	1.7	6.3	25.7	1.7	4.4
2.5	13.6	0.7	1.8	6.4	26.2	1.7	4.5
2.6	13.6	0.7	1.9	6.5	26.2	1.7	4.5
2.7	14.1	0.8	2.0	6.6	26.7	1.7	4.6
2.8	14.6	0.8	2.1	6.7	27.2	1.7	4.6
2.9	14.6	0.8	2.1	6.8	27.6	1.7	4.7
3.0	15.0	0.9	2.2	6.9	28.1	1.7	4.7
3.1	15.5	0.9	2.3	7.0	28.6	1.8	4.8
3.2	15.5	0.9	2.4	7.1	29.1	1.8	4.8
3.3	16.0	1.0	2.5	7.3	29.6	1.8	4.9
3.4	16.5	1.0	2.5	7.4	30.0	1.8	5.0
3.5	16.5	1.0	2.6	7.5	30.6	1.8	5.0
3.6	17.0	1.0	2.7	7.6	31.0	1.8	5.1
3.7	17.5	1.1	2.7	7.7	31.5	1.8	5.1
3.8	17.9	1.1	2.8	7.8	32.0	1.8	5.2
4.0	18.4	1.2	3.0	7.9	32.5	1.9	5.2
4.2	18.9	1.2	3.1	8.0	33.0	1.9	5.3
4.3	19.4	1.2	3.2	8.2	33.5	1.9	5.4
4.4	19.4	1.3	3.2	8.3	34.0	1.9	5.4
4.5	19.9	1.3	3.3	8.4	34.4	1.9	5.4
4.6	20.4	1.3	3.4	8.5	35.0	1.9	5.5
4.7	20.4	1.3	3.4	8.6	35.4	1.9	5.5
4.8	20.9	1.4	3.5	8.8	35.9	1.9	5.6
4.9	21.3	1.4	3.6	8.9	36.4	1.9	5.6
5.0	21.3	1.4	3.6	9.0	36.9	1.9	5.7
5.1	21.8	1.4	3.7	9.1	37.3	1.9	5.7
5.2	22.3	1.4	3.8	9.2	37.8	1.9	5.8
5.3	22.3	1.5	3.8	9.3	38.3	1.9	5.8
5.4	22.8	1.5	3.9	9.4	38.8	1.9	5.8
5.5	23.3	1.5	4.0	9.6	39.3	1.9	5.9
5.6	23.3	1.5	4.0	9.7	39.8	1.9	5.9
5.7	23.8	1.5	4.1				

Adapted from Mayden KL, Tortora M, Berkowitz RL et al: Am J Obstet Gynecol 144:289, 1982.

posterior position (fetal orbits directed up), orbital distances can also be determined. In this view the orbital rings, lens, and nasal structures can be demonstrated (Fig. 23-13). Measurements of the inner orbital distance (IOD) should be made from the medial border of the orbit to the opposite medial border while the outer orbital distance (OOD) is measured from the lateral border of one orbit to the opposite lateral wall[105] (Fig. 23-11 to 23-13). Nomograms for orbital distance spacing have been reported (Table 23-3).[79,105]

Hypotelorism. Hypotelorism is a fetal condition in which there is a reduced distance between the orbits (Fig. 23-9) that is highly associated with additional fetal anomalies and genetic syndromes.[105,129] Hypotelorism in the fetus can range from cyclopia (single fused orbit) to varying degrees of hypotelorism (cebocephaly and eth-

mocephaly). Ultrasound has proven to be useful in detecting the most severe forms of hypotelorism.[26,105] Measurements of the IOD and OOD will define fetuses with orbital distances outside of the normal ranges and therefore suspicious for hypotelorism. Fetal conditions that may demonstrate hypotelorism include several forms of holoprosencephaly, microcephaly, and phenylketonuria (PKU).

Hypertelorism. Hypertelorism is characterized as abnormally wide-spaced orbits. Fetal hypertelorism can be diagnosed by orbital distances that fall significantly above normal ranges for gestational age. Hypertelorism has been noted in a number of abnormal fetal conditions, genetic syndromes, and chromosomal anomalies. Fetuses exposed to phenytoin (Dilantin) during pregnancy may manifest signs of hypertelorism as part of the fetal phenytoin syndrome (microcephaly; growth abnormalities; cleft lip/palate; cardiac, genitourinary, central nervous system, and skeletal anomalies). In Pfeiffer and Apert syndromes, hypertelorism and brachycephaly (see Chapter 21) have been described[129] as a result of abnormal closure of the cranial sutures (craniosynostosis). In both syndromes, ventriculomegaly may be identified. Other conditions that manifest with hypertelorism and unusual cranial contours include Crouzon disease cephalosyndactyly, acrocephalopolysyndactyly, and oculodentodigital dysplasia.[129]

As demonstrated with hypotelorism, the recognition of hypertelorism may provide evidence for a particular genetic syndrome or concurrent anomalies of the fetus. Median cleft face syndrome was diagnosed in a fetus with ventriculomegaly based on the sonographic findings of hypertelorism and cleft lip[31] (Fig. 23-14).

Evaluation of the orbits in the fetus with ventriculomegaly cannot be overemphasized. In addition, orbital studies are highly useful in evaluation of fetuses at risk for craniofacial malformations.[116]

Abnormalities of the nose, maxilla, lips, and palate

The normal anatomy of the fetal nose, maxilla, and lips have been described (see Chapter 20). Evaluation of this facial complex can be achieved by placement of the transducer in a lateral coronal plane, sagittal profile plane, and in modified tangential maxillary views[8] (inferior-superior projection) (Fig. 23-15). In the lateral coronal view the integrity of the nasal structures in relationship to the orbital rings and maxillae can be appreciated. In a profile plane the contour of the nose, upper and lower lips, and chin can be delineated. This is an important view in assessing the presence or absence of the nose, lips, and chin. Absence of the nose can be detected in this scanning plane. Irregularities in the contour of the nose may indicate a particular syndrome. Tangential cuts with the transducer angled inferiorly to superiorly through the maxilla will demonstrate the nasal septum, openings of the nostrils, and nares. Congenital absence of the nose or a single or atypical nostril placement may be identified in this view. In fetuses with holoprosencephaly, careful scrutiny of this area should be sought, as anomalies of the nose are frequent.

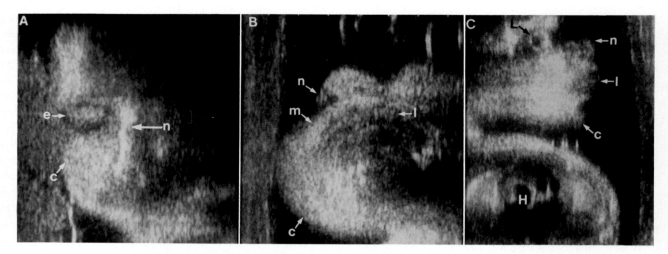

Fig. 23-15. **A,** Coronal section of the face illustrating the eyelid, *e,* cheek, *c,* and nasal bones, *n.* **B,** Tangential plane demonstrating nares, *n,* maxillae, *m,* lips, *l,* and chin, *c.* **C,** Profile scan outlining ocular lens, *L,* soft tissue of the nose, *n,* lips, *l,* and chin, *c.* H, Heart.

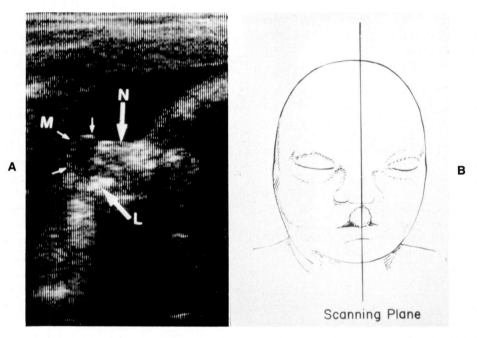

Fig. 23-16. **A,** Sagittal scan showing fetal profile and relationship of mass to nose and lip. *L,* lip; *N,* nose; *M,* mass. **B,** Demonstration of scanning plane. (From Chervenak FA, Tortora M, Mayden KL, et al: Am J Obstet Gynecol 149:94, 1984.)

Evaluation of the nasal triad should include assessment of (1) nostril symmetry, (2) nasal septum integrity, and (3) continuity of maxilla and upper lip to exclude cleft lip and palate (Fig. 23-16).

The fetal maxilla is a highly reflective structure during the fetal period and therefore amenable to sonographic study. Because the maxilla represents the posterior border of the nasal structures, it is an important landmark in the assessment of the fetus at risk for premaxillary protuberance as seen in Robert syndrome[63] and clefting of the fetal face (cleft lip and palate).

Improvements in imaging have permitted the antenatal diagnosis of cleft lip and palate. Seeds and Cefalo[134] are credited with the first report of bilateral cleft lip and palate by antenatal ultrasound. The diagnosis of facial clefting can be determined by evaluating the fetal nose, nasal septum, maxilla, and lips. Scanning views as detailed earlier are used to evaluate the morphology of the face.

Clefts of the face may occur along different facial planes because of defects in development or maturation of the embryonic facial structures.[135] Defects range from clefting of the lip alone to frequent involvement of the hard and soft palate, which can extend to the nose and, in rare cases, to the inferior border of the orbit. In addition, clefts can occur as unilateral (one side of lip) or bilateral (both sides of lip) lesions.

Cleft lip is the most common facial clefting abnormality and occurs due to the absence or lack of development of embryonic tissues. Cleft palate results from a lack of fusion of the sides of the palate. Cleft lip can occur with or without cleft palate; cleft palate can also occur as an isolated anomaly. The etiology of these facial malformations appears to be related to heredity and environmental factors.[135] Clefting of the face occurs as often as 1 per 600 births,[33,139] and therefore an expected increase in the frequency of patients referred for exclusion of these lesions can be expected in ultrasound laboratories. The association of other fetal anomalies has been found in fetuses with cleft lip and palate.[135]

With improved resolution, continued prenatal diagnoses will be made in regard to structural facial defects; however, it should be stressed that evaluation of the fetal face is extremely difficult and is dependent on equipment and operator sophistication, the amount of amniotic fluid, and fetal position. Even under optimal circumstances, facial scanning is not an infallible screening modality for lesions of the face. Severe clefting defects may be sonographically detected; however, small lesions and those that may be hidden by bone shadowing may be missed by sonography.[116] With these caveats in mind, the sonographer should attempt to become familiar with the embryologic development of the facial structures to fully appreciate the intricacies of abnormal facial morphology. The future of prenatal diagnosis will certainly witness a continued and dedicated interest in the scanning of these minute details of the face.

Abnormalities of the oral cavity and mandible

Although few congenital malformations of the oral cavity exist, evaluation of this area should be included in the comprehensive evaluation of the face, as defects may be present in the anomalous fetus. The normal fetus can exhibit various behavioral patterns such as swallowing, protrusion and retrusion of the tongue, and hiccoughing. An abnormal positioning of the tongue may be indicative of a mass of the oral cavity or an obstructive process.

The antenatal sonographic diagnosis of epignathus has been reported.[32] An epignathus is a teratoma located in the area of the oropharynx. These masses may be highly complex and contain solid, cystic, or calcified components. In fetuses with epignathus swallowing may be impaired, resulting in polyhydramnios. In these cases a small stomach may be present.

The fetal mandible (chin) can be seen in the majority of fetuses. The texture of the triangular-shaped mandible resembles that of the maxilla. A rare anomaly that causes a reduction of the chin (micrognathia) has been detected by prenatal sonographic investigation.[116]

It is important to remember that polyhydramnios is a common feature in fetuses with craniofacial malformations, and difficulties in swallowing may explain the excessive amounts of amniotic fluid.

Meticulous scanning should ensue whenever a mass is found to originate from the fetal face. Attempts should be made to identify the origin of the mass to allow optimal

counseling concerning prognosis, mode of delivery, and neonatal management.

ABNORMALITIES OF THE NECK

Neck abnormalities can be detected during evaluation of the ventral, dorsal, and lateral surfaces of the neck. The neck is often difficult to assess when amniotic fluid is decreased, when the fetus is in an unfavorable position, or when the neck is in close proximity to the placenta. Nonetheless, evaluation of the neck should be routinely attempted. The anatomic description of fetal neck structures has been discussed (see Chapter 20).

Anomalies of the fetal neck are rare but when present may represent life-threatening disorders.

Fetal cystic hygromas result from malformations of the lymphatic system that lead to single or multiloculated lymph-filled cavities, which are most commonly seen in the area of the fetal neck. Failure of the lymphatic system to properly connect with the venous system results in distension of the jugular lymph sacs and the accumulation of lymph in fetal tissues.[76,146] This abnormal collection of lymph frequently causes gross distension of lymph cavities, causing fetal hydrops and even fetal death. Cystic hygromas are believed to occur from a developmental defect of the lymphatic vessels. Normally the lymphatic vessels empty into two sacs lateral to the jugular veins (jugular lymph sacs). These sacs communicate with the venous system and form the right lymphatic duct and thoracic duct (Fig. 23-17, A).[2]

Cystic hygromas may be small and regress because of alternate routes of lymph drainage. With this type of hygroma, webbing of the neck and swelling of the extremities may be appreciated after birth. These features are frequently seen in neonates with Turner's syndrome (XO karyotype). Cystic hygromas can present as isolated small cystic cavities with or without septations[24] and can arise from the anterior, lateral, or posterior fetal neck. Small hygromas may be associated with other fetal anatomic defects.

Large fetal cystic hygromas have a typical sonographic appearance (Fig. 23-17, B). Bilateral large cystic masses are noted at the posterolateral borders of the neck, which in severe cases completely surround the neck and head. Typically a dense midline septum divides the hygroma with septations identified within the dilated lymph sacs. Because of an accumulation of lymph in fetal tissues, fetal hydrops results. Pericardial or pleural effusions, edema of thoracic and abdominal skin, ascites, and limb edema are frequent (Fig. 23-18). Heart failure commonly results in intrauterine death.

Chervenak and associates[24] demonstrated a high incidence of large cystic hygromas with Turner's syndrome. An association of cystic hygromas with other chromosomal anomalies was noted. The prognosis for fetuses with cystic hygromas and hydrops was uniformly dismal. Because other fetal malformations are common, a careful study of fetal anatomy is necessary whenever a hygroma has been detected.

Additional criteria for identification of a cystic hygroma

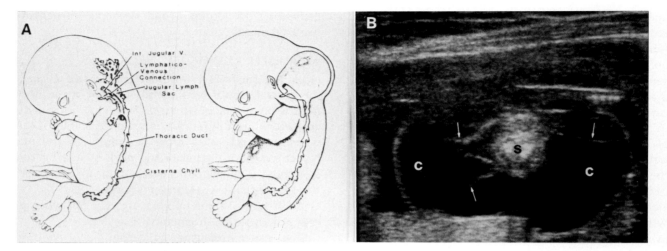

Fig. 23-17. A, Lymphatic system in a normal fetus *(left)* with a patent connection between the jugular lymph sac and the internal jugular vein and a cystic hygroma and hydrops from a failed lymphaticovenous connection *(right)*. **B,** Transverse view through fetal neck demonstrating large cystic structures, *c,* surrounding fetal neck representing cystic hygroma in a fetus with Turner syndrome, *XO.* Note the multiple septations within the hygroma *(arrows). s,* Cervical spine. (**A** From Chervenak FA, Isaacson G, Blakemore KJ, et al: N Engl J Med 309:822, 1985.)

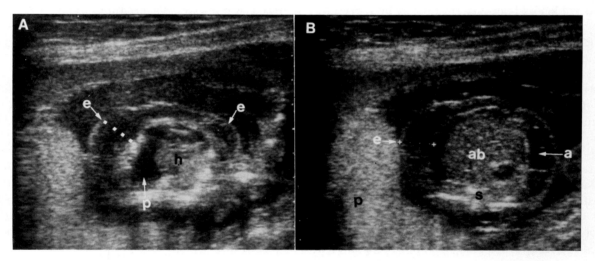

Fig. 23-18. A, Cross-section through chest in fetus in (Fig. 23-17, *B*) with cystic hygroma demonstrating pleural effusion, *p,* and tissue edema, *e,* due to heart failure. *h,* Heart. **B,** At a lower level, abdominal ascites, *a,* and tissue edema, *e,* are evident. *p,* Placenta; *ab,* abdomen; *s,* spine.

include a normal-appearing fetal skull and spine, the presence of cysts and septations, a consistent position of the cystic mass, and the absence of solid structures within the mass.

The differential diagnosis for cystic hygroma includes meningomyelocele, encephalocele, nuchal edema, branchial cleft cyst, cystic teratoma, or an empty sac of a blighted twin, hemangiomas, fetal edema, and thyroglossal duct cysts.

Other fetal neck lesions diagnosable by ultrasound are teratomas of the neck. These masses are typically complex in appearance. Cystic, solid, and calcified components can be found in these masses, which are usually large and atypically located.[27,129] If neck teratomas are large, they may interfere with fetal swallowing, and hydramnios may be evident. Recognition of this lesion is imperative, as resuscitative support after delivery is critical to the care of affected neonates.

Reports of sonographically detected goiters are found in the literature.[3,151] During ultrasound a fetal goiter will appear as a solid mass arising from the anterior fetal neck in the region of the fetal thyroid gland. A bilobed appearance may be visualized.[3] Obstruction of the esophagus by a goiter may occur, resulting in hydramnios and a small or absent stomach. Follow-up studies of fetuses identified with a goiter should include size estimations of the goiter, presence and size of the fetal stomach, and the amount of amniotic fluid.

Most masses of the fetal neck will be found in the low-risk obstetric patient, thereby necessitating evaluation of the fetal neck on a routine basis in an attempt to recognize cervical masses that may compromise neonatal survival.

ABNORMALITIES OF THE VERTEBRAL COLUMN

Evaluation of the fetal vertebral column remains one of the most technically difficult examinations confronting the sonographic team. The fetal spine is challenging to evaluate because of flexion of the cervical and lumbosacral spine and the large surface area requiring study.

Patients are referred most often for the detection of spina bifida. Sacrococcygeal teratomas are usually diagnosed during basic obstetrical studies. Fetuses at risk for caudal regression syndrome (occurring in fetuses of insulin-dependent mothers—see Chapter 22) are often referred for comprehensive studies of the spine.

Although ultrasound techniques may be limited in the detection of all spinal lesions, the comprehensive spinal study has proven to be a reliable tool in the detection of spina bifida. Comprehensive sonography is used to evaluate the spine when elevations of α-fetoprotein are found in amniotic fluid and, in some centers, as the primary diagnostic tool for exclusion of spina bifida following maternal serum α-fetoprotein elevations.[115]

Spina bifida

Spina bifida encompasses a wide range of vertebral defects. The term spina bifida means bifid (cleft or split in two) spine. Spinal defects vary in size and severity, and in the least severe form represent a failure of the dorsal vertebrae to fuse together.[93] This causes a defect or opening in the vertebral column.

When a spinal defect is covered by skin or hair, it is referred to as spina bifida occulta. These lesions are associated with a normal spinal cord and nerves with normal neurologic development.[93] Occulta defects are extremely difficult to detect antenatally. The skin covering in occulta defects prevents the leakage of α-fetoprotein into amniotic fluid or maternal serum.

When spinal defects involve more than one vertebral segment, the meninges can then protrude through the opening. A skin-covered sac can be found extending from the posterior wall of the fetus. This lesion is termed a meningocele.[93]

Defects may be more extensive with protrusion of both meninges and spinal cord/nerves (meningomyelocele). A meningomyelocele appears as a protruding sac containing echogenic structures representing neural tissue.[22,45] Neurologic impairment from minor anesthesia to complete paralysis are found with meningomyeloceles. In fetuses with myelomeningoceles, cranial malformations are common. The medulla and cerebellum herniate into the foramen magnum, which results in ventriculomegaly because of these prolapsed structures. These associated cranial problems are referred to as the Arnold-Chiari malformation.[93]

A myelocele or rachischisis pertains to an extensive and severely exposed open spinal defect.

Ultrasound examination for spina bifida. The contour of the normal fetal spine can be appreciated on sagittal sections of the vertebral column. The cervical, thoracic, lumbar, and sacral components can be distinguished and assessed in this plane. The fetal skin will be seen along with the parallel nature of the laminae or transverse processes. Frequently an additional central line of densities representing the spinous processes are noted[81,128] The cervical spine normally widens at the entrance of the spine into the fetal cranium, whereas the sacral spine tapers at the tip of the vertebral column.

On transverse sections the vertebrae appear as bony circles (ossification centers) encompassing the spinal cord. The ossification centers visualized are the pedicles, the center of the vertebral body, and the posterior ossification center.[55] The posterior ossification echo (vertebral arch) is absent in fetuses with spina bifida. The pedicles will appear to be splayed in a V, U, or C-shaped appearance[55] (Figs. 23-19 and 23-20).

Spinal defects most commonly involve the lumbosacral region. The sonographic examination for exclusion of a spinal defect uses a series of transverse and longitudinal scans of the spine. On transverse sections each vertebral segment is studied to check for the circular (O-shaped) configuration perpendicular to the sagittal plane of the spine. Vertebrae are examined from the occiput (cervical spine) to the sacrum. It is crucial that the transducer angle is positioned at right angles to the long axis of the spine because improper transducer angles can erroneously suggest a spinal defect. The vertebral column should appear as a closed circle throughout the entire length of the spine.

After repeated sweeps of the spine in a transverse orientation, longitudinal sections should be performed. The proper section to assess the integrity of the spine includes a plane that contains both transverse processes running in parallel to each other.[81] An equal amount of fetal tissue should be identified on each side of the transverse processes. Examinations of the spine by ultrasound are lengthy, requiring on the average 1 hour to perform.

Following are sonographic characteristics of an open spinal defect:

TRANSVERSE SECTIONS

1. Splaying of the vertebral pedicles with loss of the posterior ossification echo (incomplete spinal circle) (Figs. 23-19 and 23-20)
2. V, C, or U-shaped appearance of the vertebral pedicles (Figs. 23-19 and 23-20)
3. Presence of protruding saclike structure:
   a. Meningocele (echo-free sac)
   b. Meningomyelocele (meninges and spinal cord within sac) (Figs. 23-19 to 23-22)
4. Disruption in the continuity of the covering skin

LONGITUDINAL SECTIONS

1. Loss in continuity of spinal contour (apparent "break" in spine) (Fig. 23-20).
2. Widening of transverse process with absent spinous process (Fig. 23-21)
3. Presence of protruding saclike structure (meningocele, meningomyelocele) (Figs. 23-19 to 23-22)

The sonographer should be aware of several technical points when evaluating the fetal spine. Examinations of the spine should only be attempted when the fetus is lying on the side or is spine up. The spine cannot be ade-

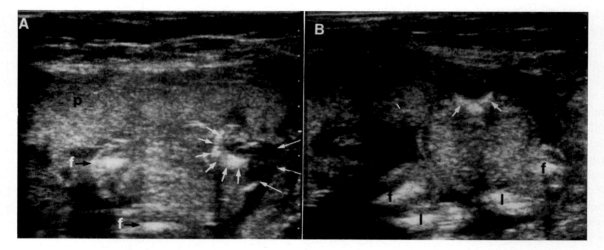

Fig. 23-19.   A, Transverse scan demonstrating wedge-shaped (C,V,U) defect *(arrows)* of the lumbar spine in a 21-week fetus with an open spinal defect. Note the protruding neural components contained within the meningomyelocele sac *(long white arrows). p,* Placenta. **B,** Defect *(arrows)* identified, in same patient, with the fetus in a spine-up position. *f,* Femurs; *l,* lower legs.

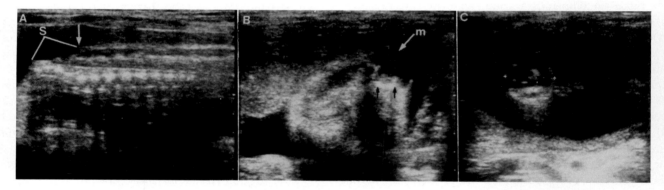

Fig. 23-20.   A, Sagittal scan of lumbosacral spine identifying a "break" *(arrow)* in the contour at the sacrum in a 26-week fetus. The posterior spinal surface is absent. *S,* Sacral spine. **B,** Transverse section of sacrum, in same patient, depicting defect *(arrows).* A meningomyelocele sac, *m,* is noted protruding from the defect. **C,** Tangential scan through the sacrum localizing the 2.5 cm meningomyelocele. Echogenic interfaces representing neural components are visible.

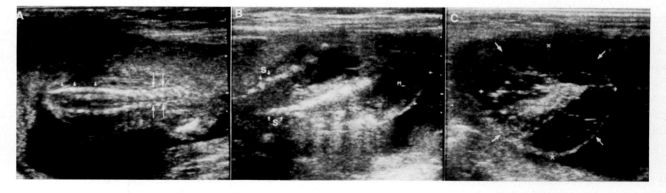

Fig. 23-21.   A, Sagittal scan denoting the splaying of the thoracic, lumbar, and sacral spine in a fetus with a large spinal defect *(small arrows). Long arrows,* upper thoracic spine. **B,** Magnified view of spinal defect demonstrating marked widening of the spine, *s,* and protruding meningomyelocele sac, *M.* **C,** Tangential view of 7 cm meningomyelocele *(arrows)* with multiple neural components.

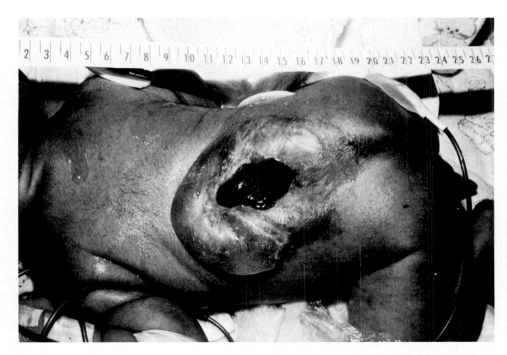

Fig. 23-22.   Photograph of neonate with large (7 cm) spinal defect as depicted sonographically in Fig. 23-21.

quately studied when the fetus is lying on the back.

It is crucial to align the transducer along the transverse processes of the spine (in longitudinal scans) and at right angles (on transverse scans).

Spinal flexion makes evaluation of the spine difficult. This clinical limitation is encountered when evaluating the spine in the late second and third trimesters of pregnancy. The optimal time to study the fetal spine is from 19 to 23 weeks of gestation. At this time the fetus is mobile and unflexed and surrounded by large pockets of amniotic fluid, which optimizes spinal imaging.

In fetuses with ventriculomegaly, investigation of the spine is always warranted. Spinal defects and ventriculomegaly are often associated (Arnold-Chiari malformation).

The spine may not be amenable for sonographic investigation in pregnancies complicated by breech lies, oligohydramnios, and maternal obesity.

It is important to meticulously inspect the sacrum of the fetus. Small sacral defects are easy to miss. A cephalad angulation directed toward the tip of the sacrum is often necessary to visualize a small sacral defect (Fig. 23-20). Even in experienced hands, small spinal defects may be undetected.

After a spinal defect has been identified, the investigators should determine (1) the level and extent of the defect, (2) the presence or absence of neural components contained within the protruding sac, and (3) whether dilated cerebral ventricles are present.

Spinal defects are associated with cephaloceles, cleft lip and palate, hypotelorism, and hypertelorism.[81] In addition, congenital heart defects and genitourinary anomalies have been reported. Biparietal diameter measurements may be reduced in fetuses with spina bifida.

The comprehensive examination of the fetal spine is technically difficult for novice investigators. Repeated identification of normal spinal anatomy on all obstetrical scans and specialized training with experienced scanners will aid the sonographer in developing the skills necessary to detect spinal malformations.

Caudal regression syndrome

The caudal regression syndrome is a developmental disorder most frequently afflicting fetuses of diabetic mothers.[96] Comprehensive fetal studies are performed in pregnancies complicated by insulin-dependent diabetes to search for lesions typical of this condition. In caudal regression syndrome the sacrum and lower extremities are hypoplastic (underdeveloped).[113] In these patients the sacrum should be carefully examined and the contour, length, and morphology of each limb assessed.

Sacrococcygeal teratoma

A sacrococcygeal teratoma is a mass arising from the sacrum and coccyx of the fetus. They are usually benign and can reach extremely large sizes, which may interfere with vaginal delivery.[130]

A sacrococcygeal teratoma is a soft-tissue mass containing cystic, solid, and calcified structures (Fig. 23-23). The tumor may protrude from the coccyx or may be more extensive, extending into the fetal pelvis or into the abdomen.[130] Serial sonograms are used to monitor the size of the teratoma. Teratomas may rapidly increase in size; therefore careful follow-up of the lesions is necessary in the management and delivery of these fetuses. Polyhydramnios and hydrops may accompany sacrococcygeal teratomas.

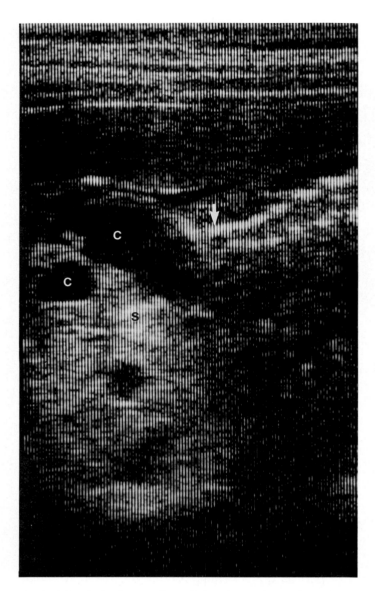

Fig. 23-23.   Sagittal scan of sacral area *(arrow)* revealing a large complex mass (cystic, *C,* and solid components, *S*) consistent with a sacrococcygeal teratoma. (From Grannum PAT, Tortora M, Mayden KL, et al: Obstetrics. In Taylor KJW, editor: Atlas of ultrasonography, ed 2, New York, 1985, Churchill Livingstone.)

When a teratoma is found, a meticulous search for additional fetal malformations is warranted. Coexisting anomalies may involve the musculoskeletal, renal, and central nervous systems.

A sacral meningomyelocele may mimic a sacrococcygeal teratoma; however, meningomyeloceles are largely cystic, whereas sacrococcygeal teratomas are predominantly soft-tissue masses. The complex appearance of a teratoma further distinguishes this lesion.

ABNORMALITIES OF THE THORACIC CAVITY

The fetal thoracic cavity has become more accessible for sonographic evaluation of masses involving the lungs, heart, and diaphragm. The detection of thoracic defects is important, since many lesions may compromise fetal breathing and require surgery in the immediate neonatal period.

Abnormalities of the lungs

The sonographic evaluation of the fetal lungs is important in the routine obstetrical assessment and is essential in fetuses at high risk for lung masses. Normal fetal lung texture appears homogeneous. They serve as medial borders for the heart and as inferior borders for the diaphragm. The peripheral boundaries are the chest walls. The mediastinum is difficult to clearly define by current ultrasound techniques; however, the identification of mediastinal masses is possible. The fetal lungs are filled with fluid and therefore are highly visible by sonography.

Evaluation of the fetal lungs to exclude masses should include a thorough investigation of lung texture and homogenicity. Masses of the lung are separate from the heart and are located above the level of the diaphragm. Lesions of the lungs may be cystic, solid, or complex. Lung masses should be studied to determine their relationship to the fetal heart and diaphragm. Fetal echocardiography is beneficial in excluding cardiac involvement, and evaluation of an intact diaphragm is necessary to exclude a diaphragmatic hernia. Abnormalities in cardiac rhythm and fetal hydrops may be present in fetuses with lung masses due to compression of venous return and cardiac failure. Frequently, pleural effusions are identified in conjunction with masses of the lung.

Cystic lung masses

Lung cysts are echo-free masses that replace normal lung parenchyma. Lung cysts may vary in size, ranging from small isolated lesions to large cystic masses that can cause marked shifts of intrathoracic structures. Cystic lung masses appear as echo-free areas within lung tissue (Fig. 23-24, *A*). Simple cysts can be surgically excised after delivery.

Pleural effusions are accumulations of fluid wtihin the pleural cavity that may present as isolated lesions or as a part of complex fetal abnormalities. Pleural effusions may result from immune (e.g., Rh disease) or nonimmune causes or from congestive heart failure. Effusions may also occur in fetuses with chromosomal abnormalities or in the fetus with a cardiac mass.

Sonographically, pleural effusions will appear as echo-free masses on one or both sides of the fetal heart (Fig. 23-18). The effusions will conform to the thoracic cavity and often compress lung tissue. Compression of lung parenchyma may cause lung hypoplasia, which often represents a life-threatening consequence for the neonate. Ultrasound will show the lungs to be small. Once a pleural effusion has been discovered, a careful search for lung, cardiac, and diaphragmatic lesions should be attempted. Likewise, evaluation for signs of hydrops (ascites, scalp edema, and tissue edema) should be undertaken. Correlation with clinical parameters is warranted to exclude immunologic causes for pleural effusions.

Solid lung masses

Solid tumors of the fetal lungs have been reported by ultrasound,[52,106] appearing as echo-dense masses in the lung tissue. Pulmonary sequestration and certain types of

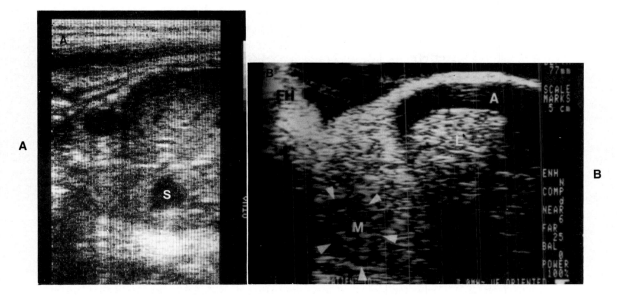

Fig. 23-24. **A,** Longitudinal section through fetal chest demonstrating cystic mass in the lung *(arrow).* Note relationship of stomach, *S,* to this mass. A benign bronchogenic cyst was noted after birth. **B,** Longitudinal scan identifying bulky echo-filled mass, *M,* in thorax consistent with congenital cystic adenomatoid malformation (III). Abdominal ascites, *A,* is present. *FH,* Fetal head; *L,* liver. (From Mayden KL, Tortora M, Chervenak FA, et al: Am J Obstet Gynecol 148:349, 1984.)

adenomatoid malformations appear as solid lung masses.

Extra pulmonary tissue is present within the same pleural sac as the lung (intralobar) or is connected to the inferior border of the lung with its own pleural cavity (extralobar).[52,124] This tissue is nonfunctional and receives its blood supply from systemic circulation. During ultrasound an echo-dense mass resembling lung tissue is demonstrated. In addition, a hypoplastic or small lung on the affected side may be noted. Hydrops is a frequent finding. Associated diaphragmatic hernias, gastrointestinal anomalies, and lung anomalies may be found.

Three forms of adenomatoid malformations have been described.[143] In type I malformations, large cysts replace lung tissue (single or multiple cysts measuring more than 2 cm); type II lesions contain multiple small cystic structures (measuring less than 1 cm).[143] Type II lesions may be associated with fetal anomalies involving the renal, gastrointestinal, and diaphragmatic regions. Type III malformations are characterized as bulky, large noncystic lesions that appear as echo-dense masses[52,106] (Fig. 23-24, *B*). Shifts of mediastinal structures (heart and lungs) can compress lung tissue. In these instances hydrops may be present. Polyhydramnios may be seen as a result of compression of the esophagus, preventing normal swallowing.

When a cystic or solid lung mass has been identified, sonographic investigation should attempt to (1) determine the number and size(s) of cystic structures, (2) check for presence or absence of a mediastinal shift, (3) identify and assess the size of the lungs, (4) look for fetal hydrops, (5) exclude cardiac masses, and (6) search for other fetal anomalies. Based on these findings, an appropriate prognosis and management plan can be instituted. Differentiation of the type of cystic adenomatoid malformations is imperative, as prognosis varies depending on the type of lesion. Type I lesions have favorable outcomes, whereas type II and III lesions have poor prognoses.[143]

Complex lung masses

The internal components of complex lung masses are cystic and solid and thus appear heterogeneous. At times, compressed adjacent thoracic organs further complicate determination of the type of lesion (pleural effusion surrounding lungs and heart). Congenital dilatation of the bronchial tree may have both cystic and solid characteristics.[106]

Abnormalities of the heart

Congenital cardiac defects can be detected during routine obstetrical examinations by evaluation of cardiac size, rhythm, and anatomy. The four-chamber view of the heart should be used, when possible, to detect gross cardiac malformations. Comprehensive studies of the fetal heart for exclusion or confirmation of cardiac lesions are performed by a specialized echocardiographic team (sonographers, sonologists, pediatric cardiologists) trained in the detection of fetal cardiac anomalies. Fetal echocardiography is discussed in Chapter 36.

Abnormalities of the diaphragm

The diaphragm is an important landmark separating the thoracic cavity from the abdomen. It is a significant anatomic structure that should be recognized on all obstetric scans. The normal diaphragm has been described in a previous section (see Chapter 20). The diaphragm is specifically studied in fetuses at risk for congenital defects of the diaphragm. In the normal fetus the diaphragm should appear as a curvilinear structure coursing anteriorly to pos-

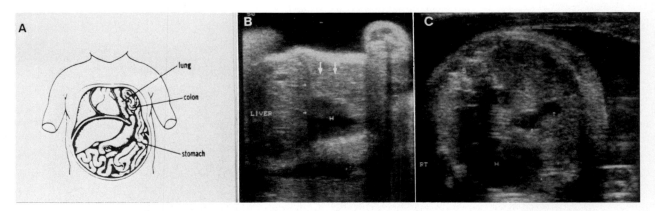

Fig. 23-25.   A, Schema demonstrating hernia of intestinal loops and part of stomach into left pleural cavity. The heart and mediastinum are frequently pushed to the right while the left lung is compressed. **B,** Sagittal view in a fetus with a diaphragmatic hernia. The heart, *H,* is displaced to the right side of fetal thorax by herniated bowel *(large arrows). Small arrows,* diaphragm. **C,** Transverse section, in same patient, showing the herniated stomach *(arrows)* at the level of the heart, *H. S,* Spine. (**A** From Langman J: Medical embryology, ed 3, Baltimore, 1975, Williams & Wilkins, Co.)

teriorly. The fetal stomach and liver should be identified caudal to the diaphragm with the lungs and heart positioned cephalad. Failure to recognize these landmarks should prompt the sonographer to search for diaphragmatic defects.

Diphragmatic hernias are common anomalies in the newborn and therefore present in the fetus during gestation. With this defect there is an opening in the pleuroperitoneal membrane (membrane dividing pleural cavity from the peritoneal cavity).[92] This opening permits the abdominal organs to enter the fetal chest (Fig. 23-25). The most common type of diaphragmatic defect occurs posteriorly and laterally in the diaphragm (herniation through foramen of Bochdalek).[36] These hernias are usually found on the left side of the diaphragm, and left-sided organs (stomach, spleen, and portions of the liver) will enter the chest through the opening. The abnormally positioned abdominal organs shift the heart and mediastinal structures to the right side of the chest. Defects on the right side of the diaphragm will allow the right-sided abdominal viscera (liver, gallbladder, intestines) to enter the chest. As a consequence of herniated abdominal organs, the lungs are compressed and may be hypoplastic. At birth, respiration can be severely compromised, which frequently results in death of the newborn.[57]

Diaphragmatic hernias can occur anteriorly and medially in the diaphragm (through foramen of Morgagni) and may communicate with the pericardial sac.[36] In anteromedial defects the heart may be normally positioned and surrounded by fluid, and the fetal stomach may be located in the abdomen.

Thinning of the diaphragm *(eventration)* may give rise to sonographic characteristics similar to diaphragmatic hernias.[36]

Sonographic criteria suggestive of diaphragmatic hernias include:

1. Shift of the heart and mediastinal structures (right shift in left-sided defects; left shift in right-sided defects) (Fig. 23-25)
2. Mass within the thoracic cavity (liver, stomach, spleen, and large bowel in left-sided defects; liver, gallbladder, intestines in right-sided defects) (Fig. 23-25)
3. Small abdominal circumference due to herniated abdominal structures
4. Obvious anatomic defect in the diaphragm

It is important to note that when a diaphragmatic hernia is present, the stomach may not be filled if there is concomitant oligohydramnios or if the fetus is swallowing abnormally. The only clue to a diaphragmatic hernia in this situation may be evidence of a solid mass in the chest. Peristalsis within the herniated intestines may be an additional diagnostic sign.

Caution should be exerted in evaluating the fetus at risk for a diaphragmatic hernia. The sonographer should scan in a carefully aligned transverse plane to correctly determine the true relationship between the stomach and diaphragm. Oblique angles of the transducer will incorrectly demonstrate the stomach at the level of the fetal heart.

When the sonographer cannot demonstrate the stomach bubble in the normal anatomic location after repeated observations, a search for a diaphragmatic hernia should be attempted. Polyhydramnios is a frequent finding in fetuses with congenital diaphragmatic hernias.

Lung and mediastinal masses, in particular, cystic adenomatoid malformations may be difficult to distinguish from diaphragmatic hernias. Careful evaluation of the fetal abdomen to identify normally positioned peritoneal organs may be of benefit in these cases.

As with all anomalies, a search for additional malformations is warranted.

Fetal surgery for diaphragmatic hernia. Attempts to surgically correct diaphragmatic hernias have been investigated in animal models.[57] Correction of this defect in

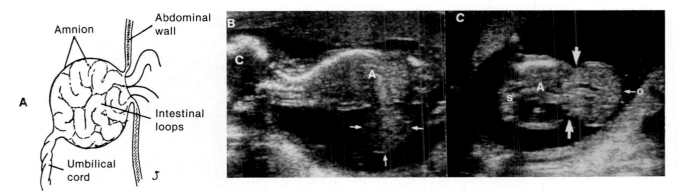

Fig. 23-26. A, Schema of omphalocele—failure of the intestinal loops and/or liver to return to the abdominal cavity. The herniated loops are surrounded by a membranous sac formed by the amnion. **B,** Sagittal scan of 18-week fetus in a spine-up position with evidence of a contained mass projecting from the anterior abdominal wall representing an omphalocele *(arrows)*. *C,* Cranium; *A,* abdomen. **C,** Transverse plane, in same patient, localizing herniation of liver in the omphalocele, *o.* Note the portal vessel within the herniated liver. *s,* Spine; *large arrows,* first border of omphalocele; *A,* abdomen. (**A** from Langman J: Medical embryology, ed 3, Baltimore, 1975, Williams & Wilkins Co.)

utero may allow for normal development of the lungs, thereby preserving lung tissue and preventing pulmonary hypoplasia.

ABNORMALITIES OF THE ANTERIOR ABDOMINAL WALL

Evaluation of the fetal ventral wall is critical in every obstetrical ultrasound examination. Defects of the anterior abdominal wall are usually obvious on sonography. Abdominal wall defects can be identified during the second trimester of pregnancy, allowing for further testing and options for clinical management. Anterior abdominal wall defects are commonly found by ultrasound following elevations of α-fetoprotein from maternal serum or amniotic fluid.

Early recognition of abdominal wall defects is important, as their presence significantly affects clinical management. Ventral wall defects are classified according to the type and size of the defect and associated anomalies. Fetuses with these defects need to be delivered in centers with access to immediate pediatric care. This will prevent heat and water loss and expedite surgical correction of the defect during the neonatal period.

Omphalocele and *gastroschisis* represent the most common defects amenable to antenatal detection. The normal contour of the abdominal wall can be appreciated on longitudinal and transverse scans as a well-defined curvilinear border (see Chapter 20). In fetuses with a defect of the anterior wall a mass can be seen protruding from the anterior surface of the abdomen.

An omphalocele is a defect characterized by the herniation of abdominal organs into the umbilical cord. In early embryonic development (around 7 to 8 weeks' gestation) intestinal loops of bowel move into the extraembryonic portion of the umbilical cord.[91] These normally herniated bowel loops, however, should return to the abdominal cavity by 11 weeks of gestation. When the intestines fail to return to the abdominal cavity, an omphalocele results. Omphaloceles commonly contain bowel and liver and, when extensive, the stomach and spleen may protrude through the defect (Fig. 23-26). As the organs are shifted into the cord, they are covered by a membrane originating from the umbilical cord, which accounts for the characteristically smooth and regular contour of this mass. This membrane protects the abdominal organs from the amniotic fluid.

The umbilical cord can often be identified as it enters the anterior wall of the omphalocele. The size of omphaloceles range from small to "giant" defects (greater than 5 cm).[111]

Omphaloceles are associated with malformations of other organ systems. When an omphalocele has been identified, defects of the fetal heart, kidneys, bladder, and central nervous system (neural tube defects) should be excluded, since these lesions occur frequently. Omphaloceles are commonly found in fetuses with chromosomal abnormalities; therefore genetic amniocentesis is offered.

Frequently ascites is noted with an omphalocele, which may confuse the ultrasound picture. As a result, the omphalocele may appear to be floating in amniotic fluid. This condition needs to be differentiated from gastroschisis defects. Infrequently omphaloceles can rupture in utero and may mimic gastroschisis defects.

Omphalocele defects may be extensive, involving the epigastric structures (sternum, diaphragm, and heart— pentalogy of Cantrell) to bladder protrusion (exstrophy) and colon abnormalities.[16] Omphaloceles may occur in conjunction with diaphragmatic hernias and as part of the Beckwith-Wiedemann syndrome (omphalocele, organomegaly, enlarged tongue).

In gastroschisis there is an opening in the skin adjacent to the fetal cord insertion in which abdominal organs protrude through the opening and are exposed to the amniotic fluid. The eviscerated abdominal organs are not cov-

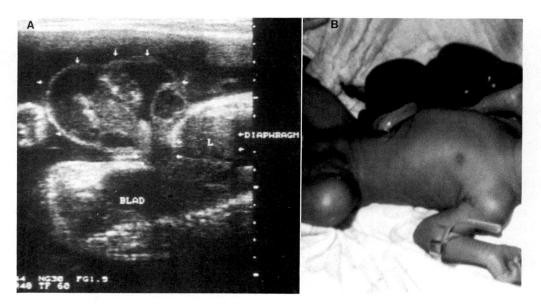

Fig. 23-27.   A, Sagittal scan demonstrating anterior abdominal wall defect with protrusion of the entire small bowel in a fetus with a gastroschisis *(arrows)*. Note the obstructed (cystic) components of small bowel. *L,* Liver. **B,** Gastroschisis defect in same patient after birth. Note the normal cord insertion.

ered by a membrane and therefore appear to float freely in the amniotic fluid.[111] In contrast to omphaloceles, gastroschises are sonographically irregular in appearance and often assume the shape of the organ that has eviscerated (Fig. 23-27). A normal cord insertion is found in fetuses with gastroschisis; therefore attempts should be made to identify its normal location. Most gastroschisis defects occur to the right of the midline, and the normal cord insertion can be identified to the left of the mass. When the fetus is lying with its right side down, the insertion site can be evaluated. Typically the intestines herniate from the defect and are easily identified by ultrasound. The bowel may appear echogenic due to inflammation and edema as the intestines are exposed to and irritated by the amniotic fluid. When the gastroschisis is large, the fetal stomach, bladder, and uterine/adnexal structures may herniate. The liver rarely protrudes in gastroschisis.

Gastroschisis usually is not associated with life-threatening malformations as compared to omphaloceles; however, there is a higher incidence of intrauterine growth retardation (IUGR) and gastrointestinal complications.[16]

Included in the differential diagnosis of fetal abdominal wall defects is a congenital umbilical hernia (may contain liver)[99] and amniotic band syndrome. In amniotic band syndrome, bands from the amnion can interfere with the development of fetal organs and may amputate portions of the fetus. Defects due to amnion rupture result in gross defects of the face, limbs, central nervous system, and anterior abdominal wall.[109,111]Amputations of the limbs, extensive herniations of viscera, and amniotic bands can be identified by prenatal sonography. Care should be taken to distinguish this lesion from an omphalocele or gastroschisis.

The sonographic team must attempt to characterize the abdominal wall defect as the prognosis is directly re-

lated to the type of lesion, size and extent of the lesion, the presence of coexisting fetal anomalies, and intestinal obstruction due to the ventral wall defect.

ABNORMALITIES OF THE HEPATOBILIARY SYSTEM

Anomalies of the liver, gallbladder, pancreas, and spleen are rare. Detection of abnormal morphology is beneficial since many lesions may be undetected in the newborn period.

The fetal liver, although involved in several congenital anomalies (diaphragmatic hernia, omphalocele), is rarely affected by isolated hepatic lesions. Liver parenchyma cysts and hemangiomas[117] of the liver have been reported. The liver enlarges in fetuses with Rh-immune disease in response to increased hematopoiesis (red blood cell production in the liver) (see Chapter 22).

Situs inversus represents the reverse positioning of the liver and stomach (liver on the left side of the fetus; stomach on the right side). Careful evaluation of the location of the liver and stomach on their respective sides should be assessed in all fetuses to identify the fetus with this condition.

Anomalies of the gallbladder may be detected using prenatal sonographic techniques. Cholelithiasis (gallstones) can be identified in the fetus when calcifications are found within the gallbladder.[5] A choledochal cyst (dilatation of the common bile duct) may be diagnosed when a cystic mass is identified adjacent to the fetal stomach[43] and gallbladder. Choledochal cysts may be confused with malformations of the stomach or bowel.

Pancreatic cysts can present as midline cystic masses in the fetal abdomen.

Evaluation of the fetal spleen for exclusion of splenic anomalies is possible. Asplenia (absence of the spleen) may be amenable to antenatal identification. Splenic cysts, hypoplasia of the spleen, and enlargement of the spleen, which occurs in several abnormal fetal states, may be identifiable using sophisticated ultrasound techniques.[131] The spleen, like the liver, may enlarge in fetuses with Rh-immune disease.

ABNORMALITIES OF THE GASTROINTESTINAL TRACT

The majority of gastrointestinal malformations are correctable after birth; consequently, recognition of a gastrointestinal anomaly before delivery can avoid the complications of dehydration, bowel necrosis, and respiratory difficulties,[10] which can occur when these lesions are not suspected at delivery.

The normal upper esophagus can frequently be seen following the swallowing of amniotic fluid by the fetus. This imbibed fluid passes through the esophagus and empties into the fetal stomach. Obstruction of the normal swallowing sequence can occur due to an atretic or obstructive process. In atresia a membrane covers the lumen of the intestine. The intestinal loops enlarge above the obstruction, and the bowel loops below the atresia are narrowed (stenotic). This enlargement of the bowel proximal to the obstruction is readily apparent on ultrasound.[10] Blockage of this system results in the back-up of amniotic fluid, resulting in hydramnios. Therefore, in pregnancies with polyhydramnios, anomalies of the gastrointestinal system should be sought.

Anomalies of the esophagus are infrequent. Atresia (absence of a normal opening) of the esophagus is difficult to diagnose by ultrasound; however, several signs may be suggestive of this condition.[10,11] In esophageal atresia a connection is usually established from the trachea to the distal esophagus (tracheoesophageal fistula), which allows swallowed amniotic fluid to pass into the stomach. In this condition, normal stomach secretions may contribute to fluid in the stomach.[66] In some instances, however, a fistula is not present, and fluid will not reach the stomach; hence the stomach will not be visualized by ultrasound. The combination of polyhydramnios and an absent stomach over repeated studies may be suggestive of esophageal atresia.[66] Esophageal atresia will not be diagnosable in the majority of cases due to a tracheoesophageal fistula.

In duodenal atresia the duodenum is blocked or obstructed. Normally, swallowed amniotic fluid passes through the stomach and into the duodenum. In duodenal atresia the amniotic fluid cannot move beyond the blocked site, and consequently, amniotic fluid backs up in the duodenum and stomach. Two echo-free structures (stomach and duodenum) are found in the upper fetal abdomen, which communicate with each other. This sonographic appearance is termed the "double bubble" sign (Fig. 23-28). Polyhydramnios is almost always seen with duodenal atresias.

Thirty percent of fetuses with duodenal atresia have trisomy 21 (Down syndrome). Cardiovascular anomalies are frequent, and therefore fetal echocardiography is invaluable in excluding cardiac lesions. Genitourinary anomalies (horseshoe kidney, ectopic kidneys) may coex-

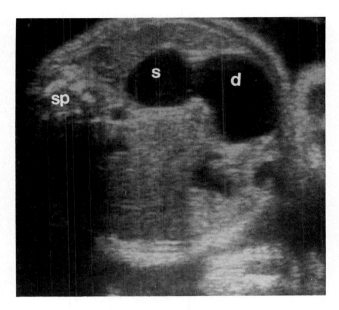

Fig. 23-28. Transverse section demonstrating dilated stomach, *s,* and duodenum, *d,* typical of the "double bubble" sign in duodenal atresia. *sp,* Spine.

ist with this condition. Other gastrointestinal abnormalities, such as imperforate anus and atresia of the small bowel, may be present.[11]

Symmetric growth retardation commonly occurs in fetuses with duodenal atresia. A careful analysis of fetal growth parameters is necessary to discover abnormal growth profiles in these fetuses.[10] Amniotic fluid α-fetoprotein values are commonly elevated in fetuses with duodenal atresia. When patients are referred for ultrasound examination because of an elevated α-fetoprotein level, duodenal atresia should be excluded.

The entire length of the bowel is subject to obstruction. Blockage of the jejunum and ileal bowel segments (jejunoileal atresia) will appear as multiple cystic structures (more than two) within the fetal abdomen. As these structures are high in the abdomen, polyhydramnios may be present. Sonographically, intestinal obstructions appear as cystic bowel loops (Fig. 23-29). It is important to remember that normal bowel loops can be identified in the third trimester of pregnancy. Commonly, normal bowel loops will contain meconium and appear filled with internal echoes. Fetal intestinal obstructions should be suspected when clear cystic structures are found. In some instances, echoes within the bowel may be identified in intestinal obstructions (Fig. 23-29, *B* and *C*).

Several intestinal obstructions have been identified by prenatal ultrasound. Meconium ileus, cystic fibrosis, and Hirschprung's disease[147] should be considered in the differential diagnosis. Meconium peritonitis is a condition in which meconium is expelled, forming calcifications within the abdomen. Conditions of congenital microcolon and the malrotation syndrome should be considered when dilated loops of intestine are noted in the lower fetal pelvis.

Intestinal obstructions that occur in the caudal intesti-

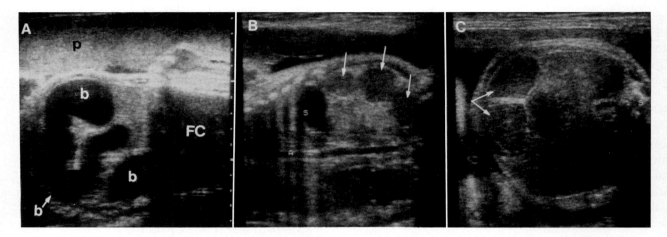

Fig. 23-29. **A,** Sagittal scan in a fetus with a bowel obstruction secondary to a gastroschisis. Note the tubular shape of the cystic bowel loops, *b. p,* Placenta; *FC,* fetal chest. **B,** Sagittal scan in a fetus with cystic fibrosis. In contrast to **A,** the dilated bowel loops are filled with echoes *(arrows).* *A,* Aorta; *S,* stomach. **C,** Echo-filled dilated bowel loops, in same patient, in a transverse direction *(arrows).* *S,* Spine.

nal tract generally are not associated with polyhydramnios (amniotic fluid is absorbed within the bowel). In anal atresia, dilated loops of bowel are found in the lower abdomen.

Included in the differential diagnosis of bowel obstructions are omental and ovarian cysts. Misinterpretation of dilated ureters or cystic kidneys for an intestinal obstruction should be avoided.

MISCELLANEOUS CYSTIC MASSES OF THE ABDOMEN

Cystic masses of the lower fetal abdomen are frequently found on ultrasound. As demonstrated previously, cystic dilatations of many organ systems can occur during the fetal period. It is important for the sonographic team to determine (1) the precise location of the mass, (2) the size of the mass, and (3) resultant compression of other organ systems (hydronephrosis, hydroureter, fetal hydrops).

When a cystic mass is discovered, attempts should be made to determine the characteristics of the mass. A description of the mass should include the components of the structure such as (1) an echo-free versus an echo-filled mass, (2) presence or absence of septations, and (3) coexisting fetal anomalies. The investigator should systematically investigate all abdominal organ systems to determine the anatomic origin of the mass. The hepatic system (liver, gallbladder, spleen, and pancreas areas) should be evaluated as well as the gastrointestinal system (esophagus, stomach, intestines) and genitourinary system (kidneys, ureters, and bladder). Occasionally cysts can arise from the urachus (dilatation of remnant allantoic stalk between umbilicus and bladder), fetal ovary, or omentum. Ovarian and omental cysts are generally isolated and well circumscribed. Determination of the fetal sex is beneficial when an ovarian mass is suspected. If abdominal masses are large, they may occupy the entire lower fetal pelvis, making a specific intrauterine diagnosis impossible.

ABNORMALITIES OF THE URINARY TRACT

Urinary tract abnormalities commonly affect all components of the urinary system. The kidneys, ureters, bladder, and urethra may be affected, or individual sites may be diseased. Renal malformations can be divided into two categories: (1) those involving a congenital disease of a specific organ and (2) those resulting from an obstructive process.

The consequences of renal malformations vary, depending on the type of lesion or extent of the obstruction. Amniotic fluid volume is a significant factor in the outcome of affected pregnancies.

As detailed in a previous section, amniotic fluid is a critical marker in the assessment of renal function. After the eighteenth to twentieth week of gestation, the production of fetal urine accounts for the majority of amniotic fluid within the uterus. In fetuses with severe renal disease the amount of amniotic fluid is reduced, and in the most severe malformations it is virtually absent. When severe oligohydramnios is found, usually both kidneys or ureters and the urethra are malformed. Unilateral obstructions may yield a normal amount of amniotic fluid, since the contralateral kidney frequently can produce urine. It is therefore important to study the kidneys, ureters, and bladder in all pregnancies with significantly reduced amniotic fluid volumes.

The recognition of urinary tract anomalies is of great importance, since several fetal conditions are incompatible with life. In unilateral obstructions of the urinary tract, early delivery of the fetus is often warranted to salvage the normally functioning kidney. Recently, intrauterine decompression of the obstructed urinary tract (posterior urethral valve syndrome) has been performed.[48] This surgical treatment is employed to relieve the obstructed urinary tract and compression of the lungs (to prevent pulmonary hypoplasia). Therefore recognition of specific renal anomalies is necessary to provide adequate information that can be used to make critical decisions regarding the management of the pregnancy.

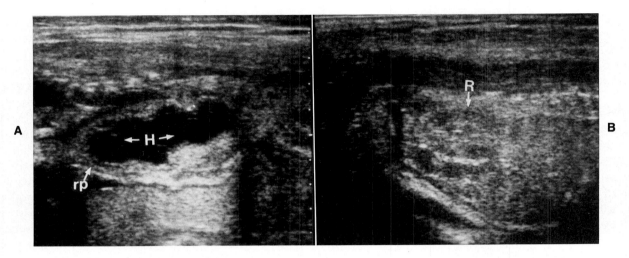

Fig. 23-30. A, Sagittal section of kidney in a fetus with a unilateral ureteropelvic junction obstruction, *UPJ,* demonstrating hydronephrosis, *H.* It is important to identify remaining renal parenchyma, *rp.* **B,** Contralateral kidney, in same fetus, demonstrating normal renal architecture, *R.*

Table 23-4   Mean Fetal Kidney Circumference/Abdominal Circumference Ratios and the Standard Deviations

	Gestational Age (weeks)					
	≤16 (n=9)	17–20 (n=18)	21–25 (n=7)	26–30 (n=11)	31–35 (n=19)	36–40 (n=25)
Mean	0.28	0.30	0.30	0.29	0.28	0.27
Standard Deviation	0.02	0.03	0.02	0.02	0.03	0.04

Adapted from Grannum PAT, Bracken M, Silverman R, and Hobbins JC: Am J Obstet Gynecol 136:2, 1980.

Ultrasound examination of the urinary tract

There are several important concepts the sonographer should be familiar with when evaluating the urinary tract. The reader is referred to the description of normal anatomic structures to fully appreciate abnormal urinary tract anatomy (see Chapter 20).

The kidneys should be evaluated by assessing kidney anatomy, texture, and size. The normal anatomic structures of the kidney are the renal cortex, parenchyma, pyramids and calyces, and renal pelvis. Marked deviations of anatomy should alert the sonographer to investigate the urinary tract more extensively. It is important to remember that a small amount of urine can be seen in the renal pelvis in the normal fetus (calicectasis). This should not be misinterpreted as an abnormal collection of urine within the pelvis (hydronephrosis) (Fig. 23-30; see Chapter 20).

The texture of the kidney is important to study. The homogeneous pattern of renal echoes should be identified in all fetal kidneys evaluated by ultrasound. Kidney texture that appears significantly enhanced should be studied to exclude renal anomalies.

The size of the fetal kidneys can be assessed using the kidney circumference to abdominal circumference (KC/AC) ratio as described by Grannum et al.[53] On a transverse scan the KC is obtained using anteroposterior (AP) and transverse diameters (technique similar to calculation of the AC). The KC is divided by the AC (obtained at conventional level) (see Chapter 21) to determine the KC/AC ratio. This ratio is constant throughout pregnancy and considered abnormal when the value exceeds 2 SD above the mean (Table 23-4).

The normal fetal ureters are usually not visualized on ultrasound. When the ureters are pathologically dilated, they will become visible by ultrasound, presenting as tortuous cystic masses in the midportion of the lower fetal pelvis (Fig. 23-31). Abnormally dilated ureters are referred to as hydroureters.

The fetal bladder is normally visualized in all fetuses. Failure to identify the bladder over repeated observations (2 to 3 hours) may indicate a severe renal abnormality. Severe renal anomalies are almost always accompanied by significant oligohydramnios; therefore careful assessment of amniotic fluid volume is essential in these cases.

The urethra, like the ureters, is usually unidentifiable in the normal fetus. Dilatation of the posterior urethra is highly suspicious for an obstructive process necessitating the careful study of the fetus for a urinary tract obstruction.

Obstructions of the urinary system can originate anywhere along the urinary tract. The consequences of an obstruction will depend on the origin of the blockage. For example, in fetuses with posterior urethral valves, urine cannot pass through the urethra and into the amniotic fluid. Consequently, urine backs up in the posterior urethra, bladder, ureters, and often extends to the kidneys.

Blockage of the ureters may result in distention of the ureters alone or may involve the kidney, causing hydronephrosis. Therefore cystic dilatations of the urinary system must be characterized in regard to the level and extent of obstruction.

Abnormalities of kidney development

Developmental disturbances in the formation of the kidneys may result in serious and frequently life-threatening malformations of the kidneys. Renal agenesis and severe infantile polycystic kidney disease are fetal conditions incompatible with life. Multicystic dysplastic kidneys, when bilateral, will result in immediate neonatal death. Recognition of these fetal disorders is critical in the antenatal pe-

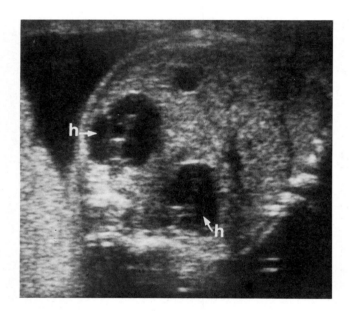

Fig. 23-31. Bilateral hydroureters, *h*, noted in axial scan of pelvis in fetus with intermittent obstruction of posterior urethra. Note coiled appearance of obstructed ureters.

riod. It is important to provide information that will aid in distinguishing lethal conditions from those with good outcomes.

Renal agenesis means the absence of the kidneys. The kidneys are absent and will not be identified sonographically (Fig. 23-32, *A*). Amniotic fluid will be absent, since the production of urine does not take place. The bladder will not be filled with urine and consequently will be unobserved. The combination of these findings are highly suggestive of this lethal disorder. It is important to remember that in the early stages of renal agenesis, amniotic fluid may be visible as it is produced from other fetal sources. In renal agenesis the adrenal glands may be large and may mimic the kidneys. A careful search in the lower fetal pelvis should be performed when the kidneys cannot be found in their normal locations. Ectopically located kidneys should be excluded when the kidneys cannot be found in their typical retroperitoneal location.

Infantile polycystic kidney disease (IPKD) is an autosomal recessive disorder (25% chance of recurrence) that affects the fetal kidneys and liver. This disease has varying presentations. Most commonly, abnormal kidneys can be seen with occasional liver cysts. The most severe forms of IPKD are those that antenatal sonography will detect.

In this disease the collecting tubules of the kidney are dilated.[60] During ultrasound, individual cysts are not identified; instead the kidneys are massively enlarged due to the hundreds of dilated tubules (Fig. 23-32, *B*). Enlargement of the kidneys may not occur until the twentyfourth week of gestation; therefore serial studies of at-risk fetuses are recommended.[60] Performance of the KC/AC ratio may be helpful in determining enlarged kidneys in these fetuses. A KC/AC ratio greater than 2 SD can be expected with the severe forms of IPKD. Enhanced renal tissue echogenicity is charcteristic because of the multiple interfaces created by the dilated cystic tubules. Enhanced sound transmission will be apparent because of the cystic nature of the kidneys.

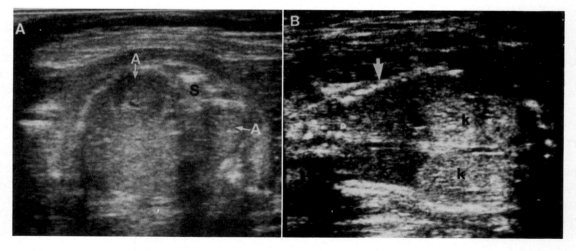

Fig. 23-32.   **A,** Renal agenesis at 29 weeks of gestation revealing enlarged adrenal glands, *A,* in the kidney spaces. Oligohydramnios and an absent bladder were also found. **B,** Sagittal scan of enlarged dense kidneys, *k,* in infantile polycystic kidney disease. Note the enhanced transmission of sound through the kidneys due to the large number of dilated cystic tubules characteristic of this disease. Oligohydramnios and an absent bladder were also found. *Arrow,* thorax.

In the most severe cases of IPKD, renal failure occurs with oligohydramnios and an absent urinary bladder.[60,125] In some cases the kidneys are so massive that they occupy the entire fetal abdomen. In view of the high recurrence rate and dismal prognosis in severe IPKD, recognition of this defect is important. IPKD may occur as part of a genetic syndrome (i.e., Meckel syndrome). The intrauterine diagnosis of IPKD should only be considered when the following characteristics are found: (1) family history of IPKD, (2) enlarged kidneys on both sides, (3) highly echogenic kidney texture, (4) significant oligohydramnios, and (5) inability to identify the fetal bladder.[125]

The third nonobstructive renal disease diagnosable by ultrasound is multicystic dysplastic kidney disease. In this condition the kidney tissue is replaced by cysts of varying sizes that are found throughout the kidney[60] (Fig. 23-33). It is often difficult to clearly define the borders of the kidney because of the distorted renal outline. The affected kidney is nonfunctional.[60] When a multicystic kidney has been identified, a careful search for anomalies of the opposite kidney should be undertaken. A multicystic kidney needs to be distinguished from hydronephrosis and calyceal dilatation. Serial scans of the fetus with a multicystic kidney are often requested to follow the normal kidney. Hydronephrosis of the functioning kidney may warrant early delivery. Remember that if the fetal bladder is visualized and the amount of amniotic fluid is normal, renal function of the unaffected kidney is usually present. When oligohydramnios is found, pursuit of other renal malformations should ensue. When both kidneys are found to be multicystic, oligohydramnios and an absent bladder are expected. A rare form of multicystic dysplastic kidneys, presenting as hydronephrosis of the kidney, has been described.[60]

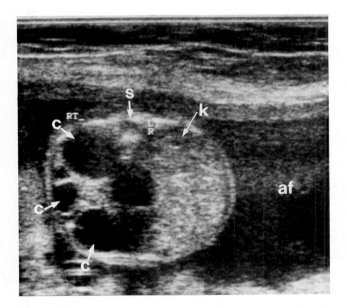

Fig. 23-33. Unilateral right multicystic kidney *(arrows)* at 21.5 weeks of gestation. Note the varying sizes of the cysts, *c,* and the normal contralateral kidney, *k.* Amniotic fluid, *af,* is normal due to the functioning left kidney. *S,* Spine.

Obstructive urinary tract abnormalities

The sonographic appearance of urinary tract obstructions differ, depending on the site and extent of blockage. Dilatation of the renal pelvis (hydronephrosis) occurs in response to a blockage of urine at some point in the urinary system. This blocked urine cannot pass the obstructed site, and while urine is constantly produced, quantities of urine back up in the kidney. Hydronephrosis commonly occurs when there is an obstruction in the ureter, bladder, or urethra. Hydronephrosis is generally the end result of an obstruction at a lower level in the urinary tract.

The ultrasound appearance of hydronephrosis varies according to the severity of the underlying obstruction. The dilated renal pelvis is centrally located and distended with urine, which often communicates with the calyces. The remaining renal tissue can be identified in all but the most severe cases of hydronephrosis.

Fetal hydronephrosis can occur as a unilateral or bilateral process. Unilateral renal hydronephrosis commonly occurs due to an obstruction at the junction of the renal pelvis and the ureter. This is called a ureteropelvic junction obstruction. In these cases a cystic structure, located medially in the renal pelvis, communicates with the calyces. The ureter, bladder, and amniotic fluid are usually normal.[60] Ureteropelvic junction obstruction can be severe.

Posterior urethral valve obstruction results in hydronephrosis, hydroureters, dilatation of the bladder, and posterior urethra. This entity occurs only in male fetuses and is manifested by the presence of valve(s) in the posterior urethra. As a result, urine cannot pass through the urethra and into the amniotic fluid. This causes a back-up of urine in the bladder, ureter, and, in the most severe cases, the kidneys. Oligohydramnios is a classic finding in the most severe forms. The following sonographic signs are suggestive of posterior urethral valve obstructions[60,69]:

1. Dilated bladder (thickening of the bladder wall commonly occurs) (Fig. 23-34, *A*)
2. Dilated posterior urethra
3. Oligohydramnios (Fig. 23-34)
4. Hydroureters (Fig. 23-34, *B*)
5. Hydronephrosis (Fig. 23-34, *B*)
6. Fetal ascites (some cases)
7. Distension of fetal abdomen (urethral obstruction malformation complex—Prune-Belly syndrome)[60]
8. Male fetus

When these sonographic signs occur in the female fetus, abnormalities of the sacrum (caudal regression anomalies) should be considered.[60]

Fetal surgery in obstructive uropathy

As the prognosis of the posterior urethral valve syndrome is invariably fatal in fetuses with severe oligohydramnios, investigators have attempted to relieve the dilated urinary tract by placing a shunt into the dilated fetal bladder.[59] This shunt drains the blocked urine into the amniotic fluid (Fig. 23-35). When the urinary tract is completely blocked, oligohydramnios and the features of Potter syn-

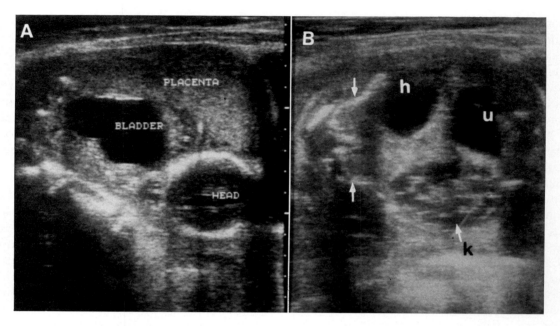

Fig. 23-34. **A,** Sagittal scan at 17 weeks of gestation demonstrating absent amniotic fluid and an abnormally distended bladder in a fetus with posterior urethral valve syndrome. **B,** In same patient at 21 weeks, a small thoracic cavity *(arrows),* hydronephrosis, *h,* hydroureter, *u,* and enlargement and early hydronephrosis of the contralateral kidney, *k,* are noted.

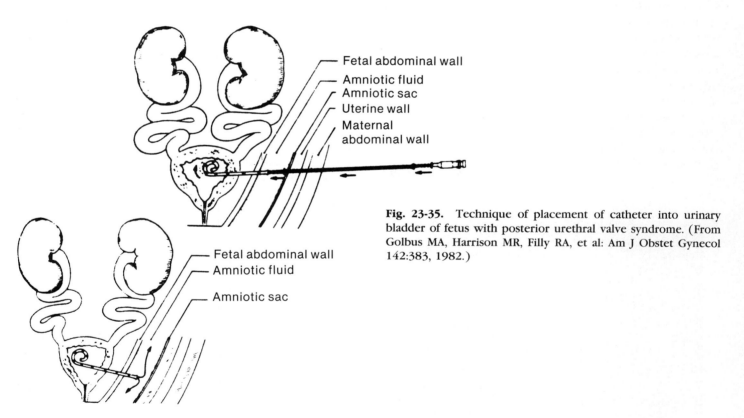

Fig. 23-35. Technique of placement of catheter into urinary bladder of fetus with posterior urethral valve syndrome. (From Golbus MA, Harrison MR, Filly RA, et al: Am J Obstet Gynecol 142:383, 1982.)

drome occur.[6] Potter syndrome includes pulmonary hypoplasia, abnormal fetal facies, malformed hands and feet, and growth problems. Intrauterine shunting procedures therefore attempt to direct urine into the amniotic cavity, thereby reducing renal damage and the devastating effects of oligohydramnios. These techniques are limited, since frequently irreversible damage to the kidneys has occurred prior to shunt placement.

Other urinary anomalies

Rare disorders such as *urethral atresia* can cause a massively dilated bladder. Duplication of the renal complexes and ectopic ureteroceles have been described.[132] Dilatation of the ureters may occur as isolated lesions (primary megaureters) resulting from atresia of the distal ureter.[41] These disorders are generally associated with adequate to increased amounts of amniotic fluid and a normal bladder.

Infrequently, renal pelvis hydronephrosis may occur. Megaureters are benign and usually do not require therapy after birth. The antenatal diagnosis of crossed renal ectopia (both kidneys fused on one side) has been reported.[56] Failure to identify a kidney should prompt the sonographer to check for this condition as well as pelvic kidneys (located ectopically in the pelvis) or unilateral renal agenesis.

Tumors of the fetal kidney are rare.[42] Masses of the kidney should be suspected when the contour of the kidney is distorted or replaced by a mass and the pelviocalyceal echoes are absent.

The reader is referred to comprehensive sources for further discussion relating to urinary tract malformations.*

ABNORMALITIES OF THE GENITALIA

Identification of fetal genitalia has previously been described (see Chapter 20). Although congenital malformations of the genital organs are rare, the sonographic team may be requested to determine the sex of the fetus when a sex-linked disorder is considered (hemophilia, aqueductal stenosis).[62] As these conditions only occur in male fetuses, identification of male genitalia aids in counseling and diagnostic testing. Likewise the demonstration of abnormal fetal genitalia may be indicative of syndromes of the endocrine and genital systems.[83]

Abnormalities of the female genital tract may be observed during the antenatal period. *Hydrometrocolpos*[40,60] (abnormal collection of fluid within the vagina and uterus) should be considered when a cystic mass is found in the lower pelvis. These masses may be predominantly cystic, may contain midlevel echoes, or may be fluid-debris levels.[127] Echoes within these masses may result from mucous secretions caused by this abnormality. Russ and associates[127] have described hydrometrocolpos in conjunction with a double uterus and septated vagina (vagina divided by a septum into two components). Ovarian masses may occur as described in a previous section.

Abnormalities of the male external genitalia may be recognized by antenatal sonography. *Hydroceles* (accumulation of serous fluid surrounding the testicle resulting from a communication with the peritoneal cavity) are frequently identified[83] (Fig. 23-36). They may occur as unilateral or bilateral lesions and are generally benign.

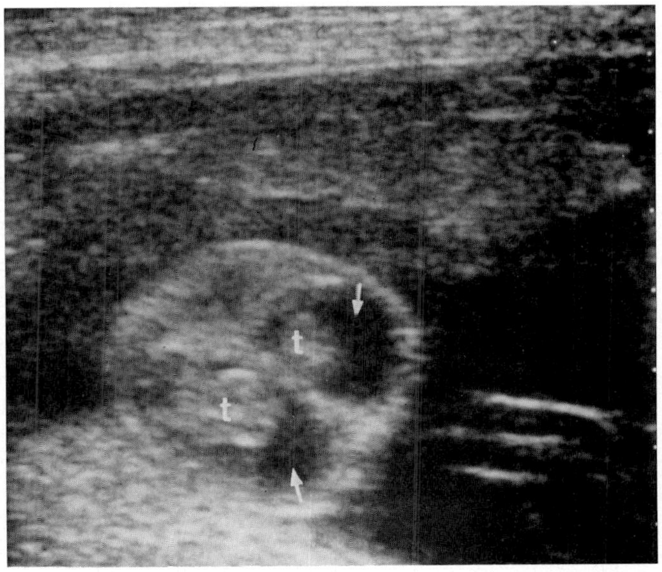

ABNORMALITIES OF THE EXTREMITIES

Evaluation of the fetal long bones is important in the estimation of fetal age and growth and in the detection of skeletal dysplasias (abnormal growth and development of limbs). Ultrasound plays a significant role in attempting to characterize different types of limb deformities. By sonography, one is able to determine the length of individual bones and assess the shape and echogenicity patterns of the bones. High-resolution ultrasound equipment allows

*References 6, 41, 42, 56, 59, 60, 69, 125, 132.

Fig. 23-36. Transverse scan demonstrating mild hydroceles bilaterally *(arrows).* The testicles, *t,* are clearly outlined.

for the identification of subtle defects of the fetal hands and feet, which often permits the specific diagnosis of certain skeletal dysplasias.

Many skeletal dysplasias can be diagnosed by the antenatal investigation of fetuses at risk for limb dysplasias. In the majority of sonographically visible dysplasias there is a marked reduction in the length of the long bones. By comparing the length of an abnormally shortened bone to one appropriate for gestational age, one can detect a limb-reduction abnormality. A skeletal dysplasia is only considered when the limb lengths are significantly shorter than normal (2 SD below the mean)[54] (Tables 23-5 and 23-6). Each skeletal dysplasia has differing clinical manifestations, and therefore a knowledge of the type of skeletal dysplasia to be sought is critical prior to sonographic evaluation. Certain skeletal dysplasias will affect different limb bones (proximal bones, femur and humeri or medial bones, lower legs and forearms). In addition, other fetal organs will be affected, depending on the type of disorder. In some dysplasias the cranium will be enlarged or may display signs of ventriculomegaly. Facial anomalies may provide valuable information (prominent maxillae or forehead), or the size and shape of the chest may aid in specific differentiation. Therefore a thorough evaluation of potentially affected body systems must be studied regarding the suspected skeletal dysplasia. A limb-reduction anomaly may be found on routine obstetrical exams, and therefore an effort must be made to determine the type of dysplasia.

Several skeletal dysplasias are lethal disorders or may be of autosomal recessive (25% recurrence risk) or autosomal dominant (50% recurrence risk) inheritance. High-risk ultrasound laboratories are frequently asked to evaluate pregnancies at risk for specific skeletal dysplasias based on family history of a disorder because of the high recurrence risks and dismal prognoses in some conditions.[64]

Table 23-5 Length of the Bones of the Leg: Normal Values

Week No.	Tibia Percentile				Fibula Percentile		
	5th	50th	95th		5th	50th	95th
12	—	7	—	:	—	6	—
13	—	10	—	:	—	9	—
14	7	12	17	:	6	12	19
15	9	15	20	—:—	9	15	21
16	12	17	22	:	13	18	23
17	15	20	25	:	13	21	28
18	17	22	27	:	15	23	31
19	20	25	30	:	19	26	33
20	22	27	33	:	21	28	36
21	25	30	35	:	24	31	37
22	27	32	38	:	27	33	39
23	30	35	40	:	28	35	42
24	32	37	42	:	29	37	45
25	34	40	45	—:—	34	40	45
26	37	42	47	:	36	42	47
27	39	44	49	:	37	44	50
28	41	46	51	:	38	45	53
29	43	48	53	:	41	47	54
30	45	50	55	:	43	49	56
31	47	52	57	:	42	51	59
32	48	54	59	:	42	52	63
33	50	55	60	:	46	54	62
34	52	57	62	:	46	55	65
35	53	58	64	—:—	51	57	62
36	55	60	65	:	54	58	63
37	56	61	67	:	54	59	65
38	58	63	68	:	56	61	65
39	59	64	69	:	56	62	67
40	61	66	71	:	59	63	67
	mm	mm	mm		mm	mm	mm

From Jeanty P and Romero R, editors: Obstetrical ultrasound, New York, 1984, McGraw Hill Book Co.

Table 23-6 Length of the Bones of the Arm: Normal Values

Week No.		Ulna Percentile				Radius Percentile		
		5th	50th	95th		5th	50th	95th
12	:	—	7	—	:	—	7	—
13	:	5	10	15	:	6	10	14
14	:	8	13	18	:	8	13	17
15	—:—	11	16	21	—:—	11	15	20
16	:	13	18	23	:	13	18	22
17	:	16	21	26	:	14	20	26
18	:	19	24	29	:	15	22	29
19	:	21	26	31	:	20	24	29
20	:	24	29	34	:	22	27	32
21	:	26	31	36	:	24	29	33
22	:	28	33	38	:	27	31	34
23	:	31	36	41	:	26	32	39
24	:	33	38	43	:	26	34	42
25	—:—	35	40	45	—:—	31	36	41
26	:	37	42	47	:	32	37	43
27	:	39	44	49	:	33	39	45
28	:	41	46	51	:	33	40	48
29	:	43	48	53	:	36	42	47
30	:	44	49	54	:	36	43	49
31	:	46	51	56	:	38	44	50
32	:	48	53	58	:	37	45	53
33	:	49	54	59	:	41	46	51
34	:	51	56	61	:	40	47	53
35	—:—	52	57	62	—:—	41	48	54
36	:	53	58	63	:	39	48	57
37	:	55	60	65	:	45	49	53
38	:	56	61	66	:	45	49	54
39	:	57	62	67	:	45	50	54
40	:	58	63	68	:	46	50	55
		mm	mm	mm		mm	mm	mm

From Jeanty P and Romero R, Obstetrical ultrasound, New York, 1984, McGraw-Hill Book Co.

The role of the sonographic team is to define the extent of limb shortening (which long bones are affected), the degree of shortening (some skeletal dysplasias do not become apparent until late in the second trimester, e.g., heterozygous achondroplasia), the contour and shape of the bones (intrauterine bowing and fractures of the long bones may be seen, e.g., *osteogenesis imperfecta*), the echogenicity of bones (several disorders will demonstrate a decrease in the mineralization of the bones and will not produce an acoustic shadow, e.g., osteogenesis imperfecta, *hypophosphatasia*), the involvement of hands and feet (irregular formation of these structures may indicate specific disorders, e.g., *polydactyly*), and coexisting malformations (cranial enlargement, abnormally shaped chests, and ventriculomegaly may be present in some dysplasias).

The intent of this discussion is to familiarize the sonographer with the most common skeletal dysplasias that can be diagnosed by current sonographic techniques. The reader is referred to comprehensive texts on this subject for a more detailed description of individual skeletal dysplasias.[51]

Thanatophoric dysplasia

Thanatophoric (death-bringing) dysplasia is generally a lethal skeletal dysplasia marked by severe reduction in the length of the long bones.[21,68,101]

Following are characteristic sonographic features of thanatophoric dysplasia:

1. Shortening of long bones (2 SD below the mean)
2. Enlargement of the cranium (greater than the 95th percentile as determined by head circumference; head/abdomen ratio)
3. Dilatation of the cerebral ventricles (commonly occurs)
4. Clover-leaf skull deformity (14% of cases)[101]
5. Prominent forehead
6. Hypertelorism

7. Narrow, pear-shaped chest (decreased thoracic diameter TC and TC/AC
8. Protuberant abdomen (determined by AC measurements)
9. Soft-tissue redundancy (thick limb buds)[68,101]
10. Nonimmune hydrops
11. Polyhydramnios

The specific diagnosis of thanatophoric dysplasia is difficult to differentiate from other disorders with shortened limbs. The specific diagnosis of thanatophoric dysplasia can be made when a dwarfed fetus is found with a cloverleaf skull deformity.[101]

Achondroplasia

Achondroplasia represents a defect in the development of cartilage at the epiphyseal centers of the long bones, which produces short and squat bones.[51] Achondroplasia has two different inheritance patterns. *Homozygous achondroplasia* is the lethal form of this disorder. There is significant shortening of the limbs and narrowing of the thoracic cavity while the cranium may be disproportionately large compared to the abdomen.

In *heterozygous achondroplasia*, skeletal abnormalities may not be apparent until the late second trimester of pregnancy. Kurtz and associates[89] noted that in fetuses with heterozygous achondroplasia, when femur length was compared to the growth of the biparietal diameter, growth of the femur was initially normal and fell outside normal limits by 27 weeks of gestation. In fetuses with heterozygous achondroplasia there may be sonographic evidence of a protuberant forehead. Measurements of the femurs and humeri should be performed in fetuses at risk for achondroplasia to appreciate the proximal (rhizomelic) shortening predominantly of the upper extremities.[51] The fetal cranium should be studied to exclude cranial enlargement and ventriculomegaly.

Achondrogenesis

Achondrogenesis is a lethal short-limbed dwarfism with an autosomal recessive inheritance pattern. This form of dwarfism is characterized by shortening of the long bones and trunk, "flipperlike" appendages,[51] a decrease in the echogenicity of the bones, absence of spinal echoes, and a prominent forehead.[68]

Osteogenesis imperfecta

Osteogenesis imperfecta is a severe metabolic disorder involving the collagen system of the fetus. Osteogenesis imperfecta presents in four forms.[136] Osteogenesis imperfecta tarda levis (type I) is an autosomal dominant disease that is difficult to identify by ultrasound. Fetuses with this form of osteogenesis imperfecta may display signs of bowing of the long bones, fractures, a decrease in acoustic shadowing late in gestation, and a ribbonlike appearance of the bones.[29] Fractures of the bones frequently occur after birth. Type II osteogenesis imperfecta congenita is an autosomal recessive disease that is incompatible with life. Fetuses with this disorder are severely affected at birth with characteristic signs of multiple fractures of the long bones, spine, and ribs and poorly mineralized crania, which may be collapsed or fractured. Blue sclera will be evident at birth.

Type II disorders are amenable to antenatal sonographic detection. Bowed or fractured limbs have been identified. The limbs may appear broad and thickened and will be markedly shortened in length (Fig. 23-37). The ribs and spine should be inspected for evidence of fractures. Occasionally the thorax can be collapsed late in gestation.

Type III osteogenesis imperfecta (autosomal recessive) is a progressively severe form of the disease with normal sclera, fractures, and bowing of the limbs. Type IV disease is characterized as a mild form of the disease (susceptible to fractures and bowing of the ribs and long bones).

In fetuses at risk for osteogenesis imperfecta, the following areas should be studied[68]:

1. Cranium (exclude hypomineralization, collapsed or fractured crania) (Fig. 23-38, *B*)
2. Ribs and clavicles (exclude fractures)
3. Spine (exclude fractures and displacement of spinal components)
4. Thorax (exclude small thoracic cavity) (Fig. 23-38, *A*)
5. Long bones (measure length of long bones, determine echogenicity, and exclude bowing/fractures) (Fig. 23-37)

Hypophosphatasia and other dysplasias

This bone disorder is hallmarked by a lack of mineralization in the bones (causing weak, fragile, ribbonlike bones), resulting in bowing of the lower extremities, a small thoracic cage, and a poorly calcified cranium.[51] The abnormalities of this disorder vary in severity. In the most severe form, neonates die in the early neonatal period due to respiratory insufficiency. This disorder may be difficult to differentiate from osteogenesis imperfecta.[68]

Several other skeletal dysplasias can be diagnosed by ultrasound. These disorders may mimic other short-limbed dysplasias, but may be differentiated by subtle characteristics specific for each disorder. Asphyxiating thoracic dysplasia (Jeune syndrome) may be identifiable by shortened limbs and marked narrowing of the thoracic cavity.[138] In campomelic dysplasia the fetal long bones will appear severely bowed or bent in configuration.[68] Chondroectodermal dysplasia (Ellis-van Creveld syndrome) may be suspected when polydactyly (addition of finger or toe) is present.[102] Hitchhiker thumbs may be indicative of diastrophic dysplasia.[103] In Robert syndrome there may be an absence of limbs or deformed limbs (tetraphocomelia), microcephaly, hand and foot anomalies, and hypotelorism.[68] In the thrombocytopenia absent radii (TAR) syndrome, absence or aplasia of the radii may be diagnostic of this disorder.

Abnormalities of the hands and feet may occur in conjunction with skeletal dysplasias, in fetuses with congenital anomalies, or as isolated anatomic defects. Fingers and toes may be missing, fused (syndactyly or lobster-claw), or excessive (polydactyly). Whenever a hand or foot aberration is discovered, a careful search for additional fetal malformations (i.e., skeletal dysplasia) should be per-

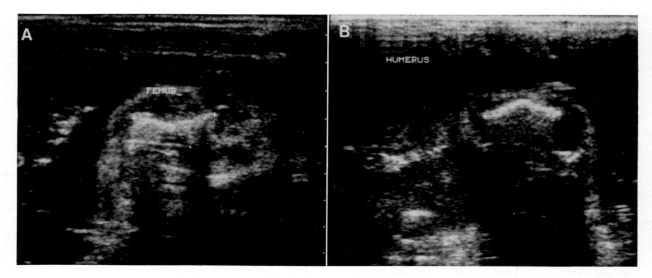

Fig. 23-37.   A, Femur length that is significantly shortened in a fetus with osteogenesis imperfecta. The femur measured 2.9 cm at 30 weeks of gestation. **B,** Bowing of humerus, in same fetus, with osteogenesis imperfecta. Humeral length measured 2.7 cm at 30 weeks of gestation.

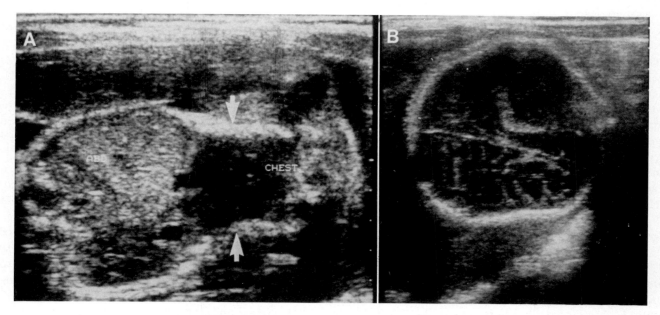

Fig. 23-38.   A, Sagittal scan demonstrating small thoracic cavity in a fetus with osteogenesis imperfecta *(arrows). ABD,* Abdomen. **B,** Transverse scan through fetal cranium showing a decrease in calcification (thin skull) with enhanced visualization of brain anatomy.

formed. The hands should be studied in coronal sections to count the number of digits and in sagittal sections to individually evaluate the contour of the digits and metacarpals.

Clubfoot (talipes) is frequently found in fetuses with spinal defects, skeletal dysplasias, chromosomal anomalies, or as isolated lesions. By ultrasound, a clubfoot (feet) may be recognized by the persistent abnormal inversion of the foot perpendicular to the lower leg (Fig. 23-39).

Other foot anomalies that have been described include (1) rockerbottom feet, (2) clinodactyly (permanent flexion of a finger over another finger), and (3) symbrachydactyly (fused short fingers).[84]

ABNORMALITIES OF THE UMBILICAL CORD

The normal human umbilical cord consists of the single umbilical vein and the smaller paired umbilical arteries. Absence of an umbilical artery (single umbilical artery) is one of the most common congenital abnormalities found in 1% of neonates.[46] In this condition the umbilical cord contains the umbilical vein and a single umbilical artery (two-vessel cord).[77,144] This can easily be visualized on sagittal or transverse scans (Fig. 23-40).

Single umbilical artery is associated with congenital anomalies[77] (skeletal and gastrointestinal most frequent), intrauterine growth retardation, and a higher incidence of perinatal mortality. Evaluation of the umbilical cord

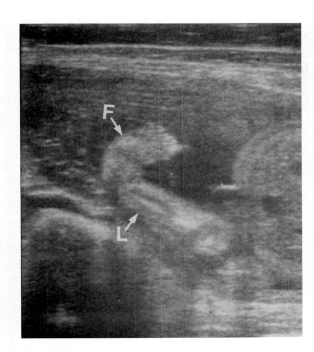

Fig. 23-39.   Clubfoot identified during a routine obstetrical scan in a 19-week fetus. Additional anomalies detected included cystic hygroma, ventriculomegaly, and ascites. Note the medial inversion of the foot, *F,* in relationship to the lower leg, *L.*

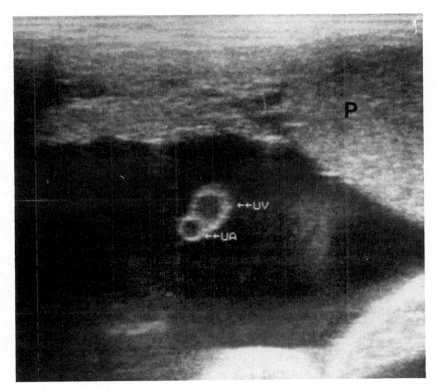

Fig. 23-40.   Transverse scan of a two-vessel umbilical cord depicting a single umbilical artery, *UA,* and umbilical vein, *UV,* associated with duodenal atresia. *P,* Placenta.

should be performed to assess the number of cord vessels in view of the prevalence of associated fetal malformations. Oligohydramnios may preclude adequate visualization of the umbilical cord vessels.

CONCLUSION

In the past ten years, ultrasound operators have been able to detect major and minor malformations of the fetus. Recognizing fetal birth defects aids in providing optimal clinical management and further allows timely deliveries

in tertiary centers equipped to handle high-risk neonates. Early detection of anomalies further affords options to attempt intrauterine surgical therapy to correct fetal lesions during the antepartum period..

ACKNOWLEDGMENTS

The author is grateful to John C. Hobbins, MD; Marge Tortora, BS, RDMS; Richard L. Berkowitz, MD; Peter A. Grannum, MD; and Frank A. Chervenak, MD for stimulating her interest and encouraging her to pursue studies of fetal malformations. Gratitude is also extended to Ms. Maria Fuentes for her skillful assistance in the preparation of this manuscript.

SUMMARY

1. Ultrasound has made a tremendous impact on the detection of congenital malformations during the antenatal period. The sophistication of comprehensive ultrasound examinations to detect anomalies has placed a considerable demand on sonographers. A working knowledge of pertinent obstetrics and genetics is necessary.

2. α-Fetoprotein (AFP) is an important fetal protein that can be studied in maternal serum and in amniotic fluid. Elevated α-fetoprotein can be detected in fetuses with neural tube defects. α-Fetoprotein values differ at each gestational age; therefore accurate menstrual dating and/or sonographic estimation of gestational age is crucial to maternal serum screening protocols. Underestimation sof gestational age are frequently found to be the reason for elevations of α-fetoprotein.

3. Chorionic villus sampling (CVS) is an ultrasound-directed procedure that permits the biopsy of fetal tissue from the chorionic villi. CVS procedures will detect the same chromosomal, metabolic, or blood disorders that can be detected by amniocentesis.

4. Comprehensive ultrasound examinations pertain to specialized scans of the fetus that are performed to detect or confirm a fetal anomaly, to evaluate the fetus at risk for an anomaly, and to follow the fetus with a known anomaly during pregnancy.

5. An abnormal volume of amniotic fluid may infer an underlying congenital malformation. Considerable operator experience is necessary to differentiate between normal and abnormal amniotic fluid states.

6. Several cranial malformations alter the contour of the fetal cranium while many affect intracranial brain structures.

7. The fetal brain structures most commonly associated with intracranial anomalies are the cerebral ventricles. Meticulous evaluation of the fetal ventricles is critical during all obstetrical examinations but most important in the fetus at risk for cranial abnormalities.

8. Ventriculomegaly is the abnormal accumulation of cerebrospinal fluid within the cerebral ventricles, resulting in their dilation. Once ventriculomegaly has been identified, the sonographic team must diligently scrutinize the fetus for sonographically de-tectable defects by evaluating all the major organ systems to identify those fetuses with single or multiple lesions.

9. Remarkable enhancements in sonographic imaging have generated a tremendous interest in the imaging of the facial structures of the fetus. A knowledge of normal anatomic facial structures is imperative to detect minute abnormalities of facial architecture.

10. Orbital architecture has become increasingly important in the evaluation of craniofacial anomalies. Both anatomic and biometric evaluation of fetal orbits should be attempted in fetuses at risk for orbital malformations.

11. The fetal thoracic cavity has become more accessible for sonographic evaluation of masses involving the lungs, heart, and diaphragm. The detection of thoracic defects is important since many lesions may compromise fetal breathing and require surgery in the neonatal period.

12. Evaluation of the fetal vertebral column remains one of the most technically difficult examinations confronting the sonographic team. It is challenging to evaluate because of flexion of the cervical and lumbosacral spine and the large surface area that needs to be studied.

13. Early recognition of abdominal wall defects is imperative. Fetuses with ventral wall defects need to be delivered in centers with access to immediate pediatric care to prevent heat and water loss and to expedite surgical correction of the defect.

14. Obstruction of the normal swallowing sequence can occur due to an atretic or obstructive process, resulting in a back-up of amniotic fluid. In pregnancies with hydramnios, anomalies of the gastrointestinal system should be sought.

15. Renal malformations are categorized into those that result from a developmental abnormality or from an obstructive process. The consequences of renal malformations vary, depending on the type of lesion or extent of obstruction. Amniotic fluid volume is a significant factor in the outcome of affected pregnancies.

16. Evaluation of the fetal long bones is important in the estimation of fetal age and growth and in the detection of skeletal dysplasias.

17. Identification of fetal anomalies by ultrasound allows optimal clinical management as well as timely deliveries with access to immediate and specialized care for the neonate, and affords options to attempt in utero surgical correction of fetal lesions.

REFERENCES

1. Alter BP, Friedman S, Hobbins JC et al: Prenatal diagnosis of sickle cell anemia and alpha g-Philadelphia. A study of a fetus also at risk for HBS/B+thalassemia, N Engl J Med 294:1040, 1976.
2. Arey LB: The vascular system. In Arey LB, editor: Developmental anatomy, ed 7, Philadelphia, 1974, WB Saunders Co.
3. Barone CM, VanNatta FC, Kourides IA, and Berkowitz RL: Sonographic detection of fetal goiter, an unusual cause of hydramnios, J Ultrasound Med 4:625, 1985.
4. Benacerraf BR and Frigoletto FD: Amniocentesis under continuous ultrasound guidance: a series of 232 cases, Obstet Gynecol 62:760, 1983.
5. Beretsky I and Lankin DH: Diagnosis of fetal cholelithiasis using real time high resolution imaging employing digital detection, J Ultrasound Med 2:381, 1983.
6. Berkowitz RL, Glickman MG, Walker-Smith GJ et al: Fetal urinary tract obstruction: what is the role of surgical intervention in utero? Am J Obstet Gynecol 144:367, 1982.
7. Bevis DCA: Composition of liquor amnii in haemolytic disease of newborn, Lancet 2:443, 1950.
8. Birnholz JC: Fetal portraiture helps to align ultrasound with traditional medicine, Diagnostic Imaging, September 1986.
9. Birnholz JC and Frigoletto FD: Antenatal treatment of hydrocephalus, N Engl J Med 303:1021, 1981.
10. Bovicelli L, Rizzo N, Orsini LF, and Pilu G: Prenatal diagnosis and management of fetal gastrointestinal abnormalities, Sem Perinatol 7:109, 1983.
11. Bowie JD: Sonography of fetal abdominal abnormalities. In Sanders RC, editor: The principles and practice of ultrasonography in obstetrics and gynecology, ed 3, Norwalk, Conn, 1985, Appleton-Century-Crofts.
12. Callen PW Chooljian D: The effect of ventricular dilatation upon biometry of the fetal head, J Ultrasound Med 5:17, 1986.
13. Callen PW, Hashimoto BE, and Newton TH: Sonographic evaluation of cerebral cortical mantle thickness in the fetus and neonatal with hydrocephalus, Ultrasound Med 5:251, 1986.
14. Campbell S, Johnstone FD, Holt EM, and May P: Anencephaly: early ultrasound diagnosis and active management, Lancet 2:1226, 1972.
15. Campbell S and Thoms A: Ultrasonic measurement of fetal head to abdomen circumference ratio in the assessment of growth retardation, Br J Obstet Gynecol 84:165, 1977.
16. Carpenter MW, Curci MR, Dibbins AW, and Haddow JE: Perinatal management of ventral wall defects, Obstet Gynecol 64:646, 1984.
17. Chang H, Hobbins JC, Cividalli G et al: In utero diagnosis of hemoglobinopathies in

fetal red cells, N Engl J Med 290:1067, 1974.
18. Chervenak FA, Berkowitz RL, Romero R, et al: The diagnosis of fetal hydrocephalus, Am J Obstet Gynecol 147:703, 1983.
19. Chervenak FA, Berkowitz RL, Tortora M, and Hobbins JC: The management of fetal hydrocephalus, Am J Obstet Gynecol 151:933, 1985.
20. Chervenak FA, Blakemore KJ, Isaacson G et al: Antenatal sonographic findings of thanatophoric dysplasia with cloverleaf skull, Am J Obstet Gynecol 146:948, 1983.
21. Chervenak FA, Blakemore KJ, Isaacson G: Antenatal sonographic findings of thanatophoric dysplasia with cloverleaf skull, Am J Obstet Gynecol 146:984, 1983.
22. Chervenak FA, Duncan C, Ment L et al: Perinatal management of meningomyelocele, Obstet Gynecol 63:376, 1984.
23. Chervenak FA, Duncan C, Ment LR et al: Outcome of fetal ventriculomegaly, Lancet 2:179, 1984.
24. Chervenak FA, Isaacson G, Blakemore KJ et al: Fetal cystic hygroma: cause and natural history, N Engl J Med 309:822, 1983.
25. Chervenak FA, Isaacson G, Mahoney MJ et al: Diagnosis and management of fetal cephalocele, Obstet Gynecol 64:86, 1984.
26. Chervenak FA, Isaacson G, Mahoney MJ et al: The obstetrical significance of holoprosencephaly, Obstet Gynecol 63:115, 1984.
27. Chervenak FA, Isaacson G, Touloukian et al: Diagnosis and management of fetal teratomas, Obstet Gynecol 66:666, 1985.
28. Chervenak FA, Jeanty P, Cantraine F et al: The diagnosis of fetal microcephaly, Am J Obstet Gynecol 149:512, 1984.
29. Chervenak FA, Romero R, Berkowitz RL et al: Antenatal sonographic findings of osteogenesis imperfecta, Am J Obstet Gynecol 143:228, 1982.
30. Chervenak FA, Tortora M, and Hobbins JC: Antenatal sonographic diagnosis of clubfoot, J Ultrasound Med 4:49, 1985.
31. Chervenak FA, Tortora M, Mayden KL et al: Median cleft face syndrome: ultrasonic demonstration of cleft lip and hypertelorism, Am J Obstet Gynecol 149:94, 1984.
32. Chervenak FA, Tortora M, Moya FR, and Hobbins JC: Antenatal sonographic diagnosis of epignathus, J Ultrasound Med 3:235, 1984.
33. Chung CS and Myrianthopoulos NC: Factors affecting risks of congenital malformations. I. Epidemiological analysis, Birth Defects 11:1, 1975.
34. Clewell WH, Johnson ML, Meier PR et al: A surgical approach to fetal hydrocephalus, N Engl J Med 306:1320, 1982.
35. Clewell WH, Manco-Johnson M, and Manchester DK: Diagnosis and management of fetal hydrocephalus, Clin Obstet Gynecol 29:514, 1986.

36. Comstock CH: The antenatal diagnosis of diaphragmatic hernia, J Ultrasound Med 5:391, 1986.
37. Comstock CH and Boal DB: Enlarged fetal cisterna magna: Appearance and significance, Obstet Gynecol 66:255, 1985.
38. Comstock CH, Culp D, Gonzalez J, and Boal DB: Agenesis of the corpus callosum in the fetus: Its evolution and significance, J Ultrasound Med 4:613, 1985.
39. Crane JP and Kopta MM: Genetic amniocentesis: impact of placental position upon the risk of pregnancy loss, Am J obstet Gynecol 150:813, 1984.
40. Davis GH, Wapner RJ, Kurtz AB et al: Antenatal diagnosis of hydrometrocolpos by ultrasound examination, J Ultrasound Med 3:371, 1984.
41. Dunn V and Glasier CM: Ultrasonographic antenatal demonstration of primary megaureters, J Ultrasound Med 4:101, 1985.
42. Ehman RL, Nicholson SF, and Machin GA: Prenatal sonographic detection of congenital mesoblastic nephroma in a monozygotic twin pregnancy, J Ultrasound Med 2:555, 1983.
43. Elrad H, Mayden KL, Gleicher N et al: Prenatal diagnosis of choledochal cyst, J Ultrasound Med 4:553, 1985.
44. Firshein SI, Hoyer LW, Lazarchick J et al: Prenatal diagnosis of classic hemophilia, N Engl J Med 300:937, 1979.
45. Fiske CE and Filly RA: Ultrasound evaluation of the normal and abnormal fetal neural axis. In Callen PW, editor: Ultrasonography in obstetrics and gynecology, Philadelphia, 1983, WB Saunders Co.
46. Froehlich LA: Significance of a single umbilical artery: report from the collaborative study of cerebral palsy, Am J Obstet Gynecol 94:274, 1966.
47. Glick PL, Harrison MR, Nakayama DK et al: Management of ventriculomegaly in the fetus, J Pediatr 105:97, 1984.
48. Golbus MS, Harrison MR, Filly RA et al: In utero treatment of urinary tract obstruction, Am J Obstet Gynecol 142:383, 1982.
49. Golbus MS, Loughman WD, Epstein CJ et al: Prenatal genetic diagnosis in 3000 amniocenteses, N Engl J Med 300:157, 1979.
50. Golbus MSA, Sagebiel RW, Filly FA et al: Prenatal diagnosis of congenital bulbous ichthyosiform erythroderma (epidermolytic hyperkeratosis) by fetal skin biopsy, N Engl J Med 302:93, 1980.
51. Goodman RM and Gorlin RJ: Genetic syndromes: skeletal dysplasias. In The malformed infant and child: an illustrated guide, New York, 1983, Oxford University Press.
52. Graham D and Sanders RC: Sonographic evaluation of the fetal chest. In Sanders RC, editor: The principles and practice of ultrasonography in obstetrics and gynecology, ed 3, Norwalk, Conn, 1985, Appleton-Century-Crofts.

53. Grannum P, Bracken M, Silverman R, and Hobbins JC: Assessment of fetal kidney size in normal gestation by comparison of ratio of kidney circumference to abdominal circumference, Am J Obstet Gynecol 136:249, 1980.

54. Grannum PA and Hobbins JC: Prenatal diagnosis of fetal skeletal dysplasias, Sem Perinatol 7:125, 1983.

55. Gray D, Crane J, and Rudolff M: Origin of midtrimester vertebral ossification centers as determined by sonographic waterbath studies of a dissected fetal spine, Presented at AIUM Annual Meeting, September 16-19, 1986, Las Vegas.

56. Greenblatt AM, Beretsky I, Lankin DH, and Phelan L: In utero diagnosis of crossed renal ectopia using high-resolution real-time ultrasound, J Ultrasound Med 4:105, 1985.

57. Harrison MR, Golbus MS, and Filly RA: Congenital diaphragmatic hernia. In The unborn patient, Orlando, Fla., 1984, Grune and Stratton.

58. Harrison MR, Golbus MS, and Filly RA: Congenital hydrocephalus. In The unborn patient: prenatal diagnosis and treatment, Orlando, Fla., 1984, Grune and Stratton.

59. Harrison MR, Golbus MS, and Filly RA: Congenital hydronephrosis. In Harrison MR, Golbus MS, and Filly RA, editors: In The unborn patient: prenatal diagnosis and management, Orlando, Fla., 1984, Grune and Stratton.

60. Harrison, MR, Golbus MS, and Filly RA: Ultrasonography. In The unborn patient: prenatal diagnosis and treatment, Orlando, Fla., 1984, Grune & Stratton.

61. Harrison R, Campbell S, and Craft I: Risks of fetomaternal hemorrhage results from amniocentesis with and without ultrasound placental localization, Obstet Gynecol 46:389, 1975.

62. Hobbins JC: Determination of fetal sex in early pregnancy, N Engl J Med 309:942, 1983.

63. Hobbins JC: Ultrasound can diagnose fetal malformations, Contrib. Ob/Gyn 19:99, 1982.

64. Hobbins JC, Bracken MB, and Mahoney MJ: Diagnosis of fetal skeletal dysplasias with ultrasound, Am J Obstet Gynecol 142:306, 1982.

65. Hobbins JC, Grannum PA, Romero R et al: Percutaneous umbilical blood sampling, Am J Obstet Gynecol 152:1, 1985.

66. Hobbins JC, Grannum PAT, Berkowitz RL et al: Ultrasound in the diagnosis of congenital anomalies, Am J Obstet Gynecol 134:331, 1979.

67. Hobbins JC and Mahoney MJ: In utero diagnosis of hemoglobinopathies: techniques for obtaining fetal blood, N Engl J Med 290:1065, 1974.

68. Hobbins JC and Mahoney MJ: Skeletal dysplasia. In Sanders RC, editor: The principles and practice of ultrasonography in obstetrics and gynecology, ed 3, Norwalk, Conn., 1985, Appleton-Century-Crofts.

69. Hobbins JC, Romero R, Grannum P et al: Antenatal diagnosis of renal anomalies with ultrasound. I. Obstructive uropathy, Am J Obstet Gynecol 148:868, 1984.

70. Hobbins JC and Venus I: Congenital anomalies in diagnostic ultrasound in obstetrics. In Hobbins JC, editor: Clinics in diagnostic ultrasound, New York, 1979, Churchill Livingstone.

71. Hobbins JC, Venus I, Tortora M et al: Stage II ultrasound examination for the diagnosis of fetal abnormalities with an elevated amniotic fluid alpha-fetoprotein concentration, Am J Obstet Gynecol 142:1026, 1982.

72. Hobbins JC, Winsberg F, and Berkowitz RL: Ultrasonography in obstetrics and gynecology, ed 2, Baltimore, 1983, Williams and Wilkins Co.

73. Hohler CW and Ouetel TA: Comparison of ultrasound femur length and biparietal diameter in late pregnancy, Am J Obstet Gynecol 141:759, 1981.

74. Hook EB and Chambers GM: Estimated rates of Down syndrome in live births by one year maternal age intervals for mothers aged 20–49 in a New York state study: implications of the risk figures for genetic counseling and cost-benefit analysis of prenatal diagnosis programs, Birth Defects 13(3a):123, 1977.

75. Hytten FE and Lind T: Diagnostic indices in pregnancy, Basel, Switzerland, 1973, Ciba-Geigy.

76. van der Putte, SC: Lymphatic malformation in human fetuses: a study of fetuses with Turner's syndrome or status: Bonnevie-Ullrich, Virchows Arch [A] (Pathol Anat) 376:233, 1977.

77. Jassani MN, Breunam JN, and Merkatz IR: Prenatal diagnosis of single umbilical artery by ultrasound, J Clin Ultrasound 8:447, 1980.

78. Jeanty P, Cantraine F, Cousaert E et al: The binocular distance: a new parameter to estimated fetal age, J Ultrasound Med 3:241, 1984.

79. Jeanty P, Dramaix-Wilmet M, and Van-Gansbeke D: Fetal ocular biometry by ultrasound, Radiology 143:513, 1982.

80. Jeanty P, Rodesch F, Romero R et al: How to improve your amniocentesis technique, Am J Obstet Gynecol 146:593, 1983.

81. Jeanty P and Romero R: Is there a neural tube defect? In Jeanty P and Romero R, editors: Obstetrical ultrasound, New York, 1984, McGraw-Hill Book Co.

82. Jeanty P and Romero R: Is there a normal amount of amniotic fluid? In Obstetrical ultrasound, New York, 1984, McGraw-Hill Book Co.

83. Jeanty P and Romero R: The sex of the fetus. In Jeanty P and Romero R, editors: Obstetrical ultrasound, New York, 1984, McGraw-Hill Book Co.J

84. Jeanty P, Romero R, d'Alton M et al: In utero sonographic detection of hand and foot deformities, J Ultrasound med 4:595, 1985.

85. Jeffrey MF: The role of ultrasound in chorionic villus sampling: a review, J Diagn Med Sonogr 3:135, 1986.

86. Johnson ML, Dunne MG, Mack LA et al: Evaluation of fetal intracranial anatomy by static and real-time ultrasound, J Clin Ultrasound 8:311, 1980.

87. Kalter H and Warkany J: Congenital malformations: etiologic factors and their role in prevention (first of two parts), N Engl J Med 308:424, 1983.

88. Kapp LE, Smith DW, Omenn GS et al: Use of ultrasound in the prenatal exclusion of primary microcephaly, Gynecol Invest 5:311, 1974.

89. Kurtz AB, Filly RA, Wapner RJ et al: In utero analysis of heterozygous achondroplasia: variable time of onset as detected by femur length measurements, J Ultrasound Med 5:137, 1986.

90. Kurtz AB, Wapner RJ, Rubin CS et al: Ultrasound criteria for in utero diagnosis of microcephaly, J Clin Ultrasound 8:11, 1980.

91. Langman J: Caudal part of the foregut. In Langman J, editor: Medical embryology, Baltimore, 1975, Williams and Wilkins Co.

92. Langman J: Hindgut. In Langman J, editor: Medical embryology ed 3, Baltimore, 1975, Williams and Wilkins Co.

93. Langman J: Spinal cord. In Langman J, editor: Medical embryology, ed 3, Baltimore, 1975, Williams and Wilkins Co.

94. Laurence KM: Antenatal detection of neural tube defects. In Barson AJ, editor: Fetal and neonatal pathology, New York, 1982, Praeger Publishers.

95. Lenke RR, Platt LD, and Koch R: Ultrasonic failure of early detection of fetal microcephaly in maternal phenylketonuria, J Ultrasound Med 2:177, 1983.

96. Lenz W and Maier E: Congenital malformations and maternal diabetes, Lancet 2:1124, 1964.

97. Lorber J and Schofield JK: The prognosis of occipital encephalocele, Z Kinderchir 28:347, 1979.

98. Luthy DA, Ashwood ER, and Cheng E: The Society of Perinatal Obstetricians, January 30–February 1, 1986, San Antonio, Texas.

99. Mack L, Gottesfeld K, and Johnson ML: Antenatal detection of ectopic fetal liver by ultrasound, Clin Ultrasound 6:215, 1978.

100. Mahoney B, Callen P, Filly R et al: The fetal cisterna magna, Radiology 153:773, 1984.

101. Mahoney BS, Filly RA, Callen PW, and Golbus MS: Thanatophoric dwarfism with the cloverleaf skull: a specific antenatal sonographic diagnosis, J Ultrasound Med 4:151, 1985.

102. Mahoney MJ and Hobbins JC: Prenatal diagnosis of chondroectodermal dysplasia (Ellis-van Creveld syndrome) with fetoscopy and ultrasound, N Engl J Med 297:258, 1977.

103. Manatagos S, Weiss RR, Mahoney M, and Hobbins JC: Prenatal diagnosis of diastrophic dwarfism, Am J Obstet Gynecol 139:111, 1981.

104. Manning FA: International Fetal Surgery

Registry: 1985 Update, Clin Obstet Gynecol 29:551, 1986.

105. Mayden KL, Tortora M, Berkowitz RL et al: Orbital diameters: a new parameter for prenatal diagnosis and dating, Am J Obstet Gynecol 144:289, 1982.

106. Mayden KL, Tortora M, Chervenak FA, and Hobbins JC: The antenatal, sonographic detection of lung masses, Am J Obstet Gynecol 148:349, 1984.

107. McCormack MK: AFP, Clin Teratol 28:153, 1983.

108. Michejda M, Queenan JT, and McCullough D: Present status of intrauterine treatment of hydrocephalus and its future, Am J Obstet Gynecol 155:873, 1986.

109. Miller ME, Graham JM, Higginbottom MC, and Smith DW: Compression-related defects from early amnion rupture: evidence for mechanical teratogenesis, J Pediatr 98:292, 1981.

110. Milunsky A and Sapirstein VS: Prenatal diagnosis of open neural tube defects using the amniotic fluid acetylcholinesterase assay, Obstet Gynecol 59:1, 1982.

111. Nakayama DK: Management of the fetus with an abdominal wall defect. In Harrison MR, Golbus MS, and Filly RA, editors: The unborn patient—prenatal diagnosis and treatment, Orlando, Fla., 1984, Grune & Stratton.

111a. Nicolaides KH, Gabbe SG, Campbell S et al: Ultrasound screening for spina bifida: cranial and cerebellar signs, Lancet 2:72, 1986.

112. Nicolaides KH and Rodeck CH: Future muscle wasting: greatest hope lies in gene therapy, Gen Practit Dec. 3, 1982, p. 44.

113. Ober C and Simpson JL: Diabetes mellitus: preventing anomalies through maternal metabolic intervention, Clin Obstet Gynecol 29:558, 1986.

114. Osathanondh R and Birnholz JC: Ultrasonically guided transabdominal encephalocentesis, J Reprod Med 25:125, 1981.

115. Pearce JM, Little D, and Campbell S: The diagnosis of abnormalities of the fetal central nervous system. In Sanders RC, editor: The principles and practice of ultrasonography in obstetrics and gynecology, ed 3, Norwalk, Conn., 1985, Appleton-Century-Crofts.

116. Pilu G, Reece EA, Romero R et al: Prenatal diagnosis of craniofacial malformations with ultrasonography, Am J Obstet Gynecol 155:45, 1986.

117. Platt LD, Devore GR, Benner P et al: Antenatal diagnosis of a fetal liver mass, J Ultrasound Med 2:521, 1983.

118. Pretorius DH, Drose JA, and Manco-Johnson ML: Fetal lateral ventricular ratio determination during the second trimester, J Ultrasound Med 5:121, 1986.

119. Reece AE and Hobbins JC: Ultrasound's role in diabetic pregnancies, Contemp Ob/Gyn 23:87, 1984.

120. Rodeck CH and Campbell S: Umbilical cord insertion as a source of pure fetal blood for prenatal diagnosis, Lancet 1:1244, 1979.

121. Rodeck CH, Morsman JM, Nicolaides KH et al: A single-operator technique for first trimester chorion biopsy. Lancet 2:1340, 1983.

122. Rodeck CH and Nicolaides KH: Ultrasound guided invasive procedures in obstetrics, Clin Obstet Gynecol 10:515, 1983.

123. Rodeck CH, Patrick AD, Pembrey ME et al: Fetal liver biopsy for prenatal diagnosis of ornithine carabanyl transferase deficiency, Lancet 1:297, 1982.

124. Romero R, Chervenak FA, Kotzen J et al: Antenatal sonographic findings of extralobar pulmonary sequestration, J Ultrasound med 1:131, 1982.

125. Romero R, Cullen M, Jeanty P et al: The diagnosis of congenital renal anomalies with ultrasound. II. Infantile polycystic kidney disease, Am J Obstet Gynecol 150:259, 1984.

126. Romero R, Jeanty P, Reece EA et al: Sonographically monitored amniocentesis to decrease intraoperative complications, Obstet Gynecol 65:426, 1985.

127. Russ PD, Zavitz WR, Pretorius DH et al: Hydrometrocolpos, uterus didelphys and septate vagina: an antenatal sonographic diagnosis, J Ultrasound Med 3:371, 1984.

128. Sanders RC: Fetal anomalies. In Clinical sonography: a practical guide, Boston, 1984, Little, Brown and Co.

129. Sanders RC: Ultrasonic assessment of the face and neck. In Sanders RC, editor: The principles and practice of ultrasonography in obstetrics and gynecology, Norwalk, Conn., 1985, Appleton-Century-Crofts.

130. Sanders RC: Ultrasonic assessment of genitourinary anomalies in utero. In Sanders RC, editor: The principles and practice of ultrasonography in obstetrics and gynecology, Norwalk, Conn., 1985, Appleton-Century-Crofts.

131. Schmidt W, Yarkoni S, Jeanty P et al: Sonographic measurements of the fetal spleen, J Ultrasound Med 4:667, 1985.

132. Schoenecker SA, Cyr DR, Mack LA et al: Sonographic diagnosis of bilateral fetal renal duplication with ectopic ureteroceles, J Ultrasound Med 4:617, 1985.

133. Scrimgeour JB: Amniocentesis: technique and complications. In Emery AEH, editor: Antenatal diagnosis of genetic disease, Baltimore, 1973, Williams & Wilkins Co.

134. Seeds JW and Cefalo RC: Techniques of early sonographic diagnosis of bilateral cleft lip and palate, Obstet Gynecol 62:2S, 1983.

135. Shafer WG, Hine MK, and Levy BM: Developmental disturbances of oral and paraoral structures. In A textbook of oral pathology, ed 3, Philadelphia, 1974, WB Saunders Co.

136. Sillence DO, Seen A, and Danks DM: Clinical heterogeneity in osteogenesis imperfecta, J Med Genet 16:101, 1979.

137. Simoni G, Brambati B, Danesino C et al: Efficient direct chromosome analyses and enzyme determinations from chorionic villi samples in the first trimester of pregnancy, Hum Genet 63:349, 1983.

138. Skiptunas S and Weiner S: Early prenatal diagnosis of asphyxiating thoracic dysplasia (Jeune's syndrome) value of fetal thoracic measurement, J Ultrasound Med 6:41, 1987.

139. Slavkin HC: Congenital craniofacial malformations: issues and perspectives, J Prosthet Dent 51:109, 1984.

140. Smidt-Jensen S and Hahnemann N: Transabdominal fine needle biopsy from chorionic villi in the first trimester, Prenat Diag 4:163, 1984.

141. Smithells RW, Sheppard S et al: Possible prevention of neural tube defects by periconceptual vitamin supplements, Lancet 1:339, 1980.

142. Special report: the status of fetoscopy and fetal tissue sampling, Prenat Diag 4:79, 1984.

143. Stocker JT, Madewell JE, and Drake RM: Congenital cystic adenomatoid malformations of the lung, Hum Pathol 8:155, 1977.

144. Tortora M, Chervenak FA, Mayden K, and Hobbins JC: Antenatal sonographic diagnosis of single umbilical artery, Obstet Gynecol 63:693, 1984.

145. United Kingdom collaborative study on alpha-fetoprotein in relation to neural tube defects: maternal serum alpha-fetoprotein measurement in antenatal screening for anencephaly and spina bifida in early pregnancy, Lancet 1:1323, 1977.

145a. van der Putte, SC; 1977. See ref. 76.

146. van der Putte SCJ: The development of the lymphatic system in man, Adv Anat Embryol Cell Biol 51:3, 1975.

147. Vermesh M, Mayden KL, Confino E et al: Prenatal sonographic diagnosis of Hirschprung's disease, J Ultrasound Med 5:37, 1986.

148. Wapner R: Technical aspects of obtaining chorionic villi, Chorionic Villus Sampling Meeting, March 22-23, 1983, Chicago.

149. Wapner RJ, Jackson LG, and Davis GH: Chorionic villus sampling: first trimester cytogenetic and biochemical fetal diagnosis, Female Patient 10:95, 1985.

150. Ward RHT, Modell B, Petrou M et al: Method of sampling chorionic villi in first trimester of pregnancy under guidance of real-time ultrasound, Br Med J 286:1542, 1983.

151. Weiner S, Scharf JI, Bolognese RJ et al: Antenatal diagnosis and treatment of a fetal goiter, J Reprod med 24:39, 1980.

152. Williamson R, Eskdale T, Coleman DV et al: Direct gene analysis of chorionic villi: a possible technique for first trimester antenatal diagnosis of haemoglobinopathies, Lancet 2:1125, 1981.

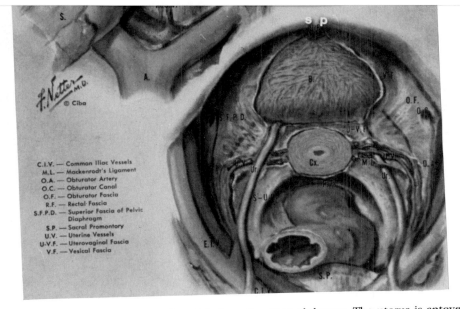

FIG. 24-1. The anatomy of the female pelvis from the open abdomen. The uterus is anteverted. *SP*, symphysis pubis. (Courtesy CIBA)

placing the real-time transducer just cephalad to the symphysis, either parallel or perpendicular to it, and focusing into the pelvis through the bladder (Fig. 24-2, *A*). The transducer is kept in firm skin contact in that location, and the deep pelvic structures are located by rocking the transducer handle around the fixed point of contact. The sonic beam is thus passed behind the symphysis, thereby avoiding its shadowing effect. Viewed from the abdomen, the pelvis is a bowl bounded on the sides by the iliac bones and acetabuli, in the deep posterior midline by the sacrum, and in the front by the pubic bones (Fig. 24-4, *A*

Soft tissue structures

The pelvic muscles. The rectus abdominus, iliopsoas, obturator internus, and piriformis comprise the four key paired muscles in a cross-section of the pelvis (Fig. 24-4). Both muscles of a pair are best seen with the broader view of a static scanner (Fig. 24-5). They can be mistaken for ovaries, fluid collections, or masses. Their symmetrical bilateral arrangement indicates that they are muscles. The rectus abdominis muscles insert on the pubic ramus and are paired parasagittal straps in the abdominal wall. The psoas muscles extend from paravertebral lumbar origins

24

Gynecologic Ultrasound

ANNA K. PARSONS AND JAMES C. RYVA

THE ROLE OF ULTRASOUND IN EVALUATION OF THE FEMALE PELVIS

The normal female pelvis contains the lower urinary tract (bladder and ureters), reproductive tract (vagina, cervix, uterus, fallopian tubes, and ovaries), and lower gastrointestinal tract (bowel and rectum) (Fig. 24-1). The bladder is anterior to the cervix and uterus, behind the symphysis pubis, and provides a useful sonic window through which the other structures can be viewed (Fig. 24-2). The vagina conveniently affords an even clearer

tion. It is used to follow follicle development and to harvest oocytes without surgery.[10,53,71,72] Other operative uses include culdocentesis or transvaginally directed needle aspiration and biopsy.[14,55] Transabdominal ultrasound can be used during difficult dilatation and curettage (D & C) to assure proper placement of the curet in the uterus. Response to treatment of children with precocious puberty has been assessed by ultrasonic observation of a decrease in uterine size as inappropriately elevated sex hormone levels decline.[62] Results of treatment of uterine my-

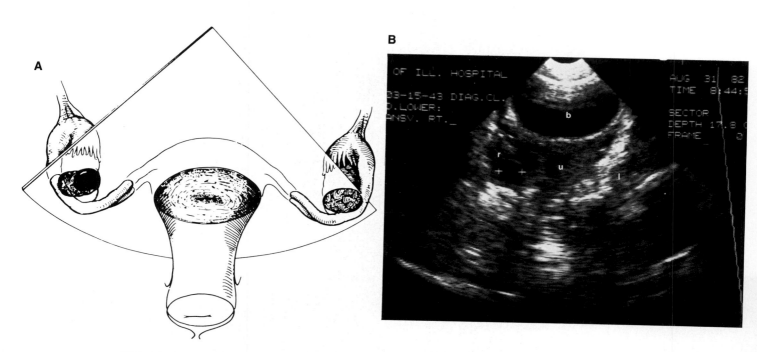

FIG. 24-2. **A,** Transabdominal (TA) transverse view (looking toward the patient's head) of the right ovary with a growing follicle, uterine fundus, and left ovary. The bladder is superior to the uterus and is not shown here. **B,** TA view of right ovary *r,* with a follicle (crosses), uterus *u,* and left ovary, *l,* comparable to **A.** The full bladder contains near-field artifacts. (**A** courtesy Linda Twomey).

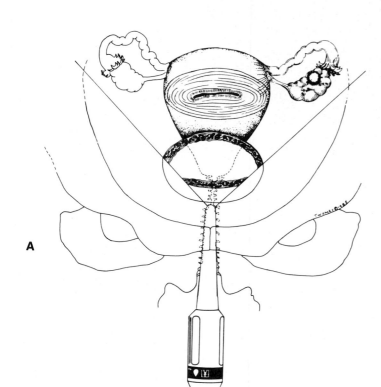

FIG. 24-3. **A,** Transvaginal (TV) view of uterus and left ovary. The transducer is in the vagina, under the symphysis pubis. The right ovary lies just below the scanning plane. The best resolution is obtained with the transducer 1 to 2 cm from the subject, which narrows the field of view.

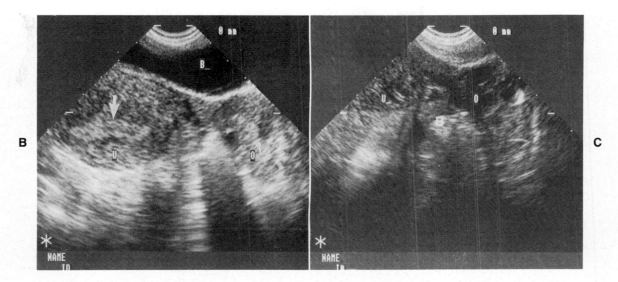

FIG. 24-3, cont'd.   B, A transverse view with the transducer placed closer, pressing on the bladder, *B.* Note the thick, bright, mid-luteal endometrium *(large arrow)* in the uterus, *U.* The left ovary, *O,* is at the tip of the *small arrow.* **C,** With the transducer moved in closer, the resolution improves further. Cornual vessels are seen in the uterus, *U.* The ovary, *O,* contains small (4 mm) cysts and is covered by bowel, *B.* (**A** Courtesy Linda Twomey.)

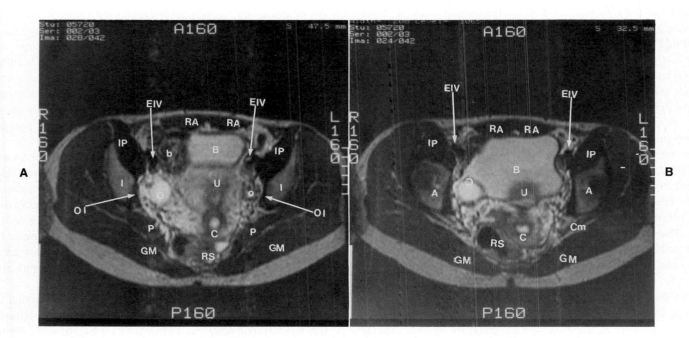

FIG. 24-4.   Magnetic resonance images of a female pelvis at the lower sacrum and coccyx, showing a uterus that is bulky, anteverted, and slightly left sided. Dotted lines in **C** denote the levels of **A** and **B,** respectively. **A,** Transverse image with a full bladder, *B,* through some of the uterine cavity, *U,* and cervix, *C.* The external iliac vessels, *EIV,* are medial to the iliopsoas, *IP.* The uterus and cervix are surrounded by a plexus of bright-appearing vessels from the internal iliac. *b,* bowel; *RA,* rectus and abdominal muscles; *I,* ilium; *P,* pyriformis muscle; *GM,* gluteus maximus; *O,* ovary (right one contains a 2.5 cm cyst); *RS,* rectosigmoid; *OI,* a thin strip of the obturator internus, which lines much of the pelvic sidewall. **B,** A transverse section somewhat lower than **A.** This level demonstrates the ribbon-like coccygeus muscle, *Cm,* on the left posterior sidewall. Compare with Fig. 24-5.   *Continued.*

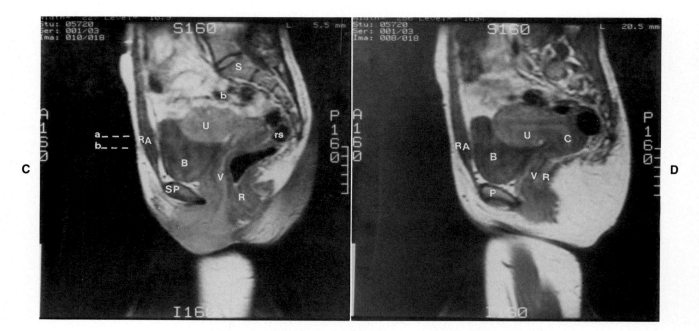

FIG. 24-4, cont'd.   C, Sagittal view of the midline, showing a lateral section of the right side of the uterus, with urine in the bladder appearing slightly darker. The vagina, *V,* is clearly seen next to rectum, *R.* Gas in the rectosigmoid, *rs* appears black here. It often obscures the sacrum, *S,* on ultrasound. *SP,* symphysis pubis; *b,* bowel; *RA,* rectus and abdominal muscles. **D,** The left-sided uterus, *U,* and cervix, *C,* are better demonstrated, with a clear endometrial cavity. The bladder is very full and pushes the uterine fundus cephalad.

abdominal ultrasound at the superior lateral bladder borders and may even bulge slightly into the bladder wall if well developed (Fig. 24-5, *C*). They are usually discrete because of their low-level homogeneous echoes, which should not be mistaken for cystic structures. The iliac vessels divide across the iliopsoas. The external iliac (femoral) vessels run along the medial border of the muscle. The internal iliac vessels diverge from them medially to run beneath the ovaries en route to the uterus.

The obturator internus muscles lie in the anterior lateral pelvis and can be seen along the lower lateral border of the bladder in transverse transabdominal views (Fig. 24-5, *D*). Farther posterior and medial in the pelvis, lateral and posterior to the uterus on a transverse transabdominal view, the wedge-shaped piriformis muscles are visible if there is not excessive bowel gas (Fig. 24-5, *D*).

The bladder and ureters. The cystic, highly sonolucent bladder is the sonographer's signpost and transabdominal pathway to the pelvis. It displaces bowel and freely transmits sound waves to the underlying tissues. The bladder is a thin-walled regular structure that is oblong in the axial plane when well filled. It is a round-edged triangle in the longitudinal view. Its inferior cephalic border outlines the anteverted uterine corpus and fundus. The bladder will define the fundus of a retroverted or very anteverted uterus when slightly overfilled, using the transabdominal approach (Fig. 24-6, *A* and *B*). However, if the uterus is displaced by a huge bladder, normal relationships may be distorted (Fig. 24-6, *C*).

Urine in the bladder can be used as a standard of clear fluid by comparing it with other cystic structures at various gain settings. When overfilled, the bladder may com-

press the uterus and adnexa into sonographic oblivion, while when underfilled, it loses transmittance. The benefits of using only a minimally distended bladder, the vaginal wall, or both as the sonic windows to structures that are within 1 to 5 cm from a vaginal transducer are obvious to any woman who has had to adjust her bladder volume during a lengthy transabdominal exam. A few drops of urine in the bladder are useful but not necessary as a landmark for transvaginal scanning. A slightly more distended bladder will allow a better image of a sharply anteverted uterus with transvaginal technique.

When seen transabdominally, a normal uterus or an unusually distended rectum may indent the posterior bladder wall gently. Any real distortion of the normal profile is due to a mass (Fig. 24-7, *A*). Occasionally it is necessary to empty the bladder. This will allow a distinction to be made between it and a large cystic mass that cannot be entirely imaged by the sector scanner. A long linear array transducer or a static scanner will also demonstrate the relationship (Fig. 24-7, *B*).

The ureters are found posterior and slightly medial to the ovary, coursing to the bladder. In a transverse oblique transabdominal scan each appears as a bright-walled anechoic-centered tube between the ovary and internal iliac vessels (Fig. 24-8, *A*). They enter the bladder lateral and anterior to the cervix on each side of the urethra. The turbulence of the urine created at their orifices is visible in the bladder (Fig. 24-8, *B* and *C*). Ureteral peristalsis has been described as "intermittent sparkling" in the tubular structure.[51] Ureteral dilation resulting from compression by pelvic masses is identified by following the sausage-like structure to the kidney.   *Text continued on p. 531.*

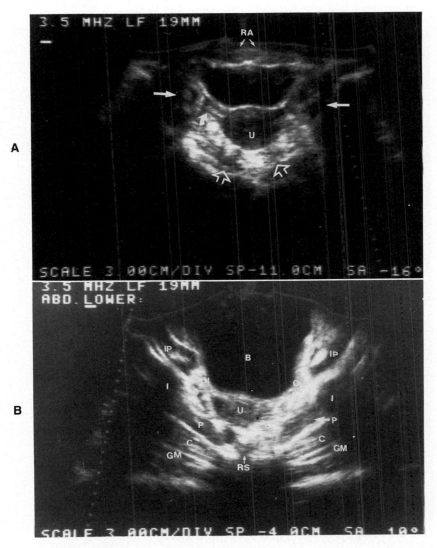

FIG. 24-5. **A,** Transverse static scan of the pelvis with a partially full bladder at the level of S5, showing anterior rectus abdominis muscles, *RA,* and lateral iliopsoas muscles *(long arrows),* which could be mistaken for ovaries. The piriformis muscles *(open arrows)* are deep to the uterus, *U,* and part of the broad ligaments are visible at each side of the uterus, which looks normal. **B,** Static transverse view of the deep pelvic muscles, obtained by angling the transducer at the symphysis cephalad toward the sacral hollow. The iliopsoas muscles, *IP,* form the anterolateral "brim" of the pelvic bowel and contain the external iliac vessels and femoral nerve sheath along their medial surfaces. The obturator internus, *OI,* muscles sheath the iliac bones, *I,* forming a bright reflective interface at the bony surface along the lateral wall of the bladder. Thin sections of piriformis muscles, *P,* are seen superior to the ribbon-like coccygeus muscles, *C,* which attach to the coccyx. The contents of the rectosigmoid, *RS,* produce a midline shadow beneath it. *B,* bladder; *U,* uterus; *O,* right ovary; *GM,* gluteus maximus.   *Continued.*

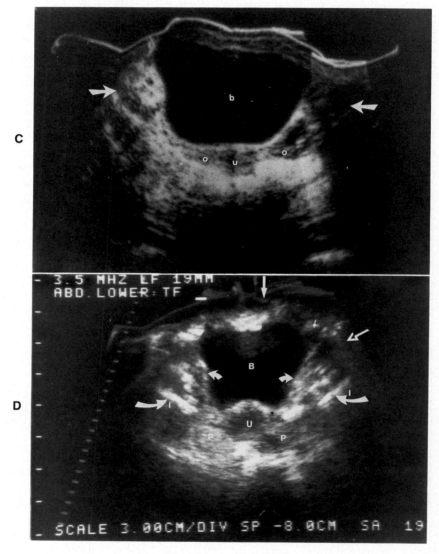

FIG. 24-5, cont'd.   C, Well-developed iliopsoas muscles *(arrows)* of varying consistency due to the aim of the transducer: when aimed through the bladder, *b,* the tissue is enhanced and looks like a solid mass, as on the left. The right iliopsoas appears cystic due to the almost perpendicular angle of the sound waves and their attenuation in soft tissue. The right ovary, *o,* contains a cyst. **D,** Well-developed obturator internus muscles *(short curved arrows)* near the lower uterus, *U,* with the transverse scanning plane angled cephalad from above the symphysis. The iliopsoas on the right *(open arrow)* demonstrates external iliac vessels *(tiny arrow).* The arrow indicates the right rectus muscle. The bright reflection of the obturator fascia *(large curved arrows)* is seen over the iliac bones, *I. P,* piriformis internus muscles.

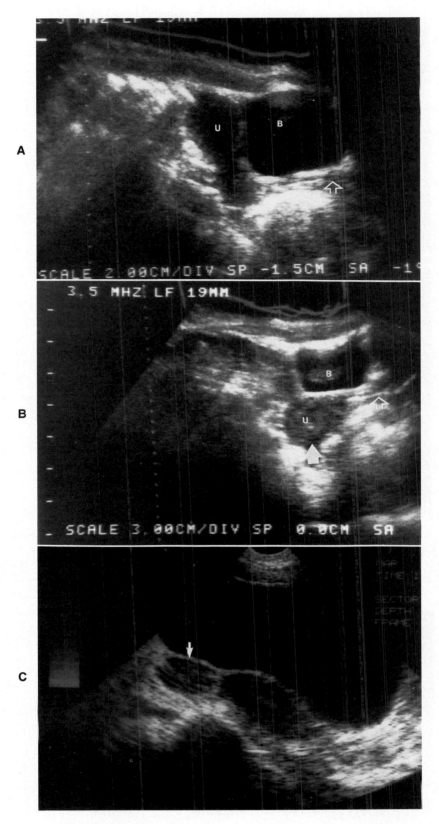

FIG. 24-6.   A, Static sagittal scan with very anteverted uterus, *U,* outlining the vaginal canal *(open arrow).* Objects below the bladder are brighter due to high transmittance of sound waves. The angle of the uterus is improved by the overfilled bladder, *B.* **B,** This retroverted uterus has also been reoriented by a full bladder, which elevated the fundus *(arrow). Open arrow* indicates vagina. **C,** Sagittal TA scan of a normal left ovary *(arrow)* above a midline uterine fundus, with an overfilled bladder. Viewed sagittally, the bladder should not extend much above the fundus.

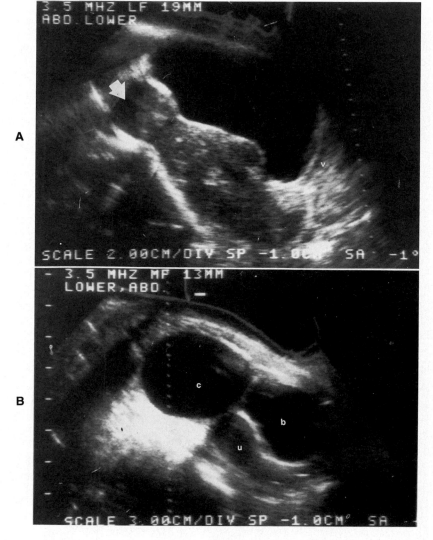

FIG. 24-7. **A,** Sagittal static view of a uterus with an 8 cm myoma in the fundus *(arrow)* and another smaller anterior myoma bulging into the bladder. *v,* Vaginal canal. **B,** An 8 × 11 cm ovarian cyst, *c,* is seen above the uterus, *u,* on a sagittal static scan. This would be easier to see with the bladder, *b,* empty using a TV or TA sector scanner.

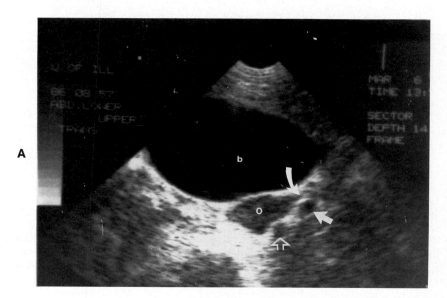

FIG. 24-8. **A,** Transverse TA view of a left ovary, *O,* with ovarian vessels (infundibulopelvic ligament) at its lateral edge *(curved arrow)*, crossing an internal iliac vessel *(solid arrow)* and the ureter *(open arrow)*. The sector transducer is in the midline and aimed at the pelvic sidewall. The ureter has a thicker wall than do blood vessels.

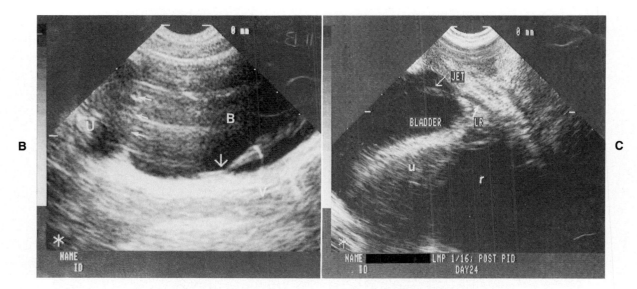

FIG. 24-8, cont'd.   B, TA view of a bladder, *B,* filled with artefact and the left ureteral orifice with a jet of urine streaming from it *(arrow).* The very anteverted left-sided uterine fundus, *U,* is outlined by the tiny arrows, and the lateral vagina, *V,* lies below the bladder. The transducer is 4 cm medial and parallel to the inguinal ligament. **C,** Sagittal oblique TV view of lateral edge of bladder, showing urine jet emanating from ureter, *UR,* lateral to uterus, *u.* The transducer is parallel to and beneath the inguinal ligament. The rectosigmoid, *r,* is lost in a shadow.

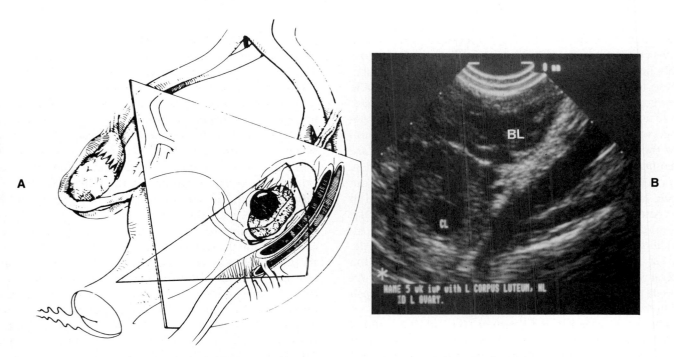

FIG. 24-9.   A, Line drawing of the orientation of TA view of the external iliac vessels (large sector) and that required for a transvaginal view (small sector). **B,** TV view of external iliac vein and branch near an ovary with a typical corpus luteum of pregnancy, *CL.* This patient is 5 weeks pregnant, and the transducer is probing a dilated broad ligament plexus of vessels, *BL.* (**A** courtesy Linda Twomey.)

The pelvic vessels. Blood vessels are thin-walled sonolucent pulsatile sinuous structures that range from 1 mm to over 1 cm in diameter. The abdominal aorta and inferior vena cava (IVC) to its right are easily identified in the midline sagittal transabdominal view. Turning the transabdominal transducer in a midline-to-hip oblique angle will help to find the external iliacs (Fig. 24-9). The internal iliacs appear posterior to the ovaries and become

the uterine arteries, which approach the lateral cervix at right angles (Fig. 24-10). They are useful landmarks by which to identify the ovary. These large vessels are frequently near at hand during transvaginal ovarian follicle aspirations, but are so visible that they are easily avoided.

Parametrial and cevical branches of the uterine arteries run north and south, respectively, along the lateral uterus and cervix. They are often well seen in transabdominal

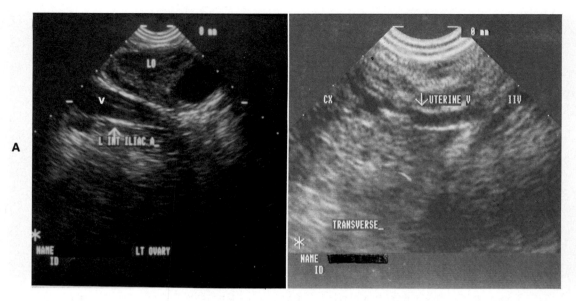

Fig. 24-10. **A,** sagittal TV of the left ovary, *LO,* with a preovulatory follicle, the internal iliac artery, and its vein, *V,* above it. **B,** The uterine vein enroute to the uterocervical isthmus, *CX,* as it branches from the internal iliac or hypogastric vein, *IIV.* This is a TV transverse view from a lateral vaginal fornix.

transverse as well as transvaginal coronal and sagittal views (Fig. 24-11, *A* and *B*). Branches of these vessels join with branches of the ovarian arteries around the tube. These form a network of broad ligament vessels visible between ovary and fundus. They are most obvious at midcycle and in pregnancy. These vessels should not be confused with the ovary (Fig. 24-11, *C*). The tubal vessels follow the inferior (mesenteric) surface of the tube and are seen near the uterus in transverse transvaginal views (Fig. 24-11, *D*). The ovarian arteries arise from the aorta and circle laterally and down the posterior abdominal wall in the retroperitoneal space. The ovarian vessels leave the sidewall in a cable, termed the ovarian suspensory or infundibulopelvic ligament, which leads to the ovary (Fig. 24-12). They can be seen as pulsatile small vessels on the lateral superior surfaces of the ovaries (Fig. 24-12). All vessels should be demonstrated lengthwise to distinguish them from small cysts.

The rectosigmoid and bowel. Gas- and fluid-filled bowel loops are poorly defined, echo-free mobile structures, that usually demonstrate peristalsis under observation. Solid material in the bowel is hyperechoic and may produce shadowing, as does gas (Fig. 24-13, *A*). Empty bowel can look like an irregular bull's eye with a thin, sharp, hypoechoic outline on cross section. When rectal gas obscures the cul-de-sac, a saline or water enema can clearly delineate rectosigmoid, posterior uterus, and cul-de-sac in a transabdominal view (Fig. 24-13, *B*). Fluid-filled small bowel loops can appear cystic but are easily identified by their swirling activity. Fluid may accumulate in the small bowel as well as in the cul-de-sac with rapid oral hydration. A transvaginal search for ovaries is aided by the fact that the movements of bowel can outline the relatively immobile ovaries even if their sonic consistency

is similar to that of intestine (Fig. 24-13, *C*). Immobile, dilated, or distorted bowel should be investigated (Fig. 24-13, *D*). Bowel should move freely and collapse when probed with the transvaginal transducer.

The uterus and tubes. The uterus is a very mobile, inverted, pear-shaped structure more or less in the midline. It is fixed in the vagina at the cardinal ligament and suspended in the pelvis by its peritoneal attachments. The domelike top of the uterus is the fundus, and on its superior lateral horns, or cornua, are the tubes (Fig. 24-1). Anterior to them, the round ligaments traverse the anterior cul-de-sac to enter the internal inguinal ring lateral to the symphysis pubis. Inferior to the tubes and posterior to the round ligament are the uteroovarian ligaments, attaching the medial pole of the ovary to the uterus. These can often be identified in the transverse or coronal planes as 1 to 3 cm long sonodense connections between uterus and ovary (Fig. 24-3, *B* and *C*). The muscular, hollow uterus consists of the globular fundus, which tapers slightly at the corpus, then narrows at the isthmus into the cylindrical, densely fibrous cervix (Figs. 24-14 and 24-15). This opens into the vagina at the external cervical os. The part of the cervix protruding into the vagina is the portio vaginalis (Fig. 24-16). A cycling woman's uterus measures roughly 8 cm in length from external cervical os to the fundus, 3 to 4 cm in width, and 3 to 4 cm in the anteroposterior dimension. These dimensions vary widely, being slightly larger after pregnancy. The prepubertal uterus, which has not been exposed to estrogen, lacks fundal enlargement. In a sagittal view an infantile uterus looks like a tiny banana and is mostly cervix (Fig. 24-17, *A*). In a female under age 7, the anteroposterior diameter of the cervix sometimes appears thicker than that of the fundus.[22,41] The uterine dimensions are about 2.5 × 1.5 × 1.0 cm be-

Text continued on p. 537.

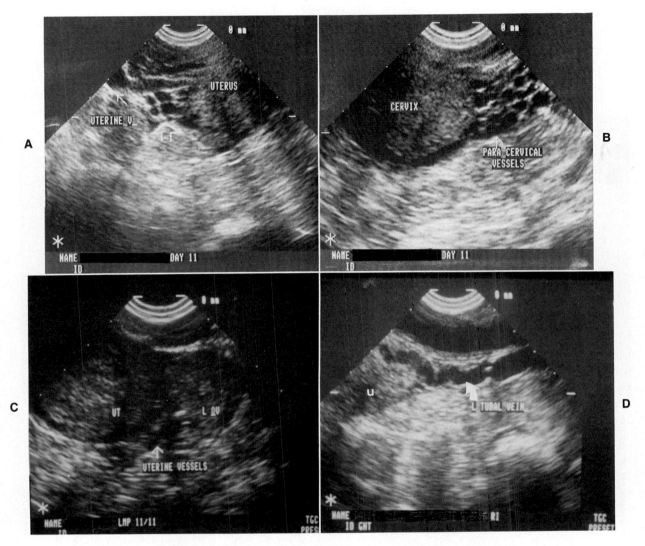

Fig. 24-11. **A,** The uterine vein at the uterocervical isthmus and parametrial branches in cross-section *(open arrow)* as they run north along the uterus, a transverse TV view, at midcycle. **B,** The paracervical plexus of vessels, a cross-section (transverse) TV view in the same patient, mid-cycle. **C,** The broad ligament uterine-ovarian anastomoses (uterine vessels) between the uterus and ovary, *LOV,* in a 9-week pregnancy, a transverse TV view. Verification of vessels seen in cross-section is made by turning the transducer until the length of the vessel is observed. **D,** The tubal vessels run parallel to the tube in the mesosalpinx. This transverse TV view was taken following a hysterosalpingogram with lymphatic uptake of high osmolar contrast medium, producing venous congestion. The tube itself is in a slightly superior plane and not imaged. The bladder is seen above the vessel. *U,* uterine cornu.

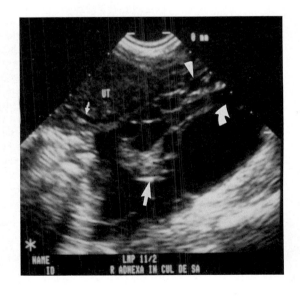

Fig. 24-12. View of a left ovary *(arrow)* in a fluid-filled cul-de-sac, the transducer aiming toward the lower sacrum through the cornu of a retroverted uterus, *UT.* The ovarian vessels leave the hilum at the *curved arrow.* The utero-ovarian ligament is not seen. The uterine vein *(tiny arrow)* can be followed off the cornua into the tubal branch *(arrowhead).* There are four small follicles (5 mm size) and an irregular cyst in the ovary (day 4 of the cycle). The hyperechoic bowel is below the uterus, and the pelvic sidewall is to the right of the ovary.

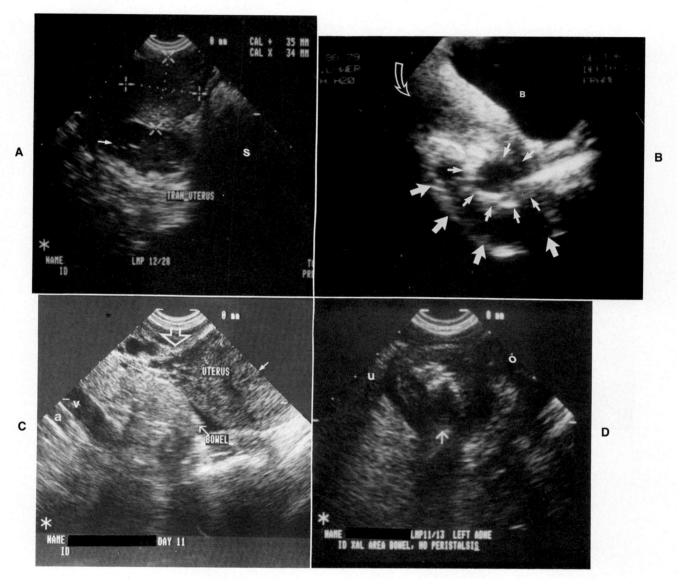

Fig. 24-13. **A,** Posterior TV transverse view through a uterus into the cul-de-sac in a case of severe pelvic inflammatory disease. The uterus is outlined by calipers. There is a mild ileus and fluid-filled bowel *(arrow)* behind the uterus. Gas- and solid-filled bowel cast a shadow, *S,* on the right side of the image. **B,** TA view of a cystic mass *(small arrows)* behind a sagittal uterus *(curved arrow),* outlined by saline in the rectosigmoid *(large arrows).* Bladder, *B,* outlines the anteverted uterus. **C,** Transverse TV view of the fundus, showing the broad ligament and its vessels at one cornu *(open arrow)* anterior to homogeneous-looking sonodense bowel, which could be seen moving freely. The internal iliac artery, *a,* and vein, *v,* are seen along the pelvic sidewall. Endometrium *(small arrow)* is visible in the uterus. **D,** An immobile, tender, uncompressible section of sigmoid *(arrow)* positioned between a normal ovary, *o,* and uterus, *u,* in a 24-year-old woman with an adnexal mass. The thickened, edematous bowel wall appears dark, and there is a solid echogenic 1.5 cm mass in the lumen, which did not demonstrate peristalsis under observation. Barium enema and transrectal biopsy revealed an advanced colonic cancer.

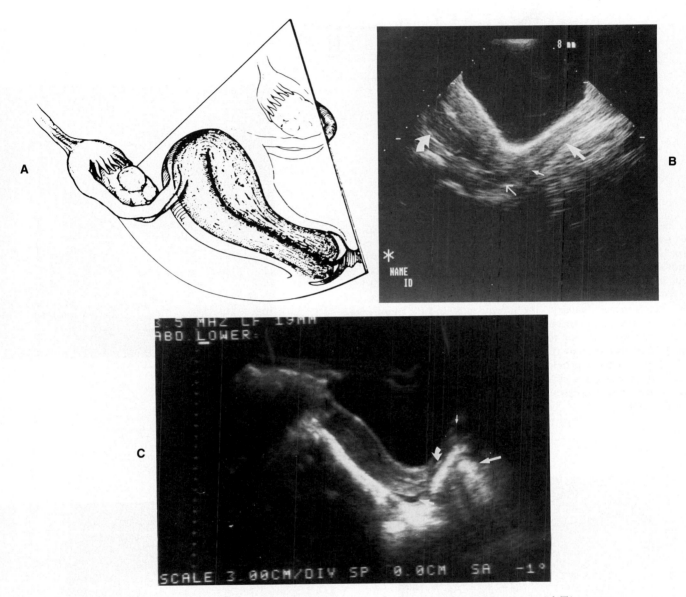

FIG. 24-14. Sagittal views of the uterus using different techniques. **A,** Conventional TA sector scanning from just above the symphysis through the bladder (not shown). The uterus is slightly anteflexed. The ovaries, which are normally below and behind the tubes, are not in the ultrasonic field of view. **B,** Ultrasound view of **A** of a midluteal sagittal uterus, with anteverted fundus *(curved arrow),* with rectosigmoid behind it *(arrow),* cervix at the *tiny arrow,* and vagina at *bold arrow.* Note the dense endometrium. **C,** The most comprehensive view is obtained with a static scanner, despite its cumbersome technique and fixed image. This is a post-menstrual uterus with a small amount of fluid in the posterior cul-de-sac *(short arrow)* and a thin, sharp endometrium. The *curved arrow* points to the vagina, and the *long arrow* indicates rectosigmoid and contents. The urethra is seen at the *tiny arrow.* (**A** courtesy Linda Twomey.)

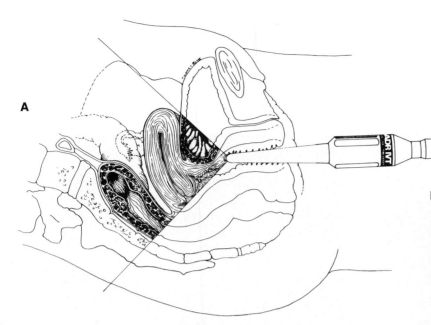

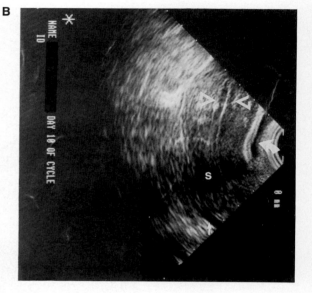

FIG. 24-15. A, Line drawing of the following sagittal vaginal view, except that the transducer is not in close contact with the uterus. Moving it closer narrows the field of view but allows beautiful resolution of texture. **B,** TV view of the anteverted uterus just before ovulation. The endometrium is thick and lucent with a sharp, bright, central mucus line *(arrowheads).* The transducer is perpendicular to the uterine axis, and the picture is turned to match the orientation of the other studies. A thin rim of bladder is anterior to the fundus *(curved arrow),* and scant fluid is also seen in the posterior cul-de-sac, behind the cervix. The transducer is held firmly against the anterior vaginal wall, and the uterovesicle reflection plus the vaginal mucosa create a shadow, *S,* across the uterocervical isthmus. (**A** courtesy Linda Twomey.)

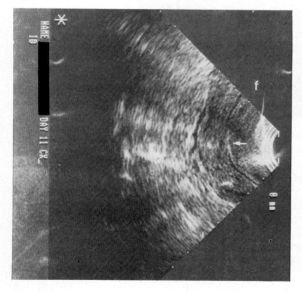

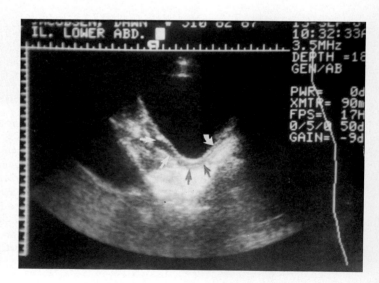

FIG. 24-16. TV view of the cervix, with an arrow at the internal os, and the uterine fundus at *f.* There is a very thin lucent rim of fluid behind the isthmus in the posterior cul-de-sac. The photo is turned to match orientation in Figs. 24-14 and 24-15.

FIG. 24-17. Sagittal TA view of a prepubertal uterus with a typically thin fundus *(white arrows)* and comparable cervix *(gray arrows),* ending in a vaginal stripe *(curved arrow).* The sigmoid contains fluid, and the bladder is full. This is the infantile uterus of a patient with Turner's syndrome, who has never been exposed to estradiol.

tween the ages of 1 and 7 years. Menopausal uteri are miniature versions of cycling organs (roughly 4 × 3 × 2 cm) (Fig. 24-17, *B* and *C*).

The bladder is attached to the lower anterior uterus and cervix. Peritoneal attachments of the uterus drape fore and aft to the pelvic floor in two sheets, lining the anterior and posterior cul-de-sacs. The posterior cul-de-sac or pouch of Douglas is in the hollow of the sacrum (Figs. 24-1; 24-15, *B*; 24-16). This drape of peritoneum extends laterally off the tubes or salpinges and runs to the pelvic sidewall. In the bases of these two sheets of peritoneum run the uterine arteries and veins, which cross the ureter 2 cm lateral to the cervix (Fig. 24-10, *B*). These peritoneal wings on either side of the uterus, and their vascular contents, are the broad ligaments. They occasionally contain cysts, which may be remnants of the embryonic wolffian ducts (vestigial male structures), of the paramesonephric ducts (remnant female structures), or which are simple peritoneal cysts. These distinctions are made with a microscope. Transvaginal ultrasound may enable broad ligament cysts to be diagnosed by clearly separating them from ovarian tissue. Absolute identification may be difficult, and surgery may be required for diagnosis and removal. These cysts can also continue down into the lateral walls of the vagina. In this case they are called Gartner's duct cysts and are palpable and visible on vaginal inspection.

At the pelvic sidewall the broad ligaments narrow to surround the ovarian arteries and veins as they turn cephalad. These peritoneum-covered cables of vessels are the infundibulopelvic ligaments or suspensory ligaments of the ovary (see Fig. 24-1).

The uterine axis varies widely—from anteverted and perpendicular to the abdominal wall to sharply retroverted, with varying degrees of flexion of the fundus from the cervical axis. A retroverted, retroflexed uterus will attenuate the sound waves reaching the fundus, making it appear cystic in a transabdominal scan. Overdistension of the bladder solves the problem by elevating the fundus (Fig. 24-6, *B*). A transvaginal approach is preferred. Most uteri are perpendicular to the vaginal axis when the bladder is empty.

The central canal of the uterus and cervix are continuous with the vagina. The endometrium is slightly less echogenic than the myometrium in the first half of the cycle. It is more echogenic in the second half. The endometrium and a bright central line of mucus produce the uterine stripe, which is an essential landmark. This is best seen and measured in the longitudinal plane (Fig. 24-18). It is surrounded by a hypoechoic "halo," which has been identified as a vascular compact layer or junctional zone of myometrium bordering the endometrium. The echogenicity and thickness of the endometrium change with the hormonal effects of the menstrual cycle.[16,17] In the estrogen-dominant proliferative phase it is more sonolucent than myometrium and sharply defined by a bright central mucus layer. As estrogen levels rise approaching ovulation, the sharp mucus line thickens and the endometrium grows from 2 to around 5 mm. In the progesterone-dominant secretory phase the endometrial echo is more sonodense than myometrium and 5 to 10 mm thick. Less central mucus is seen in the fundus, and more in the cervix. The so-called ring sign just after ovulation describes a thick, fuzzy endometrium surrounding a lucent center.[18] This fills into a uniform density as the secretory phase progresses (Fig. 24-18, *C*).

Liquid blood appears hypoechoic in either the uterus or the vagina, while clots and tissue can produce a bright complex echo (Fig. 24-18, *A*). During menstruation the sonolucent cavity may be irregular, and often at least the proximal portions of the fallopian tubes are seen to contain menstrual fluid (Fig. 24-15, *A* and 24-19, *A*).

The endometrium is measured from the central canal to the border between the bright endometrial line and the more lucent junctional zone. If there is no fluid or mucus in the cavity, the entire bright endometrial line can be measured and this number can be halved to determine each wall's thickness.

Postmenopausal endometrium usually forms a very thin bright line surrounded by a prominent junctional zone or anechoic halo. The endometrium is usually less than 3 mm thick. A thickness greater than this may be due to endometrial hyperplasia, cancer, or polyps. The uteri of women who are receiving estrogen replacement appear premenopausal, with endometrial thickness of up to 5 mm (Fig. 24-19, *B* and *C*).

It has often been stated that an ultrasonically visible tube is an abnormal tube. This is no longer always the case with the high-resolution vaginal probes available. It is not unusual to visualize part of the tubal lumen during menses when it is filled with endometrium and blood (Fig. 24-19). Tubal secretions also make the proximal tube prominent at midcycle (see Fig. 24-60).

Timor-Tritsch and Rottem were the first to publish beautiful studies of the salpinx using a high-frequency (6.5 MHz) transvaginal probe. They demonstrate that the fimbriae may be visible against fluid in the cul-de-sac (see Fig. 24-55).[64-66] The tubes lie above the uteroovarian ligaments, the round ligaments, and the tuboovarian vessels. They must be distinguished from all three (see Fig. 24-56).

The ovaries. The ovaries are ovoid organs approximately 2 × 2 × 3 cm in the premenopausal cycling woman and may contain follicles or small cysts of various sizes until after menopause (Fig. 24-20). The volume of the ovary can be calculated using a rough formula for a prolate ellipsoid: $0.5 \times D_1 \times D_2 \times D_3$ where D is the longest diameter in three different planes. Human eggs or oocytes are contained in tiny follicles.[18,25] In a natural cycle, one clear cystic follicle will enlarge to a diameter of 2 to 3 cm and release its mature egg or ovum during ovulation (Fig. 24-20). The cumulus oophorus surrounding the egg itself may be visible just before ovulation (Fig. 24-21, *A*). Either transvaginal or transabdominal ultrasound is particularly accurate for follicular measurement.[25,56,74] After ovulation the remaining estrogen- and progesterone-producing cells in the follicle (the theca and granulosa cells) continue to function as a gland. This is called the

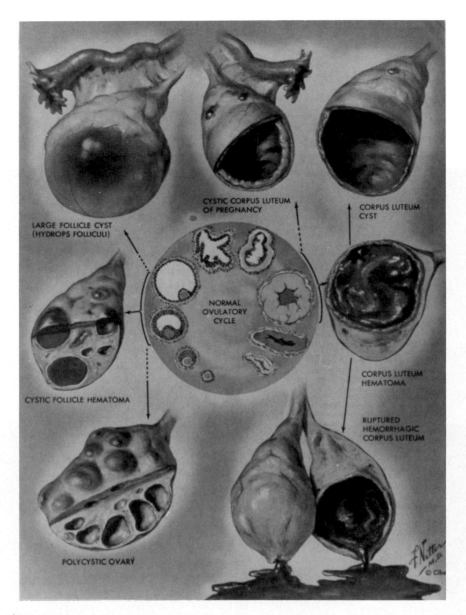

FIG. 24-20. Aberrant results (periphery) of normal ovarian function (center). (Courtesy CIBA)

corpus luteum. Disruption of the follicle and a dramatic increase of the fluid in the cul-de-sac is highly suggestive of ovulation (Fig. 24-21, *B*).

In our experience, ovulation in spontaneous cycles alternates equally from side to side. Werlin et al.[70] found it to be preferentially on one side 75% of the time in both induced and spontaneous cycles in women with various causes of infertility. The untreated, nondominant (nonovulating) ovary may have tiny follicles, but almost never contains another mature or large follicle (Fig. 24-22).

The postovulatory follicle, or corpus hemorrhagicum, may appear to be cystic with low-level internal echoes. They may also appear to be cystic and irregular, bright and irregular, or may disappear (Fig. 24-21).[18] The mature corpus luteum is best seen around 7 days after ovula-

tion as an irregular, dense-walled, webbed lucency measuring from 0.5 to (rarely) 10 cm (Fig. 24-23). The center contains a blood clot. It is usually cystic if a pregnancy ensues and generally regresses by the third trimester (Fig. 24-24).

Postmenopausal ovaries are small and dense (Fig. 24-25). They are, therefore, difficult to image in some women. Mean volumes of 4.33 cm³ ± 1.91 down to 2.5 cm³ have been considered normal.[6,19] Normal postmenopausal ovaries should be of similar size with relatively regular texture on both sides. A size limit for normal ovaries in menopausal and postmenopausal women has not yet been established. It is reasonable to assume that ovarian size will progressively decrease until well after menopause is complete.[2,48]

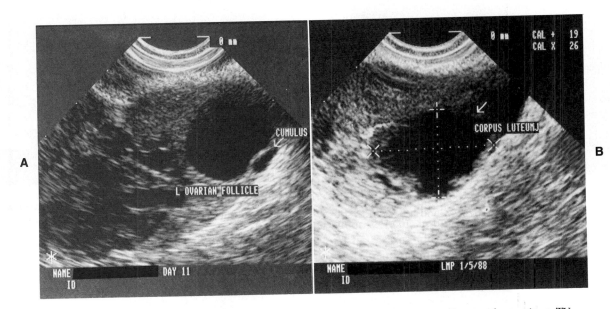

FIG. 24-21. A, Dark, preovulatory, fluid-filled follicle containing a cumulus oophorus in a TV closeup. **B,** The same follicle, 2 days later after ovulation. The wall is irregular, but the contents remain clear in this case.

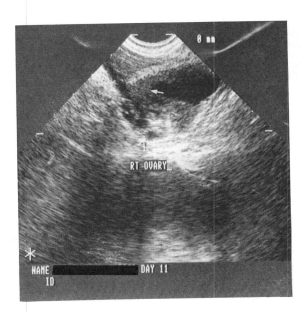

FIG. 24-22. The nondominant ovary, scanned at the same time as Fig. 24-21, *A,* above. Note the preovulatory, fluid-filled cul-de-sac and the utero-ovarian ligament *(tiny arrow),* as well as the tiny follicles in the ovary.

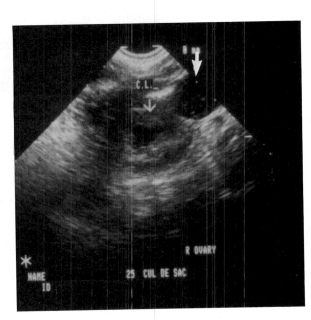

FIG. 24-23. A mature corpus luteum on day 25 *(small arrow).* Note the thick wall and central fluid-filled cyst. There is a small, blood-filled endometrioma in this ovary as well *(large arrow).*

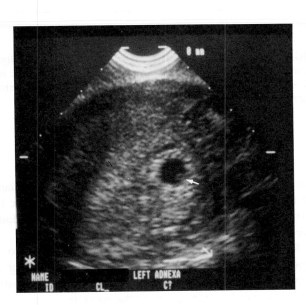

FIG. 24-37. TV transverse view of a 5½-week gestation with a faint yolk sac *(arrow).*

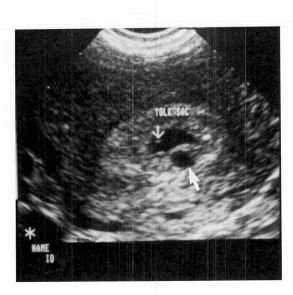

FIG. 24-38. TV transverse view of a 6-week gestation. The yolk sac is barely visible in this picture. The small amniotic cavity is starting to form *(arrow)* under the fetus.

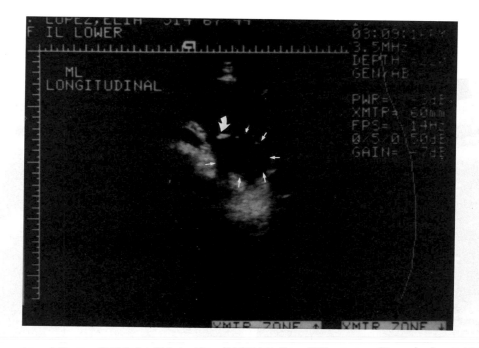

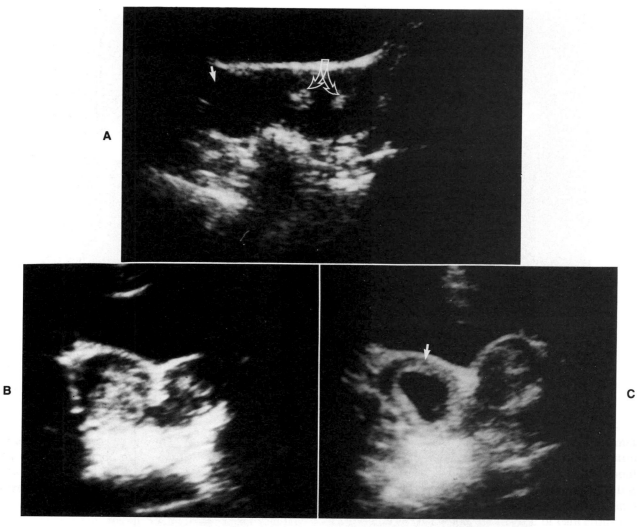

FIG. 24-51.   **A,** TA transverse view of a septate uterus, which has a normal external shape, with a heart-shaped cavity. The smooth external contour and two uterine stripes *(open arrows)* are demonstrated in cross-section. The lucent left ovary *(arrow)* is on the right side of the photo. **B,** TA transverse scan of a uterus didelphys, with two completely separate horns. **C,** TA transverse view of a similar uterus, except that one horn contains a gestational sac *(arrow).*

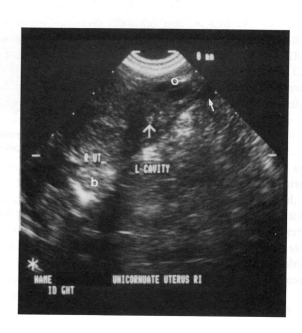

FIG. 24-52.   TV transverse view of a rudimentary, *L,* uterine horn with a tiny cavity *(arrow)* connecting to a tube *(tiny arrow).* Part of an ovary is seen with small follicles, *O.* The well-developed side of the uterus is marked *R UT* along its border. *b,* bowel.

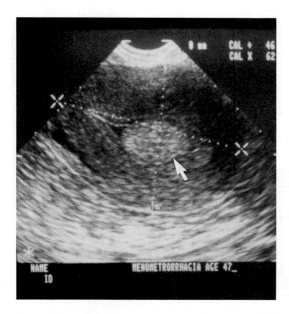

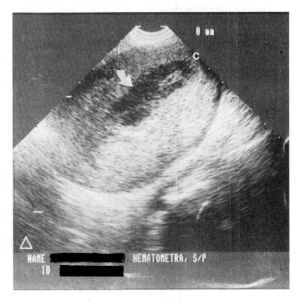

FIG. 24-53. TV sagittal view of an oval endometrial polyp *(arrow)* in the midst of secretory endometrium.

FIG. 24-54. Endometrial cancer in an 11.5 cm long uterus, a sagittal TV view not including the cervix (at area *c*), showing a dilated fluid- and tissue-filled cavity *(curved arrow)* but fairly regular myometrium in which there was less than 30% invasion.

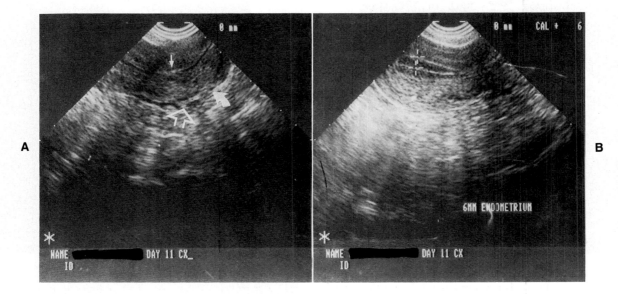

FIG. 24-55. **A,** TV sagittal view of a normal, nulliparous, midcycle cervix with a prominent endo-cervical canal and internal os *(arrow)*. The vaginal mucosa *(curved arrow)* and peritoneum *(open arrow)* divide the scant fluid in the posterior fornix from that in the posterior cul-de-sac. **B,** Same uterine fundus shows the internal os again, and the natural configuration of the midcycle (late pro-liferative) endometrium, marked with calipers at the thickest point.

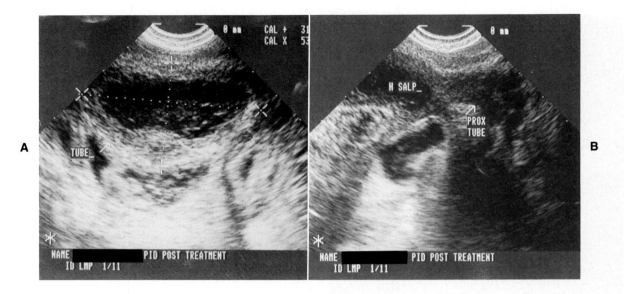

FIG. 24-66. **A,** Longitudinal section of a widely dilated, pus-filled tube (outlined by calipers) after 7 days of IV antibiotics. Echogenic pus is still inside, the walls are thick and appear nodular. The patient was clinically improved. **B,** Proximal portion of the same tube. Note where the tube widens into a sactosalpinx. The structures below the tube are loops of bowel.

clarified, as are early (4.5 weeks) intrauterine gestational sacs (Fig. 24-67). This enables early identification of ectopic pregnancies and prevention of tubal rupture with more selective use of surgery. The "discriminatory zone" of β-HCG for the transvaginal probe is about 1000 mIU/ml (2nd IS) compared with 6500 mIU/ml (IRP) originally described for transabdominal ultrasound. At that level, an identifiable gestational sac or chorionic cavity is always seen in a normal intrauterine pregnancy. If the uterine cavity appears empty with a thick endometrial stripe, a pregnancy must be sought in the tubes or elsewhere (Fig. 24-68).

To reiterate, very early pregnancy is best diagnosed with transvaginal ultrasound. There are virtually no technical limitations imposed by patient size or uterine retroversion. The scanner should always be alert for free fluid in the abdomen or the adnexal mass of an ectopic pregnancy. If the uninvolved tube is full of blood, it can be difficult to distinguish which tube carries the conceptus (Fig. 24-69).

It is important to examine the ovaries carefully, since a ruptured, bleeding corpus luteum can produce symptoms similar to a ruptured ectopic pregnancy. Frequently, women with normal early intrauterine pregnancies have unilateral discomfort from a normal cystic corpus luteum (see Fig. 24-24). The rare occurrence of simultaneous intrauterine and ectopic pregnancy has been reported to be increasing. This tends to happen more often in patients who are undergoing infertility treatments.[60]

A gestational sac and heart beat are only occasionally seen within the tube (Fig. 24-70). The criteria for ectopic pregnancy include: (1) absence of an intrauterine sac with a serum β-HCG of more than 1500 mIU/ml (IRP) or 1000 mIU/ml (2nd IS) and (2) an adnexal mass and free fluid in the abdomen.

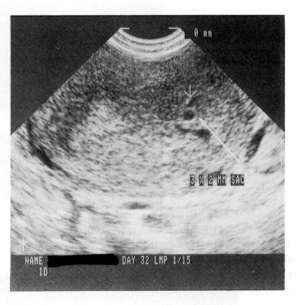

FIG. 24-67. TV view of a 4-week, 4-day pregnancy *(arrow)* after administration of clomiphene citrate. The 6 mm chorionic sac is clearly defined, and there is a thick decidual reaction. The lacunar spaces *(small arrow)* evident in the decidua are often apparent at this stage. The β-HCG was already 1800.

THE OVARIES

A woman with 40 years of fertility will ovulate nearly 400 times, and some 250,000 follicles will be stimulated to varying degrees during this time. It is not surprising that such a dynamic organ can form over 100 different types of benign or malignant tumors. Transvaginal ultrasound has evolved into the most effective means of ovarian imaging. Transvaginal scanning complements and extends the bimanual pelvic examination when it is hampered by the patient's obesity, difficult anatomy, pain, or fear.[65]

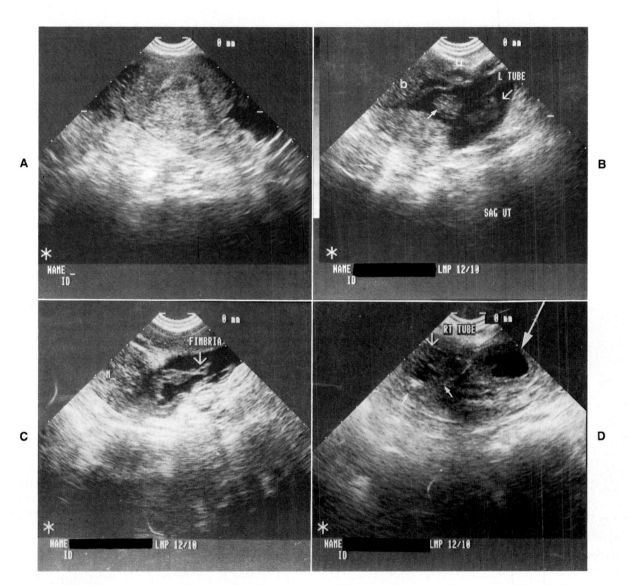

FIG. 24-68. **A,** Anatomy of a midtubal pregnancy: a TV transverse view of a uterus with a thick decidual reaction but no central lucency, at 6 weeks gestation. **B,** View into the left cul-de-sac in which a normal left tube is floating, ending in feathery fimbriae *(small arrow). u,* uterus; *b,* bowel. **C,** The midtubal 35 mm ectopic mass, *M,* seen in sagittal section with the normal-looking distal tube emanating from it. **D,** A 35 mm mass in the proximal right tube (outlined by *arrows*) next to an irregular 1.5 × 2 cm cystic corpus luteum *(long arrow).*

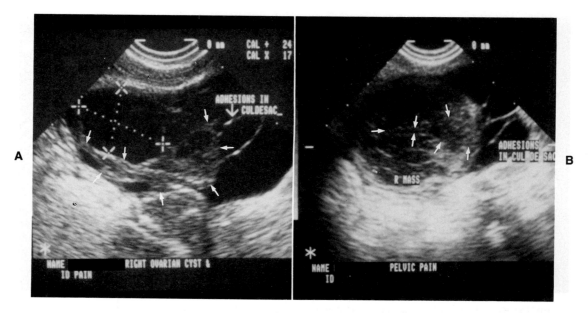

FIG. 24-72.   A, TV view of cul-de-sac showing a left ovary left in place after hysterectomy in a young woman with an apparently preovulatory follicle outlined in calipers. Filmy adhesions are easily seen in the fluid-filled cul-de-sac. The patient was started on contraceptives to suppress further follicle formation because of her pain. Normal ovarian tissue is outlined by *tiny arrows.* **B,** The same ovary 6 weeks later. Ovulation occurred and a hemorrhagic normal corpus luteum formed, giving the ovary a typical round shape and a webbed appearance of a textured solid mass. The same adhesions are seen, and a wedge of normal ovarian tissue is compressed but still evident *(arrows)* and surrounded by the hemorrhagic tissue. The patient refused further medical management, and the ovary was excised.

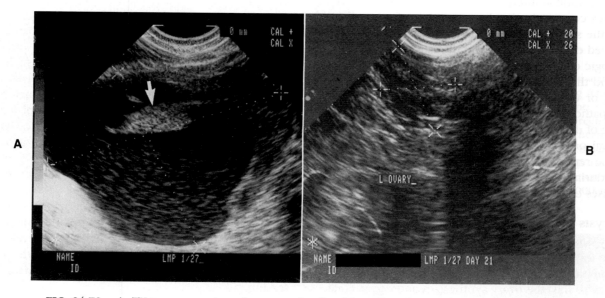

FIG. 24-73.   A, TV transverse view of an ovary (outlined by calipers) with a large, painful, cystic, ovarian mass first noted to be 8 cm on cycle day 1. It had regressed by half by day 14 (this study). It appears to be a hemorrhagic corpus luteum with a tiny, mobile blood clot *(arrow).* **B,** A remarkable resolution 1 week later, following ovulation in the opposite ovary. The ovary is outlined by calipers.

domen. Omental cysts tend to be higher in the abdomen, and urachal cysts are midline in the anterior abdominal wall. Any tumor may have cystic elements, although the following neoplasms commonly have a single, simple cyst.

Serous cystadenomas are simple cystic tumors usually occurring in menstruating women. They are a common ovarian neoplasm and are benign. One third occur bilaterally. They are thin walled, of variable size, and may have multiseptations (Figs. 24-74 and 24-75). The malignant form, serous cystadenocarcinoma, may also be cystic. However, malignancies typically have irregular textures with papillary projections. Pelvic ascites is often present with malignancies (Fig. 24-76). Mucinous cystadenoma, a

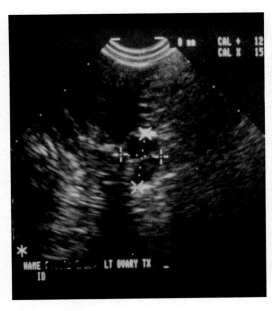

FIG. 24-74. A 1.2 × 1.5 cm double adnexal cyst in a 68-year-old woman seen incidentally by TV ultrasound proved to be a cystadenoma. The ovary is marked by calipers.

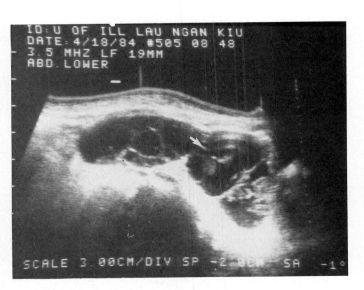

FIG. 24-75. Parasagittal static view of a large, bilobed multiseptate serous cystadenoma behind and above the bladder (*arrow* at the upper border of the bladder).

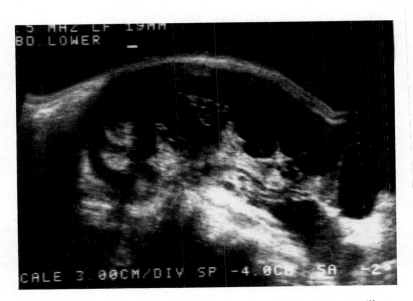

FIG. 24-76. Sagittal static view of a large cystadenocarcinoma containing papillary excrescences into the cysts. The bladder is slightly compressed (right side of photo).

benign tumor, may be unilocular and tends to be very large (Fig. 24-77).[28]

Bilateral multiseptate cystic ovaries

Bilateral multiseptate cystic ovaries are associated with excessive ovarian stimulation. These lutein cysts can occur with molar pregnancy or nonovarian choriocarcinoma. Hyperstimulation most often results from ovulation induction (Fig. 24-78). The ovaries are greatly enlarged, cystic, and multiseptate.

Polycystic ovary (Stein-Levanthal) syndrome is a relatively common cause of infertility, infrequent menses, and excessive hair growth. Polycystic ovaries are normal size or slightly enlarged. They are regular, oval, and always contain numerous tiny follicles less than 1 cm in size surrounded by thickened ovarian tissue or stroma. These tiny

cysts may not be resolved transabdominally.[42] Follicle after follicle develops partially, but fails to ovulate. The stroma produces excessive male hormones. The most extreme form of the condition is known as hyperthecosis (Fig. 24-79). Women with this may be masculinized with very high testosterone levels. Ovarian tumors, some of which produce male hormones, should be sought in these ovaries. The uterus tends to be relatively small, with thickened endometrium.

Mixed solid/cystic ovarian masses

Mixed solid/cystic ovarian masses are typical of all of the epithelial type of ovarian tumors. The most common are the benign serous cystadenoma and its malignant form, serous cystadenocarcinoma. They contain tubal type tissue and may have one or multiple cysts. The more sonograph-

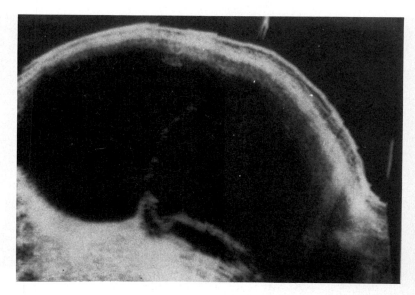

FIG. 24-77. Sagittal static view of an enormous mucinous cystadenoma. Tumors of this size can weigh about 90 lb.

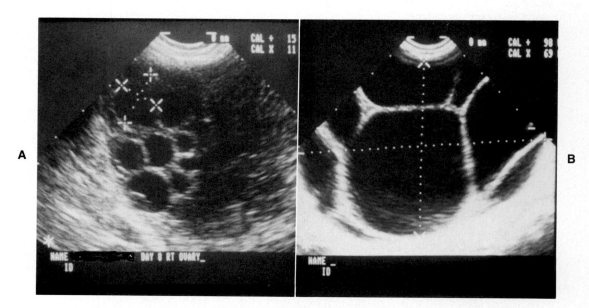

FIG. 24-78. **A,** HMG (human menopausal gonadotropin) stimulated ovary with a leading follicle (in calipers) and a number of smaller follicles, *TV.* **B,** The same ovary 11 days later after stimulated ovulation. The follicles have enlarged the ovaries to 11 cm in length and they cannot be entirely visualized transvaginally. There was no ascites.

ically complex the tumor, the more likely it is to be malignant, especially if it is associated with ascites (Fig. 24-80). One fourth of serous cystadenocarcinomas are bilateral, and most occur in women over age 40. They are large in size, around 10 cm, and often fill the pelvis (Fig. 24-77).

The second type of epithelial tumor contains the mucin-producing tissues of cervix or bowel. The benign form is a *mucinous cystadenoma,* the malignant is a *cystadenocarcinoma.* Seventy-five percent of mucinous cystadenomas are simple or septate cysts without internal papillary projections, but the mucinous fluid may produce

bright pinpoint echoes. They are typically large (15 to 30 or more centimeters in diameter), smooth tumors and have weighed more than 100 pounds. They are usually benign and unilateral, although when malignant, 10% to 20% are bilateral. Ten percent occur in postmenopausal women. A few have occurred in teenagers. A sizable cystic mass in a cycling woman is almost always a mucinous cystadenoma. Mucinous cystadenocarcinomas can become very large and are more likely than their benign counterparts to rupture. When the cyst is ruptured, the viscous contents produce massive adhesions and mucoid ascites (pseudomyxoma peritoneii). Ultrasonically the

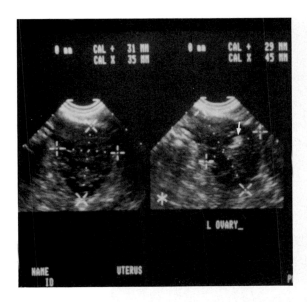

FIG. 24-79. TV transverse and longitudinal studies of a hyperthecotic ovary containing many tiny subcapsular cysts and dense central stroma. A dense 10 mm mass was incidentally seen in the sagittal view, and wedge resection at this point produced a tiny, fat-filled, dermoid cyst *(arrow)*.

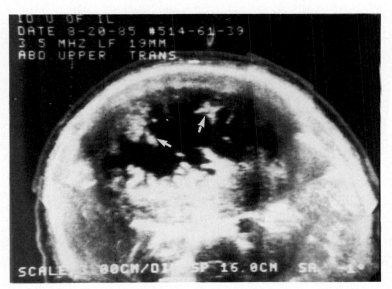

FIG. 24-80. Transverse static scan of stage III ovarian carcinoma with ascites and nodules visible on the peritoneum *(arrows)*, and a pelvis full of ill-defined cystic and solid structures.

mucoid ascites appears as hypoechoic fluid with bright echoes.[51]

The third epithelial tumor is the *endometrioid* type. It is the least common, but is usually malignant, accounting for 20% of ovarian cancers. It occurs more often in older women in the sixth decade. They range from 10 to 25 cm in diameter with varying proportions of cystic and solid tissue, which is histologically similar to endometrium.

It is usually diagnosed at an earlier stage than other epithelial tumors, giving a better prognosis. Careful attention should be given to ultrasound examination of the uterus, since an associated adenocarcinoma may be present in the endometrium.

Clear cell carcinoma consists of moderately enlarged cystic tumors with solid protrusions into the cyst. Five percent are bilateral, and over 50% are confined to the ovary at diagnosis.

Carcinomatosis can occur with any of these tumors with widespread peritoneal involvement, and usually produces ascites (Fig. 24-80). Since one cannot distinguish between tumors with mixed components, an abdominal survey is always indicated, as is laparotomy and exploration. It is essential that the sonographer, for his or her own enlightenment, obtain the pathologic details on the nature of every pelvic mass that is detected. Most clinicians are delighted to correlate their findings with ultrasonic information to steadily improve diagnostic accuracy.

One of the more common ovarian tumors with mixed components is a germ cell derivative, the *dermoid cyst.* It is a very common, usually benign, teratoma frequently found in young women. Dermoid tumors tend to lie anterior or superior to the uterus (Fig. 24-81) and consist of scrambled tissues that may include skin with long, matted

sometimes reaching 20 to 30 cm in the longest dimension (Fig. 24-87, *B*). Massive fluid shifts produce ascites, hypovolemia, and hemoconcentration, which may result in blood clot formation, hypercoagulability, or renal failure. Any trauma, including pelvic examination, could rupture the fragile ovaries and produce hemorrhage. Treatment entails bed rest, electrolyte correction, and IV fluid hydration and observation. The syndrome is more likely to occur in polycystic ovaries and with pregnancy. It will not occur if the ovulatory dose of HCG is withheld. Ultrasonographic evidence of more than two or three stimulated follicles, or a serum estradiol level of more than 2000 pg/ml will prevent many clinicians from administering HCG. The symptoms (more than 10 lb weight gain, abdominal distension, and prostration) will occur 7 to 10 days after ovulation and will resolve within a week without pregnancy. If pregnancy occurs, a month or more may be required. Even gentle pelvic examination may rupture the fragile vascular ovaries, increasing the risk of hemorrhage.

Gentle serial ultrasound examinations provide information that is preventative, diagnostic, and helpful in following the progress of the syndrome when physical palpation is unwise.

Understanding the nature and causes of ovulatory defects requires painstaking serial observation of follicle appearance, corpus luteum formation, and correlation of hormone levels. Several abnormal patterns of follicle growth in both spontaneous and treated cycles have been detected.[13,33]

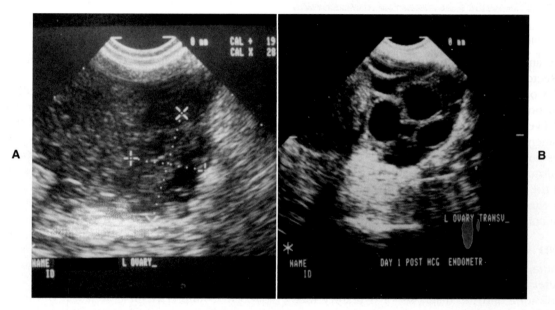

FIG. 24-87. **A,** A normal ovary, outlined by calipers, measuring 1.9 × 2.8 cm. **B,** The same ovary, 10 days later, after stimulation with HMG and hCG.

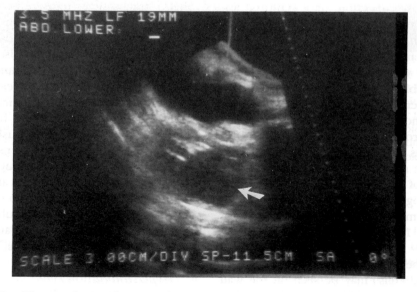

FIG. 24-88. TA sagittal view showing a hematoma *(arrow)* in the pelvis following hysterectomy.

POSTOPERATIVE USES OF ULTRASOUND

Pain and masses following pelvic surgery can indicate complications such as postoperative bleeding, hematomas, or abscess formation. Postoperative masses are not always dangerous. More than one surgeon has made the diagnosis of severely distended bladder by ordering an ultrasound for a postoperative pelvic mass. Ultrasound can be used to demonstrate these fluid collections (Figs. 24-88 and 24-89) and to visualize the operative site (Fig. 24-90). The ability to palpate specific structures with the transvaginal probe and avoidance of the abdominal wound is valuable in determining the site of pain in a postoperative pelvis. Resolving hematomas (1 week postoperative) often appear to be of a solid consistency and can be followed as they shrink (Fig. 24-91).

Ultrasonically guided needle drainage of abscesses and stable hematomas, either through the abdominal wall or the vagina, is diagnostic and therapeutic. Recurrent tumor masses may be biopsied in a similar fashion. The transvaginal ultrasound and needle guide make entering the anterior or posterior cul-de-sacs safer and easier for pelvic fluid aspiration, biopsies, or radiation needle placement.[14,57]

An expert combination of transvaginal and transabdominal techniques is essential as new gynecologic applica-

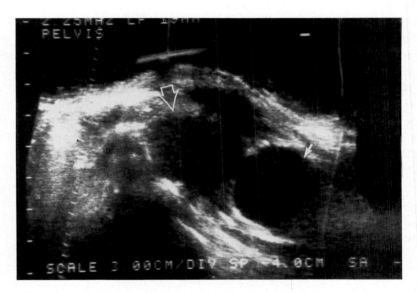

FIG. 24-89. TA longitudinal view of postcesarean section abscess between the bladder, peritoneum, and the uterus where the uterine incision was made. The uterus *(open arrow)* is still enlarged from pregnancy, and the bladder lies below the abscess *(arrow)*.

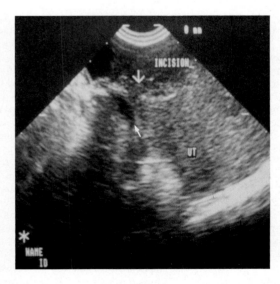

FIG. 24-90. TV sagittal normal postoperative uterine scan following a low transverse incision in the uterus just above the cervix. Bright echoes on either side of the arrow are sutures. The bladder is in the near field on the left side of the photo. There is a tiny accumulation of fluid between the bladder and uterus *(tiny arrow)*.

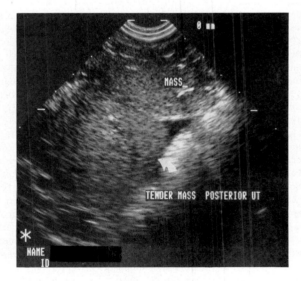

FIG. 24-91. TV transverse view into the cul-de-sac of a hematoma *(MASS)* behind a uterus following termination of a 14-week gestation by D & C. The clot is well organized and is the same consistency as the uterus *(curved arrow)*.

tions of ultrasound continue to be found in the screening, diagnosis, and therapy of pelvic pathology in female fetuses, children, and adults.

ACKNOWLEDGMENT
The authors gratefully acknowledge the expert assistance of Irma Lopez in preparation of the manuscript and the generosity of the Ultrasound Department of Blodgett Memorial Medical Center, Grand Rapids, Michigan.

SUMMARY

1. Ultrasound is most often used to delineate the size, consistency, and structure of origin of pelvic masses. It also supplies information about the function and morphology of abnormal organs when the pelvic examination is unremarkable or difficult.

2. The three current methods of pelvic sonography in use are transabdominal static scanning, transabdominal real-time scanning, and transvaginal real-time scanning.

3. Accurate imaging from the narrow suprapubic site through the bladder is most easily accomplished with a real-time sector transducer, and correct interpretation is more likely if the sonologist observes the scan or a videotape of it.

4. It is sometimes helpful to combine bimanual or digital vaginal examination with transabdominal ultrasound to define structures and to manipulate the uterus and/or mass and establish their relationship and mobility.

5. Transvaginal ultrasonography of the female pelvis has been in use since 1983. It is an important technique that allows superb definition of pelvic contents without sound wave deflection by bowel gas or attenuation by a thick abdominal wall.

6. Commonly called "fibroids," myomas in the uterus are easily demonstrated by their distortion of bladder and uterine contours and texture changes either by transvaginal or transabdominal ultrasound.

7. Transabdominal ultrasound is fairly specific in diagnosing unexpected anomalies with double uterine cavities, but is less likely to detect abnormalities with essentially single cavities. It is also excellent for evaluating vaginal obstruction.

8. The diagnosis of ectopic pregnancy is greatly simplified by the use of pelvic ultrasound and β-HCG levels. Transvaginal transducers substantially clarify tubal anatomy and early (4.5 weeks) intrauterine gestational sacs. This enables early localization, more selective use of laparoscopy or laparotomy, and prevention of tubal rupture.

9. Although the premier role of ultrasound in women is still obstetrical, its use is becoming pervasive in gynecology, especially in the evaluation and treatment of infertility.

REFERENCES

1. Andolf E, Svalenius E, and Astedt B: Ultrasonography for early detection of ovarian carcinoma. Br J Obstet Gynecol 93:1286, 1986.
2. Barber HR and Graber EA: The PMPO syndrome (postmenopausal palpable ovary syndrome), Obstet Gynecol 38:6:921, 1971.
3. Bernaschek G, Deutinger J, Bartl W, et al: Endosonographic staging of carcinoma of the uterine cervix, Arch Gynecol 239:21, 1986.
4. Blumenfeld Z, Rottem S, Elgali S, et al: Transvaginal assessment of early embryologic development. In Timor-Trisch IE and Rottem S, editors: Transvaginal ultrasonography, New York, 1988, Elsevier Science Publishing Co.
5. Bordt J, Hanker JP, and Schneider HPG: Ultrasound controlled gonadotropin therapy of anovulatory infertility, Fertil Steril 46:818, 1986.
6. Campbell S, Goessens L, Goswamy R, et al: Real-time ultrasonography for determination of ovarian morphology and volume: a possible early screening test for ovarian cancer? Lancet 1:425, 1982.
7. Davis JA: Fluid in the female pelvis: cystic patterns, J Ultrasound Med 5:75, 1986.
8. Dawood MY: Endometriosis: endocrine disorders in the female. In Gold J and Josimovich J, editors: Gynecologic endocri-

nology, ed. 4, New York and London, 1986, Plenum Medical Book Co., p 387.
9. DeCherney AH, Romero R, and Polan ML: Ultrasound in reproductive endocrinology, Fertil Steril 37:323, 1982.
10. Dellenbach P, Nisand I, Morean L, et al: Transvaginal sonographically controlled ovarian follicle puncture for egg retrieval [letter], Lancet 1:1467, 1984.
11. Dellenbach P, Nisand I, Moveau L, et al: Transvaginal sonographically controlled follicle puncture for oocyte retrieval, Fertil Steril 44:656, 1985.
12. DuBose TJ, Hill LW, Hennigan HW, et al: Sonography of arcuate uterine blood vessels, J Ultrasound Med 4:229, 1985.
13. Eissa MF, Sawers RS, Docker MF, et al: Characteristics and incidence of dysfunctional ovulation patterns detected by ultrasound, Fertil Steril 47:603, 1987.
14. Feichtinger W and Kemeter P: Transvaginal sector scan sonography for needle guided transvaginal follicle aspiration and other applications in gynecologic routine and research, Fertil Steril 45(5):722, 1986.
15. Fleischer AC, Dudley BS, Entman SS, et al: Myometrial invasion by endometrial carcinoma: sonographic assessment, Radiology 162:307, 1987.
16. Fleischer AC, Kalemeris GC, Machin JE et al: Sonographic depiction of normal and abnormal endometrium with histopatho-

logic correlation, J Ultrasound Med 5:445, 1986.
16a. Fossum GT, Davajan V, and Kletzky O: Early detection of pregnancy with transvaginal ultrasound, Fertil Steril 49:788, 1988.
17. Giorlandino C, Gleicher N, Nanni C, et al: The sonographic picture of endometrium in spontaneous and induced cycles, Fertil Steril 47:508, 1987.
18. Hackeloer BJ and Sallam HN: Ultrasound scanning of ovarian follicles, Clin Obstet Gynecol 10:611, 1983.
19. Hall DA, McCarthy KA, and Kopans DB: Sonographic visualization of the normal postmenopausal ovary, J Ultrasound Med 5:9, 1986.
20. Haning RV, Austin CW, Kuzma DL, et al: Ultrasound evaluation of estrogen monitoring for induction of ovulation with menotropins, Fertil Steril 37:627, 1982.
21. Herrmann UJ Jr, Locher GW, and Goldhirsch A: Sonographic patterns of ovarian tumors prediction of malignancy, Obstet Gynecol 69:777, 1987.
22. Ivarsson SA, Nilsson KO, and Persson PH: Ultrasonography of the pelvic organs in prepubertal and postpubertal girls, Arch Dis Child 58:352, 1983.
23. Janssen-Caspers HAB, Kruitwagen RFP, Wladimiroff JW, et al: Diagnosis of luteinizing unruptured follicle by ultrasound and steroid hormone assays in peritoneal

fluid: a comparative study, Fertil Steril 46:823, 1986.

24. Kadar N, DeVore G, and Romero R: The discriminatory hCG zone: its use in the sonographic evaluation for ectopic pregnancy, Obstet Gynecol 58:156, 1981.

25. Kerin JF, Edmunds KD, Warnes GM, et al: Morphological and functional relations of graafian follicle growth to ovulation in women, using ultrasonographic, laparoscopic and biochemical measurements, Br J Obstet Gynecol 88:81, 1981.

26. Killick S, Eyong E, and Elstein M: Ovarian follicular development in oral contraceptive cycles, Fertil Steril 48:409, 1987.

27. Kim DS, Sung RC, Park MI, and Kim YP: Comparative review of diagnostic accuracy in tubal pregnancy: a 14-year survey of 1040 cases, Obstet Gynecol 70:547, 1987.

28. Knapp RC and Berkowitz RS: Gynecologic oncology, New York, 1986, MacMillan Publishing Co.

29. Lenz S and Lauritsen JG: Ultrasonically guided percutaneous aspiration of human follicles under local anesthesia, Fertil Steril 38:673, 1982.

30. Lewin A, Margoliath EJ, Rabinowitz R, et al: Comparative study of ultrasonographically guided percutaneous aspiration with local anesthesia and laparoscopic aspiration of follicles for IVF, Am J Obstet Gynecol 151:621, 1985.

31. Liebman AJ, Druse B, and McSweeney MB: Transvaginal sonography: comparison with transabdominal sonography in the diagnosis of pelvic masses, 151:89, 1988.

32. Lindeque BG, DuToit JP, Muller LM, and Deale JCD: Ultrasonographic criteria for the conservative management of antenatally diagnosed fetal ovarian cysts, J Reprod Med 33:196, 1988.

33. Liukkonen S, Koskimies AI, Tenhunen A, et al: Diagnosis of luteinized unruptured follicle syndrome by ultrasound, Fertil Steril 41:26, 1984.

34. Malini S, Valdes C, and Malinak LR: Sonographic diagnosis and classification of anomalies of the female genital tract, J Ultrasound Med 3(9):397, 1984.

35. Marinbo AO, Sallam HN, Goessens LK, et al: Real time pelvic ultrasonography during the periovulatory period of patients attending an artificial insemination clinic, Fertil Steril 37:633, 1982.

36. Mendelson B, Bohm-Velez M, Joseph N, and Neiman H: Gynecologic imaging: comparison of transabdominal and transvaginal sonography, Radiology 166:321, 1988.

37. Morimoto N, Noda Y, Takai I, et al: Ultrasonographic observation of follicular development via vaginal route, Nippon Sanka Fujinka Gakkai Zasshi 35(2):151, 1983.

38. Najarian KE and Kurtz AB: New observations in the sonographic evaluation of intrauterine contraceptive devices, J Ultrasound Med 5:205, 1986.

39. Nicolini V, Bellotti M, Bonazzi B, et al: Can ultrasound be used to screen uterine malformations? Fertil Steril 47:89, 1987.

40. Nyberg DA, Filly RA, Filho DLD, et al: Abnormal pregnancy: early diagnosis by US and serum chorionic gonadotropin levels, Radiology 158:393, 1986.

41. Orsini LF, Salardi S, Pilu GL, et al: Pelvic organs in premenarcheal girls: real-time ultrasonography, Radiology 153:113, 1984.

42. Orsini LF, Venturoli S, Lorusso R, et al: Ultrasonic findings in polycystic ovarian disease, Fertil Steril 43:709, 1985.

43. Platt D, Manning A, and Hill A: Simultaneous real-time ultrasound scanning and pelvic examination in assessment of pelvic disease, Am J Obstet Gynecol 136:693, 1980.

44. Randolph JR, Ying YK, Maier DB, et al: Comparison of real-time ultrasonography, Hysterosalpingography, and laparoscopy/hysteroscopy in the evaluation of uterine abnormalities and tubal patency, Fertil Steril 46:828, 1986.

45. Reeves R, Drake TS, and O'Brien WF: Ultrasonographic vs clinical evaluation of a pelvic mass, Obstet Gynecol 55:551, 1980.

46. Renaud RL, Macler J, Dervain I, et al: Echographic study of follicular maturation and ovulation during the normal menstrual cycle, Fertil Steril 33:272, 1980.

47. Rubin D, Graham MF, Cronhelm C, et al: Echogenic hematometra mimicking endometrial carcinoma, J Ultrasound Med 4:47, 1985.

48. Rulin MC and Preston AL: Adnexal masses in postmenopausal women, Obstet Gynecol 70:578, 1987.

49. Russ PD, Zaritz WR, Pretorious DH, et al: Hydrometrocolpos, uterus didelphys, and septate vagina: an antenatal sonographic diagnosis, J Ultrasound Med 5(4):211, 1986.

50. Sallam HN, Marincho AO, Collins WP, et al: Monitoring gonadotrophin therapy by real-time ultrasonic scanning of ovarian follicles, Br J Obstet Gynaecol 89:155, 1982.

51. Sanders RC and James AE: The principals and practice of ultrasonography in obstetrics and gynecology, ed 3, Norwalk, Conn, 1985, Appleton-Century-Crofts.

52. Schulman JD, Dorfmann A, Jones SL, et al: Laparoscopy for in vitro fertilization: end of an era, Fertil Steril 44:713, 1985.

53. Schulman JD, Dorfmann A, Jones SL, et al: Outpatient in vitro fertilization using transvaginal oocyte retrieval and local anesthesia, N Engl J Med 312:1639, 1985.

54. Schulman JD, Dorfmann AD, Jones SL, et al: Outpatient in vitro fertilization using transvaginal ultrasound guided oocyte retrieval, Obstet Gynecol 69:665, 1987.

55. Schwimer SR and Lebovic J: Transvaginal pelvic ultrasonography, J Ultrasound Med 3:381, 1984.

56. Schwimer SR and Lebovic J: Transvaginal pelvic ultrasonography: accuracy in follicle and cyst size determination, J Ultrasound Med 4:61, 1985.

57. Schwimer SR, Marik J, and Lebovic J: Percutaneous ovarian cyst aspiration using continuous transvaginal ultrasonographic

monitoring, J Ultrasound Med 4:259, 1985.

58. Seidler DS, Laing FL, Jeffery RB, and Wing VW: Uterine adenomyosis: a difficult sonographic diagnosis, J Ultrasound Med 6:345, 1987.

59. Shapiro BS, Cullen M, Taylor JW, and DeCherney A: Transvaginal ultrasonography for the diagnosis of ectopic pregnancy, Fertil Steril 50:425, 1988.

60. Simpson EL, Coleman BG, and Sondheimer SJ: In vitro fertilization and embryo transfer complicated by simultaneous ectopic and intrauterine twin gestation, J Ultrasound Med 5:49, 1986.

61. Smith DH, Picker RH, Sinosich M, and Saunders DM: Assessment of ovulation by ultrasound and estradiol levels during spontaneous and induced cycles, Fertil Steril 33:387, 1980.

62. Styne DM, Harris DA, Egli CA, et al: Treatment of true precocious puberty with a potent luteinizing hormone-releasing factor agonist: effect on growth sexual maturation, pelvic sonography, and the hypothalamic-pituitary-gonadal axis, J Clin Endocrinol Metab 1:142, 1985.

63. Swayne LC, Rubenstein JB, and Mitchell B: The Mayer-Rokitansky-Kuster-Hauser syndrome: sonographic aid to diagnosis, J Ultrasound Med 5(5):287, 1986.

64. Timor-Tritsch IE: A close look at early embryonic development with the high frequency transvaginal transducer, abstract #15, Eighth Annual Meeting of the Society for Perinatal Obstetricians, Las Vegas, Feb. 3, 1988.

65. Timor-Tritsch IE and Rottem S: Transvaginal ultrasonographic study of the fallopian tube, Obstet Gynecol 70:424, 1987.

66. Timor-Trisch IE and Rottem S, editors: Transvaginal sonography, New York, 1988, Elsevier Science Publishing Co.

67. Valdes C, Malini S, and Malinak LR: Ultrasound evaluation of female genital tract anomalies: a review of 64 cases, Am J Obstet Gynecol 149:285, 1984.

68. Wade RV, Smyth AR, Watt GW, et al: Reliability of gynecologic sonographic diagnosis 1978-1984, Am J Obstet Gynecol 153:186, 1985.

69. Walsh JW, Taylor KJW, and Rosenfield AT: Gray scale ultrasonography in the diagnosis of endometriosis and adenomyosis, AJR 132:87, 1979.

70. Werlin LB, Weckstein LW, Weathersbee PS, et al: Ultrasound: a technique useful in determining the side of ovulation, Fertil Steril 46:814, 1986.

71. Wikland M, Enic L, Hammarberg K, and Nilsson L: Use of a vaginal transducer for oocyte retrieval in an IVF/ET program, J Clin Ultrasound 15:245, 1987.

72. Wikland M, Lennart E, and Hamberger L: Transvesical and transvaginal approaches for the aspiration of follicles by use of ultrasound, Ann NY Acad Sci 442:182, 1985.

73. Winer S, Spirtos T, Platt L, and Mans RP: Vaginal realtime ultrasound for diagnosis of ectopic pregnancies, abstract, The

American Fertility Society Meeting, Sept. 27, 1986.

74. Yee B, Barnes RB, Vargyas JM, and Marrs RP: Correlation of transabdominal and transvaginal ultrasound measurements of follicle size and number with laparoscopic findings for in vitro fertilization, Fertil Steril 47:828, 1987.

75. Yeh HC and Rabinowitz J: Amniotic sac development: ultrasound features of early pregnancy—the double bleb sign, Radiology 66:97, 1988.

76. Ying YK, Daly DC, Randolph JF, et al: Ultrasonographic monitoring of follicular growth for luteal phase defects, Fertil Steril 48:433, 1987.

Part Six

CARDIOLOGY

25

Anatomic and Physiologic Relationships Within the Thoracic Cavity

This chapter will introduce the student to the anatomic features of the thoracic cavity. However, the primary concentration will be on the cardiac anatomic and physiologic relationships.

THORAX

The thorax constitutes the upper part of the body. The thoracic cavity lies within the thorax and is separated from the abdominal cavity by the diaphragm (Figs. 25-1 to 25-3). The diaphragm reaches upward as high as the mid-axillary level of the seventh rib. Superiorly the upper thoracic cavity gives access to the root of the neck. It is bounded by the upper part of the sternum, the first ribs, and the body of the first thoracic vertebra. Anteriorly the sternum consists of three parts: the manubrium, the corpus sterni (body), and the xyphoid. The junction between the manubrium and the body of the sternum is a prominent ridge; together they form the angle of Louis. This palpable landmark is important in locating the superior mediastinum or the second rib cartilages, which articulate with the sternum at this point.

The greater part of the thoracic cavity is occupied by the two lungs, which are enclosed by the pleural sac. To understand the pleural sac, imagine a deflated plastic bag covering your fist. Both sides of the bag should be reflected onto your fist to simulate the pleural sac. The internal layer, or *visceral pleura,* is adherent to each lobe of the lung. The external layer, or *parietal pleura,* is adherent to the inner surface of the chest wall *(costal pleura),*

diaphragm *(diaphragmatic pleura),* and mediastinum *(mediastinal pleura)* (Fig. 25-4).

The *costophrenic sinus* is the pleural reflection between the costal and diaphragmatic portions of the parietal pleura. This space lies lower than the edge of the lung and, in most cases, is never occupied by lung. When pleural fluid accumulates, its most common location is in the costophrenic sinus. On a radiographic examination, the costophrenic angle in blunted by the presence of pleural effusion.

The *mediastinum* is the median partition of the thoracic cavity. The mediastinum is a movable, thick structure and extends superiorly to the thoracic inlet and the root of the neck and inferiorly to the diaphragm. It extends anteriorly to the sternum and posteriorly to the twelfth thoracic vertebra. Within the mediastinum are found the remains of the thymus, the heart and great vessels, the trachea and esophagus, the thoracic duct and lymph nodes, the vagus and phrenic nerves, and the sympathetic trunks.

The mediastinum may be divided into superior and inferior mediastina by an imaginary plane from the sternal angle to the lower body of the fourth thoracic vertebra. The inferior mediastinum is subdivided into three parts: (1) middle, which contains the pericardium and the heart; (2) anterior, which is a space between the pericardium and sternum; and (3) posterior, which lies between the pericardium and vertebral column.

It is useful to remember the following major mediasti-

580

FIG. 25-1. Anterior view of the thorax. Manubrium of the sternum, *1;* right clavicle, *2;* thyroid gland, *3;* trachea, *4;* left common carotid artery, *5;* left internal jugular-vein, *6;* left phrenic nerve, *7;* superior and inferior lobes of the right lung, *8;* pericardium, *9;* xyphoid process, *10;* diaphragm, *11.* (From Hagen-Ansert SL: The anatomy workbook, Philadelphia, 1986, JB Lippincott Co.)

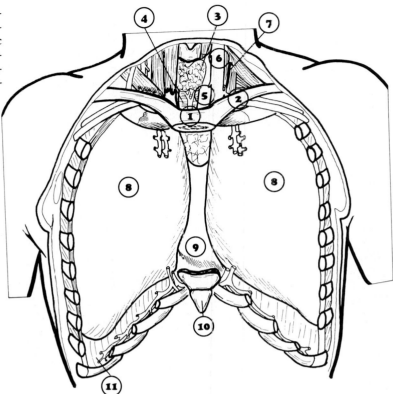

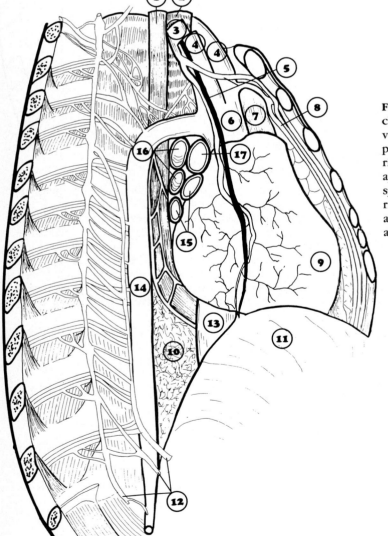

FIG. 25-2. Right lateral view of the thorax. Esophagus, *1;* trachea, *2;* brachiocephalic artery, *3;* right and left brachiocephalic veins, *4;* right phrenic nerve and inferior thoracic artery, *5;* superior vena cava, *6;* ascending aorta, *7;* inferior thoracic vein, *8;* right surface of the pericardium, *9;* pleura of the left side, *10;* diaphragm pulled inferiorly, *11;* greater, lesser, and lowest splanchnic nerves, *12;* inferior vena cava, *13;* azygos vein, *14;* right pulmonary veins, *15;* right bronchus, *16;* right pulmonary artery, *17.* (From Hagen-Ansert SL: The anatomy workbook, Philadelphia, 1986, JB Lippincott Co.)

FIG. 25-3. Left lateral view of the thorax. Trachea, *1;* esophagus, *2;* left common carotid and subclavian veins, *3;* left brachiocephalic vein, *4;* left phrenic nerve, *5;* internal thoracic vessels, *6;* left surface of the pericardium, *7;* diaphragm, *8;* greater and lesser splanchnic nerves, *9;* hemiazygos vein, *10;* descending aorta, *11;* left pulmonary vein, *12;* left bronchus (divided), *13;* left pulmonary artery, *14;* aortic arch, *15.* (From Hagen-Ansert SL: The anatomy workbook, Philadelphia, 1986, JB Lippincott Co.)

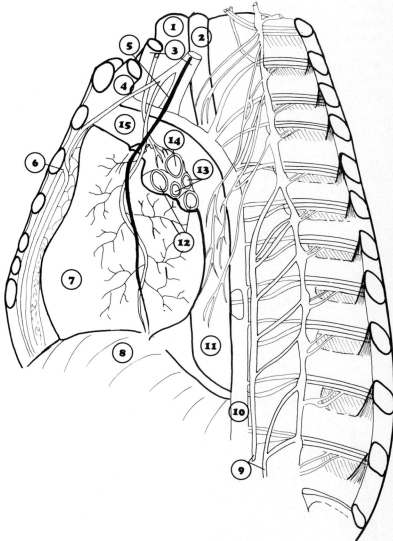

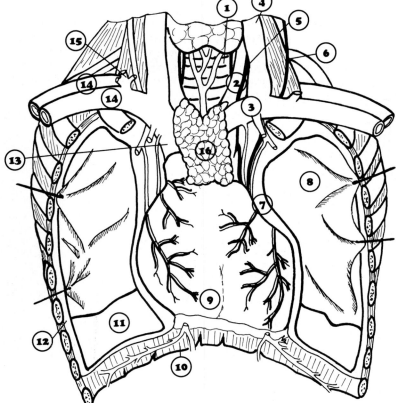

FIG. 25-4. Anterior view of the thorax with the lungs removed. Trachea, *1;* left common carotid artery, *2;* left brachiocephalic (innominate) vein, *3;* left internal jugular vein, *4;* left vagus nerve, *5;* left phrenic nerve, *6;* mediastinal pleura, *7;* left lung, *8;* pericardium, *9;* diaphragm, *10;* diaphragmatic pleural space, *11;* costal pleural space, *12;* superior vena cava, *13;* right subclavian artery and vein, *14;* right external jugular vein, *15;* thymus gland, *16.* (From Hagen-Ansert SL: The anatomy workbook, Philadelphia, 1986, JB Lippincott Co.)

nal structures are arranged in the following order from anterior to posterior:

Superior Mediastinum	Inferior Mediastinum
Thymus	Thymus
Great veins	Heart within the pericardium with the phrenic nerves on either side
Great arteries	
Trachea	
Esophagus and thoracic duct	Esophagus and thoracic duct
Sympathetic trunks	Descending aorta
	Sympathetic trunks

THE HEART

The heart lies obliquely in the chest, posterior to the sternum, with the greater portion of its muscular mass lying slightly to the left of midline. The heart is protected within the chest by the sternum and rib cage anteriorly and the vertebral column and rib cage posteriorly. The other structures within the thoracic cavity in close approximation to the heart are the lungs, esophagus, and descending thoracic aorta.

Contrary to most simplified anatomic illustrations, the heart is not situated with its right chambers lying to the right and its left chambers to the left. It may be better considered as an anteroposterior structure with its right-sided chambers located more anterior than its left-sided chambers. As we look at the embryologic development, the heart forms as a tubular right-to-left structure. However, as development continues, the right side becomes more ventral and the left side remains dorsal. In addition, another change in axis causes the apex (or the inferior surface of the heart) to tilt anteriorly. The final development of the heart presents the right atrium anterior to and to the right of the sternum; while the right ventricle presents anterior and beneath or slightly to the left of the sternum. The left atrium becomes the most posterior chamber to the left of the sternum; while the left ventricle swings its posterior axis slightly toward the anterior chest wall.

The heart has three surfaces: sternocostal (anterior), diaphragmatic (inferior or apex), and base (posterior) (Fig. 25-5). The right atrium forms the right border of the heart to the right of the sternum. The left border is formed by the left ventricle and atrium. The right and left ventricles are separated by the anterior interventricular groove. The diaphragmatic surface of the heart is formed principally by the right and left ventricles separated by the posterior interventricular groove (Fig. 25-6). A small part of the inferior surface of the right atrium also forms this surface. The base of the heart is formed by the left atrium, into which the four pulmonary veins enter from the lungs. The right atrium contributes a small part to this posterior surface (Fig. 25-7). The left ventricle forms the apex of the heart, which can be palpated at the level of the fifth intercostal space, about 9 cm from the midline.

Pericardial sac

The heart and roots of the great vessels lie within the pericardial sac. Like the pleura of the lungs, the pericardium is a double sac. The *fibrous pericardium* limits the

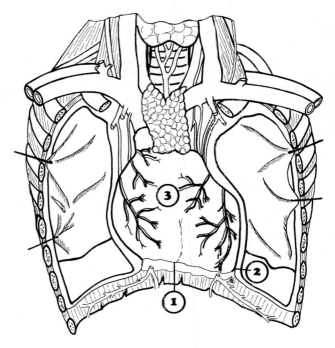

FIG. 25-5. Three surfaces of the heart. *1*, Diaphragmatic surface; *2*, apex; *3*, sternocostal surface. (From Hagen-Ansert SL: The anatomy workbook, Philadelphia, 1986, JB Lippincott Co.)

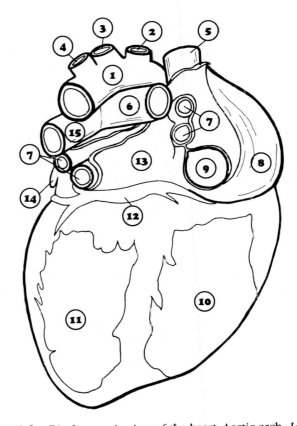

FIG. 25-6. Diaphragmatic view of the heart. Aortic arch, *1;* brachiocephalic artery, *2;* left common carotid artery, *3;* left subclavian artery, *4;* superior vena cava, *5;* right pulmonary artery, *6;* pulmonary veins, *7;* right atrium, *8;* inferior vena cava, *9;* right ventricle, *10;* left ventricle, *11;* coronary sinus, *12;* left atrium, *13;* left auricle, *14;* left pulmonary artery, *15.* (From Hagen-Ansert SL: The anatomy workbook, Philadelphia, 1986, JB Lippincott Co.)

FIG. 25-7. Posterior (basal) view of the heart. Aortic arch, *1;* right auricle, *2;* superior vena cava, *3;* right superior pulmonary vein, *4;* right inferior pulmonary vein, *5;* left superior pulmonary vein, *6;* left inferior pulmonary vein, *7;* right atrium, *8;* inferior vena cava, *9;* right ventricle, *10;* right pulmonary artery, *11;* left pulmonary artery, *12;* left auricle, *13;* left atrium, *14;* pericardial reflection, *15;* coronary sinus, *16;* left ventricle, *17.* (From Hagen-Ansert SL: The anatomy workbook, Philadelphia, 1986, JB Lippincott Co.)

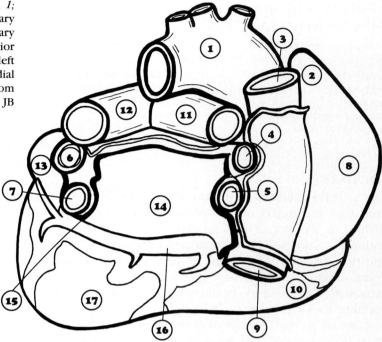

movement of the heart by attaching to the central tendon of the diaphragm below and the outer coats of the great vessels above. The sternopericardial ligaments attach it in the front. The *serous pericardium* is divided into parietal and visceral layers. The parietal layer lines the fibrous pericardium and is reflected around the roots of the great vessels to become continuous with the visceral layer of serous pericardium. The visceral layer is very closely applied to the heart and is often called the *epicardium.* The slit between the parietal and visceral layers is the pericardial cavity. This cavity normally contains a very small amount of fluid that lubricates the heart as it moves.

The pericardial sac provides the heart protection against friction. If the serous pericardium becomes inflamed, *pericarditis* will develop, or if too much pericardial fluid, fibrin, or pus develops in the pericardial space, the visceral and parietal layers may adhere to one another.

The pericardial sac does not totally encompass the heart. On the posterior left atrial surface of the heart, the reflection of serous pericardium around the pulmonary veins forms the recess of the oblique sinus. This may be an important landmark in the echocardiographic separation of pericardial effusion from pleural effusion. The transverse sinus lies between the reflection of serous pericardium around the aorta and pulmonary arteries and between the reflection around the pulmonary veins.

The lining of the heart

The chambers of the heart are lined by three layers: the endocardium, the myocardium, and the epicardium.

The *endocardium* is the intimal lining of the heart and is continuous with the intima of the vessels connecting to it. The endocardium is very similar to the intima of blood vessels. It also forms the valves that lie between the filling (atria) and pumping (ventricle) chambers of the heart, as well as along the bases of the two great arterial trunks leaving the heart (the aorta and pulmonary artery).

The muscular part of the heart, the *myocardium,* is a special type of cardiac muscle found only in the heart and great vessels. This cardiac muscle is equivalent to the media of a blood vessel. The cardiac muscle is very complex as compared to other muscular fibers. Although it is striated like voluntary muscle, the fibers of the cardiac muscle so branch and anastomose that it is impossible to determine the limits of a fiber. The myocardium of both ventricles is one continuous muscle mass, as is the myocardium of both atria. Because of this continuity, an impulse for contraction originating in the atrium can spread throughout the atrial musculature; similarly, an impulse originating in a ventricle can spread throughout the ventricular musculature. A special bundle of fibers connects the atria to the ventricles. The unique feature of cardiac muscle is the ability to possess intrinsic rhythmic contractility. It is this rhythmicity that keeps the heart contracting: with nerve impulses modifying rather than initiating the heart beat.

Since the atria work at very low pressures, the musculature of the atria is very thin in comparison to the ventricle wall mass. The primary purpose of the atria are filling chambers that serve to drive the blood into the relaxed ventricular cavity. In contrast, the myocardium of the ventricles is much greater than the atria. The left ventricle has the greatest muscle mass, since is must pump blood to all of the body while the right ventricle only needs enough pressure to pump the blood to the lungs.

The outside layer of the heart is the *epicardium,* or the visceral layer of the serous pericardium. The outer surface of the epicardium is a single layer of mesothelial cells continuous with the serous (inner) surface of the pericardium.

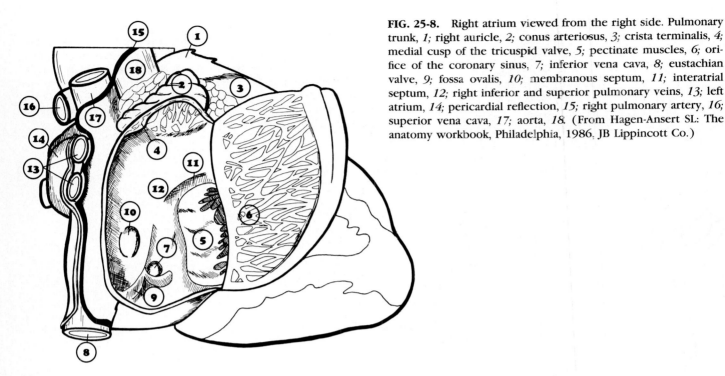

FIG. 25-8. Right atrium viewed from the right side. Pulmonary trunk, *1;* right auricle, *2;* conus arteriosus, *3;* crista terminalis, *4;* medial cusp of the tricuspid valve, *5;* pectinate muscles, *6;* orifice of the coronary sinus, *7;* inferior vena cava, *8;* eustachian valve, *9;* fossa ovalis, *10;* membranous septum, *11;* interatrial septum, *12;* right inferior and superior pulmonary veins, *13;* left atrium, *14;* pericardial reflection, *15;* right pulmonary artery, *16;* superior vena cava, *17;* aorta, *18.* (From Hagen-Ansert SL: The anatomy workbook, Philadelphia, 1986. JB Lippincott Co.)

Right atrium

The right atrium forms the right border of the heart. The superior vena cava enters the upper posterior border, and the inferior vena cava enters the lower posterior lateral border (Fig. 25-8). The posterior wall of the right atrium is directly related to the pulmonary veins (which flow from the lungs to empty into the left atrium). The medial wall of the right atrium is formed by the interatrial septum. The septum angles slightly posterior and to the patient's right, so the atrium lies in front and to the right of the left atrium. The central ovale portion of the septum is thin and fibrous. Just superior and in front of the opening of the inferior vena cava lies a shallow depression, the *fossa ovalis.* Its borders are the *limbus fossae ovalis* and the primitive *septum primum.* The *foramen ovale* lies under the most superior part of the limbus fossae. The limbus fossae ovalis is the remainder of the atrial septum and forms a ridge around the fossa ovalis.

The atrioventricular part of the membranous septum separates the right atrium and left ventricle. Atrial septal defects can occur in this area, causing blood to flow from the high-pressured left ventricle into the right atrial cavity.

The anterior and lateral walls of the right atrium are ridged by the *pectinate muscles.* The superior portion of the right atrium, the right atrial appendage, contains the most prominent pectinate muscles. The posterior and medial walls are smooth, probably due to the continual flow of blood from the inferior and superior venae cavae and coronary sinus.

The inferior vena cava is guarded by a fold of tissue called the *eustachian valve* while the coronary sinus is guarded by the *thebesian valve* (Fig. 25-9).

The coronary sinus drains the blood supply from the heart wall. It is bordered by the fossa ovalis and the tricuspid valve.

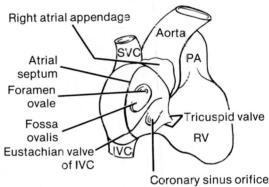

FIG. 25-9. Right atrium featuring the foramen ovale, fossa ovalis, and eustachian valve. (From Hagen-Ansert SL: The anatomy workbook, Philadelphia, 1986. JB Lippincott Co.)

Right ventricle

The base of the right ventricle lies on the diaphragm whereas the roof is occupied by the *crista supraventricularis,* which lies between the tricuspid and pulmonary orifices. The right ventricle is essentially divided into two parts: the posteroinferior inflow portion (containing the tricuspid valve) and the anterosuperior outflow portion (containing the origin of the pulmonary trunk). The demarcation between these two parts is by a number of prominent bands—*parietal band, supraventricular crest, septal band, and moderator band.* (Fig. 25-10). Together these bands form an almost circular orifice that normally is wide and forms no impediment to flow.

The inflow tract of the right ventricle is short and heavily trabeculated. It extends from the tricuspid valve and merges into the trabecular zone. This zone is known as the body of the right ventricle. The trabeculae carneae enclose an elongated ovoid opening. The inflow tract unites with the outflow tract, which extends to the pul-

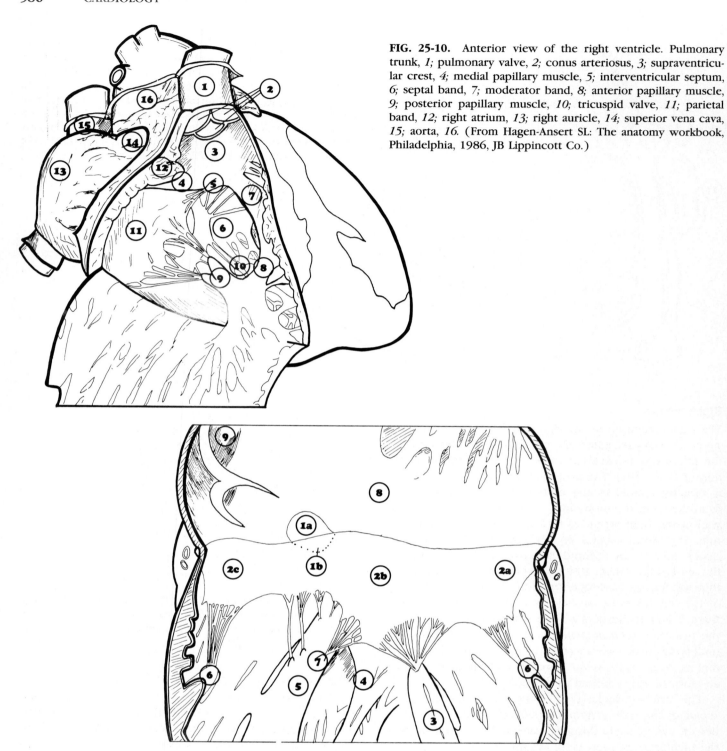

FIG. 25-10. Anterior view of the right ventricle. Pulmonary trunk, *1;* pulmonary valve, *2;* conus arteriosus, *3;* supraventricular crest, *4;* medial papillary muscle, *5;* interventricular septum, *6;* septal band, *7;* moderator band, *8;* anterior papillary muscle, *9;* posterior papillary muscle, *10;* tricuspid valve, *11;* parietal band, *12;* right atrium, *13;* right auricle, *14;* superior vena cava, *15;* aorta, *16.* (From Hagen-Ansert SL: The anatomy workbook, Philadelphia, 1986, JB Lippincott Co.)

FIG. 25-11. Anatomy of the tricuspid valve. Membranous septum, *1;* atrioventricular part, *1a;* interventricular part (behind valve), *1b;* tricuspid valve, *2;* posterior cusp, *2a;* anterior cusp, *2b;* medial cusp, *2c;* anterior papillary muscle, *3;* parietal band, *4;* septal band, *5;* posterior papillary muscles (sectioned), *6;* medial (conal) papillary muscle, *7;* right atrium, *8;* inferior vena cava, *9.* (From Hagen-Ansert SL: The anatomy workbook, Philadelphia, 1986, JB Lippincott Co.)

monary valve. The outflow portion of the right ventricle, or *infundibulum,* is smooth walled and contains few trabeculae.

The right ventricle has two walls, an anterior (corresponding to the sternocostal surface) and a posterior (formed by the ventricular septum).

Tricuspid valve. The tricuspid valve separates the right atrium from the right ventricle. It has three leaflets: anterior, septal, and inferior (or mural) (Fig. 25-11). The

septal leaflet may be maldeveloped in association with such conditions as ostium primum defect or ventricular septal defect. The leaflets are attached by their bases to the fibrous atrioventricular ring. The chordae tendineae attach the leaflets to the papillary muscles. As these muscles contract with ventricular contraction, the leaflets are pulled together to prevent their being pulled into the atrial cavity. The septal and anterior leaflets are connected to the same papillary muscle, which helps in this process.

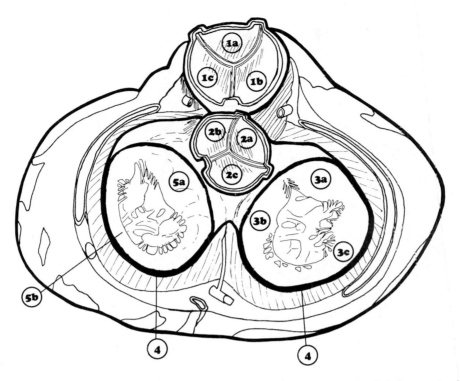

FIG. 25-12.   Pulmonary valve viewed from the base with the atria removed. Pulmonary valve, *1;* anterior cusp, *1a;* right cusp, *1b;* left cusp, *1c;* aortic valve, *2;* right coronary cusp, *2a;* left coronary cusp, *2b;* noncoronary cusp, *2c;* tricuspid valve, *3;* anterior cusp, *3a;* medial (septal) cusp; *3b;* posterior cusp, *3c;* annulus fibrosus, *4;* mitral valve, *5;* anterior cusp, *5a;* posterior cusp, *5b.* (From Hagen-Ansert SL: The anatomy workbook, Philadelphia, 1986, JB Lippincott Co.)

Pulmonary valve and trunk. The pulmonary valve lies at the upper anterior aspect of the right ventricle. It has three cusps: anterior, right, and left (Fig. 25-12). The wall of the pulmonary artery bulges our adjacent to each cusp to form pockets known as the pulmonary *sinuses of valsalva.*

The pulmonary trunk passes posterior and slightly upward from the right ventricle. It bifurcates into the right and left pulmonary arteries just after leaving the pericardial cavity. The *ligamentum arteriosum* connects the upper aspect of the bifurcation to the anterior surface of the aortic arch. (The ligamentum arteriosum is a remnant of the fetal ductus arteriosus).

Left atrium

The left atrium is a smooth-walled circular sac that lies posterior in the base of the heart. Two pulmonary veins enter posterior on either side of the cavity (Fig. 25-13). Occasionally these veins unite prior to entering the atrium, and sometimes there are more than two veins on either side. The veins may also be congenitally defective and enter the right atrium or other areas in the thoracic cavity. This absence of pulmonary veins entering the left atrial cavity is known as *total anomalous pulmonary venous return.*

The septal surface of the atrium is fairly smooth. A somewhat irregular area indicates the position of the fetal valve of the foramen ovale. The left auricle, or left atrial appendage, is a continuation of the left upper anterior part of the left atrium. Small pectinate muscles are located within its lumen.

Left ventricle

The left ventricle is conical or egg shaped. The smaller end of the ventricle represents the apex of the heart whereas the larger end, near the orifice of the mitral valve, is considered near the base of the heart (Fig. 25-14). The left ventricle has a short inflow tract from the mitral valve to the trabecular zone that merges with the outflow tract extending to the aortic valve. Unlike the right side of the heart (where there is no continuity between the tricuspid and pulmonary valves), the anterior leaflet of the mitral valve is continuous with the posterior aortic wall, and the left side of the interventricular septum is continuous with the anterior aortic wall.

The left ventricle has several wall segments that can be recognized in relation to their surrounding structures. The medial wall is formed by the ventricular septum. The lateral wall, posterior wall, posterior-basal wall, and apex are all formed by their relative locations in the heart. The lateral wall is covered with trabeculae, which are finer and more numerous than those found in the right ventricle.

As mentioned previously, the wall of the ventricle is composed of three layers: the endocardium, the myocardium, and the epicardium. This wall thickness is two to three times greater than the thickness of the right ventricular wall due to the increased pressures in the left ventricular cavity.

Interventricular septum

The septum is somewhat triangular in shape, with its apex corresponding to the apex of the heart and its base fusing posteriorly and superiorly with the atrial septum. The

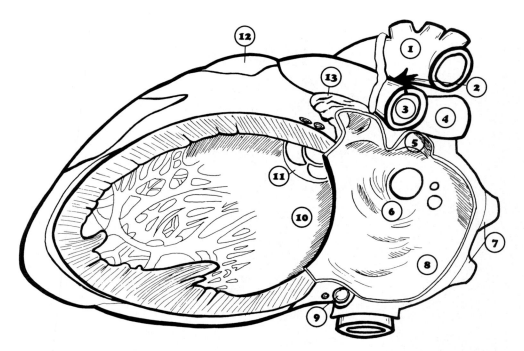

FIG. 25-13. Posterolateral view of the left atrium and ventricle. Aortic arch, *1;* ligamentum arteriosum, *2;* left pulmonary artery, *3;* right pulmonary artery, *4;* left superior pulmonary vein, *5;* valve of the foramen ovale, *6;* right pulmonary veins, *7;* left atrium, *8;* coronary sinus, *9;* mitral valve (cut away), *10;* aortic valve, *11;* conus arteriosus, *12;* left auricle, *13.* (From Hagen-Ansert SL: The anatomy workbook, Philadelphia, 1986, JB Lippincott Co.)

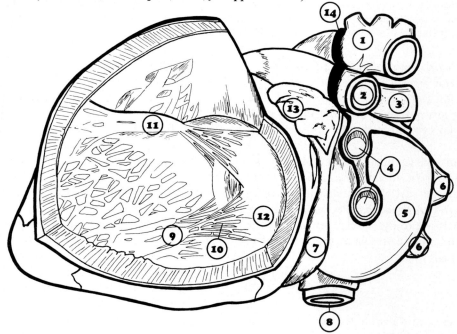

FIG. 25-14. Posterolateral view of the left ventricle. Aortic arch, *1;* left pulmonary artery, *2;* right pulmonary artery, *3;* left pulmonary veins, *4;* left atrium, *5;* right pulmonary veins, *6;* coronary sinus, *7;* inferior vena cava, *8;* posterior papillary muscle, *9;* chordae tendineae, *10;* anterior papillary muscle, *11;* mitral valve, *12;* left auricle, *13;* pericardial reflection, *14.* (From Hagen-Ansert SL: The anatomy workbook, Philadelphia, 1986, JB Lippincott Co.)

ventricular septum is formed of four parts: membranous, inflow, trabecular, and infundibular. These parts arise from the endocardial cushions, the primitive ventricle, and the bulbous cordis. The membranous septum varies in size and shape. It merges into the tissue at the aortic root and infundibular septum, but is sharply demarcated from the muscular portion of the septum.

Most of the interventricular septum is muscular and thicker than the membranous portion of the septum (Fig.

25-15). The muscular septum comprises about two thirds of the septal length, with the membranous septum located just inferior to the aortic root in the area of the left ventricular outflow tract. Most interventricular septal defects occur in this thin, membranous part of the septum.

The muscular septum consists of two layers, a thin layer on the right side and a thicker layer on the left side. The major septal arteries run between these layers. The muscular portion of the septum has approximately the

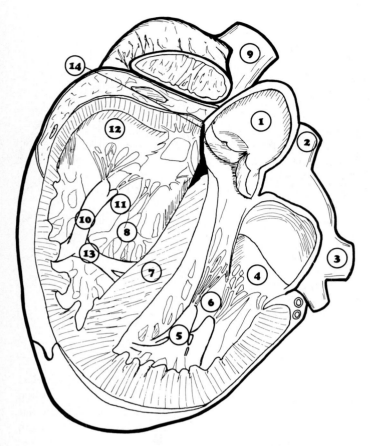

FIG. 25-15. Parasagittal long axis view of the interventricular septum. Ascending aorta, *1;* right pulmonary vein, *2;* left pulmonary vein, *3;* mitral valve, *4;* posterior papillary muscle, *5;* left ventricle, *6;* muscular interventricular septum, *7;* right posterior papillary muscle, *8;* superior vena cava, *9;* septal band, *10;* right ventricle, *11;* tricuspid valve, *12;* moderator band, *13;* membranous interventricular septum, *14.* (From Hagen-Ansert SL: The anatomy workbook, Philadelphia, 1986, JB Lippincott Co.)

same thickness as the left ventricular wall. (In patients with concentric hypertrophy, the septal wall and posterior ventricular wall thicken symmetrically, whereas in patients with hypertrophic cardiomyopathy there is asymmetric septal thickening).

Mitral valve

The mitral valve separates the left atrium from the left ventricle. It consists of two large principle leaflets (anterior and posterior) and two small commissural cusps (which usually merge with the posterior leaflet). The anterior leaflet is much longer and larger than the posterior leaflet. It projects downward into the left ventricular cavity. The leaflets are thick membranes that are trapezoidal with fine irregular edges (Fig. 25-16). They originate from the *anulus fibrosus* and are attached to the papillary muscles by *chordae tendineae.* The functions of the chordae tendineae are to prevent the opposing borders of the leaflets from inverting into the atrial cavity, to act as mainstays of the valves, and to form bands or foldlike structures that may contain muscle.

Aortic valve

The aortic valve lies at the root of the aorta and has three cusps: right, left, and posterior (or noncoronary) (Fig. 25-17). The wall of the aorta bulges slightly at each cusp to form the sinus of Valsalva. The main coronary arteries arise from the right and left coronary cusp. At the center of each cusp is a small fibrous nodule, *Arantius's nodule,* which aids in preventing leakage of blood from the left ventricle when the aortic cusps are closed. Often it becomes the site of calcification in patients in whom arteriosclerosis develops.

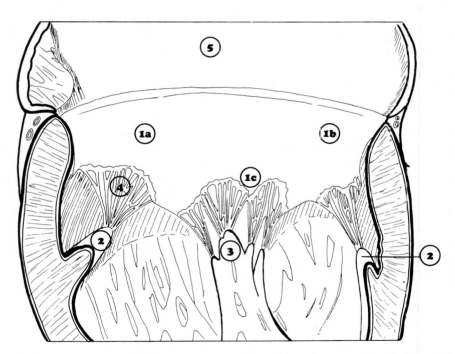

FIG. 25-16. Anatomy of the mitral valve. Mitral valve, *1;* anterior cusp, *1a;* posterior cusp, *1b;* commissural cusps, *1c;* anterior papillary muscle, *2;* posterior papillary muscle, *3;* chordae tendineae, *4;* left atrium, *5.* (From Hagen-Ansert SL: The anatomy workbook, Philadelphia, 1986, JB Lippincott Co.)

FIG. 25-17.   Three cusps of the aortic valve. Ascending aorta, *1;* aortic valve, *2;* left cusp, *2a;* posterior cusp, *2b;* right cusp, *2c;* orifice of the left coronary artery, *3;* anterior mitral valve leaflet, *4;* muscular interventricular septum, *5;* membranous septum, *6;* interventricular part, *6a;* artioventricular part, *6b;* orifice of the right coronary artery, *7;* aortic sinuses of Valsalva, *8.* (From Hagen-Ansert SL: The anatomy workbook, Philadelphia, 1986, JB Lippincott Co.)

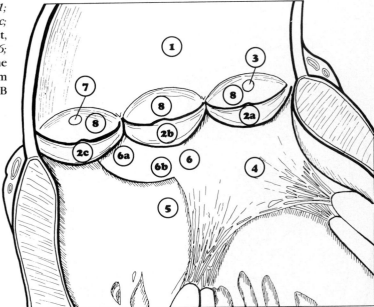

THE CARDIAC CYCLE

The heart is a muscular pump that propels blood to all parts of the body. It is able to act in definite strokes or beats and in the normal adult beats 70 times per minute on the average. The cardiac cycle is the series of changes that the heart undergoes as it fills with blood and empties. Rhythmic contraction of the heart causes blood to be pumped through the chambers of the heart and out through the great vessels. The forceful contraction of the cardiac chambers is "systole," and the relaxed phase of the cycle is "diastole."

We shall consider the systematic events of the heart beat starting from the diastolic phase, when the muscle is relaxed. During this phase venous blood enters the right atrium from the superior and inferior venae cavae. At the same time the oxygenated blood returns from the lungs through the pulmonary veins to enter the left atrium. At this point the atrioventricular valves (tricuspid and mitral) between the atria and ventricles are open so the blood may flow from the atria into the ventricles. The next phase allows atrial contraction to squeeze the remaining blood from the atria into the ventricles. The combination of atrial contraction and increased pressure of the full atrial cavities ultimately drains the atrial blood into the ventricles.

Shortly after this phase the ventricles contract (ventricular systole). The rising pressure in the ventricular cavity closes the atrioventricular valves. As the pressure increases in the ventricles, the semilunar valves (pulmonary and aortic) open so that blood can be forced into the lungs and body, respectively.

The ventricles relax when contraction is completed (ventricular diastole). The blood in the aorta is under very high pressure, and the decreased pressure in the ventricles would cause it to flow backward into the ventricle. However, the semilunar valves prevent this reverse flow. The blood fills the sinuses of Valsalva and forces the valves to close. During ventricular contraction the atria relax and the venous blood starts to fill them again. When the ventricles are completely relaxed, the atrioventricular valves open and blood flows into the ventricles to begin the next cardiac cycle.

Heart valves

Surface anatomy (Fig. 25-18). The tricuspid valve lies behind the right half of the sternum opposite the fourth intercostal space. The mitral valve lies behind the left half of the sternum opposite the fourth costal cartilage. The pulmonary valve lies behind the medial end of the third left costal cartilage and the adjoining part of the sternum. The aortic valve lies behind the left half of the sternum opposite the third intercostal space.

Auscultation. Heart sounds are associated with the initiation of ventricular systole, closing of the atrioventricular valves, and opening of the semilunar valves (Fig. 25-19).

The first sound is lower in pitch and longer in duration than the second. Both sounds can be heard over the entire area of the heart, but the first sound, "lubb," is heard most clearly in the region of the apex of the heart.

The second sound, "dupp," is sharper and shorter and has a higher pitch. It is heard best over the second right rib, for the aorta approaches nearest the surface at this point. The second sound is caused mainly by the closing of the semilunar valves during ventricular diastole. Following the second sound there is a period of silence. Thus the sequence sounds like this—lubb, dupp, silence, lubb, dupp, silence, and so on.

Defects in the valves can cause excessive turbulence or regurgitation of the blood. These are extra abnormal sounds and are called murmurs or clicks. If the valves fail to close tightly and blood leaks back, a hissing murmur is heard. The hissing sound is heard in the area of the affected valve; thus if the mitral valve is affected, it will be

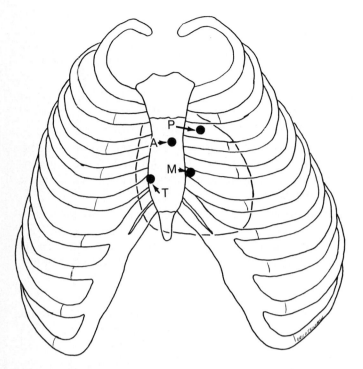

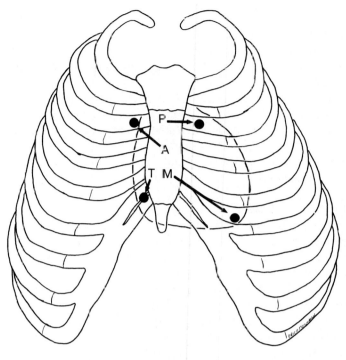

FIG. 25-18. Surface anatomy of the four cardiac valves. *P,* pulmonic valve; *A,* aortic valve; *M,* mitral valve; *T,* tricuspid valve. (From Hagen-Ansert SL: The anatomy workbook, Philadelphia, 1986, JB Lippincott Co.)

FIG. 25-19. The valve opening and closing sounds may be heard best with the least interference at the location of the *arrows.* (From Hagen-Ansert SL: The anatomy workbook, Philadelphia, 1986, JB Lippincott Co.)

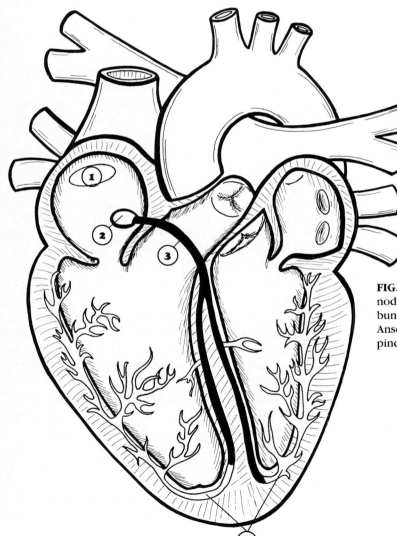

FIG. 25-20. Electrical conducting system of the heart. Sinus node, *1;* atrioventricular node, *2;* penetrating atrioventricular bundle (bundle of His), *3;* Purkinje fibers, *4.* (From Hagen-Ansert SL: The anatomy workbook, Philadelphia, 1986, JB Lippincott Co.)

heard in the first sound. Another condition giving rise to an abnormal sound is stenosis or stiffening of a valve orifice. In this case a rumble is heard in the area of the affected valve.

It is beyond the scope of this text to present an in-depth approach to auscultation, and the reader is referred to the Bibliography for additional reading on this subject. An understanding of auscultation will help in understanding the cardiac physiology and echocardiographic differential diagnosis.

Electrocardiography

Upon stimulation of a muscle or nerve, the cell membranes are depolarized, and on recovery they are repolarized. These electrical events are spread throughout the body and can be detected with suitable instruments applied to the skin surface at considerable distances from the sites of origin. The study of the heart's electrical activity is termed electrocardiography.

The electrodes (or leads) are made of metal and are slightly concave so as to make good contact with the skin in the regions of the wrists and ankles. A gel containing an electrolyte is rubbed over the surface of the skin to facilitate conduction of the impulse from the skin through the electrode attached at this area to the machine.

In echocardiography examinations lead 1 is used for the ECG tracing. An ECG lead is attached to the patient's right and left wrists, with a ground on the ankle. The ECG has three components: P, QRS, and T waves.

P wave. The impulse is initiated by the sinoatrial (SA) node and spreads over the atria. The P wave represents the electrical activity associated with the spread of the impulse over the atria (i.e., the wave of depolarization or activity of the atria).

QRS complex. The wave of depolarization spreads from the SA node over the bundle branches (His) and Purkinje system to activate both ventricles simultaneously. The QRS complex is the result of all electrical activity occurring in the ventricles (Fig. 25-20).

P-R interval. This is measured from the beginning of the P wave to the beginning of the QRS complex. It indicates the time that elapses between activation of the SA node and activation of the AV node.

T wave. This represents ventricular repolarization.

SUMMARY

1. The thoracic cavity lies within the thorax and is separated from the abdominal cavity by the diaphragm.

2. The junction between the manubrium and the body of the sternum is a prominent ridge; together they form the angle of Louis.

3. The lungs are enclosed by the pleural sac. The internal layer, or visceral pleural, is adherent to each lobe of the lung. The external layer, or parietal pleura, is adherent to the inner surface of the chest wall, diaphragm, and mediastinum.

4. The costophrenic sinus is the pleural reflection between the costal and diaphragmatic portions of the parietal pleura.

5. The mediastinum is a movable, thick structure and extends superiorly to the thoracic inlet and the root of the neck and inferiorly to the diaphragm.

6. The heart lies obliquely in the chest, posterior to the sternum, with the greater portion of its muscular mass lying slightly to the left of midline.

7. The right atrium forms the right border to the heart, and the left border is formed by the left ventricle and atrium. The left ventricle forms the apex of the heart.

8. The heart and roots of the great vessels lie within the pericardial sac. This is a double sac: fibrous pericardium and serous pericardium. The serous pericardium is divided into parietal and visceral layers.

9. The reflection of the serous pericardium around the pulmonary veins form the recess of the oblique sinus. The transverse sinus lies between the reflection of serous pericardium around the aorta and pulmonary arteries and between the reflection around the pulmonary veins.

10. The chambers of the heart are lined by three layers: the endocardium, myocardium, and epicardium.

11. The musculature of the atria is very thin in comparision to the ventricular wall mass. Their primary purpose is filling chambers. The ventricular muscle mass is much greater, with the left ventricle having the greatest mass.

12. In the right atrium the superior vena cava enters the upper posterior border, and the inferior vena cava enters the lower posterior lateral border. The medial wall is formed by the interatrial septum. Just superior and in front of the opening of the inferior vena cava lies a shallow depression, the fossa ovalis. The inferior vena cava is guarded by a fold of tissue called the Eustachian valve.

13. The base of the right ventricle lies on the diaphragm, whereas the roof is formed by the crista supraventricularis. The ventricle is divided into two parts: the posteroinferior inflow portion and the anterosuperior outflow portion. The demarcation between these two parts is by a number of prominent bands.

14. The tricuspid valve separates the right atrium from the right ventricle. The three leaflets are attached by their bases to the fibrous atrioventricular ring. The chordae tendineae attach the leaflets to the papillary muscles.

15. The pulmonary valve lies at the upper anterior aspect of the right ventricle. It has three cusps. The wall of the pulmonary artery bulges adjacent to each cusp to form the sinuses of Valsalva. The pulmonary trunk bifurcates into the right and left pulmonary arteries.

16. The left atrium is a smooth-walled circular sac that lies posterior in the base of the heart. Two pulmo-

nary veins enter posteriorly on either side of the cavity.

17. The left ventricle is conical or egg-shaped. The short inflow tract from the mitral valve to the trabecular zone merges with the outflow tract extending to the aortic valve. The anterior leaflet of the mitral valve is continuous with the posterior aortic wall. The left side of the interventricular septum is continuous with anterior aortic wall.

18. The ventricular septum is formed of four parts: membranous, inflow, trabecular, and infundibular. Most of the septum is muscular and thicker than the membranous portion of the septum.

19. The mitral valve separated the left atrium from the left ventricle. The two leaflets originate from the anulus fibrosus and are attached to the papillary muscles by chordae tendineae.

20. The aortic valve lies at the root of the aorta and has three cusps. The sinus of Valsalva is located at the bulge of each cusp. The main coronary arteries arise from the right and left coronary cusp.

21. The cardiac cycle is the series of changes the heart undergoes as it fills with blood and empties. The forceful contraction of the cardiac chambers is systole, and the relaxed phase of the cycle is diastole.

22. Heart sounds (auscultation) are associated with the initiation of ventricular systole, closing of the atrioventricular valves, and opening of the semilunar valves. Defects in the valves can cause excessive turbulence or regurgitation of the blood (called murmurs or clicks).

23. Electrocardiography is the study of the heart's electrical activity. An ECG lead is attached to three points on the patient's body. The ECG has three components: P wave, QRS complex, and the T wave, which all correspond to different phases of diastole and systole.

26

Echocardiographic Techniques and Evaluation

The evaluation of cardiac structures by echocardiography has many important parameters that must be fully understood and used in daily practice. Previously M-mode (time-motion mode) echocardiography had been employed and regarded as an essential diagnostic tool for the practice of cardiology. The reason for its widespread use was its noninvasive, reproducible, and accurate assessment of cardiac structures in the evaluation of cardiac disease. The M-mode technique is limited, however, in that it provides only a one-dimensional or "icepick" view of the heart. The advent of two-dimensional echocardiography has allowed cardiac structures to be visualized in a real-time fashion. Thus observation of contractility, assessment of intracardiac lesions, and the estimation of valvular function can all now be accomplished by the echocardiographer. The combination two-dimensional and M-mode studies provides an extremely accurate means of evaluating wall thickness, valvular orifice and chamber size, and contractility of the left ventricle.

To perform a diagnostic echocardiogram examination the sonographer must be aware of anatomic and pathophysiologic parameters of the heart as well as understand the physical principles of sonography. These parameters will be discussed relative to M-mode and two-dimensional techniques. The standard M-mode examination will be presented first and followed by the evaluation of the heart by combined two-dimensional and M-mode techniques.

TRANSDUCERS

Several types of transducers are available for echocardiographic techniques. Ideally one should use as high a fre-quency as possible to improve the resolution of returning echoes. However, the higher the frequency, the less the penetration; therefore compromises will have to be made in an effort to obtain the best possible image.

Many adult echocardiographers use a 3.5 MHz transducer with a medium focus. The larger patient may require a 2.25 MHz transducer while a barrel-chested, emphysematous patient will need a 1.6 MHz transducer. The pediatric patient generally requires a 5.0 or a 7.5 MHz transducer for improved resolution and near-field definition.

Although many transducers are internally focused to improve resolution by shaping the beam and reducing distortion, most cardiac transducers are of medium focus to concentrate the maximum resolution in the area of the mitral valve.

The smaller crystal or diameter of the transducer allows better skin contact between the rib interspaces and also gives more freedom to "sweep the beam." Thus the transducer remains in one interspace, but the beam angle is swept obliquely from the right shoulder to the left hip to record cardiac structures.

Specially designed transducers may be advantageous, depending on the specific examination required. An aspiration transducer may be useful in the localization of pericardial effusion for pericardiocentesis. This transducer has a single crystal with a permanent hole drilled in the center for needle placement. The transducer may be gas sterilized and thus held over the area of interest to permit accurate placement of the needle within the pericardial sac. The other special transducer is a small suprasternal crystal

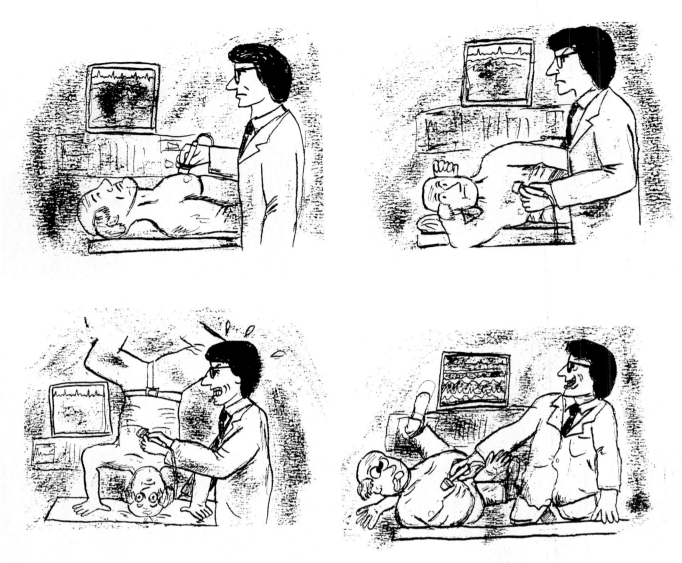

FIG. 26-1. Sometimes the cardiac sonographer thinks it is impossible to find the correct cardiac window in the standard position; however, with moderate manipulations, success will be obtained. (Illustration by Richard E. Rae.)

that is angled approximately 45 to 90 degrees to just fit into the suprasternal notch. This transducer is useful for evaluating the left atrium, the pulmonary veins, the left brachial cephalic vein, the ascending aorta, or for the detection of a dissecting aneurysm in the aortic arch, or the presence of left atrial thrombi.

DISPLAY OF NORMAL HEART PATTERNS

The patient is generally examined in the supine or left lateral semidecubitus position (Fig. 26-1). The cardiac window is usually found between the third to fifth intercostal space, slightly to the left of the sternal border. The cardiac window may be considered that area on the anterior chest where the heart is just beneath the skin surface, free of lung interference (Fig. 26-2). With initial high gain settings we have found it more advantageous to cover a larger area along the sternal border in the search for typical echocardiographic patterns in an effort to determine which intercostal space is the best window. When the transducer is placed along the left sternal border, the examiner should "run" the transducer up and down (be-

tween the third to fifth intercostal spaces) the chest wall to define the pericardial echo with the strongest or loudest echo reflection. After the pericardium is defined, one can search for the mitral and aortic valve patterns and determine which interspace is best for demonstrating the continuity of the cardiac structures.

The cardiac sonographer must keep in mind that different body shapes will require variations in transducer position. An obese patient may have a transverse heart, and thus a slight lateral movement from the sternal border may be needed to record cardiac structures. A thin patient may have a long and slender heart, requiring a lower, more medial transducer position. Barrel-chested patients may present with echographic difficulties because of the lung absorption interference. It may be necessary to turn these patients completely on their left side or even prone to eliminate this lung interference. Sometimes the upright or slightly "bent-forward" position is useful in forcing the heart closer to the anterior chest wall.

The following techniques are guidelines for the aver-

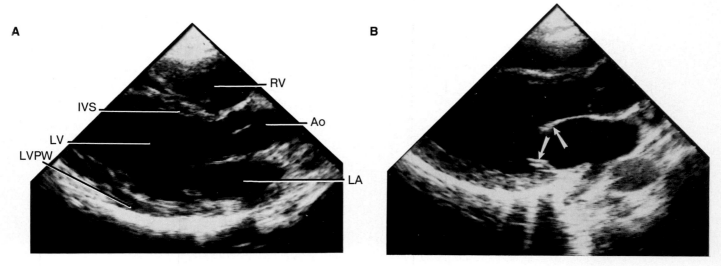

FIG. 26-2. **A,** Generally it is best to localize the maximum excursion of the mitral leaflet by the cardiac sweep from the left ventricle to the aortic leaflet area. The tip of the mitral valve is seen in early diastole just before the minor axis of the left ventricle is visualized. *RV,* right ventricle; *IVS,* interventricular septum; *Ao,* aorta; *LV,* left ventricle; *LA,* left atrium; *LVPW,* left ventricular posterior wall. **B,** The mitral valve has fully opened and is starting to close in mid-diastole.

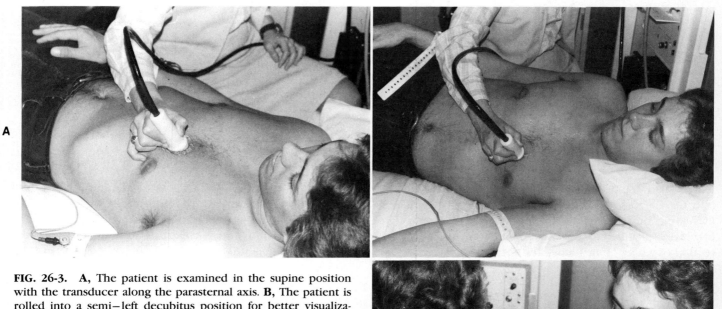

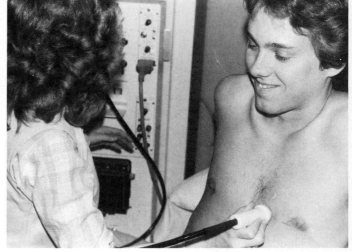

FIG. 26-3. **A,** The patient is examined in the supine position with the transducer along the parasternal axis. **B,** The patient is rolled into a semi–left decubitus position for better visualization of the cardiac structures along the parasternal axis. **C,** An alternate view is the upright position. In some patients this view permits the cardiac structures to fall against the chest wall and thus avoid lung-air interference.

age patient. In the initial echocardiographic study, moving the transducer freely along the left sternal border until all the cardiac structures are easily identified is a better practice than restricting it to one interspace. This saves time and gives the examiner a better understanding of cardiac relationships. If there is difficulty examining the patient in the supine position, a semidecubitus position should be used (Fig. 26-3). Sometimes, if the heart is actually very medial, the best study is performed with the patient completely on the left side. If too much lung interference clouds the study, the patient should exhale for as long as possible. This will usually give the examiner enough time to record pieces of a valid study.

The gain or power settings are usually increased for the initial search period and then decreased to obtain a clear tracing. The highest gain will be used in the area of the left ventricle and mitral valve, with the more anterior structures such as the aorta, tricuspid, and pulmonary valves requiring less gain. Table 26-1 contains approximate locations and characteristics of intracardiac structures as seen by M-mode echocardiography.

Normal mitral valve

The bicuspid atrioventricular valve located between the left atrium and left ventricle is the mitral valve. The posterior leaflet of the mitral valve is continuous with the endocardial layer of the left atrial wall, while the anterior leaflet of the mitral valve is continuous with the posterior wall of the aortic root. The mitral ring or anulus is the superior border of the valvular structure, and the multiple sail-like chordae tendineae attach the anterior and posterior leaflets to the papillary muscle of the left ventricular heart wall.

Echographically, the mitral valve is one of the easiest cardiac structures to recognize. The transducer should be directed perpendicular to the patient's chest wall, slightly away from the left sternal border, in approximately the fourth intercostal space. With proper gain settings, the M-mode tracings are often the most sensitive recorder of initial mitral valve motion. The cardiac sonographer may recognize the initial echo of the right ventricular wall, the echo-free cavity of the right ventricular cavity, the anterior and posterior walls of the interventricular septum, and, finally, the mitral valve apparatus as shown in the left atrial or left ventricular cavity (depending on transducer angulation) (Fig. 26-4). The mitral valve pattern is usually seen 6 to 9 cm from the patient's skin surface. It has the greatest amplitude and excursion and can be unquestionably recognized by its "double" or biphasic kick. This is caused by the initial opening of the valve in ventricular diastole and the atrial contraction at end diastole.

As diastole beings, the anterior mitral leaflet executes a rapid anterior motion, coming to a peak at point "e." As the ventricle fills rapidly with blood from the left atrium, the valve drifts closed at point "f." The rate at which this movement takes place represents the rate of left atrial emptying and serves as an important indicator of altered mitral function. As the left atrium contracts, the mitral valve opens in a shorter anterior excursion and terminates at "a" point, which occurs just after the "P" wave on the electrocardiogram. This is followed by a rapid posterior movement from point "b" to point "c," which coincides with the QRS systolic component on the electrocardiogram produced by the left ventricular contractility closing the valve.

Normal aortic valve and left atrium

The aorta has many subdivisions as it leaves the left ventricle. The base of this vessel is the aortic root, which has three cusps to prohibit a free flow of blood to the rest of the body. The ascending aorta arises from the aortic root and begins its posterior descent at the arch of the aorta (Fig. 26-5). The descending aorta then proceeds posteriorly to pierce the diaphragm and enter the abdominal cavity.

To examine the aortic root, semilunar cusps, and left atrial cavity, the transducer should be directed cephalad toward the right shoulder, from the landmark area of the mitral valve (Fig. 26-6). The cardiac sonographer should be able to identify the anterior leaflet of the mitral valve blending with the posterior aortic wall at the same time as the interventricular septum blends into the anterior aortic wall. Often there is a double parallel echo appearance along the anterior and posterior aortic walls, denoting wall thickness. Care should be taken to record both wall echoes to ensure proper measurement of the aortic root dimensions. Adjustment of the near-gain control allows excellent visualization of the anterior wall. The echoes recorded from the aortic root should be parallel, moving anteriorly in systole and posteriorly in diastole.

As the transducer is angled slightly medial, two of the three semilunar cusps can be visualized. On M-mode tracings, the right coronary cusp is shown anterior and the noncoronary cusp posterior (Fig. 26-7). When seen, the left coronary cusp is shown in the midline between the other two cusps. The onset of systole causes the cusps to open to the full extent of the aortic root. The extreme force of blood through this opening causes fine flutter to occur during systole. As the pressure relents in the ventricle, the cusps begin to drift to a closed position until they are fully closed in diastole.

Chang[1] states that the anterior "humping" of the aortic valve following its closure is a common occurrence in patients with efficient cardiac outputs. It may be a total displacement of the aortic root anteriorly following systolic completion and does not seem to denote an abnormality.

The chamber posterior to the aortic root is the left atrium, which can be recognized by its immobile posterior wall. As one sweeps from the mitral apparatus medially and superiorly, the left ventricular wall blends into the atrioventricular groove and finally into the left atrial wall (Fig. 26-8). Thus the sweep demonstrates good contractility in the left ventricle, with anterior wall motion in systole to the atrioventricular area where the posterior wall starts to move posteriorly in systole, and then to the left atrium, where there is no movement.

Sometimes it is possible to record the left pulmonary vein within the left atrial cavity. This appears as a thin,

Table 26-1 Approximate Locations of Intracardiac Structures

Structure	Distance from transducer (cm)	Transducer position	Characteristics
Posterior heart wall (PW)	9 to 12	Usually found in third, fourth, and fifth interspace with transducer directed perpendicular to chest wall	Strong pulsating echo complex Pericardium strongest reflection in cardiac cavity Three layers of posterior heart wall, endocardium, myocardium, epicardium, are seen anterior to pericardium
Anterior leaflet of mitral valve (ALMV)	6 to 9	Transducer perpendicular to chest wall; may need slight medial or lateral angulation	Biphasic kick (M pattern seen on M-mode) Moves at least 2 to 3 cm in A- or M-mode Strong reflector
Posterior leaflet of mitral valve (PLMV)	9 to 10	From ALMV, angle *slightly* inferiorly and laterally (must maintain part of ALMV and watch for "clapping hands" movement of ALMV and PLMV moving opposite one another)	W pattern on M-mode Weak echo (be careful reject is not turned up to wipe out this echo)
Aortic root	4 to 6	From MV, angle transducer superiorly and medially toward right shoulder	Parallel echo movement on A-mode Anterior part of aorta comes off IVS Posterior part of aorta comes off ALMV Normal aortic valve size: 1.2 to 1.9 cm
Cusps		Slight angulations to record cusp movement (may be medial, lateral inferior, or superior); if there is trouble recording noncoronary cusp, move slightly down and laterally or have patient stop breathing; may have to move up an interspace or roll patient to left side to see cusps	Internal echo seen within parallel echo complex on A-mode When both noncoronary and right coronary cusps recorded, box pattern is seen on M-mode Third cusp (left coronary) moves throughout center of box
Tricuspid valve (TV)	2 to 4	From aortic root, angle inferiorly and slightly medially or from MV, angle medially	Similar in appearance to MV (biphasic kick, wide excursion) Because of location under sternal border, difficult to record completely; usually initial opening recorded
Right ventricle (RV)	1 to 3	Right ventricle seen anterior to IVS and MV, aortic root with transducer on left sternal border	Anterior side of RV can be identified as first moving structure beyond crystal artifact and chest wall Posterior surface anterior side of IVS Normal size less than 2 to 3 cm

Structure	Distance from transducer (cm)	Transducer position	Characteristics
Interventricular septum (IVS)	2 to 4	Usually seen with transducer perpendicular to chest wall or angled inferiorly and lateral to MV	Should be able to identify both sides of septum well by using near gain (suppression) and delay; if too many echoes in RV, turn gear gain up; If not enough, turn near gain down (counterclockwise) (delay should be increased until it breaks off at anterior edge of septum) Should equal posterior wall thickness (ratio 1.3:1)
Left ventricular wall (LVW) (endocardium, myocardium, epicardium, pericardium)	9 to 12	Inferior and lateral to ALMV	Extremely important to sweep from ALMV to left ventricle Chordae tendineae may be demonstrated anterior to LVW (appears as denser echo than endocardium and has less excursion); endocardium has characteristic notch Chordae tendineae Endocardium By decreasing gain, three layers of LVW may be demonstrated, with pericardial echo remaining as strongest moving reflection (demonstration of pericardial effusion is done by this method if fluid layer would dampen movement of pericardium)
LV and IVS		Transducer inferior and lateral to ALMV, but may angle slightly superiorly to this position to record IVS (use care to record IVS movement in correct position; when transducer is angled toward aorta, paradoxical motion may be seen)	For LV dimensions important to record IVS and LVW together (in systole they contract, in diastole they relax, and normal movement requires IVS and LVW to move toward one another); conversely, paradoxical septal motion means IVS moving opposite LV in systole
Pulmonary valve (PV)	1 to 3	From aortic root, angle superiorly and laterally toward left shoulder; may have to move up on interspace	Parallel movement on A-mode Cusp echo may be seen within echo complex Usually only posterior cusp seen, which moves posteriorly with systole

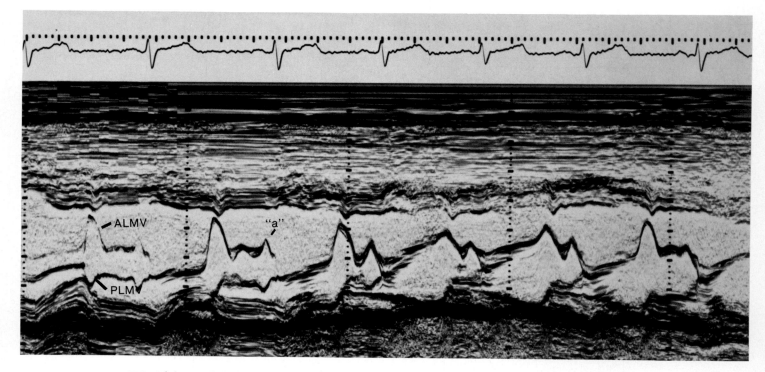

FIG. 26-4. Both leaflets of the mitral valve are clearly seen in this patient. The systolic segment moves slightly anteriorly until diastole begins, which causes the anterior leaflet, *ALMV,* to sweep anteriorly while the posterior leaflet, *PLMV,* dips posteriorly. Atrial contraction gives rise to the smaller *a* kick until the valve closes at end diastole.

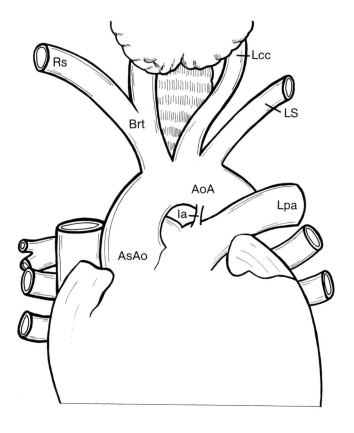

FIG. 26-5. Schema of the ascending aorta with its branch arteries. *Lcc,* left common carotid; *Ls,* left subclavian; *AoA,* aortic arch; *la,* ligamentum arteriosum; *Lpa,* left pulmonary artery; *AsAo,* ascending aorta; *Brt,* brachiocephalic trunk; *Rs,* right subclavian artery. (From Hagen-Ansert SL: The anatomy workbook, Philadelphia, 1986, JB Lippincott Co.)

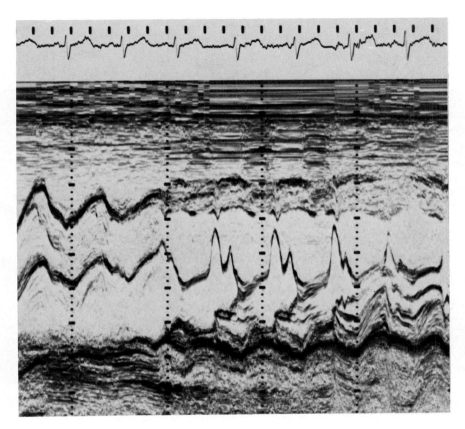

FIG. 26-6.   The anterior wall of the aortic root is continuous with the interventricular septum, and the posterior wall is continuous with the anterior leaflet of the mitral valve.

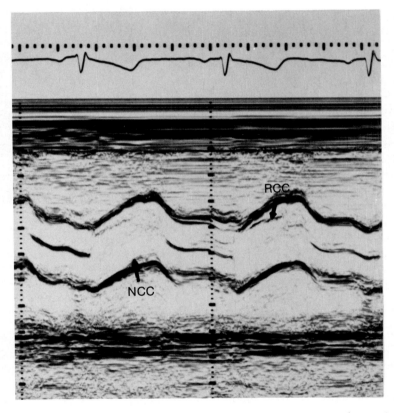

FIG. 26-7.   The right coronary cusp, *RCC,* is the most anterior cusp seen in the aortic sweep, and the noncoronary cusp, *NCC,* is the most posterior. The left coronary cusp is sometimes seen in the middle of the other two cusps.

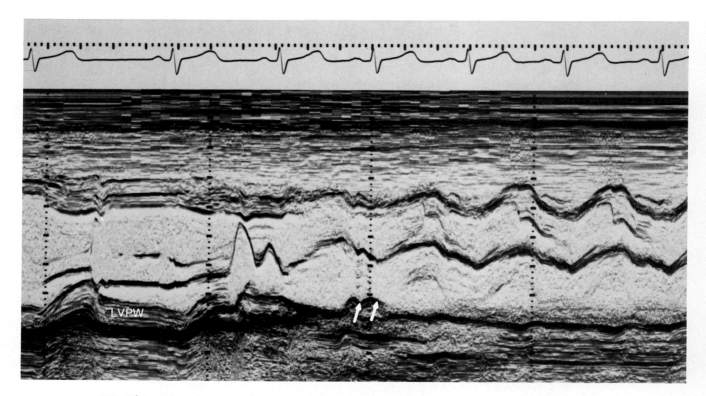

FIG. 26-8.   M-mode sweep from the left ventricle through the mitral valve to the aorta and left atrium demonstrates the changing movement of the posterior wall of the left ventricle, *LVPW,* as it passes the mitral valve at the atrioventricular junction *(arrows).* The left atrial wall should be an immobile line contiguous with the posterior heart wall.

double-walled vessel and can be a problem in determining left atrial measurements. Care should be taken to sweep from the mitral valve to the aortic root and back to the mitral apparatus several times to note the continuity of the posterior ventricular wall to the left atrial wall to avoid confusion. The pulmonary vein will never appear continuous with the left ventricular wall.

Other structures posterior to the left atrial cavity that may lead to confusion in the identification of the left atrial wall are the left atrial appendage and descending aorta. The left atrial appendage may appear very prominent posterior to the left atrial wall if there is severe enlargement of the left atrial cavity (especially seen in patients with severe mitral valve disease). Real-time evaluation with the transducer in the apical four-chamber position will clarify the atrial appendage as a separate structure (Fig. 26-9). The descending aorta may also be recognized as a parallel pulsating tubular structure posterior to the left atrial cavity (Fig. 26-10). The aorta will not be continuous with the left ventricular wall as the left atrial wall is, thus the cardiac sonographer should be able to distinguish this echo reflection as normal anatomy.

Interventricular septum

The interventricular septum divides the right ventricle from the left ventricle. Its right side is contiguous with the anterior aortic root. At this junction the movement of the septum is influenced by the movement of the aorta, and thus it may appear to move abnormally or paradoxically in relation to the posterior heart wall. As the trans-

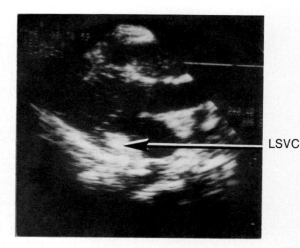

FIG. 26-9.   Other structures that may be misleading when one tries to evaluate the left atrial cavity are the pulmonary veins and a persistent left superior vena cava, *LSVC.* In this patient the "cloud" of echoes within the left atrial cavity is filled with saline that has been injected into the patient's arm. The left superior vena cava quickly fills with saline, followed by saline echoes within the right ventricular cavity.

ducer is angled slightly inferior and lateral to the mitral valve, the septum moves somewhat anteriorly in early systole and posteriorly at the end of systole and early diastole (Fig. 26-11). Both sides of the septum should move symmetrically. If they do not, the transducer should be placed more medial on the chest wall or the patient should be rolled into a slightly steeper decubitus position.

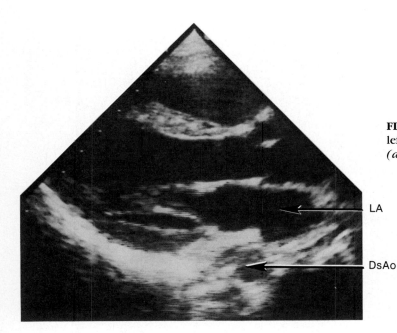

LA

DsAo

FIG. 26-10. The descending aorta, *DsAo*, flows posterior to the left atrial, *LA*, cavity and is shown as a pulsatile tubular structure *(arrow)* on the parasternal long-axis view.

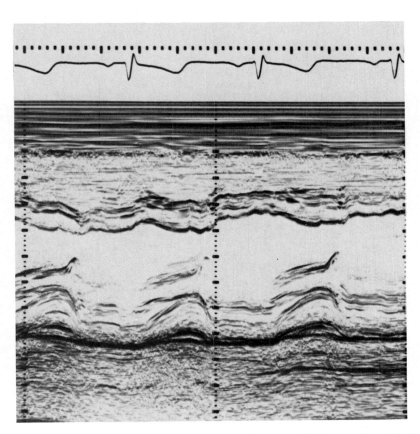

FIG. 26-11. M-mode tracing of a normal septum moving posteriorly at end systole to contract with the posterior left ventricular wall.

Echo reflections from the chordae tendineae of papillary muscle apparatus in the right heart may be mistaken for the right side of the septum, and care should be used to accurately identify the true right side of the septum (Fig. 26-12).

The septum thickens in systole at the midportion of the ventricular cavity. The measurement and evaluation of septal thickness and motion should be made at this point.

Normal septal thickness should match that of the posterior left ventricular wall and not exceed 1.2 cm.

Left ventricle

The determination of left ventricular volume and function may be made with a routine M-mode sweep. The patient is generally examined in the left semidecubitus position to best define septal motion and left ventricular posterior

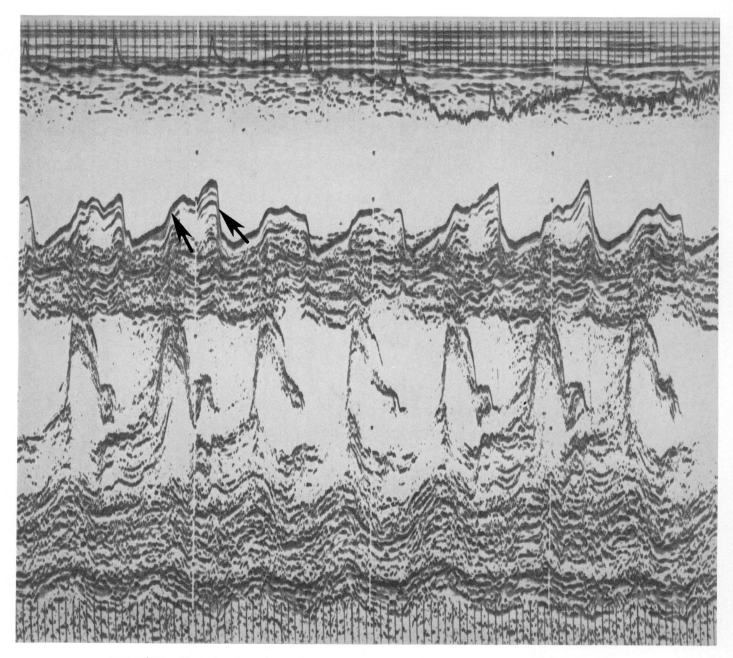

FIG. 26-12.   M-mode of a catheter *(arrows)* within the right ventricle, which makes it difficult to determine the location of the right side of the septum. With careful angulation, the beam can be directed to image the right septal wall more clearly.

wall motion. The anterior leaflet of the mitral valve should first be located and then the beam angled slightly inferior and lateral (toward the left hip) to record the left ventricular chamber. Correct identification of this chamber may be made when both sides of the septum are seen to contract with the posterior heart wall (Fig. 26-13). If the septum is not well defined or does not appear to move well, a more medial placement of the transducer along the sternal border with a lateral angulation may permit better visualization of this structure.

The three layers of the posterior heart wall—endocardium (inner layer), myocardium (middle layer), and epicardium (outer layer)—should be identified separately

from the pericardium (Fig. 26-14). Sometimes it is difficult to separate the epicardium from the pericardium until the gain is reduced. The myocardium usually has a fine scattering of echoes throughout its muscular layer. The endocardium may be a more difficult structure to record since it reflects a very weak echo pattern. Sometimes the multiple chordae tendineae are difficult to separate from the endocardium, and careful evaluation of the posterior wall must be used. The chordae are much denser structures than the endocardium. They generally are shown in the systolic segment along the anterior surface of the endocardium. As the ventricle contracts, the endocardial velocity is greater than the chordae tendineae velocity.

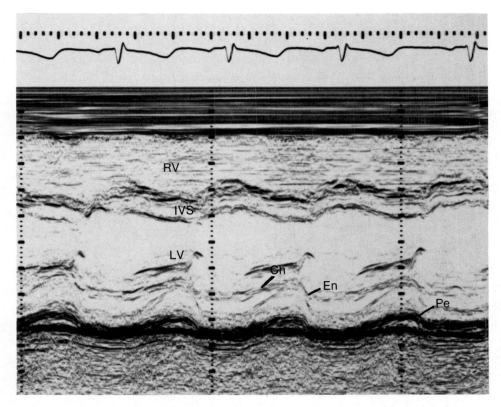

FIG. 26-13. M-mode recording in the left ventricular cavity. *RV,* right ventricle; *IVS,* interventricular septum; *En,* endocardium; *Pe,* pericardium; and *Ch,* chordae.

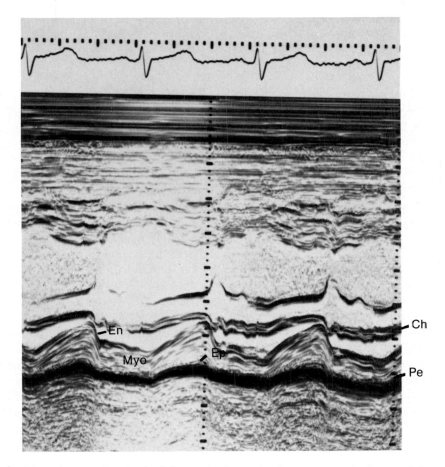

FIG. 26-14. M-mode recording in the left ventricular cavity demonstrates the layers of the posterior heart wall: endocardium, *En,* myocardium *Myo,* epicardium, *Ep,* pericardium, *Pe,* and chordae, *Ch.* The distinction between the endocardium and chordal structures may be made by assessing the velocity of the two structures. The normal endocardial velocity is always much greater than the chordal velocity.

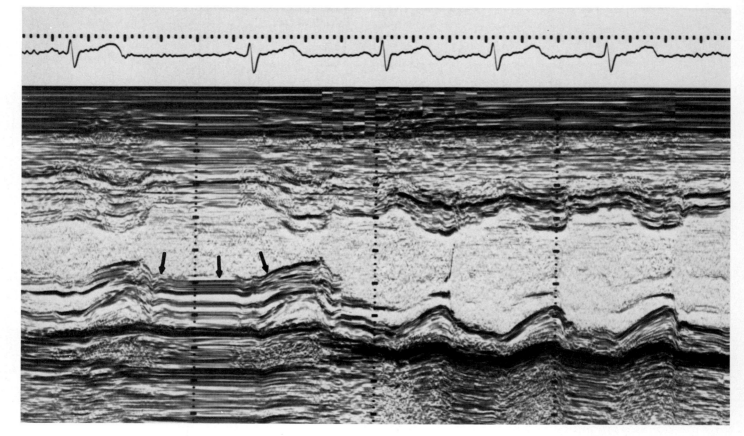

FIG. 26-15. M-mode tracing of the left ventricular cavity. As the beam is swept from the mid-apex of the cavity, the coarse echoes *(arrows)* represent reflections from the papillary muscles and chordal structures anterior to the posterior heart wall.

Small pieces of the mitral apparatus seen in the left ventricle ensure that the correct dimension is being evaluated. Posterior papillary muscles are shown near the apex of the ventricle. These appear as a dense, fuzzy echo band and make it difficult to evaluate the posterior wall clearly (Fig. 26-15). If the ventricular volume is to be determined, these muscles are a clue that the transducer is directed too far inferior to the desired point of measurement and the cavity size would be underestimated.

Right ventricle

The right ventricle is the most anterior chamber of the heart. Its anterior wall may be demonstrated with proper near-gain settings adjusted so the first moving echo shown after the immobile main bang and chest wall echoes represents the right ventricular wall (Fig. 26-16). If this echo is not clearly defined, Popp has suggested an arbitrary measurement of 0.5 cm from the last nonmoving echo to serve as the right ventricular wall for right ventricular size determination. Most ventricular measurements are made in the supine position and thus must be slightly adjusted if the patient is examined in an upright or decubitus position.

Right atrium

The right atrium is best seen on the longitudinal, subcostal, two-dimensional display as the inferior vena cava empties into it (Fig. 26-17). It may also be seen on the parasternal long-axis two-dimensional view as the cardiac sonographer angles the transducer medially from the level of the mitral valve to visualize the right ventricle, tricuspid valve, and right atrial cavity. The apical four-chamber view is another excellent position for evaluating the size of the right atrium.

Often fine linear echoes may be recorded within the right atrial cavity, which most likely represent remnants of the Chiari network (these linear echoes are located near the interatrial septum) and the eustachian valve (the valve found at the exit of the inferior vena cava) (Fig. 26-18).

Normal tricuspid valve

The tricuspid valve is not as easily identified as the mitral valve because of its substernal location in most patients. Recordings are easily made if the right ventricle is slightly enlarged or if the heart is rotated to the left of the sternum. When the transducer has recorded the mitral apparatus, the beam should be angled slightly medially, under the sternum, to record the tricuspid valve (Fig. 26-19). It is fairly easy to identify the whipping motion of the anterior valve in systole and early diastole. However, the complete diastolic period reveals the pathologic changes of stenosis and regurgitation; and careful angulation may allow this phase to be recorded. An alternate method of re-

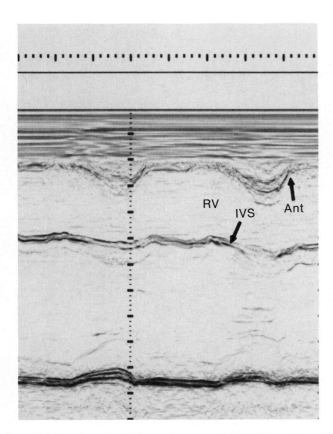

FIG. 26-16. M-mode of the right ventricular, *RV,* cavity with the gain decreased to demonstrate the right side of the anterior heart wall, *Ant,* and the right side of the septum, *IVS.*

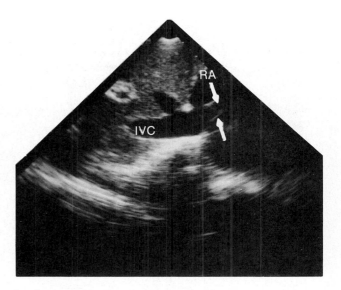

FIG. 26-17. Sagittal image of the inferior vena cave, *IVC,* as it enters into the right atrial cavity, *RA.* The arrows point out the eustachian valve that lies at the junction of the IVC and RA. This valve can be very prominent in some patients.

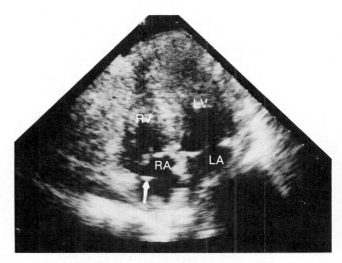

FIG. 26-18. The Chiari network *(arrow)* can be seen within the right atrium, *RA,* and is generally located near the base of the atrium. It can be redundant and "swirl" within the cavity. It can be differentiated from thrombus by its fine, linear type echo pattern (thrombus is usually thicker and fluffier). This apical four-chamber view demonstrates the right atrium, *RA,* right ventricle, *RV,* left atrium, *LA,* and left ventricle, *LV.*

cording the valve is to locate the aortic root. The transducer beam should sweep inferiorly and medially toward the patient's right foot to record the valve leaflet.

Sometimes on M-mode scan it may be confusing to differentiate the tricuspid valve from the pulmonary valve. In the normal person the tricuspid valve is always inferior and medial to the aortic root whereas the pulmonary valve is superior and lateral to the aorta. The other difference is that the tricuspid valve moves anteriorly with atrial contraction while the pulmonary valve dips posteriorly.

Normal pulmonary valve

The pulmonary valve was the last of the four cardiac valves to be adequately visualized by ultrasound. Gramiak and Nanda[4] were the first to document its echographic pattern through the aid of contrast studies. Although it is a semilunar three-cusp valve, only the left or posterior cusp can be adequately demonstrated echocardiographically.

A slow sweep from the aortic valve area, laterally and superiorly toward the left shoulder, should allow visualization of the pulmonary valve area. The parallel aortic echoes serve as a landmark in the sweep to the pulmonary valve. The anterior aortic root forms the posterior boundary of the pulmonary valve area. There should be a 2 to 4 cm space beneath the anterior chest wall and in

front of this posterior border in which to visualize the pulmonary valve. Gramiak[3] identified these posterior structures as the junction of the right ventricular outflow tract with the pulmonary artery and the atriopulmonary sulcus (with the left atrium posterior).

When this structure complex is identified, small adjustments in beam position and direction will usually pass the beam through the left pulmonary valve cusp. The appearance of the cusp is similar to that of the aortic cusp and requires very slight angulations of the beam to demonstrate fully (Fig. 26-20). We have not found it easier to lo-

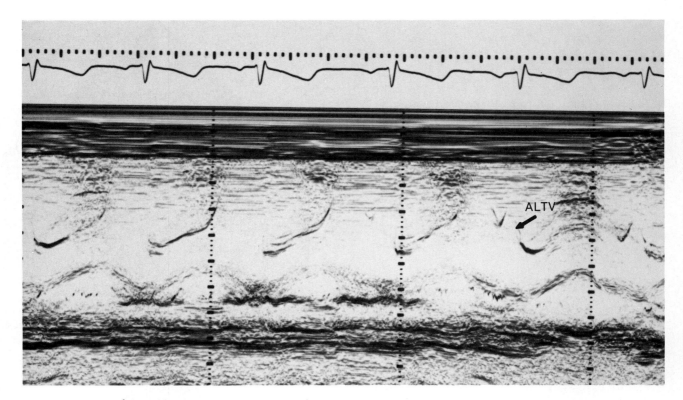

FIG. 26-19. The tricuspid valve in young children, adolescents, and slim adults is easy to record. In most cases the transducer may be held directly over the sternum, or the patient may be rolled into a left decubitus or lateral position to allow the right side of the heart to be viewed. As one sweeps medial and slightly caudal from the mitral valve, the tricuspid valve is demonstrated. *ALTV,* anterior leaflet tricuspid valve.

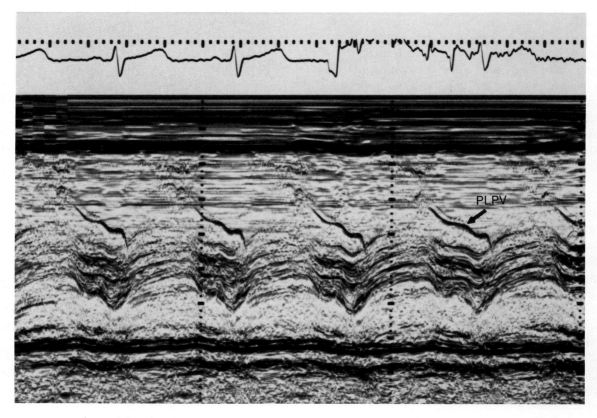

FIG. 26-20. The lateral cephalic angulation from the aortic position is used to record echoes from the pulmonary valve's posterior cusp. *PLPV,* posterior leaflet pulmonary valve.

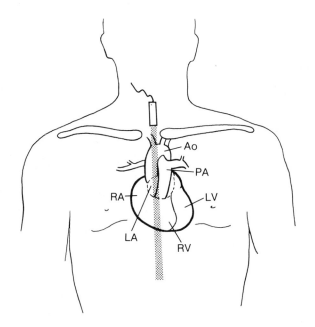

FIG. 26-21.   Schema of the suprasternal approach. The ascending aorta, *Ao,* is anterior to the pulmonary artery, *PA. RA,* right atrium; *RV,* right ventricle; *LA,* left atrium; and *LV,* left ventricle.

cate this valve in one particular position. Generally we search for the cusp with the patient in a semidecubitus position. With two-dimensional capabilities, the optimal view is generally a high-parasternal short-axis view with a slight angulation of the beam toward the left shoulder.

Gramiak[3] described the physiologic parameters as shown on the M-mode echocardiogram. At the beginning of diastole, the pulmonary valve is displaced downward and is represented anteriorly on the ultrasound recording. The low transducer position with upward beam angulation, together with the vertical inclination of the pulmonary ring, results in the examination of the valve from below. All elevations of the pulmonary valve in the stream of flow are represented as posterior movements on the echo. Likewise, downward movements are represented by anterior cusp positions on the trace.

The valve begins to move posteriorly, points *e* to *f,* in a gradual manner as the right ventricle fills in diastole. Atrial systole elevates the valve and produces a 3 to 7 mm posterior movement *a* dip. The valve completes the opening, points *b* and *c,* and at the *c* to *d* point, the valve moves upward with ventricular systole.

Other methods of echocardiographic examination

In a small percentage of the patients scanned, the examiner will not be able to record adequate information from the conventional left sternal approach. This may be a function of lung interference, an unusual angulation of the cardiac structures, or relational pathology surrounding the cardiac structures. Therefore other useful approaches should be employed to obtain the echographic information.

Suprasternal approach. The suprasternal technique was first described by Goldberg.[2] A special angulated transducer is placed in the suprasternal notch with the beam directed caudad toward the aortic arch (Fig. 26-21). The transducer beam passes through the left brachiocephalic artery, aortic arch, right pulmonary artery, and left atrium (Fig. 26-22). This technique has proven useful in the further detection of aneurysmal growth, tumor invasion, and in determining accurate great vessel dimensions.

Subxiphoid approach. Chang[1] first described the subxiphoid approach as an alternative method in the evaluation of cardiac structures obscured by lung tissue. The transducer is directed in a cephalic angulation from the subxiphoid approach (Fig. 26-23). Recordings can then be made of the left ventricular wall, mitral valve, and aortic valve. Although measurements cannot be obtained from this tangential approach and compared with "normal" measurements from the semidecubitus approach, this method has proven a useful technique in ruling out certain cardiac problems such as valvular disease, pericardial effusion, and tumor formation.

EVALUATION OF THE HEART WITH TWO-DIMENSIONAL ECHOCARDIOGRAPHY

The widespread clinic acceptance of the real-life two-dimensional image has tremendously aided the diagnostic results of a typical echocardiographic examination. Improved transducer design, resolution capabilities, focus parameters, gray-scale differentiation, gain control factors, cine loop functions, and other computer capabilities have aided the cardiac sonographer in the attempt to record consistent, high-quality images from the multiple scan planes necessary to obtain a composite image of the cardiac structures. In addition, most two-dimensional transducers have the combined function to image as well as to select one crystal to perform an M-mode or a Doppler study simultaneously. Thus the addition of these functions has increased the accuracy of the M-mode and Doppler

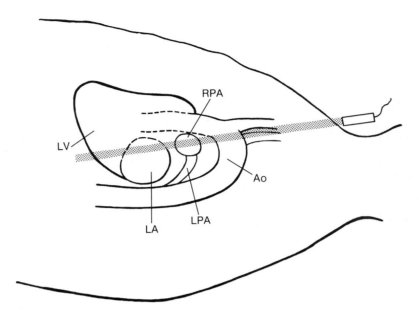

FIG. 26-22. Suprasternal approach demonstrating the aortic arch, *Ao,* right pulmonary artery, *RPA,* left pulmonary artery, *LPA,* left atrium, *LA,* and left ventricle, *LV.*

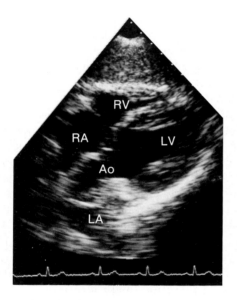

FIG. 26-23. Subxyphoid technique is used for patients with too much lung interference in the conventional echographic approach, or as an alternative window for the apical four-chamber view. *RA,* right atrium; *RV,* right ventricle; *Ao,* aorta; *LA,* left atrium; *LV,* left ventricle.

studies. The ability to actually image the cardiac anatomy has also improved the speed with which an M-mode study can be performed. Most equipment has the capability of computing dimensions of various cardiac structures in either two-dimensional or M-mode. More advanced echocardiographic equipment has the added feature of combined pulsed-wave (PW) and continuous-wave (CW) Doppler capabilities, with the further ability to actually "steer" the CW Doppler beam.

The recent addition of color-flow (CF) Doppler has added a new dimension for the cardiac sonographer in the detection of intracardiac shunt flow, mapping out regurgitant pathways, and in determining obstructive flow pathways. This will be discussed further at the end of this chapter.

Two-dimensional echocardiography

Nomenclature and image orientation. The Committee on Nomenclature and Standards in Two-Dimensional Echocardiography of the American Society of Echocardiography recommends the following nomenclature and image orientation standards for transducer locations:

suprasternal Transducer placed in the suprasternal notch.
subcostal Transducer located near body midline and beneath costal margin.
apical Transducer located over cardiac apex (at the point of maximal impulse) (Fig. 26-24).
parasternal Transducer placed over the area bounded superiorly by left clavicle, medically by sternum, and inferiorly by apical region (Fig. 26-25).
imaging planes These planes are described by the manner in which the two-dimensional transducer transects the heart.
long axis Transects heart perpendicular to dorsal and ventral surfaces of body and parallel with long axis of heart (Fig. 26-26).
short axis Transects heart perpendicular to dorsal and ventral surfaces of body and perpendicular to long axis of heart (Fig. 26-27).
four chamber Transects heart approximately parallel with dorsal and ventral surfaces of body (Fig. 26-28).

Sectional cardiac anatomy

To perform an adequate two-dimensional examination of the heart the cardiac sonographer must have a very good understanding of cardiac anatomy as it is visualized in several different imaging planes. Thus the superficial understanding of cardiac anatomy that was useful in the M-

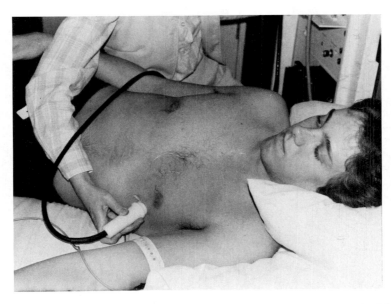

FIG. 26-24. The apical four-chamber view is performed after the posterior maximal impulse, *PMI*, is felt along the far left lateral chest wall. The beam is directed in a sharp cephalic direction to record the four cardiac chambers.

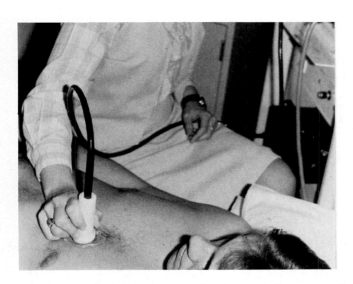

FIG. 26-25. Transducer position for the typical parasternal views of the cardiac structures.

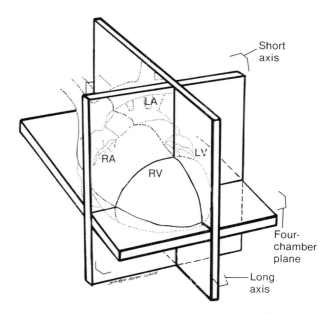

FIG. 26-26. Schema of the parasternal long and short axis, and apical four-chamber views of the heart. *RV,* right ventricle; *RA,* right atrium; *LV,* left ventricle; *LA,* left atrium.

mode examination now is expanded as the two-dimensional examination has become the primary echocardiographic study. The cardiac sonographer should try to spend time in a gross anatomy laboratory to really gain an understanding of the interrelationships within the heart. Most equipment provides excellent resolution and so can image very small coronary arteries and other structures that were not recognized previously by echo.

The following serial cross-sections are taken throughout the thoracic cavity to provide the cardiac sonographer with a basic understanding of cardiac anatomy. One must remember, however, that anatomic sections vary slightly in each person, and thus relationships should be relied on more than particular anatomy seen in a certain section.

Level 1. This section is taken at the level of the fourth thoracic vertebra. The aortic arch is cut along its lower border. The ascending and descending aorta is shown in part. The right and left pulmonary arteries originate in the lower portion of this section. The superior vena cava is shown as it enters the right atrium. The pericardium is reflected to show a portion of the pericardial cavity. The trachea is shown to the right of the mesial plane. The bronchi begin to subdivide in the body of this section (Fig. 26-29).

Level 2. This section is taken at the level of the fifth

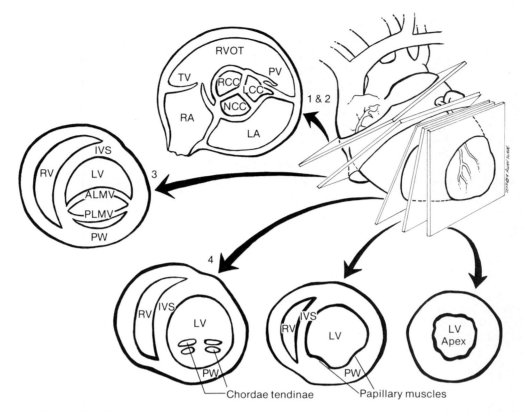

FIG. 26-27. The short-axis plane may be used to evaluate cardiac structures at the level of the right ventricular outflow tract and pulmonary artery; the right ventricle, septum, mitral valve, and left ventricle; the left ventricle, septum, and right ventricle; or at the apex of the ventricle.

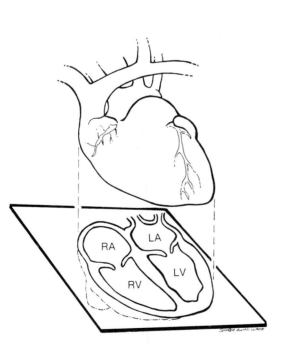

FIG. 26-28. Schema of the apical four chambers of the heart. *RA,* right atrium; *RV,* right ventricle; *LA,* left atrium; *LV,* left ventricle.

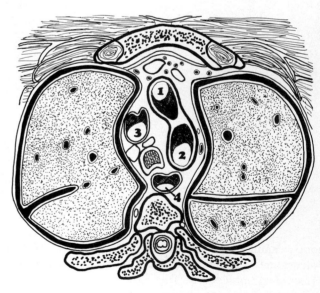

FIG. 26-29. Thoracic cross-section, level 1. This section is taken at the level of the fourth thoracic vertebra. The aortic arch is cut along its lower border. The ascending, *1,* and descending, *2,* aorta is shown in part. The right and left pulmonary arteries originate in the lower portion of this section. The superior vena cava, *3,* is shown as it enters the right atrium. The pericardium is reflected to show a portion of the pericardial cavity. The trachea, *4,* is shown to the right of the mesial plane. The bronchi begin to subdivide in the body of this section. (From Hagen-Ansert SL: The anatomy workbook, Philadelphia, 1986, JB Lippincott Co.)

thoracic disc. The ascending and descending parts of the aorta are shown. The superior vena cava enters the right atrium in the lower portion of this section and the upper portion of level 1. The pulmonary valves are shown in the pulmonary artery. The atrial appendages are seen within this section, as is the conus arteriosus. The trachea has bifurcated, and the bronchi are seen. The esophagus lies in the midline (Fig. 26-30).

Level 3. This section is taken at the upper part of the seventh thoracic vertebra. The right atrium is shown at the entrance of the superior vena cava. The left atrium is shown just below the entrance of the right superior pulmonary vein. The right inferior pulmonary vein enters the atrium within this section. The left superior pulmonary vein is cut at its entrance into the left atrium. The left inferior pulmonary vein enters the left atrium within this section. The foramen ovale is slightly open in the interatrial septum. The aortic valve and the sinuses of Valsalva are shown. The right ventricle shows the chordae tendineae, which are attached to the tricuspid leaflets. The pulmonary valve lies anterior to and to the left of the aortic valve. The mitral valve lies partly in this section and partly in level 2. The right coronary artery is shown as it arises from the right coronary cusp (Fig. 26-31).

Level 4. This section is taken at the level of the eighth thoracic vertebra. The diaphragm extends into the lower portion of this section, and the right and left atria and

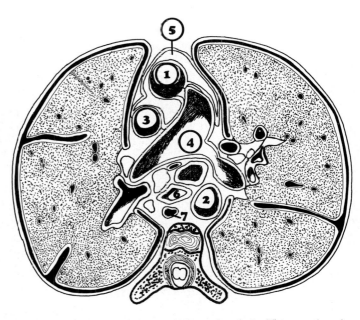

FIG. 26-30. Thoracic cross-section, level 2. This section is taken at the level of the fifth thoracic disc. The ascending, *1,* and descending, *2,* aorta is shown. The superior vena cava, *3,* enters the right atrium in the lower portion of this section and the upper portion of level 1. The pulmonary valves are shown in the pulmonary artery, *4.* The conus arteriosus is seen, *5.* The esophagus, *6,* and azygos vein, *7,* are shown anterior to the spine. (From Hagen-Ansert SL: The anatomy workbook, Philadelphia, 1986, JB Lippincott Co.)

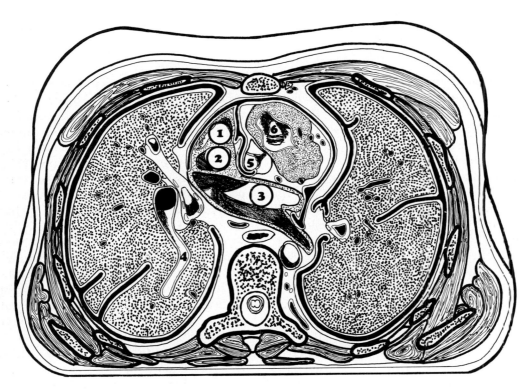

FIG. 26-31. Thoracic cross-section, level 3. This section is taken at the upper part of the seventh thoracic vertebra. The right atrium, *1,* is shown at the entrance of the superior vena cava, *2.* The left atrium, *3,* is seen just below the entrance of the right superior pulmonary vein, *4.* The right inferior pulmonary vein enters the atrium within this section. The left superior pulmonary vein is cut at its entrance into the left atrium. The foramen ovale is slightly open in the interatrial septum. The aortic valve, *5,* and sinuses of Valsalva are shown. The right ventricle, *6,* shows chordae tendineae, which are attached to the tricuspid leaflets. The mitral valve lies partly in this section and partly in level 2. (From Hagen-Ansert SL: The anatomy workbook, Philadelphia, 1986, JB Lippincott Co.)

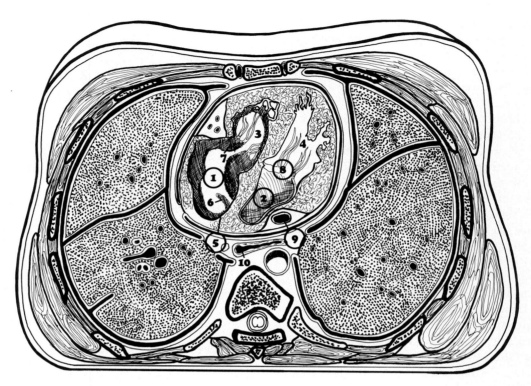

FIG. 26-32. Thoracic cross-section, level 4. This section is taken at the level of the eighth thoracic vertebra. This diaphragm extends into the lower portion of this section, and the right, *1,* and left, *2,* atria and ventricle, *3* and *4,* are shown as is the opening of the inferior vena cava, *5,* into the right atrium. The eustachian valve, *6,* of the orifice of the inferior vena cava can be seen. The tricuspid valve, *7,* and mitral valve, *8,* are both shown as they separate the atria from the ventricular chambers. The coronary sinus, *9,* opens into the right atrium at the *arrow.* The esophagus, *10,* is shown slightly to the left of midline. (From Hagen-Ansert SL: The anatomy workbook, Philadelphia, 1986, JB Lippincott Co.)

ventricles are shown, as is the opening of the inferior vena cava into the right atrium. The eustachian valve of the orifice of the inferior vena cava can be seen. The tricuspid valve and mitral valves are both shown as they separate the atria from the ventricular chambers. The coronary sinus opens into the right atrium at the arrow. The esophagus is shown slightly to the left of midline (Fig. 26-32).

Level 5. This section is taken at the level of the ninth intervertebral disc. The pleural surface of the diaphragm is seen on the right. On the left, oblique fibers of the diaphragm are shown. The right atrium and left ventricles are seen. The pericardium, epicardium, and pericardial cavity are shown. The hepatic vein is shown to enter the inferior vena cava at the level of the diaphragm (Fig. 26-33).

The two-dimensional examination

A routine two-dimenstional examination for the adult and pediatric patient usually begins with the patient in a semi—left lateral decubitus position. This position allows the heart to move away from the sternum and closer to the chest wall, thus allowing a better cardiac window.

Parasternal long-axis view. The parasternal long-axis (PLA) view should be used first in the echographic examination. An attempt should be made to record as many of the cardiac structures as possible (from the base

of the heart to the apex). Generally this is accomplished by placing the transducer slightly to the left of the sternum in about the fourth intercostal space. When the bright echo reflection of the pericardium is noted, the transducer is gradually rotated until a long-axis view of the heart is obtained. If it is not possible to record the entire long axis on a single scan, the transducer should be gently rocked cephalad to caudad in an "ice-pick" fashion to record all the information from the base to the apex of the heart (Fig. 26-34).

The cardiac sonographer should observe the following structures and functions in the PLA view:
1. Composite size of the cardiac chambers
2. Contractility of the right and left ventricles
3. Thickness of the right ventricular wall
4. Continuity of the interventricular septum with the anterior wall of the aorta
5. Pliability of the atrioventricular and semilunar valves
6. Coaptation of the atrioventricular valves
7. Presence of increased echoes on the atrioventricular and semilunar valves
8. Systolic clearance of the aortic cusps
9. Presence of abnormal echo collections in the chambers or attached to the valve orifice
10. Presence and movement of chordal-papillary muscle structure
11. Thickness of the septum and posterior wall left ventricle

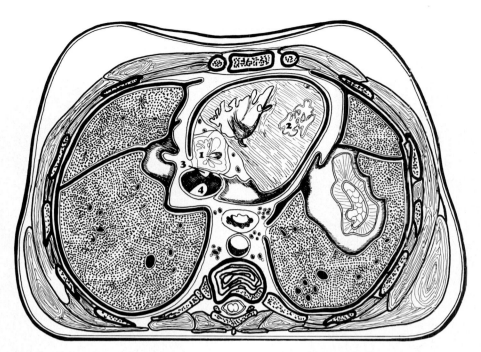

FIG. 26-33. Thoracic cross-section, level 5. This section is taken at the level of the ninth intervertebral disc. The pleural surface of the diaphragm is seen on the right. At left, oblique fibers of the diaphragm are shown. The right atrium, *1,* and left ventricle, *2,* is seen. The pericardium, epicardium, and pericardial cavity are shown. The hepatic vein, *3,* is shown to enter the inferior vena cava, *4,* at the level of the diaphragm. (From Hagen-Ansert SL: The anatomy workbook, Philadelphia, 1986, JB Lippincott Co.)

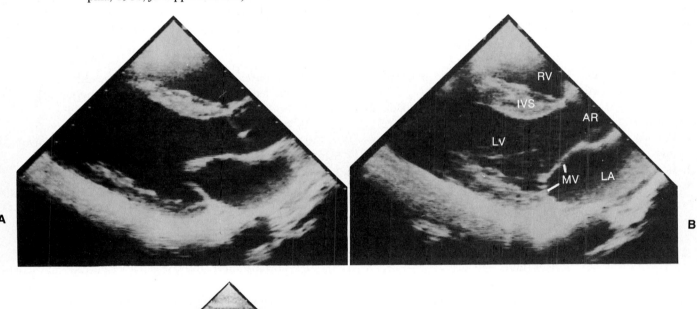

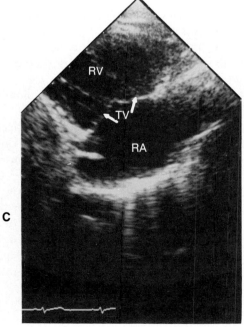

FIG. 26-34. The two-dimensional parasternal long-axis view of the heart in, **A,** early diastole and, **B,** end systole. *RV,* right ventricle; *IVS,* interventricular septum; *LV,* left ventricle; *MV,* mitral valve; *LA,* left atrium; *AR,* aortic root. **C,** Parasternal long-axis view of the tricuspid valve, *TV,* as it separates the right ventricle, *RV,* from the right atrium, *RA.*

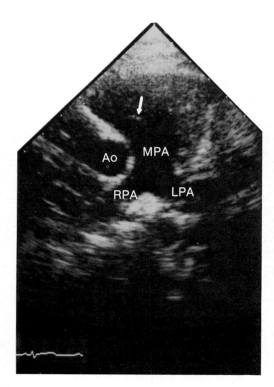

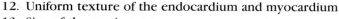

FIG. 26-35. High parasternal short-axis view of the aorta, *Ao*, pulmonary cusp *(arrow)*, main pulmonary artery, *MPA*, right pulmonary artery, *RPA*, and left pulmonary artery, *LPA*.

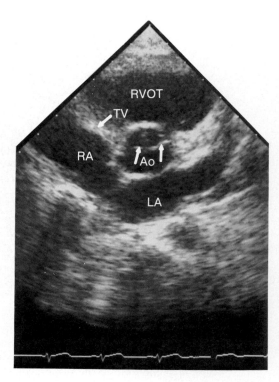

FIG. 26-36. High mid-parasternal short-axis view of the right ventricular outflow tract, *RVOT*, tricuspid valve, *TV*, right atrium, *RA*, aorta, *Ao*, aortic cusp *(arrow)*, and left atrium, *LA*.

12. Uniform texture of the endocardium and myocardium
13. Size of the aortic root

Respective M-mode tracings should then be made in these areas:

1. Record the aortic root at the level of the cusp opening.
2. Record the size of the left atrium.
3. Sweep the beam from the aortic root to the mitral valve:
   a. Demonstrate right side of interventricular septum to anterior aortic wall continuity.
   b. Demonstrate posterior aortic wall to anterior leaflet mitral valve continuity.
   c. Show transition from left atrial wall to atrioventricular groove to posterior wall left ventricle.
4. Record the anterior leaflet mitral valve at the "tip" of the leaflet.
5. Record both leaflets of the mitral valve.
6. Record the left ventricle at an area inferior to the tip of the mitral valve apparatus and superior to the papillary muscles.

Parasternal short-axis view. The transducer should be rotated 90 degrees from the parasternal long-axis view to obtain multiple transverse short-axis views of the heart at particularly these four levels:

1. High PSA view to demonstrate the pulmonary valve, right ventricular outflow tract, and aorta (Fig. 26-35):
   a. Typical "sausage-shaped" right ventricular outflow tract and pulmonary artery draped anterior to circular aorta

   b. Similunar cusp thickness and mobility
   c. Presence of calcification or extraneous echoes or both in right ventricle or valve areas
   d. Pulmonary valve mobility and thickness

Respective M-mode tracings should then be made in these areas:

1. Record the mobility of the pulmonary cusps.
2. Moderate to high PSA view to demonstrate the right ventricle, tricuspid valve, aortic cusps, coronary arteries, right and left atria (Fig. 26-36):
   a. Size of right ventricle and left atrium
   b. Presence of mass lesions in right or left atrium
   c. Mobility and thickness of tricuspid and aortic valves
   d. Continuity of interatrial septum
   e. Right ventricular wall thickness
   f. Presence of trileaflet aortic valve

Respective M-mode tracings should then be made in these areas:

1. Record the right ventricular outflow tract, aorta with cusps, and left atrial size.
2. Record the right ventricle and tricuspid valve.
3. Mid PSA view to demonstrate the right ventricle, left ventricular outflow tract, and anterior and posterior leaflets of the mitral valve (Fig. 26-37):
   a. Size of the left ventricular outflow tract
   b. Size of the septum and posterior wall
   c. Presence of mass lesions in left or right ventricle
   d. Mobility and thickness of the mitral valve
   e. Presence of a flutter on the septum or anterior leaflet mitral valve or both

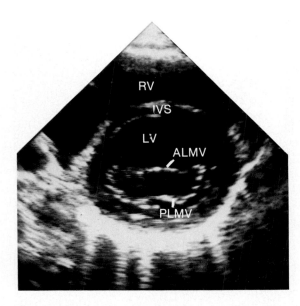

FIG. 26-37.   Mid-parasternal short-axis view of the right ventricle, *RV*, interventricular septum, *IVS*, anterior leaflet mitral valve, *ALMV*, posterior leaflet mitral valve, *PLMV*, and left ventricle, *LV*.

f. Systolic apposition of mitral valve leaflets
g. Contractility of septum and posterior wall

Respective M-mode tracings should then be made in these areas:

1. Record the right ventricle, interventricular septum, anterior leaflet mitral valve, and left ventricle.
2. Record both leaflets of the mitral valve in the left ventricular cavity.

4. Low PSA view should demonstrate the right ventricle, left ventricle, and papillary muscles (chordal echoes may also be seen) (Fig. 26-38):
    a. Contractility of the septum and posterior wall of the left ventricle.
    b. Thickness of the septum and posterior wall.
    c. Size of the left ventricle.
    d. Presence or absence of mural thrombus or other mass.
    e. Presence or absence of pericardial fluid, constriction, or restriction.
    f. Presence of increased echo density in posterior wall.
    g. Number of papillary muscles and their location within the left ventricular cavity.

Respective M-mode tracings should then be made in these areas:

1. Record the right ventricle, interventricular septum (chordae tendineae), left ventricle, endocardium, myocardium, epicardium, and pericardium. Reduce gain to show bright pericardial echo reflection.
2. Sweep from left ventricle to mitral valve to aorta.

Apical views. Two apical views are very useful: the four-chamber view and the apical long-axis view, or two-chamber view. The cardiac sonographer should palpate

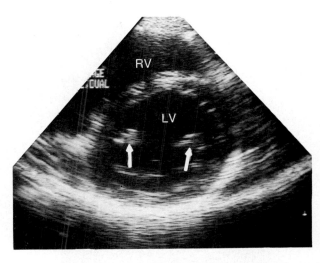

FIG. 26-38.   Low parasternal short-axis view of the right ventricle, *RV*, left ventricle, *LV*, and posterior papillary muscle *(arrows)*.

the patient's chest to detect the posterior maximal impulse (PMI). The transducer should then be directed in a "transverse" plane at the PMI and angled sharply cephalad to record the four chambers of the heart. If there is too much lung interference, then the proper cardiac window has not been found and care should be taken to adjust the patient's position or the transducer position to adequately see all four chambers of the heart. Many laboratories have found it useful to use a very thick mattress with a large hole cut out of the mattress at the level of the apex of the heart. This allows the transducer more flexibility in recording the four-chamber view.

This view is excellent for assessing cardiac contractility, size of cardiac chambers, presence of mass lesions, alignment of atrioventricular valves, coaptation of atrioventricular valves, septal or posterior wall hypertrophy, chordal attachments, and the presence of pericardial effusion. It is not a good view to evaluate the presence of an atrial septal defect since the beam is parallel to the thin foramen ovalae and the septum commonly appears as a "defect" in this view. The subcostal four-chamber view is much better to evaluate the presence of such a defect.

Generally no M-mode tracings are made in the apical views; therefore the cardiac sonographer should observe the following structures (Fig. 26-39):

1. Size of the cardiac chambers
2. Contractility of right and left ventricles
3. Septal and posterior wall thickness, contractility, and continuity
4. Coaptation of atrioventricular valves
5. Alignment of atrioventricular valves
6. Presence of increased echoes on valve apparatus
7. Presence of mass or thrombus in cardiac chambers
8. Entrance of pulmonary veins into left atrial cavity
9. Size of left ventricular outflow tract, signs of obstruction, mobility of aortic cusps, absence of subaortic membrane
10. Entrance of inferior and superior vena cava into right atrium

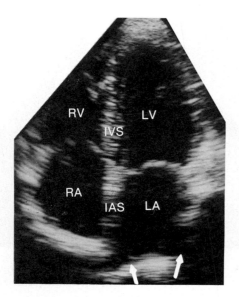

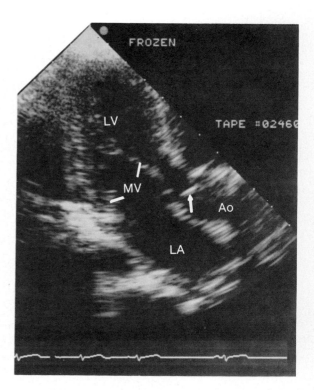

FIG. 26-39. Apical four-chamber view. *RA,* right atrium; *RV,* right ventricle; *IAS,* interatrial septum; *IVS,* interventricular septum; *LA,* left atrium; *LV,* left ventricle; pulmonary veins *(arrows).*

The apical long-axis view is very useful to evaluate the left ventricular cavity and aortic outflow tract (Fig. 26-40). Once the apical four-chamber view is obtained, the transducer should be rotated 90 degrees to visualize the left ventricle, left atrium, and aorta with cusps. This view permits the cardiac sonographer to evaluate the wall motion of the posterior basal segment of the left ventricle, the anterior wall, and the apex of the left ventricle. It also permits another view of the left ventricular outflow tract, which may be useful in determining aortic cusp motion or the presence of a subvalvular membrane.

Subcostal view. This view also has multiple windows in the four-chamber and short-axis planes. Many of the views are only available in the pediatric patient (because of the flexible stomach muscles) and therefore will be discussed in detail in Chapter 35. The subcostal four-chamber view is generally a useful view in many adults and may serve as an alternate view if the apical four-chamber view is unobtainable. The transducer should be placed in the subcostal space, and with a moderate amount of pressure, angled steeply toward the patient's left shoulder. The plane of the transducer is transverse to visualize the four chambers of the heart.

It is usually easy to follow the inferior vena cava into the right atrium of the heart. With careful angulation, the interatrial septum may be visualized between the anterior right atrial chamber and the posterior left atrial chamber. It usually is more difficult to "open" up the right ventricular cavity in this view; therefore no size assessment should be made. This view is usually very good to evaluate the presence of pericardial effusion, especially since it surrounds the anterior segment of the right heart (Fig. 26-41).

Suprasternal view. The transducer is directed transversely in the patient's suprasternal notch and angled steeply toward the arch of the aorta. This view is only

FIG. 26-40. Apical two-chamber view of the left ventricle, *LV,* left atrium, *LA,* aorta, *Ao,* aortic cusp *(arrow),* and mitral valve, *MV.*

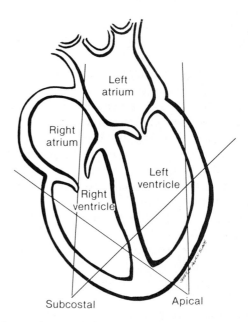

FIG. 26-41. Schema of the transducer positions for an apical and subcostal view of the four chambers of the heart.

useful if the design of the transducer is small enough to fit well into the suprasternal notch. The patient is best prepared if several towels or a pillow is placed under the shoulders in an effort to flex the neck enough to avoid interference with the neck of the transducer and cable. The patient's head should be turned to the right, again to avoid interference with the cable. With careful angulation, the cardiac structures visualized are the aortic arch, bra-

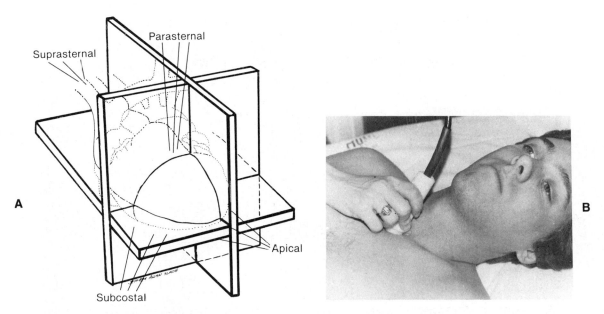

FIG. 26-42. **A,** Schema of the four transducer positions for the two-dimensional echocardiogram: suprasternal—transducer is placed in the suprasternal notch; subcostal—transducer is located near the midline and beneath the costal margin; apical—transducer is located over the cardiac apex; and parasternal—transducer is located in the fourth intercostal space just to the left of midline. **B,** Suprasternal transducer position for visualizing the aortic arch, brachiocephalic vessels, right pulmonary artery, and left atrium.

chiocephalic vessels, right pulmonary artery, left atrium, and left main bronchus (Fig. 26-42).

This view is especially useful in determining supravalvular enlargement of the aorta, coarctation of the aorta, or dissection of the aorta.

DOPPLER APPLICATIONS AND TECHNIQUE

The Doppler effect, first described by Christian Johann Doppler, is demonstrated on an echocardiogram as red blood cells move from a lower frequency sound source at rest toward a higher frequency sound source. The change in frequency is called the Doppler shift in frequency, or the Doppler frequency.

The Doppler shift depends on the angle between the ultrasonic beam and the direction of the blood velocity. In many instances, this angle is unknown. To measure the blood velocity through the heart valves, it is possible to place the transducer so the angle is small (ideally, it should be close to zero) to quantify the results.

There are four different types of Doppler used in the echocardiographic study: pulsed wave (PW), continuous wave (CW), high pulsed-range frequency (PRF), and color flow.

The PW Doppler is range directed and is best used for lower blood velocities. The maximum velocity that can be measured is limited because of a phenomenon called frequency aliasing. When this velocity limit is exceeded, the Doppler shifts are mapped out as the opposite sign. Thus a patient with aortic stenosis, when examined from the apical four-chamber view with PW Doppler, would show the high-frequency shift away from the transducer, as well as the "wraparound" or alias toward the trans-

ducer (Fig. 26-43). To clarify this Doppler shift, a CW Doppler should be used.

The CW Doppler does not have the aliasing limitation and therefore is useful in recording the higher velocities in the heart. This transducer does not have the range resolution found in the PW Doppler.

The high PRF Doppler is a modification of PW Doppler. It takes advantage of the fact that only a fraction of the ultrasound energy is backscattered at the region of sampling; and much of the remaining energy continues along the path of the beam and can be used for sampling. The high PRF sampling approach allows faster sampling rates, thereby avoiding signal aliasing.

Color flow (CF) Doppler uses multiple range gates along individual lines of sight, with parallel processing of Doppler information from the individual gates. By sweeping the ultrasound beam electronically across an examining sector and determining Doppler information at multiple range gates along each of these different lines of sight, Doppler information can be derived from a sector of interrogation. The corresponding Doppler velocities can then be mapped spatially and displayed as an overlay along with the corresponding two-dimensional image. Thus different colors are used for velocities moving toward and away from the transducer. (Usually red is used toward the transducer, and blue is used away from the transducer.) Various degrees of brightness of each color are used to code for the relative velocities. Since CF Doppler is a pulsed technique, the color mapping is limited by aliasing, and thus quantitation demands that this be integrated with conventional CW or high PRF waveforms. (Some manufacturers color code this aliasing pattern with yellows and greens so that the alias can be readily inter-

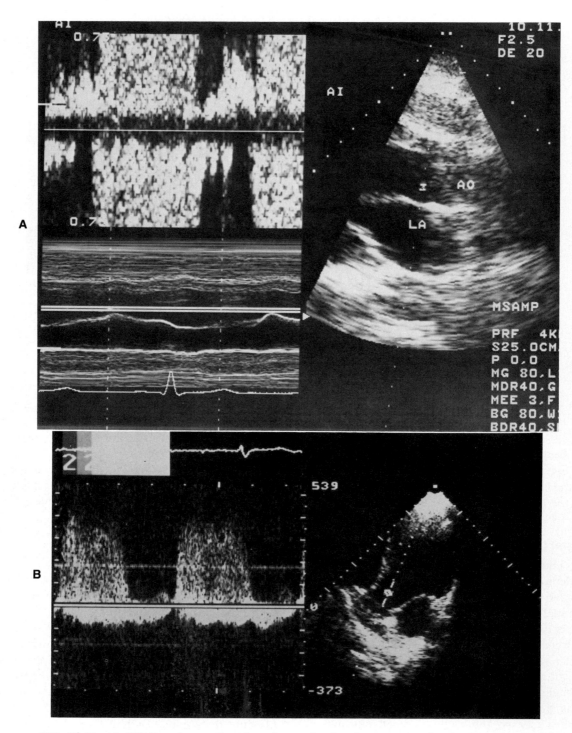

FIG. 26-43. **A,** PW Doppler tracing of an abnormal valve demonstrates the aliasing pattern seen when the velocities are over 2 m/s. **B,** CW Doppler tracing of the same valve allows higher velocities to be recorded so the maximum flow velocity pattern can be obtained.

preted.) Color flow mapping provides spatial orientation and allows demonstration of the spatial distribution of flow through stenotic valves and septal defects or of regurgitant flow disturbances.

Doppler applications

Doppler has a number of important clinical applications and is generally used routinely on all patients in our laboratory. Volume flow can be determined by measuring the

average velocity and duration of flow as well as the cross-sectional flow area. This approach requires that flow be laminar, that the profile of velocities be relatively blunt so that the instantaneous Doppler velocities are representative of the spatial average velocity across the area of interest, and that the cross-sectional flow area can be measured accurately.

Pressure differences across many kinds of intracardiac defects can be determined from the velocity of blood flow

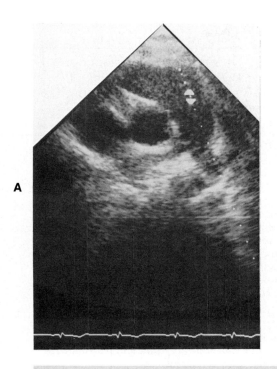

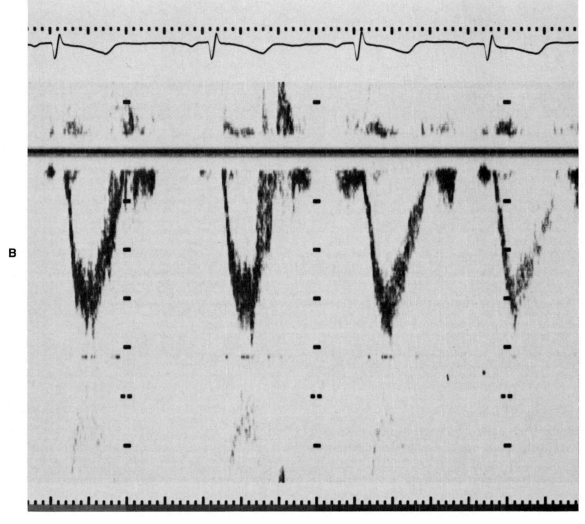

FIG. 26-44. A, High to mid-parasternal short-axis view is used to obtain pressures in the pulmonary artery. The Doppler sample volume *(large arrows)* is placed in the proximal pulmonary artery. The beam is then gently rocked anteroposterior and mediolateral to obtain the best sound as well as the sharpest flow profile. **B,** Pulmonary artery blood flow tracing in a normal subject. The presystolic blood flow velocity shift occurs prior to the QRS complex (which is synchronous with the *a* dip on the pulmonary valve M-mode).

through the defect. A modification of the Bernoulli equation is used to relate the measured blood velocity (V) to the pressure gradient (P). The energy used to propel blood flow through a discrete narrowing is expended in several ways; however, the most useful to the clinical setting is the energy required to accelerate the blood through the narrowed area. This acceleration can be estimated from the flow velocity using the modified Bernoulli equation $P = 4(V)^2$. This approach has allowed accurate estimation of instantaneous pressure gradients across the stenotic cardiac valves and across other discrete obstructions in the cardiac chambers or vessels. A similar approach allows determination of instantaneous pressures across regurgitant valves.

Doppler technique

A typical Doppler examination in our laboratory is performed after the two-dimensional and M-mode examination has been completed. A PW Doppler transducer is then used to listen for normal/abnormal flows across each of the cardiac valves. A high parasternal short-axis view is best used for detecting pulmonary valve flow. The range gate on the PW transducer should be placed just above the pulmonary valve, in the main pulmonary artery, to listen and record the normal velocity (Fig. 26-44). The range gate could then be moved to the level of the valve opening to listen and record the presence of pulmonary insufficiency.

The other cardiac valves are best recorded from the apical four-chamber view (Table 26-2). The atrioventricular valves are examined next with the range gate located approximately at the anulus level (Figs. 26-45 and 26-46). The beam is then repositioned to the outflow portion of the valve and then moved back into the atrial cavity to record the inflow portion of the valve. If flows are normal at these levels, no further investigation is made along the interventricular septum or interatrial septum to listen for shunt flow. To record velocities from the left ventricular outflow tract and aorta, the beam should be directed just inferior to the aortic outflow tract (Fig. 26-47) (the two-dimensional image is now directed slightly anterior from the position of the atrioventricular valves to see the aortic root and left ventricular outflow tract).

If adequate velocities are not obtained from the aorta in the apical four-chamber view, then the suprasternal notch is an excellent view to Doppler the ascending and descending aortic flow. If it is difficult to position the PW transducer in the suprasternal notch, then the smaller CW transducer can be used for this view.

Protocol for the Doppler examination

The typical Doppler examination will include imaging and listening for the best Doppler signal from several different cardiac planes. The cardiac sonographer needs to determine which window is the best for the proper Doppler recording. The following windows are guidelines that may be used to listen for these valvular and septal flow patterns:

Table 26-2 Maximal Velocities Recorded with Doppler in Normal Individuals (cm/s)

	Children	Adults
Mitral flow	80-130	60-130
Tricuspid flow	50-80	30-70
Pulmonary artery	70-110	60-90
Left ventricle	70-120	70-110
Aorta	120-180	100-170

From Hatle L: Doppler ultrasound in cardiology, Philadelphia, 1982, Lea & Febiger.

Apical window
Mitral valve
Tricuspid valve
Left ventricular outflow tract
Aortic valve
Pulmonary vein inflow
Superior vena cava inflow
Interventricular septum

Parasternal short-axis window
Pulmonic valve
  Main pulmonary artery, right and left branches
  Patent ductus arteriosus flow
Tricuspid valve

Suprasternal notch window
Ascending aorta
Descending aorta
Patent ductus arteriosus flow
Right pulmonary artery

Subcostal window
Interatrial septum
Interventricular septum
Inferior vena cava flow
Superior vena cava flow

Parasternal long-axis window
Mitral regurgitation
Tricuspid regurgitation
Aortic regurgitation

Right parasternal window
Ascending aorta

SUMMARY

1. The combination of two-dimensional and M-mode studies provides an accurate means of evaluating wall thickness, valvular orifice and chamber size, and contractility of the ventricles.

2. The transducer should be as high as possible to improve the resolution of returning echoes.

3. The cardiac window is usually found between the third to fifth intercostal space, slightly to the left of the sternal border.

4. Mitral valve: the transducer should be directed perpendicular to the patient's chest wall, slightly away from the left sternal border, in approximately the

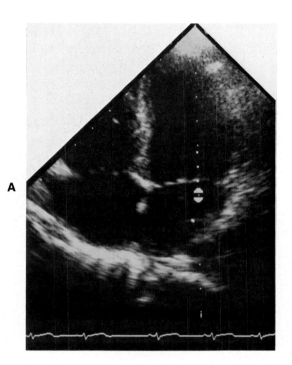

FIG. 26-45.   A, The apical four-chamber view is used to record pressures from the mitral valve. The Doppler sample volume can initially be placed at the level of the mitral anulus, away from the left ventricular outflow tract and aortic flows. The beam is then directed slightly lateral since most regurgitant leaks seem to flow toward the lateral left atrial wall. The sample volume should be gradually moved to the inflow of the mitral valve as well as into the left atrial cavity to record pressures of flow velocities. **B,** Mitral valve blood flow in a normal subject. The pattern is biphasic, similar to the pattern on the M-mode.

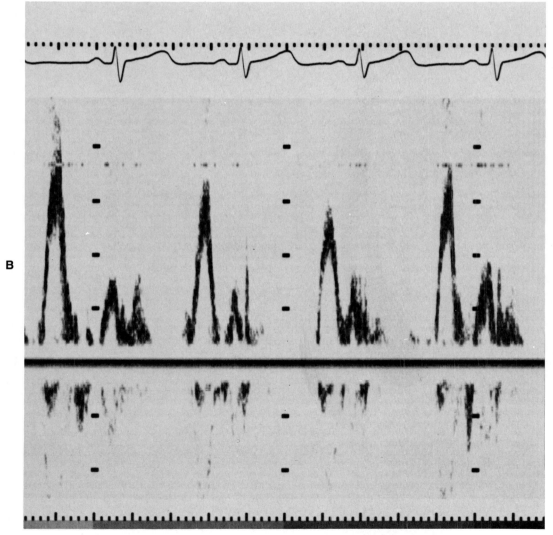

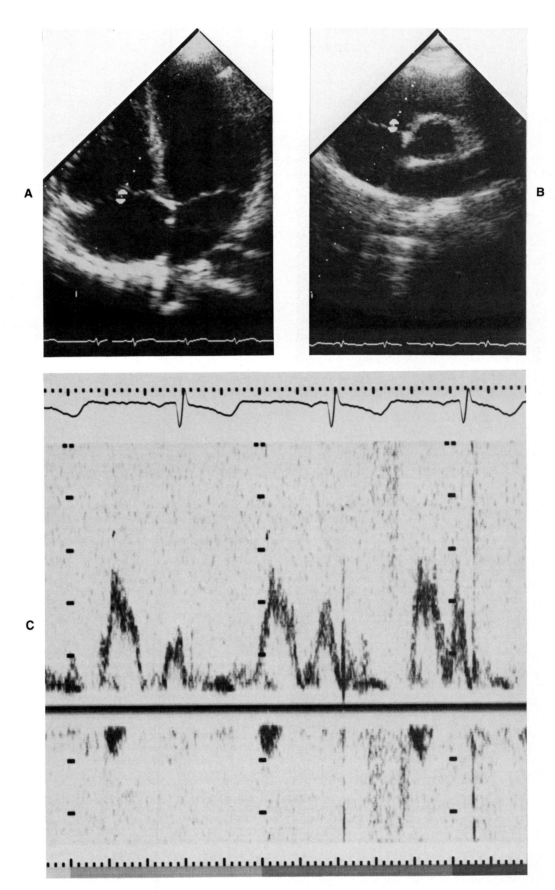

FIG. 26-46. **A,** The apical four-chamber view is also used to record blood flow velocities from the tricuspid valve. The Doppler sample volume can be placed at the level of the anulus and then carefully directed medially and laterally to record abnormal blood flow patterns. Generally the regurgitant jets seem to flow toward the interatrial septum, and careful attention should be made to that area. Like the mitral valve, the inflow pattern should be investigated as well as the flow pattern in the right atrium. **B,** The mid-parasternal short-axis view is another window often used to record tricuspid velocities. **C,** Tricuspid valve blood flow in a normal subject.

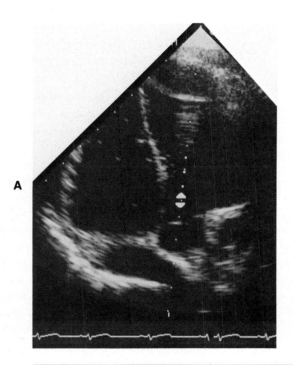

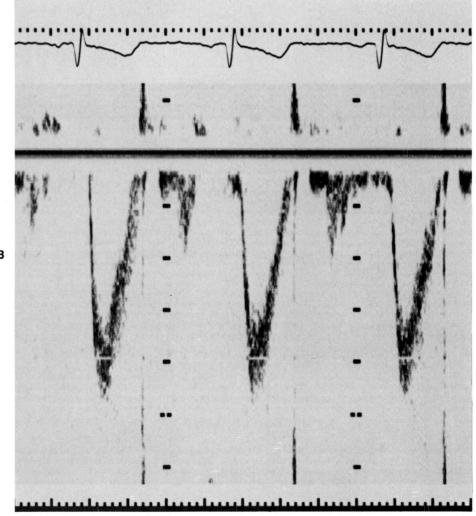

FIG. 26-47.   A, The apical "five"-chamber view is used to record blood flow velocities from the left ventricular outflow tract and aortic root. This is obtained after an apical four-chamber view has been demonstrated; the transducer is then carefully angulated in an anterior direction to record the aorta with cusps. The Doppler sample volume can be placed just beneath the aortic cusps, close to the interventricular septum. **B,** Aortic valve flow pattern in a normal subject.

fourth intercostal space. The mitral valve pattern is usually seen 6 to 9 cm from the patient's skin surface. The greatest amplitude and excursion should be found.

5. Aorta and left atrium: the transducer should be directed cephalad toward the right shoulder, from the landmark area of the mitral valve. The anterior leaflet of the mitral valve should blend with the posterior aortic wall as the interventricular septum blends into the anterior aortic wall. As one sweeps the transducer from the mitral valve medially and superiorly, the left ventricular wall blends into the atrioventricular groove and finally into the left atrial wall.

6. Interventricular septum: both sides of the septum should move symmetrically. The septum thickens in systole at the midportion of the ventricular cavity.

7. Left ventricle: the anterior leaflet of the mitral valve should first be located and then the beam angled slightly inferior and lateral toward the left hip, to record the left ventricular chamber. The three layers of the posterior heart wall are the endocardium, myocardium, and epicardium.

8. Right ventricle: the anterior wall is demonstrated with proper near-gain settings.

9. Right atrium: this is best seen on the longitudinal subcostal view since the inferior vena cava empties into this chamber.

10. Tricuspid valve: the transducer is angled medially and slightly inferior from the mitral valve.

11. Pulmonary valve: the transducer is swept laterally and superiorly from the aortic valve toward the left shoulder.

12. Suprasternal notch: the transducer is directed caudally toward the aortic arch, right pulmonary artery, and left atrium.

13. The two-dimensional echo has improved transducer design, resolution capabilities, focus parameters, gray-scale differentiation, gain control factors, cine loop function, and color-flow capabilities.

14. Transducer locations for two-dimensional imaging include suprasternal, subcostal, apical, and parasternal.

15. The Doppler effect is demonstrated on an echocardiogram as red blood cells move from a lower frequency sound source at rest toward a higher-frequency sound source. If the cells move away from a source, the frequency at the source will be lower. The change in frequency is called the Doppler shift. The shift depends on the angle between the beam and the direction of blood velocity.

16. There are four different types of Doppler displays: the pulsed wave (PW), continuous wave (CW), high pulsed-range frequency (PRF), and color flow (CF).

17. The typical Doppler examination will include imaging and listening for the best Doppler signal from several different cardiac planes.

REFERENCES

1. Chang S: M-mode echocardiographic techniques and pattern recognition, Philadelphia, 1976, Lea & Febiger.
2. Goldberg BB: Suprasternal ultrasonography, JAMA 215:245, 1972.
3. Gramiak R: Cardiac ultrasonography: a review of current applications, Rad Clin North Am 9:469, 1971.
4. Gramiak R and Nanda NC: Cardiac ultrasound, St Louis, 1972, The CV Mosby Co.

Echocardiographic Measurements

The ability to evaluate echographic data has been of great interest to the clinicians and investigators involved in echographic techniques. Early pioneers in echocardiography were able to correlate their data consistently with data from other diagnostic studies to confirm the validity of ultrasonic measurements. To have meaning, the data must be evaluated along with the patient's clinical history and symptoms. Although many laboratories have discontinued certain echocardiographic measurements, we have found the echocardiogram a very useful teaching tool. Instructing students how to evaluate the study by using measurements improves their technique and sharpens their skills in echo interpretation. We have also found that "eyeballing" a study can mislead an inexperienced cardiac sonographer to overread or underread a particular study.

Therefore this chapter is devoted to echocardiographic measurements and their explanation. This data has been accumulated from various investigators in the field with specific references to normal valves. An example of the echocardiographic report form has been included within this chapter to give the reader an idea of how the information can be presented to the clinician. An outline of specific diseases and their echocardiographic significance (with chamber enlargement) is provided in Table 27-1.

To fully evaluate the cardiac patient, we have found it useful to perform the conventional M-mode, two-dimensional, and Doppler examination on every patient in whom pathology was demonstrated. Thus when calculations are performed on the echo tracing, the added dimension of the two-dimensional image adds to the understanding of the total picture of cardiac function and contractility.

The use of calipers facilitates the measurement process and should be employed for uniformity and accuracy in data accumulation. The echographic tracings and data sheets are then reviewed by the cardiologist for final interpretation.

MITRAL VALVE

Normal appearance. The anterior and posterior leaflets of the mitral valve are assigned specific letters corresponding to their systolic and diastolic components as timed on the ECG. The systolic component consists of *c* and *d* points. The diastolic component has *e, f, a,* and *b* points (Fig. 27-1). Each letter point coincides with a specific ECG function. The QRS on the ECG marks the onset of systole and coincides with the *c* point on the mitral leaflet. The T wave on the ECG coincides with the *d* point, signifying the end of systole. Shortly thereafter (the onset of diastole), the *e* point is shown and the ventricle starts to relax at the *f* point. The P wave on the ECG triggers atrial contraction and the *a* "kick" is then seen on the mitral valve. Normally the *b* point is not identified in patients without elevated end diastolic pressure and occurs just prior to the QRS.

c-d amplitude (Fig. 27-2). This is a measurement from the *c* point to the *d* point. It is the closed systolic position during which the valve leaflets move with the mitral anulus. It normally has little to do with the valve itself and relates to the heart movement. These structures may be an important indicator of a systolic anterior motion (SAM) or mitral valve prolapse (posterior bulging into the atrial cavity). The normal valve is 20 to 30 mm.

c-d slope. This measurement depicts the rate of movement of the valve leaflets as the anulus moves anteriorly in systole. The slope is measured by extending the line through points *c* and *d* and is a time-distance measurement. The normal value is 35 mm/s.

Table 27-1   Echocardiographic Structures

Disease	LA	LV	LVO	RV	Mitral valve (anterior and posterior)
MV stenosis	↑			? ↑	↓ E-F slope (<35 mm/s) ↓ C-E amplitude (severe) No *a* kick (usually) PLMV moves anterior (usually)
MV regurgitation	↑	↑	↑		e point touches IVS ↑ C-E amplitude E-F slope >180 mm/s Flutter ALMV
MV prolapse	↑ (MR)	↑ (MR)	↑ (MR)		Posterior motion in systole (3 to 5 mm)
Aortic insufficiency		↑	↑		↓ E-F slope Flutter of ALMV
Aortic stenosis					↓ E-F slope ? Calcified mitral anulus
CCM	↑	↑	↑	↑	↓ Amplitudes ALMV/PLMV clearly recorded
IHSS or HOCM	? ↑ MR		↓		e point touches IVS ↓ E-F slope SAM (obstructive)
Vegetations	↑ MR	↑ AI	↑ AI	↑ TR	Multilayered thickening Coarse diastolic flutter (MV veg.)
Normal heart	1.9 to 4.0 cm; 1:1 LA/Ao	4.0 to 5.5 cm	20 to 35 cm	0.7 to 2.6 cm	M shape of ALMV PLMV moves posterior E-F slope 80 to 150 mm/s C-E amplitude 20 to 35 mm

Code:

MR	= Mitral regurgitation		ALMV	= Anterior leaflet mitral valve
CCM	= Concentric cardiomyopathy		SAM	= Systolic anterior motion
IHSS	= Idiopathic hypertrophic subaortic stenosis		AR	= Aortic root
HOCM	= Hypertrophic cardiomyopathy		PHW	= Posterior heart wall
AI	= Aortic insufficiency		PLMV	= Posterior leaflet mitral valve
TR	= Tricuspid regurgitation		LA index	= Left atrial size/Body surface area

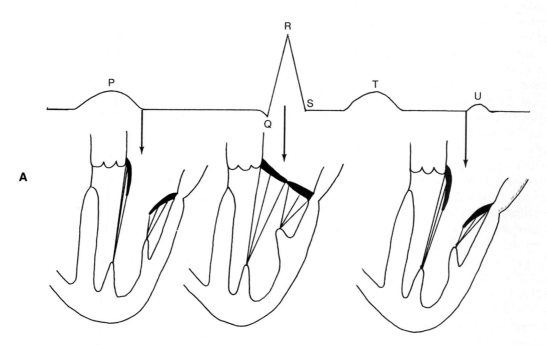

FIG. 27-1.   A, The onset of systole (QRS on the ECG) shows the closure of the mitral leaflets. At the onset of diastole (end of the T wave on the ECG), the mitral leaflets open fully. They start to close until the atrium contracts (the P wave on the ECG). The leaflet opens, but not as fully as it did in early diastole.

Aortic valve	IVS	Posterior heart wall	Other
	Hyperdynamic		Calcification (thickening) Prolapse? "Hump" in pericardial effusion (pseudoprolapse)
	↑ Amplitude (may have) ? Flutter IVS		
Calcified walls ↓ Systolic septal wall motion	↑ Thickness	Concentric hypertrophy	Bicuspid (eccentric cusps)
Decreased motion	Thin Poor contractility	Thin Poor contractility	Cardiomegaly; pericardial effusion
Midsystolic closure	1.8 to 2.0 cm IVS/PHW < 1.3 cm		Pseudo-SAM in hypertension
Coarse diastolic flutter (AR veg.)			Vegetations 2 to 3 mm thick
Box shape	0.6 to 1.2 cm IVS/PHW 1.3	1.1 cm	
Systolic separation 1.5 to 2.6 cm			
LA index <2.2			

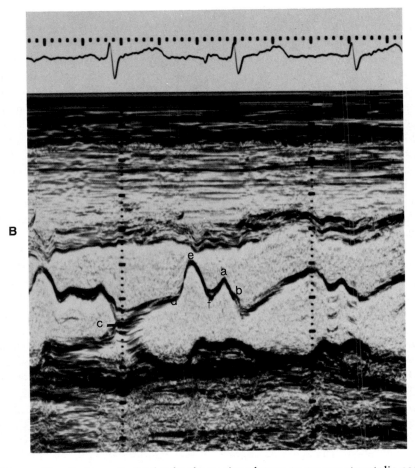

FIG. 27-1, cont'd. **B,** The mitral valve has been given letters to represent systolic components, *c* and *d*, and diastolic components, *d, e, f, a, b,* and *c.* (Note that the *c* point represents end diastole, onset of systole; the *d* point represents end systole, onset of diastole.)

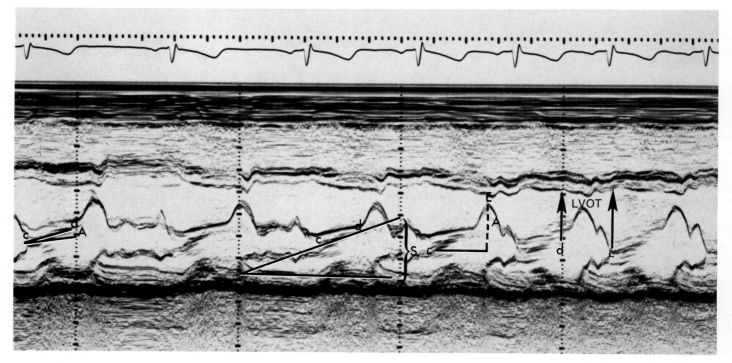

FIG. 27-2. For an explanation of *c-d* amplitude, *A,* slope, *S, c-e* amplitude, and left ventricular outflow tract, *LVOT,* at *c* and *d,* see text.

c-e amplitude. This is a measurement from the *c* point to the *e* point. It denotes the amplitude at which the mitral valve is opening. The *e* point is the most anterior excursion. The normal value is 20 to 33 mm.

Left ventricular outflow tract at the c point. Measure the left ventricular outflow tract from the left side of the septum to the *c* point on the mitral valve. The normal value is 20 to 33 mm.

Left ventricular outflow tract at the d point. Measure from the left side of the septum to the *d* point on the mitral valve. The normal value is 12 to 33 mm.

d-e slope (Fig. 27-3). This measurement signifies the opening movement of the mitral valve in early diastole. The slope is measured by extending the line through points *d* and *e*. This may be an indicator of left ventricular failure and elevated end-systolic volume with a decreased *d-e* slope. The normal value is 240 to 380 mm/s.

d-e amplitude. This is a measurement of the maximum excursion of the anterior mitral valve following early diastolic opening. The measurement is taken from the *d* point to the *e* point. It may be an important indicator of mitral regurgitation. The normal value is 17 to 30 mm.

e-f slope (Fig. 27-4). This measures the rate of motion of the cusp in early distole and expresses the rate of left atrial emptying. Since a slope is being measured, extend the line connecting the *e* and *f* points through one second in time. Draw a line from the bottom of the time line (at the point of intersection) and measure the distance along the vertical axis from the end of the completed line to the beginning of the time line. The normal value is 50 to 180 mm/s.

a-c slope. This depicts the rate of systolic closure of the mitral valve. The measurement is made by extending a slope line through points *a* and *c*. A decreased rate of closure may indicate elevated left ventricular end diastolic pressure or poor ventricular performance. The normal value is 350 to 360 mm/s.

PR-ac interval. This is a measurement to detect premature closure of the mitral valve (acute aortic insufficiency). It is taken from the beginning of the P wave on the ECG to the beginning of the Q wave on the ECG (for the PR component); the *ac* component is from the *a* point to the *c* point on the mitral valve. The interval is then determined by subtracting the ac from the PR interval. Time line of 0.04 s is used for this calibration; normal values are less than 0.06 s.

Fluttering of the leaflet. Flutter may be seen as a fine oscillation of the anterior leaflet of the mitral valve in diastole. It may be secondary to aortic insufficiency, vegetations, or, if a coarse flutter, to atrial fibrillation.

Systolic anterior motion. With this abnormality, the anterior leaflet moves anterior after the onset of systole and then returns to its normal position just before diastole. Often it is seen with obstructive hypertrophic cardiomyopathy, and the degree of obstruction is directly related to the size of the systolic motion.

Pseudosystolic anterior motion may be seen when the chordal structures move anterior in systole and mimic the motion of SAM as seen with obstructive disorders. One can distinguish pseudo-SAM from obstructive SAM by following the systolic segment of the mitral leaflet. In pseudo-SAM this segment remains in its normal position, and the chordal reflections move "over" the systolic seg-

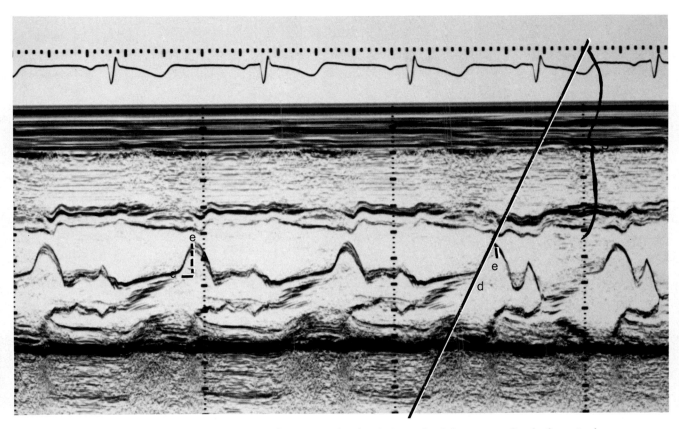

FIG. 27-3. Some laboratories use the *d-e* amplitude, *A,* instead of the *c-e* amplitude for mitral valve excursion. See text for explanation.

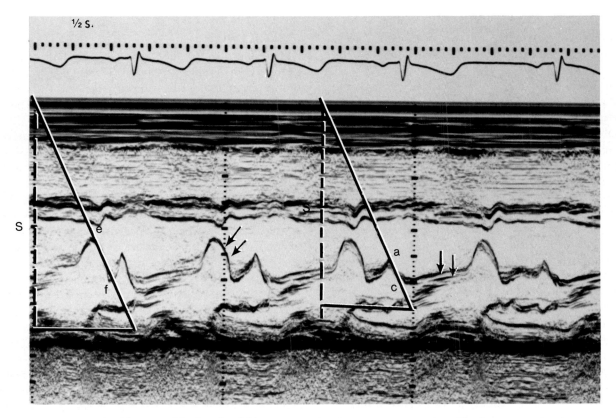

FIG. 27-4. The mitral leaflet should be measured at its greatest excursion. The best excursion is normally below the aorta near the tip of the leaflet (the posterior leaflet may also be seen at this point). In determining the *e-f* slope, the steepest slope should be measured. See text for the explanation of *a-c* slope, flutter, and SAM.

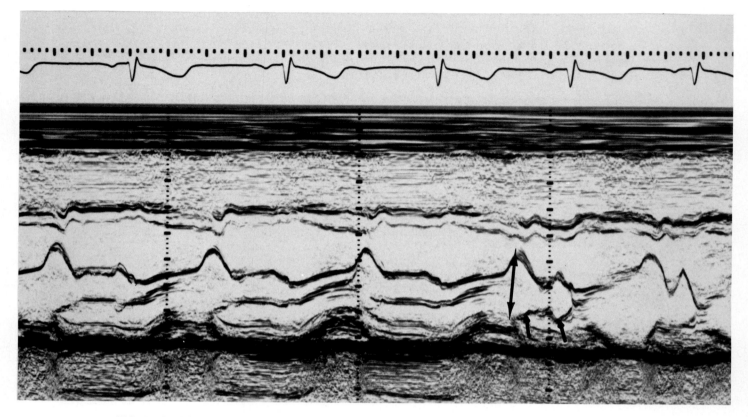

FIG. 27-5. The posterior leaflet is a mirror image of the anterior leaflet in ventricular diastole. The anterior and posterior leaflets should meet in systole at points *c* and *d*. See text for explanation of mitral valve separation, thickening, and multiple echoes in diastole.

ment. In obstructive SAM the motion is actually caused by the systolic segment of the mitral *c-d* portion of the leaflet.

Multiple echoes. In the absence of calcification, the mitral complex is a thin, single reflection.

Thickening. Multiple bright echoes due to fibrosis or calcification may be seen on either the anterior or the posterior leaflet. The degree of thickening or calcification is a function of the amount of multiple echoes seen and may be an indication of a rheumatic process.

Posterior leaflet of mitral valve (Fig. 27-5). Designate whether the posterior leaflet moves posterior in diastole (normal) or anterior (as seen in rheumatic disease such as mitral stenosis).

Posterior bulging. Posterior bulging is indicated when the anterior, the posterior, or both leaflets are displaced posteriorly in systole. The normal *c-d* slope is interrupted by a posterior movement, usually 3 to 5 mm, and is an indication of prolapse.

Space beneath the mitral valve clear. Echoes posterior to the mitral valve in diastole that do not disappear as the gain is decreased are abnormal. If there is an echo-free space in early diastole followed by an increased mass of echoes, this most likely represents a myxoma or tumor.

***Amputated* e, *prominent* a.** This occurs with elevated left ventricular end diastolic pressure. The *e* point is diminished, and the *a* point is accentuated. (It is often seen in gross aortic insufficiency.)

AORTIC ROOT

Dimension. Measure at the end of diastole at the onset of the first rapid deflection of the QRS complex from the leading edge of the anterior aortic root to the leading edge of the posterior aortic root (Fig. 27-6). The normal value is 20 to 37 mm.

Thickening. Abnormal thickness with an increase in the amount of echoes or brightness of the aortic walls usually is due to calcification. A decrease in wall motility may be noted.

Wall amplitude. This is a measurement of the anterior motion of the posterior aortic wall during ventricular systole. It is obtained by drawing a horizontal line between the external boundaries of the posterior aortic wall in diastole and then measuring the maximal vertical distance from this line to the external boundary of the aortic wall during ventricular systole. Decreased values indicate low cardiac output and a reduced stroke volume.

AORTIC VALVE

Normal appearance. The characteristic feature of the normal valve is the "box-like" configuration that presents as a linear echo pattern formed by the right and noncoronary aortic cusps as they open in ventricular systole (Fig. 27-7). The closed position in diastole presents as a dominant echo pattern in the middle of the aortic root.

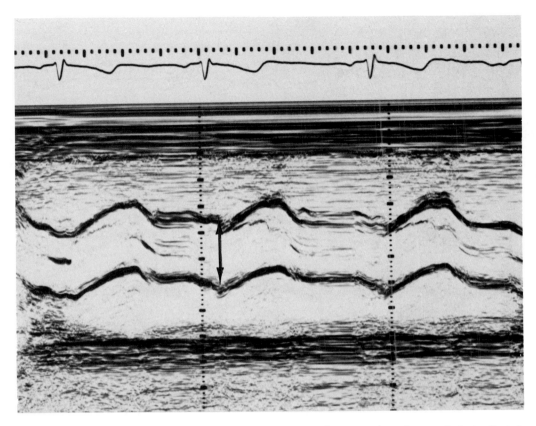

FIG. 27-6. The parallel bond of echoes that moves anteriorly in systole and posteriorly in diastole delineates the walls of the aorta. The leading edge to leading edge is measured because it is a finite and initial point (according to Popp), and there should be little difficulty in separating the walls from the lumen of the aorta.

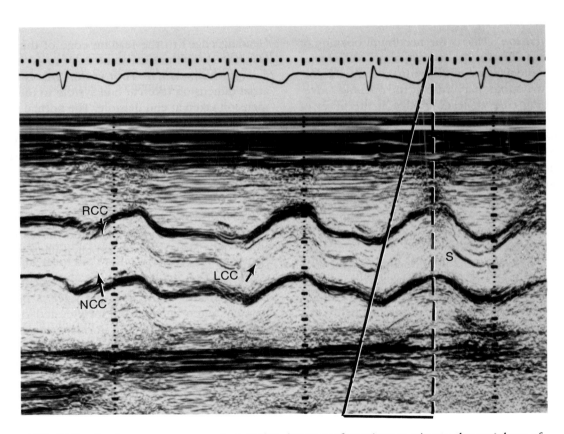

FIG. 27-7. Aortic cusps are recognized as thin, linear configurations moving to the periphery of the aorta in systole and occupying a midaortic position in diastole. The right and noncoronary cusps, *RCC* and *NCC*, show significant systolic movement in the opposite direction and produce a boxlike configuration. The left coronary cusp, *LCC*, is normally not visualized, since it lies at right angles to the sonic beam. See text for systolic opening rate. *S,* slope.

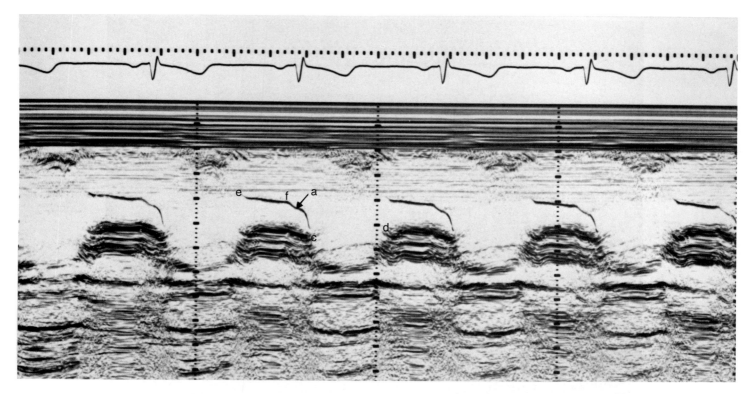

FIG. 27-10. The pulmonic valve is recorded as the beam is swept lateral and slightly cephalic from the aortic valve toward the left shoulder. *e,* onset of diastole; *f,* relaxation of ventricle; *a,* atrial contraction; *c,* end diastole, beginning systole; *d,* end systole, beginning diastole; *b,* relaxation of ventricle in diastole.

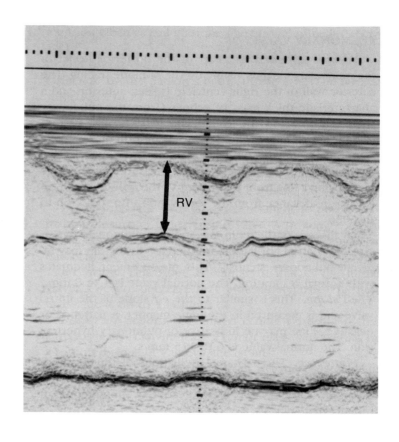

FIG. 27-11. If the right ventricular wall echo cannot be visualized, an estimate of 0.5 cm posterior to the last nonmoving chest wall echo as the location of the right ventricular wall can be made. The right ventricle, *RV,* will appear slightly enlarged as the patient assumes the semi-decubitus position because of the tangential angulation of the transducer.

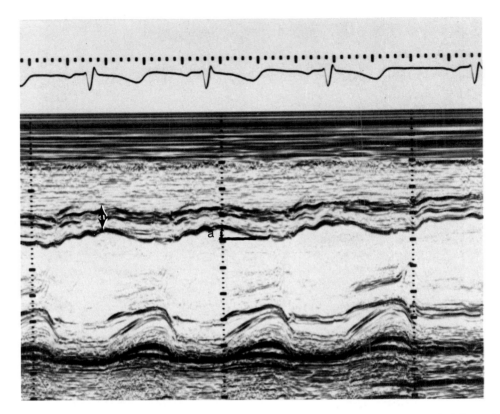

FIG. 27-12. The interventricular septum is identified as two parallel echoes recorded from the right and left sides of the septum. The membranous portion of the septum is continuous with the anterior wall of the aorta. Therefore the basal portion moves anteriorly in systole and posteriorly in diastole. This is "paradoxical motion" because the septum moves like the left ventricle (which is normal in the basal portion of the septum). The septal motion and measurements are evaluated at the muscular portion of the septum, which is much thicker than the membranous septum and moves anteriorly in diastole and posteriorly in systole. See text for discussion of septal wall thickness, septal wall amplitude, and motion. *a*, amplitude.

onset of the QRS. It should be made from leading edge to leading edge (Fig. 27-12). Abnormal thickening may be seen in patients with obstructive or concentric hypertrophy. The normal value is 6 to 11 mm.

Wall amplitude. This is a measurement of the posterior motion of the left ventricular side of the septum. It is obtained by drawing a horizontal line between the most posterior point of the septum during systole and then measuring the maximal vertical distance from this line to the septum just before the septum moves posteriorly in systole. The normal value is 5 to 12 mm.

Wall motion. Normally the septum moves posteriorly after the onset of systole (as the posterior wall moves anteriorly). Following is a breakdown of common septal abnormalities:

1. Exaggerated septal motion may indicate hyperdynamic contractility—as seen in aortic or mitral insufficiency, ventricular septal defect, patent ductus arteriosus, increased cardiac output, or coronary artery disease—and implies left ventricular volume overload.
2. Paradoxical septal motion (the septum and posterior wall move anteriorly after the onset of systole) may be caused by left bundle branch block, ventricular aneurysm, atrial septal defect, or pulmonary or tricuspid in-

sufficiency. It is indicative of right ventricular volume overload.
3. Flattened septal motion is suggested when the left side of the septum moves poorly or not at all in systole. This indicates possible left anterior descending coronary artery disease, or it may be due to technical problems connected with patient positioning.

LEFT VENTRICLE

The left ventricle measurements should be made on an M-mode tracing that was recorded just inferior to the tip of the mitral leaflet that includes a portion of the chordae tendineae. The interventricular septum and three layers of the posterior heart wall should be distinct and continuous throughout the cardiac cycle. The technique should involve a sweep with a decrease in gain to visualize the dense chordae from the endocardial surface of the posterior heart wall and the bright reflector of the pericardium from the posterior heart wall.

End diastolic dimension (Fig. 27-13). EDD is a measurement of the maximal left ventricular size in diastole. The vertical distance is measured from the left side of the septum to the endocardial surface of the posterior heart

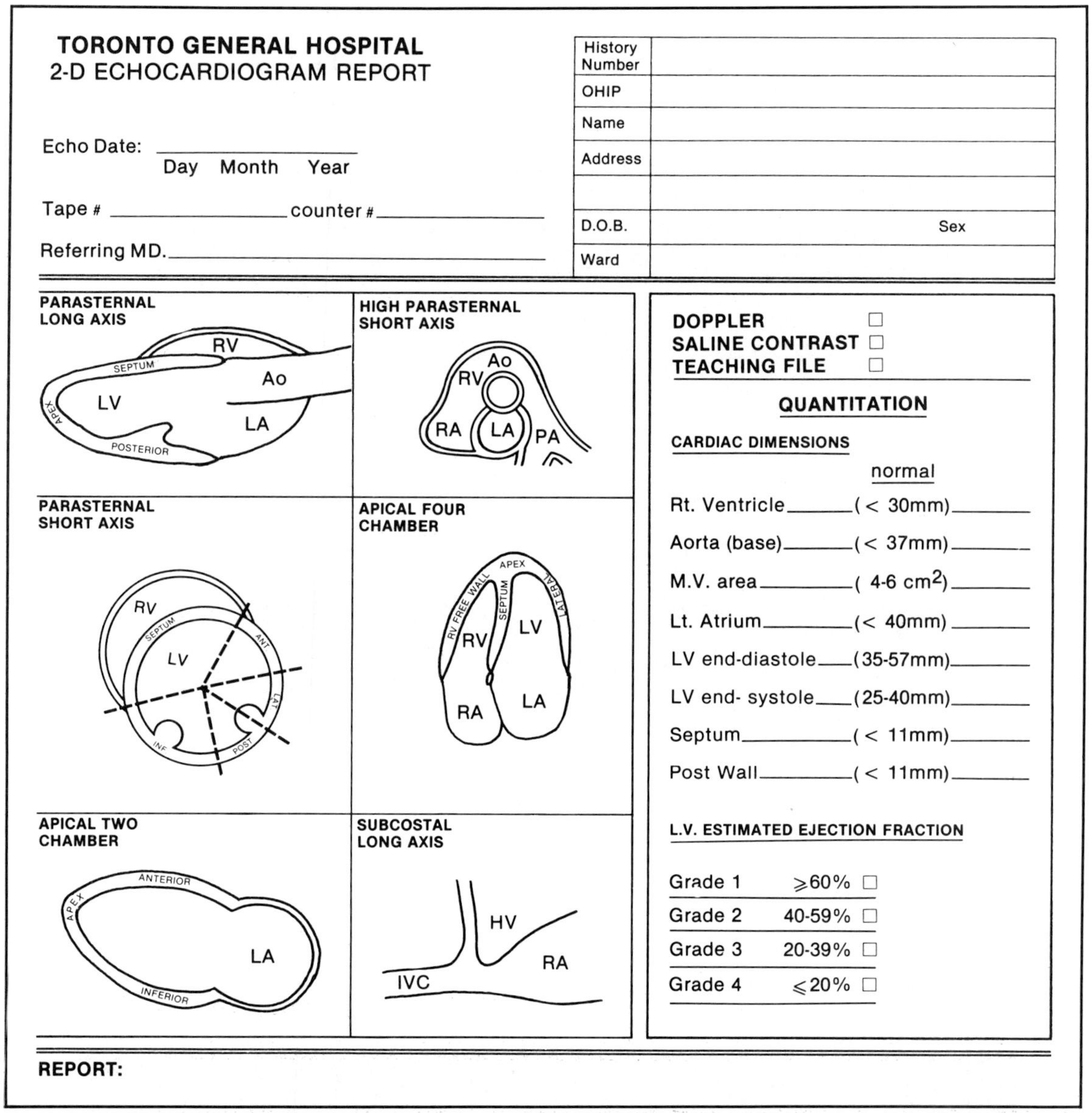

TORONTO GENERAL HOSPITAL
2-D ECHOCARDIOGRAM REPORT

Echo Date: _____
　　　　　　Day　Month　Year

Tape # _____ counter # _____

Referring MD. _____

History Number	
OHIP	
Name	
Address	
D.O.B.	Sex
Ward	

PARASTERNAL LONG AXIS

RV
SEPTUM
Ao
LV
APEX
LA
POSTERIOR

HIGH PARASTERNAL SHORT AXIS

Ao
RV
RA　LA　PA

PARASTERNAL SHORT AXIS

RV
SEPTUM
ANT
LV
LAT
INF
POST

APICAL FOUR CHAMBER

APEX
RV FREE WALL
SEPTUM
LATERAL
RV　LV
RA　LA

APICAL TWO CHAMBER

APEX
ANTERIOR
LA
INFERIOR

SUBCOSTAL LONG AXIS

HV
RA
IVC

DOPPLER　☐
SALINE CONTRAST　☐
TEACHING FILE　☐

QUANTITATION

CARDIAC DIMENSIONS

　　　　　　　　　　　normal

Rt. Ventricle _____ (< 30mm) _____

Aorta (base) _____ (< 37mm) _____

M.V. area _____ (4-6 cm^2) _____

Lt. Atrium _____ (< 40mm) _____

LV end-diastole _____ (35-57mm) _____

LV end-systole _____ (25-40mm) _____

Septum _____ (< 11mm) _____

Post Wall _____ (< 11mm) _____

L.V. ESTIMATED EJECTION FRACTION

Grade 1	≥60% ☐
Grade 2	40-59% ☐
Grade 3	20-39% ☐
Grade 4	≤20% ☐

REPORT:

Cardiac output. CO is an estimated measurement of the amount of blood ejected from the left ventricle per minute in liters:

$$CO = (HR \times SV)/1000$$

where HR is heart rate.

Ejection fraction. EF is the estimated measurement of the percentage of blood filling the left ventricle in diastole that is ejected in systole:

$$EF = \frac{EDD^3 - ESD^3}{EDD^3} \times 100$$

ΔD measures the performance of the left ventricle by:

$$\Delta D = \frac{LVD - LVS}{LVD}$$

Left ventricular mass. This mass is a measurement of the weight of the left ventricle and may be determined by:

$$LV \text{ mass} = (EDD + \text{Septal thickness} + \text{Posterior wall thickness})^3 - EDD^3$$

NOTE: These measurements are made in diastole and are invalid when asymmetric hypertrophy is present.

SUMMARY

1. The echocardiographic data must be evaluated along with the patient's clinical history and symptoms.

2. To fully evaluate the cardiac patient, an M-mode, two-dimensional, and Doppler examination (with or without color flow mapping) should be performed on each patient.

3. The use of electronic or hand-held calipers facilitate the measurement process and should be employed for uniformity and accuracy in data accumulation.

Acquired Valvular Heart Disease

This chapter will deal primarily with acquired valvular heart disease, specifically to include rheumatic heart disease, degenerative sclerosis, and prosthetic heart valves.

RHEUMATIC HEART DISEASE

Rheumatic fever is probably the primary cause of valvar stenosis and regurgitation problems in the heart. Rheumatic disease follows an infection caused by group A hemolytic streptococcal bacteria and is actually secondary to the infection. The patient with rheumatic fever becomes hypersensitive to antibodies made by his or her own system. A continuing reaction develops in all tissues between the *Streptococcus* organism, its poisons, and the antibodies. This constitutes the beginning of rheumatic fever. The interaction between antigens and antibodies keeps the inflammation of rheumatic fever going in many tissues of the body. The inflammation is found in the joints, tissues, brain, heart, and under the skin. Masses of these inflamed areas form and heal, but the most dangerous characteristic of the disease is its tendency to leave scar tissue as it heals.

The clinical history of a patient who has rheumatic fever may include a streptococcal throat infection with fever, joint tenderness and pain, carditis, chorea (uncontrollable twitching of arms, legs, and face), a skin rash, or subcutaneous nodules.

Rheumatic fever may cause three forms of carditis: endocarditis, myocarditis, and pericarditis. Endocarditis is an acute inflammation that affects the valves and the inner lining of the heart (endocardium). It may involve all the valves or primarily the left-side valves. Small vegetations develop on the affected leaflets, and damage results from the healing of inflamed areas, leaving scar tissue and destroying the valve tissue. *Myocarditis* causes the muscles to become weak and balloon outward. Myocardial failure eventually results. *Pericarditis* represents the severest form of the disease in which large pericardial effusions of serum and fibrin are found in the pericardial space.

Whereas 1 out of 100 individuals will contract rheumatic fever, in only about half of these patients will heart disease develop. The mitral valve is attacked by the disease in 65% of the patients, the aortic valve in 30%, and the tricuspid and pulmonary valves in less than 5%. Healing may be complete, or progressive scarring may develop over time due to the subacute or chronic inflammation.

A pericardial effusion may be detected in the acute phase of the disease; however, echocardiography is not yet sensitive enough to detect the small granular infections on the valve in the early stages. As the scar tissue increases and causes a permanent heart valve deformity, echocardiography may assess the thickness and pliability of the affected valve. Echocardiography may also be sensitive in the detection of thrombus secondary to the rheumatic infection.

FIG. 28-1. **A,** Parasternal long-axis view of a patient with rheumatic heart disease. The mitral valve, *MV,* is thickened and assumes a "bent knee" appearance in diastole. There is left atrial enlargement secondary to mitral stenosis and regurgitation. The aortic leaflets are thickened with restricted opening. *RV,* right ventricle; *LV,* left ventricle; *LA,* left atrium; *MV,* mitral valve; *AV,* aortic valve. **B,** M-mode tracing of mitral valve. The *e-f* slope is reduced. The amplitude of the mitral leaflet is restricted, and the posterior leaflet moves in an anterior direction with the anterior leaflet.

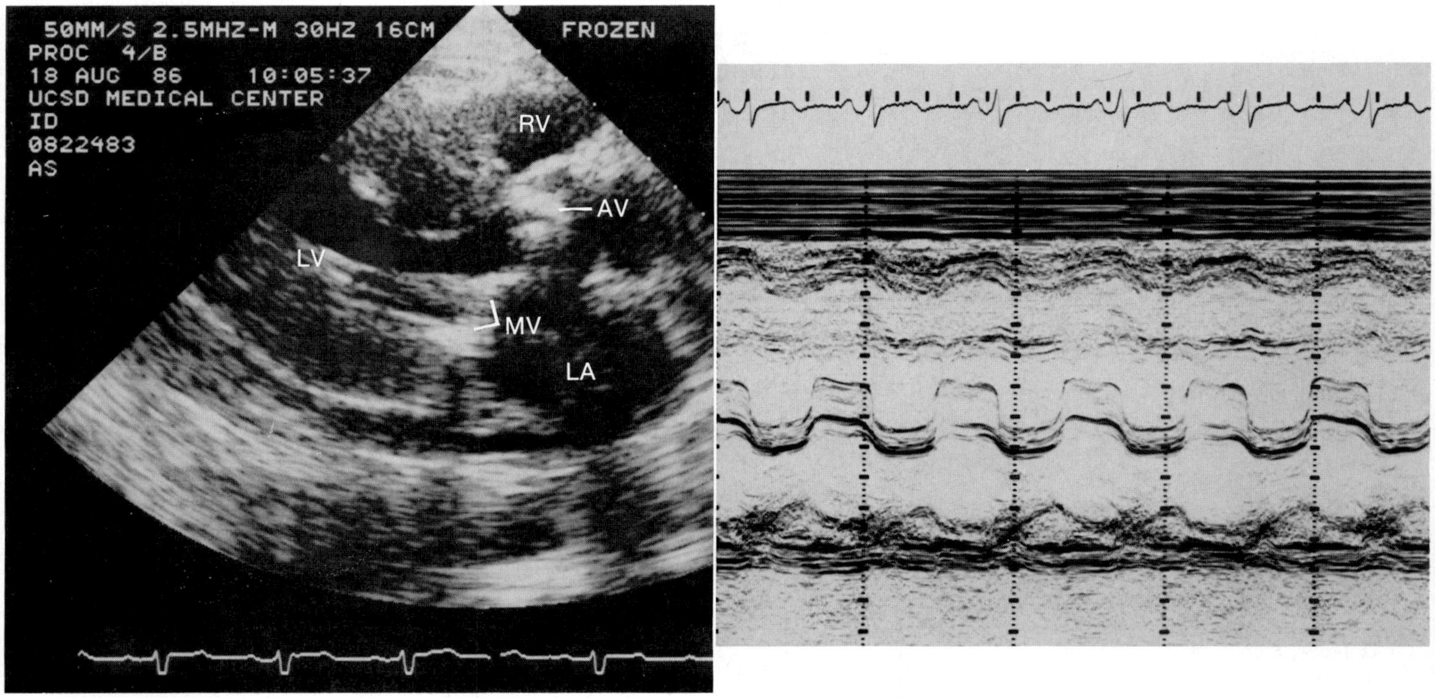

MITRAL STENOSIS

Obstruction at the mitral valve orifice can be acquired, congenital, or obstructed secondary to a tumor mass. This discussion will concentrate primarily on the acquired obstruction of the leaflet secondary to rheumatic fever.

The presence of rheumatic fever may cause several changes to occur on the valve leaflets. These changes will progress with scarring and calcification. The leaflets may be diffusely thickened by fibrous tissue or calcium deposits, or the commissures may be fused. The chordae tendineae may be shortened and fused together. Sometimes the chordae are so retracted that the leaflets appear to insert directly into the posterior papillary muscle. When this occurs, the stenosis is always severe because the interchordal spaces are obliterated. In other cases the chordae inserting into one papillary muscle may be well preserved whereas those inserting into the opposite muscle will be completely fused.

In a normal heart the cross-sectional area of the mitral valve orifice is about 5 cm^2. When stenosis is present, this orifice measurement is decreased. A valve area of 2.5 cm^2 represents mild stenosis, whereas an area of 1 cm^2 represents moderately severe stenosis.

Several studies have found that patients with *e-f* slopes of less than 10 mm/s by M-mode criteria would be considered to have severe mitral stenosis (Fig. 28-1).[1,4] However, when these patients were evaluated by the short-

axis real-time technique, only two thirds could be expected to have severe mitral stenosis with the criteria of a mitral valve area measuring less than 1.3 cm^2. Kisslo and Cope[1,4] found that for slopes higher than 10 mm/s the M-mode could not predict the severity of the lesion with any certainty.

Evaluation of the mitral orifice (leaflet pliability, thickening, and restriction of motion) should be made in two planes, the short and long axis (Fig. 28-2). The orifice is assessed in the short-axis plane first, and a planimeter measurement is taken at its narrowest point, near the leaflet tips in diastole (Fig. 28-3). The gain settings are then reduced to eliminate reverberations produced by the fibrosis and thickening. Often the mitral orifice will be found to have an irregular configuration, so care must be taken to record the accurate orifice opening.

Obstruction to the flow of blood from the left atrium into the left ventricle will cause an increase in the left atrial pressure that extends backward into the pulmonary veins, from there into the pulmonary capillaries, and from there into the pulmonary arteries. The resultant condition is pulmonary hypertension, which in turn will lead to pulmonary hypertrophy.

Echographically, the most consistent finding in mitral stenosis is the reduction of the *e-f* slope of the anterior leaflet of the valve; that is, the velocity of the *e-f* slope measures less than 35 mm/s (Fig. 28-4). Since this slope is

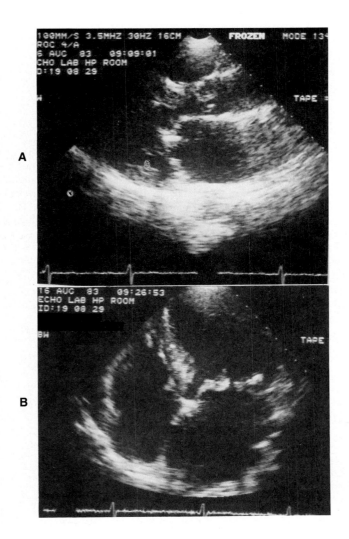

FIG. 28-2. The evaluation of the mitral leaflet pliability, thickening, and restriction of motion should be made in at least two planes (parasternal long axis, *A,* and the short axis). The apical four-chamber view, **B,** is often very useful in assessing the amount of thickening and dilatation of cardiac chambers.

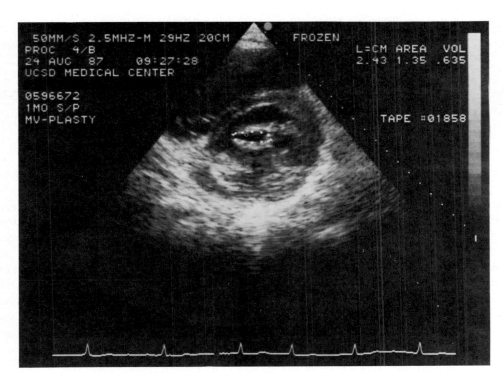

FIG. 28-3. The parasternal short-axis view is used to measure the relative size of the mitral valve orifice. The planimeter measurement is made at the narrowest opening of the anterior and posterior mitral valve, near the leaflet tips in diastole. The gain settings should be reduced to eliminate erroneous measurement calculations.

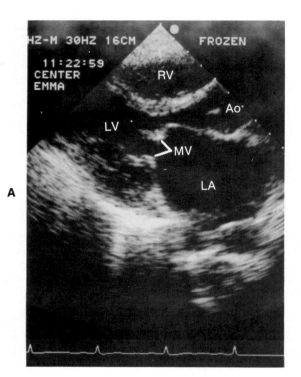

A

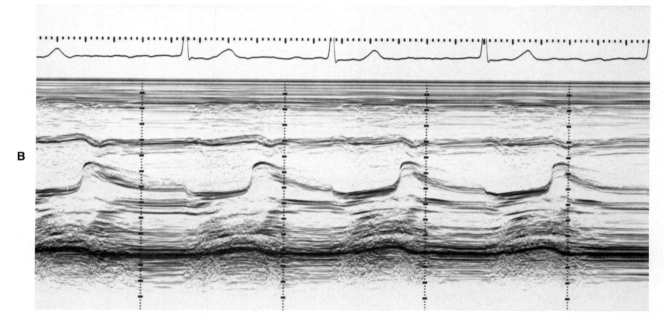

B

FIG. 28-4. **A,** Parasternal long-axis view of a patient with combined valvular disease. The left atrium is enlarged secondary to mitral regurgitation. The anterior leaflet has restricted mobility and is thickened at the tips of the leaflet. *RV,* right ventricle; *LV,* left ventricle; *LA,* left atrium; *Ao,* aorta; *MV,* mitral valve. **B,** The most consistent M-mode finding in mitral stenosis is the reduction of the *e-f* slope of the anterior leaflet, with decreased *c-e* excursion of the valve.

an indicator of the rate of left atrial emptying, in mitral stenosis the decreased slope signifies an obstruction caused by the stenosis orifice.

In addition to the decreased *e-f* slope, the posterior leaflet moves in the same direction as the anterior leaflet because of commissural fusion (Fig. 28-5). In very mild cases of mitral stenosis with little thickening or calcification, the posterior leaflet may move in its normal posterior position.

The amplitude, or *c-e* excursion, of the valve measures the degree of mobility or restriction on the leaflet. In a heavily calcified valve this amplitude is reduced. To assess the maximum mobility of the valve, the examiner must angle the transducer carefully. When the leaflet is demon-

strated, a search is made for its greatest excursion by slight additional angulations of the transducer or by moving the beam up or down an interspace.

Increased echoes on the mitral apparatus indicate thickening or the presence of calcification. The gain settings must be carefully adjusted so calcification can be distinguished from reverberation. When the posterior leaflet is well shown, the sensitivity should be gradually reduced to assess the degree of calcification from the remaining echoes.

In approximately 50% of the patients with mitral stenosis, atrial fibrillation develops (Fig. 28-6). This complication is usually serious because there is a loss of atrial contraction. (The atrial contraction may contribute 15%

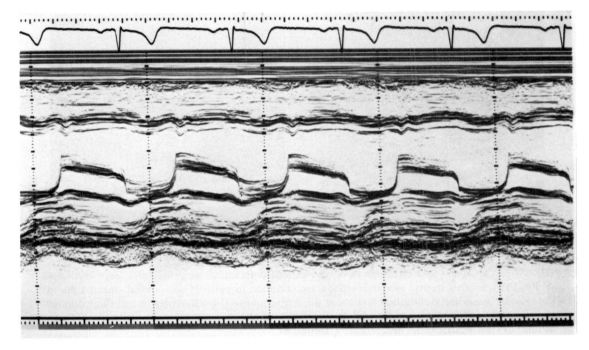

FIG. 28-5. The posterior and anterior mitral leaflets become fused with calcification and thus both move together in an anterior direction during the onset of diastole.

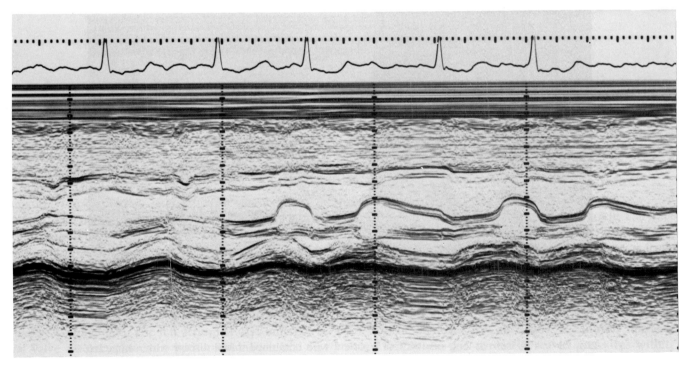

FIG. 28-6. In approximately 50% of the patients with mitral stenosis, atrial fibrillation develops.

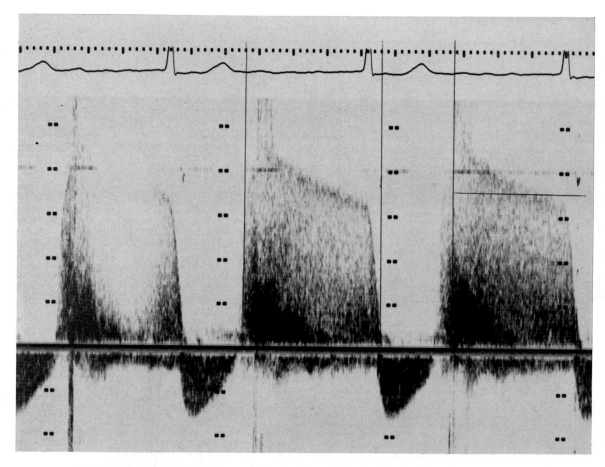

FIG. 28-15. Pressure halftime calculation for mitral stenosis. See text for explanation.

Thus the velocity representing half the initial pressure gradient is established by dividing the peak velocity by 1.4. This point is marked on the tracing, and a horizontal line representing that velocity is drawn.

3. To estimate the pressure halftime, a line is drawn along the slope of the maximum velocities, and a vertical line drawn where the calculated velocity crosses the outline. The distance between the two vertical lines is measured, and the time is then calculated from the timing marks at the edge of the trace (Fig. 28-16).

4. Estimating valve orifice area; pressure halftime remains relatively constant for an orifice over a wide range of flows. For a valve area of 1 cm^2, the pressure halftime ($P\frac{1}{2}$) is 220 milliseconds (ms). The effective orifice can be obtained by dividing the actual $P\frac{1}{2}$ into 220:

$$\text{Area}\,(\text{cm}^2) = \frac{220}{P\frac{1}{2}}$$

This measurement technique should be performed with high paper speeds (50 to 100 m/s). If the patient is in sinus rhythm, an average of 3 to 5 beats should be used for measurements. If the patient is in atrial fibrillation, then one should use at least 5 to 10 beats to obtain a more accurate measurement.

Mean mitral valve presssure gradient. These calculations can be performed by dividing the diastolic flow into five to nine equally spaced segments, averaging all the velocities, and then calculating the gradient using the average velocity. This can be done at rest and with exercise.

The Doppler tracings are generally made initially with the PW crystal in an effort to record the sharp spectral outline of the stenotic valve and the presence of mitral regurgitation (Fig. 28-17). To combine the higher velocities with a cleaner spectral pattern the CW crystal should be used. This tracing will show more spectral broadening and will be useful in recording the maximum velocities from both the stenotic and regurgitant mitral valve (Fig. 28-18).

The use of color-flow mapping can be very helpful in detecting the turbulent flow across the stenotic mitral orifice. The color flow will allow the cardiac sonographer to actually see the width and extent of the jet caused by the obstructed valve, and thus a simultaneous Doppler tracing can then be placed at the ideal site to record the maximum velocities across the valve. The presence and extent of mitral regurgitation is also well demonstrated with the color-flow technique.

MITRAL REGURGITATION

The inability of the mitral leaflets to close completely or to appose precisely in systole can be due to a variety of lesions. The leaflets may be damaged by rheumatic fever,

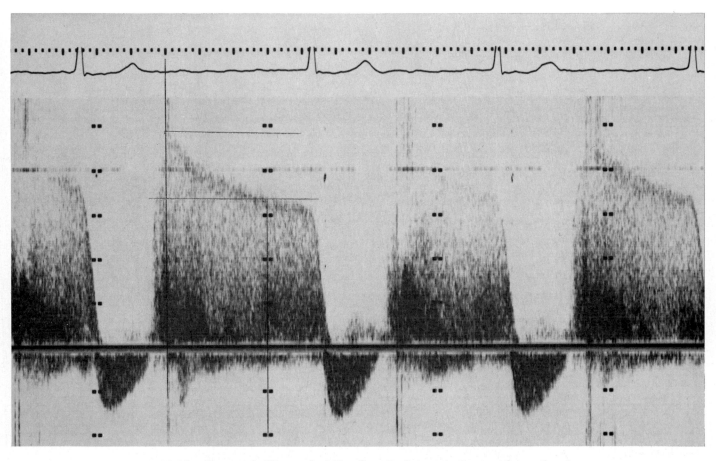

FIG. 28-16. Pressure halftime calculation for mitral stenosis. See text for explanation.

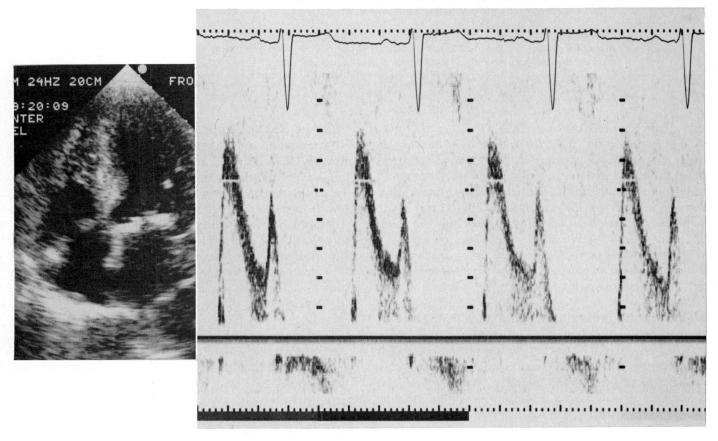

FIG. 28-17. The Doppler tracings are generally made with the PW crystal in an effort to record the sharp spectral outline of the stenotic mitral valve and the presence of mitral regurgitation. This patient has mild mitral stenosis with velocities of 120 cm/s.

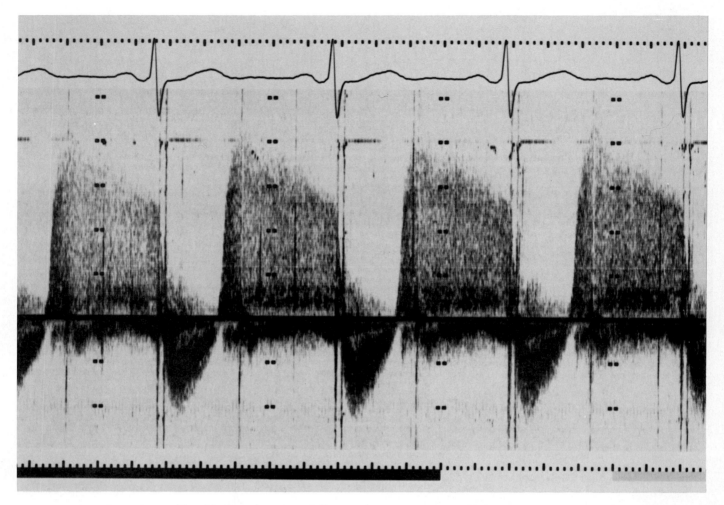

FIG. 28-18. The CW Doppler tracing allows one to record the higher-velocity flow pattern. In this tracing, each vertical marking represents 50 cm of flow; thus the mitral velocity is 2 m/s of forward flow (stenosis) and 1 m/s of reversed flow (regurgitation).

whose effects could cause regurgitation due to leaflet thickening, distortion, and calcification, thus allowing insufficient tissue for apposition or shortening of the chordae tendineae (pulling the cusps into the ventricle). Other causes are a ruptured papillary muscle, mitral valve prolapse, or hypertrophic cardiomyopathy. These conditions may give rise to mitral valve dysfunction and cause regurgitation into the left atrial cavity. Further regurgitation may be due to infective endocarditis, congenital deformity of the valve, increased diameter of the anulus, or rupture of a chordae tendineae.

The magnitude of the leakage is determined by the area of the valve orifice that remains open during systole. The regurgitation of blood into the left atrial cavity causes an increased volume in the left atrium, with a rise in left atrial pressure. This, in turn, causes a stronger atrial contraction (Starling's law) and a longer period of flow. The increased output of the left atrium increases the diastolic volume and pressure in the left ventricular cavity, which leads to dilatation and hypertrophy.

Because of the mitral regurgitation, the compensation of the left atrium and the left ventricle is achieved by an increased workload of both chambers. In an effort to maintain cardiac output, the ejection time of the left ventricle shortens and the peripheral vascular resistance decreases. Such changes enhance the forward flow of blood and diminish the regurgitant jet.

Distinction may be made between acute and chronic forms of mitral regurgitation. In "acute" forms such as a ruptured chordae tendineae, a sudden rise in left atrial pressure is noted with resulting pulmonary edema. In "chronic" cases there is left ventricular failure with reduced cardiac output and an increased ventricular diastolic pressure. The left ventricular failure may cause right ventricular failure and systemic congestion in the patient.

Echographic visualization of mitral regurgitation. Echographically, patients with rheumatic mitral regurgitation manifest findings similar to those of patients with mitral stenosis since both have thickening of the leaflets. The left atrial cavity is very enlarged, as is the left ventricular cavity (Fig. 28-19). The cardiac function is hypercontractile. Chronic cases of regurgitation will exhibit right ventricular hypertrophy with pulmonary hypertension.

On M-mode tracings the *c-e* amplitude is increased and, because of its wide excursion, may reach the left side

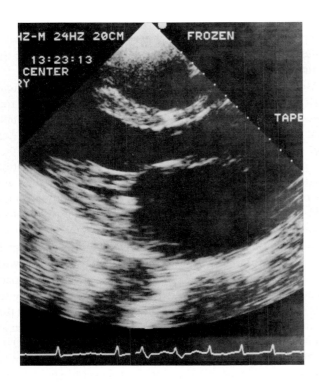

FIG. 28-19. Parasternal long-axis view of a patient with primary mitral regurgitation. The left atrial cavity is very large, as is typically seen in valvular disease.

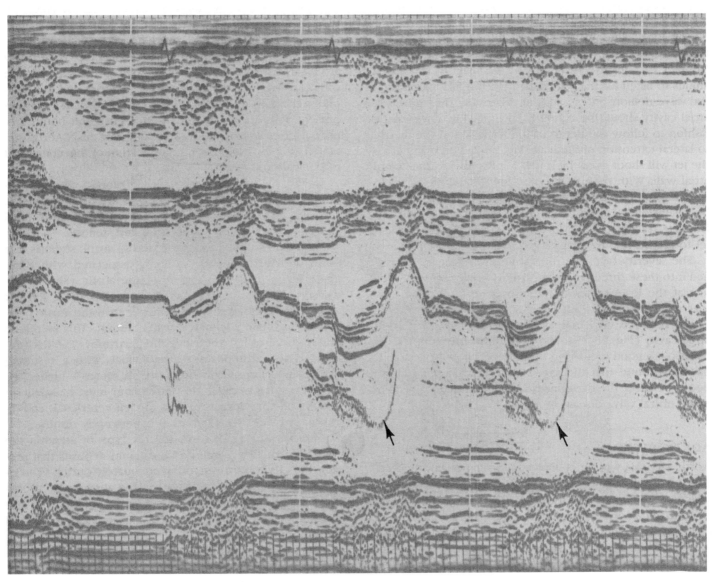

FIG. 28-20. Mitral valve prolapse is one of the more common lesions to cause primary mitral regurgitation without rheumatic involvement. Doppler has been very useful in detecting the presence of even mild forms of regurgitation with prolapse.

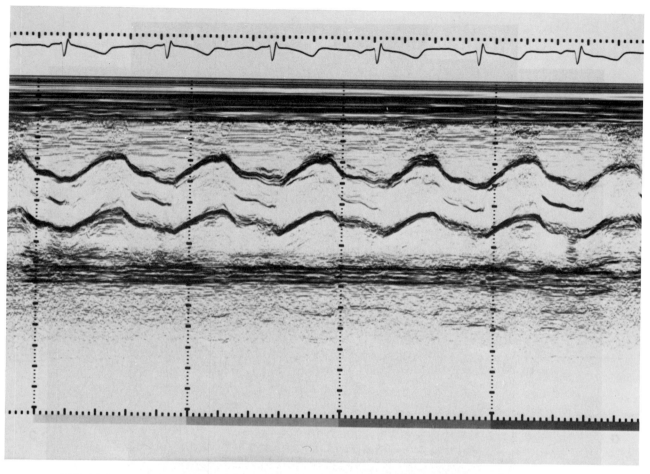

FIG. 28-28. Normal M-mode sweep of the aortic root demonstrates the motion of the aorta as it moves anterior in systole and posterior in diastole.

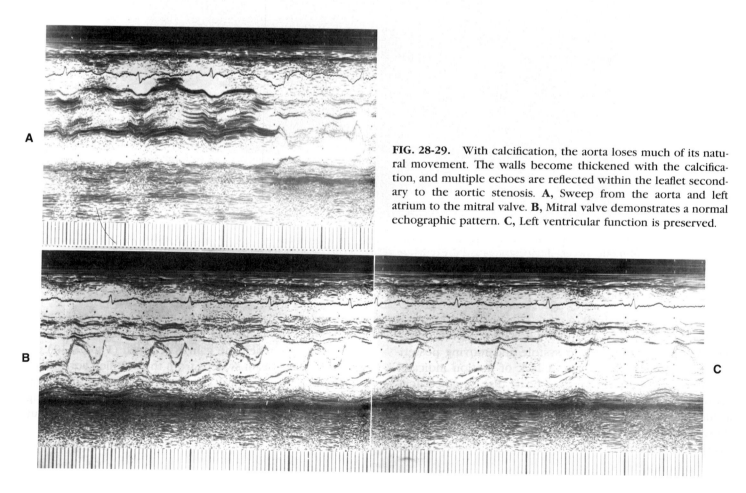

FIG. 28-29. With calcification, the aorta loses much of its natural movement. The walls become thickened with the calcification, and multiple echoes are reflected within the leaflet secondary to the aortic stenosis. **A,** Sweep from the aorta and left atrium to the mitral valve. **B,** Mitral valve demonstrates a normal echographic pattern. **C,** Left ventricular function is preserved.

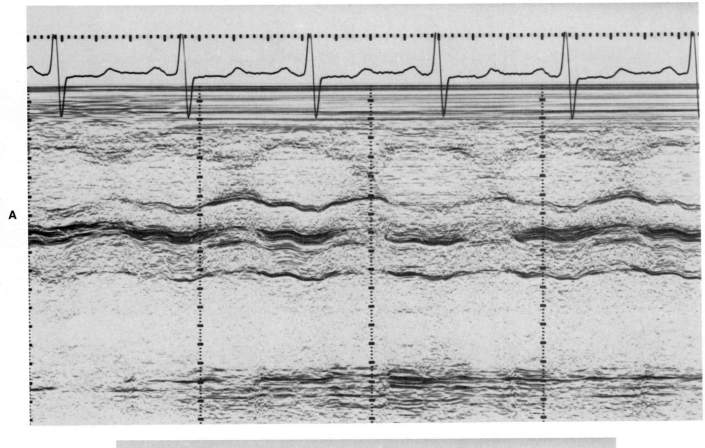

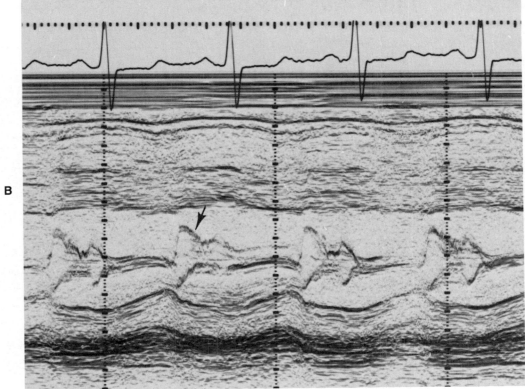

FIG. 28-30. **A,** M-mode tracing of severe aortic stenosis. Without the ECG tracing, it would be difficult to distinguish diastole from systole since the aortic cusps do not open fully. **B,** Flutter on the anterior leaflet of the mitral valve is shown due to aortic insufficiency.   *Continued.*

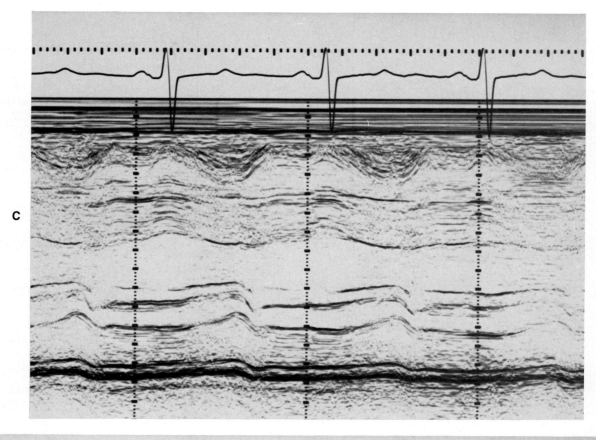

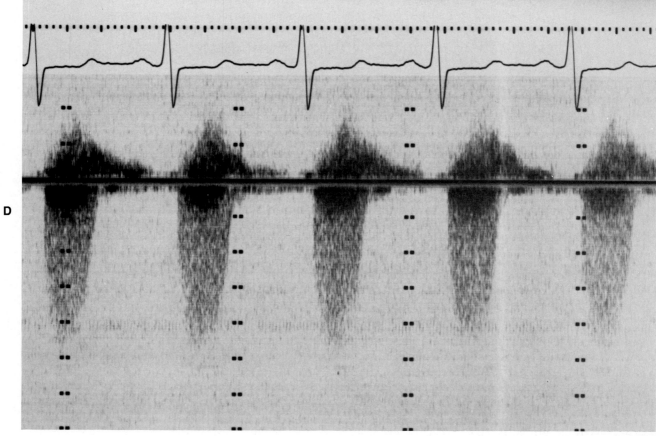

FIG. 28-30, cont'd. **C,** The left ventricular function is preserved, although there is left ventricular hypertrophy. **D,** CW Doppler tracing shows 4.5 m/s gradient across the aortic valve.

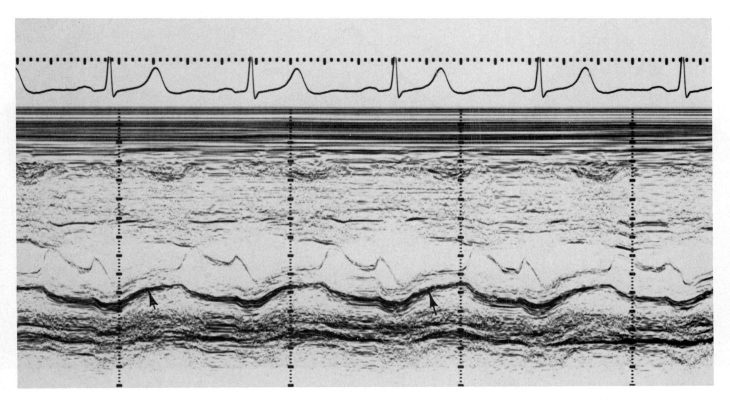

FIG. 28-31. It is common for the calcification of the aortic root to extend into the anulus of the mitral valve. This calcification is recognized as a bright, continuous echo shown posterior to the mitral valve and just anterior to the endocardial surface (see *arrows*).

within the aortic root (Fig. 28-32). With thickening and fibrosis, these echoes increase their intensity and lose their characteristic flutter. The wide systolic opening of the cusps diminishes with the degree of calcification. If the valve is severely calcified, the systolic component of the aortic cusp will be difficult to separate from the diastolic since there are so many increased echoes within the aortic root (Figs. 28-33 to 28-35).

Although the mitral valve is often pathologically unaffected by aortic stenosis, changes can be shown on the echo that result from increased pressures in the left ventricle. The amplitude of the mitral valve becomes reduced, and the *e-f* slope flattens according to the severity of the stenosis. The posterior leaflet of the mitral valve continues its normal posterior motion, and the *a* kick of the anterior leaflet is generally still apparent.

Concentric hypertrophic changes in the left ventricle have also been noted in patients with severe aortic stenosis and increased left ventricular pressure. The left ventricle exhibits decreased contractility with decompensation.

BICUSPID AORTIC VALVE. The cusps of the normal aortic valve close concentrically in diastole whereas those of the bicuspid valve close eccentrically (Fig. 28-36). It is important to record the aortic cusps in various positions to ascertain whether this abnormal condition is present. It is well known that the beam angulation can cause the normal cusps to appear to close eccentrically. We always evaluate the patient in a supine and left decubitus position and carefully search for the aortic root area to determine the accurate appearance of the aortic cusps.

As the bicuspid valve becomes calcified, ascertaining whether it is normal or bicuspid is difficult because of the increased echoes within the aortic root. The possibility that a valve is bicuspid cannot be ruled out completely by echo; but if the eccentricity is demonstrated and only two cusps are shown on the two-dimensional image, the valve is most likely bicuspid.

The two-dimensional study provides an additional method of evaluating aortic cusp closure. In the normal patient the short-axis view will show normal trileaflet cusp motion (simulating an inverted Mercedes-Benz insignia), whereas the bicuspid valve will clearly demonstrate eccentric cusp closure.

Doppler evaluation of aortic stenosis

Doppler techniques have been very useful in the evaluation of aortic stenosis; however, the severity of valvular stenosis has been more easily applied in younger patients than in adults because of the secondary effects of decreased left ventricular function as a result of the aortic disease.

The CW Doppler is the most useful crystal to use in the estimation of high-velocity flows across the calcified cusp tissue. The patient should be examined from at least two of these three windows: the apical "five"-chamber view (this is the apical four-chamber view with the transducer directed slightly more anterior to record the left ventricular outflow tract, the aorta, and aortic cusps), the suprasternal notch to sample the ascending and descend-

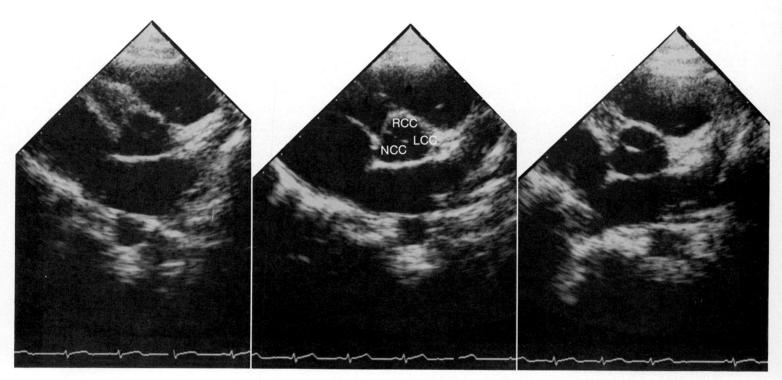

FIG. 28-32.   Multiple frames of the parasternal short-axis view of the normal aorta with the three leaflets: right coronary cusp, *RCC;* left coronary cusp, *LCC;* and noncoronary cusp, *NCC.*

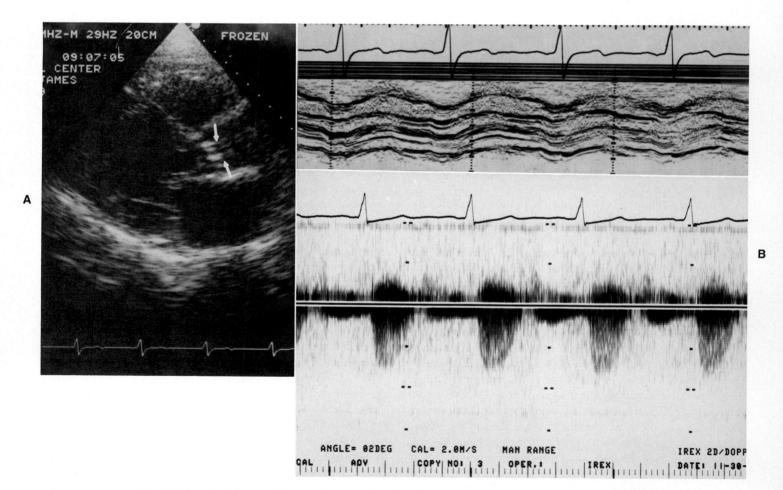

FIG. 28-33.   A, Parasternal long-axis view of the thickened and immobile aortic leaflets *(arrow).* **B,** M-mode tracing through the calcified aortic leaflets. **C,** The CW Doppler tracing made from the apical five-chamber view just beneath the aortic cusps shows a gradient of 3 m/s.

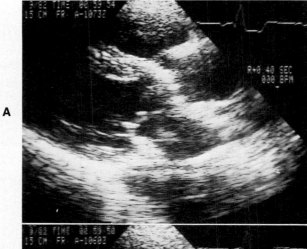

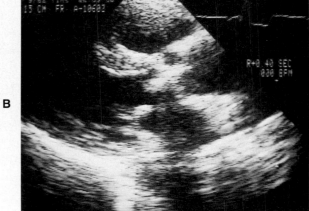

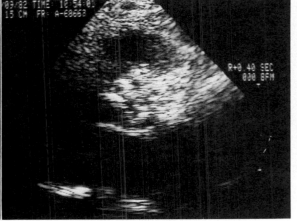

FIG. 28-34. A and **B,** Parasternal long-axis view of a patient with aortic stenosis with extension to the mitral anulus. There is mild concentric hypertrophy of the left ventricle. **C,** Parasternal short-axis view of the very thickened aortic valve. **D,** M-mode tracing of the aorta shows decreased excursion of the cusps with calcification throughout systole and diastole.

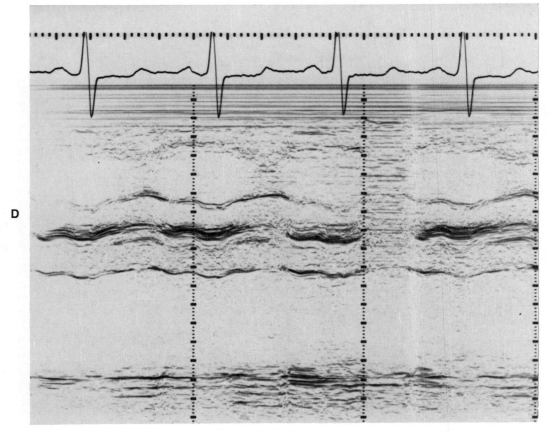

Continued.

E

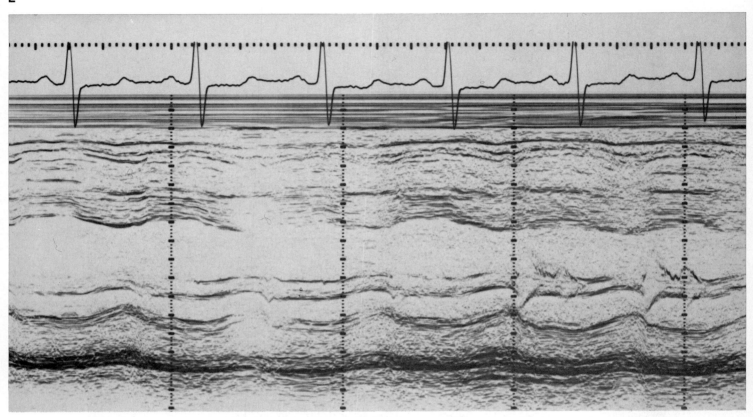

FIG. 28-34, cont'd. **E,** M-mode tracing shows the good left ventricular function with mild concentric hypertrophy.

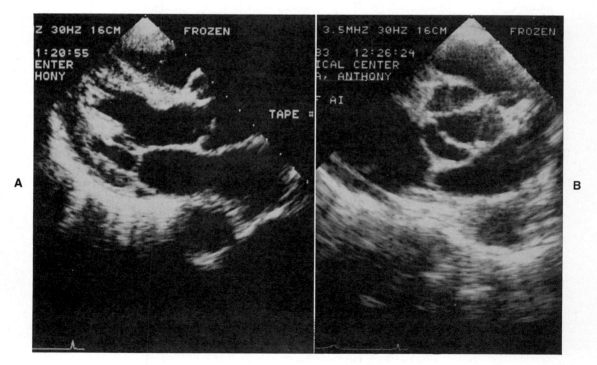

FIG. 28-35. **A,** Parasternal long-axis of the dilated aorta with slight thickening of the aortic cusps. **B,** Short-axis view of the aorta shows the trileaflet aorta with thickening along the leaflets.

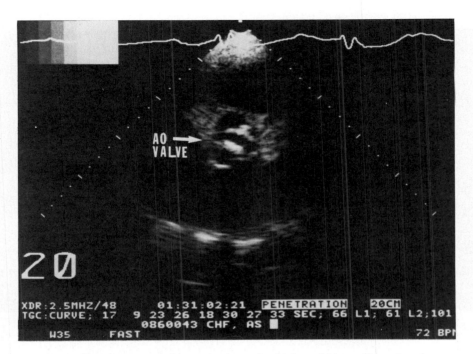

FIG. 28-36. Parasternal short-axis view of a thickened bicuspid aortic valve.

ing aortic flow, and, if possible, the right parasternal long-axis view (Fig. 28-37).

Once the highest velocity is recorded, the modified Bernoulli equation may be applied to calculate the transvalvular gradient:

$$\text{Gradient} = 4(V_{max})^2$$

For example, if a patient has a velocity of 3 m/s, one would substitute $V = 3$, thus:

$$\text{Gradient} = 4(3)^2$$
$$\text{Gradient} = 4(9)$$
$$\text{Gradient} = 36 \text{ m/s}$$

During performance of this examination it is important to keep several key points in mind. The angle of incidence is very important to record the maximum velocity. It may be difficult to find the direction of flow through the stenotic aortic valve, and thus underestimate the maximum flow. With the use of color-flow Doppler the Doppler beam may be placed in the exact maximum flow velocity pattern, and thus the actual gradient will coincide closer to the cardiac catheterization data than with just the conventional two-dimensional or blind CW probe. It is also important to remember that Doppler measures the peak instantaneous gradient (Figs. 28-38 and 28-39), and cardiac catheterization measures the "peak" pressure gradients (this is where the peak aortic pressure is subtracted from the peak left ventricular pressure). Thus a transvalvular gradient of 50 mmHg represents significant aortic stenosis. The finding of a gradient less than 50 mm Hg does not rule out the diagnosis, since the patient may have severe left ventricular dysfunction, and thus the aortic gradient would be underestimated.

AORTIC INSUFFICIENCY

The causes of aortic insufficiency include rheumatic fever, bacterial endocarditis, syphilis, aneurysm of the ascending aorta, ruptured aortic cusp, myxomatous degeneration of the aortic cusps, and hypertensive dilatation of the aortic root.

A number of factors play a role in determining the significance of aortic regurgitation: the size of the diastolic aperture, the compensation and diastolic stretchability of the left ventricle, and the peripheral resistance.

During diastole, if there is aortic valve regurgitation, the left ventricle competes with the peripheral vascular resistance for the blood in the aorta. During systole it must eject whatever extra blood it has received. Critical aortic regurgitation is present when the amount of leak is two to four times the effective cardiac output and the orifice size is 0.3 to 0.7 cm^2.

Rheumatic fever may directly involve the aortic cusps, leaving them shrunken and fibrotic. The aortic insufficiency appears secondarily on the anterior leaflet of the mitral valve as fine flutter during diastole (Fig. 28-40). The amplitude and *e-f* slope of the mitral valve decrease secondarily to the increased pressures in the left ventricle. If the mitral apparatus is calcified, the fine flutter will be difficult to detect by echo and may be seen on the left side of the septum.

Left ventricular dilation will be present in aortic insufficiency, with a hyperdynamic contractile state (Fig. 28-41). Other findings may include dilation of the aortic root (as seen in cystic medial necrosis and Marfan's syndrome) and premature closure of the anterior leaflet of the mitral valve secondary to acute aortic insufficiency (Fig. 28-42). In such patients the PR-*ac* interval would be

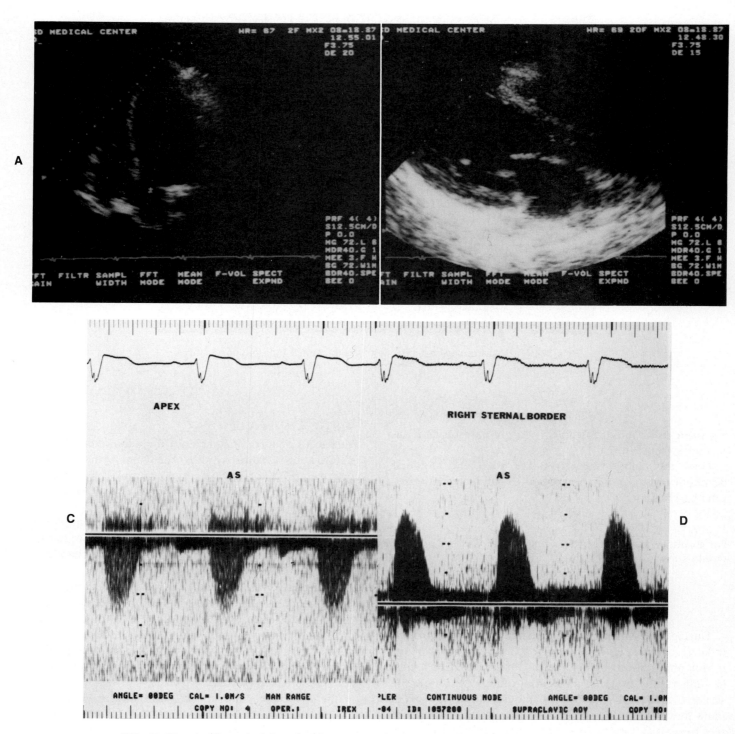

FIG. 28-37. **A,** The apical five-chamber view is best to record Doppler flow patterns from the aorta. The sample volume should be placed initially at the level of the cusps, then slowly moved into the left ventricular outflow tract (to listen for aortic insufficiency), and back into the ascending aorta (to record turbulence from aortic stenosis). **B,** The parasternal long-axis view may also be used to record the presence of aortic insufficiency. The sample volume is placed at the level of the cusps and then swept into the left ventricular outflow tract in a slight anterior-to-posterior movement. **C,** CW Doppler tracing made at the level of the aorta with the transducer placed at the apex. The flow velocity measures 2.5 m/s. The turbulent pattern is shown within the aorta. The borders of the flow profile are smooth, indicating the transducer is in the main flow stream. **D,** An alternative transducer position for aortic velocities is along the right sternal border. The velocity should be recorded in at least two different windows if possible, and the maximum velocity should be used to determine the gradient. Another window that can be useful is the suprasternal notch. The small circular "stand alone" transducer is made to fit into the sternal notch and directed caudally to record flows from the ascending and descending aorta.

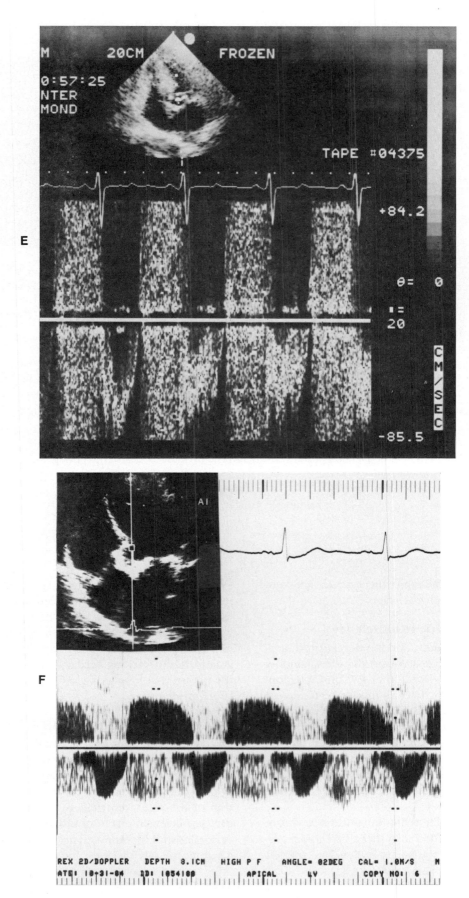

FIG. 28-37, cont'd.   E, The PW Doppler tracing may be used to record the high-pitched flows seen with aortic insufficiency, but to accurately ascertain the flow velocity, the CW recording must be made. **F,** This CW tracing shows slightly increased velocities in the ascending aorta (1.5 m/s). The diastolic flow from the aortic insufficiency is harsh and extends throughout the diastolic cycle.

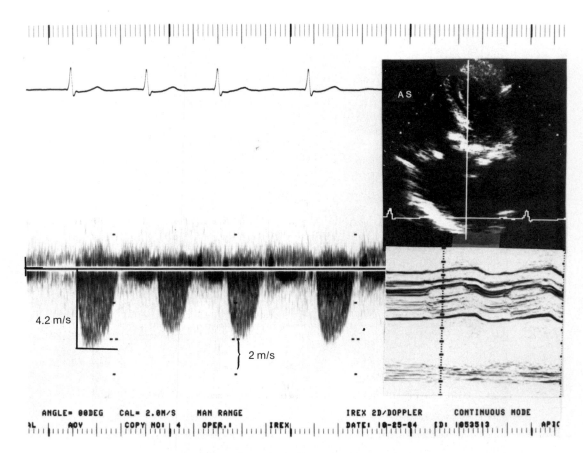

4.2 m/s

2 m/s

ANGLE= 00DEG   CAL= 2.0M/S   MAN RANGE   IREX 2D/DOPPLER   CONTINUOUS MODE

FIG. 28-38. Gradient conversion of the velocity to peak pressure. Measure the peak gradient and substitute into the formula:

$$Gradient = 4\,(V_{max})^2$$
$$(V \text{ is velocity; in this case } V = 4.2 \text{ m/s})$$

Thus
$$= 4\,(4.2)^2$$
$$= 68 \text{ mmHg}$$

foreshortened, indicating the rapid increase in left ventricular pressure from the valve leakage.

Doppler evaluation of aortic insufficiency

Doppler is a sensitive technique for the detection of aortic insufficiency. As with aortic stenosis, the ideal window is the apical "five"-chamber view. Either PW or CW Doppler may be used, although if there is moderate to severe insufficiency, the CW probe will record the maximum velocity better than the PW probe (Fig. 28-43). Aortic insufficiency is recorded as a diastolic flow reversal in the left ventricular outflow tract or ascending aorta. One may also see increased systolic aortic velocities of 1.5 to 2.5 m/s with increased velocities beginning in the left ventricular outflow tract.

With conventional Doppler techniques the severity of the insufficiency may be graded into three categories:
1. Mild: extends just below the aortic leaflets into the left ventricular outflow tract
2. Moderate: extends midway to the septum into the left ventricle
3. Severe: extends to the apex of the left ventricle

With CF Doppler one can precisely record the severity of the flow by mapping out the exact velocity pattern as it

extends into the left ventricle. The path of the regurgitant jet will be influenced by the amount of calcification on the aortic leaflets, thus while most jets "hug" the septal wall, many will take bizarre pathways into the left ventricular cavity and may be seen with multiple transducer angulations and various cardiac windows. In some patients the parasternal long-axis view is the best to see a particular regurgitant jet.

TRICUSPID STENOSIS AND INSUFFICIENCY

Tricuspid valve disease is usually present in approximately 25% of the patients with severe rheumatic heart lesions. However, clinically significant disease is present in only about 5% to 10% of these patients. Because dilation of the right ventricle is a common result of pulmonary hypertension from mitral and aortic valve disease, severe tricuspid incompetence may occur in the absence of a significant valve lesion.

Tricuspid stenosis

Most cases of tricuspid stenosis are of rheumatic origin, with the mitral and aortic valves being affected first. Other causes are congenital defects, systemic lupus erythematosus, and carcinoid tumors. The stenotic leaflets

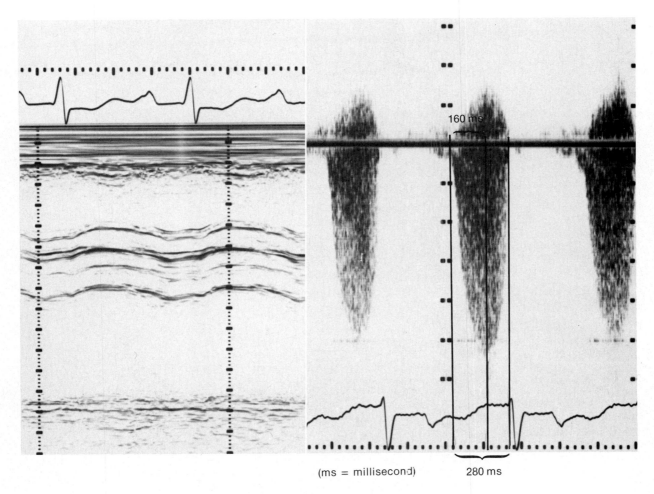

(ms = millisecond)   280 ms

FIG. 28-39. Time to peak velocity measurement in systole.

$$\frac{\text{Time to peak velocity}}{\text{Left ventricular ejection time}}$$

$$\frac{160 \text{ ms}}{280 \text{ ms}} = 0.50$$

Time to peak values: Mild obstruction = <0.50; severe obstruction = >0.55

usually fuse, leaving a roundish hilum in the central area of the leaflets and some degree of incompetence of the valve. Right atrial hypertrophy occurs, and cardiac output falls when the right ventricular filling is impaired because of further narrowing of the valve orifice.

Tricuspid insufficiency

There are two types of tricuspid insufficiency: functional and organic. Functional insufficiency is the result of right ventricular failure, which causes right ventricular dilatation. This dilatation causes the tricuspid ring also to dilate, producing tricuspid valve regurgitation (Fig. 28-44). Organic regurgitation is caused by rheumatic disease, congenital lesions of Ebstein's disease and endocardial cushion defects, or bacterial endocarditis. The right atrium enlarges with regurgitant flow from the tricuspid valve (Fig. 28-45). Likewise, during diastole the right ventricle receives this blood from the right atrium in addition to that reaching the right atrium from the great veins, causing hypertrophy and dilation. The dilated right side of

the heart permits easy visualization of the tricuspid valve echographically.

The tricuspid leaflet opens and closes as the mitral leaflet does, with no fluttering motion. If fine flutter is noted, there are several possible causes, the most common is pulmonary insufficiency. The regurgitation from the pulmonary valve acts the same as aortic insufficiency does on the mitral apparatus. The backflow of blood strikes the tricuspid leaflet, causing high-frequency flutter.

Doppler evaluation of the tricuspid valve

Generally the most common lesion seen is tricuspid insufficiency. The best window to record velocities from the tricuspid valve is the apical four-chamber window or the left parasternal long-axis window (Figs. 28-46 and 28-47). Sometimes the velocities may be recorded from the parasternal short-axis window; as one demonstrates the aortic valve and right ventricular outflow tract, the transducer is angled slightly inferior to record the leaflets

Text continued on p. 678.

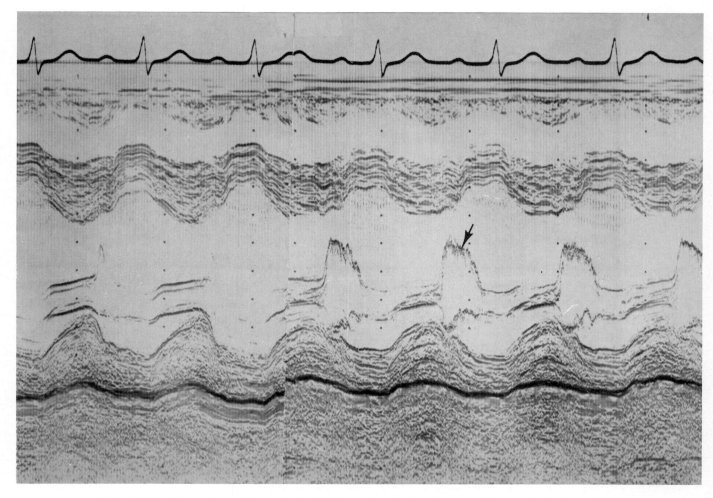

FIG. 28-40. The patient with aortic insufficiency shows a fine flutter on the anterior leaflet of the mitral valve as the regurgitant jet from the incompetent aortic cusp hits the leaflet. There is also dilatation of the left ventricular cavity.

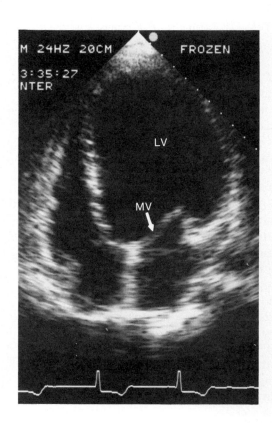

FIG. 28-41. Apical four-chamber view of the dilated left ventricular cavity and decreased opening of the anterior leaflet of the mitral valve in a patient with aortic insufficiency. *LV,* left ventricle; *MV,* mitral valve.

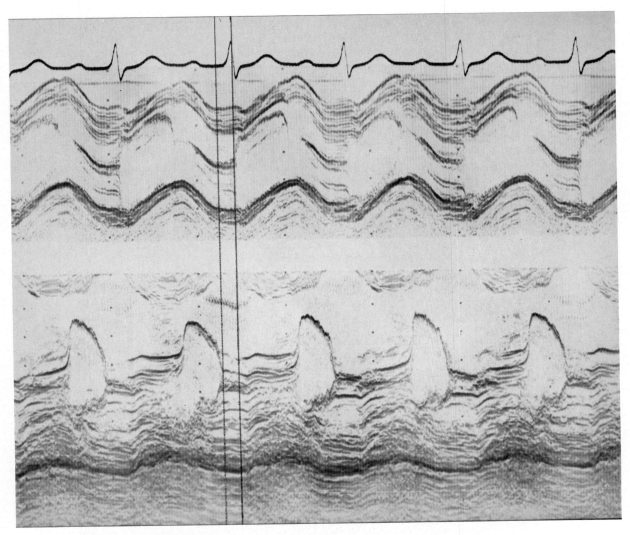

FIG. 28-42. Premature closure of the mitral valve secondary to acute onset of aortic insufficiency. The PR-*ac* interval is foreshortened, indicating the rapid increase in left ventricular pressure from the jet.

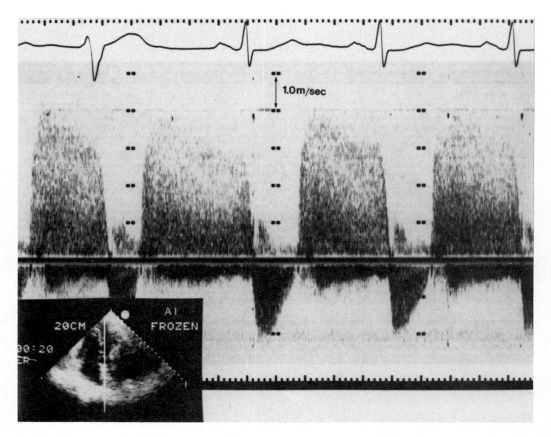

FIG. 28-43. Aortic insufficiency is recorded as a diastolic flow reversal in the left ventricular out-flow tract or ascending aorta.

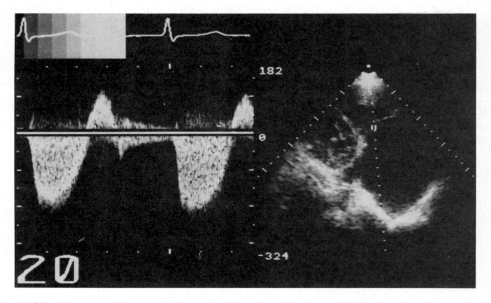

FIG. 28-44. Parasternal long-axis view over the tricuspid valve with CW Doppler shows the flow reversal of insufficiency.

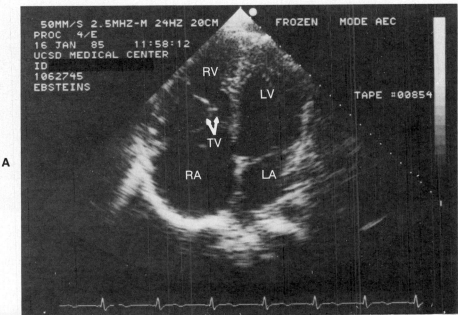

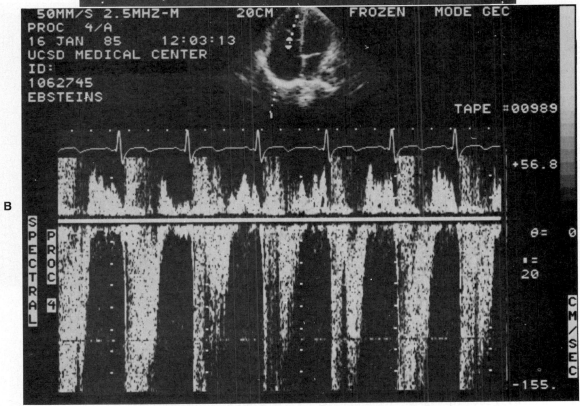

FIG. 28-45. A, Apical four-chamber view of a patient with organic tricuspid regurgitation from Ebstein's malformation of the tricuspid valve. The valve is displaced apically and has an abnormal closure, causing the regurgitant jet into the right atrial cavity. *RA,* right atrium; *RV,* right ventricle; *TV,* tricuspid valve; *LV,* left ventricle; *LA,* left atrium. **B,** PW tracing of the tricuspid regurgitation.

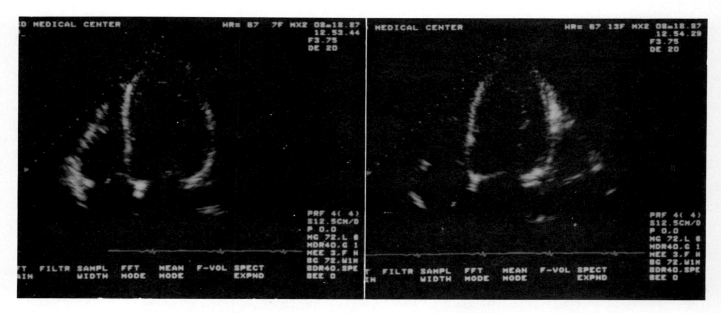

FIG. 28-46. The tricuspid velocities may be recorded from several different windows. If the apical four-chamber view is used, the sample volume is placed at the level of the tricuspid valve and then is slowly moved into the right atrial cavity, usually near the interatrial septum, since this is where most regurgitant jets flow.

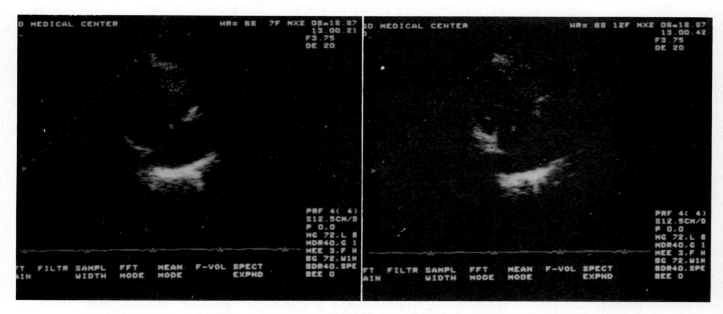

FIG. 28-47. An alternative window for tricuspid velocities is the parasternal long-axis view over the tricuspid leaflets. The sample volume is placed at the level of the leaflets and then is slowly moved into the right atrial cavity.

of the tricuspid valve with the right atrial chamber (Fig. 28-48).

The severity of the insufficiency is classified in terms of mild, moderate, and severe. The mild form is seen just at the anulus level. The moderate form extends midway into the right atrial cavity, and the severe form extends to the base of the right atrium. As with other valves, the strength of the Doppler signal, the position and width of the velocity, and the sound of the velocity differential will help the examiner determine the classification of the regurgitant jet.

Color-flow mapping has shown us that not all regurgitant jets are shown to flow from the tricuspid anulus to the medial wall of the interatrial septum. The path of the jet will depend on the deformity of the valve and thus may dart in a lateral pathway, or even directly into the atrial cavity.

Systolic pressure gradient. It is possible to calculate the systolic pressure gradient across the tricuspid valve by using the regurgitant velocity and the Bernoulli equation formula ($P_1 - P_2 = 4V^2$) to give an accurate estimate of the systolic pressure difference between the right

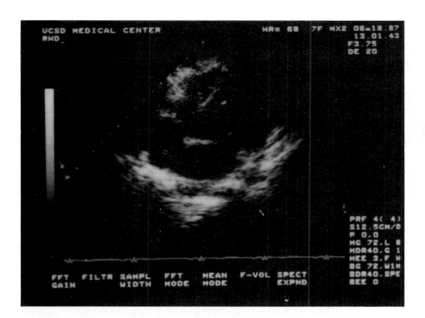

FIG. 28-48. The modified four-chamber view (which is somewhat in between a short-axis and apical view) is also useful in many patients to record adequate tricuspid flows.

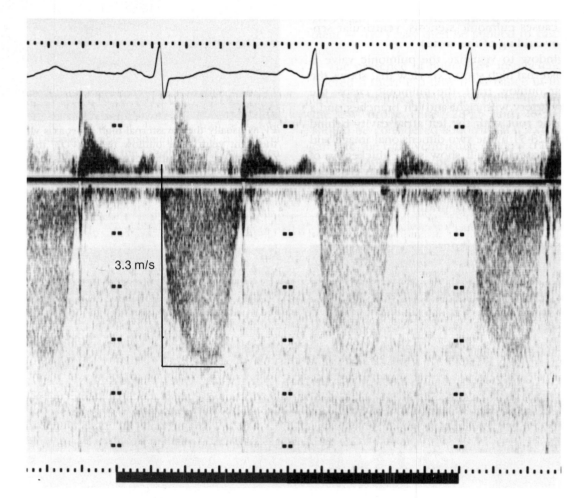

3.3 m/s

FIG. 28-49. Right ventricular systolic pressure.
RVSP: Right ventricular systolic pressure
RA: Right atrial pressure (Constant of 5 mm Hg used for right atrial pressure in systole. Normal range is 0 to 5 mm Hg.)

$$4(V_{max})^2 - \text{Tricuspid regurgitation velocity}$$
$$\text{RVSP} = \text{RA} + 4\,(V_{max})^2$$
$$= 5\,\text{mm Hg} + 4\,(3.3)^2$$
$$= 5\,\text{mm Hg} + 44$$
$$= 49\,\text{mm Hg}$$

creasing depths, loss of signal strength because of attenuation may make distinction of signal from background noise quite difficult; failure to detect Doppler signals from significant depths may be a function of attenuation rather than absence of flow abnormality. Doppler techniques are to some extent limited by their relative insensitivity to differences in flow profiles across regions of interest: pulsed techniques may be subject to sampling errors if flow profiles are not blunt, and continuous-wave techniques are best suited to showing the highest (rather than the spatial average) velocities.

Flow velocities are dependent on volume flow rates, so that conditions that alter flow rates from normal (ventricular dysfunction, valvular regurgitation, intracardiac shunting) may reduce or elevate the measured velocities.

The last pitfall is important when one is comparing Doppler data to independent invasive measurements—results from the dynamics of hemodynamics. Cardiac pressures and flows clearly can vary substantially over time, even from beat to beat, and these variations are not always accompanied by overt changes in the clinical state of the patient.

Thus as one bears in mind these pitfalls and attempts to avoid them when performing the Doppler examination, the information obtained from a Doppler examination can be very useful in the clinical management of patients with valvular heart disease.

PROSTHETIC VALVES

When a patient develops rheumatic heart disease, progressive degeneration and calcification of the valvular structures causes heart failure. To relieve the narrowing of these valves, it becomes necessary to replace the damaged tissue with a prosthetic heart valve to relieve the heart of this burden. There are several types of prosthetic valves: caged-ball, caged-disk, tilting disk, and bioprosthesis. It is important for the sonographer to know the type of prosthetic valve the patient has implanted for adequate recording of its most perpendicular axis.

There are three basic parts to each type of mechanical valve: the disk or ball, the strut or cage, and the sewing ring or seating of the valve (the upper and lower round attachment of the valve). Any of these components is subject to changes. The Starr-Edwards ball is composed of silicon and is subject to ball variance or a grooving irregularity. This ball variance is not seen in the Teflon disk valves. Some of the valves are cloth covered and not as subject to thrombus formation.

The incidence of thrombosis with good anticoagulation is 30%. The upper and lower seating is frequently subject to thrombus, which in turn narrows the valve. The lower seating thrombosis interferes with closure of the valve and eventually can lead to regurgitation. In addition to these problems with thrombosis, the sutures around the area of the valve can come loose, causing regurgitation.

The evaluation of defects in the valve is sometimes difficult. Most patients are asymptomatic. Some demonstrate signs of fatigue. Some go into congestive heart failure because of a sticking poppet. Embolism to various organs may be seen as a result of thrombus formation on the valve. Bacterial endocarditis is one complication of prosthetic valves because the malfunctioning valve is a seedbed for bacteria.

The disk and hinge valves can be used interchangeably in the aorta and mitral valve by reversing their positions. During auscultation the valves should make two noises during one cycle. At the onset of systole the mitral valve should have a closing click, whereas the aortic valve should have an opening click. Likewise, during diastole the mitral valve should have an opening click and the aortic valve a closing click. With the valve in the aortic area there is normally a slight gradient. In the mitral area there is a small gradient as the blood flows from a low pressure to a high pressure, giving rise to the mid-diastolic murmur. The various valves have different intensities in their opening and closing clicks. For example, a Bjork-Shiley prosthesis has a soft opening and a loud closing.

The presence of a systolic murmur in the mitral valve area is abnormal and is frequently attributed to a paravalvular leak. If there is a clot inside the cage, it causes the valve to close improperly, and regurgitation is the inevitable result.

Diagnostic studies useful in assessing prosthetic function are chest radiography, fluoroscopy, angiography, and echocardiography.

Chest radiography can determine cardiac enlargement or the position of the prosthesis. Fluoroscopy is helpful if there is a detachment of the valve or a paravalvular leak, causing the valve to tilt in the mitral position (i.e., into the left atrium). With the aortic valve, movement is usually very dramatic; if there is a problem, side-to-side "flipping" of the valve can be recorded.

Angiography can detect leakage, but since there is a slight degree of regurgitation with the prosthesis, it may be more difficult. Diagnostic regurgitation is physiologic in the mitral valve area. In pathologic regurgitation the dye will be seen to go into the ventricle during systole.

Echocardiography has proven to be a useful technique in the assessment of valve function because of the strong reflecting interface between the artificial valve and the surrounding structures. The exact model and size of the prosthesis are noted prior to recording the valve movement. If the examiner is not careful, only the supporting structures of the cage may be recorded without disk or ball movement. By angling the transducer so the beam is more perpendicular to the prosthesis, one can record the proper echoes. This transducer angle is critical in the assessment of valvar motion and excursion. The motion of the prosthesis is determined by valve characteristics and the entire cardiac structure. To provide the most accurate assessment of valve function, recordings should be made shortly after surgery and followed at specific time intervals.

Mitral valve prosthesis

The best mitral recording will clearly record the valve opening and closure and most closely approximate the valve's normal excursion. Disk or hinge valves can gener-

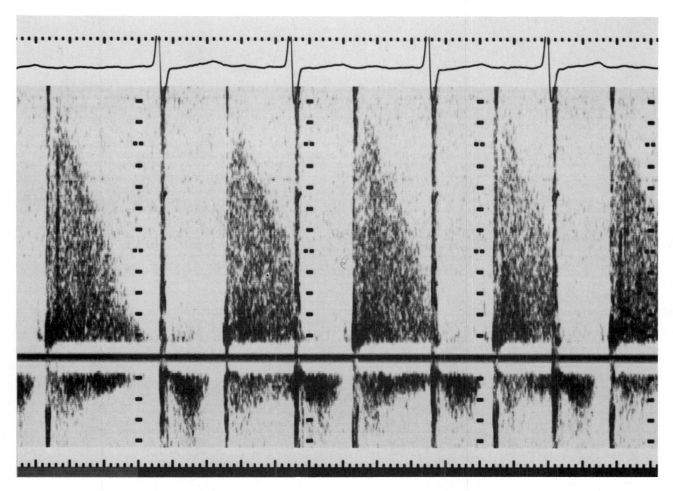

FIG. 28-57. CW Doppler tracing of a Braunwald Cutter mechanical prosthesis in the mitral valve position. Using real-time ultrasound, the valve appeared to be well seated with normal valve ball motion. The peak velocity across the prosthetic mitral valve is 2.0 to 2.5 m/s, which suggests a mitral valve area of approximately 1.1 cm². No mitral insufficiency was seen.

ally be recorded in their usual mitral position (Fig. 28-57). However, it may be necessary to locate the Starr-Edwards valve position on the radiographic film for proper transducer angulation. Often the sonographer must move to the apex of the heart and angle the transducer severely cephalad to record the valve at its most perpendicular angle (Fig. 28-58).

The actual thrombus formation is difficult to distinguish by echo, but the altered valve motion may be recorded. Sometimes there is a delay in the valve opening, or there is no opening at all during some cycles. Decreased amplitude of valve opening must be assessed with the transducer in various angles to ascertain the maximum excursion. Because of the intense echo reflection of the valve apparatus, there often appears to be large clumps or "ring-down" echoes behind the open valve. This should not be confused with thrombus and usually can be eliminated by slight transducer angulations or a reduction in the sensitivity of the equipment.

Johnson[3] described the actual measurement of the older type of ball valves by echo and has mutliple charts available for analysis of individual tracings. He also discov-ered that the Starr-Edwards ball was made of Silastic rubber, a slower sound conduction material. Thus when recordings are made from such a valve, it appears that the posterior edge of the ball is actually beyond its posterior cage. A correction factor of 0.64 can be applied to the measurement of the ball diameter to adjust for this factor.

Doppler assessment of mitral valve dysfunction. Most prosthetic valves result in a slight to moderate obstruction of flow, which results in increased velocity across the prosthetic valve (Fig. 28-59). With this increased velocity, a pressure drop can be calculated from the increase in velocity as in valve stenosis. The velocity and pressure drop depend on the valve area, heart rate, flow across the valve, cardiac output, and regurgitant flow. Hatle[2] states that pressure halftimes are slightly longer than across normal valves (i.e., under 60 ms), usually between 70 and 120 ms, varying with the type and size of prosthesis.

It is difficult to record regurgitant flow velocity with the disk-type prosthesis. If there is leakage around the valve (paravalvular), it may be more easily recorded by Doppler, and certainly easier to record with color-flow

Text continued on p. 690.

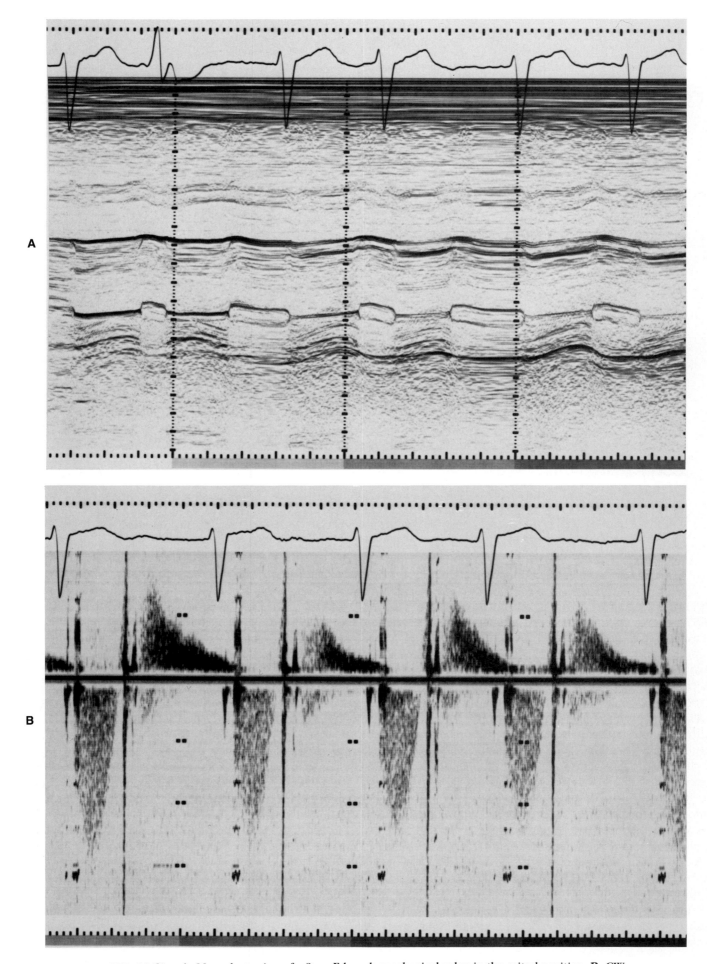

FIG. 28-58. **A,** M-mode tracing of a Starr-Edwards mechanical valve in the mitral position. **B,** CW Doppler tracing of the valve. Mild to moderate mitral regurgitation is present.

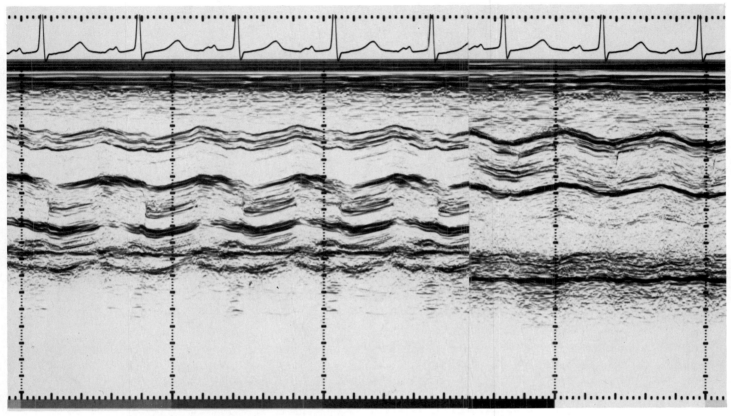

A

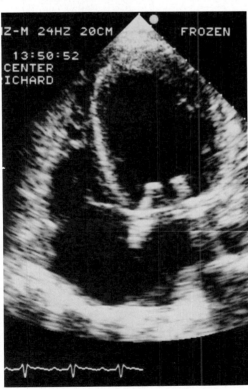

B

FIG. 28-59. **A,** M-mode sweep in a patient with a porcine mitral and aortic valve. **B,** Apical four-chamber view showing the mitral prosthesis. *Continued.*

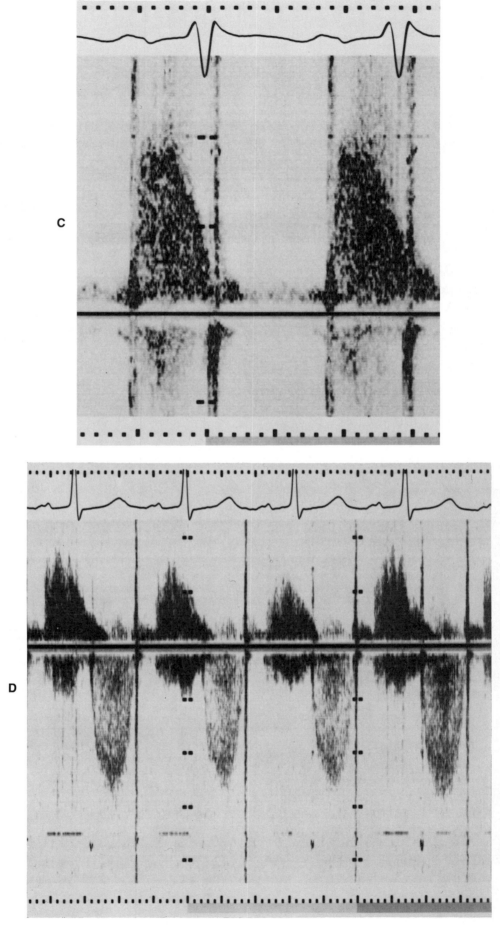

FIG. 28-59, cont'd.   C, CW Doppler of the normal mitral valve flow. **D,** CW Doppler of the aortic valve flow with some aortic insufficiency.

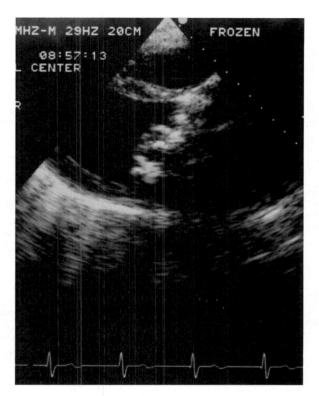

FIG. 28-60. Parasternal long-axis of the mitral and aortic prosthesis. The strong reflections from the prosthetic device make it difficult to determine the presence of vegetation or thickening.

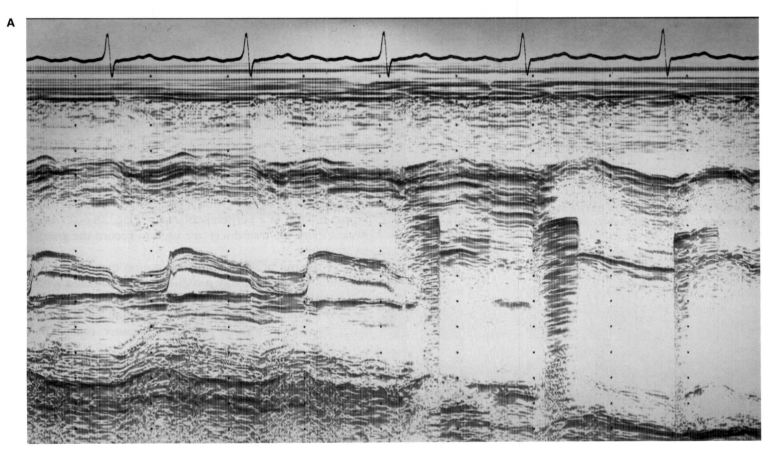

FIG. 28-61. **A,** M-mode tracing of a patient with an aortic prosthesis. Note the strong reflections from the hinge of the prosthetic device as they "ring" into the left atrial cavity.   *Continued.*

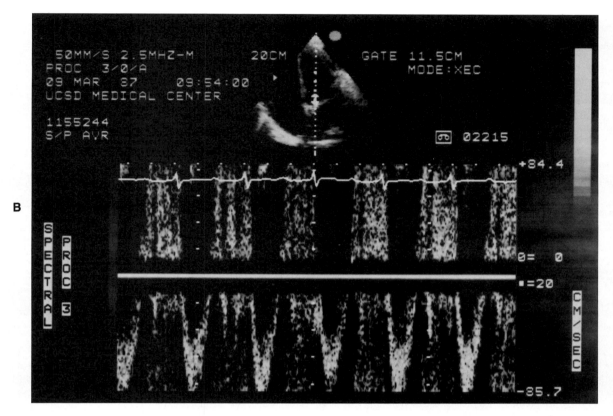

FIG. 28-62, cont'd.   B, PW Doppler shows the presence of aortic insufficiency along the septum and near the right coronary cusp.

Tricuspid valve

It is often confusing to evaluate a patient with two or three prosthetic valves, and careful examination must be done to separate each of the valves. With routine cardiac sweeps, the transducer may record the individual valves to help the sonographer evaluate the most perpendicular axis. Then the transducer can be moved to the tricuspid area or to the apex of the heart to record the maximum amplitude of the valves.

Doppler assessment of tricuspid valve function. The Doppler evaluation of tricuspid prosthetic valve dysfunction would be approached in a manner similar to that for the mitral valve evaluation (Fig. 28-63). Care must be taken to avoid the reflections from the prosthetic device so they will not interfere with the Doppler reflections.

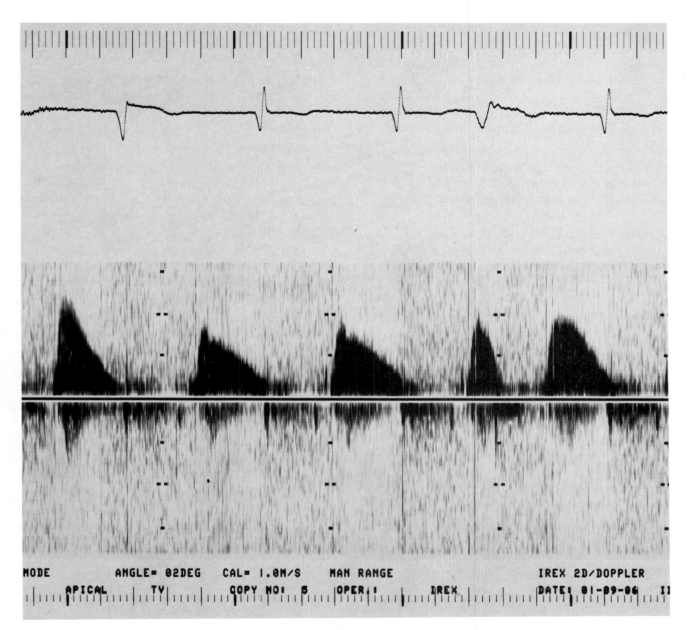

FIG. 28-63. CW Doppler tracing in a patient with a porcine heterograft in the tricuspid position. The valve appeared to be well seated. There was no evidence for tricuspid regurgitation. The half-time calculation of the tricuspid valve orifice area gave an estimate of 1.3 cm.

SUMMARY

1. Rheumatic fever is probably the primary cause of valvar stenosis and regurgitation problems in the heart. The fever may cause three forms of carditis: endocarditis, myocarditis, and pericarditis.

2. Obstruction at the mitral valve orifice can be acquired, congenital, or obstructed secondary to a tumor mass.

3. The presence of rheumatic fever may cause several changes to occur on the valve leaflets. Changes will progress with scarring and calcification. Leaflets may be diffusely thickened by fibrous tissue or calcium deposits, or the commissures may be fused.

4. Echographically: (Mitral stenosis) reduction of the *e-f* slope of the anterior leaflet of the mitral valve, posterior leaflet moves anteriorly, reduced amplitude, increased echoes due to calcification, atrial fibrillation, enlarged left atrium, systemic emboli.

5. "Pseudo" stenosis may be caused by aortic stenosis, hypertrophic cardiomyopathy, or tumor mass.

6. In patients with mitral stenosis, the Doppler velocity would be greater than 1 m/s, and there would be a slower deceleration of blood velocity after the early diastolic filling phase. The severity of the stenosis can be estimated by calculating the mitral valve orifice by either the pressure halftime method or by

measuring the mean pressure gradient across the valve.

7. Color-flow Doppler allows the width and extent of the jet caused by the obstructed valve to be seen.

8. The inability of the mitral leaflets to close completely or to appose precisely in systole can be due to a variety of lesions.

9. The magnitude of regurgitation is determined by the area of the valve orifice that remains open during systole. The regurgitation of blood into the left atrial cavity causes an increased volume in the left atrium.

10. Doppler is a specific and very sensitive method to diagnose mitral regurgitation. The severity is classified into three categories: mild, moderate, and severe.

11. Aortic stenosis may be related to one of three entities: isolated stenosis, acquired stenosis, and congenital lesions of the aorta.

12. Echographically the aortic valve thickens and fibrose. Concentric hypertrophy may develop with pressure overload in the left ventricle.

13. CW Doppler is the most useful technique to evaluate the severity of the stenosis. The modified Bernoulli equation is used to calculate the gradient across the valve.

14. Causes of aortic insufficiency are rheumatic fever, bacterial endocarditis, syphilis, aneurysm of the ascending aorta, ruptured aortic cusp, myxomatous degeneration of the aortic cusps, and hypertensive dilatation of the root.

15. Aortic insufficiency is recorded on Doppler as a diastolic flow reversal in the left ventricular outflow tract or ascending aorta.

16. The severity of the insufficiency is graded in three categories: mild, moderate, and severe.

17. Color-flow Doppler shows the path of the regurgitant jet.

18. Most cases of tricuspid stenosis are of rheumatic origin. Other causes are congenital defects, systemic lupus erythematosus, and carcinoid tumors.

19. There are two types of tricuspid insufficiency: functional and organic. The severity is classified as mild, moderate, or severe.

20. Color-flow Doppler shows the path of the jet as it moves into the right atrial cavity.

21. Systolic pressure gradient may be calculated by using the regurgitant velocity and the Bernoulli equation formula to give an accurate estimate of the systolic pressure difference between the right ventricle and right atrium.

22. The occurrence of pulmonary stenosis is more frequently seen in the neonate and pediatric patient. The most common cause is residual stenosis after a tetralogy of Fallot repair.

23. Doppler flow velocities are dependent on volume flow rates, so conditions that alter flow from normal may reduce or elevate the measured velocities.

24. A prosthetic valve is used to relieve the narrowing of the diseased cardiac valves.

25. Several types of prosthetic valves: caged-ball, caged-disk, tilting disk, and bioprosthesis.

26. There are three basic parts to each type of mechanical valve: the disk or ball, the strut or cage, and the sewing ring or seating of the valve.

27. The incidence of thrombosis with good anticoagulation is 30%.

28. Echographically the transducer angle is critical in the assessment of prosthetic valvular motion and excursion.

29. Most prosthetic valves result in a slight to moderate obstruction of flow, which results in increased velocity across the prosthetic valve.

REFERENCES

1. Cope GD, Kisslo JA, Johnson ML, et al.: A reassessment of the echocardiogram in mitral stenosis, Circulation 52:664, 1975.
2. Hatle L: Doppler ultrasound in cardiology, Philadelphia, 1982, Lea & Febiger.
3. Johnson ML: Echocardiographic evaluation of prosthetic heart valves. In Gramiak R and Waag RC, editors: Cardiac ultrasound, St. Louis, 1975, The CV Mosby Co.
4. Kisslo J: Two-dimensional echocardiography, New York, 1980, Churchill Livingstone.
5. Pearlman AS: Pitfalls in Doppler evaluation of valvular disease, Fourth Curriculum on Color Flow Mapping and Cardiac Doppler, Washington DC, Nov. 7-10, 1985.

Other Valvular Abnormalities

This chapter concentrates on acquired valvular abnormalities such as atrioventricular valve prolapse, Marfan's syndrome, bacterial endocarditis, rupture of the chordal structures or papillary muscles, papillary muscle dysfunction, calcification of the mitral anulus, and supravalvular and subvalvular aortic stenosis.

ATRIOVENTRICULAR VALVE PROLAPSE

The exact cause of prolapse of the mitral valve is a topic of controversy. Numerous studies have been conducted in an effort to relate information about prolapse with other clinical data. One acknowledged condition is a change in the consistency of the leaflet or papillary muscle. Clinical investigations have reported that a myxomatous degeneration of the mitral apparatus can lead to prolapse of the leaflet.[2] Elongation of the anterior leaflet is a common finding in prolapse and causes the valve to sag and close beyond the mitral anulus into the left atrial cavity.

Barlow et al.[1] demonstrated that a midsystolic click and late systolic murmur did, in fact, result from a billowing or prolapse of the mitral leaflet, referred to as Barlow's syndrome. He noted that these particular patients had mitral regurgitation during the latter part of systole. Some patients had unusual anatomic deformities of the mitral valve apparatus characterized by mid to late systolic prolapse. The cause of such a floppy valve could not be totally explained, but several investigators believed it was a genetic factor.

A high percentage of patients with prolapse have clinical symptoms of chest pain, fatigue, and ventricular arrhythmias at some point in their clinical course. This fact supports the belief that the syndrome of a prolapsed mitral valve is a significant component of left ventricular disease.

The disease frequently is found in young adults and has been probably more often discovered with the echo examination. The prolapsed leaflet generally becomes elongated, redundant, and thickened by the myxomatous degeneration (Fig. 29-1). The chordae become elongated and thus allow the mitral apparatus to buckle into the left atrium (producing the click on auscultation). The timing and intensity of the click and murmur (of mitral regurgitation) vary with volume changes of the left ventricle induced by posture changes, or with the Valsalva maneuver, or with amyl nitrite.

The major complications of prolapse include mitral regurgitation, spontaneous chordal rupture, increased tendency to develop infective endocarditis, or, infrequently, sudden death.

Echography of the mitral apparatus can be very sensitive for prolapse if certain criteria are met. The systolic posterior displacement of the anterior or posterior leaflet is one of the primary findings in prolapse. Prolapse can occur throughout systole (holosystolic or pansystolic), in midsystole, or in late systole. Normally the c-d segment of the mitral apparatus moves slightly anterior in systole. However, in prolapse the d point stays 2 to 3 mm behind the c point into the left atrial cavity (Fig. 29-2). The midsystolic click coincides with this posterior movement.

The valve may also show several echoes throughout systole and diastole that may represent thickening, degeneration, or redundancy of the leaflet (Fig. 29-3).

The holosystolic bowing of the mitral apparatus was

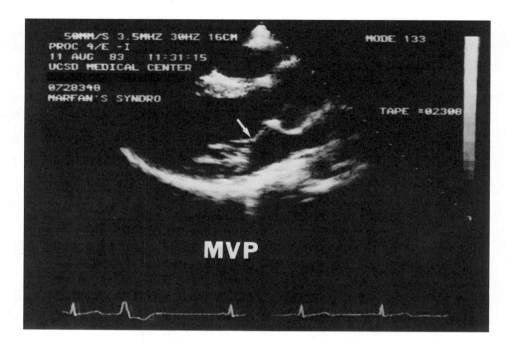

FIG. 29-6. Often it is easier to identify a patient with prolapse with the two-dimensional image rather than the M-mode image because more of the valve leaflet may be visualized in many different windows. The parasternal long-axis view is probably the best view to identify a prolapse pattern. The leaflet may appear to be longer than normal (show redundancy), appear thicker than normal, or prolapse into the left atrial cavity. In addition, one should search for chordal attachments to rule out the possibility of a torn chordae tendineae. The *arrow* points to the anterior leaflet of the mitral valve as it sags into the left atrial cavity.

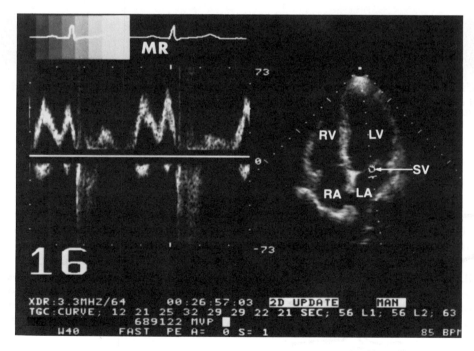

FIG. 29-7. Associated mitral regurgitation is usually present in patients with mitral valve prolapse. The Doppler sample volume should initially be placed at the level of the mitral anulus, and then carefully moved into the atrial cavity to listen for the regurgitant jet flow. With color-flow Doppler, one can easily map the jet with the turbulent color pattern in the left atrial cavity. *RV,* right ventricle; *RA,* right atrium; *LV,* left ventricle; *LA,* left atrium; *SV,* sample volume; *MR,* mitral regurgitation.

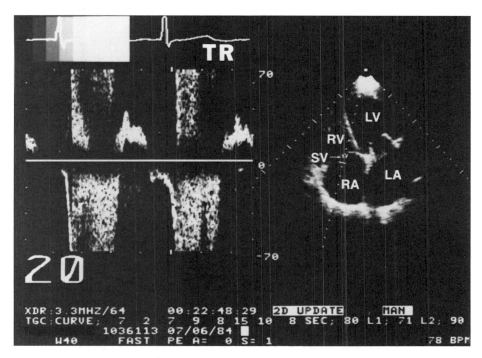

FIG. 29-8. The tricuspid valve should also be carefully interrogated in patients with mitral valve prolapse, as the myxomatous degeneration may affect both valve leaflets. This sample volume, *SV*, is placed at the anulus of the tricuspid valve to record the regurgitant jet flow in the apical four-chamber view. *RV*, right ventricle; *RA*, right atrium; *LV*, left ventricle; *LA*, left atrium.

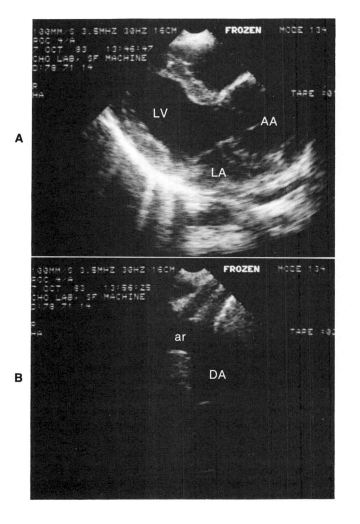

FIG. 29-9. In patients with Marfan's syndrome, the mitral valve is abnormal (redundant with prolapse), and the aortic root is very dilated. This dilatation may extend into the ascending aorta, to the arch, and to the descending aorta, depending on the extent of the disorder. Thus careful evaluation of the aorta from the parasternal and suprasternal windows is essential to note the size of the aorta. These patients tend to develop a dissection of the aorta, and careful follow-up should be made with the echo to detect changes in the aortic diameter. **A,** Parasternal long-axis view. **B,** Suprasternal view. *LV,* left ventricle; *Ao,* aorta; *LA,* left atrium; *ar,* arch; *DA,* descending aorta; *AA,* ascending aorta.

ascending aorta in more severe cases) and myxomatous degeneration of the aortic and mitral valves with resultant redundancy, prolapse, and insufficiency (Figs. 29-9 and 29-10). As the insufficient valve becomes more severe, the left ventricle dilates to assume the hemodynamic overload, which may then progress to left ventricular dysfunction (Fig. 29-11). The dilated aortic root may become very thin with increased dimensions and may lead to a dissection of the aorta (Figs. 29-12 and 29-13).

FLAIL MITRAL APPARATUS OR RUPTURED PAPILLARY MUSCLE

A rupture of the papillary muscle occurs from a myocardial infarction and death of the papillary muscle, or from a chest injury. As a result, massive acute mitral regurgitation will occur, and if not surgically corrected, may result

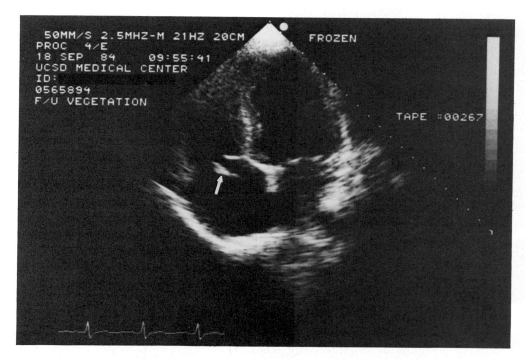

FIG. 29-30. Apical four-chamber view of a drug addict with fever of unknown origin. The right heart is enlarged and a pliable mass was seen in the area of the tricuspid valve *(arrow)*. Echo can be very useful in patients with known lesions, as they can be followed with weekly to monthly echoes as the clinical treatment progresses to see the regression of the vegetation.

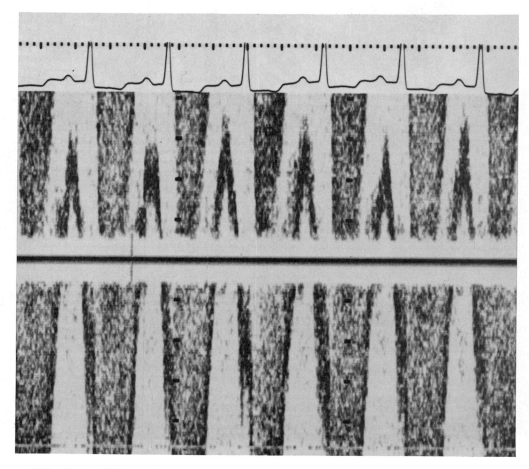

FIG. 29-31. PW Doppler of a patient with tricuspid regurgitation shows the jet to alias.

A

B

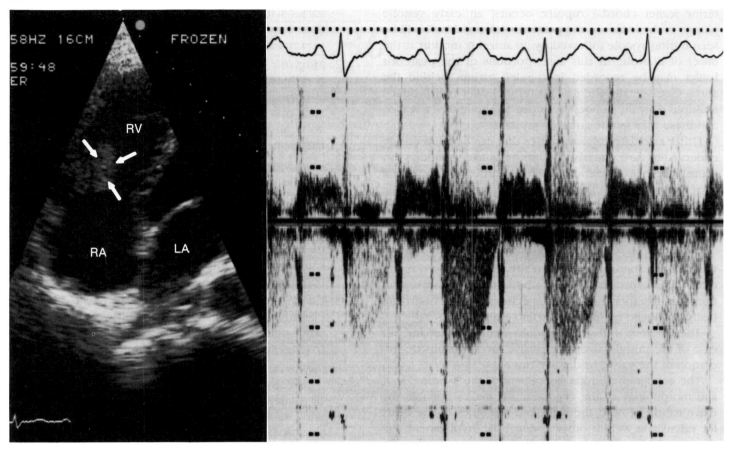

FIG. 29-32. A, Apical four-chamber view of a patient with a huge vegetative lesion of the anterior leaflet of the tricuspid valve *(arrows)*. *RV,* right ventricle; *RA,* right atrium; *LA,* left atrium. **B,** CW Doppler of the regurgitant jet recorded at maximum velocity of 2.4 m/s.

Table 29-1   Criteria for Echocardiographic Diagnosis of Endocarditis

Location	Findings
Aortic valve	Shaggy nonuniform thickening in systole or diastole with unrestricted leaflet motion
	Dense shaggy echoes moving across valve and into LVOT
	Flail or ruptured cusps
	Fine diastolic fluttering on ALMV secondary to aortic insufficiency
	Mitral valve preclosure secondary to acute aortic insufficiency
Mitral valve	Thick shaggy echoes attached to or moving behind leaflets demonstrating unrestricted motion
	Systolic flutter of prolapsing segments of mitral valve
	Fuzzy leaflet echoes in left atrial cavity during systole (differentiate from myxoma)
Tricuspid and pulmonary valves	Shaggy thickening of leaflets, demonstrating unrestrictive motion
	Mass of echoes moving with leaflets (dependent motion)
	Rupture of tricuspid chordae
Prosthetic valve	Thick shaggy collection located behind site of attachment of prosthesis to valve ring
	Evidence of severe regurgitation

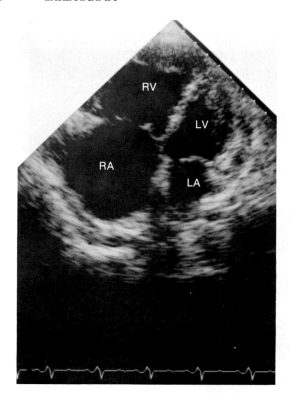

FIG. 30-6. Apical four-chamber view in a patient with pulmonary hypertension shows a dilated dysfunctioning right ventricular cavity on multiple views with hypertrophy of the right heart wall. *RV,* right ventricle; *RA,* right atrium; *LV,* left ventricle; *LA,* left atrium.

nary artery pressure. If the patient develops right ventricular failure, the "a" dip may reappear as the pressure in the right heart diminishes. One of the more specific findings is that of mid-systolic notching of the pulmonary valve (also termed the "flying W" sign) (Fig. 30-8).

Because the pulmonary artery dilates in hypertensive patients, the Doppler often reveals pulmonary insufficiency (Fig. 30-9).

The tricuspid valve may secondarily reflect changes due to the right ventricular dysfunction and dilatation. As seen on the left side of the heart with increased pressures, the tricuspid valve may show abnormal patterns of diastolic motion (i.e., decreased diastolic opening excursion, "B" notch, or decreased diastolic closure rate). With the Doppler, evidence of tricuspid insufficiency may be present (Fig. 30-10).

A striking feature of pulmonary hypertension is seen on the interventricular septum. As the right ventricular overload increases, the septum begins to bulge toward the left ventricle or "pancake" (flatten) with increased pressures (Fig. 30-11). Thus the right ventricle becomes more circular in shape and the left ventricle becomes more crescent shaped (as seen in the normal right ventricle).

The M-mode tracing shows displaced posterior septal motion toward the left ventricle during diastole. During systole, the left ventricular pressure momentarily exceeds right ventricular pressure and forces the septum anteri-

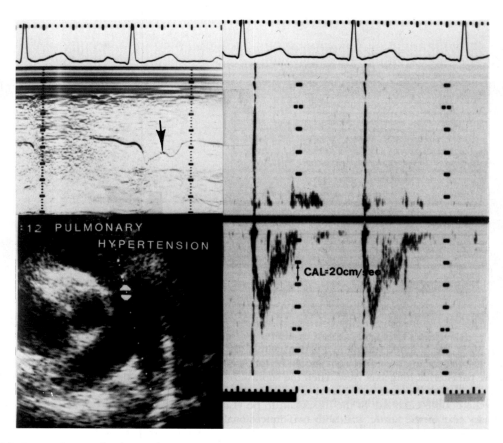

FIG. 30-7. A typical echographic pattern of pulmonary hypertension is the dilated pulmonary artery, midsystolic closure of the pulmonic cusp *(arrow),* and early closure of the flow pattern as seen on PW Doppler.

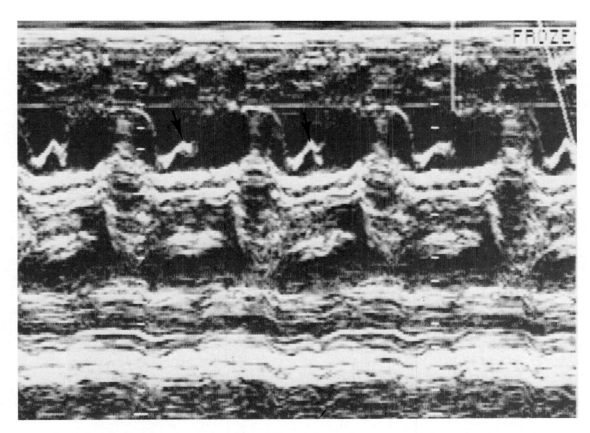

FIG. 30-8.   M-mode tracing in a patient with pulmonary hypertension shows the decreased *c-e* slope and midsystolic notching (flying W) of the cusp *(arrows)*.

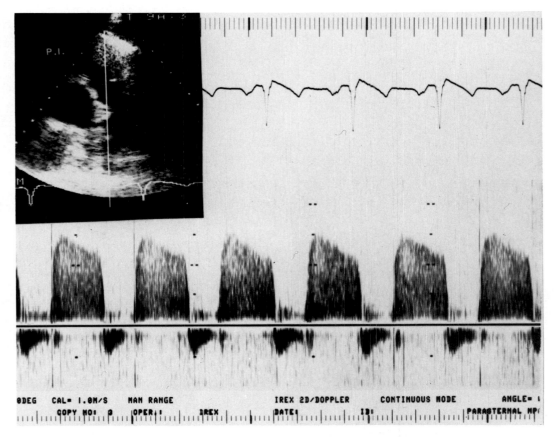

FIG. 30-9.   Doppler tracing in a patient with pulmonary hypertension shows a dilated pulmonary anulus, leading to pulmonary insufficiency. This is a CW tracing.

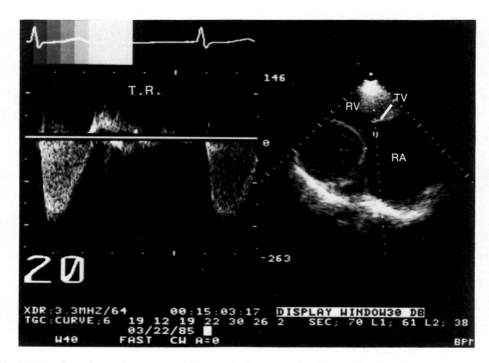

FIG. 30-10.   Doppler and parasternal long-axis view over the tricuspid valve also may show signs of insufficiency due to the secondary right ventricular dysfunction and dilatation in patients with pulmonary hypertension. *RV,* right ventricle; *TV,* tricuspid valve; *RA,* right atrium.

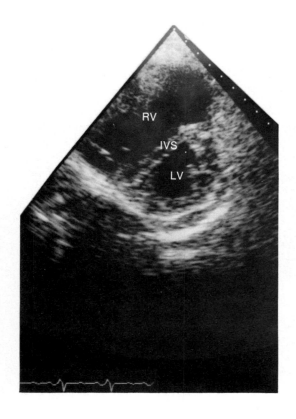

FIG. 30-11.   Parasternal short-axis view of a patient with pulmonary hypertension shows a pancake effect of the interventricular septum secondary to the increased pressures in the right heart. Sometimes the pressure can be so great that the septum actually bulges into the left ventricle. *RV,* right ventricle; *IVS,* interventricular septum; *LV,* left ventricle.

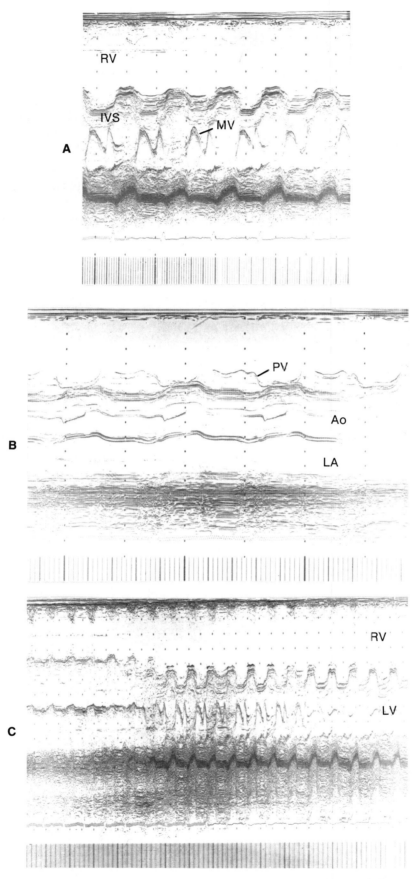

FIG. 30-12. M-mode tracings of a patient with pulmonary hypertension and abnormal septal motion secondary to increased right heart pressures. **A,** Dilated right ventricle, *RV,* abnormal septal motion, *IVS,* and mitral valve, *MV.* **B,** Dilated right ventricular outflow tract with some pulmonary valve, *PV,* aortic root, *Ao,* and left atrium, *LA.* **C,** Sweep from the aorta into the left ventricular cavity, *LV.* Note the markedly abnormal septal motion.

orly. **This pattern may be quite pronounced and, with right-sided overload, appear very accentuated** (Fig. 30-12).

SUMMARY

1. Systemic hypertension is an abnormal condition in which the arterial blood pressure is above normal limits when taken under normal conditions.

2. Hypertension may be grouped under two classifications: primary, or essential, and secondary.

3. Vascular complications of hypertension can be considered to be either hypertensive or atherosclerotic.

4. With echocardiography, hypertension presents with a concentrically thickened myocardium that is stiff and noncompliant.

5. Cystic medial necrosis of the aorta may develop with hypertension due to the increased stress caused by increased ventricular pressure.

6. There are numerous causes for pulmonary hypertension: increased resistance to pulmonary venous drainage, increased resistance to flow through the pulmonary vascular bed, increased resistance to flow through the pulmonary arteries, hypoventilation, and miscellaneous causes.

7. Echographically, hypertension shows a dilated and dysfunctioning right ventricular cavity with hypertrophy of the right heart wall. The pulmonic valve motion is abnormal with the loss of the "a" dip and flattening of the *c-e* slope.

REFERENCES

1. Grossman W, Alpert JS, and Braunwald E: Pulmonary hypertension. In Braunwald E, editor: Heart disease, vol 1, Philadelphia, 1984, WB Saunders.
2. Harrigan P and Lee R: Principles of interpretation in echocardiography: systemic and pulmonary hypertensive disease, New York, 1985, J Wiley & Sons.
3. Kaplan NM: Systemic hypertension: mechanisms and diagnosis. In Braunwald E, editor: Heart disease, vol 1, Philadelphia, 1984, WB Saunders.

31

Cardiomyopathy

CRIS D. GRESSER

Cardiomyopathy refers to a heterogeneous group of diseases characterized by an abnormality in the structure or function of the myocardium.[7] Diseases of the heart that may secondarily involve the myocardium (e.g., hypertension, coronary insufficiency, valvular malfunction, or rheumatic heart disease) are excluded by this definition.

M-mode and two-dimensional echocardiography have played important roles in the identification and characterization of the three types of cardiomyopathies. Doppler and color-flow Doppler techniques have added a new dimension in allowing the quantitation of regurgitant lesions and the measurement of the magnitude of the gradients. The future development of tissue characterization and three-dimensional echocardiography may help us to further classify these conditions.

CLASSIFICATION

Cardiomyopathies may be classified as primary or secondary. Primary cardiomyopathies are those in which the cause of the heart disease is unknown and is not part of a disease affecting other organs.[5,10] Secondary cardiomyopathies are conditions in which the myocardial abnormality is but one manifestation of a systemic disease process (e.g., sarcoid).[2] Cardiomyopathies are divided into three types: (1) congestive, (2) hypertrophic, or muscular subaortic stenosis, and (3) infiltrative or restrictive (Table 31-1).

Table 31-1   Echo Findings in Cardiomyopathies

	LVED	RVED	LVPW	RVAW	LVSF	RVSF	LVDF	RVDF
Congestive	↑	N/↑	↑	N/↓	↑	N/↓	N	N
Hypertrophic	N/↓	N/↓	N/↑	N	N/↓	N	N/↓	N
Infiltrative	N	N	↑	↑	N	N	↓	↓

LVED, Left ventricular end diastolic dimension; RVED, Right ventricular end diastolic dimension; LVPW, Left ventricular posterior wall dimension; RVAW, Right ventricular anterior wall dimension; LVSF, Left ventricular systolic function; RVSF, Right ventricular systolic function; LVDF, Left ventricular diastolic function; RVDF, Right ventricular diastolic function.

Congestive cardiomyopathy. Congestive cardiomyopathy (CCM) is a syndrome characterized by cardiac enlargement and congestive heart failure. The congestive cardiomyopathies demonstrate impairment principally of systolic function. Ejection fraction is decreased, and both the end diastolic and end systolic volumes are increased.[2] Although a toxin can cause a congestive cardiomyopathy (e.g., alcohol,[12] cobalt,[11] or radiation[1]), in many cases the cause is unknown, although viral infections have been postulated.

Hypertrophic cardiomyopathy. Hypertrophic cardiomyopathy (HCM) or muscular subaortic stenosis (MSS) may be defined as ventricular hypertrophy without identifiable cause that is usually associated with microscopic evidence of myocardial fiber disarray.[17] This disease is thought in some instances to be hereditary.

Infiltrative or restrictive cardiomyopathy.
Restrictive or infiltrative cardiomyopathy is an infiltrative myocardial disease. In patients with restrictive cardiomyopathy, there is concentric left ventricular hypertrophy. The left ventricular filling is impaired, which causes a reduction of left ventricular emptying secondary to a decreased contractile performance.

CONGESTIVE CARDIOMYOPATHY
Clinical manifestations

The symptoms of cardiomyopathy are those of heart failure: dyspnea, fatigue, palpitations, and chest pain. Because of the decreased cardiac function, thrombi may form in the apex of the left ventricle, resulting in systemic embolization. The diagnosis of this disease may require myocardial biopsy.

Treatment

Medical treatment of this disease is that for congestive heart failure (i.e., digitalis, diuretics, and afterload manipulation). For end-stage cardiomyopathy the surgical treatment is cardiac transplantation.

Echocardiographic features

Along with gross cardiac dilatation, there is decreased amplitude of the mitral valve. In many cases the anterior and posterior leaflets assume the same small amplitude, termed the "double diamond" pattern (by M-mode) (Fig. 31-1). This ability to record both leaflets simultaneously is due to the ventricular dilatation and slight cardiac rota-

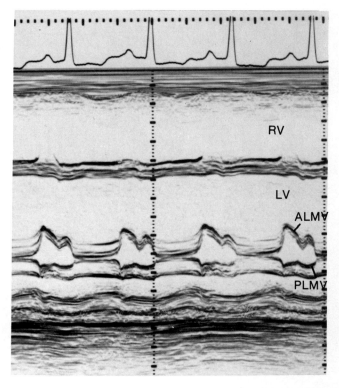

FIG. 31-1. M-mode tracing of the anterior and posterior leaflets of the mitral valve in a patient with cardiomyopathy. The leaflets have assumed nearly the same amplitude, termed the "double diamond" appearance by echo. The left ventricular cavity is dilated with poor contractility. *RV,* right ventricle; *LV,* left ventricle; *ALMV,* anterior leaflet mitral valve; *PLMV,* posterior leaflet mitral valve.

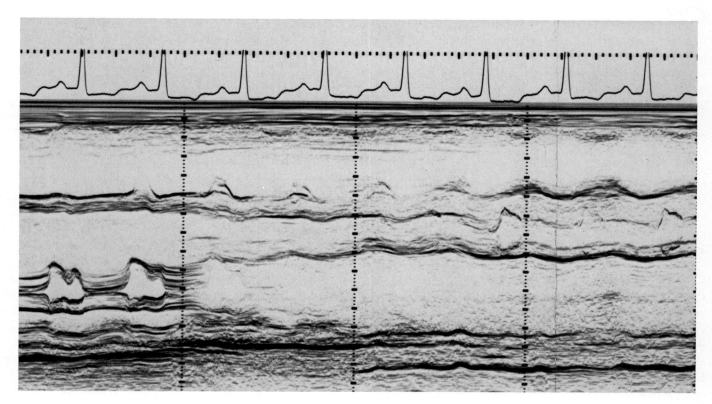

FIG. 31-2. M-mode sweep from the mitral valve to the aortic root in a patient with congestive cardiomyopathy. Note the dilated cardiac chambers as well as the increased distance from the *e* point on the anterior leaflet of the mitral valve to the septum.

tion. In addition, multiple echoes that arise from the chordal structures are recorded in the systolic and diastolic segments. The systolic *c-d* segment is flattened. The distance from the *e* point on the anterior leaflet to the interventricular septum is increased (Fig. 31-2). The aortic root motion is decreased, and the cusps do not open as wide, secondary to decreased cardiac output (Fig. 31-3). The right-sided structures, tricuspid and pulmonary valves, are easily recorded because of chamber hypertrophy.

The two-dimensional image shows a greater area of the left ventricular cavity and thus has been useful in distinguishing areas of global hypokinesis from segmental asynergy as seen in patients with coronary artery disease. It has also provided a means of recognizing left ventricular mural thrombi, which frequently may be associated with congestive cardiomyopathy (Fig. 31-4).

2D FEATURES

1. Four-chamber enlargement.
2. Generalized biventricular hypokinesis is common, although in some instances the right ventricle is not involved. This global nature of hypokinesis may distinguish CCM from coronary artery disease, which demonstrates a segmental pattern. However, end-stage coronary disease of any etiology may present with these features.
3. Occasionally a pericardial effusion is present.
4. Mural thrombi are found at the apex of the left ventricle in approximately 60% of the patients with CCM.

M-MODE FEATURES

1. Typical findings associated with decreased cardiac output:
   a. Decreased excursion of the aortic root
   b. Closing drift of the aortic cusps in systole
   c. A "double diamond" mitral valve pattern
   d. Increased "e" point—septal separation (more than 1 cm)
2. A mitral valve *b* notch (indicating abnormal closure of the mitral valve) due to increased left ventricular end diastolic pressure (LVEDP) (Fig. 31-5)
3. Increased left ventricular and left atrial size
4. Decreased excursion of the interventricular septum and left ventricular posterior wall (Fig. 31-6)

DOPPLER FINDINGS[8]

1. Mitral regurgiation secondary to left ventricular enlargement with dilatation of the mitral anulus.
2. Tricuspid regurgitation secondary to (Fig. 31-7)
   a. Passive pulmonary hypertension
   b. Right ventricular dysfunction
   c. Right ventricular enlargement with dilatation of the anulus (Fig. 31-8).
3. Decreased velocity of ejection and increased ejection time in the left ventricular outflow tract.
4. A typical pattern of pulmonary hypertension may be present (Fig. 31-9).
5. The diastolic flow across the mitral valve may suggest abnormalities of relaxation.

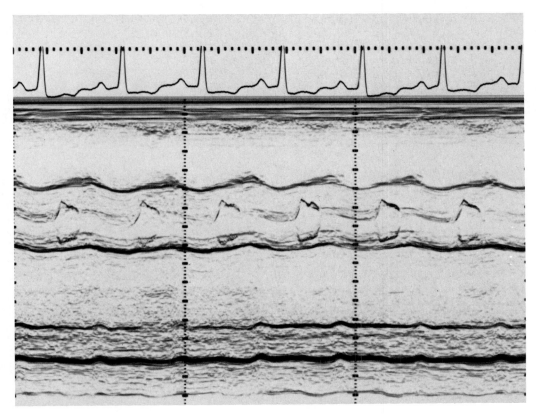

FIG. 31-3. M-mode tracing of the same patient with cardiomyopathy. The aortic root shows a decreased motion, with decreased opening of the cusps secondary to decreased cardiac output.

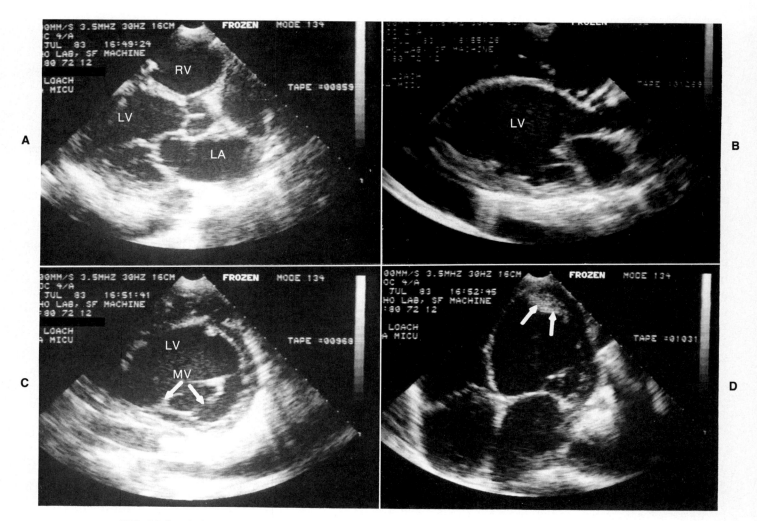

FIG. 31-4. **A,** Parasternal long-axis view of a patient with congestive cardiomyopathy. The right ventricle, *RV,* left ventricle, *LV,* and left atrium, *LA,* are dilated. **B,** Parasternal long-axis view of the dilated, poorly functioning left ventricular cavity, *LV.* **C,** Parasternal short-axis view of the dilated left ventricle, *LV,* with the anterior and posterior mitral leaflets, *MV.* **D,** Apical four-chamber view of the dilated four chambers of the heart. The global hypokinesis leads to the formation of mural thrombi, usually along the apex of the left ventricle *(arrows).*

FIG. 31-5. M-mode tracing of a patient with elevated end diastolic pressure leads to the *b* notch *(arrows)* on the closing motion of the anterior leaflet of the mitral valve.

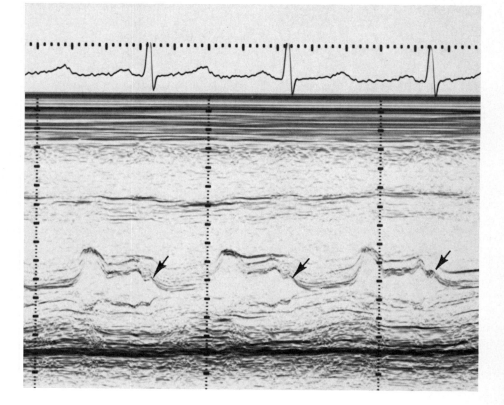

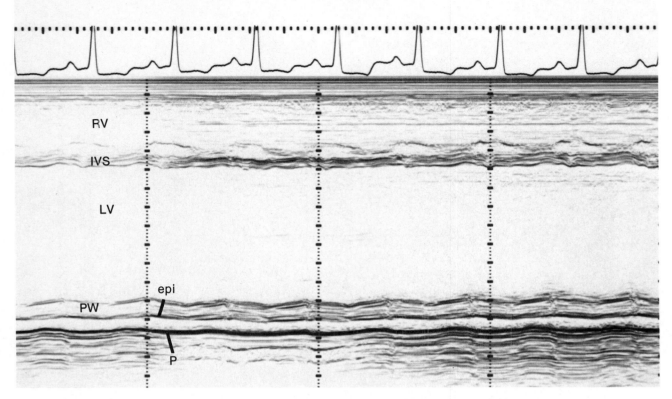

FIG. 31-6. M-mode tracing of the dilated left ventricle shows decreased excursion of the interventricular septum and posterior heart wall. In addition, a small pericardial effusion is shown posterior to the epicardial surface. *RV,* right ventricle; *IVS,* interventricular septum; *LV,* left ventricle; *PW,* posterior heart wall; *epi,* epicardium; *P,* pericardium.

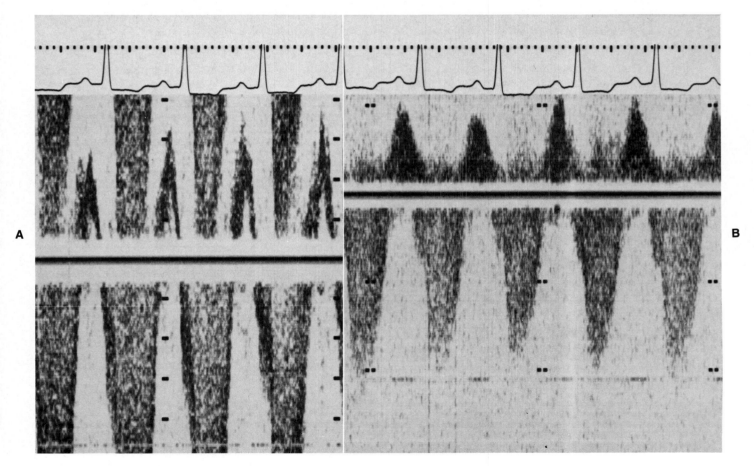

FIG. 31-7. Patients with cardiomyopathy often have regurgitation of some or all their cardiac valves. **A,** The PW Doppler tracing is recorded over the tricuspid valve area. The velocity of the tricuspid valve indicates reduced cardiac output, while the systolic jet represents the regurgitation present. **B,** The CW Doppler tracing records the tricuspid regurgitation without an alias pattern. At least 2 m/s of jet flow is recorded in this dilated cavity.

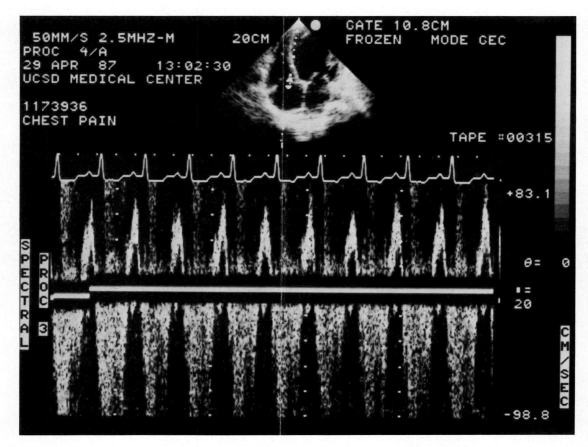

FIG. 31-8. PW Doppler tracing over the tricuspid valve shows a regurgitant jet at the level of the dilated anulus. The jet should be followed into the atrial cavity to see how far back the regurgitation is seen and heard.

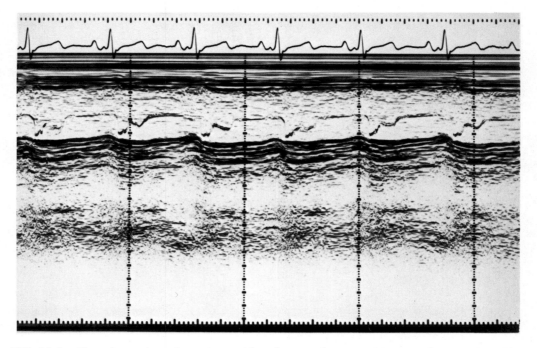

FIG. 31-9. M-mode tracing of a patient with pulmonary hypertension secondary to congestive cardiomyopathy. The typical "flying W" pattern is seen in systole as the valve begins to close early.

HYPERTROPHIC CARDIOMYOPATHY

Hypertrophic cardiomyopathy is characterized by symmetric or asymmetric hypertrophy of the left and/or right ventricles. It is a primary disorder of the heart muscle in which the site and extent of the hypertrophic process are important in determining the disease manifestations.[13]

Classification

Hypertrophic cardiomyopathy will be discussed under the following classifications:

1. Ventricular asymmetric septal hypertrophies:
   a. Resting obstructives
   b. Latent obstructives
   c. Nonobstructives
2. Midventricular cavity obstructives
3. Asymmetric apical hypertrophies

The disease may be hereditary, so it is important to screen family members of patients with known hypertrophic cardiomyopathy. The manifestation, prognosis, and therapy is different for the various subgroups, so it is important to distinguish one from the other. In general, patients with extensive hypertrophy are more likely to manifest the abnormalities of systolic and diastolic function, as well as being more prone to atrial and ventricular arrhythmias and sudden death.[16] The two-dimensional, M-mode, and Doppler findings of these patients vary with their respective classifications.

In discussing the hypertrophies, three terms need to be defined: asymmetric septal hypertrophy (ASH), systolic anterior motion (SAM) of the mitral valve, and Venturi mechanism.

Asymmetric septal hypertrophy. The hypertrophy of the base of the interventricular septum at end diastole is asymmetric (i.e., there is a disproportionate ratio of thickening of the base of the interventricular septum as compared to the left ventricular posterior wall of 1.3:1 or greater (Fig. 31-10). (Some authors suggest a ratio of 1.5:1 or greater.[17])

Systolic anterior motion. Systolic anterior motion refers to the movement of either leaflet tip of the mitral valve toward the interventricular septum, which, depending on its extent, may or may not cause obstruction to the left ventricular outflow (Fig. 31-11). Several mechanisms have been proposed for this phenomenon; the most commonly accepted is the Venturi mechanism.[15]

Venturi mechanism. Because ASH narrows the left ventricular outflow tract, the path of the blood ejecting from the left ventricle passes closer to the anterior mitral leaflet than is normal. This high-velocity flow passing close to the anterior mitral valve leaflet "sucks" the leaflet forward in systole toward the interventricular septum, causing variable degrees of obstruction.[3,4]

Clinical manifestations

The clinical manifestations of HCM are varied. Patients without left ventricular outflow tract obstruction may be completely asymptomatic, whereas patients with some form of obstruction have symptoms that may include dizziness, syncope, fatigue, chest pain, and shortness of breath. The symptoms increase with the use of the Valsalva maneuver or with the inhalation of amyl nitrite, since these tend to increase the degree of obstruction. (It is important to note that amyl nitrite should not be used in patients with significant aortic stenosis, or in those patients with resting obstruction, since complete obstruction of the left ventricular outflow tract could be catastrophic.)

Treatment

Medical treatment of these patients includes therapy to decrease the left ventricular outflow tract gradient (e.g., beta blockers and antiarrhythmic drugs to prevent sudden death). The incidence of arrhythmias and sudden death in these patients seems to be proportional to the extent of hypertrophy. The group of patients with resting obstruction who are unresponsive to maximal medical therapy are commonly referred for surgical treatment.

Surgical treatment includes a myectomy wherein a piece of the basal septum is removed, which widens the left ventricular outflow tract and reduces the obstruction to ventricular ejection.

Echocardiographic features of ventricular asymmetric septal hypertrophy

Ventricular asymmetric hypertrophy is the most common form of HCM and is characterized by abnormalities of systolic and diastolic function as well as rhythm disturbances (Fig. 31-12). Systole is characterized by the presence of an intraventricular pressure gradient, which may be persistent (gradient at rest), labile (not always present, but spontaneously variable), or latent (not always present, but provocable).[8,13] Diastole is characterized by abnormalities of ventricular relaxation[4] and increased chamber stiffness.[16]

Resting obstructives. With the use of M-mode criteria, the degree of resting obstruction can be described as: severe—where SAM contacts the septum for greater than 30% of systole; moderate—when the distance between SAM and the septum is less than 10 mm; and mild—when the distance between SAM and the septum is greater than 10 mm (Fig. 31-13).

Aortic valve notching is present in resting obstructives and correlates with the degree and onset of SAM and therefore the degree of outflow tract obstruction (Fig. 31-14). It is due to the fact that during ejection, as the dynamic obstruction increases, outflow decreases and the aortic valve starts to close. Later in systole, the obstruction decreases and the valve reopens.

All patients with resting obstruction have mitral regurgitation and, therefore, secondarily left atrial enlargement.

The echographic examination is described by the following parameters.

M-MODE FINDINGS

1. Asymmetric septal hypertrophy. (Note: Care must be taken to measure from the leading edge of the right septal wall to the leading edge of the left septal wall and not include the tricuspid chordal structures or the right ventricular papillary muscle located near the right septal wall.)

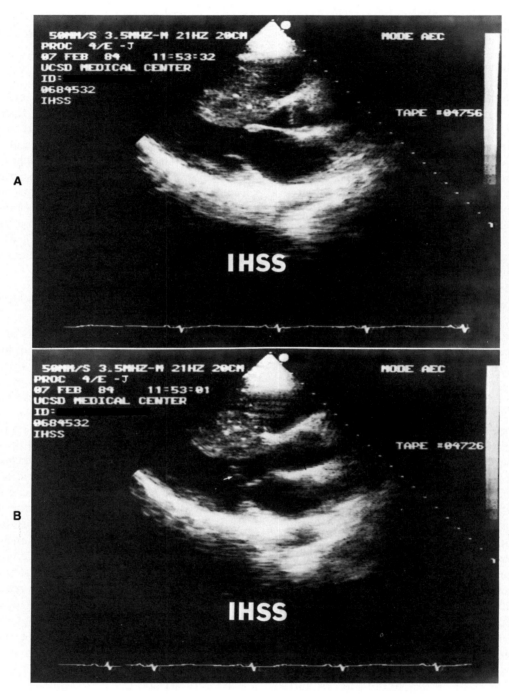

FIG. 31-10.   A, Parasternal long-axis view of a patient with asymmetric septal hypertrophy. The hypertrophy of the base of the interventricular septum at end diastole is asymmetric (i.e., there is a disproportionate ratio of thickening of the base of the septum as compared to the left ventricular posterior wall of 1.3:1 or greater. (IHSS) idiopathic hypertrophic subaortic stenosis. **B,** Parasternal long-axis view of the same patient. The *arrow* points to the systolic anterior movement (SAM) as seen in patients with IHSS.

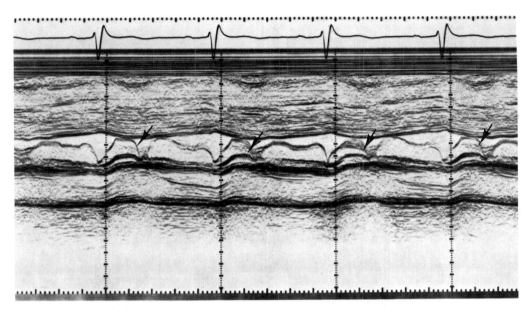

FIG. 31-11. M-mode tracing of a patient with IHSS with severe obstructive disease. The systolic anterior motion *(arrows)* refers to the movement of either leaflet tip of the mitral valve toward the interventricular septum.

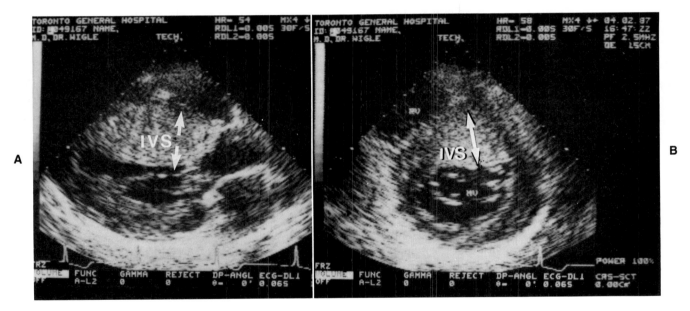

FIG. 31-12. **A,** Parasternal long-axis view of a patient with extreme asymmetric septal hypertrophy *(arrow)*. The left ventricular outflow tract is narrowed considerably due to this condition. **B,** Parasternal short-axis view of the hypertrophic cardiomyopathy. The septal thickness *(arrow)* is well demarcated. Often the septum is slightly brighter than is normally seen. It also loses its mobility with increased hypertrophy. *IVS,* interventricular septum.

2. Systolic anterior motion is recorded, and the distance between SAM and the septum should be noted to describe the degree of obstruction. (Note: SAM can be differentiated from "pseudo" SAM, which is caused by chordal anterior motion, since true SAM comes back to the baseline before the mitral valve opens.)

3. The aortic cusps can be interrogated for systolic notching, since notching coincides with the onset of SAM,

causing outflow tract obstruction and thus systolic closure of aortic leaflets.

4. Left atrial size can be reliably measured.

2D FEATURES

1. Subjective evaluation of septal to posterior wall thickness is allowed on the parasternal long- and short-axis views (Fig. 31-15).

2. SAM to septal distance can be subjectively assessed.

PERICARDIAL EFFUSION

Pericardial effusion is characterized by an enlarged cardiac silhouette and may be confused with cardiac dilation as seen in valvular heart disease or cardiomyopathy. Clinical findings can include distant heart sounds (muffled by the fluid accumulation) and a low-voltage electrocardiogram (ECG). The speed with which the fluid accumulates largely determines the subsequent clinical manifestations: a rapid accumulation of 200 to 300 ml may lead to tamponade and shock from acute cardiac insufficiency, whereas a slower accumulation of 1000 ml may produce no evidence of cardiac insufficiency.

The pericardium is able to adapt to large collections of fluid if permitted to do so over a long period of time. Cardiac tamponade may result from trauma, a ruptured aneurysm, or pericarditis. With tamponade, the systemic venous pressure increases while the arterial pressure decreases, and thus the acute cardiac insufficiency develops.

Echographic examination

Echography is the procedure of choice for evaluating the patient with pericardial effusion. If effusion is present, then serial examinations of the patient may be made with echo to follow the decrease or increase in the fluid accumulation.

The evaluation of a patient with pericardial effusion should be performed carefully and systematically. A routine parasternal long-axis scan is made to locate the aorta, left atrium, and mitral apparatus. The transducer is then directed inferior and slightly lateral (toward the left hip of the patient), off the tip of the mitral leaflet, to record the layers of the posterior left ventricular wall and pericardium. The contractility of the ventricle should be followed throughout the cardiac cycle for any compensation or decompensation factors that may be due to the rapid accumulation of fluid. The pericardial echo reflection is the strongest reflection in the normal heart and thus is easily recognized on the M-mode and two-dimensional recordings as the brightest echo reflector (Fig. 32-1). The three layers of the posterior wall (endocardium, myocardium, and epicardium) must be defined so these echoes can be separated from the pericardial echo (Fig. 32-2).

Various gain settings are used to define these structures. A high gain will allow visualization of the right ventricular wall, septum, posterior layers of the left ventricular wall, and pericardium. As the gain is reduced, the finer, less dense echoes of the chordae and endocardium are not recorded. Further reduction in gain allows only the bright pericardial reflection to remain. Thus the sweep from the aortic root to the left ventricular cavity must be made at the same time the gain is increased and decreased to distinguish the presence of fluid separating the epicardium from the pericardium (Fig. 32-3). In addition to this technique, careful observation of the continuity of the left atrial wall with the pericardium must be made. Normally the left atrial wall will be motionless; however, in the presence of a large effusion or in a hypercontractile heart, there will be an abrupt anterior movement of the left atrial wall (Fig. 32-4).

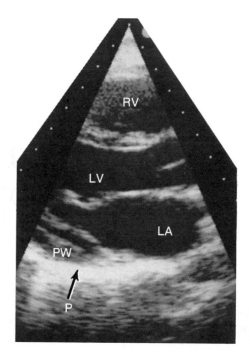

FIG. 32-1. Parasternal long-axis view of the left ventricle. The pericardium is recognized as the brightest reflector in this image. This is because there is such a definite acoustic impedance change as the echo signal passes through the left ventricle, chordae tendineae, and layers of the posterior heart wall to the pericardium. Thus recognition of the pericardial echo becomes relatively easy with both two-dimensional or M-mode methods. *RV*, right ventricle; *LV*, left ventricle; *LA*, left atrium; *PW*, posterior heart wall; *P*, pericardium.

In pericardial effusion the separation of the pericardium from the epicardium will cause the cardiac pulsations to be dampened by the time they reach the pericardium. Thus one of the more obvious features of an effusion is a nonmobile pericardium, separated from the posterior heart wall by fluid (Fig. 32-5). Sometimes the amount of fluid is so small that these pulsations are transmitted slightly to the pericardium, in which case the sonographer will see diminished motion of the pericardium.

Fluid generally accumulates in the most posterior-dependent area of the heart, accounting for the visualization of a posterior effusion before any anterior effusion is seen.

Small effusions may produce an echo-free space behind the epicardium in systole but disappear in diastole. Many echocardiographers prefer to see the separation in diastole before they report a small effusion. A systolic separation of 5 to 10 mm may indicate a small effusion of approximately 100 ml (Fig. 32-6).

Moderate effusions will produce an echo-free space in systole and diastole in the anterior and posterior pericardial space (Fig. 32-7). Usually a separation of 10 mm in systole means the patient has a moderate-sized effusion of approximately 200 to 300 ml.

A large effusion of 500 ml or greater will exhibit wide spaces anteriorly and posteriorly with a systolic separa-

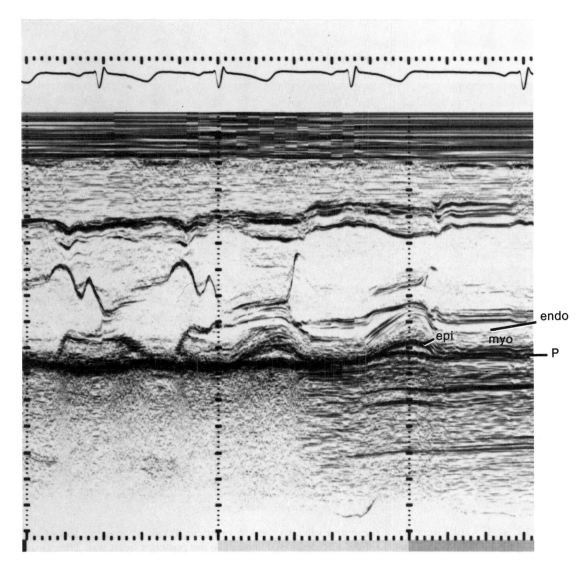

FIG. 32-2.   The three layers of the posterior heart wall: endocardium, *endo,* myocardium, *myo,* and epicardium, *epi,* must be shown as separate structures from the pericardium, *P.*

tion of at least 15 to 20 mm (Fig. 32-8). Such large effusions may seem to extend posterior to the left atrium (in the area of the oblique sinus). The erratic motion of the cardiac silhouette may be exhibited in large effusions that go on to cardiac tamponade.

As reported by Nanda and Gramiak,[2] the heart may "swing" in the pericardial effusion space, with a resultant change in the pattern of wall motion. Normally the right ventricular wall moves posteriorly in systole and anteriorly in diastole. When the heart "swings," it may move posteriorly in one cardiac cycle and anteriorly in the next, so that it is physically nearer the chest wall with every other beat. This form of cardiac "swinging" is associated with the phenomenon of electrical alternans and is seen in patients with cardiac tamponade. Tamponade occurs when the intrapericardial pressure reaches a sufficient level to compromise the filling of the heart (Fig. 32-9). An emergency pericardiocentesis, with or without ultrasound guidance, must be performed to relieve the intrapericardial pressure.

Pericardiocentesis

The removal of fluid from the pericardium may serve a therapeutic or diagnostic purpose. Needle aspiration of the pericardium is best performed with the patient in a semiupright position, for the fluid tends to gravitate anteriorly and inferolaterally. The apical or subxiphoid approach is generally used. The cardiac sonographer may locate the position of maximum fluid accumulation and, with a special aspiration transducer, guide the clinician as the fluid is withdrawn from the pericardial space. The needle may be followed on the two-dimensional and M-mode tracing so perforation of the ventricular wall is avoided (Fig. 32-10).

Pseudo-SAM and pseudoprolapse

The sonographer should be careful not to evaluate other cardiac structures in the presence of pericardial effusion. The atrioventricular valves may exhibit pseudo-SAM (due to chordal structures) or pseudoprolapse patterns in systole. The semilunar valves show late systolic collapse of

Text continued on p. 756.

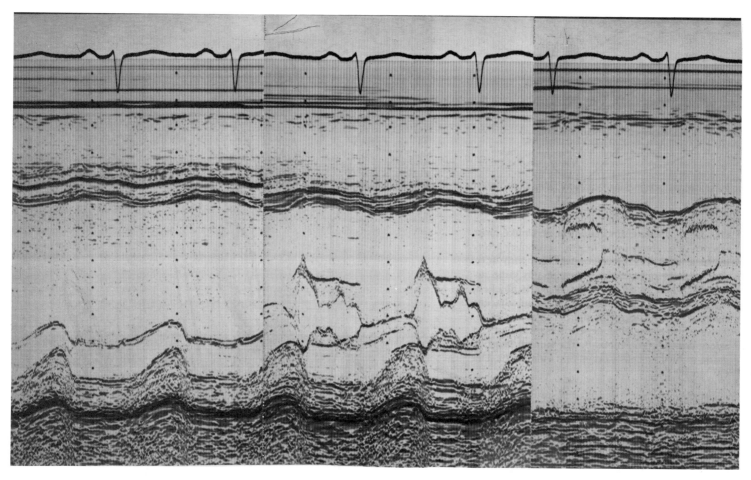

FIG. 33-4. M-mode sweep from the left ventricle, through the mitral valve, to the aorta and left atrial cavity showing a dilated left ventricle with decreased septal motion indicative of an anterior myocardial infarction. The posterior wall of the left ventricle shows normal to slightly exaggerated septal motion to compensate for the infarcted septal wall.

carefully examine the myocardial segments for the presence of aneurysm formation or bright echo reflectors, which may represent infarcted scar tissue from the infarct.

The true anterior left ventricular wall may be examined echographically in a parasternal long-axis view by sliding the transducer in a linear fashion toward the left hip. This allows the sonographer to move away from the interventricular septum and record the wall of the left ventricle. When the anterior wall of the left ventricle is best seen, there is no right ventricular cavity shown, as there is in the plane when the septum is recorded.

Indirect evidence of segmental left ventricular disease may be seen in exaggerated wall motion of the opposing nonischemic area of the left ventricle.

Another indirect clue to the presence of a hypokinetic wall segment is a cloud of intracavitary echoes adjacent to the poorly moving wall. Normally the left ventricular cavity is echo free, but if there are intracavitary echoes, they are uniformly distributed throughout the cavity or appear as a series of straight lines. The echoes frequently accumulate next to a hypokinetic or dyskinetic segment of the ventricle.

An additional indirect sign is a prominent, somewhat exaggerated, right ventricular wall motion. It is unusual for the amplitude of the right ventricular wall echoes to exceed the amplitude of septal motion, except in patients with coronary artery disease.

If the interventricular septal motion is abnormal, there is probably a proximal left anterior descending or left main coronary artery obstruction. However, normal septal motion in no way precludes the possibility of obstruction in these arteries. The septal motion correlates better with the myocardial perfusion of the septum than with anatomic obstructions of the coronary artery.

The two-dimensional echo again offers a better visualization to myocardial contractility than does the M-mode echo. The M-mode echo allows one to visualize only a small "icepick" portion of the myocardial segment, and it is difficult to adequately assess myocardial function on a global basis. Especially important are the apical four-chamber and apical long-axis views, as well as the parasternal long- and short-axis views in judging wall motion and thickness patterns. Thus the two-dimensional image can record the medial, lateral, basal, and apical portions of the left ventricle (Fig. 33-6).

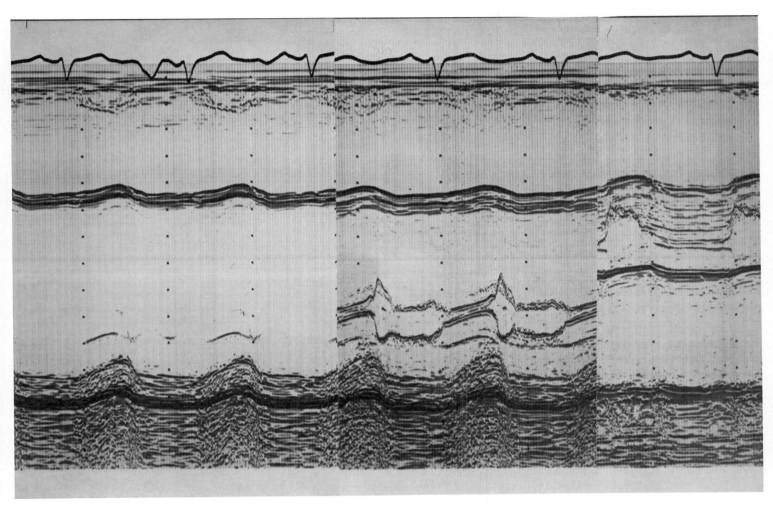

FIG. 33-5. M-mode sweep of a patient with an anterior myocardial infarction. The left ventricle is dilated, septal motion is decreased, and there is increased distance from the *e* point of the mitral valve to the septum, indicating left ventricular dysfunction.

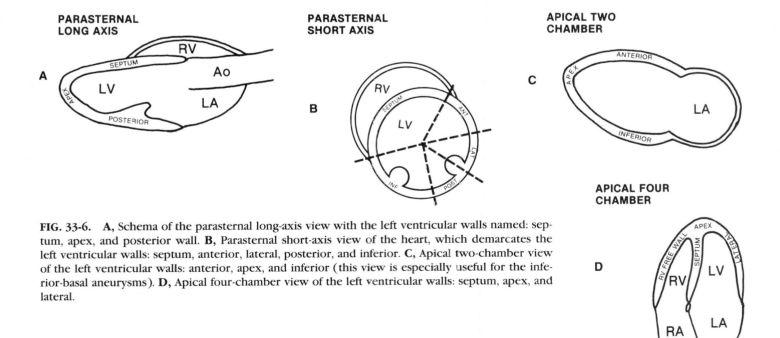

FIG. 33-6. A, Schema of the parasternal long-axis view with the left ventricular walls named: septum, apex, and posterior wall. **B,** Parasternal short-axis view of the heart, which demarcates the left ventricular walls: septum, anterior, lateral, posterior, and inferior. **C,** Apical two-chamber view of the left ventricular walls: anterior, apex, and inferior (this view is especially useful for the inferior-basal aneurysms). **D,** Apical four-chamber view of the left ventricular walls: septum, apex, and lateral.

Wall thickening

Any given segment of the ventricle is influenced by its movement of the adjacent muscle to which it is attached. It may be hypokinetic in one area and be influenced by hyperkinesis in another. Thus by merely looking at wall motion on echo, one usually overestimates the amount of ischemic muscle when looking just for motion abnormalities. A more specific finding for ischemic muscle is the alteration in systolic thickening.

With acute ischemia or infarction one may record systolic thinning whereby the thickness of the left ventricular wall is greater in diastole than in systole. The affected wall segment exhibits not only the paradoxical motion but also the systolic thinning, which is probably more specific for ischemia. Systolic thinning almost always occurs with a dyskinetic segment and is usually associated with acute myocardial infarction. Decreased thickening occurs in both chronic and acute ischemia.

Change in acoustic properties

The healing process of an acute myocardial infarction involves the deposition of collagen and the formation of a scar. These changes produce a decrease in the thickness of the affected wall segment. The second effect, scar formation, is a change in the acoustic properties of the segment. Collagen and scar both change the reflective properties of the wall, although fibrosis is a much stronger reflector of ultrasound than is the normal myocardium.

In efforts to judge wall thickness, motion, and reflective properties, careful technique must be used to image the interventricular septum. The entire width and length of the septum must be recorded in the long-axis and apical views. The gain setting must be adjusted so the echoes do not appear to be more reflective than they really are.

Quantitation of ischemic muscle

If all the left ventricular segments move abnormally, one can expect to find extensive ischemic damage. However, if no abnormal muscle is recorded, then the damage is considerably less.

In efforts to map out the areas of ischemia in the left ventricle, the cavity can be divided into specific areas: the long-axis view records the anterior and posterior segments along with the cardiac apex; the short-axis view shows the anterior, posterior, medial, and lateral walls of the ventricle; the apical view shows the apex, medial, and lateral walls of the left ventricle (Figs. 33-7 to 33-10). If one assumes that each segment is equal in area, the number of abnormal segments can be totaled and the percentage of surface area or percentage of mass of the left ventricle that is abnormal can be calculated.

Elevated end diastolic pressure

Patients with coronary artery disease often have higher left ventricular end diastolic pressure that is primarily a result of an elevated atrial component of ventricular pressure. Such an alteration in pressure, and possibly to some extent abnormal ventricular contraction, changes the manner in which the mitral valve closes. On the M-mode

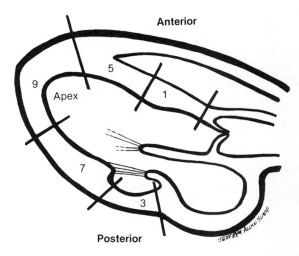

FIG. 33-7.   Parasternal long-axis schematic view of the left ventricle shows the nine segments of the wall. *1,* Anterior; *3,* posterior; *5,* anterior; *7,* posterior; *9,* apex. (Adapted from Heger J, Weyman A, Wann L, et al: Cross-sectional echocardiography in acute myocardial infarction: detection and localization of regional left ventricular asynergy, Circulation 60:531, 1979.)

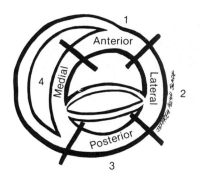

FIG. 33-8.   Parasternal short-axis view of the wall segments. *1,* Anterior; *2,* lateral; *3,* posterior; *4,* medial. (Adapted from Heger J, Weyman A, Wann L, et al: Cross-sectional echocardiography in acute myocardial infarction: detection and localization of regional left ventricular asynergy, Circulation 60:531, 1979.)

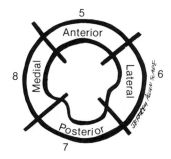

FIG. 33-9.   Parasternal short-axis view of the wall segments slightly inferior from Fig. 33-8. *5,* Anterior; *6,* lateral; *7,* posterior; *8,* medial. (Adapted from Heger J, Weyman A, Wann L, et al: Cross-sectional echocardiography in acute myocardial infarction: detection and localization of regional left ventricular asynergy, Circulation 60:531, 1979.)

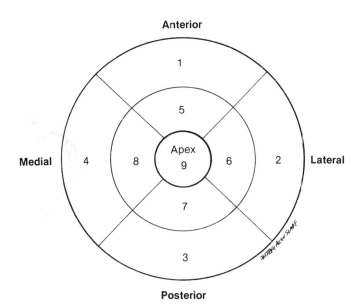

FIG. 33-10. Method used to depict the location of asynergy in acute myocardial infarction. All nine segments are displayed as a series of concentric rings. See text for further explanation. (Adapted from Heger J, Weyman A, Wann L, et al: Cross-sectional echocardiography in acute myocardial infarction: detection and localization of regional left ventricular asynergy, Circulation 60:531, 1979.)

tracing, a notch is recorded between the *a* and *c* points and is termed the B notch. This notch may also be a function of poor contractility of the left ventricle.

In addition, the aortic valve may reveal a gradually diminishing systolic opening excursion secondary to the decreased contractility. Doppler measurements taken at the site of the aortic valve in this instance would not truly reflect aortic ejection.

Ventricular aneurysm

An aneurysm is a common complication of myocardial infarction. A true aneurysm may form at the site of the infarcted myocardium where the wall is thinned and scarred. With systole, the aneurysmal myocardium expands outward to exhibit a dyskinetic motion in systole. Mural thrombi may occur at this aneurysmal site.

If an M-mode strip at slow speed is obtained with a ventricular aneurysm, one will see an increase in distance between the left side of the septum and the posterior endocardium as the apex is approached. The two-dimensional echo is probably a better method for examining the left ventricular cavity, and since the common site for aneurysm formation is the apex of the heart, the apical four-chamber view is the most sensitive (Fig. 33-11). The aneurysmal dilation can be seen in diastole, with expansion in systole, and may be visible in almost any part of the ventricle.

Another common site of aneurysm formation is the basal segment of the left ventricle near the atrioventricular groove. This is best imaged with the parasternal long-axis or apical two-chamber view (Figs. 33-12 to 33-15). The transducer should be carefully angled in a medial to

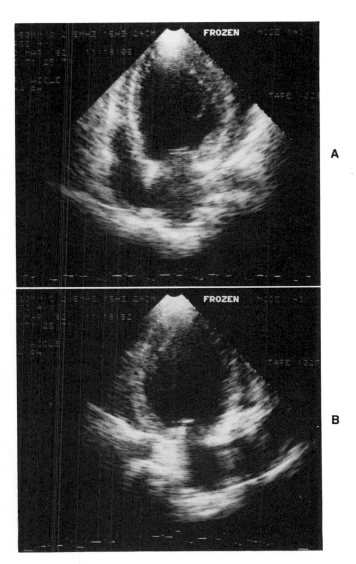

FIG. 33-11. Two-dimensional echocardiography is a very sensitive method for evaluating a patient with an aneurysm formation, especially at the apex of the heart. The aneurysm can be seen in diastole, with expansion in systole, and may be visible in almost any apical window. **A,** Apical four-chamber view. **B,** Modified apical four-chamber view.

lateral direction to record the basal segment of the ventricle.

Left ventricular thrombi

The formation of thrombi is another common complication of myocardial infarction. The thrombi occur adjacent to the dyskinetic or akinetic area, which frequently is dilated and aneurysmal (Figs. 33-16 to 33-19). The sluggish blood flow present in low flow states establishes a favorable environment for the stacking of the red blood cells into clumps. These clumps hypothetically may become large enough to be visualized on a two-dimensional image resulting in a low-level haze of echoes adjacent to an akinetic segment (Harrigan, page 298). The risk of embolization is increased with the formation of mural thrombi, and two-dimensional echo becomes a clinically useful modality in following the regression of thrombi. Generally the

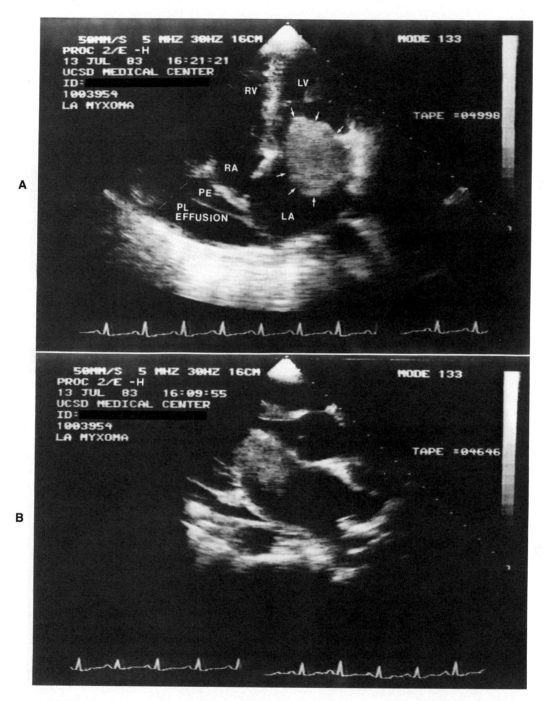

FIG. 34-5. For the past several years this 59-year-old woman has experienced brief episodes of lightheadedness without syncope. During the preceding 6 months she had increasing fatigue and dyspnea. She then lost consciousness and was sent to the hospital for evaluation. The echo demonstrated a large prolapsing atrial myxoma from the left atrial cavity to the left ventricular cavity. The left heart was slightly enlarged secondary to mitral regurgitation. **A,** Apical four-chamber view of the atrial myxoma *(arrows)* as it prolapses into the left ventricle. Also noted are the presence of a small pericardial effusion, *PE,* and pleural effusion, *PL. RV,* right ventricle; *RA,* right atrium; *LV,* left ventricle; *LA,* left atrium. **B,** Parasternal long-axis view of the myxoma. The pericardial effusion is shown to end just anterior to the descending aorta.

C

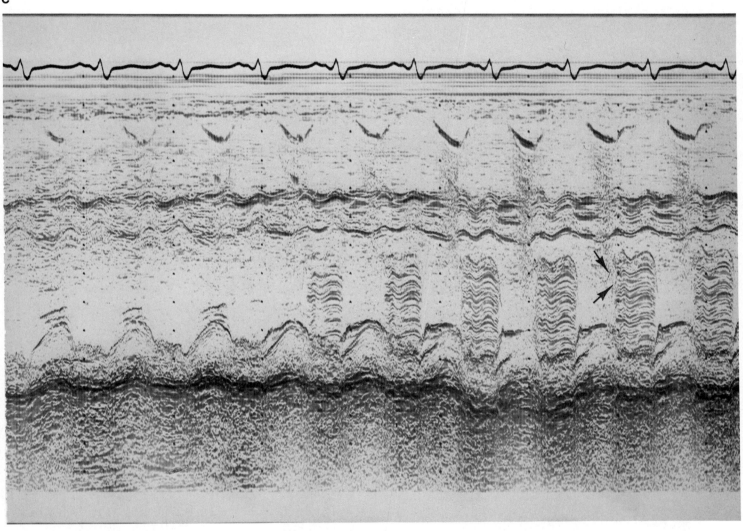

FIG. 34-5, cont'd. C, M-mode tracing of a left atrial myxoma as it prolapses posterior to the mitral leaflet. There is a small diastolic filling space as it takes a few milliseconds for the valve to open and the tumor to prolapse into the left ventricular cavity *(arrows)*.

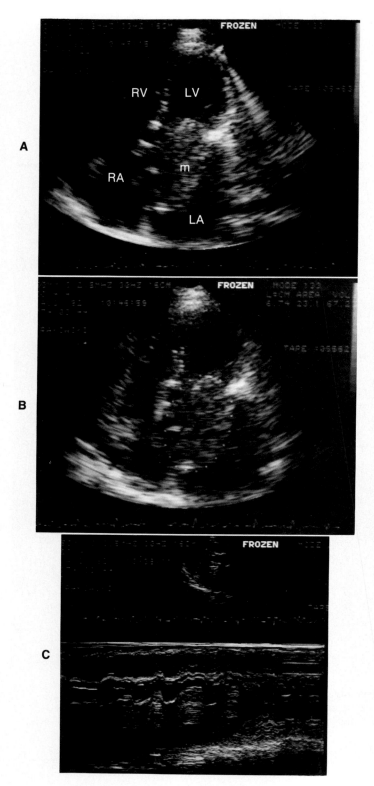

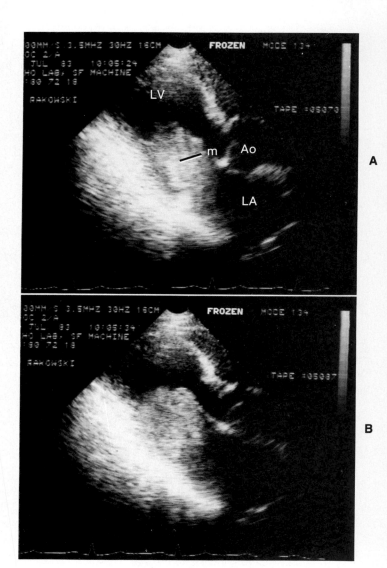

FIG. 34-6. **A** and **B,** Apical four-chamber view of a patient with a left atrial myxoma attached by a stalk to the left atrial septum. **C,** M-mode sweep from the left atrium to the left ventricle shows the progression of the tumor flop as the beam is swept through its large mass. *RV,* right ventricle; *RA,* right atrium; *LV,* left ventricle; *LA,* left atrium; *m,* myxoma.

FIG. 34-7. **A** and **B,** Parasternal long-axis view of a patient with a left atrial myxoma. The gain settings are high to visualize the complex nature of this tissue mass. *LV,* left ventricle; *LA,* left atrium; *Ao,* aorta; *m,* myxoma.

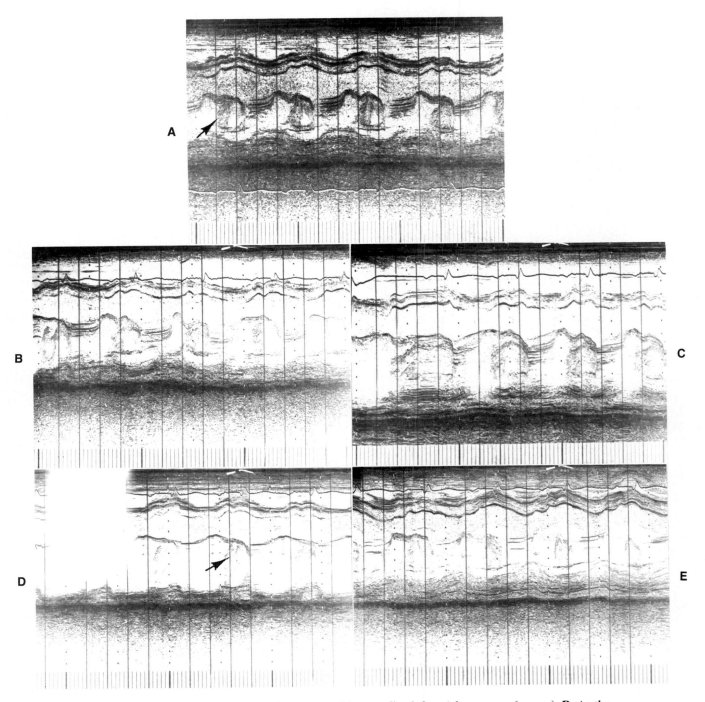

FIG. 34-8. **A,** M-mode tracing of a patient with a smaller left atrial myxoma *(arrow)*. **B,** As the beam is moved into the left ventricle, the myxoma becomes more difficult to visualize. **C,** Sweep from the left atrial cavity into the mitral valve/left ventricular cavity shows the appearance of the myxoma. **D,** Left atrial cavity shows a hint of a mass lesion *(arrow)*. **E,** Left ventricle shows the myxoma just posterior to the mitral valve.

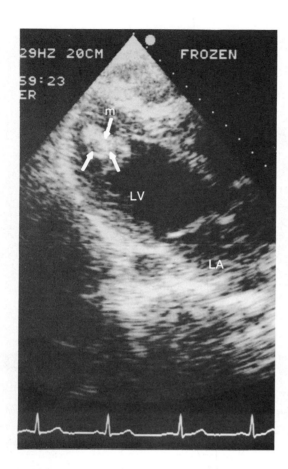

FIG. 34-9. Parasternal long-axis view of a patient with osteosarcoma shows a mass in the apex of the left ventricle most likely representing a metastatic lesion. *LV,* left ventricle; *LA,* left atrium; *m,* mass.

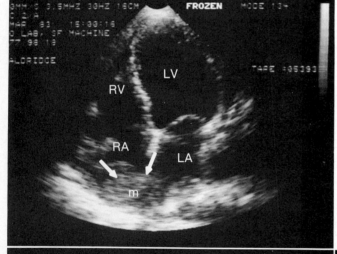

A

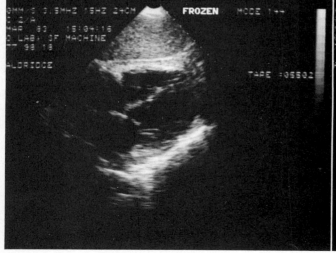

B

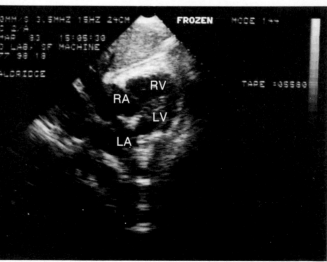

C

FIG. 34-10. Multiple windows should be used to evaluate a patient with suspected metastatic disease involving the heart. **A,** The apical four-chamber view shows a large mass at the base of the right atrial cavity. In the subcostal window, **B** and **C,** the mass is not well demonstrated. With careful angulation the mass can be seen to move independently within the atrial cavity. *RV,* right ventricle; *RA,* right atrium; *LV,* left ventricle; *LA,* left atrium; *m,* mass.

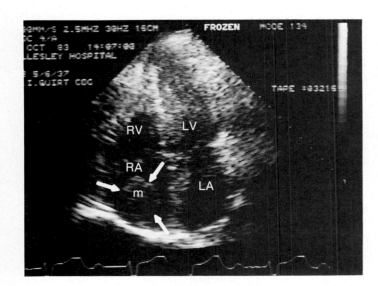

FIG. 34-11. Patient with malignant melanoma with a lesion shown in the right atrial cavity *(arrows)*. This is a modified apical four-chamber view used to demonstrate the mass. *RV,* right ventricle; *RA,* right atrium; *LV,* left ventricle; *LA,* left atrium; *m,* mass.

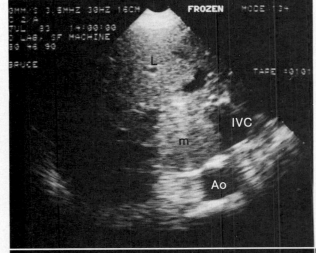

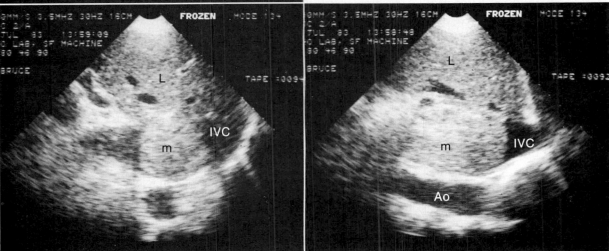

Fig. 34-12. If a patient is known to have a renal tumor (especially on the right), the inferior vena cava should be carefully evaluated to see if the tumor extends into this vessel. The best view to visualize the inferior vena cava is a sagittal abdominal view with a sharp angulation as the cava flows from the right atrial cavity. Careful "sweeping" of the inferior vena cava will allow maximal visualization of the tumor mass. **A,** Transverse cross-section of the upper abdomen shows the dilated inferior vena cava filled with tumor mass. *L,* liver; *IVC,* inferior vena cava; *Ao,* aorta; *m,* mass. **B,** Sagittal view of the liver and inferior vena cava showing the dilated vessel with the huge tumor mass. **C,** Sagittal view of the liver and inferior vena cava with a slight lateral angulation showing a greater extent of the tumor mass in the vessel.

ments of flowing blood. After the thrombus forms, part or all of it may break loose to create an embolus that travels downstream to lodge at a peripheral site. The potential consequence of a thrombosis or embolism is ischemic necrosis of these peripheral cells and tissue, which is termed infarction.

Mural thrombi occur in the lumina of the heart or aorta and attach to one of the walls, usually in the area of infarction. Other sites for mural thrombi are the atrial appendages and left ventricular walls juxtaposed to myocardial infarcts. In the aorta they attach to previously damaged areas such as atherosclerosis or to the syphilitic aortic aneurysm.

Emboli. An embolism is the occlusion of some part of the cardiovascular system by the impaction of a foreign mass transported to the site through the bloodstream. Thromboembolism is the term used for an embolus that is a part or a whole thrombus that has become dislodged and carried downstream to occlude a smaller vessel.

EVALUATION BY ECHOCARDIOGRAPHY

The evaluation of left atrial or ventricular thrombi in patients with suspected myocardial infarction or calcific rheumatic heart disease may be performed by two-dimensional echo using the apical and subxiphoid four-chamber approach.

The cardiac apex is a frequent location for most ventricular thrombi (Fig. 34-13 and 34-14). This area must be carefully assessed for abnormal masses and separated from large papillary muscles or artifactual masses due to side lobes. It is more difficult to detect all left atrial thrombi; possibly the pressure to which the left atrial thrombi are subjected causes the organizing ventricular thrombi to be firmer and better reflective targets than the left atrial thrombi, which are not subjected to the same type of pressure (Figs. 34-15 to 34-17).

Martin[1] further states five points to remember in detecting left ventricular thrombi by echo:

1. Left ventricular thrombi are often closely adherent to

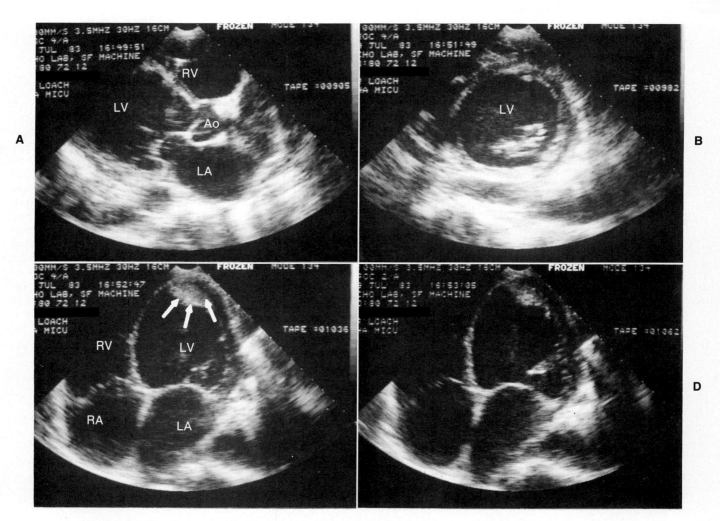

FIG. 34-13.   Patients with dilated cardiac chambers and decreased cardiac function are ideal candidates for thrombus formation, generally at the apex of the ventricle. This patient has congestive cardiomyopathy with very poor contractility. **A,** Parasternal long-axis view of the dilated right ventricle, *RV,* left ventricle, *LV,* left atrium, *LA,* and aorta, *Ao.* **B,** Parasternal short-axis view of the dilated left ventricle, *LV,* with mitral valve apparatus. **C** and **D,** Apical four-chamber view of the dilated cardiac chambers with the apical clot *(arrows).*

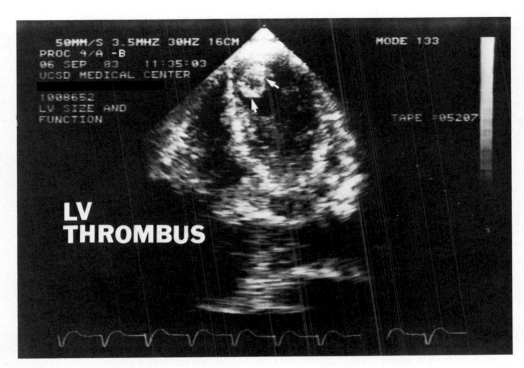

FIG. 34-14. Modified apical four-chamber view of a patient with a thrombus at the apex of the left ventricle. *RV,* right ventricle; *LV,* left ventricle; thrombus *(arrow).*

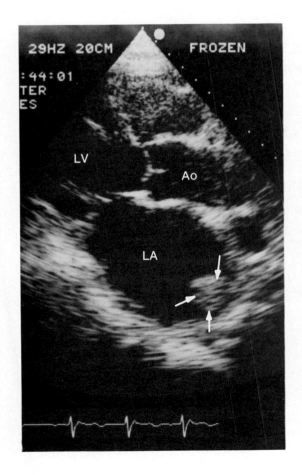

FIG. 34-15. Parasternal long-axis view of a patient with valvular heart disease. The dilated left atrial cavity shows a small thrombus located near the base of the atrium. *LV,* left ventricle; *LA,* left atrium; *Ao,* aorta; thrombus *(arrows).*

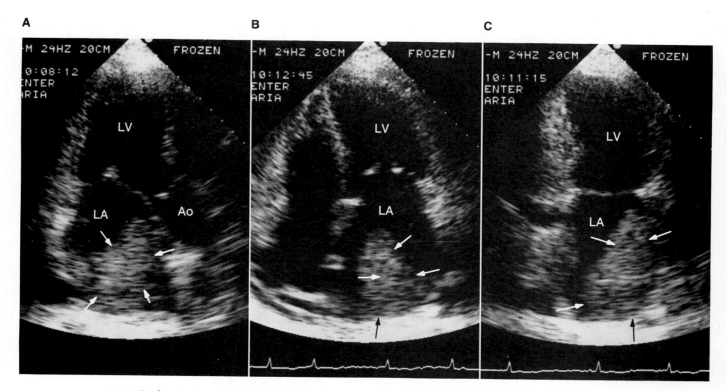

FIG. 34-16. Patient with rheumatic heart disease showing mitral stenosis, a very dilated left atrial cavity with decreased flow, thus allowing the formation of a huge atrial thrombus at the base of the atrium. **A,** Apical two-chamber view. **B,** Apical four-chamber view. **C,** Modified apical two-chamber view. *LV,* left ventricle; *LA,* left atrium; *Ao,* aorta; thrombus *(arrows).*

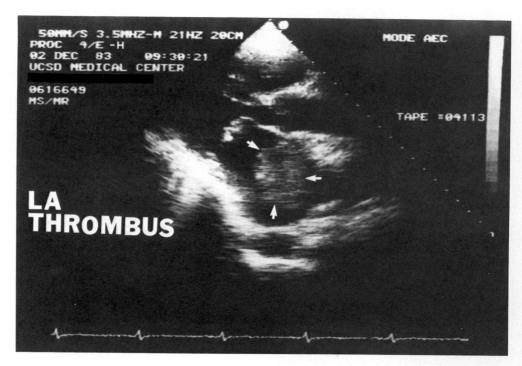

FIG. 34-17. Patient with mitral stenosis and a dilated left atrial cavity with a huge left atrial thrombus *(arrows).* If the gain is not turned up high enough, it may be possible to overlook the thrombus formation since echo reflections are weaker with a thrombus in the left atrium than in the left ventricle.

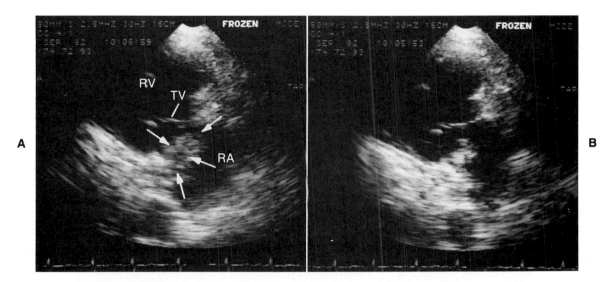

FIG. 34-18. **A** and **B,** Parasternal long-axis view over the right side of the heart shows the right ventricle, *RV,* tricuspid valve, *TV,* and right atrial cavity, *RA.* The thrombus is seen along the medial wall of the right atrial cavity *(arrows).* This mass should be correlated with the patient's clinical history to differentiate whether it is thrombus formation or another type of mass lesion.

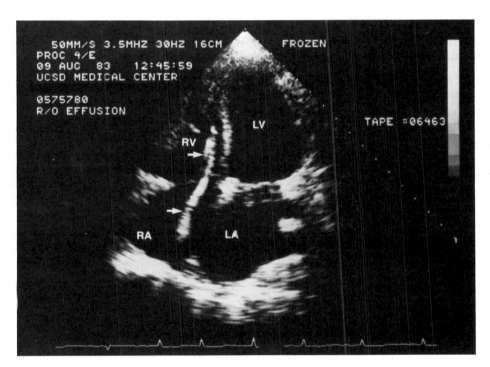

FIG. 34-19. A catheter within the cardiac chambers is shown as a reflective echo pattern. As the transducer is carefully rotated, the full extent of the catheter may be shown. This technique can be useful in defining the end of the catheter in an effort to direct exact placement for the clinician. The echoes from the catheter are "thicker" along its stint, but are uniformly thick, with no clot formation *(arrows).* RV, right ventricle; RA, right atrium; LV, left ventricle; LA, left atrium.

the endocardial surfaces of the ventricle but have a distinct margin or site of origin from the surrounding endocardial echoes.

2. Whereas the myocardium often appears as a dark structure with bright endocardial surfaces, left ventricular thrombis frequently have a granular appearance quite different from that of the surrounding myocardium.

3. The site of the mass lesion is often near the cardiac apex, so the apical and subxiphoid transducer positions are best for detecting ventricular thrombi.

4. Mural thrombi appear to have a motion synchronous with that of the adjacent ventricular walls.

5. Left ventricular thrombi can arise on a short stalk (adjacent to the akinetic-dyskinetic area) or appear as a large, firmly adherent mass of echoes.

Thus echo may prove to be a valuable procedure in the

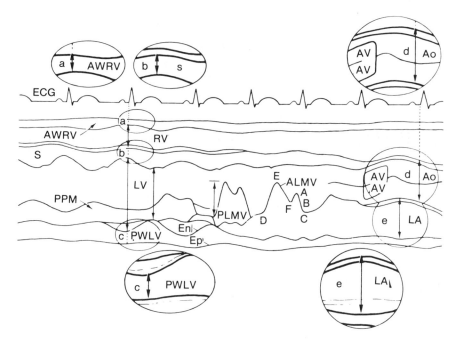

FIG. 35-1. Schema of M-mode echocardiogram sweep showing the recommended criteria for measurement. Diastolic measurements are made at the onset of the QRS complex. Cavities and walls are measured at the level of the chordae below the mitral valve. The illustration and the elliptical inserts, **A** to **E**, show the leading-edge method of measurement (i.e., the diameter is taken from the leading edge of one structure to the leading edge of another structure). The usual M-mode measurements include the diameter of the anterior wall of the right ventricle, *AWRV,* right ventricular cavity, *RV,* interventricular septum, *S,* left ventricle in diastole and in systole, *LV,* posterior wall of left ventricle, *PWLV,* the diameter of the aorta, *Ao,* and the left atrium, *LA. PPM,* posterior papillary muscle; *ALMV* and *PLMV,* anterior and posterior leaflets of the mitral valve; *En,* endocardium; *Ep,* epicardium. Points A to F of mitral valve. (Modified from Sahn DJ et al: Circulation 58:1072, 1978. Used with permission of the American Heart Association.)

Transducer selection

Since an infant's chest is very small and the structures to be visualized are somewhat superficial, it is important to use a transducer with the best possible resolution. This is achieved by the use of high-frequency focused transducers. The transducers available in our laboratory include the following: 10 MHz short focus for premature infants, 7.5 MHz medium focus for neonates, 5.0 MHz short to medium focus for toddlers and slim adolescents, and 3.5 MHz medium focus for adolescents and slim adults. We also occasionally use a 2.25 MHz medium focus for heavier adolescents. To optimize the recording, various transducers are often employed during the study.

Measurements

Measurement sites for neonates and small children may differ slightly from the standards set by the American Society of Echocardiography (ASE) shown in Fig. 35-1. Because the posterior leaflet of the mitral valve hangs further down in the body of the left ventricle, the minor axis along which the ventricular measurements are made is more accurately represented by a perpendicular M-mode line dropped in the plane of the posterior leaflet (Fig. 35-2).

The left atrial measurement has significance in neonates and infants since an increase in the ratio of left atrial to aortic root size (LA/Ao, normally 0.7 to 0.85) is an in-

dicator of a left-to-right shunt (Fig. 35-3). The left atrial size of premature infants must be related to their body weight. Echoes occurring within the left atrium, which could be confused with those from the left atrial posterior wall, have been attributed to entering pulmonary veins or beam width artifacts from the mitral anulus, and can be eliminated by decreasing the gain or altering the transducer position.

The true left atrial wall can be identified by its "motion" as well as its depth. During ventricular systole the left atrial wall moves posteriorly (i.e., away from the transducer) and the ventricular wall moves anteriorly. A sweep from the mitral to aortic valve should show the left atrial posterior wall continuous with the endocardium of the left ventricle (Fig. 35-4). A depth measurement from the crystal artifact to each of these structures should normally show them at the same level. In some instances (e.g., sternal retractions with respiratory distress, in which the anteroposterior plane is flattened), the left atrial dimension may be underestimated. In this case the suprasternal notch view, which cuts through the transverse aortic arch, right pulmonary artery, and left atrium, provides a more representative left atrial dimension. This view is also helpful in lesions in which an increased pulmonary blood flow may cause dilatation of the right pulmonary artery. The transverse aortic arch dimension increases with obstructive lesions, both proximally and dis-

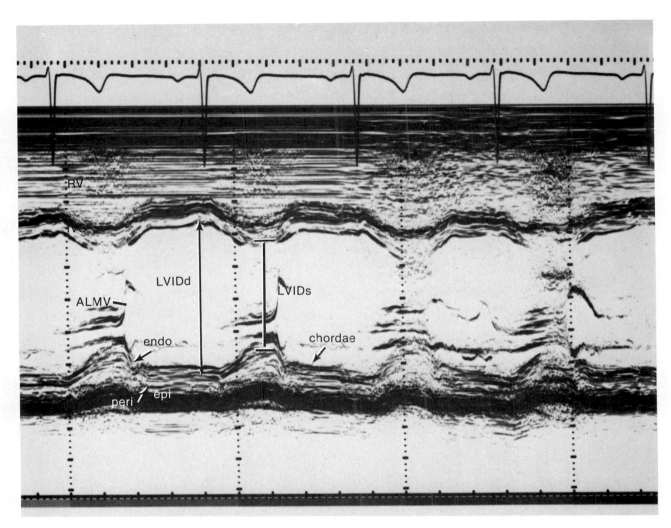

FIG. 35-2.   M-mode tracing of the systolic and diastolic measurements of the left ventricular cavity. *RV,* right ventricle; *IVS,* interventricular septum; *ALMV,* anterior leaflet of mitral valve; *LVIDd,* left ventricular internal dimension in diastole; *LVIDs,* left ventricular internal dimension in systole; *endo,* endocardium; *epi,* epicardium; *peri,* pericardium.

tally, as seen with Marfan's and Turner's syndromes. A small transverse aortic arch dimension can help in confirming the diagnosis of hypoplastic left heart sydrome.

Technique

Our patients are examined with a combined two-dimensional, M-mode, and Doppler ultrasound technology. Many of the abnormal cases are also studied with color-flow Doppler. Each patient is approached in a routine, systemized manner, no matter what the pathology may be.

The initial view is the parasternal long axis in which we demonstrate relative cardiac relationships (Fig. 35-5). The right ventricle should be smaller than the left ventricle in this view. There should be good contractility of the interventricular septum and posterior heart wall. The size of the septum and posterior heart wall should be symmetric and within normal limits for the patient's height and weight. There should be continuity of the anterior aortic wall to the septum as well as continuity between the posterior aortic wall and the anterior leaflet of the mitral valve. The ratio of the aorta to the left atrial cavity should

be approximately 1:1. The aortic cusps should be thin and open to the full extent of the aortic root; there should be symmetric closure of the cusps in diastole. The mitral valve should be thin and mobile, with closure in a plane aligned with the aortic cusps and atrioventricular groove (to rule out prolapse). The chordal structures and papillary muscles should be examined.

From the parasternal long-axis view, the transducer is rotated 90 degrees to a short-axis view (Fig. 35-6). The high short-axis view demonstrates the right ventricular outflow tract, the tricuspid valve, the right atrium, the pulmonary cusps, the main pulmonary artery, the right and left pulmonary arteries, the patent ductus arteriosus (if present), the aorta with its three cusps, the right and left coronary arteries, and the left atrium. Often it is necessary to angle slightly, or rotate the patient's position slightly, to record the more subtle anatomy such as the cusps or the coronary arteries.

The transducer is then directed in a more perpendicular manner, while remaining in the short-axis position. At this level, the right ventricle, interventricular septum, mi-

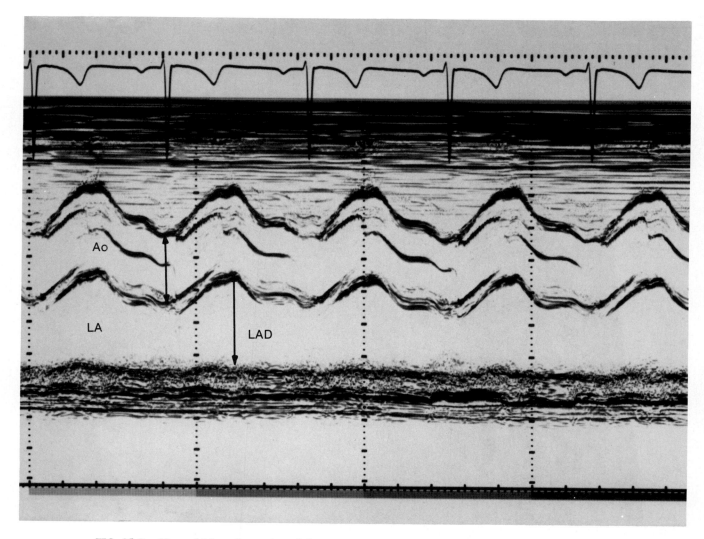

FIG. 35-3.   Normal M-mode tracing of the aorta, *Ao,* and left atrium, *LA,* showing the characteristic left atrial posterior wall motion. Note that the transducer beam projects two of the aortic valve leaflets (the right cusp is anterior, and the noncoronary cusp is posterior; the left is often not seen well but projects into the middle of the "box" when shown). The standard sites for measurement are shown. The aortic diameter is measured at the onset of the QRS from leading edge to leading edge. The left atrial dimension, *LAD,* is calculated in diastole, from the widest point, from leading edge to leading edge.

tral valve orifice, and left ventricular cavity are well seen (Fig. 35-7). This is a good view to evaluate the mitral valve; one should look for redundancy of the leaflet, as well as for a split in the anterior leaflet to signify a cleft mitral valve. The septum should move posteriorly in systole and anterior in diastole. There should be no septal flattening (as occurs with increased volume in the right ventricle, such as pulmonary hypertension). The size of the right ventricle should be crescent-shaped, with the left ventricle assuming a more rounded shape.

The transducer is then angled inferior toward the apex of the heart to record the right ventricle, septum, and left ventricle with papillary muscles (care should be used to identify the two separate papillary muscles) (Fig. 35-8).

The next window is usually the apical four-chamber view to record the four cardiac chambers, the alignment of the tricuspid and mitral valves, and the continuity of the interventricular and interatrial septum (Fig. 35-9). The foramen ovalae is very thin in the mid-portion of the

interatrial septum, and thus may not be visualized well in this view (the subcostal four chamber is a better window to see the atrial septum). The pulmonary veins should enter the left atrial cavity in this view. This is a good window to evaluate cardiac function, the presence of pericardial effusion, and wall dimensions.

The alternative four-chamber view is made with the transducer in the subcostal position (Fig. 35-10). The right ventricle is shown as the anterior chamber, just beneath the liver. The interventricular septum and interatrial septum are well seen. The mitral and tricuspid valves are well seen. The right and left atrial cavities may be identified and examined for the presence of thrombus or other mass lesions.

The short-axis view in the subcostal plane is very good to image the right ventricular outflow tract, the pulmonary artery and its bifurcation, the aorta (ascending and arch), and tricuspid valve (Fig. 35-11).

The suprasternal view is excellent to evaluate the as-

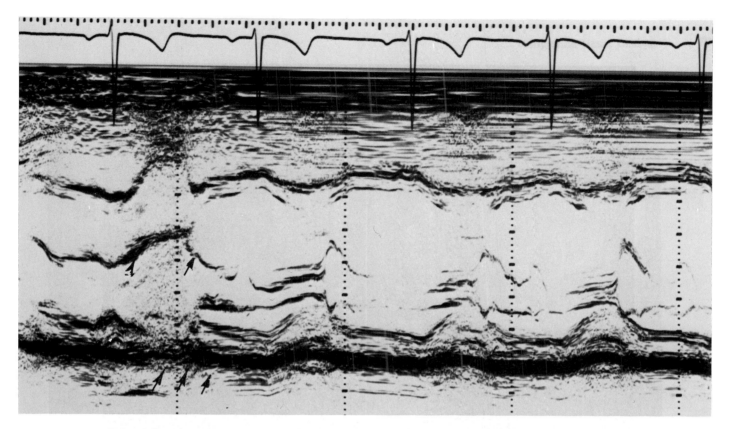

FIG. 35-4. M-mode sweep from the aorta into the left ventricular cavity shows the continuity of the posterior wall of the two chambers. The atrial wall has a slight motion when scanned at the level of the atrioventricular junction. As one scans cephalad, away from the ventricle, the atrial wall becomes motionless.

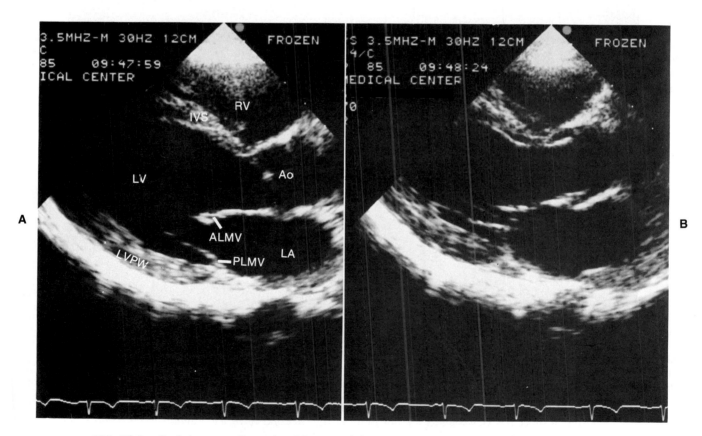

FIG. 35-5. Real-time two-dimensional images of the parasternal long-axis view of the heart in diastole, **A,** and systole, **B.** The structures identified are the right ventricle, *RV,* interventricular septum, *IVS,* the aorta, *Ao,* the left ventricle, *LV,* the left atrium, *LA,* the anterior and posterior leaflets of the mitral valve, *ALMV* and *PLMV,* and the left ventricular posterior wall, *LVPW.*

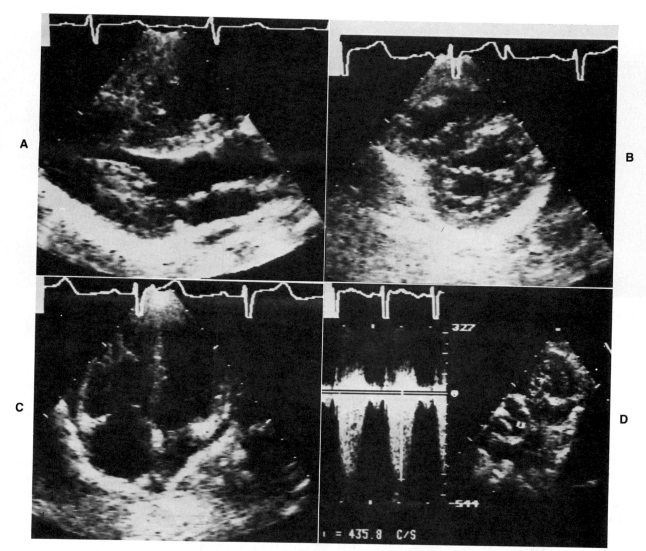

FIG. 35-14. Congenital pulmonic stenosis is seen in this young patient. **A,** Parasternal long-axis view showing a dilated, pressure-overloaded right ventricle with hypertrophy of the myocardial wall. **B,** Parasternal short-axis view showing the hypertrophied right ventricular cavity. **C,** Apical four-chamber view. **D,** Subcostal short-axis view. The aorta is to the right, pulmonary artery to the left. The pulmonary cusps are thickened with decreased mobility. The continuous-wave Doppler shows a velocity of 4.3, which corresponds to a gradient of 74, indicating severe pulmonary stenosis.

One should look for subpulmonic or suprapulmonic narrowing or hypoplasia (Fig. 35-17). If no pulmonary valve cusp motion is apparent, the valve is likely atretic.

Doppler examination of the main pulmonary artery is extremely useful in delineating the degree of stenosis present. Generally a stenotic valve will show a turbulent pattern with the PW tracing, thus the CW transducer must be used to record the maximum velocity (Fig. 35-18). The Doppler not only determines the gradient across the valve (using the modified Bernoulli formula $4V^2$) but also determines if any flow is going out the main pulmonary artery in critical pulmonary stenosis. One must be careful in the presence of other intracardiac shunts that the velocity is not overestimated because of the increased blood flow. Patients with a ventricular septal defect (or a form of tetralogy of Fallot, discussed later

in this chapter) may cause the pulmonary Doppler flow to be increased.

PULMONARY ATRESIA WITH INTACT VENTRICULAR SEPTUM

Pulmonary atresia with intact ventricular septum is characterized by a complete anatomic obstruction to forward blood flow from the right ventricle into the pulmonary trunk because the pulmonary valve is imperforate and the ventricular septum is intact.[11] An interatrial communication through the foramen ovale is the only communication with the right heart. The atretic pulmonary valve has a sealed fibrous membrane. The rest of the pulmonary trunk assumes a somewhat patent funnel shape and varies from hypoplastic to slightly larger than normal. In many

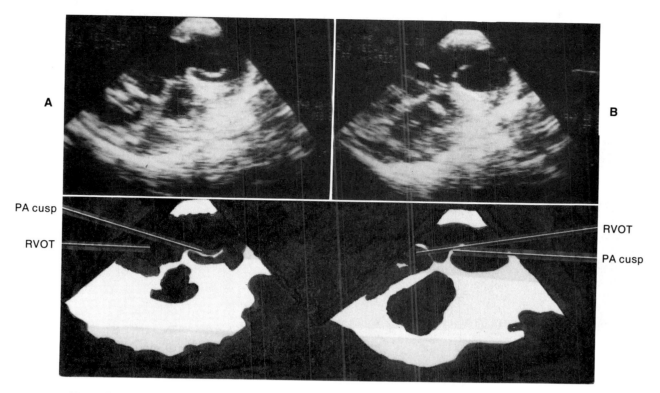

FIG. 35-15. Parasternal long-axis view of a patient with a domed pulmonary valve. The valve opens in systole and domes into the pulmonary artery, **A.** In **B,** the valve domes forward in diastole. These cusps are not thickened and the amount of pulmonary stenosis is very mild. *RVOT,* right ventricular outflow tract.

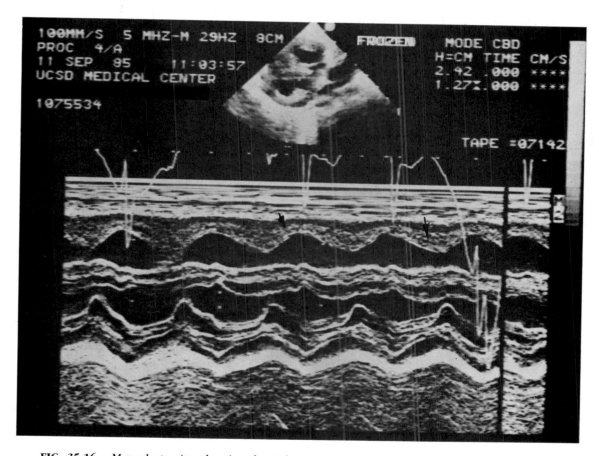

FIG. 35-16. M-mode tracing showing the right ventricular hypertrophy secondary to increased pressure in the right ventricle.

septum. The aorta does receive blood from both right

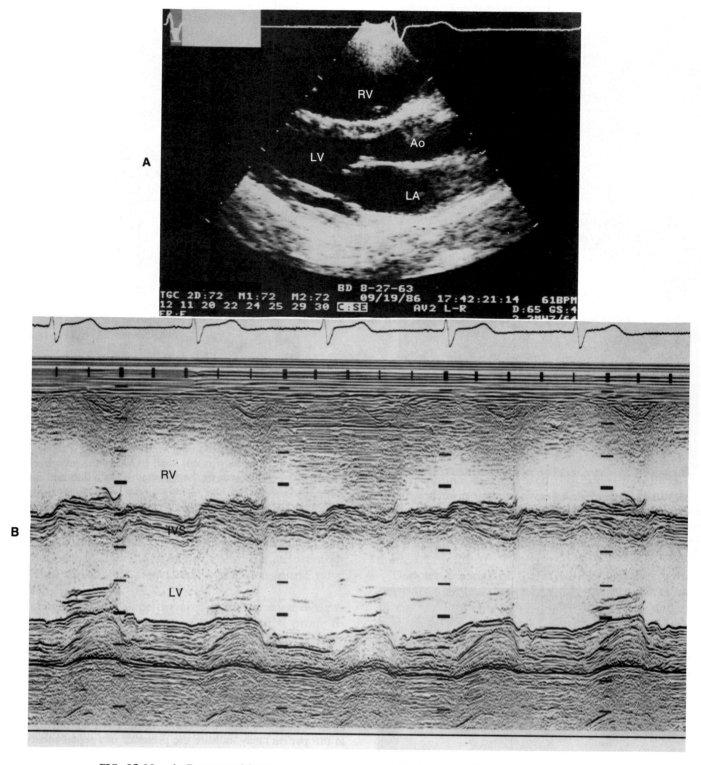

FIG. 35-33. A, Parasternal long-axis view of a patient with a large atrial septal defect. The right ventricle, *RV,* is enlarged, causing the interventricular septum to bow slightly into the left ventricle. *LV,* left ventricle. **B,** M-mode tracing of the enlarged right ventricle, and abnormal septal motion. The presence of a volume overload in the right ventricle causes the septal motion to become paradoxical or flattened (as seen in this patient). *IVS,* interventricular septum.

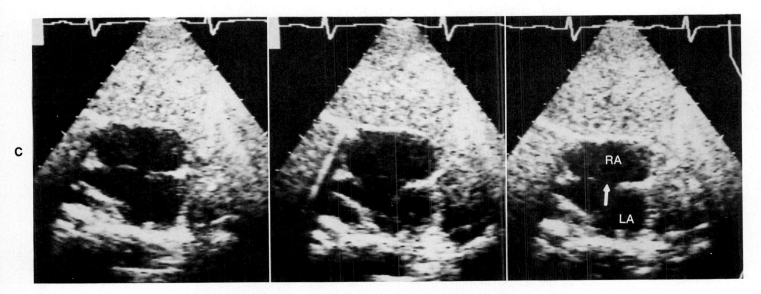

FIG. 35-33, cont'd. C, Subcostal four-chamber view of the right atrium, *RA,* and left atrium, *LA.* The presence of a large secundum-type atrial septal defect is shown in multiple frames of systole and diastole.

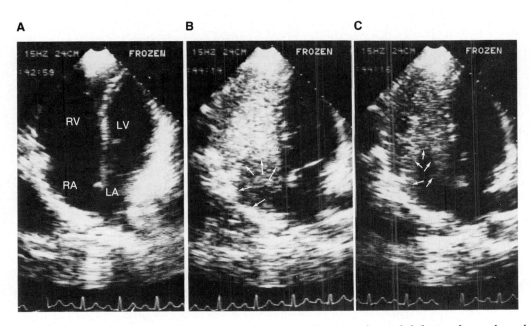

FIG. 35-34. A, Apical four-chamber view in a patient with an atrial septal defect and an enlarged right heart. **B,** Saline contrast injection into the right side of the heart through an intervenous line in the patient's arm. The saline solution is rapidly shaken before the injection is made. The injection is done with vigor, causing microbubbles to appear in the right side of the heart. The beginning of a negative contrast effect across the atrial septal defect is present *(arrows).* **C,** Negative contrast effect *(arrows)* as the blood shunts from the left to the right.

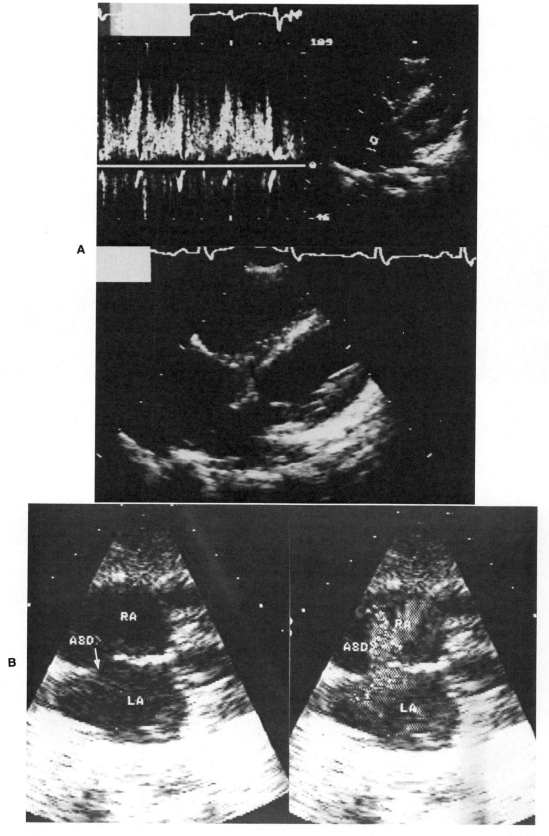

FIG. 35-35.   A, A patient with an atrial septal defect shows positive Doppler flow across the secundum defect. The Doppler sample volume is placed on the right side of the defect to record the
left-to-right shunt. The view is a subcostal four chamber. The dilated right atrium and ventricle are
well seen. **B,** Subcostal four-chamber view of a patient with an atrial septal defect, *ASD*. The image
on the right shows a black-and-white effect of color flow through the defect. In actual color, the
flow would be red, and it flows freely from the left to the right heart.

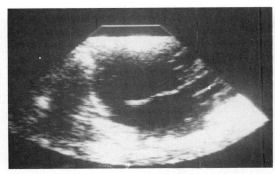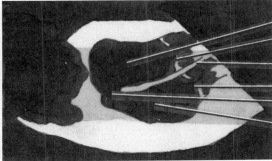

RA
TVR
IVS
MVR
asd–sin ven
LA

FIG. 35-36. Subcostal four-chamber view demonstrating a sinus venosus–type atrial septal defect. Note the signal dropout in the superior most portion of the atrial septum. The secundum and primum parts of the septum are intact. *RA*, right atrium; *TVR*, tricuspid valve ring; *IVS*, interventricular septum; *MVR*, mitral valve ring; *asd–sin ven*, atrial septal defect–sinus venosus, *LA*, left atrium.

usually associated with this type of defect, thus it is important to identify the entry site of the pulmonary veins into the left atrial cavity. Color-flow mapping is useful in this type of problem because it allows the sonographer to actually visualize the venous return to the left atrium and a flow pattern crossing into the right atrial cavity.

TOTAL ANOMALOUS PULMONARY VENOUS RETURN

Total anomalous pulmonary venous return is a condition in which all the venous blood from both lungs enters the right atrium directly or through one of its tributary veins. The anomalous veins emerge individually from the lungs and either enter directly into the right atrium or unite in the mediastinum to form a confluence. A separate vascular channel connects this confluence of veins to a systemic vein that lies either within the thorax or within the abdomen. Blood from this systemic vein finds its way into the right atrium.

The thoracic or supradiaphragmatic venous channel that receives the confluence is from one of the following: (1) the coronary sinus, (2) the left innominate vein, which communicates with the confluence via an anomalous vertical vein or a left superior vena cava, or (3) the right superior vena cava directly or via the azygous vein.

Less frequently, the pulmonary veins join the systemic venous system below the diaphragm. This vascular channel enters the abdominal cavity through the esophageal hiatus and terminates in the portal vein or its tributaries or in the ductus venosus. Other entry sites have been described, and occasionally there is more than one entry site.

One problem that occurs in this condition is the impedance of flow from the lungs. The most common cause of obstruction is drainage below the diaphragm. In the thorax the obstruction may be compressed when the channel passes between the pulmonary trunk and left bronchus as it travels to the left innominate vein.

An interatrial communication is critical in total anomalous pulmonary venous return so blood may reach the left heart. This may be a true atrial septal defect or a patent foramen ovale. The wider the defect, the more efficient the interchange between the right and left atrium.

Echographically, this diagnosis is one of the most difficult to detect (Fig. 35-37). The most common findings include an enlarged right heart (with the atrial septum bowing into the left atrial cavity), a "common" channel seen posterior to the left atrium, or by Doppler, increased flow in the right atrial cavity. Color-flow Doppler may help distinguish abnormal venous connections as they drain into the right atrial cavity.

ENDOCARDIAL CUSHION DEFECT

Endocardial cushion defects occur at a critical region where the atrial and ventricular septa joins the mitral and tricuspid valves. A complete defect means there is a primum atrial septal defect, a ventricular septal defect, and clefts in the mitral and tricuspid valves. An incomplete defect has an ostium primum atrial septal defect and a cleft mitral valve. Usually the ventricular septum is intact and the tricuspid valve is normal, although occasionally it may be cleft or underdeveloped.

The abnormal attachments to the ventricular septum displace the mitral valve leaflet into the left ventricular outflow tract, causing it to open in a superior plane. This abnormal plane of anterior leaflet motion, parallel with rather than perpendicular to the ventricular septum, makes simultaneous recording of both mitral leaflets difficult from the normal transducer position. The echo shows a long diastolic apposition of the anterior leaflet to the interventricular septum, right ventricular volume overload, and multiple mitral echoes from redundant tissue (Fig. 35-38). The parasternal long-axis view demonstrates the narrowed left ventricular outflow tract that is akin to the "gooseneck" deformity seen on cardiac catheterization.

If failure of the endocardial cushions to fuse is complete, a ventricular septal defect and abnormal tricuspid valve are seen in conjunction with a primum atrial septal defect and cleft mitral valve. The ventricular septal defect occurs just below the atrioventricular ring and is continuous with the primum atrial septal defect (Fig. 35-39). Paradoxical septal motion is not seen in a complete canal because of equalized flow and pressure between the ventricles. The Rastelli types A and B are characterized by insertion of the chordae from the cleft mitral valve and

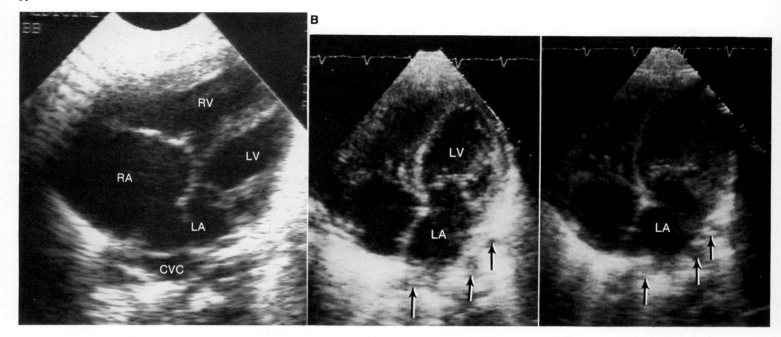

FIG. 35-37. **A,** A patient with total anomalous pulmonary venous return may be difficult to visualize with echocardiography unless extreme care is made to image the four pulmonary veins draining into the left atrial cavity. In this patient the pulmonary veins drained into a common venous chamber, *CVC,* posterior to the left atrium, *LA,* before draining into the right atrium, *RA.* Thus the right atrium is very large; the atrial septum bows to the left because of the overload in the right atrium. The left atrium and ventricle, *LV,* are small due to the reduced inflow into the heart. The ventricular function is abnormal. Color flow is useful for distinguishing venous communications and their entrance into the heart. *RV,* right ventricle. **B,** The patient has been surgically repaired, and the four pulmonary veins are now shown to drain into the left atrium. The atrial septum is no longer bowing toward the left heart. Pulmonary veins *(arrows).*

FIG. **35-38. A,** Subxiphoid four-chamber view along the coronal plane. This corresponds to the most posterior plane, *A,* on the insert. Note the position of the atrial septum. The primum septum is closest to the atrioventricular valves and the endocardial cushion. The absence of this part of the septum should alert the sonographer to search carefully for the position of the atrioventricular valves and their chordal attachments. **B,** Subxiphoid four-chamber view in a patient with a primum atrial septal defect, *asd−prim,* demonstrating the break in the atrial septal continuity *(arrow)* just above the AV ring in the primum area. Note the blunt edge of the defect. (**A,** From Sahn DJ et al: Circulation 60:1317, 1979. Used with permission of The American Heart Association.)

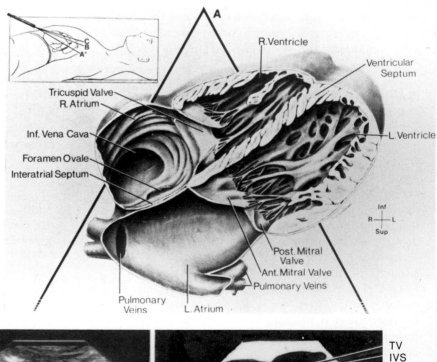

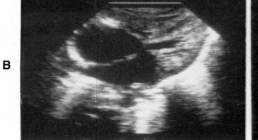

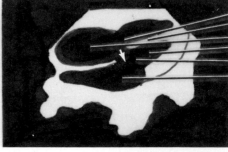

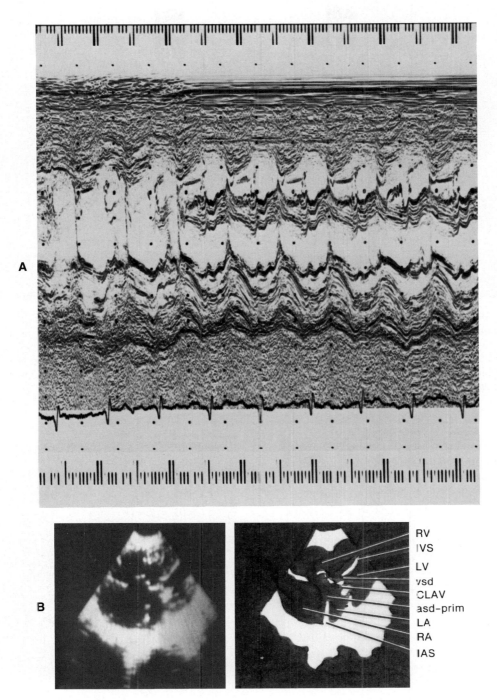

Labels on image B: RV, IVS, LV, vsd, CLAV, asd-prim, LA, RA, IAS

FIG. 35-39. A, M-mode tracing in a patient with a complete endocardial cushion defect showing the interruption of the interventricular septum as one sweeps from the ventricle to the aortic root. The common atrioventricular valve is shown to flow from the left to the right ventricle through the septal defect. **B,** Apical four-chamber view in a patient with a complete endocardial cushion defect (also called AV canal). The common AV valve leaflet can be seen stretching across the endocardial cushion defect. Note also the blunting at the edges of both defects (atrial and ventricular). There is a common leaflet of the AV valve. Careful evaluation of the atrioventricular area must be made to determine if there is one common leaflet or two leaflets present. In some cases the leaflet is atretic on one side. The demonstration of leaflet mobility, chordal attachments, and papillary muscle position should be made to determine the alignment of the AV leaflets.

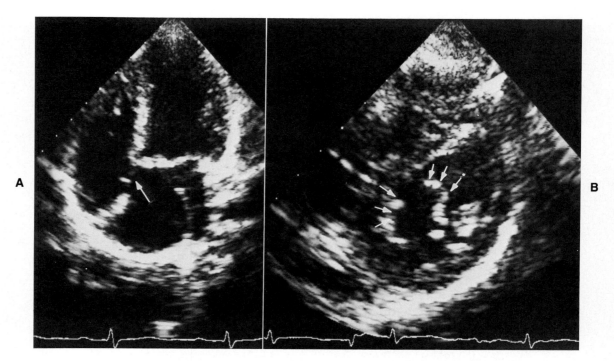

FIG. 35-40.   **A,** Apical four-chamber view of a patient with an endocardial cushion defect. The primum septum is absent *(arrow).* **B,** Parasternal two-chamber view of the abnormal mitral valve showing a break in the normal diastolic curve of the anterior leaflet, with the edges of the cleft mitral leaflet apparent *(arrows).* The anterior leaflet has two parts: one opening toward the septum, the other toward the lateral wall of the ventricle. Generally this type of valve is insufficient as well, causing the left atrium to dilate with the amount of regurgitation present.

tricuspid valve into the crest of the interventricular septum or a right ventricular papillary muscle, respectively (Fig. 35-40). Rastelli type C, the most primitive form, has a single, undivided, free-floating leaflet stretching across both ventricles. A sweep from the mitral to aortic valves shows the anterior leaflet of the mitral valve "swinging" through the ventricular septal defect in continuity with the tricuspid valve. The tricuspid valve is said to "cap" the mitral valve. Evaluation of the pulmonary valve for signs of pulmonary artery hypertension is extremely important in canal patients, since the right ventricular pressure reaches systemic levels very early.

Postoperative canal patients are evaluated for mitral insufficiency and stenosis associated with repair of the cleft mitral valve. Mitral insufficiency remains if the repaired anterior leaflet does not coapt evenly with the posterior leaflet. The Doppler and color-flow map is useful to evaluate the amount and severity of regurgitation present.

COR TRIATRIATUM

This anomaly partitions the left atrium into two compartments. The pulmonary veins drain into an accessory left atrial chamber that lies proximal to the true left atrium.[8] The accessory chamber is believed to represent the dilated common pulmonary vein of the embryo so that cortriatriatum has also been called stenosis of the common pulmonary vein.[3]

The distal compartment communicates with the mitral valve and contains the left atrial appendage and fossa ovalis.[8] The muscular band that partitions the left atrium has

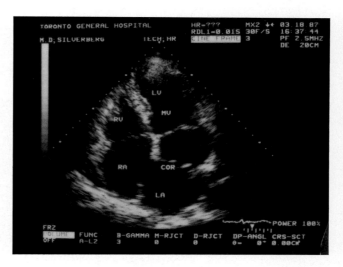

FIG. 35-41.   Apical four-chamber view of a patient with a cor triatriatum. The linear structure "dividing" the left atrium represents this anomaly. The pulmonary veins drain into the accessory left atrial chamber that lies proximal to the true left atrium. There is usually one or more openings within this muscular band that determine the amount of atrial obstruction.

one or more openings, and the size of these openings determines the degree of atrial obstruction.[9]

By echo, the membrane within the left atrial cavity may be seen on the long-axis or apical four-chamber view as the beam is carefully swept through the atrial cavity (Fig. 35-41). Associated problems of atrial septal defect and pulmonary hypertension may also be seen with echo. Doppler studies in the area would show an obstructive type of flow through the orifice as the sample volume is placed near the fibromuscular band. Color-flow Doppler would show a turbulent pattern in the left atrial cavity, especially at the site of the diaphragmatic band.

CONGENITAL MITRAL STENOSIS

There are several different types of congenital mitral stenosis.[10] One form shows the leaflets to be thickened, nodular and fibrotic without calcification; the commissures are very small to absent; the chordae tendineae are shortened, thickened and fused; and the papillary muscles are fibrosed. The valve is somewhat tunnel shaped. The presence of endocardial fibroelastosis may be found in the left ventricle and atrium.

Another form is a "parachute" deformity of the valve.[10] In this condition, normal leaflets and commissures are drawn into close apposition by shortened chordae tendineae that converge and insert into a single large papillary muscle. The interchordal slit-like spaces provide the only access to the left ventricle.

A rare form of congenital stenosis occurs when the papillary muscles are the cause of the obstruction. The muscles become so thickened that they encroach on the subvalvular area.

Another form of stenosis occurs when the mitral leaflets are normal but the inlet of the left ventricle is encroached on by a circumferential supravalvular ridge of connective tissue that arises at the base of the atrial aspect of the mitral leaflets.[10] This defect may occur alone or with other obstructive lesions (supravalvular ring of the left atrium, parachute mitral valve, subaortic stenosis, and coarctation of the aorta).

Echographically, the thickened mitral valve is shown to dome on multiple long-axis and four-chamber views (Fig. 35-42). The short-axis view shows the narrow orifice of the anterior and posterior leaflet. The left atrium will be enlarged, and with insufficiency, enlargement of the left ventricle will also be present. Doppler flow studies should be carefully performed with the sample volume placed at the inlet of the valve and moved slowly into the left ven-

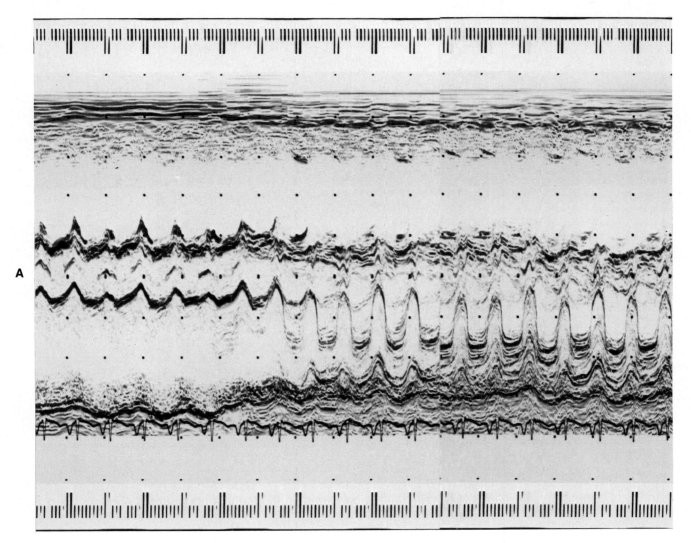

FIG. 35-42.   A, M-mode tracing in a patient with congenital mitral stenosis. The left atrium is enlarged secondary to the narrowed orifice of the mitral valve and regurgitation. The amplitude of the mitral leaflet is good. The posterior leaflet moves anteriorly with the anterior leaflet, typical of stenotic valves.

Continued.

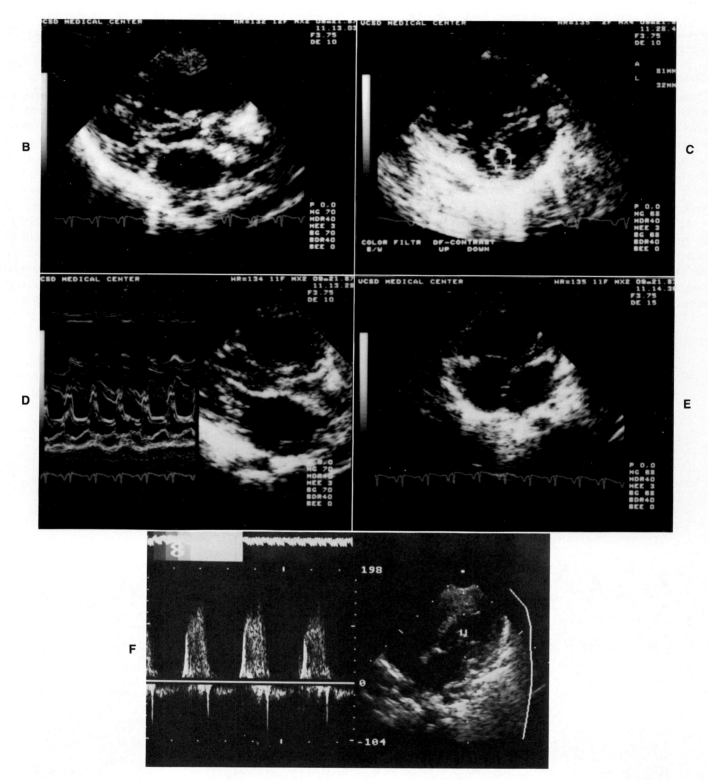

FIG. 35-42, cont'd.   B, Parasternal long-axis view of a patient with congenital mitral stenosis. The thickened mitral leaflet is seen. The left atrium is enlarged. The right ventricle is enlarged secondary to pulmonary hypertension. **C,** M-mode tracing of the mitral valve shows an abnormal pattern. The posterior leaflet moves anterior with the anterior leaflet. The septal motion is typical of pulmonary hypertension—volume overload of the right ventricle. **D,** Parasternal short-axis view of the enlarged right ventricle and flattened septal motion. The mitral orifice is small. **E,** Apical four-chamber view showing the enlarged right heart. There is tricuspid insufficiency secondary to pulmonary hypertension. The abnormal mitral valve is seen. **F,** Doppler flow patterns of the mitral valve inflow show a turbulent pattern with a diminished *e-f* slope.

tricle to note the velocity changes with the CW tracing. The left atrium should be evaluated for the amount and severity of regurgitation present. Color-flow studies are typical for valvular disease. Turbulence in the area of the narrowing will demonstrate the stenosis; while the jet stream into the left atrium will be easily demonstrated on the four-chamber and long-axis views.

LEFT VENTRICULAR OUTFLOW TRACT OBSTRUCTION

Left ventricular outflow tract obstruction can occur at three levels: (1) supravalvar, (2) valvar, and (3) subvalvar. The stenosis can be either fixed or dynamic in nature. Because auscultation often cannot localize either the site or the severity of a left ventricular outflow tract obstruction two-dimensional echocardiography, with its ability to visualize many planes of the heart, has become very important for qualitative, if not quantitative (with Doppler), assessment of the condition.

Supravalvar aortic obstruction

Supravalvar aortic obstruction occurs as a narrowing of the aortic root lumen, from both anterior and posterior walls, just above the level of the aortic valve. It is best visualized in the parasternal long-axis, apical four-chamber, and subcostal views.

M-mode has proved unreliable in the assessment of valvar aortic stenosis, for the limited M-mode view may not cut through the tips of the domed aortic valve. Two-dimensional echo, with its ability to visualize the domed aortic leaflets in systole, was used by Weyman[14] to quantitate the severity of valvar aortic stenosis in children. He compared the ratio of maximum aortic cusp separation to aortic root diameter against the aortic valve gradients obtained during cardiac catheterization and found that the MAoCS/AoD must be below 0.5 to predict a significant gradient.

Valves that open superiorly into the aortic root, rather than anteriorly and posteriorly, during systole and show a diagonal sagging diastolic closure pattern warrant more vigorous examination to ensure that significant stenosis is not missed. Dilation of the ascending aorta (poststenotic dilation) is another indicator of obstruction.

The Weyman technique described above is not applicable to all patients with stenotic aortic valves. Increased echo return from calcified leaflets results in an artificially small maximum aortic cusp separation. The aortic orifice in postoperative patients has been difficult to evaluate reliably. Also a dilated aortic root is found in Marfan's and Turner's syndromes invalidates this technique since it makes the denominator artificially large.

Congenital aortic stenosis

The aortic valve itself may be malformed to give rise to the obstruction in the left ventricular outflow tract (Fig. 35-43). The valve may be unicuspid or bicuspid with restricted mobility.

A bicuspid aortic valve may be the cause of aortic obstruction. The aorta should be carefully evaluated to record the presence of the number of cusps and the opening excursion of such cusps. Depending on how the cusps are divided, the M-mode tracing may show eccentricity in the diastolic segment.

Subvalvar aortic stenosis

Subvalvular aortic stenosis is a less common type of ventricular tract obstruction. It can occur as a discrete ridge or membrane below the aortic root, a diffuse long tunnel involvement, or a dynamic obstruction due to systolic motion of the anterior leaflet of the mitral valve. The parasternal long-axis view (Fig. 35-44) and the apical four-chamber view are probably the best views to visualize this subaortic area. On M-mode studies, early closure of the aortic valve may be seen in systole. There may be concentric hypertrophy of the left ventricle secondary to the pressure overload.

The Doppler study can be extremely useful to evaluate the patient with aortic stenosis. As explained in Chapter 28, the Bernoulli equation allows one to access the velocity and thus determine the gradient across the stenotic area. The best view is generally the apical "five"-chamber view with the CW sample volume placed at the level of the aortic valve and then carefully moved from the left ventricular outflow tract into the ascending aorta (Figs. 35-43, E, and 35-45, C and D).

Alternate views useful for aortic stenosis include the suprasternal approach and subcostal view (Fig. 35-45, A and B) In the suprasternal approach the transducer is placed in the suprasternal notch just to the right of the midline (Fig. 35-46). The patient's head should be turned to the left to allow better contact of the transducer and sternal notch (Fig. 35-47). A steep angulation of the transducer is necessary to record the ascending aorta, aortic arch, and descending aorta. If high velocities are recorded, the CW "stand-alone" transducer should be used as it is much smaller in diameter and may fit very well into the suprasternal notch. This transducer does not allow the simultaneous two-dimensional visualization of structures, but with the harsh sound and typical aortic stenosis waveform in the Doppler pattern, the sonographer can determine when the maximum velocity is obtained. The tracing should be smooth and well defined along its maximum border. The audible "sound" should be turbulent and harsh in its sound when the best window has been found to record the maximum velocity.

Color-flow Doppler is useful in patients with aortic valve disease. The turbulent pattern is well demonstrated with the color mapping, thus the Doppler may be placed in the correct jet stream to record the maximum velocity tracing.

Hypoplastic left heart syndrome

Hypoplastic left heart syndrome represents the most severe form of left ventricular outflow tract obstruction (Fig. 35-48). This may be due to severe tubular hypoplasia of the arch, severe aortic stenosis, or aortic atresia during fetal development. This causes the left-sided develop-

Text continued on p. 829.

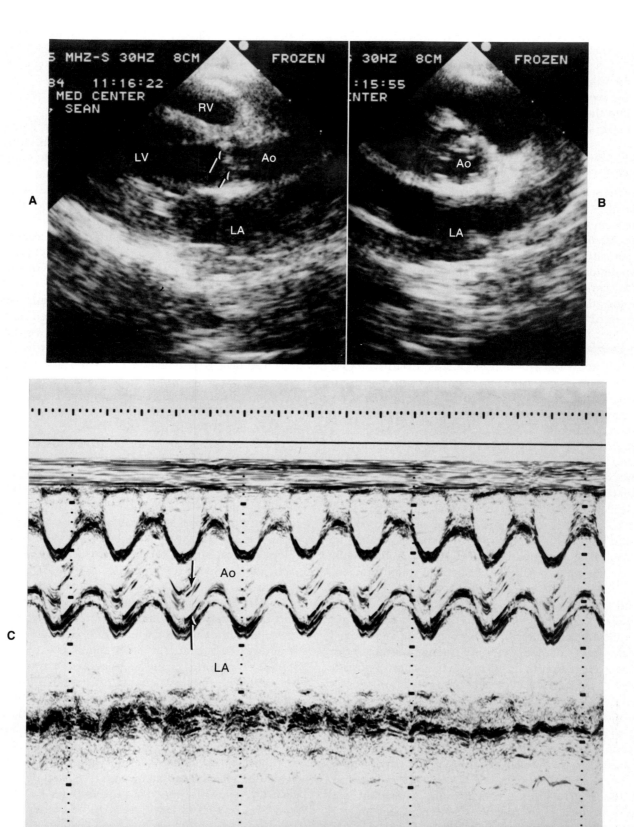

FIG. 35-43.   A, Parasternal long-axis view in a patient with congenital aortic stenosis. The cusps are thickened and show reduced excursion. *LV,* left ventricle; *RV,* right ventricle; *LA,* left atrium; *Ao,* aorta. **B,** The parasternal short-axis view shows the valve to be bicuspid with reduced orifice size. **C,** M-mode tracing of the aorta and left atrium showing the aortic valve to open with reduced excursion *(arrows).* There is eccentricity of the cusps in diastole, representing the bicuspid nature of the valve.

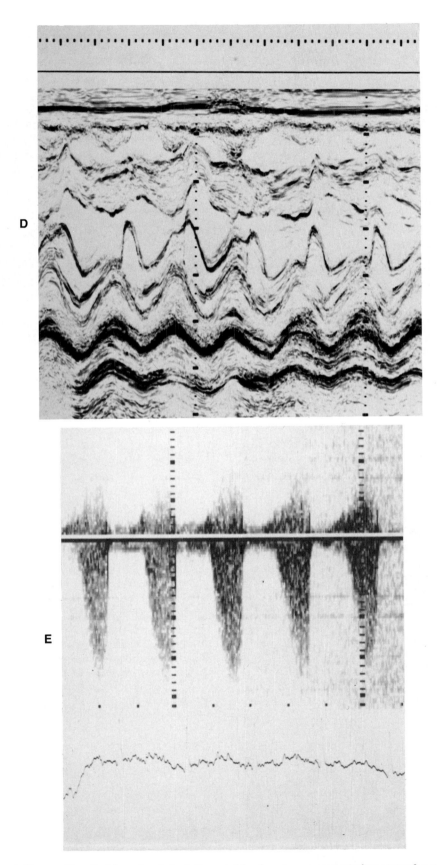

FIG. 35-43, cont'd.   D, M-mode of the left ventricle showing concentric hypertrophy of the interventricular septum and posterior heart wall, which occurs when there is a pressure overload in the left ventricle. **E,** Continuous-wave Doppler tracing taken from the apical five-chamber view at the level of the aortic valve showing a velocity of 3.2 m/s, which corresponds with a gradient of 41, representing moderate aortic stenosis.

A

B

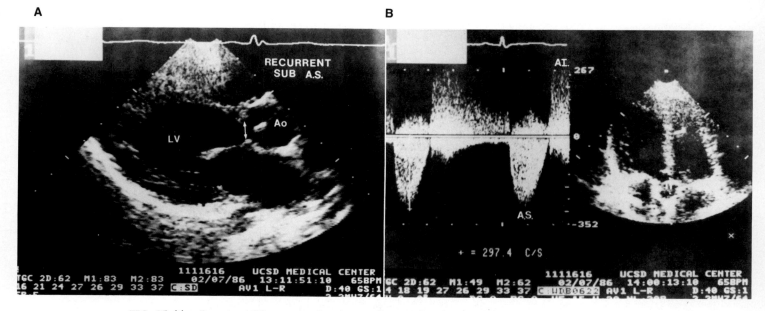

FIG. 35-44.   Parasternal long-axis view in a patient with subaortic stenosis *(arrows)*. **A,** Reduced orifice of the ventricular outflow tract due to a thickened ridge in the interventricular septum just below the aortic valve. **B,** M-mode of the early systolic notching of the aortic valve.

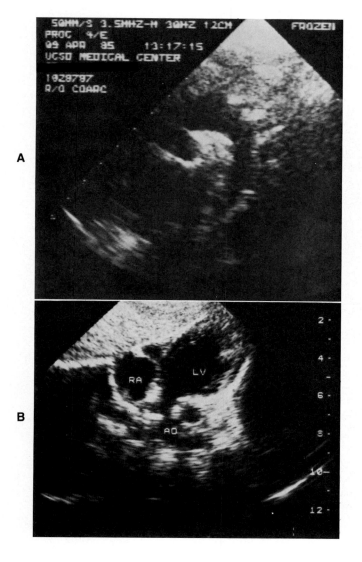

FIG. 35-45.   Alternate views to image the left ventricular outflow tract and record aortic velocities other than the apical five-chamber view include, **A,** suprasternal view of the ascending, arch, and descending aorta, and **B,** subcostal four-chamber view with anterior angulation of the transducer to record the ascending aorta and arch. This view is especially useful in neonates and toddlers.

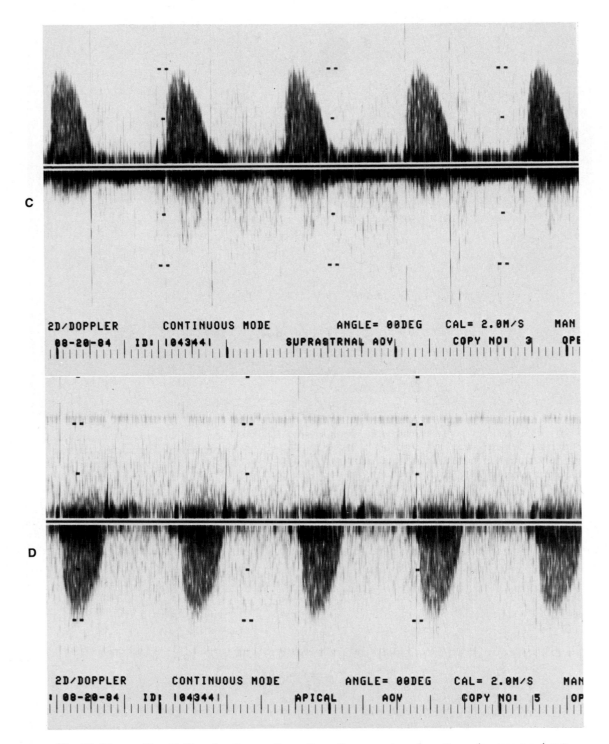

Fig. 35-45, cont'd.   **C,** Doppler flow patterns from the suprasternal aortic arch measure 4 m/s, representing a gradient of 64. **D,** Doppler flow from the apical five-chamber view in the same patient with aortic stenosis. The velocity should be recorded from at least two separate windows.

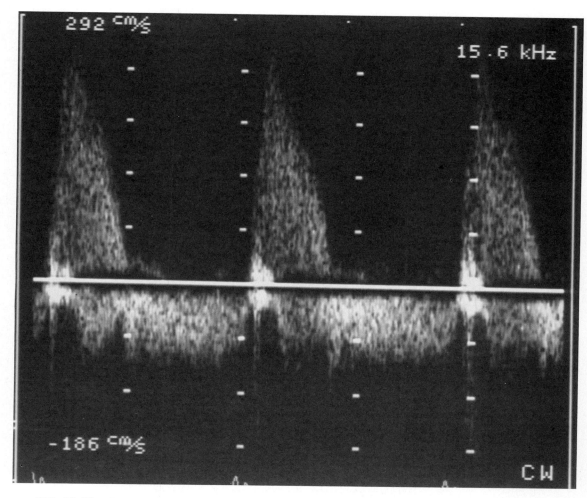

FIG. 35-46.   Suprasternal tracing with continuous-wave Doppler in a patient with aortic stenosis shows a velocity of 2.6 m/s. The flow is above the baseline as the transducer is placed in the suprasternal notch and is directed toward the ascending aorta. Thus the aortic flow is anterior, toward the transducer.

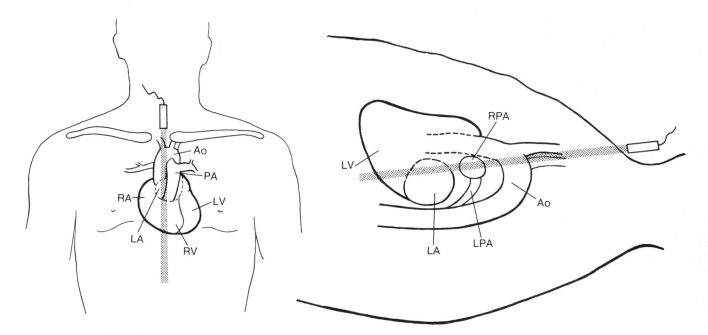

FIG. 35-47.   The beam from a transducer placed in the suprasternal notch transects the transverse aortic arch, right pulmonary artery, and left atrium. (From Goldberg S et al: Pediatric and adolescent echocardiography, ed 2, Chicago, 1980, Year Book Medical Publishers, Inc.)

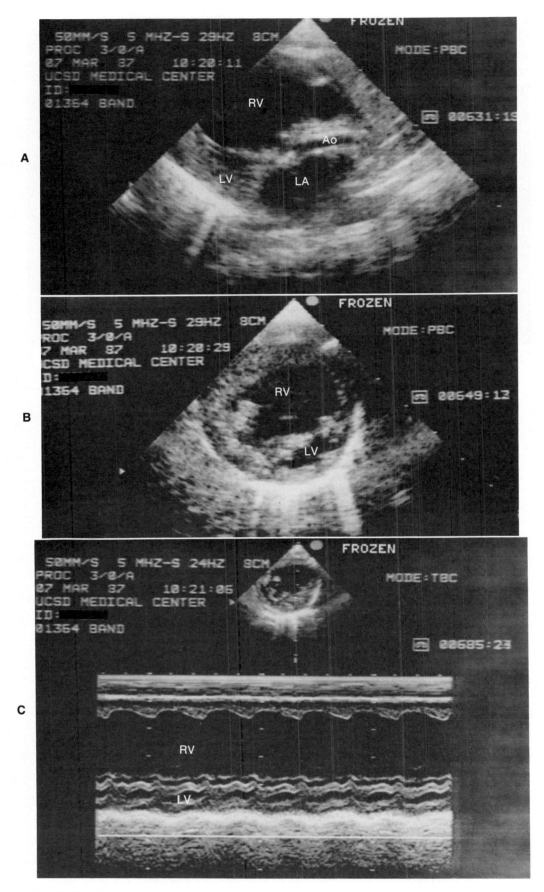

FIG. 35-48.   Parasternal long-axis, **A**, and short-axis, **B**, views of a patient with hypoplasia of the ascending aorta and hypoplastic left heart syndrome. The right ventricle, *RV*, is huge with the septum bulging into the small left ventricular cavity. *LV*, left ventricle; *LA*, left atrium; *Ao*, aorta. **C**, M-mode tracing of the huge right ventricle and small left ventricular chamber.

Continued.

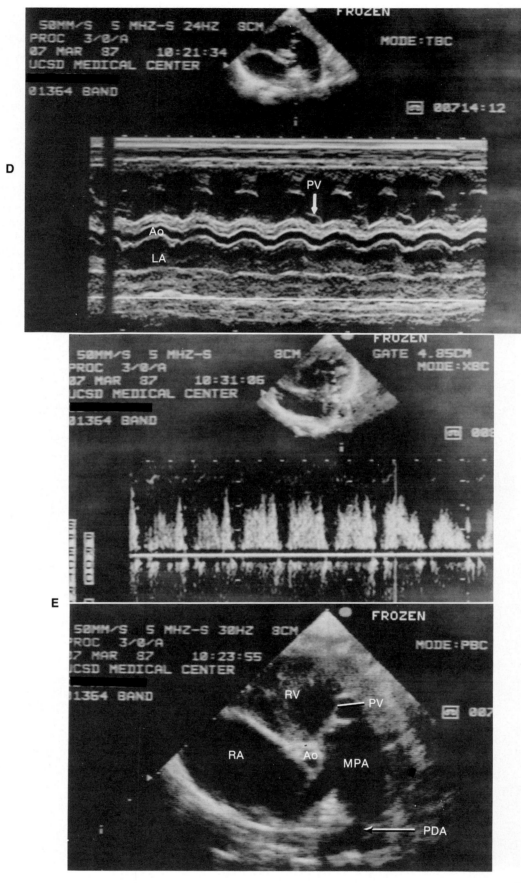

FIG. 35-48, cont'd. **D,** M-mode of the hypoplastic aortic root. The dilated pulmonary artery is anterior to the aorta. *PV,* pulmonary vein. **E,** The patent ductus arteriosus, *PDA,* was still open, and left-to-right flow was seen in the main pulmonary artery, *MPA,* secondary to the ductus. *RA,* right atrium.

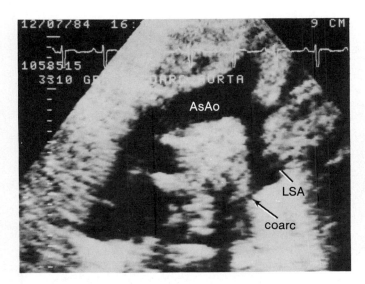

FIG. 35-49. Suprasternal view of a patient with a coarctation of the aorta *(coarc)*. The area of narrowing is just inferior to the left subclavian artery, *LSA*. A shelf of tissue is shown at the site of the patent ductus. When the ductus begins to close, this shelf constricts and causes the obstruction to the descending aorta.

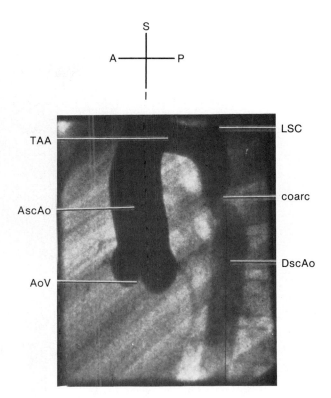

FIG. 35-50. Angiographic demonstration of coarctation of the aorta in the lateral projection. The coarctation occurs in the usual site, just distal to the takeoff of the left subclavian artery. *AoV,* aortic valve; *Asc Ao,* ascending aorta; *TAA,* transverse aortic arch; *LSA,* left subclavian artery; *DscAo,* descending aorta.

ment to be atretic and hypoplastic with poor contractility. (The mitral valve may also be atretic or abnormal in this disease.) The ascending aorta is usually the smallest part of the aorta while the descending aorta is larger, since systemic cardiac output is maintained via blood ejected from the right ventricle passing right to left through a persistent patent ductus arteriosus.

COARCTATION OF THE AORTA

The anatomic defect in coarctation of the aorta is a localized deformity of the media of the aortic wall, which is shown by a curtainlike infolding that eccentrically narrows the aortic lumen.[3] The area of coarctation is usually located just distal to the origin of the left subclavian artery at the site of the ductus.[12] At other times the coarctation occurs as a diffusely narrowed aortic segment that begins distal to the innominate artery and ends in a localized constriction just beyond the left subclavian (termed "preductal" or infantile coarctation).[5]

Echographically, the site of the coarctation is best visualized from the suprasternal notch window (Fig. 35-49). The angle of the notch is obtained by propping a pillow or rolled towel under the child's neck so the head falls back. The transducer is placed in the suprasternal notch and beamed toward the feet to obtain a plane passing between the right nipple and left scapular tip, yielding a long-axis view of the suprasternal notch. By angling the beam posteriorly or anteriorly, a plane should be produced in which the transverse arch and its brachiocephalic vessels, right pulmonary artery, right main bronchus, and descending aorta are visualized.

A right- versus a left-sided aortic arch differentiation is made by noticing whether the beam passes through the right or left side of the sternum as the arch is visualized. The arch should be visualized completely to beyond the

subclavian artery to rule out the presence of a coarctation (Fig. 35-50). The sonographer must be careful not to mistake the echo reflections from the bronchus, right pulmonary artery, or left subclavian artery as a narrowed "shelf" within the arch. The site of the suspected coarctation should be consistent throughout several cardiac cycles if it is indeed a narrowing. The incidence of aortic valve disease (bicuspid valve) is increased with the presence of a coarctation.

Doppler flow patterns are characteristic in the area of the coarctation. The velocities may be normal to slightly increased in the ascending aorta, with increased velocity occurring as one moves the sample volume closer to the narrowing (Fig. 35-51). At the site of the coarctation the velocity becomes very turbulent with a dropoff in velocity during the latter part of systole and extending into the diastolic segment.

Color-flow Doppler has been extremely helpful in visualizing the more distal segments of the coarctation. Often it is difficult to see the descending aorta with routine two-dimensional imaging, and thus with the color-flow Doppler, one can follow the turbulent velocity pattern through the site of the narrowing.

CORONARY ARTERIES: KAWASAKI DISEASE

In the late 1960s the initial description of mucocutaneous lymph node syndrome was described by a Japanese physician, Kawasaki. This syndrome is today known as Kawasa-

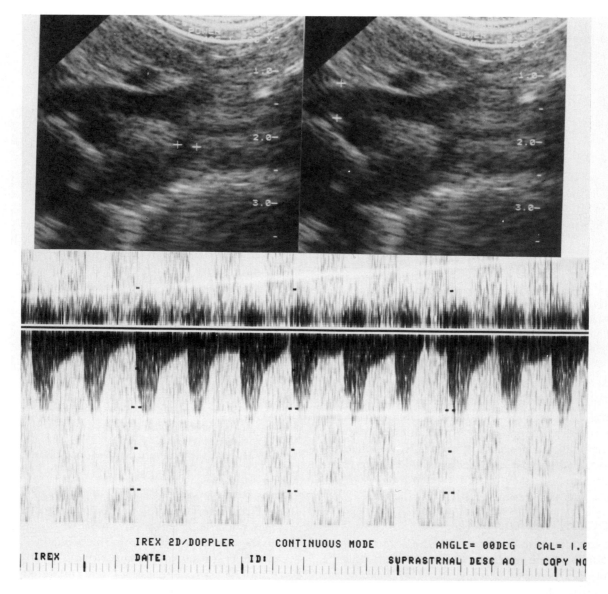

FIG. 35-51. Suprasternal views of a patient with a coarctation of the isthmus of the aorta. The CW Doppler tracing in the descending aorta shows a slightly increased flow across the area of the coarctation. The flow continues throughout the cardiac cycle.

ki's disease and occurs predominately in children, with 50% of the cases occurring in children under the age of 2. The criteria for the diagnosis of Kawasaki's disease are fever unresponsive to antibiotics, skin lesions, cracked, reddened lips and tongue, swollen lymph nodes, conjunctival injection, and edema and rashes of the hands and feet. At least 10% of children affected have lesions of the cardiac and peripheral vascular system.

Cardiac manifestations include myocardial changes suggestive of myocarditis. There may be tachycardia and gallop rhythm during the acute phase. Microvessel disease and pancarditis are also seen during this phase. This microvessel disease may advance to macrovessel inflammation or formation of coronary artery aneurysms in the course of the disease. The formation of thrombus may occur in these aneurysms, and thus careful evaluation must be made during these early phases.

Echographically one is able to demonstrate the coro-

nary arteries as they arise from the right and left aortic cusp. The right coronary artery may be seen on the parasternal long-axis view as it arises from the aorta and flows along the septal wall (Fig. 35-52). The high parasternal short-axis view shows the right coronary artery to arise about the 11 o'clock position. Another view for the right coronary artery is the modified apical four-chamber view (Fig. 35-53). As the transducer is swept along the rim of the tricuspid anulus, the long segment of the artery may be seen.

The left main coronary artery arises from the left coronary cusp at the 4 o'clock position, and with careful angulation, this artery may be followed to its point of bifurcation into the circumflex and left anterior descending branches (Fig. 35-54). A modified short-axis view with extreme angulation toward the pulmonary artery will demonstrate a long segment of the pulmonary artery (with cusp) and just below will be the left anterior descending

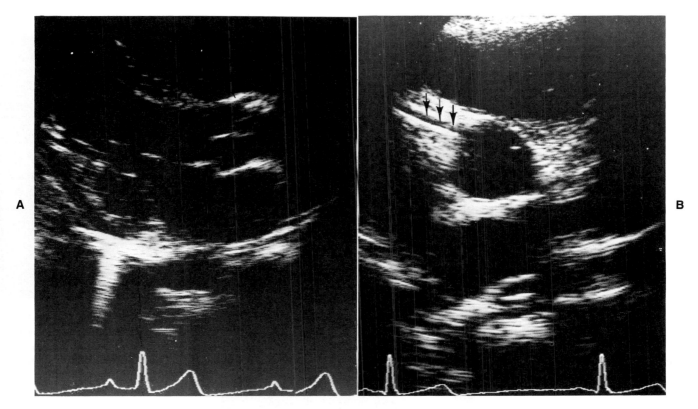

FIG. 35-52.   A, The right coronary artery may be seen on the parasternal long-axis view as it arises from the aorta and flows along the septal wall. **B,** Parasternal short-axis view of the right coronary artery as it arises from the wall of the aorta *(arrows).*

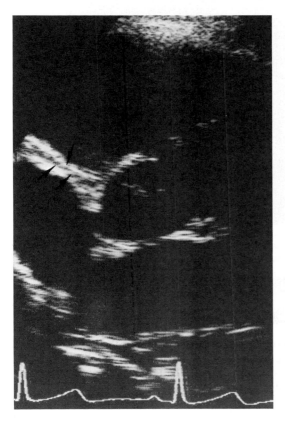

FIG. 35-53.   Modified apical four-chamber view with an anterior sweep showing the long segment of the right coronary artery at the level of the tricuspid anulus.

artery (Fig. 35-55). The pulmonic cusp marks the distinction between the proximal and distal segments of the vessel.

The left posterior descending artery is sometimes seen with a modified apical to subcostal four-chamber view. As the septum is brought into view, the transducer is gradually swept back and forth until the vessel is seen to flow along the posterior surface of the left side of the septum.

The coronary arteries should assume a smooth, tubular course as they arise from the aorta. Generally vessels under 3 mm in diameter are considered within normal limits. The presence of an aneurysm may appear to encompass a long segment or short segment of the vessel; they may be single or multiple; and they may occur at any segment of the coronary artery (Figs. 35-56 and 35-57). Thus it is very important to carefully record as much of the proximal and distal segments of each of the coronaries as possible. If an aneurysm is found, the cardiac echo is an excellent method in following the dilation until subsequent resolution of the normal size is obtained.

Doppler evaluation of the mitral and aortic valves is also recorded to document evidence of regurgitation. This is best done in the apical four-chamber view of the level of the mitral and aortic valves.

Evaluation of the cardiac function and wall motion is also important to assess contractility and the presence of myocarditis. The presence of pericardial effusion should be evaluated in the parasternal and apical windows.

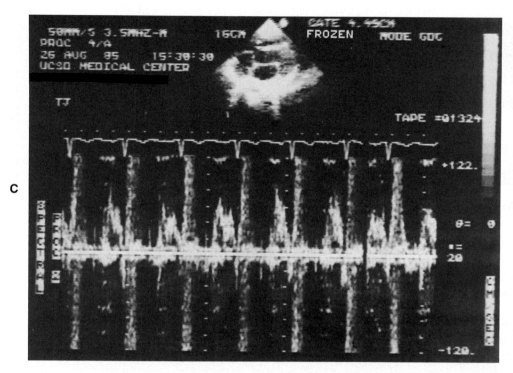

FIG. 35-59, cont'd. C, Doppler tracing in the short-axis view showing a systolic left-to-right flow from the septal defect.

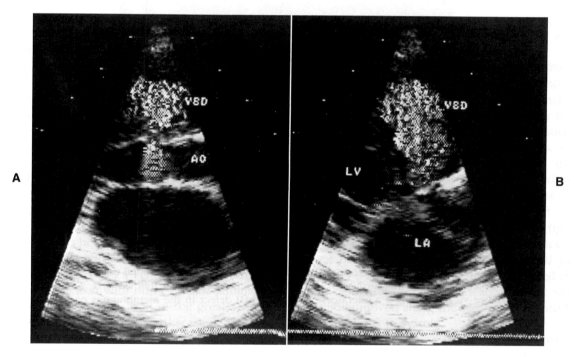

FIG. 35-60. Parasternal long-axis, **A,** and subcostal four-chamber, **B,** views of a patient with a membranous septal defect. The black-and-white color picture shows a communication between the left ventricle and right heart. The color flow would be red, yellow, and orange through this small defect.

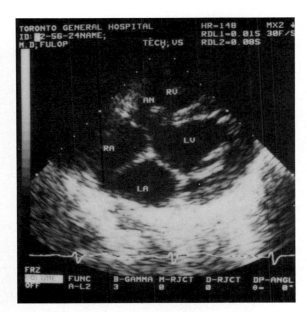

FIG. 35-61. Subcostal four-chamber view of the large ventricular septum defect with aneurysm formation.

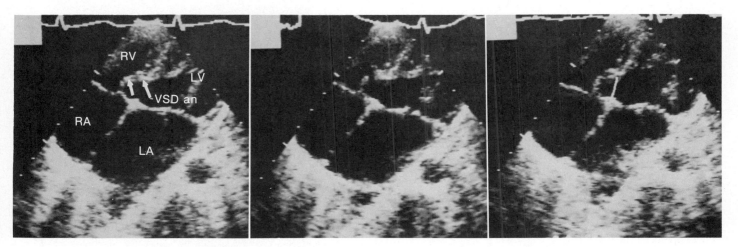

FIG. 35-62. Multiple frames of a patient with a ventricular septal defect aneurysm, *VSDan*. The middle frame shows a slight defect in the aneurysm in which there was still a left-to-right communication of blood flow. The Doppler was positive for a shunt. The color-flow study is useful in these patients to determine the site of the leak. It is especially useful in postsurgical ventricular septal defect patients to determine the site of shunt leakage when a murmur has been detected.

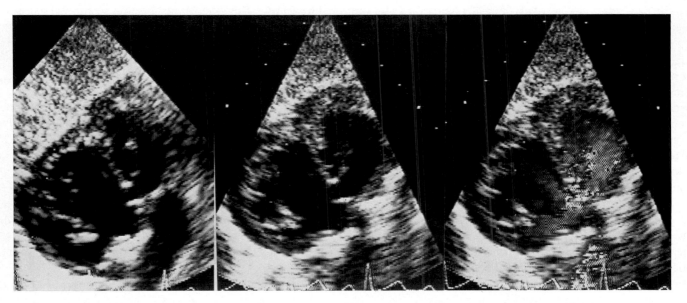

FIG. 35-63. Muscular septal defects are more difficult to image with real-time equipment. This is a particularly large defect and is easily seen. The blunt edges are evident at either end of the defect. The last frame is a black-and-white color image showing flow from the left to the right ventricle.

able to tell exactly where the shunt is flowing. Color allows one to actually see the turbulent pattern jet into the cavity, and then record the shunt flow.

COMPLETE TRANSPOSITION OF THE GREAT VESSELS

The anatomic findings in complete transposition of the great vessels are the following[10]: two ventricles are present (a ventricular septal defect may occur), the aorta and coronary arteries arise from the right ventricle, while the pulmonary trunk takes origin from the left ventricle. Both atrioventricular valves are patent and are normally located in a right-left heart arrangement. The connections of the systemic, pulmonary, and coronary veins are normal.

There is generally an interatrial communication, a ventricular septal defect, a patent ductus arteriosus, or large bronchial arteries that join the aorta to the pulmonary bed.[10]

Anatomic obstruction to the left ventricular outflow occurs as either valvular or subvalvular pulmonic stenosis.[4] If there is a defect in the ventricular septum, pulmonic stenosis is more likely to occur.

There are several varieties of transposition: those associated with single ventricle, tricuspid atresia, right ventricular aorta with biventricular pulmonary trunk, or congenitally corrected transposition. This section will only discuss the complete form of transposition.

In dextrotransposition of the great arteries (d-TGA), the truncus septates properly and then spirals in such a manner that the aorta arises from the right ventricle, anterior to and to the right of the pulmonary artery, which arises from the left ventricle.

The use of two-dimensional echocardiography allows the direct visualization of the great vessels and their relationship to one another. On the parasternal long-axis view, the aorta normally takes a straight course as it ascends into the arch; however, in transposition the pulmonary artery takes the place of the aorta as the posterior vessel and thus dips downward as it begins to bifurcate into right and left branches (Fig. 35-64).

On the short-axis view the right ventricular outflow tract normally "wraps" around the root of the aorta (referred to as the "sausage and eggs" sign) (Fig. 35-65). Since the great vessels are parallel in d-TGA rather than wrapping about each other, they appear as double circles (or "two eggs"). To visualize the anterior great vessel as a complete circle, one moves the transducer more cephalad. The vessel remains as a circle because of its natural superior course. Conversely, the pulmonary artery should bifurcate as it passes posterior to the lungs.

The subxiphoid window is also very useful in neonates to outline the ventricular outflow tract and great vessel orientation. The pulmonary artery and its bifurcation may be seen to arise from the left ventricle, while the aorta, the arch, and its descending branch are seen to arise from the right ventricle.

An interatrial communication generally exists, and it is important to record how much of a patent foramen or

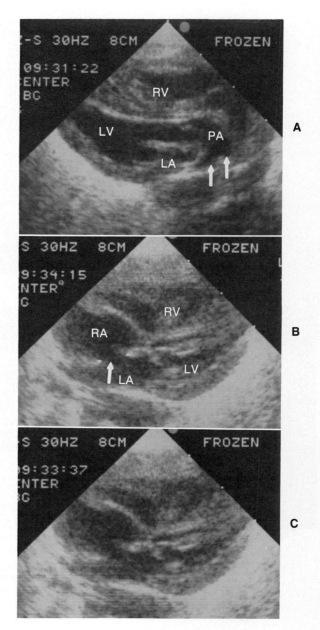

FIG. 35-64. This cyanotic neonate was sent to the special care nursery to evaluate the presence of congenital heart disease. **A,** The parasternal long-axis view may be useful in determining the presence of transposition of the great arteries. Normally the aorta arises in an anterior direction from the ventricle. However, when transposition is present, the pulmonary artery, *PA*, arises from the ventricle, and as one follows the ascension of the artery, the bifurcation of the vessel is shown. *RV,* right ventricle; *LV,* left ventricle; *LA,* left atrium. **B** and **C,** Subcostal four-chamber views showing the patent foramen ovale is open, with flow going from the left to right heart. *RA,* right atrium.

atrial septal defect is present (Fig. 35-66). If necessary, a balloon septostomy may be performed during the cardiac catheterization to open the atrial communication wider so that adequate mixing of systemic and pulmonic flow may occur.

On a normal M-mode scan, the pulmonary artery is the anterior great vessel and is located by angling the transducer anterior and toward the patient's left shoulder from

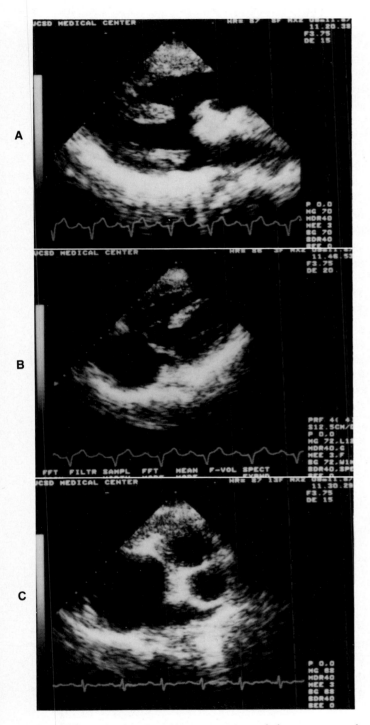

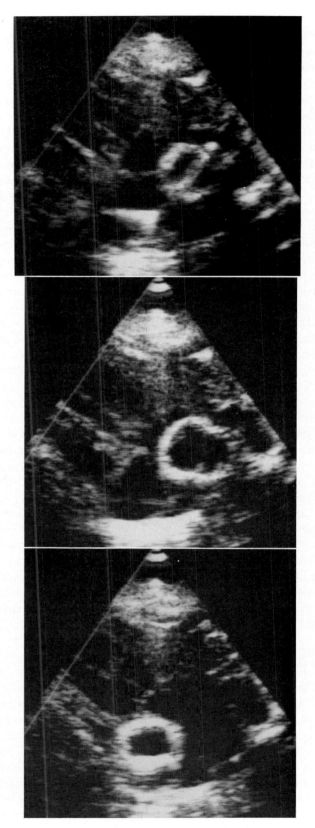

FIG. 35-65. A patient with transposition of the great vessels showing the presence of a ventricular septal defect, **A** and **B**. The short-axis view shows the abnormal position of the great arteries. The pulmonary artery is posterior and to the right, while the aorta is anterior and to the left, **C.**

FIG. 35-66. In patients with transposition of the great vessels, a communication must exist between the atrial chambers for the blood to mix adequately. If this is not present, a balloon atrial septostomy may be done while the patient is undergoing a cardiac catheterization. In these subsequent scans, the balloon is placed across the patent foramen into the left atrium. The balloon is then inflated and quickly pulled across the foramen to tear the septum so a better mixture of blood flow can be obtained. It is useful to perform an echo study during the time of the septostomy since it aids in the placement of the balloon and in defining the size of the defect.

a transducer position that reveals the aorta (or posterior great vessel). If it is not apparent toward the left shoulder, but instead is located by angling toward the right shoulder, a diagnosis of d-TGA should be considered. Another technique is the ability to simultaneously record both great vessels from the same transducer position.

The surgical repair of choice in uncomplicated d-TGA is the Mustard procedure. This involves creation of a new atria. A patch is sewn over the superior and inferior vena caval orifices and, depending on the technique, usually over the coronary sinus as well.[11] This baffle directs both superior and inferior vena caval return toward the mitral valve. As a result systemic venous blood flows into the left ventricle, to the pulmonary artery, and to the lungs.[11] The pulmonary veins and their drainage pass around and over the baffle from left to right, directed toward the tricuspid valve. Baffling is performed after most of the native atrial septum has been surgically removed.[11]

The turbulence created by these altered flow paths will create flutter on both atrioventricular valves and can be detected on the M-mode. Because the right ventricle is carrying the systemic pressure, it will become thick-walled and dilated. The left ventricle may now be relatively smaller and appear pancaked or flattened on the short-axis view.

The baffle can be seen in the apical four-chamber view. The systemic baffle takes a horizontal course across the atrial chambers, while the pulmonic baffle takes a "dog-leg" course from the pulmonary venous inflow into the tricuspid orifice.

Obstruction may occur at either the caval-systemic venous atrial junction or at the pulmonary vein entry sites, and thus careful Doppler recordings should be taken in these areas. Color-flow mapping helps in locating the site of turbulence within the baffle so an accurate Doppler tracing can be made. The suprasternal notch window is sometimes helpful to image the superior vena caval—right atrial junction area.

CORRECTED TRANSPOSITION OF THE GREAT ARTERIES

If the anterior great vessel is to the left of the pulmonary artery, L-TGA should be suspected. This occurs when the great arteries are transposed, but because of ventricular inversion, the circulatory pattern is hemodynamically correct. Each ventricle keeps its respective atrioventricular valve when it inverts. Thus the right atrium empties via the mitral valve into a right-sided morphologic (smooth-walled) left ventricle, which ejects through a posterior pulmonary artery. The left atrium empties via a tricuspid valve into a left-sided morphologic (heavily trabeculated) right ventricle, which ejects through an anterior leftward aorta.

Since the crista supraventricularis separates the aorta from the tricuspid valve, continuity is not seen on the long-axis view between the left-sided atrioventricular valve and the semilunar valve. Visualization of the septal insertion sites of the atrioventricular valves in the four-chamber view identifies the inverted ventricles. If the tri-

cuspid valve, which inserts into the septum more inferiorly, is on the left side in the four-chamber view, that left-sided ventricle is identified as a morphologic right ventricle. Ebstein's malformation of the left-sided tricuspid valve, ventricular septal defect, and pulmonary stenosis are findings commonly associated with this anomaly.

DOUBLE OUTLET RIGHT VENTRICLE

In double outlet right ventricle the pulmonary artery arises in its normal position, but the aorta arises entirely from the right ventricle. A ventricular septal defect provides the only outlet for the left ventricle. There may be coexistent pulmonic stenosis.

Echographically the apical four-chamber view is probably the best window to outline both great vessels as they arise from the right ventricle. The subcostal view may also be useful to delineate the great vessel orientation. The parasternal long-axis view may allow one to outline both great vessels as they assume their parallel course from the right ventricle; in this case a large ventricular septal defect would also be seen just below the transposed pulmonary artery (Fig. 35-67).

TRUNCUS ARTERIOSUS

Truncus arteriosus is a congenital anomaly in which a single great vessel leaves the base of the heart through a single semilunar valve (Fig. 35-68). There is a ventricular septal defect present. The truncal vessel receives blood from both ventricles. The coronary arteries arise from the truncal vessel. Generally there are multiple leaflets within the vessel.

Edwards et al.[3] have classified truncal variations into four categories:

Type 1: a short pulmonary trunk emerges from the truncus arteriosus and gives rise to the right and left pulmonary arteries.

Type 2: the right and left pulmonary arteries arise directly from the posterior wall of the truncus.

Type 3: the right and left pulmonary arteries originate from the lateral walls of the truncus.

Type 4: the pulmonary arteries are absent altogether and the arterial supply to the lungs is through bronchial arteries.

Echographically, one would see a very large great vessel with multiple leaflet echoes within. It may be difficult to distinguish the truncal vessel from a tetralogy of Fallot with severe pulmonary stenosis. To do this with certainty, one should see the multiple cusps' echoes as well as identify the truncal origin of the pulmonary artery.

There is increased pulmonary blood flow in types 1 and 2, in which the pulmonary arteries arise from the truncus.[11] Thus the presence or absence of a pulmonary valve is an important differential between tetralogy of Fallot and truncus arteriosus. The subxiphoid right ventricular outflow tract would not be obtainable in truncus arteriosus, but a left ventricular outflow tract scanned superiorly might reveal the pulmonary artery arising from the truncus. A second differential point is that the left atrium is enlarged in truncus due to an increased flow through

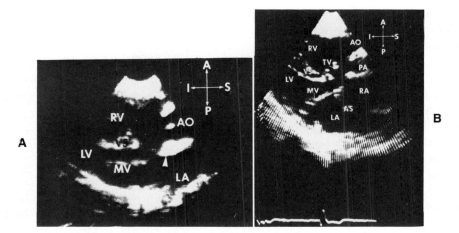

FIG. 35-67. Echocardiographic appearance of a double outlet right ventricle. **A,** Parasternal long-axis view showing a posterior aorta displaced anteriorly and separated from the mitral valve by a conus *(arrowhead)*. Note the aorta is almost entirely committed to the right ventricle and the subaortic ventricular septal defect is the only left ventricular outlet. **B,** Parasternal long-axis view with the posterior great vessel displaced superiorly and separated from the mitral valve by a conus of elongated dense echoes *(two arrowheads)*. If a line is projected superiorly along the plane of the interventricular septum, both great arteries arise anterior to it from the right ventricle. The two great vessels are one on top of the other, with the subpulmonic ventricular septal defect as the only left ventricular outlet. (From Hagler OJ et al: Circulation 63:419, 1981. Used with permission of The American Heart Association.)

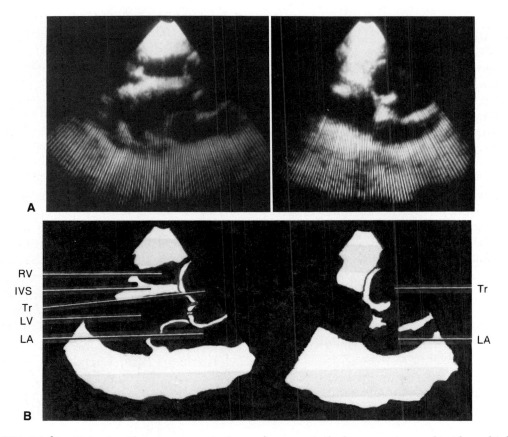

FIG. 35-68. Patient with a truncus arteriosus shows a single large great vessel with multiple cusps, **A.** In the parasternal short axis view, **B,** the large common great vessel is seen with no sign of a pulmonary artery. The multiple cusps within the great vessel make it very suggestive of a common vessel.

the lungs. Tetralogy, with its decreased flow to the lungs stemming from right ventricular outflow tract obstruction, should show a normal to small left atrium.

SINGLE VENTRICLE

The term single ventricle refers to a congenital anomaly in which there are two atria but only one ventricular chamber, which receives both the mitral and tricuspid valves.[1] Both atrioventricular valves are patent, and thus mitral and tricuspid atresia are excluded. Occasionally the mitral and tricuspid valves join to form a common atrioventricular valve.

The most common form of a single ventricle heart is a morphologic left ventricle with a small outlet chamber that represents the infundibular portion of the right ventricle[10] (with the body or inflow portion of the ventricle absent). There may be absence of the right or the left atrioventricular connection, and there may be transposition of the great arteries with the aorta arising above the small outlet chamber.[10] If transposition is present, the pulmonary artery lies posterior to the aorta. The infundibulum lies at the base of the ventricle, communicating with the aorta above and the single ventricle below.[10] If the great vessels are normal, the infundibulum communicates with the pulmonary trunk. The outlet chambers may be left-sided and anterior or right-sided and anterior, but they commonly lie high on the cardiac silhouette.[10]

The presence of pulmonary stenosis may or may not coexist. If present, the pulmonary stenosis is usually valvular or subvalvular.[10] The pulmonary trunk is usually slightly smaller than the aortic trunk.

The apical four-chamber view is probably the most useful window in delineating the cardiac anatomy. With echocardiography one should be careful not to confuse the very prominent papillary muscles with interventricular septum.[11] In a single ventricle the papillary muscles may be quite prominent. With transducer angulation the chordal structures may be traced to these structures for correct delineation. The right ventricle may be just a slit-like cavity as seen on the apical four-chamber view. The position of the great arteries should be assessed, and the aorta and pulmonary arteries should be delineated clearly. There may be regurgitant jets associated with abnormal chordal connections of the atrioventricular valves. Careful Doppler mapping should be used to outline the degree of regurgitation.

SUMMARY

1. The pediatric cardiac sonographer deals with children as well as with the complex anatomy associated with their congenital heart defects.

2. One should use a transducer with the best possible resolution (high-frequency, focused beam).

3. The left atrial measurement has significance in neonates and infants since an increase in the ratio of left atrial to aortic root size is an indicator of a left-to-right shunt.

4. Echographic technique includes all of these windows: parasternal long- and short-axis, apical four-chamber, subcostal two- and four-chambers, and suprasternal.

5. Pulmonary artery hypertension often occurs with a cardiac shunt. Pulmonary hypertension secondary to lung disease or left-sided heart disease shows a dilated pulmonary root and systolic flutter of the posterior cusp with early closure of the valve (the "a dip" is lost).

6. With pulmonary insufficiency the pulmonary cusps may be thickened, or there may be dilation of the pulmonary ring. With significant insufficiency there may be paradoxical septal motion and right ventricular volume overload.

7. The absent pulmonary valve syndrome is the failure of adequate formation of the cusps, often accompanied by a dilated pulmonary ring with aneurysmal dilatation of the main, right, and left pulmonary arteries.

8. Pulmonary valve stenosis is the most common form of right ventricular outflow tract obstruction. The valve cusps are thickened and domed, with a restricted orifice.

9. Pulmonary atresia is a complete anatomic obstruction to forward blood flow from the right ventricle into the pulmonary trunk.

10. Tetralogy of Fallot has four characteristics: (1) high membranous ventricular septal defect, (2) large anteriorly displaced aorta, (3) pulmonary stenosis, and (4) right ventricular hypertrophy.

11. Patent ductus arteriosus represents a persistence of a normal fetal vascular channel between the pulmonary artery and the aorta. The ductus is located slightly to the left of the bifurcation of the pulmonary trunk near the origin of the left pulmonary artery. The persistent patency of the ductus depends on two factors: the size of the communication and the pulmonary vascular resistance.

12. In Ebstein's anomaly portions of the tricuspid valve leaflet are apically displaced. The portion of the right ventricle underlying this valve tissue is usually quite thin and functions as a receiving chamber analogous to the right atrium. The right atrium is usually massively dilated.

13. In tricuspid atresia the tricuspid orifice is always absent, and the only outlet for right atrial blood is by means of an interatrial communication.

14. Atrial septal defects are one of three types: (1) secundum, (2) sinus venosus, and (3) primum.

15. In total anomalous pulmonary venous return all the venous blood from both lungs enters the right atrium directly or through one of its tributary veins. The anomalous veins emerge individually from the lungs and either enter directly into the right atrium or unite in the mediastinum to form a confluence.

16. Endocardial cushion defects occur where the atrial

and ventricular septa joins the mitral and tricuspid valves. A complete defect means there is a primum atrial septal defect, a ventricular septal defect, and clefts in the mitral and tricuspid valves. An incomplete defect has an ostium primum atrial septal defect and a cleft mitral valve. There may also be abnormal attachments of the mitral and tricuspid valves to the septum (overriding or straddling).

17. Cor triatriatum partitions the left atrium into two compartments. The pulmonary veins drain into an accessory left atrial chamber that lies proximal to the true left atrium.

18. There are different types of congenital mitral stenosis: one shows the leaflets to be thickened, nodular, and fibrotic without calcification; another is a "parachute" deformity of the valve; a rare form is when the papillary muscles are the cause of the obstruction; and another form occurs when the mitral leaflets are normal but the inlet of the left ventricle is encroached upon by a circumferential supravalvular ridge of connective tissue that arises at the base of the atrial aspect of the mitral leaflet.

19. Left ventricular outflow tract obstruction can occur at three levels: supravalvar, valvar, and subvalvar. The stenosis can be either fixed or dynamic.

20. Hypoplastic left heart syndrome represents the most severe form of left ventricular outflow tract obstruction. This is due to severe tubular hypoplasia of the arch, severe aortic stenosis, or aortic atresia.

21. The anatomic defect in coarctation of the aorta is a localized deformity of the media of the aortic wall, which is shown by a curtain-like infolding that eccentrically narrows the aortic lumen. The area of coarctation is usually located just distal to the origin of the left subclavian artery, at the site of the ductus.

22. Kawasaki's disease includes cardiac problems such as pericarditis, myocarditis, and microvessel disease that may advance to macrovessel inflammation or formation of coronary artery aneurysms in the course of the infection.

23. The most common congenital lesion of the heart is the ventricular septal defect. These defects lie either above or below the crista supraventricularis. They may be membranous or muscular, single or multiple.

24. Anatomic findings in complete transposition of the great vessels include the following: two ventricles are present (may have a ventricular septal defect); the aorta and coronary arteries arise from the right ventricle, while the pulmonary trunk takes origin from the left ventricle. There is usually an interatrial communication, a ventricular septal defect, a patent ductus arteriosus, or large bronchial arteries that join the aorta to the pulmonary bed. Anatomic obstruction to the left ventricular outflow occurs as either valvular or subvalvular pulmonic stenosis.

25. In corrected transposition of the great vessels, the great arteries are transposed, but due to ventricular inversion the circulatory pattern is hemodynamically correct.

26. Double outlet right ventricle has the pulmonary artery and aorta both arising from the right ventricle. A ventricular septal defect provides the only outlet for the left ventricle. There may be coexistent pulmonic stenosis.

27. Truncus arteriosus is a congenital anomaly in which a single great vessel leaves the base of the heart through a single semi-lunar valve. A ventricular septal defect is present. The truncal vessel receives blood from both ventricles.

28. A single ventricle implies that two atria are present with only one ventricular chamber that receives two atrioventricular valves. The most common type of single ventricle is the morphologic left ventricle with a small outlet chamber that represents the infundibular portion of the right ventricle.

REFERENCES

1. Anselmi G, Armas SM, dela Cruz MV, et al: Diagnosis and classification of single ventricle, Am J Cardiol 21:813, 1968.
2. Cleland WP: Ventricular septal defect, Proc Roy Soc Med 54:785, 1961.
3. Edwards JE, Carey LS, Neufeld HN, and Lester RG: Congenital heart disease, Philadelphia, 1965, WB Saunders Co.
4. Elliott LP, Neufeld HN, Anderson RC, et al: Complete transposition of the great vessels. I. An anatomic study of sixty cases, Circulation 27:1105, 1963.
5. Elliott LP and Schiebler GL: X-ray diagnosis of congenital cardiac disease, Springfield, Ill, 1968, Charles C Thomas.
6. Grosse-Brockhoff F and Loogen F: Ventricular septal defect, Circulation 38:iv, 1968.
7. Larsen KA and Noer T: Cardiac aneurysm of the membranous portion of the interventricular septum, Acta Med Scand 166:401, 1960.
8. Lucas RV Jr, Anderson RC, Ampltatz K, et al: Congenital causes of pulmonary venous obstruction, Pediatr Clin North Am 10:781, 1963.
9. Niwayama G: Cortriatriatum, Am Heart J 59:291, 1960.
10. Perloff JK: The clinical recognition of congenital heart disease, Philadelphia, 1970, WB Saunders Co.
11. Sahn DJ and Anderson FA: Two dimensional anatomy of the heart, New York, 1982, J Wiley & Sons.
12. Tawes RL, Aberdeen E, Waterson DJ, and Bonham-Carter RE: Coarctation of the aorta in infants and children, Circulation 39(suppl 1):173, 1969.
13. Tikoff G, Echgaray HM, Schmidt AM, and Kuida H: Patent ductus arteriosus complicated by heart failure, Am J Med 46:43, 1969.
14. Weyman AE, Feigenbaum H, Hurwitz RA, et al: Cross-sectional echocardiographic assessment of the severity of aortic stenosis in children, Circulation 55:773, 1977.
15. Willius FA and Keys TE: Classics of cardiology, New York, 1961, Dover Publications.

36

Fetal Echocardiography

The development of high-resolution, real-time sonography has enabled the sonographer to visualize the anatomic structures of the fetal heart as early as 16 weeks of gestation. This ability to visualize detailed cardiac anatomy has aided in the prenatal diagnosis of congenital heart disease. The incidence of congenital heart disease is about 8%, or 30,000 infants per year in the United States.[3]

The early investigation of the fetal heart used combined M-mode and B-mode techniques; transducer development at that time was not adequate for obtaining a high-resolution image, thus the technique was not very useful in the early to midtrimester pregnancy. Thus the development of high-resolution mechanical, phased array, and annular array transducers permitted adequate visualization of the smallest structures within the fetal cardiac chambers. These transducers, complete with M-mode and Doppler capabilities, enable the sonographer to perform a complete fetal echocardiogram on obstetric patients in their 16th week of pregnancy up until the time of delivery. Although fetal heart motion may be seen within the gestational sac as early as 6 to 8 weeks of gestation, structural information is seen at 14 to 16 weeks of gestation, with detailed information shown at 16 weeks to 40 weeks.

FETAL CIRCULATION

Blood flow in the fetus is slightly different than in the neonatal stage (Fig. 36-1). Communication is open between the right and left sides of the heart, as well as between the aorta and the pulmonary artery. It is useful to know these communications to appreciate the intracardiac function of the fetal heart.

Before birth the oxygenated blood returns by way of the umbilical vein from the placenta to the heart. Approximately half of the blood passes through the hepatic sinusoids, while the remainder bypasses the liver to go through the ductus venosus into the inferior vena cava.

Blood flows from the inferior vena cava and enters the right atrium. Blood in the right atrium is less oxygenated than blood in the umbilical vein. Blood from the inferior vena cava is directed by the lower border of the septum secundum (the crista dividens) through the foramen ovale into the left atrium. It mixes with a small amount of deoxygenated blood returning from the lungs via the pulmonary veins into the left atrium. The blood then flows into the left ventricle and leaves through the ascending aorta.

A small amount of oxygenated blood from the inferior vena cava is diverted by the crista dividens and remains in the right atrium to mix with deoxygenated blood from the superior vena cava and coronary sinus. This blood flows into the right ventricle and leaves through the pulmonary artery. Most of the blood passes through the patent ductus arteriosus into the aorta. Only a very small amount goes to the lungs. Most of the mixed blood in the descending aorta passes into the umbilical arteries and is returned to the placenta for reoxygenation. The remainder of the blood circulates through the lower part of the body.

After birth, the circulation of the fetal blood through the placenta ceases, and the neonatal lungs begin to function. The fetal cardiac structures that no longer are needed are the foramen ovale, the ductus arteriosus, the ductus venosus, and the umbilical vessels (Fig. 36-2). Omission of the placental circulation causes an immediate fall of blood pressure in the newborn's inferior vena cava and right atrium. As the lungs expand with air, there is a fall in the pulmonary vascular resistance. This causes an increase in pulmonary blood flow and a progressive thinning of the walls of the pulmonary arteries. Thus the pressure in the left atrium becomes higher than that in the right atrium. This causes the foramen ovale to close. With time, complete closure of the foramen occurs from the adhesion of the septum primum to the left margin of the septum secundum. The septum primum forms the floor of the fossa ovalis. The lower edge of the septum secundum

844

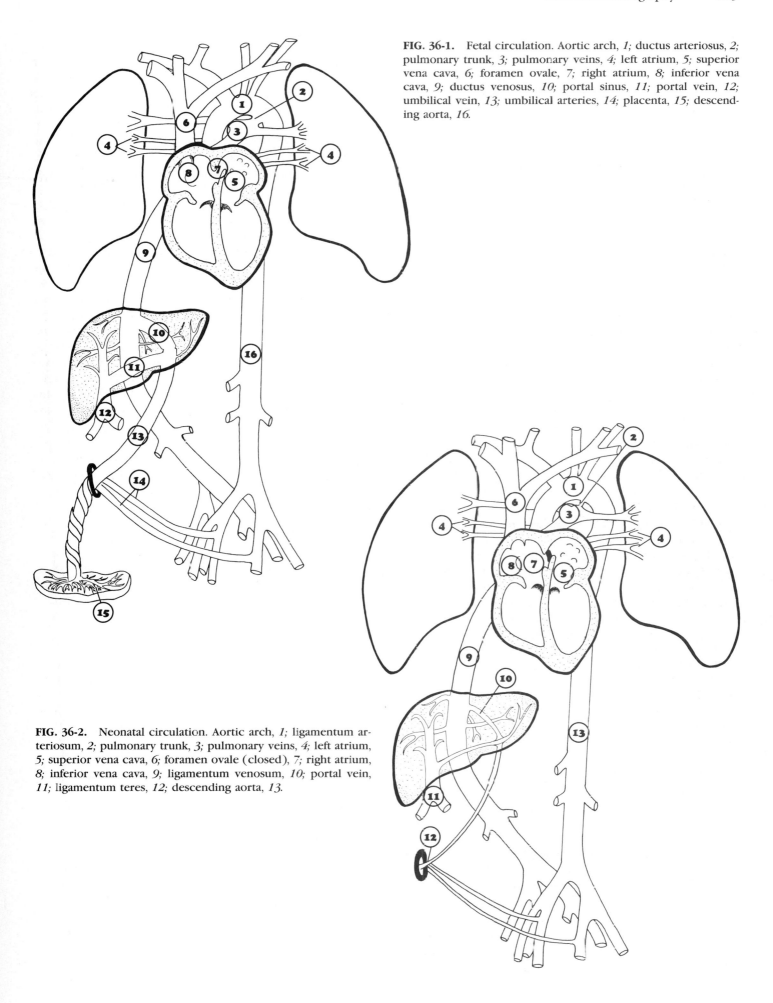

FIG. 36-1.   Fetal circulation. Aortic arch, *1;* ductus arteriosus, *2;* pulmonary trunk, *3;* pulmonary veins, *4;* left atrium, *5;* superior vena cava, *6;* foramen ovale, *7;* right atrium, *8;* inferior vena cava, *9;* ductus venosus, *10;* portal sinus, *11;* portal vein, *12;* umbilical vein, *13;* umbilical arteries, *14;* placenta, *15;* descending aorta, *16.*

FIG. 36-2.   Neonatal circulation. Aortic arch, *1;* ligamentum arteriosum, *2;* pulmonary trunk, *3;* pulmonary veins, *4;* left atrium, *5;* superior vena cava, *6;* foramen ovale (closed), *7;* right atrium, *8;* inferior vena cava, *9;* ligamentum venosum, *10;* portal vein, *11;* ligamentum teres, *12;* descending aorta, *13.*

forms the limbus fossae ovalis, which demarcates the former cranial boundary of the foramen ovale.

The ductus arteriosus usually constricts shortly after birth, once the left-sided pressures exceed the right-sided pressures. Often there is a small shunt of blood from the aorta to the pulmonary artery until these pressures adjust to neonatal life. The ductus turns into the ligamentum arteriosum in the neonate. This ligament passes from the left pulmonary artery to the arch of the aorta.

The umbilical arteries also constrict after birth to prevent blood loss from the neonate. The umbilical vein may remain patent for some time after birth.

RISK FACTORS INDICATING FETAL ECHOCARDIOGRAPHY

Specific risk factors indicate that the fetus is at a higher than normal risk for congenital heart disease to warrant a fetal echocardiogram. These may be divided into three categories: fetal risk factors, maternal risk factors, and familial risk factors.[2] Fetal risk factors include the presence of intrauterine growth retardation, cardiac arrhythmias, abnormal amniocentesis indicating a trisomy, and other anomalies as detected by the sonogram, such as hydrops fetalis.

Maternal risk factors include heart disease (congenital or acquired), drug ingestion, polyhydramnios or oligohydramnios, diabetes mellitus (incidence of hypertrophic cardiomyopathy), Rh sensitization, collagen vascular disease, and preeclampsia.

Familial risk factors include genetic syndromes or the presence of congenital heart disease in a previous sibling. The recurrence risk cited given a sibling with one of the most common cardiovascular abnormalities (ventricular septal defect, atrial septal defect, patent ductus arteriosus, tetralogy of Fallot) varies from 2.5% to 3%.[2] Similar data given one parent with a congenital heart defect suggest that for the common defects listed above the recurrence risk ranges from 2.5% (atrial septal defect) to 4% (ventricular septal defect, patent ductus arteriosus, tetralogy of Fallot).[2]

EQUIPMENT

Transducer selection. A high-frequency transducer such as a 5.0 MHz with a medium focus generally is ideal for the typical pregnancy in the second trimester. If adequate penetration is not obtained, then the 3.5 MHz transducer with a medium to long focus may be used. Some equipment allows the sonographer to decide between a linear array and sector array. We have found the sector allows a little better image in the obese patient; otherwise a linear array transducer is used.

Type of equipment. The linear array with a variable focus or transmit zone is the ideal piece of equipment. It should have a high-power resolution zoom capability, variable depth control, individual (TGC) gain control panel, a simultaneous M-mode with range expansion (and preferably a strip chart recorder for arrhythmias), and simultaneous Doppler capacity with PW and CW flow profiles.

TECHNIQUE

To perform a fetal echocardiogram, certain sonographic data should be obtained. The sonographer should localize the position of the fetus (to determine if the spine is up or down and to determine anatomical structures to define right from left), and the position of the fetal skull should be ascertained so measurements may be made across the biparietal diameter to obtain data to measure the gestational age of the fetus (Fig. 36-3). The position of the placenta and the fetal extremities should also be noted so the best window may be used to visualize the cardiac structures. It will be much easier to identify all the cardiac structures if the fetus is lying face up (spine down).

If the fetus is particularly difficult to image well, it is usually because of the position in which the fetus is lying. Rotation of the mother sometimes is helpful in efforts to cause the fetus to mobilize and change positions. Other times slight transducer manipulation will cause the fetus to roll around into a more photogenic position. If the amniotic fluid appears normal and the fetus is still difficult to image well, the best thing to do is to wait until the fetus changes position to fully examine the cardiac structures.

Difficulties are encountered when there is oligohydramnios, maternal obesity, unusual fetal position, early gestation of the fetus, or when equipment without high-resolution capabilities is used. If fetal pathology is already present (i.e., diaphragmatic hernia, pleural effusion, or absent lung), then the cardiac structures may be deviated from their normal position.

IMAGING FETAL CARDIAC ANATOMY

Since the fetal liver occupies a large percentage of the fetal abdomen, this organ is extremely useful in the cardiac evaluation (Fig. 36-4). The transducer is angled through the homogeneous fetal liver to visualize the four-chamber view of the heart. The heart is slightly more transverse than is seen in neonatal life, thus the view through the liver is very accessible.

Once the sonographer has become oriented to the position of the fetal head, spine, and stomach, the routine cardiac views may be used to identify anatomy.

A normal study should include at least these views (Figs. 36-6 to 36-14):
1. Parasternal long-axis view
2. Suprasternal view of the aortic arch
3. Parasternal short-axis view
4. Four-chamber view
5. "Five"-chamber view of aorta and left ventricular outflow tract

Parasternal long-axis view

These structures should be visualized:
1. Right ventricle (moderator band)
2. Interventricular septum
3. Left ventricle
4. Mitral valve leaflets
5. Aorta with leaflets
6. Left atrium

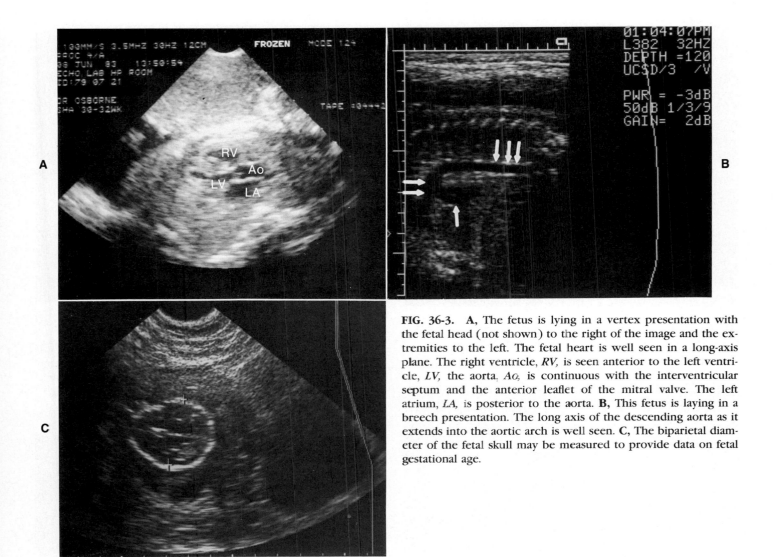

FIG. 36-3. **A,** The fetus is lying in a vertex presentation with the fetal head (not shown) to the right of the image and the extremities to the left. The fetal heart is well seen in a long-axis plane. The right ventricle, *RV,* is seen anterior to the left ventricle, *LV,* the aorta. *Ao,* is continuous with the interventricular septum and the anterior leaflet of the mitral valve. The left atrium, *LA,* is posterior to the aorta. **B,** This fetus is laying in a breech presentation. The long axis of the descending aorta as it extends into the aortic arch is well seen. **C,** The biparietal diameter of the fetal skull may be measured to provide data on fetal gestational age.

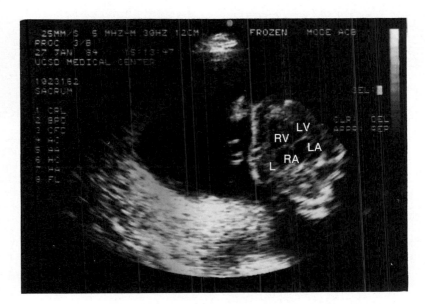

FIG. 36-4. In the transverse plane the fetal liver, *L,* is useful to use as an acoustic window to image the fetal cardiac structures. The four chambers of the heart are well demonstrated. The fetal spine is posterior and rotated slightly to the right. *RV,* right ventricle; *LV,* left ventricle; *RA,* right atrium; *LA,* left atrium.

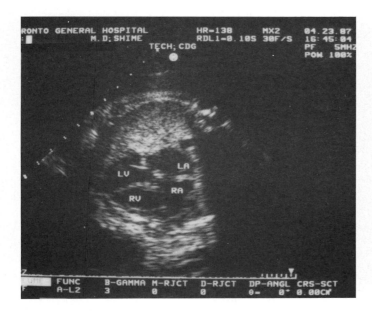

FIG. 36-5. The right side of the heart is slightly larger than the left side of the heart during the fetal development stage.

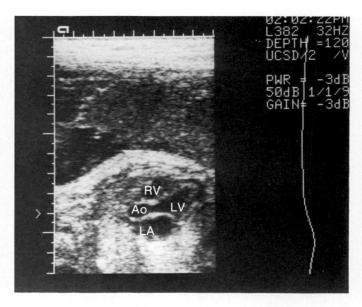

FIG. 36-6. Parasternal long-axis view of the heart. The fetal skull (not shown) is located to the left of the screen. This is a good view to rule out aortic override or an outlet ventricular septal defect. There is symmetry between the septum and posterior heart wall. *Ao,* aorta; *RV,* right ventricle; *LV,* left ventricle; *LA,* left atrium.

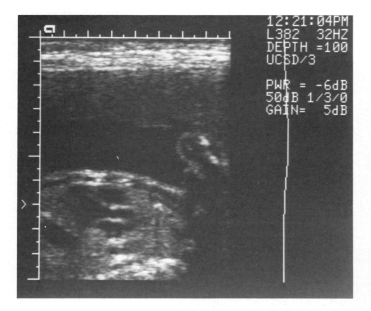

FIG. 36-7. Parasternal long-axis view is also good to evaluate the ventricular function and relative size of the cardiac chambers.

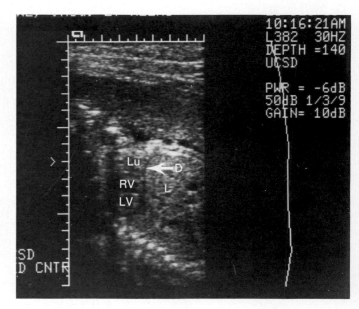

FIG. 36-8. Other fetal structures may be identified in the parasternal long-axis view. The fetal liver, *L,* is shown inferior to the diaphragm, *D.* The right and left ventricles, *RV* and *LV,* are seen just above the diaphragm. *LU,* lung.

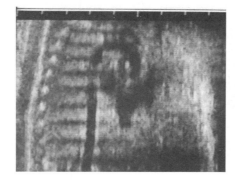

FIG. 36-9. Parasternal long-axis view of the aortic arch. The arch is identified as the three head and neck vessels arise from this structure.

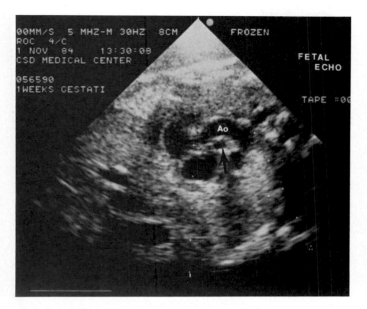

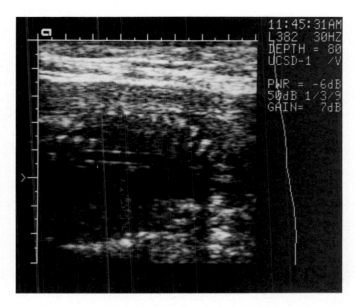

FIG. 36-10. Parasternal long-axis view of the aortic arch and right pulmonary artery *(arrow)*. This is a normal long-axis relationship.

FIG. 36-11. The descending aorta is approximately the same diameter as the aortic arch and ascending aorta.

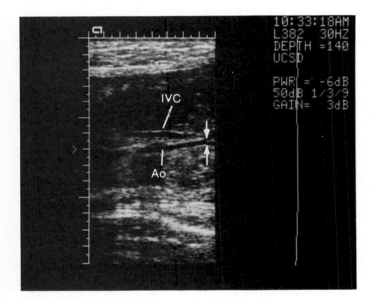

FIG. 36-12. Long-axis view of the inferior vena cava, *IVC,* the abdominal aorta, *Ao,* and the bifurcation of the aorta *(arrows)*.

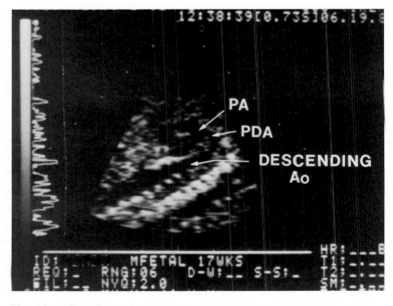

FIG. 36-13. The "ductal" arch or the patent ductus arteriosus, *PDA,* is the fetal communication between the aortic arch, *Ao,* and the pulmonary artery, *PA.* It is inferior to the aortic arch and has no head and neck vessels arising from its superior border (as the aortic arch has).

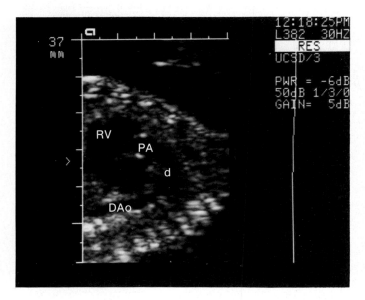

FIG. 36-14.   Parasternal long-axis view of the right ventricular outflow tract, *RV,* the main pulmonary artery, *PA,* and the patent ductus arteriosus, *d,* as it communicates with the descending aorta, *DAo.*

In the parasternal long-axis view the size of the right and left ventricles and left atrial cavity should be assessed to obtain an overview of cardiac disease and function. The left atrial cavity is generally about the same size as the aortic root and is anechoic. The right ventricle is slightly larger than the left ventricle in fetal life (this is more pronounced on the four-chamber view). The moderator band is usually seen near the apex of the right ventricle, which helps identify it from the left ventricle. The contractility of both ventricles may be assessed from this view, as well as from the four-chamber view.

The thickness of the interventricular septum may be assessed from this view. The septum is thin along its short membranous portion (just inferior to the aortic root) and thickens in its muscular component, which comprises two thirds of the septum. The septum and the posterior left ventricular wall are generally the same thickness. The thickness of the ventricular walls are best seen in the long-axis view where the beam is perpendicular to the ventricular walls and septum rather than in the apical four-chamber view. (There is better axial resolution of the transducer in this plane.)

The diabetic fetus has been reported to occasionally show an increased septal thickness with or without associated anterior motion of the mitral valve. This may be due to edema in the myocardium, since the septal thickness returns to normal within a few months after birth.

There are a few rare diseases that cause concentric hypertrophy of the septum and posterior heart wall (i.e., hypertrophic cardiomyopathy, aortic stenosis, aortic hypoplasia), and these may be abnormal when the thickness does not correspond with the normal cardiac data when compared with other fetal measurements (BPD, femur length, abdominal circumference).

The continuity of the right side of the septum with the anterior wall of the aortic root is important to rule out the presence of a membranous ventricular septal defect (VSD), conal truncal abnormality (truncus, endocardial cushion defect), or tetralogy of Fallot (VSD, override of aorta with anterior wall of the interventricular septum, pulmonic stenosis, and right ventricular hypertrophy). The interventricular septum should be evaluated to rule out the presence of a membranous or muscular VSD. A very small VSD may not be visualized at this stage, depending on the resolution of the equipment and quality of visualization of the fetus. Usually we use the guideline that if the defect is the size of the aorta, adquate visualization is possible. A repeat study in 4 to 6 weeks is recommended to observe a patient with a history of a previous child with a septal defect.

The size of the aorta should be assessed. A patient with a hypoplastic left heart syndrome would show a very hypoplastic (underdeveloped) aortic root. A patient with a truncus arteriosus (a common origin of both great vessels—aorta and pulmonary artery with multiple cusps) would show a very large single great vessel with virtually no anterior great vessel and overriding of the posterior great vessel. A patient with Marfan's syndrome (cystic medial necrosis of the arterial wall tissue) would show a dilated aortic root with possible extension into the aortic arch and descending aorta.

The aortic cusp motion should be assessed on the long- and short-axis view. Normally the three cusps open in systole to the full extent of the aortic root and close in a midposition in diastole. They do not "flop" into the left ventricular outflow tract, as is sometimes seen in various degrees with a bicuspid or unicuspid valve. The aortic root should be anechoic from its base throughout the arch and descending aorta. The presence of interluminal echoes with dilatation may indicate some degree of aortic stenosis (with poststenotic dilatation).

With careful angulation of the transducer, the base of the aorta, the ascending aorta, the arch, and the descending aorta may be assessed. The tubular dimension of this vessel should be "uniform" in nature as one follows the aorta from its base through the ascending aorta, arch, and descending aorta into the abdomen (Figs. 36-15 to 36-17). By careful sweeping back and forth, the inner "core" should be anechoic. The neck branch arteries may be seen along the arch of the aorta as they ascend into the head. As the transducer is angled slightly inferior, a second "arch"-type pattern (appearing as large as the aorta) is shown, which represents the patent ductus arteriosus (a fetal communication between the pulmonary artery and aorta).

There are numerous variations in aortic arch malformations, which will not be dealt with in detail in this section. The most common malformation of the arch is the presence of a coarctation of the aorta (a shelflike narrowing of the aorta, which may be a short segment, or may consist of a very long segment of constriction). Many coarctations occur at the level of the insertion of the patent ductus arteriosus, near the left subclavian artery in the descending aorta. There is an increased incidence of associated bicuspid aortic valve lesions in these patients.

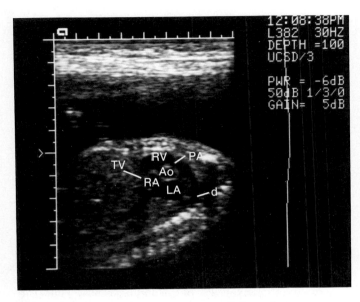

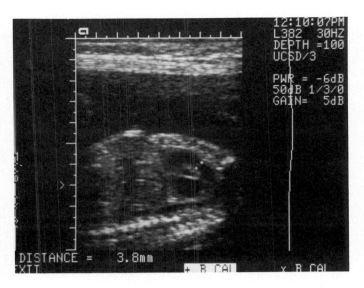

FIG. 36-15. Modified long-axis view of the pulmonary artery and aorta. This is the same view used in the neonate to evaluate the presence of a persistent ductus arteriosus. *RV*, right ventricle; *PA*, main pulmonary artery; *Ao*, aorta; *TV*, tricuspid valve; *RA*, right atrium; *LA*, left atrium; *d*, ductus arteriosus.

FIG. 36-16. The measurement of the main pulmonary artery may be made in this view and compared with the aortic measurement. The pulmonary artery is slightly larger than the aorta.

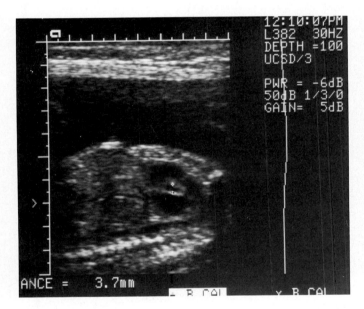

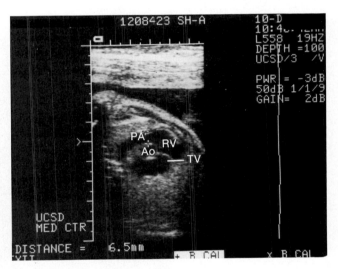

FIG. 36-18. Parasternal short-axis view of the pulmonary artery, *PA*, right ventricle, *RV*, aorta, *Ao*, and tricuspid valve, *TV*.

FIG. 36-17. Measurement of the aorta is made from the leading edge to leading edge.

Parasternal short-axis view

Once the long-axis view has been obtained, the transducer is rotated 90 degrees to the transverse or parasternal short-axis plane. The position of the spine, fluid-filled stomach, heart, and liver may help decide which is right side up from left side up. The patent foramen ovalae may also be visualized to determine the right from the left as the foramen bulges toward the left atrium in fetal life (after birth, pressures on the left increase to force the foramen to close).

Generally the transducer is slightly angled in a cephalic

direction to make this view a high parasternal short-axis view. The following structures should be visualized (Figs. 36-18 to 36-22):

1. Right ventricular outflow tract
2. Pulmonary cusps
3. Main pulmonary artery
4. Right and left pulmonary arteries
5. Aorta with cusps
6. Left atrial cavity

We chose the parasternal short-axis view to measure the diameter of the pulmonary artery and the aorta. It is also important to visualize the pulmonary branch arteries (right and left) to rule out transposition of the great vessels. (Transposition occurs when the great vessels fail to make a complete loop in early development and the anterior great vessel becomes the aorta and the posterior ves-

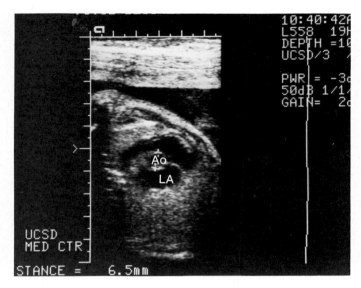

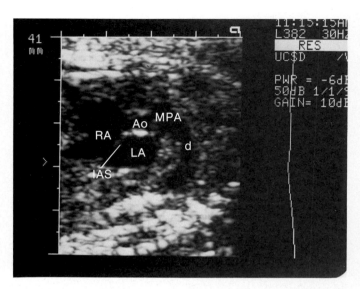

FIG. 36-19. The aorta, *Ao,* may be evaluated in this short-axis view for size, cusp opening and position of cusps, and diameter in comparison to the pulmonary artery. The left atrium, *LA,* is seen posterior to the aorta.

FIG. 36-20. Short-axis view of the aorta, *Ao,* main pulmonary artery, *MPA,* ductus, *d,* right atrium, *RA,* left atrium, *LA,* and interatrial septum, *IAS.* The opening of the ductus is generally the size of the aorta in fetal life.

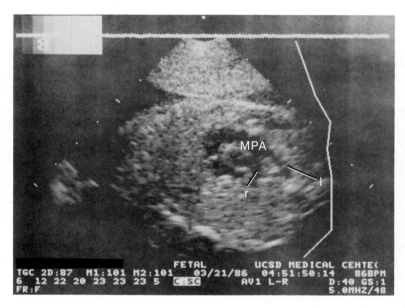

FIG. 36-21. The parasternal short-axis view is best to visualize the main pulmonary artery, *MPA,* and the bifurcation of the right, *r,* and left, *l,* pulmonary arteries.

sel the pulmonary artery.) Other conditions associated with transposition include a single ventricle (with a hypoplastic right ventricle) and a VSD. On the short-axis view, normally the right ventricular outflow tract and pulmonary artery "drape"' over the circular aorta (referred to as the "sausage and egg" pattern). In transposition, the anterior aorta is circular, as is the posterior pulmonary artery, and is called the double circle or "two egg" pattern. There are many other variations of transposition (e.g., left-sided or right-sided aortic arch), but for our purposes in fetal echo, the important fact is identifying the problem in the great vessel orientation. The extent of the disease may be evaluated further at a later date.

The trileaflet aortic cusps may be visualized in this short-axis view and an M-mode recording made (Fig. 36-23). A bicuspid aortic valve would appear as two cusps with or without eccentric closure, depending on the equal distribution of cusp tissue.

Four-chamber view

The four-chamber view is probably one of the easiest views to demonstrate cardiac anatomy. The transducer generally is angled in a cephalic direction through the fetal liver (which serves as a good window to visualize cardiac structures). The anatomy visualized should include (Figs. 36-24 to 36-33):

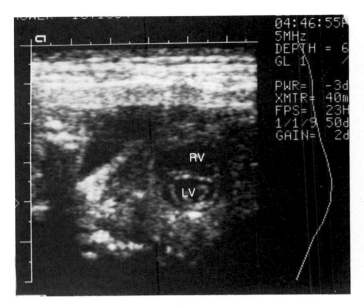

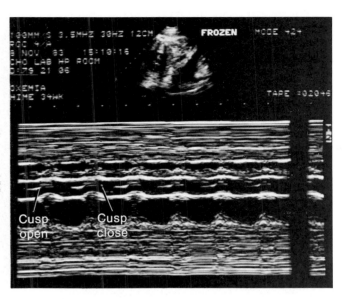

FIG. 36-22. Short-axis view of the right ventricle, *RV,* and left ventricle, *LV.* This view is good to obtain an M-mode tracing of the two ventricles, to determine wall thickness and contractility, and to determine relative size of the two chambers.

FIG. 36-23. The short-axis view is good to obtain an M-mode tracing of the aortic valve. As the aorta moves anterior, the cusps open in systole; they remain open throughout systole and close at the onset of diastole.

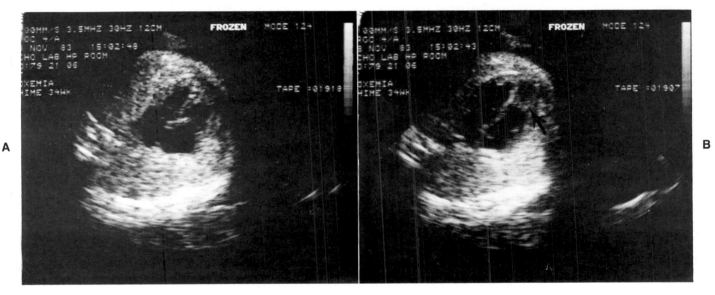

FIG. 36-24. **A,** Apical four-chamber view of the fetal heart. The right ventricle may be identified by its relative size, the presence of the moderator band located near the apex of the right ventricle (*arrow* in **B**), and the presence of the foramen ovale as it flaps open to the left atrium.

1. Right atrium
2. Right ventricle
3. Tricuspid valve
4. Left atrium
5. Left ventricle
6. Mitral valve
7. Interventricular septum
8. Interatrial septum
9. Foramen ovalae
10. Pulmonary veins as they enter into the left atrium.

General analysis of the relative size of the atria and ventricular cavities and function should be noted. As mentioned previously, the right heart is slightly larger in utero than the left heart. The right and left sides may be identified by the position of the patent foramen ovalae. In utero the foramen opens toward the left atrium; after birth the pressure in the left heart forces the foramen to close. Failure to do so results in an atrial septal defect (ASD). The moderator band can also be used to identify the right ventricle. It stretches across the right ventricle near the apex.

The position of the mitral and tricuspid leaflets (atrioventricular leaflets) should be assessed. Normally the tricuspid valve is located slightly inferior to the mitral valve. An Ebstein's malformation exists when the tricuspid valve is apically displaced. The remaining part of the right ventricle, superior to the tricuspid valve, becomes "atrial-

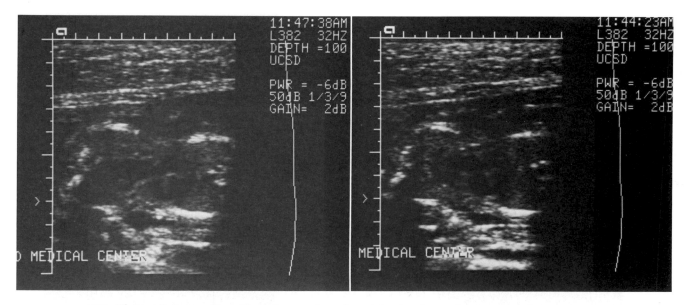

FIG. 36-40. Patient with a 22-week gestation of conjoined twins at the thorax with a significant risk for congenital heart disease. In the echocardiogram there was one single large primitive cavity identified that was shared between the two babies. The cavity had multiple septation defects. The atrioventricular valves were abnormal. There was a suggestion of transposition of the great arteries.

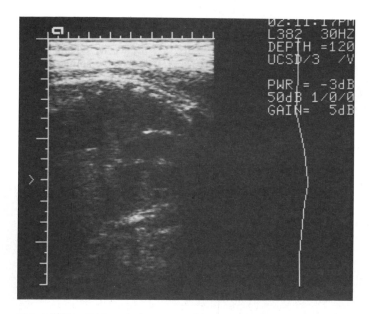

FIG. 36-41. Patient in her second trimester of pregnancy showing signs of an atrioventricular canal on the apical four-chamber view. There is evidence of a membranous ventricular septal defect and a primum atrial septal defect, and the atrioventricular valves are on the same level.

with amniotic fluid to identify it as an echo-free structure near the heart. The inferior vena cava may be followed as it passes through the fetal liver to return blood to the right atrium. The entrance of the hepatic veins may be identified at the level of the diaphragm and they enter the inferior vena cava.

The identification of the atrioventricular junction is important in establishing the presence or absence of the mitral and tricuspid valves. Valvular atresia is present when

one of the atrioventricular valves is absent. Generally this will lead to an atretic or hypoplastic ventricle because of the atretic valve. The presence of an endocardial cushion defect may cause abnormal development in the atrioventricular valves and result in formation of only one common valve. A large ventricular septal defect and primum atrial septal defect is also present in this condition. The presence of multiple chordae may be somewhat confusing in trying to separate the valve tissue from the chordal tissue. Careful angulation should show the chordal tissue attached to the papillary muscles, while the valve tissue is attached to the chordal structures and moves with systole and diastole. Generally this valve is incompetent, and the use of Doppler can determine how much regurgitation is present (Fig. 36-42). Color-flow mapping is also useful to track the path of the jet stream as it flows into the atrial cavity.

Another cardiac malformation is Ebstein's anomaly wherein the tricuspid valve is apically displaced in the right ventricle (Fig. 36-43). This is shown as a dilated right heart (the "mid-section" of the right ventricle—below the right atrium and above the displaced tricuspid valve—becomes atrialized and very dilated from the incompetent tricuspid valve).

Finally, the localization of the ventriculoarterial junction will allow one to assess abnormalities of the great vessels (the aorta and pulmonary artery). Since the pulmonary artery is slightly larger than the aorta during fetal life, an abnormal ratio of the two vessels is indicative of some form of stenosis or atresia. The pulmonary artery is best evaluated in the short-axis view as it drapes anterior to the aorta (Fig. 36-44). In some forms of pulmonary atresia (where the pulmonary artery does not connect to

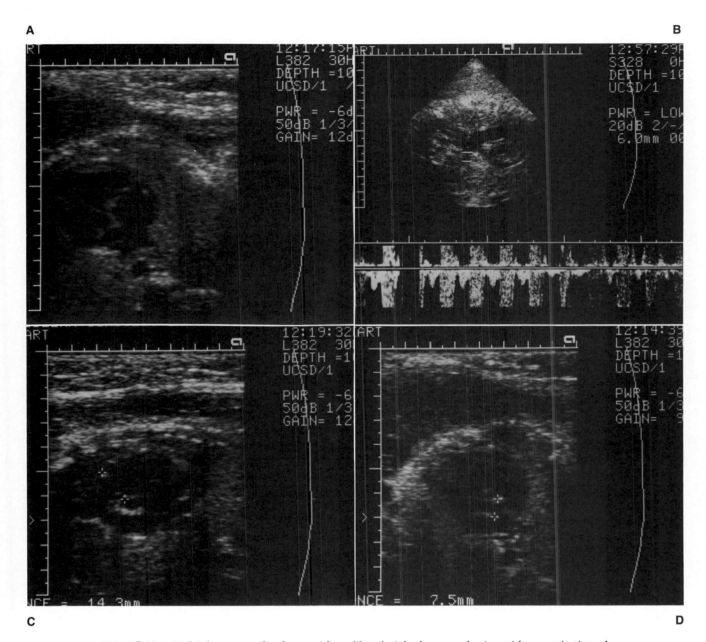

FIG. 36-42. Multiple scans of a fetus with a dilated right heart and tricuspid regurgitation. **A,** Four-chamber view showing the right heart to be much larger than the left heart. **B,** Doppler tracing of the incompetent tricuspid valve. **C,** Measurement of the pulmonary artery is 14.3 mm and compared to the aorta, **D,** which measured 7.5 mm. This most likely represents some form of pulmonary stenosis that leads to a dilated right heart and tricuspid regurgitation.

the right ventricle), the right and left branches of the pulmonary arteries become huge as they are filled by the patent ductus during fetal life. Other forms of stenosis may show a thickened valve with doming as is seen in neonatal life. Associated cardiac lesions that may be seen with pulmonary stenosis are aortic override and a ventricular septal defect.

Aortic stenosis may be identified in the same manner by visualizing the thickness of the cusp tissue or by identifying an abnormality in the cusp tissue itself (bicuspid valve or unicuspid valve). The size of the root of the vessel is important to rule out supravalvular dilatation or hypoplasia. In a fetus with severe hypoplastic left heart disease, the entire left side of the heart is underdeveloped

(Fig. 36-45). The left ventricle may be difficult to identify since the muscle is very thick and the cavity may only be a slit. The mitral valve is usually abnormal and may be atretic. The aorta is very small and may be hypoplastic throughout the ascending aorta and arch. Care must be taken to not mistake a hypoplastic left heart from a single ventricle (a single ventricle would have normal-sized great arteries, although they may be transposed) (Fig. 36-46).

The presence of transposition is more difficult to make on the fetal echocardiogram, but with perseverance the identification of the great vessels may be made. The long- and short-axis views are probably best to determine correct orientation of the aorta and pulmonary artery. One

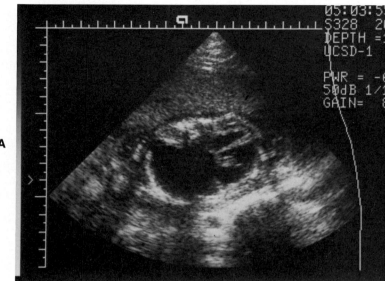

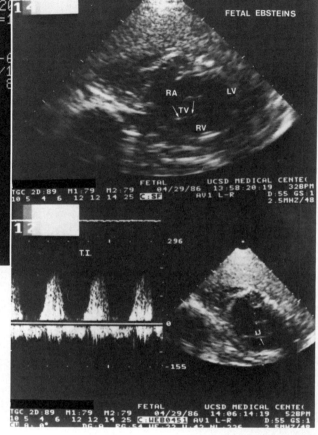

FIG. 36-43.   A and **B,** Fetal echocardiogram in a late gestation fetus showing fetal Ebstein's malformation. The tricuspid valve, *TV,* is displaced toward the apex of the right ventricle, *RV.* There is incompetence of the tricuspid valve into a dilated right atrial cavity, *RA.*

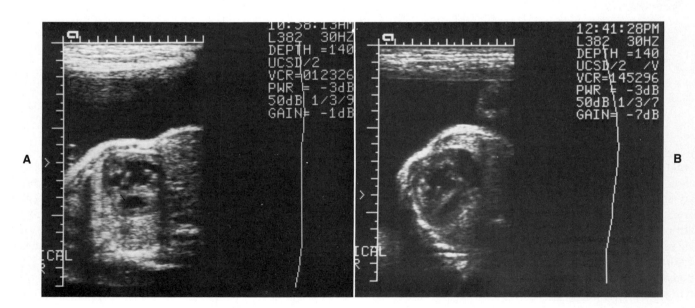

FIG. 36-44.   Multiple scans of a fetus with pulmonary atresia. The right heart is dilated. The pulmonary bifurcation is extremely dilated secondary to the pulmonary atresia. **A,** Short-axis view of the large right ventricle anterior to the left ventricle. **B,** Four-chamber view of the heart shows the very large right ventricle.

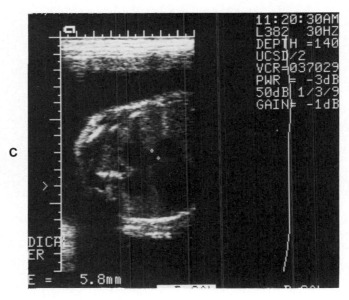

FIG. 36-44, cont'd.   C, The pulmonary arteries were also dilated as one scanned into a short-axis view.

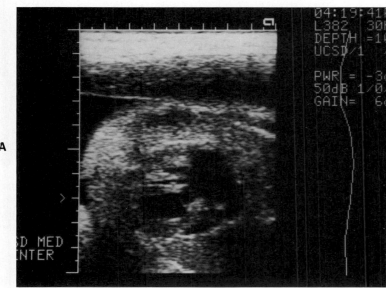

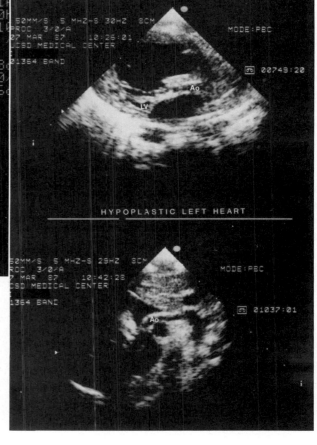

FIG. 36-45.   A, Fetal echocardiogram of a hypoplastic left heart. The left side is up and is underdeveloped in comparison to the right heart. The ascending aorta is small and hypoplastic to the arch. **B,** Neonatal echo shows the large right ventricle compressing the hypoplastic left ventricle (top). The bottom image shows the small ascending aorta to the arch.

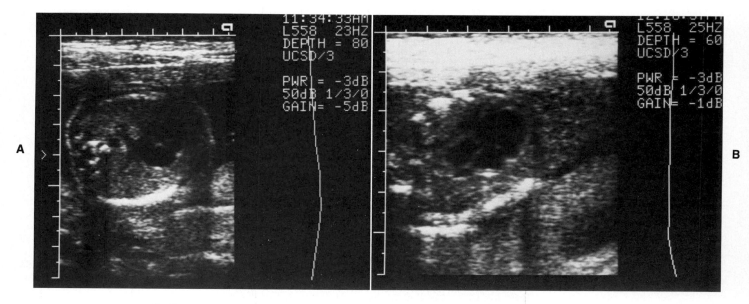

FIG. 36-46. **A,** This study was done on a fetus of 20 weeks gestation. There was a single ventricle with two atrioventricular valves emptying into the cavity. **B,** The aorta appeared to be displaced anterior, with a characteristic transposition pattern.

must see the bifurcation of the pulmonary artery as the main pulmonary artery divides into the right and left branches (usually the short-axis view is the best). On the long-axis view one may see the vessels arise in parallel orientation with the pulmonary artery anterior and to the left of the aorta. The mitral and tricuspid valves are at the same level in transposition. The great vessel from the right ventricle forms the aortic arch with head and neck vessel bifurcation, whereas the great vessel closer to the center of the heart appears to branch into the right and left pulmonary arteries.

Hypertrophy of the myocardium may be seen in some diabetic patients or in patients with hypertrophic cardio-myopathy (Fig. 36-47). It is usually detected in the second trimester and followed with subsequent echocardio-graphic scans and occasionally Doppler evaluation to rule out obstructive heart disease.

The presence of septal defects with the heart may be more difficult to assess in fetal life. An atrial septal defect cannot really be assessed unless part of the primum atrial septum is missing as is found in endocardial cushion defect. The presence of a common atrium would show a large atrial cavity with no interatrial septum. The more common secundum-type atrial septal defects that occur in the area of the fossa ovalis do not appear until after birth as the foramen is patent during fetal life.

The ventricular septal defects greater than half the size of the aortic root will be visualized by echo (Fig. 36-48 and 36-49). Since the mean aortic root size is 2 to 4 mm at 16 to 20 weeks of gestation, the resolution of most equipment is only 1 to 2 mm. Therefore after 20 weeks of gestation visualization will improve as the fetus continues to grow. The area of the membranous septum is very thin during development, and with just a slight transducer angulation, one can make a ventricular septal defect "ap-

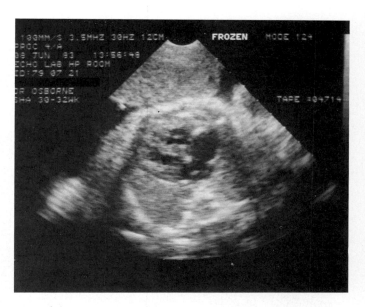

FIG. 36-47. Diabetic mothers have a slightly higher incidence of having a baby with some type of heart disease. The most common is hypertrophy of the septum and posterior wall. This hypertrophy tends to diminish several weeks to months after delivery and is easily followed with echocardiography.

pear" (Fig. 36-50). Generally, if this septal area is difficult to scan with confidence, the patient may be asked to return in 4 to 6 weeks for reevaluation. The presence of multiple small ventricular septal defects may be difficult to image with conventional ultrasound, but with color-flow Doppler may be more assessable in the second trimester.

The presence of a very bright echo within the left ventricle is sometimes seen as a normal variant. This is a reflection from the fibrous tissue of the medial papillary muscle and has no clinical significance. Of course this

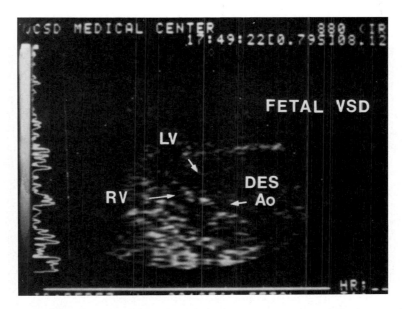

FIG. 36-48. The presence of a ventricular septal defect, *VSD*, is more difficult to make in utero. The abnormal break in echo formation along the septum is suggestive of a defect if the septal area has been carefully scanned.

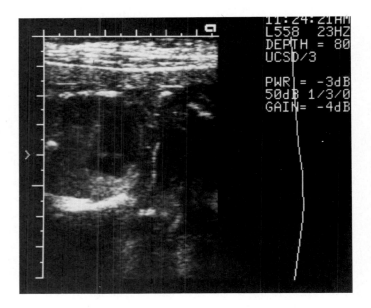

FIG. 36-49. Patients with other known congenital heart lesions may have a ventricular septal defect as part of their disease. This is a patient with transposition and a single ventricle with a septal defect.

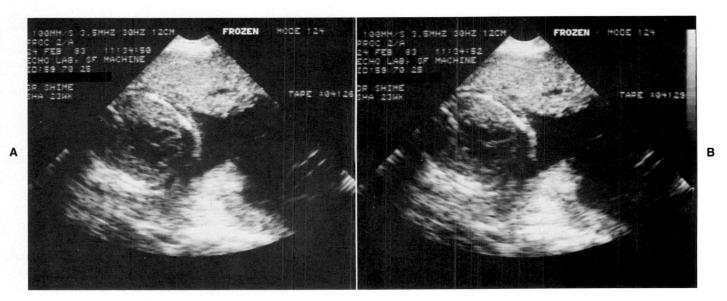

FIG. 36-50. **A,** The membranous part of the septum is very thin and sometimes difficult to image well in early pregnancy. Careful scanning should be done in multiple planes to rule out a septal defect. If the transducer is angled correctly, **B,** the apparent "defect" may disappear.

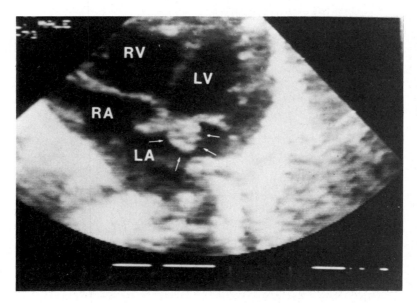

FIG. 36-51. Tumors can be located anywhere in the heart. They may be within the cardiac chamber or attached to the atrial septum, or be a part of the atrioventricular valve tissue. This patient has a dense mass attached to the anterior leaflet of the mitral valve. (Courtesy R. Bender, Kaiser Medical Center, San Diego, California.)

bright echo from the papillary muscle must be separate from that of a tumor within the heart (Fig. 36-51). Tumors can be located anywhere; they may be within the cardiac chamber or attached to the atrial septum or a part of the atrioventricular valve tissue. They may be life threatening if they obstruct blood flow.

A rarer form of cardiac disease is primary endocardial fibroelastosis. This occurs when there is hypertrophy of both ventricles with dense endocardial thickening. This may also occur secondary to obstructive lesions of the left side such as critical aortic stenosis or hypoplastic left heart.

The presence of dilated cardiac chambers with decreased function may be representative of a cardiomyopathy (Figs. 36-52 to 36-54). This condition may be life threatening within the fetus. There may be pericardial effusion surrounding the heart, indicating congestive heart failure.

ARRHYTHMIAS

The normal fetal heart rate is about 140 to 160 beats/min. It is not uncommon to notice short episodes of sinus bradycardia throughout the fetal study (the heart may actually stop beating for a few seconds during the study and then resume normal activity). Increased heart rate (sinus tachycardia) of 180 to 190 beats/min is commonly associated with fetal movement. The heart rate becomes abnormal when it is too slow (bradycardia, under 100 beats/min) or too fast (tachycardia, over 200 beats/min). If these conditions persist over several minutes, careful evaluation of the fetus must be made to monitor the fetal heart so it does not go into failure. Often medications are given to stimulate the heart into normal sinus rhythm.

If a patient is sent for a fetal echocardiogram to rule out an arrhythmia, certain procedures should be per-

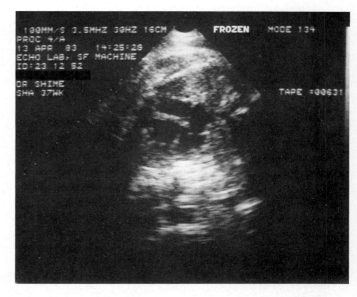

FIG. 36-52. This patient was 35 weeks pregnant and was sent for a fetal echocardiogram because of bradycardia. On real-time imaging, the four cardiac chambers were grossly dilated with very poor contractility. The heart rate was 60 beats/min. This represented a fetal cardiomyopathy.

formed to complete the study. Once cardiac anatomy has been defined, cardiac function should be evaluated to rule out failure (enalrged right ventricle, ascites, edema, pleural effusion, or pericardial effusion). The next step is to perform several M-mode studies of the simultaneous atrial and ventricular rhythm. This can be done by a four-chamber view with the M-mode cursor directed through the atrial cavity and ventricular cavity, or with a short-axis view of the aorta, cusps, and left atrium. In a normal heart, every ventricular contraction is preceded by an atrial con-

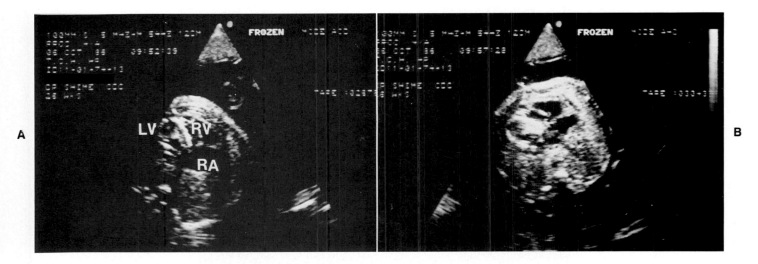

FIG. 36-53. **A** and **B**, Fetal cardiomyopathy with thrombus lining the ventricular cavity. This was confirmed at pathology. (Courtesy C. Gresser, Toronto General Hospital, Toronto, Ontario.)

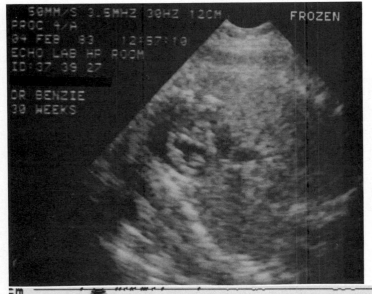

FIG. 36-54. **A,** Real-time study of a patient with fetal hydrops and a large pericardial effusion surrounding the apex of the heart. **B,** M-mode tracing of the ventricles, with pericardial effusion posterior to the ventricle *(arrows)*.

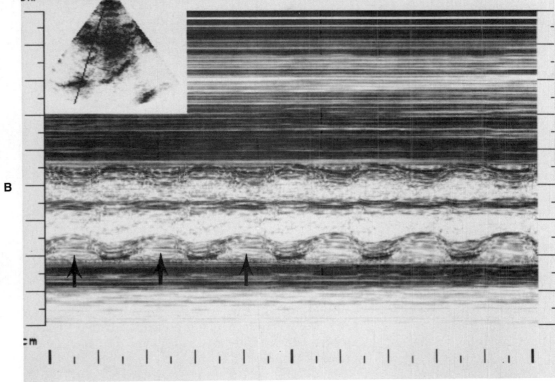

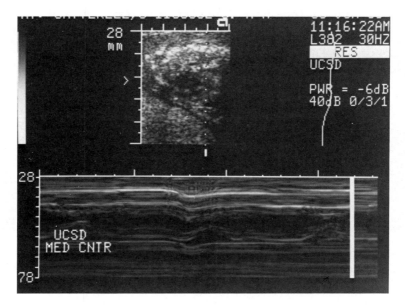

FIG. 36-55.   M-mode study of a patient with bradycardia.

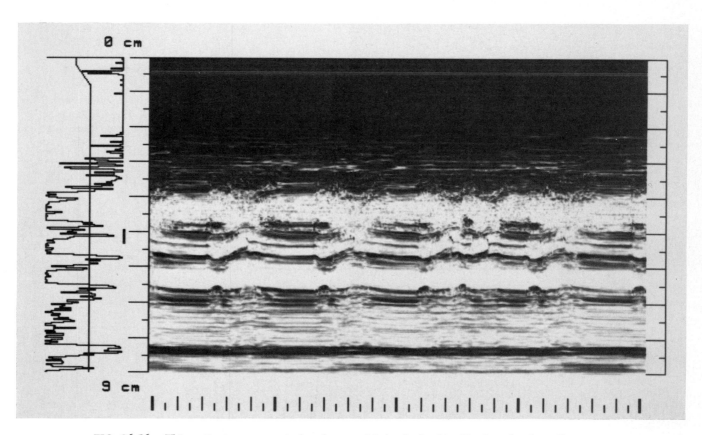

FIG. 36-56.   This patient was reported to have atrial dysrhythmia with sinus bradycardia versus silent atrial ectopic beats, resulting in a prolonged period of an effective heart rate of 70 beats/min.

traction with a fixed time relationship of less than 100 ms.[1]

Bradycardia. This condition is seen in fetal distress or in a fetus with blocked atrial ectopic beats (Figs. 36-55 and 36-56). The slow rhythm can be produced by atrial ectopic beats occurring too close to the sinus beat to transmit every beat.[1] Only every second atrial contraction produces ventricular systole. This is a benign condition.

In complete heart block the ventricular rhythm is around 50 to 100 beats/min (Figs. 36-57 and 36-58). This is totally dissociated from atrial contraction. A complete heart block with structural heart disease has a very poor prognosis. Fetal hydrops may develop with interuterine death.

Tachycardia. This is a condition where the heart beats over 200 beats/min. It is usually seen in the third trimester. Cardiac failure may be present (dilated chambers, pericardial effusion).

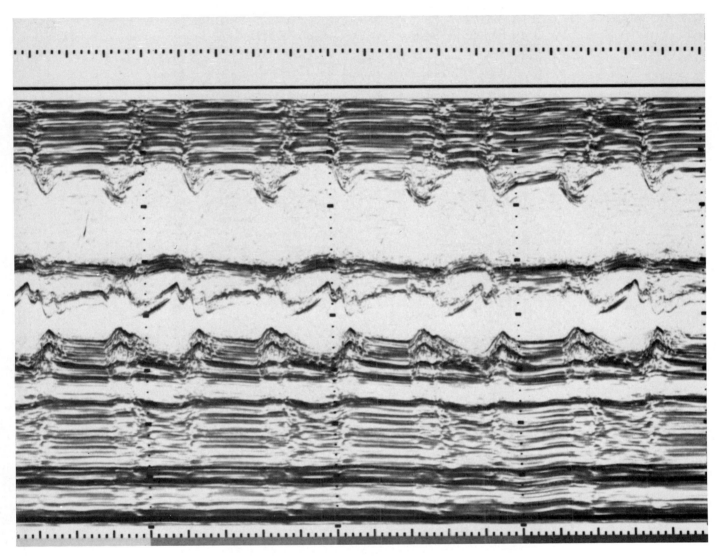

FIG. 36-57. Fetal echocardiogram shows an M-mode tracing of a fetus with a 2:1 heart block with evidence of atrial activity not being conducted to the ventricle.

In supraventricular tachycardia there is a sudden onset of rapid heart rate with a 1:1 conduction and a fixed time interval between each atrial and ventricular beat (Fig. 36-59).

Irregular rhythms. It is not uncommon to see ectopic beats, both atrial and ventricular, throughout the fetal echocardiogram. These ectopic beats are usually more common in the last trimester of pregnancy (Fig. 36-60).

Abnormalities associated with abnormal rhythms are cardiac tumors, cardiomyopathy, and Ebstein's malformation. These lesions should be ruled out by defining normal cardiac anatomy and function.

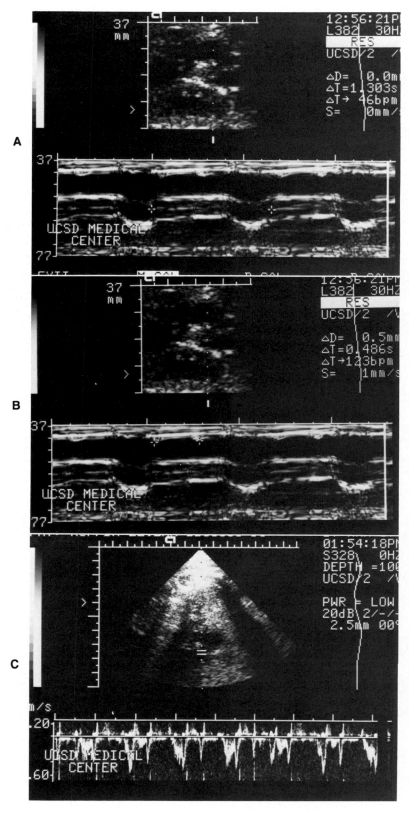

FIG. 36-58.   This patient was in her 34th week of gestation when the fetal echocardiogram was performed. There was enlargement of the ventricles with good contractility. There was complete atrial ventricular discordance with a ventricular rate of 49 and an atrial rate of 120. Doppler studies showed good cardiac output with no significant valvular insufficiency. **A,** M-mode tracing of the aorta showing a ventricular rate of 49. **B,** M-mode tracing of the atrial wall showing a rate of 120. **C,** Doppler tracing over the mitral valve showed no signs of incompetence.

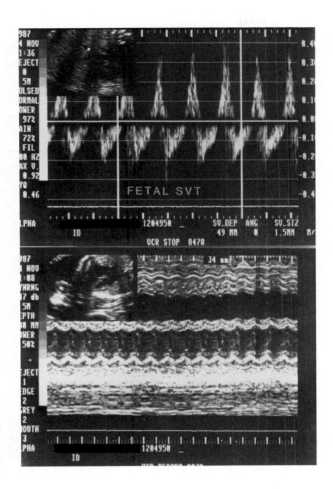

FIG. 36-59. This patient presented in her third trimester with a heart rate of 240 beats/min. This represented supraventricular tachycardia. Subsequent scans were made to see if the fetus converted with cardiac medication and to monitor the cardiac function.

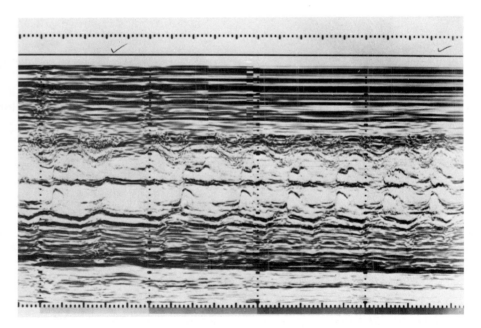

FIG. 36-60. This patient presented at 21 weeks gestation with a history of an irregular heart rate. The cardiac dimensions were normal. There were periods of irregularity consisting of early premature beats followed by a fairly long compensatory pause. There was atrial activity preceding each of the extra events. This rhythm represented an atrial-origin arrhythmia and was a benign condition for the fetus. M-mode tracing of ventricular activity showing the premature ventricular beat.

SUMMARY

1. The blood flow in the fetus is slightly different than in the neonatal stage. Communication is open between the right and left sides of the heart as well as between the aorta and pulmonary artery.

2. Before birth the oxygenated blood returns by way of the umbilical vein from the placenta to the heart.

3. Blood flows from the inferior vena cava and enters the right atrium. The blood from the inferior vena cava is directed by the lower border of the septum secundum through the foramen ovale into the left atrium. It mixes with a small amount of deoxygenated blood returning from the lungs via the pulmonary veins into the left atrium. The blood flows into the left ventricle and leaves through the ascending aorta.

4. A small amount of oxygenated blood from the inferior vena cava is diverted by the crista dividens and remains in the right atrium to mix with deoxygenated blood from the superior vena cava and coronary sinus.

5. Blood flows into the right ventricle and leaves through the pulmonary artery.

6. Most of the blood passes through the patent ductus arteriosus into the aorta.

7. A very small amount goes to the lungs.

8. Most of the mixed blood in the descending aorta passes into the umbilical arteries and is returned to the placenta for reoxygenation.

9. The remainder of blood circulates through the lower part of the body.

10. After birth, the fetal cardiac structures that no longer are needed are the foramen ovale, the ductus arteriosus, the ductus venosus, and the umbilical vessels.

11. Risk factors that indicate the fetus is at a higher than normal risk for congenital heart disease are divided into three categories: fetal, maternal, and familial.

12. Difficulties in performing a fetal echocardiogram are encountered when there is oligohydramnios, maternal obesity, unusual fetal position, or early gestation.

13. After discerning the position of the fetus, placenta, extremities, and biparietal diameter size, these cardiac windows are used: parasternal short- and long-axis views, four-chamber view, and long axis of aortic arch.

14. Identification of the atrial chambers may be made by finding the origin of the aorta and the inferior vena cava in relation to the fetal anatomy and position.

15. Identification of the atrioventricular valves is important in establishing the presence or absence of the valves.

16. Localization of the ventriculoarterial junction will allow one to assess abnormalities of the great vessels.

17. In some forms of pulmonary atresia, the right and left branches of the pulmonary arteries become huge as they are filled by the patent ductus during fetal life.

18. In aortic stenosis the thickness of the cusp tissue and the size of the root is important to rule out supravalvular dilation or hypoplasia.

19. Hypertrophy of the myocardium may be seen in some diabetic patients or in patients with hypertrophic cardiomyopathy.

20. The presence of septal defects may be more difficult to assess during fetal life. The ventricular septal defects greater than half the size of the aortic root will be visualized by echo. The area of the membranous septum is very thin during development, and with just a slight transducer angulation, one can make a ventricular septal defect "appear."

21. The presence of a very bright echo within the left ventricle is sometimes seen as a normal variant. This is a reflection from the fibrous tissue of the medial papillary muscle and has no clinical significance.

22. Primary endocardial fibroelastosis is when there is hypertrophy of both ventricles with dense endocardial thickening.

23. The presence of dilated cardiac chambers with decreased function may be representative of a cardiomyopathy. A pericardial effusion may be present if the fetus is going into heart failure.

24. The normal fetal heart rate is about 140 to 160 beats/min.

25. Abnormal conditions such as bradycardia and sinus tachycardia may be seen. If these conditions persist over several minutes, then careful evaluation of the fetus must be made to monitor the fetal heart so it does not go into failure.

REFERENCES

1. Allen L: Manual of fetal echocardiography, London, 1986, MTP Press Limited.
2. Kleinman C: Fetal echocardiography. In Sanders RC: US annual 1982, New York, 1982, Raven Press.
3. McCallum WD: Fetal cardiac anatomy and vascular dynamics, Clin Ostet Gynecol 24(3), 1981.
4. Reed KL, Anderson CF, and Shenker L: Fetal echocardiography. An atlas, New York, 1988, Alan R Liss.
5. Trudinger BJ and Cook CM: Umbilical and uterine artery flow velocity waveforms in pregnancy associated with major fetal abnormality, Br J Obstet Gynecol 152:155, 1985.

Part Seven

PERIPHERAL VASCULAR DOPPLER AND VASCULAR SONOGRAPHY

37

Doppler Principles and Instrumentation

RICHARD E. RAE II

Throughout medical history the circulatory system has been a source of great mystery and puzzlement. Many diseases and conditions in the human body have led investigators to discover a vascular etiology where a completely different diagnosis was expected. Unfortunately the source often has not been found in time to save a diseased organ or limb or has been discovered only after the patient's death.

The introduction of radiographic imaging of the arterial system in 1923 made possible accurate vascular diagnosis and greatly enhanced the potential for surgical repair of vascular lesions. The first carotid arteriogram was performed in 1927,[12] and the first translumbar aortogram in 1929.[7] Many years were required for perfection of angiographic equipment and techniques, but angiography has become the standard method for the assessment of vascular anatomy.

But how golden is this gold standard? The drawbacks of angiography are numerous. There are risks from reactions to the iodine-based contrast media. Furthermore, the examination is performed with the patient in an immobile position; needle punctures or cutdowns and rapid injections of contrast are required,[3,9] all of which contribute to patient anxiety and occasionally result in the patient's refusing the examination.

The introduction of digital subtraction angiography (DSA) was originally hailed as a breakthrough in diagnosis; it was intravenous as opposed to intraarterial and could be performed on an outpatient basis. Various studies undertaken since its introduction, however, have shown as little as a 65% overall accuracy when compared with ultrasonic noninvasive findings and the true "gold standard," the findings at surgery.[11] IVDSA has been supplanted by arterial injections in most institutions now, thus bringing the procedure full circle, back to the same risks found with conventional arteriography.

Many of the pitfalls of arteriography and DSA stem from the fact that these procedures are capable only of showing those structures that can be actively filled by the radiographic contrast material, thus meaning that only filling defects can be interpreted as suspect (Fig. 37-1). The images are in two dimensions only and lack the ability to show the vessel from more angles without reinjection and running another film series. The contrast agents can often mask underlying anatomy, or "sneak by" low-density soft plaques that do not obstruct flow. There are several noninvasive or nonarteriographic methods (not including ultrasonic methods) for assessing the circulatory system, which involve various methods and techniques depending on the vessels and location of the area of interest:

Plethysmography techniques use pressure transducers and base their measurements on changes in limb volume or pressure differences in arterial segments.

Strain-gauge plethysmography is used on limbs and digits for measuring limb volume changes based on the assumption that changes in limb volume are reflected in the limb circumference. This technique is often used on toes

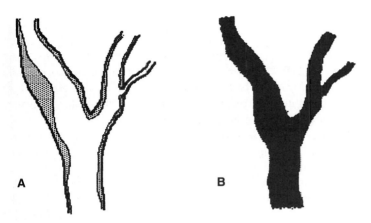

FIG. 37-1. The 50% smooth stenosis in **A** may not be adequately demonstrated by arteriography and be interpreted as normal, **B.**

and fingers for pulse-volume changes, using small mercury-in-Silastic gauges that are looped over the area to be tested, connected, and a strip-chart recording made. Comparisons are made between segments and established normal gradients.

Impedance phlebography (IPG) measures changes in limb volume before and after inflation of a thigh cuff and is used to assess venous disease and venous outflow. This test is easy to perform but is not generally quantitative, since the results are compared on a chart and are either normal or abnormal. This test is subject to pitfalls since the patient must be completely relaxed, the legs must be elevated above heart level, and the electrodes fixed to the leg are subject to poor contact if not properly maintained. Strain gauges can be used to measure calf volume and venous outflow as well and are less susceptible to the problems associated with the electrodes.

Oculoplethysmography is a technique for indirectly assessing carotid disease. This was initially performed with a water system, but the air system (GEE-OPG) has been more widely accepted and used. This system uses small cups, attached to a vacuum system, that are placed on the eyes (for the internal carotid system), and small transducers that are clipped to the earlobe (for the external carotid). Pressure differences between the internal and external carotid systems are measured. This technique more than any of the others is generally quite uncomfortable for patients (and stretches the limits of "noninvasive"). Outside of the fact that the patient must have a small cup attached to the eyeball and cannot blink comfortably, it is often disturbing that a momentary loss of vision occurs when the ophthalmic artery branches are occluded by the vacuum system. Small hemorrhages on the eyeball can often result from the pressure.

Photoplethysmography uses photocells and LEDs. The principle of PPG involves measuring the amount of ambient reflected light from the skin's vascular bed and measures blood flow proportionately. This is advantageous for monitoring digits because the transducers are simply taped to the area in question. Pitfalls of this technique are often caused by overlying vasculature, which

can cause discrepancies in the desired flow tracing, and low hemoglobin, which can affect the reflected light because of low red cell counts in the tissues and result in false readings.

These techniques are widely used with Doppler techniques. Their accuracy can vary from poor to excellent when correlated with angiographic studies and depending on the disease condition being ruled out.[3,8,9]

The ideal noninvasive vascular diagnostic method is truly noninvasive, has a high overall accuracy, is atraumatic, comfortable to the patient, can be performed quickly, and does not require bulky equipment or long setup procedures.

Doppler and high-resolution real-time ultrasonic techniques fulfill these requirements. The use of Doppler techniques has become increasingly widespread since their inception 30 years ago and as initial physician wariness has given way in response to documented accuracy. Many clinical and laboratory studies have been performed comparing Doppler methods to angiography, with 95% to 98% accuracy for some types of examination.[3,6,8,9]

The chapters in this part describe Doppler ultrasound techniques for arterial and venous examination, including the extremity vessels and the cerebrovascular system. Descriptions of spectral analysis of Doppler signals, Doppler vascular scanning, and real-time B-mode duplex sonography of the carotid system are also given. Each vascular system is considered independently, including pertinent anatomy, pathology, and equipment needs; and a complete explanation of commonly used examination procedures based on the techniques described by Barnes et al.[2,3,5] Data on examination variations, normal results, and interpretation of abnormal findings are presented as well as illustrative cases.

■ ■ ■ ■ ■

It is essential to understand the principles of a diagnostic procedure before becoming involved with it. This chapter considers the Doppler effect and how it applies to the vascular examination, along with the equipment and its use.

HISTORICAL NOTE

The Doppler ultrasound apparatus makes use of the Doppler effect, which was described by the mathematician Christian Andreas Doppler in 1842. He observed that the frequency of sound waves varied depending on the speed of the sound transmitter relative to the listener.

Two years after Doppler's equation was developed to express the phenomenon, a scientific colleague of Doppler, Christoph Buys-Ballot, devised an experiment to test the equation's validity. He assembled a small group of musicians with perfect pitch and one horn player beside a railroad track. He then had a train pull a flatcar with another horn player past these musical observers. Each horn player played the same note, and the musical observers noted that there was a difference of a half-step in tone between the note played by the musician going by on the

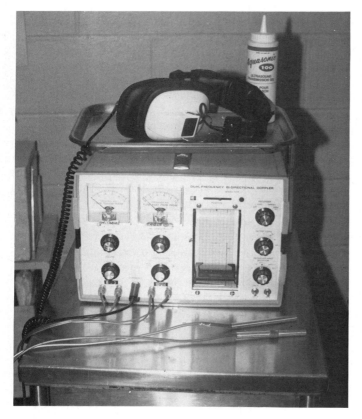

FIG. 37-2. Directional Doppler device.

flatcar and the one in the stationary group. The resulting differences proved Doppler's theory.[10]

CONTINUOUS-WAVE DOPPLER

In the continuous-wave Doppler bloodflow device (Fig. 37-2) the sound source is a small probe housing one transmitting and one receiving crystal. Red blood cells reflect ultrasound impulses, and the frequency of the reflected sound wave is shifted to either a higher or a lower pitch depending on the flow velocity. In all devices a change or shift in frequency is detected only if the flow velocity is greater than 6 cm/s; therefore an absent signal at a vascular site may imply anything from totally absent flow to flow moving at a velocity slower than 6 cm/s.[3]

In the directional Doppler device the probe is usually held so that the sound beam intersects the vessel at an angle of approximately 45 degrees to the plane of flow, which is the optimal angle for accurate measurement. Signals that do not intercept the flow at an angle other than perpendicular will not be Doppler-shifted. Angles other than 30 to 50 degrees may result in false or erroneous readings. When the probe is oriented so that the flow is toward the probe face, this is usually interpreted as *ante-grade* flow, and flow away from the probe face is usually considered *retrograde* flow (in certain circumstances and examination positions flow directions may be inverted, so sometimes the interpretation is reversed). A directional Doppler therefore is capable of showing the *direction* as well as the *relative velocity* of flow. Most equipment fea-

tures two gauges, one for *flow toward* and one for *flow away* from the probe, and these gauges are calibrated to show relative velocity of the blood flow in the direction specified. It is important that the transducer be correctly directed relative to the direction of flow in the vessel being examined so that false diagnoses of flows seeming to go in the wrong direction will be avoided.

In practice the probe is placed against the skin and is coupled by means of a water-soluble acoustic gel, which serves to eliminate air pockets and ensure optimal acoustic transmission and reception. The transmitted sound waves strike the red corpuscles and bounce back. The reflected signals are shifted in pitch, either higher or lower, depending on the relative velocity. The direction of flow also affects the reflected sound. As the reflected waveforms strike the receiving crystal, they are converted into electric signals via the piezoelectric principle. The circuitry of the Doppler device then separates the signals of increased frequency from those of decreased frequency and distinguishes between signals reflected by flow toward or away from the probe face. The signals are then fed to outputs that convert them to audible sound (heard by speakers or headphones) and also are fed to quadrature outputs for spectrum analyzers and zero-crossing strip chart devices.

Probes are available in frequencies manufactured in ranges from 2.25 to 10 MHz. The lower frequencies are usually found in fetal monitoring devices or Doppler stethoscopes intended for intraabdominal vessels, wherein sound penetration and large beam widths are desirable. The higher frequencies, from 5 to 10 MHz, are the ones most frequently used in extremity and cerebrovascular Doppler examinations. The probes also vary in size and shape, from flat transducers with a fixed beam angle used often in surgery for brachial pulse monitoring to large pocket-sized devices that incorporate the transducer and signal processors into one unit.

The most versatile probe, and the one that will be referred to exclusively in the discussion to follow, is the pencil-style probe. This probe is also available in many configurations, depending on the manufacturer. It can vary from a simple aluminum tube with the crystals epoxied into the end to a completely enclosed plastic probe with complex circuitry incorporated into the probe housing. The simpler the probe, however, the better, when maintenance and cost are prime concerns. The simple probes are light as well as practical and are easier to repair than a complex probe. Their lower cost usually means that several can be placed in reserve for the same price as one more sophisticated probe. Usually the complex probes require attached modules to allow frequency-circuit matching. The simple probes are calibrated to one set frequency and are matched to calibrated input and output jacks. The latter system has advantages in that faulty frequency-matching modules may ruin both probe and Doppler device whereas calibrated jacks and transducers require no modules between probe and Doppler system. Although the complex probe-module systems allow easier interchanging of different frequency probes,

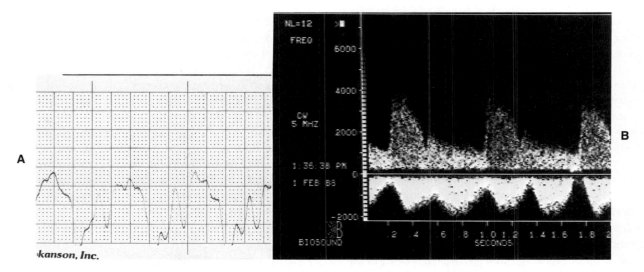

FIG. 37-3. Zero-crossing versus quadrature. Arterial and venous flow within the same beam path and in two directions is averaged together by the zero-crossing circuit, and discrimination is impossible, **A.** The same signals are easily discriminated on a spectrum analyzer and quadrature circuit, **B.**

the devices using simpler probes are optionally equipped with two sets of calibrated outlets and a selection knob so higher and lower frequencies can be used alternatively.

The audible Doppler flow information requires a method of permanent recording if later interpretation and diagnosis are required. The most commonly used system is the *strip-chart recorder.* This device has a *zero-crossing circuit,* which discriminates between antegrade and retrograde flow, much as the directional gauges in the main device do. In the standard recording format antegrade flow is placed on the positive (upward) side of a zero baseline and retrograde flow on the negative (downward) side. The examiner is thus able to determine the flow direction and flow patterns visually.

Although a zero-crossing circuit and strip-chart recorder is more than adequate in general applications, the biggest disadvantage is created when two signals in opposite directions are of equal strength. The zero-crossing circuit will average the two outputs, and the net flow signal may average out to zero, creating an erroneous chart tracing. Unlike a zero-crossing circuit, a *quadrature interface* electronically isolates antegrade and retrograde signals and resolves this problem by displaying both sets of signals simultaneously in their respective directions and respective strengths (Fig. 37-3). Quadrature circuits are almost always employed with spectrum analyzers, especially where critical flow information is important to diagnosis (see Spectral Analysis of Doppler Signals).

Some Dopplers are equipped with a signal-select switch, which can be set to show retrograde flow on the positive side of the graph when depressed. In some devices this switch can completely shut off either the right or left channel to help facilitate determination of the amount of flow reversal, or help isolate information from one particular direction of flow. Other devices have a separate knob that allows only positive, only negative, inverted net flow, or normal net flow to be recorded.

Strip charts are usually single graph, but some recorders have provisions for two readouts simultaneously. One readout is usually set for net flow and the other for antegrade flow, retrograde flow, ECG, or any other tracing that may be useful while the Doppler examination is being recorded. For most purposes one graph is sufficient, and all strip-chart examples are shown with net flow on a single-graph chart.

PULSED DOPPLER

Continuous-wave devices are useful in many applications but have a few pitfalls in resolution since everything in the path of the beam is detected. This explains why arterial and venous signals are often detected simultaneously. Another problem with this is that one cannot discriminate signals from multiple arteries in the beam path so occasional errors are often made. This is especially important when an occluded artery underlies a patent, unrelated vessel in the beam path. Pulsed Doppler devices enable discrimination to be made.

Pulsed Doppler devices are usually (but not exclusively) incorporated into real-time imaging devices and work on principles more akin to B-scan imaging than Doppler. Whereas continuous-wave Doppler is, as the name states, continuous (one transducer always sending, the other always receiving), pulsed Doppler is pulsed (i.e., a signal is sent out in a pulse and then the transducer pauses to receive the signal). The advantage here is one of depth localization, using range gating. This means that while Doppler information from all levels is being received, the range gate can be set to detect only the information at a specific level. The *sample volume,* which does this, can be located anywhere along the beam path, and is shown on an A-mode as a gate or on an imager as a box on a line that shows the beam angle on those devices with a steerable Doppler. The sample volume can also be increased or decreased in size, meaning that flow can be sampled in a vessel within as small an area as 0.5 mm or enlarged to 2 cm or more to measure flow across an entire region. The sample volume is usually elliptical in shape.

Beam angle is as critical here as it is in continuous-wave measurement; angles perpendicular to the flow will not give any useful flow-shifted information. One drawback is that the pulse repetition frequency (PRF) may often be too high to detect slow-moving flow or too low to detect very high-velocity flow, resulting in inaccurate measurement at times. If a severe stenosis results in a severe flow velocity increase and frequency shift that exceeds half the PRF (the *Nyquist* limit), then the excessive frequencies may be "cut off" or transposed as spurious frequency readings. This is known as *aliasing* (see Spectral Analysis of Doppler Signals). Pulsed Doppler is not as convenient to use as a continuous-wave device and is generally not indicated for routine examination of small peripheral vessels since both hands are usually needed to adjust all the depth and volume factors.

The best results are often obtained with a combination of pulsed and continuous-wave Doppler techniques, since the two technologies are complimentary and compensate for each modality's respective weaknesses.

HIGH-RESOLUTION DUPLEX REAL-TIME ULTRASOUND EQUIPMENT

The introduction of high-resolution small-parts scanners has proved to be a definite breakthrough in the noninvasive examination of small or difficult-to-evaluate structures in the body. In the vascular field these imaging devices are coupled with either an integral pulsed Doppler device, a continuous-wave Doppler device, or both. Units that incorporate both imaging and Doppler are generally referred to as *duplex* machines. The most obvious benefit of a duplex scanner is the ability to image a vessel, then steer the Doppler sample volume to any area on the screen and obtain a flow sample. This allows the examiner to visualize a stenosis, then obtain flow samples proximal and distal to it to determine the hemodynamic effect of the stenosis. More recent devices are able to show the flow in color superimposed over the gray-scale image (see Doppler Color-flow).

Among the many uses of duplex scanners are the following:

- Carotid artery evaluation.
- Peripheral artery evaluation.
- Peripheral venous evaluation.
- Abdominal vessel evaluation.

Most of these applications will be covered in depth later in this chapter.

Several companies manufacture small-parts scanners, and improvements in operator-oriented design and resolution are occurring constantly. Scanners used for vascular evaluation generally are either mechanical or electronically phased, and of two image format types, sector and linear. Most of these scanners use one of the following methods to obtain a real-time image of the area being examined and obtain Doppler information (Fig. 37-4).

One type of transducer uses one to three separate

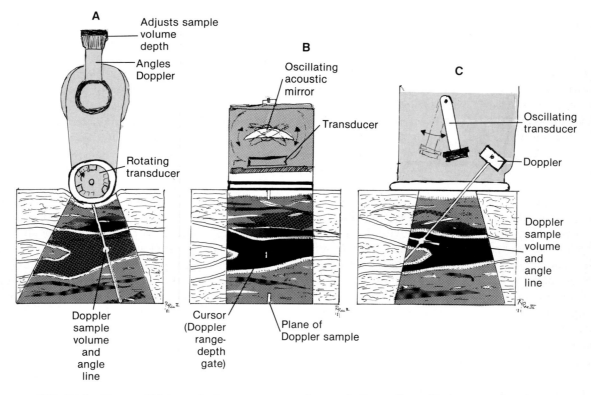

FIG. 37-4.   Types of high-resolution scanner transducers. **A,** Rotor; **B,** oscillating acoustic mirror; **C,** oscillating transducer; **D,** mechanical sector; **E,** linear phased-array/fixed Doppler; **F,** phased-array with electronically steered Doppler.

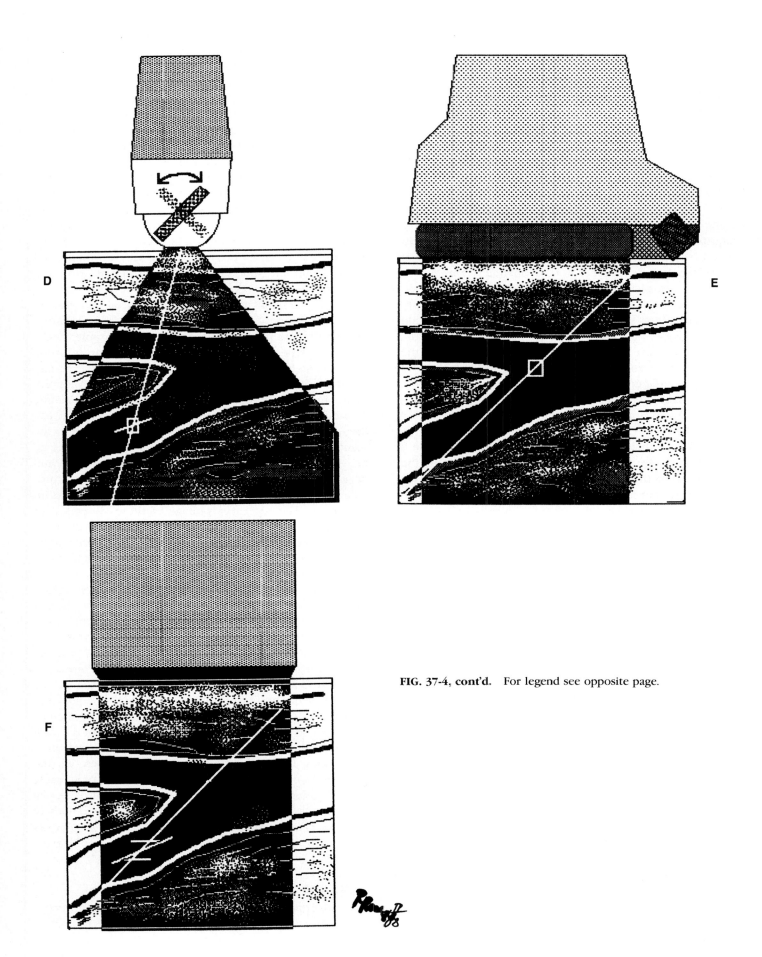

FIG. 37-4, cont'd.   For legend see opposite page.

transducers installed in a rotor assembly that rotates rapidly, sweeping the ultrasonic beam through a fluid-filled coupling head and producing a relatively flicker-free image rate. Some scanheads incorporate a 5, 7.5, and 10 MHz transducer all within the same rotor; the operator can select which of these crystals to use at a time. The selectable crystals also can give a degree of beam depth focusing in addition to different levels of penetration and resolution.

The Doppler signals are obtained by activating a 5 MHz pulsed Doppler (which uses the same transducer as the one for imaging) that can be angled relative to the scan plane of the vessel, with the sampling depth of the signal adjusted separately. One of the main disadvantages to this type of system is the fact that the image must be frozen while the Doppler information is obtained. This frozen image can usually appear in a "feedback" mode, displayed in a corner or above the spectral display, and can be updated every few seconds to help the examiner maintain the transducer position during Doppler sampling. While the frozen image still allows relative placement of the sample volume and flow angle, imaging and Doppler still are not simultaneous with this system.

A second system uses a fixed 8 MHz transducer with an oscillating acoustic mirror to sweep the beam through a fluid path.

Doppler in this system is obtained through the same 8 MHz transducer as is used for imaging. Activating the Doppler stops the mirror at the midline position and cuts in a simultaneous extended A-mode for reference when range-gating of the Doppler sample depth is being done. The examiner can thus see changes in position and move the transducer to compensate. The "steerability" of the Doppler sample is limited in this system since the mirror only traverses a 30-degree sector. The sample line can be angled 15 degrees in either direction from the centerline, however, and while angle vectoring is unavailable (see Spectral Analysis of Doppler Signals), the system is still flexible for peak frequency assessment. In addition, when the Doppler sample plane is centered, it is in the exact center of the image, and the entire probe can be angled in transverse or longitudinal positions and treated like a rather large handheld Doppler probe. The A-mode display can help with placement when the probe is used in this fashion, giving some degree of simultaneity but still not allowing a simultaneous image/Doppler display.

A third system uses an oscillating transducer at either 5 or 10 MHz for imaging and a separate offset Doppler transducer at 3 MHz. This system also allows image updates while doing Doppler and also can update the image four times a second in a "simultaneous" mode where the device continues to image at a reduced and staggered frame rate with the Doppler pulsing in the intervals when the imaging transducer is off. During this "simultaneous" phase there is usually an inordinate amount of motor noise because of the mechanical system. The system is still prone to many of the problems mentioned above and still lacks true simultaneity.

A variation of this type of system uses a fixed-angle Doppler mounted offset to the mechanical transducer. In this kind the imager does not update during Doppler evaluation because of mechanical noise.

A fourth and common type of system employs a single-crystal mechanical transducer that rocks back and forth and provides a sector image. Doppler signals are obtained with the same crystal used for imaging or an integral separate crystal in the same place as the imaging crystal. The image can be set to update periodically as in other devices, and also lacks simultaneity of Doppler and image.

A fifth type of system uses a phased-array linear probe and an offset, fixed-angle pulsed or continuous-wave Doppler transducer. In this type of system true simultaneity is possible, but the Doppler angle is fixed to about a 50-degree angle and cannot be steered. The sample volume and sample depth are still variable. The placement of the offset Doppler transducer often can interfere with scanning above the mandible area and be uncomfortable to the patient. In addition, flow in highly tortuous arteries cannot be accurately sampled because of the fixed Doppler angle.

A sixth type of system also uses a phased-array probe for imaging, but when a duplex mode is selected, certain crystals in the array can be set to provide only Doppler information, and the Doppler angle, depth, and sample volume can be electronically steered and adjusted (although one company uses a standoff block attached to the scanhead at the precise angle for Doppler acquisition), allowing the transducer to appear deceptively simple and have no mechanical parts. In addition, these systems provide true simultaneous Doppler and imaging with no interference. The biggest advantage of these systems is in the evaluation of abdominal vasculature, such as renal arteries, which can move in and out of the Doppler sample plane with each inspiration and which are almost impossible to evaluate for flow without this capability.

Most of these scanners have axial and lateral resolution capabilities of no less than 0.3 mm and can allow the image to be enlarged for evaluating the detail of the vessel walls or other area being examined. Their sizes vary from large to fairly compact, but a few of them are portable enough for use in bedside examinations. Some companies have introduced miniature versions, enabling the device to be more easily transported and providing an equivalent or better image at roughly half the cost of the larger units.

As can be seen, the differing characteristics of the various machines available demand differing examination techniques. Discussion of the examination methods and idiosyncrasies present with each type is not practicable here. A general explanation and interpretation of typical applications for these systems will be given in the body of the text, along with fairly flexible examination techniques that can be used with most of the systems currently available.

SPECTRAL ANALYSIS OF DOPPLER SIGNALS

The most common method of making a permanent record of Doppler flow signals has been through the strip-chart recorder. An organized set of flow tracings by this device also allows delayed interpretation and diagnosis of vascu-

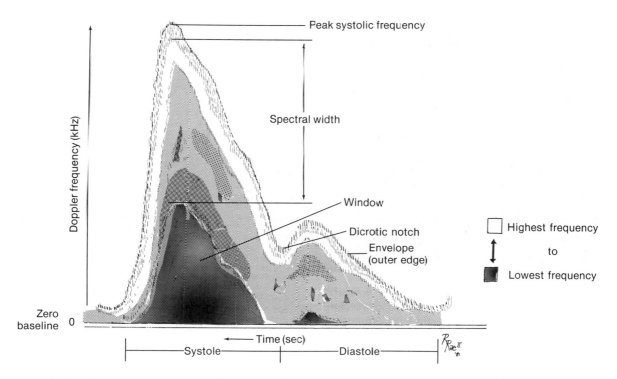

FIG. 37-5. Diagram of spectrally analyzed Doppler waveform, showing diagnostic characteristics.

lar flow abnormalities. The strip-chart tracing, however, shows only a mean flow velocity analog and does not reveal the complete range of frequencies present in the audible Doppler signal. The clinician interpreting the examination from tracings alone therefore is unable to take into account the various sounds and frequency changes in the Doppler signal that may indicate flow obstructions and stenoses. This may lead to an incorrect diagnosis, especially in the cerebrovascular system, in which normal flow is of high velocity and always above the zero baseline. Unless a lesion occludes a vessel, the high-velocity and high-frequency jet effect distal to the obstruction may often have the parameters of a normal internal carotid signal. A well-trained examiner should be able to hear these changes; unfortunately, many times the examiner and the interpreting clinician are not the same person. The examiner may note, for the benefit of the interpreting clinician, where signals that are suggestive of disease occur; but any inexperience or uncertainty can confuse the diagnosis and cause erroneous interpretation.

Sound spectral analysis of Doppler signals is a technique that allows the information lost in strip-chart recording to be permanently recorded in a visual format. This method involves analyzing the frequencies present in a Doppler-shifted signal by Fourier transformation, with subsequent *sorting* of the frequencies by a series of filters.[4,13]

The relative strengths of the sorted frequencies are assigned respective brightness levels, color codes on certain analyzers, or can be displayed as a histogram of power levels at a given moment in the waveforms as a function of time. Note that the gradients of gray or color levels do *not* signify the relative velocity; this is shown as a deflec-

tion above (and below, on bidirectional devices) a zero baseline as in the strip-chart recorder, except that antegrade and retrograde flow can be shown simultaneously. Velocity or frequency or both are shown on the vertical axis of the display; time is displayed along the horizontal axis (Fig. 37-5).

Instrumentation

The spectrum analyzer has been available in many forms for a number of years. Early devices required recording several seconds of the signal intended for analysis on a built-in tape. The waveform was traced on a paper covered rotating drum as the tape played over and over, and the process usually took a minute or longer before the sonogram was complete. This method is outdated now and had many disadvantages. The signals were not analyzed as they were being obtained (real time), and the process was not practical in a heavy case load since it meant tape recording the examination for later analysis processing. Another disadvantage was that many of the higher and lower frequencies were lost in the transfer from tape to tape. In addition, the frequency display on these older devices was extremely difficult to interpret, and is as far removed from today's spectral analysis displays as B-mode scanning with storage oscilloscopes is from today's digital gray-scale B-scanners.

Modern devices intended for Doppler flow analysis present the data in real time and allow high-quality calculations of flow velocities and frequency distribution. These devices are either incorporated into high-resolution B-scanners or are available as stand-alone units that can be attached to quadrature outputs or audio outlets defined for spectrum-analyzer use. They can display

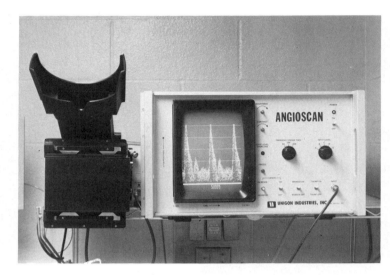

FIG. 37-8.   Typical spectral analyzer (unidirectional, gray scale).

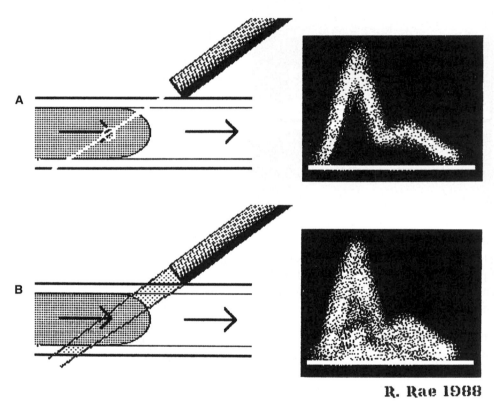

FIG. 37-9.   Pulsed vs. continuous-wave Doppler. The pulsed Doppler, **A,** allows discrete sampling of a particular flow stream from the center or edges of the vessel. The continuous-wave Doppler, **B,** samples the entire range of flow across the vessel and shows all the velocities present in the beam path at once.

concentration of flow at the baseline at peak systole and a poorly defined envelope with incresaed systolic velocity during the postsystolic/diastolic phase. This concentration corresponds with an audible *bruit* (see below).

Continuous-wave Doppler and pulsed Doppler waveforms are different on the spectral display and require modifying interpretive technique because of these differences. Continuous-wave spectrals almost always appear to have spectral broadening because flow across the entire vessel as well as any other vessels in the beam path is displayed, and the slower velocity flow along the vessel walls fills in the window. With a pulsed Doppler the sample is almost always taken from the center stream; thus the slower velocities along the walls are avoided. Pulsed Doppler spectra are inevitably cleaner and are more accurate indicators of turbulence and spectral broadening; however, continuous-wave Doppler spectra are better indicators of peak velocity/frequencies and for showing turbu-

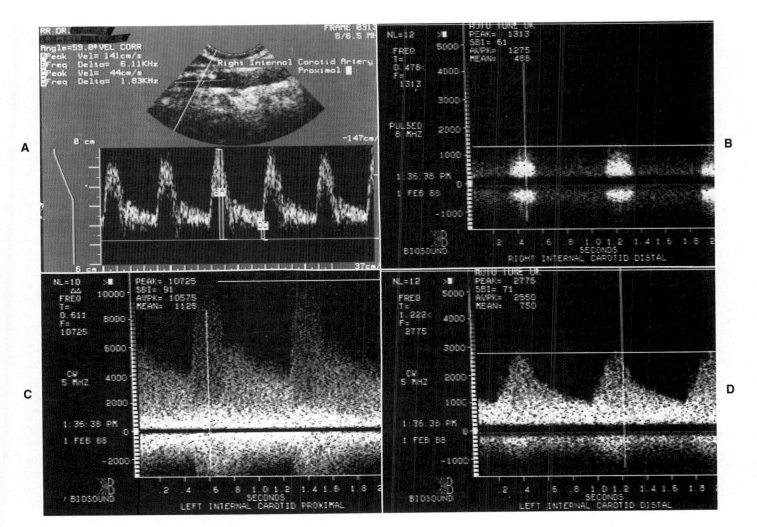

FIG. 37-10. Typical stenotic flow responses in an internal carotid artery on a spectrum analyzer. **A,** Moderate turbulence with velocity increase in a moderate stenosis. **B,** A severely turbulent and diminished pattern consistent with flow distal to a near-occlusion. **C,** Severely turbulent signal and velocity increase typical of a jet-effect response across a severe stenosis. **D,** Typical poststenotic signal 2 cm distal to the signal in **C.**

lence in the vessel, since pulsed Doppler sample placement may miss flow jets directed at areas other than where the sample is taken unless a color-flow imaging system is used, which allows the streamline to be seen (Fig. 37-9).

Note should be made that there is always some spectral broadening near a flow divider (such as the carotid bifurcation), and true flow samples should be taken at least 1 cm downstream for accurate readings.

In situations of arterial stenosis, the following diagnostic characteristics may be seen:

1. Proximal to the stenosis a normal or slightly blunted waveform may be seen. The peak frequency should be normal, and there may or may not be a rounding of the peak. The separation between the first and second components (dicrotic notch) may disappear due to vascular elastic changes along the stenosed area. The window may show some flow scattering throughout.

2. Across the stenosis an increased-frequency (higher-velocity) waveform will usually be seen. The same char-

acteristics as in the proximal waveform may be noted, and the envelope may begin to break up. The velocity will usually increase directly with the degree of stenosis. The window may also being to disappear as spectral broadening increases. A corresponding increase in pitch will be heard with the Doppler. It may help to remember that cerebrovascular flow remains nearly constant until a hemodynamically significant stenosis (at 60% to 70% luminal reduction) occurs.[1]

3. Immediately distal to the stenotic area, disturbed or turbulent flow may be found ranging from a strained burbling to a high-pitched hissing Doppler signal. Peak systolic velocity and frequency increase as the flow stream increases by the jet effect, originating at the stenosis; an area of flow stagnation immediately distal to the plaque or lesion near the artery wall may cause turbulence during systole (Fig. 37-10). The spectral waveform will have a ragged-appearing indistinct envelope, with widely distributed frequencies, and a completely absent window. The severity of the stenosis may be

judged from the level of envelope disruption and frequency distribution. Turbulence and eddy formation will cause an increase in the higher-energy intensities at the baseline[13] and in severe cases may cause a completely disrupted waveform with apparent velocity reductions *at systole* in bidirectional analyzers. Pulsatility may be absent, and the pitch may either increase or decrease with the sound becoming rough and harsh.

4. A signal obtained more distally from the stenosis, away from the turbulent region, may assume the appearance of a reduced waveform with even intensity and broadening throughout, disturbed envelope edges, and no visible flow components. The peak frequency/velocity may be markedly diminished compared with the peak of the waveform seen directly at the level of stenosis. The peak frequency may be markedly rounded. Severely diminished flow may become almost flat in appearance.

5. In total occlusion a sharp thudding or thumping sound may be heard in the patent portion of the vessel immediately proximal to the block. Flow may actually drop to or below the baseline, and a very irregular-appearing spectral waveform with no distinguishing characteristics may be seen. This is caused from flow eddies within the stump.[4] No flow should be heard in the area of occlusion, although "blips" may sometimes be seen in visibly occluded arteries; these are artifactual and can be caused by vertical motion of the vessel detected by the Doppler or by nearby pulsatile vessels if the sample volume is set too wide or placed in an atrophied vessel.

The characteristics of flow increase across a stenosis apply to extremity arteries as well. Distal to the stenosis a rounded blunt waveform will be noted, with disappearance of the window and evidence of low flow velocities. As flow decreases, a flattened signal close to the baseline will usually be found. Remember that in the extremity arteries, loss of the second retrograde component signifies stenosis or occlusion proximally, and the flow envelope may remain well defined regardless of the level of flow reduction.

DOPPLER COLOR FLOW

Within the last 5 years major advances have been made in Doppler technology toward creating a system that can superimpose a visible Doppler flow pattern in color over the standard gray-scale real-time image. While the biggest and most successful application of this technique has been in the cardiac field, much finer resolution devices have been developed for assessing the peripheral vascular system.

Existing commercial color-flow systems use linear phased-array transducers with integral pulsed-Doppler circuitry from 3.5 MHz (for abdominal applications) to 7.5 MHz. During a given moment of scanning the reflected echoes from tissue in the ultrasound beam also has as part of the reflected information Doppler-shifted flow information from the red blood cells in vascular structures in the image plane as mentioned above. The circuitry in these devices allows an examiner to show both the real-time gray-scale image information and the pulsed-Doppler velocity information from the moving blood simultaneously on the same screen. The moving blood velocities are range gated for depth localization, and returning velocities are assigned a color value proportional to their velocity and direction of flow. In most machines flow toward the transducer is assigned a shade of red and flow away from the transducer is assigned a shade of blue (this is switchable depending on probe angle). Velocity assignment runs from a dark color for slower flow to white for higher velocities for each direction. Since every element in the phased array is therefore simultaneously acting as a pulsed Doppler transducer, the effect on-screen is that of a real-time color display of blood flow superimposed over the gray-scale real-time image. High-resolution red-green-blue (RGB) color computer monitors are used to display this information.

Areas of turbulence, flow jets, direction shift, slower velocities, and areas of vascular occlusion are instantly visible and can provide an almost immediate assessment of the hemodynamics in an artery being examined. Specific velocities can be "tagged" with a green color to highlight their occurrence in a flow jet. Conventional spectrum analysis and flow sounds are also available on these machines, and sampling is more precise since the actual streamlines can be visualized and velocity vector angles can be precisely set at the flow angle of the stream seen.

These systems unfortunately have their drawbacks as well. Doppler shift information is only available in vessels parallel to the transducer face if a standoff wedge at about 18 degrees to the plane of the vessel of interest is attached to the transducer. Lesser degree angles usually result in little or no Doppler shift. The color-flow imagers currently available are extremely expensive and out of reach for nearly all but the most well-endowed medical centers (one can buy three conventional scanners for the price of one color-flow unit). Indeed, some companies often charge a premium to upgrade an existing black-and-white machine to color and charge it for *each* transducer available for the machine. There is limited reimbursement available from insurance companies for color studies at the time of writing, often making it difficult to financially justify acquiring a color-flow imager and often causing a wide variance in patient fees. The units are far from compact and cannot be easily moved, and the internal circuitry is often delicate and susceptible to shock. At this time resolution of gray-scale structures is sometimes not as fine as in noncolor machines because of the heavy computer memory required to generate color flow and the system trade-offs required to produce color. Resolution is, however, improving as manufacturers seek solutions to improve the quality. As the cost of memory chips decreases and the technology becomes more mass-produced, it is likely that color flow will eventually be in the reach of the average institution.

Following are some applications where color flow can be of value:

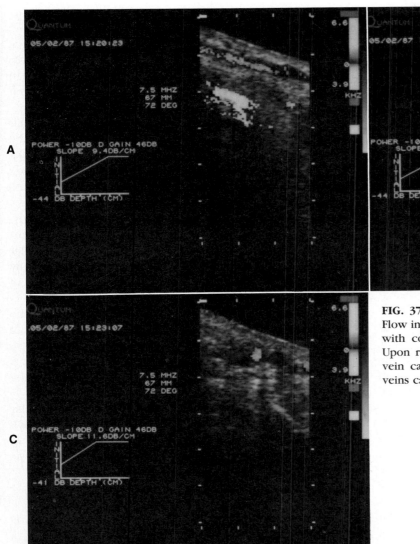

FIG. 37-11. Color-flow responses in an incompetent vein. A, Flow in the posterior tibial vein enhances (light gray and white) with compression, as does flow in a superficial collateral. B, Upon release of the compression, reflux within the superficial vein can be seen (red). C, In transverse, the posterior tibial veins can be seen flanking the posterior tibial artery.

1. *Assessment of venous function.* Color-flow devices can provide an almost immediate assessment of venous flow, valve function, reflux in veins, and presence of thrombus. Since "where there's no color, there's no flow," one can instantly pinpoint a possible thrombosis (provided angle requirements are met). Reflux through perforator veins in cases of venous insufficiency during compression is immediately seen, as is a velocity increase distal to an obstruction or in a shunting superficial vein (Fig. 37-11). Venous use of color flow shows the most significant promise among all applications, especially since extrinsic compression of a vein can be eliminated.

2. *Carotid artery hemodynamics.* Color-flow displays of turbulence, velocity jets, and diminished flow are of immense value during an exam as well as the ability to detect an internal, external, or common carotid artery occlusion or vascular steal syndrome. Nonaxial flow jets and ulcers in plaque can be instantly identified. It also allows precise velocity angles to be calculated. The ability to show minimal or absent flow in a patent internal carotid when a CVA or siphon obstruction is present also is of value. It also is of value in the follow-up of postendarterectomy patients and in cases of carotid body tumor.

3. *Abdominal vasculature.* Color flow can be used to advantage in evaluating portal vein flow, aortic flow and aneurysms, renal artery flow, renal transplant hemodynamics, and vena caval obstruction. It is excellent for enabling discrimination of residual lumen from intramural thrombus in aneurysms.

4. *Peripheral arterial evaluation.* Color flow can aid in the assessment of extremity artery stenoses as well as in evaluation of the function of bypass grafts and the presence of AV fistulas. Color flow is becoming the imaging method of choice for ruling out pseudoaneurysms, since it can instantly discriminate a hematoma with no internal flow from a pseudoaneurysm.

CONCLUSION AND GENERAL COMMENTS

Doppler techniques are accurate, sensitive, and completely noninvasive methods for evaluating the peripheral arterial and venous systems, the cerebrovascular systems, and major portions of the abdominal vascular system. The techniques are indeed somewhat involved and are often confusing to the beginner and especially the sonographers who have suddenly been told that they will "learn Doppler" and are thrown into a new environment. The techniques are often learned best by on-the-job training or attendance of any number of excellent courses that are available, often by the companies that make the equipment.

Probably the most important fact about Doppler techniques that can be stressed here is that the technologist must know the basics thoroughly. Since the physician who interprets the examination will often read it at a later time, the technologist is the direct link to the quality and accuracy of the examination. If the technologist is unable to produce an accurate and diagnostic evaluation, then the quality of care the patient receives suffers. I personally have seen many false diagnoses result from poor technique and lack of attention to the quality of the signals recorded. There is really no excuse for performing a poor-quality examination, since there are educational courses, numerous books available, and competent vascular technologists who can give helpful advice. Membership in professional organizations that deal primarily with noninvasive vascular testing can provide a wealth of knowledge and information. A typical organization is the Society of Vascular Technology (SVT), which publishes a quarterly journal for its members and has courses and seminars across the country that can help train the technologist in nearly every form of noninvasive testing available.

A technologist should thoroughly know the following before performing an examination:

1. *Vascular anatomy.* This is an absolute must. If a technologist does not know where a specific artery or vein lies and where branches are given off, then doing a Doppler study is a hopeless endeavor and is also going to be nondiagnostic or even detrimental to the patient. Study the vascular anatomy thoroughly and imagine the course of the artery or vein in question superimposed on the skin. Follow it with a Doppler to see if you envision it correctly. This simple technique can speed up the learning process immeasurably.
2. *"Knobology."* If the technologist does not know what the controls do or how the Doppler or duplex device works, then the results will show it. Take the time to read the manuals and practice whenever possible — there are simple controls on every Doppler that can do tremendous things for the quality of the examination, provided they are used. Study the examinations of others and feel free to contact an applications technologist from the company that manufactures your machine for information and help regarding image quality and equipment use.
3. *Hemodynamics.* Know the flow direction in the vessel you are examining. Be aware of what changes will occur if disease processes or collaterals are present. Learn the ranges of normal and abnormal flow velocities and frequencies. Learn the normal sound patterns and spectral appearances of arteries and veins. Learn to expect the type of flow signal that can occur if a significant-appearing stenosis is seen.
4. *Disease conditions.* Learn about the types of vascular disease and what their appearance and effect is on the circulation. Be aware of these while doing an examination so that thorough documentation of the condition is made and all appropriate arteries or veins involved are adequately assessed.

Almost all of the points above will be thoroughly covered in the following chapters. While this does not purport to be a definitive text regarding peripheral vascular Doppler and duplex vascular scanning, no text can truly be that since there are numerous ways and approaches of evaluating the vascular system and new advances are being made every day. While some techniques may become obsolete within a very short period of time, some remain the "state of the art," and it is likely that many of the techniques discussed here will remain in the latter category. A technologist can only be made a better diagnostician by knowing and practicing the material presented here.

Whether these techniques are employed by a vascular technologist or sonographer, a vascular surgeon or radiologist, remember that the ultimate beneficiary of the techniques and technology of noninvasive vascular diagnosis is the patient.

SUMMARY

1. The ideal noninvasive vascular diagnostic method is truly noninvasive, has a high overall accuracy, is atraumatic and comfortable to the patient, can be performed quickly, and does not require bulky equipment or long setup procedures. Doppler and high-resolution real-time ultrasonic techniques fulfill these requirements.

2. A directional Doppler is capable of showing the *direction* as well as the *relative velocity* of flow.

3. Although continuous-wave devices are useful in many applications, there are a few pitfalls in resolution since everything in the path of the beam is detected. Pulsed Doppler devices enable discrimination to be made.

4. A combination of pulsed and continuous-wave Doppler techniques often obtains the best results, since the two technologies are complimentary and compensate for each modality's respective weaknesses.

5. Units that incorporate both imaging and Doppler are generally referred to as duplex machines.

6. Advances in Doppler technology allow a visible, color Doppler pattern to be superimposed over the standard gray-scale real-time image. Some applications where color flow can be of value include assessment of venous function, carotid artery hemodynamics, abdominal vasculature, and peripheral arterial evaluation.

REFERENCES

1. Baker JD: Poststress Doppler ankle pressures: a comparison of treadmill exercise with two other methods of induced hyperemia, Arch Surg 113:1171, 1978.
2. Barnes RW: Axioms on acute arterial occlusion of an extremity, Hosp Med 14(6):34, 1978.
3. Barnes RW et al: Doppler ultrasonic evaluation of peripheral arterial disease, Iowa City, 1975, University of Iowa Press.
4. Barnes RW et al: Doppler ultrasonic spectrum analysis of carotid velocity signals, Richmond, 1980, Medical College of Virginia.
5. Barnes RW and Garrett WV: Intraoperative assessment of arterial reconstruction by Doppler ultrasound, Surg Obstet Gynecol 146:896, 1978.
6. Baron HC and Hiesiger E: Significance of ankle blood pressure in the diagnosis of peripheral vascular disease, Am Surg 45:289, 1979.
7. Bergan JJ and Yao JST: Gangrene and severe ischemia of the lower extremities, New York, 1978, Grune & Stratton, Inc.
8. Bernstein EF et al: Noninvasive diagnostic techniques in vascular disease, St. Louis, 1978, The CV Mosby Co.
9. Diethrich EB, editor: Noninvasive cardiovascular diagnosis, Baltimore, 1978, University Park Press.
10. Eden, A: In Aaslid R, editor: Transcranial Doppler sonography, New York, 1985, Springer-Verlag.
11. Johnson J: Angiography and ultrasound in diagnosis of carotid artery diseases: a comparison, Contemp Surg vol 20, 1982.
12. Juergens JL, Spittell JA, and Fairbairn JF: Peripheral vascular diseases, Philadelphia, 1980, WB Saunders Co.
13. Myers L, Avecilla LS, et al: Correlative studies of color-coded real-time spectral analysis of flow in model arterial systems and selected cerebrovascular pathology. Illustrative display, Bowman Gray School of Medicine (Personal communication.)

38

Arterial Sonography and Doppler Examination

RICHARD E. RAE II

The Doppler examinations pertaining to the arterial system are probably the simplest to learn and interpret. The techniques still require a high degree of examiner familiarity and a thorough knowledge of the arterial anatomy to enable confident and accurate diagnoses to be made. This section will discuss basic arterial occlusive syndromes and disease processes, Doppler signal characteristics, flow physiology, anatomy, examination of the lower and upper extremities, and related studies.

TYPES OF ARTERIAL OCCLUSIVE CONDITIONS

Occlusive diseases and other pathologic conditions are common to arteries anywhere in the body and present clinically in various manners. Extensive coverage of these is beyond the scope of this work, but several of the more common diseases and pathoses that the examiner is likely to encounter will be discussed.

Atherosclerosis accounts for the greatest percentage of occlusive diseases in which the arteries are constricted or narrowed, preventing adequate flow to the distal portion of the arterial tributaries. Atherosclerosis is distinguished from arteriosclerosis by the fact that the former is usually a focal accumulation of lipids, calcium, fibrous tissue, and blood products in the intima of an artery whereas the latter is a generalized aging process in the entire system, shown by intimal thickening, calcification, and loss of vascular wall elasticity.

Focal atherosclerotic areas are also known as *plaques*. Plaques are usually elevated lesions of the intima that can be fatty or fibrous and that project into the lumen of an artery, narrowing the flow path and reducing flow. They have amorphous, or atheromatous, cores and may calcify or become ulcerated and thromboembolic. Cast-off emboli from plaques may occlude distal capillaries and tributaries, causing ischemia (deficiency of blood) to the areas they supply. These thrombi are composed of platelet material, and it is thought that platelet secretions may interact with vessel walls and actually initiate atherosclerosis. The causes of arterial thrombosis are often related to plaque formations but may also be due to embolization from cardiac diseases, such as occurs in subacute bacterial endocarditis with vegetation formation or myocardial infarctions with an accompanying thrombus. Atherosclerosis may also be referred to in severe cases as *atherosclerosis obliterans* (ASO).[2,5,18]

Congenital arterial anomalies, such as congenital arteriovenous fistulas that cause abnormal communication between arteries and veins, can occur. Coarctation, or kinking, of an artery is also possible. Some other anomalies include variations in the anatomic course of an artery, absence of a normal vessel, and separate branches appearing in different locations or at unusual origins. The use of real-time sonography may help in questionable cases.[3,11]

Raynaud's phenomenon is related to cold and abrupt temperature changes that cause vascular spasm in the digits and resulting obstruction. Purplish fingers and toes are often seen in this disorder. Vasospasm occurring by itself is termed Raynaud's disease, whereas vasospasm resulting from another condition is Raynaud's phenomenon. The latter is often seen in lupus erythematosus, arthritis, and other diseases.[18,23]

Buerger's disease is a form of presenile spontaneous gangrene that affects the distal arteries in the digits and toes. It is caused by heavy cigarette smoking and can be distinguished from atherosclerotic disease on an arteriogram by a smooth, well-defined artery proximal to a distinct occlusion point. The fingers and toes are usually involved simultaneously, and Raynaud's phenomenon may also occur with this syndrome. The onset is much more acute than that of atherosclerotic occlusion and usually presents as a sudden total arterial occlusion. Intense rest pain may occur independently in Buerger's disease, rather than as a progressive process following claudication. (See "Symptoms of Arterial Disease.") This disease is also termed thromboangiitis obliterans (TAO). It is treated by selective amputation and/or sympathectomy in extreme cases.[8]

Frostbite involves the actual freezing of tissue. The cause of arterial occlusion has been attributed to permanent vasoconstriction in response to the cold with or without freezing of blood or fluids. The exact cause of tissue injury is not fully understood. The emergency treatment of warming the affected part is an attempt to restore circulation by relaxing the vasospasm. If flow is not restored in time to save viable tissue, necrosis of the ischemic parts will occur and amputation may be necessary.[18]

Arteritis is usually caused by collagen-related diseases. In cases such as Takayasu's syndrome the media of the artery becomes thickened and swollen, occluding the arterial lumen without changing the external configuration of the vessel itself. This process is usually detected by a diminishing pulse noted over a time. Takayasu's does not localize but usually occurs in the entire arterial system from the aortic root outward. Other types may occur in isolated vessels.[18]

Mechanical compression of an artery involves obstruction by compression of the vessel between or against another part of the body. Examples are thoracic outlet syndrome, in which the arteries, veins, and nerve plexuses are compressed against the first rib or muscle groups by arm flexion and abduction, and malignant tumors (such as chemodectomas and specifically carotid body tumors) and loculated infections that produce purulent lesions or masses, both syndromes which can compromise nearby vasculature and compress the vessels against other areas of the body.

Entrapment syndromes cause problems in a similar manner to mechanical compression syndromes but are often related to congenital anomalies or trauma and usually involve muscle fascia or ligament obstructions in areas such as the popliteal artery or the anterior compartment of the lower leg.

SYMPTOMS OF ARTERIAL DISEASE*

Claudication. This term comes from the Latin verb "to limp."[13] Patients with claudication notice tiring and pain in the limb distal to the occlusion with exertion. A walking patient may feel pain in the calf first, often within a measurable distance. The pain and tiring will progress to muscle cramping if the patient persists (e.g., for a city block). If the patient rests, the cramping and pain will resolve completely. The symptoms will resume with the onset of activity. In the arms a patient may feel pain, tiring, and cramping if extensive lifting or elevation of the affected arm is performed. In either legs or arms the affected limb may give way if too much demand is placed on it.

Dependent rubor and elevation pallor. Erythema is often seen in patients with advancing arterial disease, along with drying and flaking of skin and thickening of the nails. If the extremity is hung dependent, it will usually present puffy and red digits and even the entire forefoot or hand in advanced disease. If the limb is elevated, the redness will disappear and the limb will become increasingly pale.

Rest pain. This symptom of very severe arterial insufficiency is usually found in cases of lower-than-normal resting blood flow. The pain will be localized in specific areas of inadequate perfusion (e.g., toes, heel, calf). It is often described as a burning pain that will keep the patient awake at night. The skin is red and thin, often shiny. This symptom is a definite sign that arterial reconstruction or some other means must be undertaken to prevent loss of the limb.

Coldness of the limb. This is due to inadequate arterial flow and is readily noticed by the examiner.

Gangrene. When the disease advances to near cessation of flow, circulation to the distal portion of the digits (with the most easily occluded vessels) will often be blocked completely. The tissue will necrose and gangrene

---

*References 2, 3, 5, 8, 12, 18.

will set in, appearing as a black shriveling spot or region that progresses and from which fluids exude. Amputation is often the only course, although recent advances in hyperbaric pressure chamber medicine have enabled many largely necrosed limbs to be saved in whole or in part.

Regardless of the symptoms and signs, arterial disease is a dangerous entity. It depletes the blood flow to vital organs, impairs normal activity, and often acts as a precursor to more serious conditions.

FLOW DYNAMICS IN THE PERIPHERAL ARTERIAL SYSTEM

The normal arterial Doppler flow signal is evaluated by the chart tracing as well as by the audio signals. Both positive and negative chart deflections exist in the arterial signal, again with antegrade flow being positive and retrograde flow being negative. Probe position is critical in the arterial examination. If the sound beam is perpendicular to the direction of flow, no Doppler shift will occur and a flat tracing will result. The examiner should use the flow direction gauges and the signal strength as heard through the speakers to determine the precise angle for optimal blood flow sampling.

The normal arterial Doppler flow signal in the extremities consists of three components: a large *positive deflection* with *systole*, a period of *net flow reversal* to the *negative side* of the zero line, and a lesser *diastolic positive* deflection (Fig. 38-1). The period of reversal is due to the high resistance of the vascular bed in the extremities. In vasodilated conditions the flow will be seen primarily on the positive side, but the three deflections will still be present. The normal arterial flow signal, because of the three components, is said to be *triphasic.*[3]

In cases of arterial obstruction the flow signal begins to lose one or more components, becoming *biphasic* or *monophasic.* The flow pattern will tend to remain triphasic proximal to the obstruction but will begin to show diminished systolic components and lose the diastolic component distally, secondary to narrowing across the occlusion site and in some cases to ischemia-induced vasodilation in the distal vascular bed (Fig. 38-2).

PHYSIOLOGY OF FLOW PRESSURES[3]

Segmental blood pressure measurement in the limb is the basis of the Doppler examination in the extremities. To understand what happens, the examiner must understand some basic physiology of blood flow dynamics.

Poiseuille's law pertains to pressure gradients of fluids through arterial segments in the body. Two factors determine the flow: (1) the pressure difference across the segment and (2) the resistance of the segment. Poiseuille's law is stated as the following equation:

$$\Delta P = Q8Lv/\pi r^4$$

where the flow, Q, as determined by the length of the segment, L, viscosity of the blood, v, and radius of the segment, r, varies directly with the pressure gradient, ΔP, across the segment and indirectly with the resistance (interaction of L, v, and r) across it. ($8/\pi$ is a mathematical

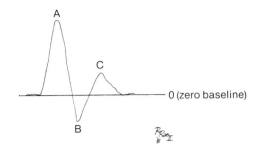

Fig. 38-1. Normal arterial waveform in the extremities. *A* is the first diastolic component, *B* the brief period of reversal, and *C* the diastolic component.

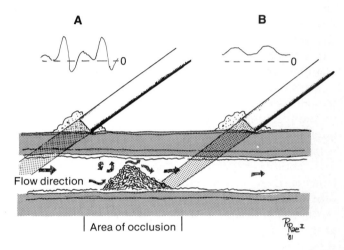

Fig. 38-2. Diagram of flow patterns proximal and distal to an occlusion. **A** shows the waveform obtained proximally, with all normal components present. **B** shows the characteristic loss of components and flow diminishing found in the segment distal to the block.

constant.) This can best be applied physiologically to arteries in which the pressure gradient across the segment can be increased by increasing the flow through the segment or decreasing the radius of the lumen.

When obstructions are present, blood is forced through collateral channels, where the resistance is higher than in the normal vessel (Fig. 38-3). Thus, as flow is forced around the obstruction and into collaterals, the pressure drop along that segment is increased. This information is important for the arterial Doppler examination since the examiner must be aware of pressure drops that can occur and must understand the mechanism of the pressure drop distal to an occlusive site.

DOPPLER LOWER EXTREMITY ARTERIAL EXAMINATION
Arterial anatomy of the lower extremities[14]

To understand the Doppler lower extremity examination, one needs to have a thorough knowledge of the vascular anatomy as it pertains to the Doppler examination. Only the arteries that are directly accessible and that figure into the examination will be discussed.

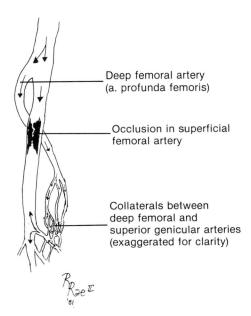

Fig. 38-3. Diagram of recovery in a segment distal to a superficial femoral occlusion due to collateralization from the profunda femoris.

Flow to the extremities comes from the *abdominal aorta*. The aorta bifurcates about the level of the umbilicus to form the *common iliac* arteries. The common iliac vessels then bifurcate into the *internal* and *external iliac* arteries. The internal iliac (hypogastric) supplies the buttock and genital area. The external iliac supplies the leg and becomes the *common femoral* artery at approximately the level of the inguinal ligament. Several branches are given off, of which the *profunda femoris* is the most important. It comes off about 2 to 5 cm below the inguinal ligament and supplies the bone and muscles of the thigh.

At this point the common femoral becomes the *superficial femoral* artery. It runs along the medial surface of the thigh and curves posteriorly behind the knee to become the *popliteal* artery.

The popliteal artery continues behind the knee joint and gives off the *anterior tibial* artery 3 to 6 cm below the popliteal fossa. The popliteal then terminates as the *posterior tibial* and *peroneal* arteries (Fig. 38-4).

The anterior tibial descends through muscles along the tibia and becomes the *dorsalis pedis* at the level of the ankle. The dorsalis pedis then runs superficially and dorsally on the medial side of the foot to terminate in the deep plantar arch between the first and second metatarsals.

The posterior tibial artery descends along the posterior surface of the tibia to run posterior to the medial malleolus.

The peroneal artery descends deeply on the fibular side of the leg and becomes accessible anterior to the lateral malleolus (Fig. 38-5).

Routine lower extremity arterial examination

There are several points that should be emphasized in connection with this examination.

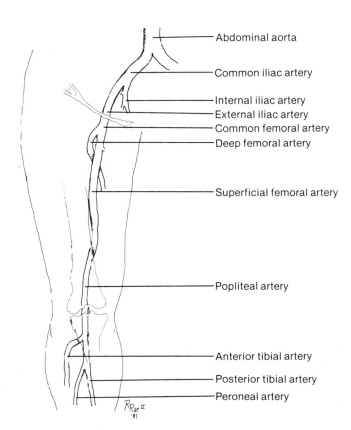

Fig. 38-4. Arterial blood supply to the lower extremity.

The first step is to obtain as complete a history as possible from the patient, the patient's chart, or both. The emphasis should be placed on the following information:

1. If the patient is *claudicating*, note whether one or both legs are affected, where the pain is felt (calf, thigh, hip, etc.), and if it is a tiring or a cramp in the muscle. The distance the patient can ambulate prior to stopping because of the pain should be noted and whether the symptoms are relieved by rest.

2. Palpate the *pulses* at the femoral, popliteal, posterior tibial, and dorsalis pedis arteries. Weak or absent pulses should be noted.

3. Check for *night cramping* or *rest pain*. Remember that simple aching or pain "at rest" may not constitute the specific diagnosis of rest pain unless the other criteria of critical ischemia are met (e.g., skin changes, absent pulses, limited mobility).

4. Note the *skin color and condition*. Check for dry skin, erythema of the toes, thickened nails, gangrenous spots, and unhealed ulcers.

5. Check for *known vascular diseases, past bypass surgeries, diabetes, cardiac disease, smoking, hypertension,* and any *family history* of these atherosclerotic risk factors. Also, when a patient states that he or she has had a "bypass," inquire further as to whether this means a *peripheral arterial bypass* in the extremity or a *coronary bypass*. This is important, since scars from the harvesting of saphenous veins for coronary surgery often appear identical to those encountered in peripheral arterial bypassing (please see **Doppler Examination of the Postoperative Patient**).

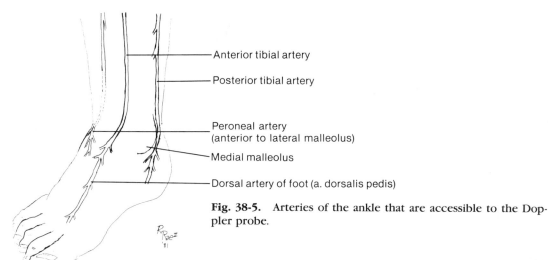

Anterior tibial artery

Posterior tibial artery

Peroneal artery
(anterior to lateral malleolus)

Medial malleolus

Dorsal artery of foot (a. dorsalis pedis)

Fig. 38-5. Arteries of the ankle that are accessible to the Doppler probe.

Blood pressure cuffs are then applied to the legs for measuring the pressure gradients (except in certain postoperative cases; see Doppler Examination of the Postoperative Patient.) The cuffs are placed in four locations on each leg: one on the *ankle,* one just below the knee on the *calf,* one just above the knee on the *lower thigh,* and one just below the groin on the *upper thigh* (Fig. 38-6).

The main requirement is that the cuffs be long enough to wrap around the patient's legs. Narrow cuffs should be used for the thigh pressures despite the higher-than-normal pressure readings that can be expected there. An aneroid sphygmomanometer can then be attached to each cuff, or one manometer or automatic cuff inflator can be easily transferred from cuff to cuff using a Luer-Lok or friction type of connector.

When the four cuffs have been placed on the legs, another one is placed on the arm to take a brachial blood pressure.

The brachial artery is examined at its site on the medial side of the antecubital fossa, and the probe is angled cephalad until the most satisfactory signal is obtained. A tracing is made of the Doppler signal. With the probe still in place, the cuff is inflated above the point at which the signal disappears. It is then deflated about 2 to 4 mm/s until the systolic pulse is heard. This breakthrough point is the systolic pressure. Deflation continues until the fourth returning sound corresponding to the diastolic antegrade component on the waveform is heard and the flow resumes its normal pattern. The point where the "slurred" sound of the third and fourth component is heard marks the diastolic pressure. Recording the pulse tracing is not necessary but can help the examiner locate the point where the flow resumes its normal pattern until proficiency or "ear training" is attained. For purposes of the Doppler examination, recording the diastolic pressure is not necessary since the systolic pressure is the only component needed for calculation of the ankle/brachial index.

The foregoing steps are repeated for the other arm. The examiner then should move to the patient's feet to

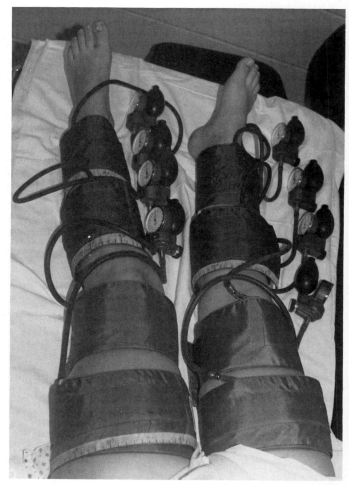

Fig. 38-6. Pressure cuffs in place on the legs for the lower extremity arterial study.

commence examination of the ankle arteries and pressures.

The posterior tibial artery is monitored and recorded at its site posterior to the medial malleolus. The probe is angled until the strongest signal is obtained. It is then kept in place, and the ankle cuff is inflated past the point where the signal disappears. Deflation begins until the systolic signal is heard, and the pressure at that point is recorded (Fig. 38-7).

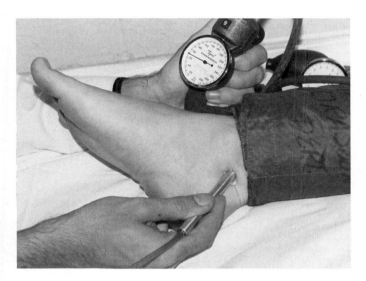

Fig. 38-7.   Examining the posterior tibial artery.

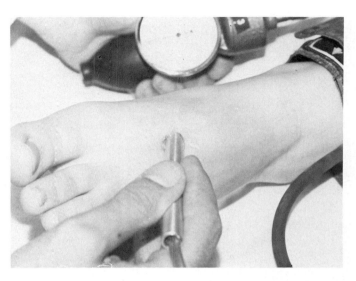

Fig. 38-8.   Examining the dorsalis pedis artery.

The examiner then moves the probe to examine the dorsalis pedis at its sites on the dorsum of the foot. Once again, the best signal is obtained and an ankle pressure is recorded in the same manner as for the posterior tibial artery (Fig. 38-8).

Before continuing, the examiner should compare waveforms and pressures of the two arteries. The artery with the higher pressure should be used to take the remaining pressures in the leg.

If flow in either the dorsalis pedis or the posterior tibial artery is unsatisfactory or absent, the peroneal artery should be examined at its site anterior to the lateral malleolus. It is examined in the same manner as were the other ankle vessels (Fig. 38-9).

The artery that is selected is then monitored. Each cuff from calf to upper thigh is inflated and deflated in turn, and the systolic blood pressure taken at each level. It is not necessary to record a tracing from the artery while the pressures are being taken. It *is* a must, however, to keep the probe stationary and motionless to prevent the systolic signal from being lost as the cuff is deflated.

When the tracings and pressures from one extremity have been taken, the procedure is repeated for the other.

After pressures have been taken at all cuff sites in both legs, the cuffs are removed. The examiner then palpates the superior border of the inguinal ligament and places the probe in position just above the ligament to determine the site for monitoring of the femoral artery (Fig. 38-10). The external iliac is actually being monitored at this level rather than the common femoral. It is better to obtain the signal here, however, than to listen below the ligament, where the bifurcation of the profunda femoris can cause confusion. The common femoral arteries are then monitored and recorded bilaterally. Some pressure on the probe may be needed to obtain a clear signal. The signals will be found lateral to the common femoral venous signals (heard as a "windstorm" sound). An arterial signal found *medial* to the vein is probably the hypogastric artery and must not be mistaken for the femoral. If

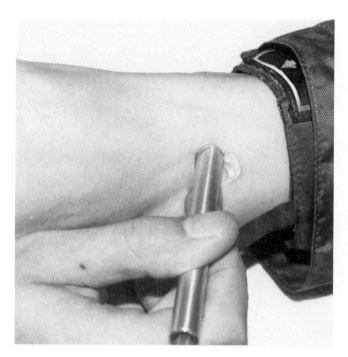

Fig. 38-9.   Examination of the peroneal artery.

in doubt, move the probe laterally and medially to locate the vein and determine the vessel's relationship. The hypogastric artery also may appear as a retrograde signal when the probe is angled cephalad.

The popliteal arteries are next to be examined and are found at their sites behind the knees. There are two methods of examining the popliteal arteries: *supine* and *prone*.

In the supine position the knees are bent to about a 75-degree angle and are relaxed laterally ("frog-leg" position) and the probe is placed in the popliteal fossa and angled cephalad (Fig. 38-11). An ample quantity of gel is required to ensure good probe-skin contact. Firm pressure may be needed to displace fat and tissue. Be careful not to occlude the artery. The probe should be angled to obtain the clearest signal with distinct waveform patterns. This

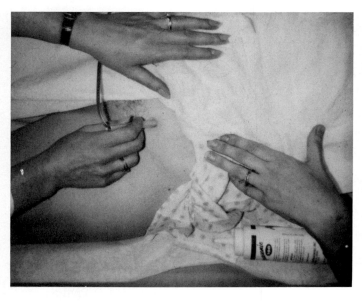

Fig. 38-10.   Examining the common femoral artery.

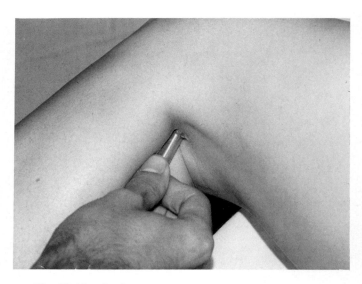

Fig. 38-11.   Supine examination of the popliteal artery.

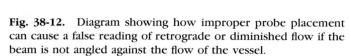

Fig. 38-12.   Diagram showing how improper probe placement can cause a false reading of retrograde or diminished flow if the beam is not angled against the flow of the vessel.

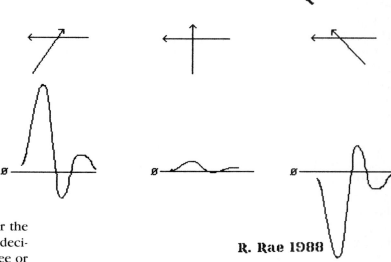

R. Rae 1988

segment of the study requires an accurate tracing, for the popliteal signal may be the determining factor in decisions as to whether an occlusion exists above the knee or in the trifurcation vessels below the knee. The best signal is obtained with the probe more toward the calf than toward the knee, to avoid catching the flow at an angle that could suggest occluded flow or even retrograde flow in the artery (Fig. 38-12).

In the prone position the patient's legs are elevated 30 to 45 degrees and are supported with a bolster or pillow (Fig. 38-13). The same basic examination technique is used as in the supine position, and the probe is angled cephalad. The advantage of this position is the ability actually to see the relationship of the popliteal fossa and the probe. It is a good position to use for the examiner-in-training.

I have found that both positions give excellent results. A major advantage of the supine position is that the patient does not need to move after the initial portion of the examination has been completed. This is especially bene-

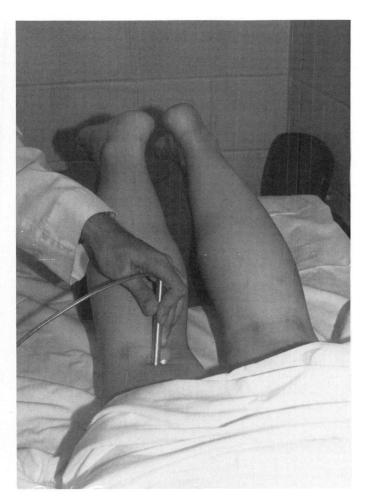

Fig. 38-13. Prone examination of the popliteal artery.

ficial to the postoperative or invalid patient who cannot turn over. The choice of examination positions is best left to the examiner's preference.

If there is a discrepancy in the signal quality between the femoral and popliteal sites, the superficial femoral artery can be examined by palpating the femur on the anterior aspect of the leg and placing the probe medial to it in the muscle groove, angling cephalad. The superficial femoral artery can be examined anywhere along the region shown in Fig. 38-14. This can help localize the level of stenosis more accurately.

In summary, these are the steps in the lower extremity arterial examination:

1. Take the patient's history, with emphasis on symptoms and past vascular disease and surgery.
2. With the patient supine, place blood pressure cuffs over the ankles, calves, lower thighs, and upper thighs bilaterally.
3. Apply cuffs to the upper arms and take bilateral brachial tracings and blood pressures.
4. Take tracings and systolic pressures from the dorsalis pedis and posterior tibial arteries at the ankle. Use the artery with the higher ankle pressure to take segmental pressures from the rest of the leg.
5. Obtain systolic pressures sequentially from the calf,

lower thigh, and upper thigh cuffs in the artery selected.
6. Examine the other leg, repeating steps 4 and 5, and remove the cuffs.
7. Check the common femoral arteries and make tracings bilaterally.
8. With the patient either supine or prone, check and record the popliteal artery pressures.
9. (Optional) If there is a loss of triphasicity between the femoral and popliteal sites, examination of the superficial femoral artery may be made at its sites in the midportion of the thigh.
10. Mount the tracings and calculate the ankle/brachial indices.

Fig. 38-14 shows the probe sites for both arterial and venous Doppler examinations. Examples of normal and abnormal examinations can be seen in the illustrative case section.

Interpretation of the lower extremity arterial examination

To determine the flow status of the extremities, one must calculate ratios of the ankle systolic pressures divided by the brachial systolic pressures. The *ankle/brachial index* is thus obtained. The higher systolic pressure of the two arteries examined at the ankle is divided by the higher systolic pressure of the two arms. This is done for each leg. The higher brachial pressure should be used for both legs to ensure uniformity.

In normal individuals the ankle/brachial index should be greater than 1.00. Patients who are asymptomatic or with slight symptoms will have indices from 0.90 to 1.00. Patients with claudication show indices of 0.50 to 0.90. Anything less than 0.50 implies rest pain or gangrene.[3,6]

Using the above criteria, the ankle/brachial ratio also can be used in *categorizing* the severity of flow impairment to the distal extremity.

- Indices running between 0.85 and 1.00 imply *mild* impairment.
- Indices running between 0.45 and 0.85 imply *moderate* impairment.
- Indices running between 0.10 and 0.45 imply *severe* impairment.

Readings falling on the borderline between categories are often interpreted as "mild to moderate," "moderate to severe," and so on.

My own experience with follow-up studies has shown that in normal individuals the ankle/brachial index can vary from 0.85 to as much as 1.10. This factor seems to depend on the relative blood pressure that a patient may have on the day of examination and whether it may change between the time the arm is checked and when the ankle pressures are taken. Therefore the examiner and interpreting physician should not expect the same index in a normal patient to be completely reproducible from examination to examination and should be aware that a lower index may not imply disease if a strong triphasic signal is found.

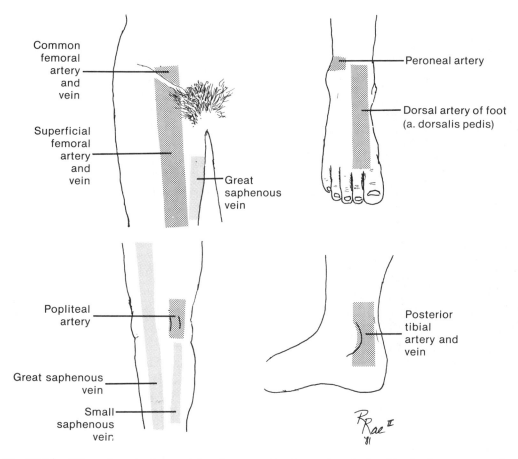

Fig. 38-14.   Sites where both arterial and venous signals can be obtained in the lower extremity.

It should also be noted that patients with calcific arteries will often have abnormally or unusually high ankle/brachial indices, such as 1.20 to 3.00. In these individuals the quality of the waveform is the best indicator of occlusion since the vessels are incompressible. Patients with extremely obese legs or diabetes also may have abnormally high indices.[8]

Further information about the circulation may be obtained by comparison of the segmental pressures. In a normal patient there will usually be no greater than 40 mm Hg of difference between any two cuffs. The pressure reading will increase as the circumference of the extremity increases. An accurate pressure at the thigh could be obtained only with an extremely wide cuff, but it is unnecessary for Doppler readings since the difference *between* cuffs is used as an indicator of a pressure drop. The upper thigh pressure should not exceed 50 mm Hg above the brachial pressure.

As mentioned, extremely high pressures (as in noncompressible arteries or other situations with pressures >300 mm Hg) in the ankle or calf imply a calcified segment. This should be noted on the report form so there will be no confusion during interpretation.

If an upper thigh pressure is significantly *less* than the brachial pressure, this implies iliac artery stenosis.

If there is a significant pressure drop between the lower and upper thigh cuffs, this implies a superficial femoral artery obstruction.

If there is a significant pressure drop between the

lower thigh and calf cuffs, a popliteal artery stenosis is implied.

If there is a significant pressure drop between the ankle and calf cuffs, this implies stenosis of the anterior tibial, posterior tibial, or peroneal arteries.

A normal arterial signal will be triphasic. Diminution or loss of any of the components implies obstruction proximal to the probe site. If flow is triphasic at the ankle, it must be triphasic at all sites above the ankle. The absence of a triphasic pattern in the popliteal artery in the presence of a normal triphasic pattern in the femoral and ankle areas implies technical error, and the artery should be rechecked.

Following is a guide to interpretation of the waveforms in cases of disease:

1. If the waveforms are triphasic in the femoral, popliteal, dorsalis pedis, and posterior tibial arteries, the flow in the leg is within normal limits.
2. If the waveforms are triphasic in the femoral and popliteal but biphasic or monophasic in either of the ankle vessels where the other is triphasic, the abnormal artery is likely the only one diseased.
3. If flow is triphasic in the femoral and popliteal but biphasic or monophasic in both ankle arteries, there is likely disease within the distal popliteal or below the popliteal involving the trifurcation vessels.
4. If flow is triphasic in the femoral but biphasic or monophasic at the popliteal and ankle vessels, this implies superficial femoral artery or popliteal artery

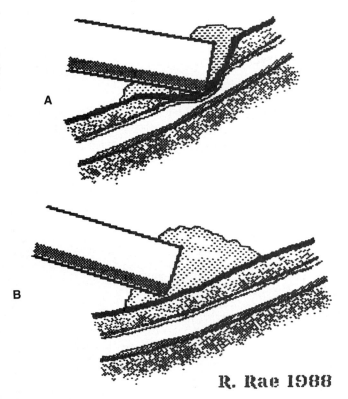

R. Rae 1988

Fig. 38-15.   Probe compression. **A,** Too much pressure with the probe can occlude a superficial artery, falsely implying an absent signal. **B,** Light contact with ample gel as a coupling window allows a signal to be obtained.

stenoses or occlusions. Examination of the proximal and distal superficial femoral artery can help locate the level of obstruction.

5. Biphasic or monophasic flow at the femoral and all sites below implies an iliac artery or distal aortic stenosis or occlusion.

6. Finally, absence of a signal in any artery with no detectable distal flow implies a complete occlusion or thrombosis of the artery. This diagnosis can be made most reliably in the trifurcation vessels; but see below.

The use of segmental pressures compared to the waveform readout and audible information is quite accurate in helping to determine the relative flow status of the extremity. However, errors in interpretation can occur and are often the result of poor examination technique. The next section will discuss these problems.

False-positive conditions and their rectification

ABSENT SIGNAL. The Doppler signal may be absent in cases of extreme atherosclerosis obliterans. The examiner must be aware, however, that absence of flow should not be observed in patients with strong pulses. The probe site should be rechecked and a careful search made for the artery by slowly moving the probe laterally and medially. Care must also be taken that an even but not extreme amount of pressure is being applied; otherwise the vessel may be occluded by the force on the probe. Careful examination is often required to register flow when there is not enough pressure in the segment to create a palpable pulse. One suggestion is to apply a generous amount of

acoustic couplant to the skin at the various probe sites along the arterial segment and place the probe within the mound of gel without actually touching the skin. The gel acts as an acoustic path, thereby allowing minimal flow information to be obtained without inadvertent pressure on the artery being examined, which might occlude it (Fig. 38-15).

FALSE DIAGNOSIS OF BIPHASIC OR MONOPHASIC FLOW AT THE POPLITEAL SITE. This is most often due to poor technique and is usually noticed because the femoral and ankle arteries exhibit normal triphasic flow. Precise positioning of the probe, careful pressure judgment, moving the probe more toward the calf than toward the thigh, and angling cephalad with respect to the course of the artery should resolve this problem. If in doubt, another attempt should be made.

FALSE DIAGNOSIS OF BIPHASIC OR MONOPHASIC FLOW AT THE FEMORAL SITE. This occurs when triphasic signals are found in the distal vessels in the postsurgical or obese patient. It is due to fatty tissue or scarring in the groin. The probe should be moved lateral to the vein and placed on either side of the scar, or with the fat held back out of the way. Angling medially or laterally into the desired area should give good results. Remember also that the beam should be 45 degrees to the *flow,* not to the skin surface. If it is impossible to obtain an accurate signal above the ligament, the report form should be noted to that effect and the proximal segment of the superficial femoral artery away from the profunda bifurcation should be obtained.

FALSE DIAGNOSIS OF RETROGRADE FLOW IN A MAJOR LIMB ARTERY. This occurs when the beam is angled through a segment at a point where flow is perceived as receding from the probe. In the femoral region the hypogastric artery can be wrongly monitored medial to the common femoral vein. The probe should be moved lateral to the vein for the correct signal. This can also occur if the probe is angled incorrectly. In the popliteal area the probe should be moved toward the calf to allow the beam to intersect flow at the correct angle.

False reversal in the posterior tibial artery and the dorsalis pedis occurs most often when flow below the knee is so reduced that pulsatility nearly vanishes and the accompanying vein sounds are mistaken for those from the artery. Careful listening is necessary to detect any trace of a pulse. The vein can be ruled out by squeezing the fleshy part of the foot and listening for a rush of flow, which will not occur in the artery.

There are several other factors that must be constantly checked to maintain accuracy. The probes must be monitored periodically for wire and electric damage, epoxy decay, or crystal damage. Manometers and cuffs should be calibrated and checked for leakage every 2 or 3 weeks.

For the examiner, concentration is required as well as practice at keeping the probe in place with one hand while inflating and releasing the cuff with the other. Cultivation of ambidextrous independence is useful to provide flexibility. Maintaining constant probe position also should be practiced to avoid losing the signal during cuff inflation and release. Experience and practice are the best ways to develop the examination technique.

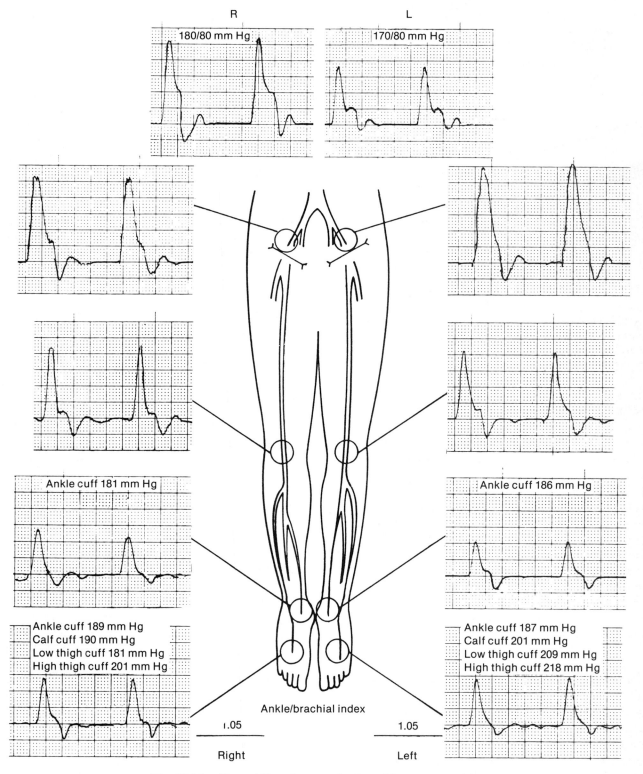

Fig. 38-16.   Normal Doppler examination of lower extremities.

Arterial lower extremity cases

CASE 1 (FIG. 38-16): NORMAL. This is an example of a normal Doppler examination of the lower extremities. Note that the waveforms are triphasic at all sites and that there are no significant segmental pressure drops between cuff sites. High thigh pressures are well above the brachial artery pressures. The ankle/brachial indices are 1.05 bilaterally, well within the normal range.

CASE 2 (FIG. 38-17): NORMAL WITH TIBIAL ARTERY STENOSIS. In this case the examination is essentially normal, as with case 1, except that there is evidence of bilateral anterior tibial artery stenoses. Note that the ankle pressures at the posterior tibial artery are slightly elevated with a slightly elevated ankle/brachial index. This patient also received a postocclusive hyperemic study (see case 2, Fig. 38-28).

CASE 3 (FIG. 38-18): RIGHT—SEVERE SUPERFICIAL FEMORAL ARTERY STENOSIS; LEFT—MILD ILIOFEMORAL ARTERY STENOSIS. In the right leg there is a relatively normal femoral signal. There is a severely turbulent signal in the right superficial femoral artery with a dramatic reduction in flow (monophasic signal) at the popliteal and anterior tibial/dorsal pedal artery. There is no signal at the right posterior tibial artery, implying possible occlusion of this vessel. The segmental pressures are consistent with the waveform analysis, as there is a significant drop in pressure between the high-thigh and low-thigh readings and distally. The right ankle/brachial index of 0.22 indicates severe impairment of flow.

In the left leg, biphasic waveforms can be seen at the femoral, popliteal, posterior tibial, and dorsal pedal sites. Pressures suggest a mild drop between the low-thigh and calf cuffs readings. The left ankle/brachial index of 0.93 is in the range of mild flow impairment.

CASE 4 (FIG. 38-19): RIGHT LEG—NORMAL. LEFT LEG—MODERATE SUBPOPLITEAL STENOSIS/TIBIAL ARTERY STENOSIS. This claudicating patient shows normal right leg waveforms, with a normal ankle/brachial index of 1.02.

The left leg, however, was symptomatic below the knee. While normal femoral and popliteal waveforms are seen, no signal was detectable in the left posterior tibial artery and there was a monophasic waveform present in the left dorsalis pedis artery. The waveform analysis coupled with the ankle/brachial index of 0.58 strongly implies a stenosis in the distal popliteal or tibial arteries with a possible posterior tibial occlusion.

CASE 5 (FIG. 38-20): DISTAL AORTA/BILATERAL ILIAC STENOSIS, MODERATE. Monophasic waveforms can be seen at all the artery sites here, and while there are no significant pressure drops within the leg, the high-thigh pressures are markedly below the systolic pressures in the brachial arteries, which is a significant finding for iliac femoral disease. Note that the ankle/brachial indices bilaterally are 0.57, in the range of low-moderate flow impairment.

CASE 6 (FIG. 38-21): DISTAL AORTA/BILATERAL ILIAC STENOSIS, SEVERE. Again, monophasic waveforms can be seen at all the artery sites here, but the amplitude is extremely low and diastole is almost flat. There are no significant pressure drops within the leg in this case either, and the high-thigh pressures are severely lower than the systolic pressures in the brachial arteries. There is additionally either bilateral anterior tibial stenosis or flow velocities in them are too slow to be detected. The ankle/brachial indices bilaterally are 0.22, in the range of severe (almost dire) impairment.

DOPPLER EXAMINATION OF THE POSTOPERATIVE PATIENT

This section will deal with the variations in the examination needed to provide adequate results in the patient who has recently undergone vascular surgery.

The basic format of the routine examination is adhered to. The brachial arteries are examined as in the routine examination unless an arterial monitor line or IV prevents it. One of the two arms is required for the ankle/brachial index determination, especially since the success or failure of the surgery often depends on the results obtained by the examiner. Again, either the higher of the two arm pressures or the single arm pressure is used. Note, however, if the only available brachial artery signal appears stenosed or occluded, the index will be inaccurate (see Doppler Upper Extremity Arterial Examination).

The history is taken, and the type of surgery and graft material (either the patient's own vein or a synthetic) is noted. If possible, a drawing of the surgical connections should be made for future reference if included in the chart, showing the vessels that were resected or ligated, the levels where the graft is attached to the artery, and the course of the graft in the extremity.

There are many different types of grafts and graft materials.* Their purpose is to shunt the main blood flow around the obstructed area to the patent sections of the artery at a lower level. Fig. 38-22 illustrates several of the most common bypasses in the lower limb.

Types of grafts and the surgical conditions for which they are used include the following:

1. *Aortoiliac.* Commonly a synthetic bifurcated graft, employed in cases of abdominal aortal aneurysm at the bifurcation of the common iliac arteries.
2. *Aortofemoral.* Also synthetic, either unilateral or bilateral, used to bypass iliac obstructions or aneurysms extending past the common iliac regions.
3. *Femorofemoral.* Synthetic, placed subcutaneously across the lower abdomen to shunt flow from a patent femoral to a point distal to the obstruction in the opposite femoral artery.
4. *Femoropopliteal.* Synthetic or autogenous saphenous vein; in the latter case the patient's own great or small saphenous vein is removed and sutured into place around superficial femoral obstructions.
5. *Femorotibial.* Same materials as in the femoropopliteal graft, but insertion is in either the anterior or the posterior tibial arteries; it is passed subcutaneously on the medial surface of the leg and may be palpated easily at the knee area; used to bypass obstructions extending through the popliteal artery and/or involving the trifurcation vessels. *Text continued on p. 907.*

Text continued on p. 907.

---

*References 4, 7, 10, 16, 19.

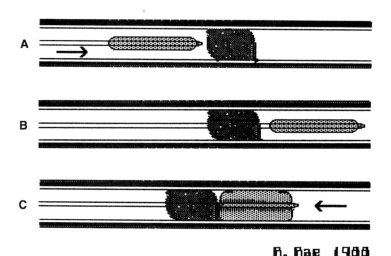

R. Rae 1988

Fig. 38-23. Embolectomy. **A,** The catheter is pushed through the embolus, and the balloon is inflated distal to it, **B.** The catheter is withdrawn, pulling the embolus with it, **C.**

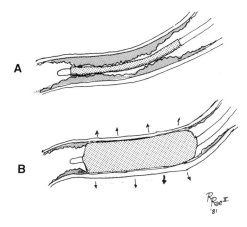

Fig. 38-24. Percutaneous transluminal angioplasty. **A,** Positioning the balloon along the diseased segment. **B,** Inflation of the balloon and dispersion of the plaque.

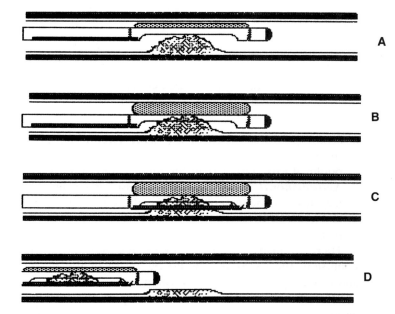

R. Rae 1988

Fig. 38-25. Atherectomy. **A,** The catheter inserted to a point where the opening approximates the plaque. **B,** The balloon forces the opening in the catheter over the plaque. **C,** The blade cuts off the section of the plaque within the catheter. **D,** The catheter with the plaque specimen is then withdrawn.

the clot with it (Fig. 38-23). When the plaque is soft and atheromatous, a technique known as percutaneous transluminal angioplasty may be used. This involves methods similar to those used for arteriography; special catheters, fluoroscopic guidance, and contrast injections are needed. A catheter designed by Dr. A. Gruntzig is used that has a balloon in its tip with the boundaries marked radiopaquely. This balloon catheter is threaded through the artery along a guide wire to the point of obstruction or stenosis. It is then threaded through the obstructed section until the balloon lies along the area marked for dilation. The balloon is inflated to a pressure of 5 atm. This compresses and disperses the plaque against the arterial walls, where it is absorbed (Fig. 38-24). The method does not work well with calcific, severe, or multiple obstructions. In some cases of focal obstruction (and often during a bypass surgery above or below the point of implantation) an *endarterectomy* may be performed. In this technique the artery is opened across the area of stenosis. An intimal elevator is used to dissect the intimal layer and area of plaque away from the walls, and this area is cut away. The loose ends of the residual intima are tacked down with sutures, remaining bits of plaque in the area are removed, and the vessel is closed.

While a direct endarterectomy is often a fairly aggressive approach, in an increasing number of these situations two newer techniques are being evaluated—the *atherectomy catheter* and the *vascular laser.*

The atherectomy catheter is thin and is somewhat similar in design to the PTA catheter, except that there is an opening on one side of the catheter and a balloon opposite. The atherectomy catheter is threaded through the negotiable lumen and is placed across the plaque section. The balloon is inflated and the opening in the catheter is forced over a portion of the plaque. Once this is done and checked under fluoroscopic guidance, a blade is passed through the catheter, slicing off the section of plaque encompassed by catheter. The catheter is withdrawn, the

specimen of plaque extracted, and repeated passes are made until the lumen is enlarged to the guiding physician's satisfaction. Usually, this can take as many as 200 passes (Fig. 38-25).

The vascular laser follows a similar technique: a guide wire is run to the area of stenosis, and the laser catheter is guided over it. It is used to systematically enlarge the lumen by vaporizing small amounts of the plaque via a bare optic tip or by using a metal tip heated by delivered laser energy. (At the time of writing, only the "hot tip" is clinically approved for nonexperimental usage.) Once the laser catheter is used to make or enlarge a lumen through a plaque, a balloon is inserted, and an angioplasty is performed as above. Risks involved include the threat of embolic phenomena and the focal heat generated by the beam, causing possible wall damage.

Both of the latter techniques are undergoing trials at the time of writing and are meeting with varying degrees of success in a number of institutions.

Of course, there are many lesions or multiple areas of stenosis or occlusion that are not amenable to any of the above techniques, and bypassing is indicated in these cases.

The Doppler examination after endarterectomy, angioplasty, thrombectomy, or atherectomy does not differ from the normal examination, except that thigh cuffs and tracings in the region of the catheterization site may be omitted if the patient is feeling tenderness in that area or if a cutdown wound would interfere with cuff placement.

EXAMINATION OF THE PATIENT WITH A FALSE-NEGATIVE DIAGNOSIS

Occasionally the examiner will encounter a patient who presents with the typical symptoms of lower extremity claudication (often severely) but has normal tracings and indices. This type of symptomatic patient is difficult to evaluate, for the pain and claudication present only with exercise. The symptoms often are due to a neuropathic rather than a vascular disorder.

In these patients either an exercise stress test or hyperemic test frequently will determine whether obstruction is present. The main aim is to increase demand for blood flow in the extremity either with exercising the patient on a treadmill or by inducing hyperemia through transient application of a tourniquet (inflated blood pressure cuff). The intention in both cases is to recreate or simulate the conditions that bring on the claudication and then measure the amount of time required for normal flow patterns to resume.

Although there are many current attitudes concerning the treadmill versus the hyperemic test,[13,17,28] I will discuss both without attempting to prove one over the other. The final decision will be left to individual opinion, and further reading is encouraged on these subjects.

Physiologic responses to exercise[3,18]

The normal response to exercise in the leg is a demand for increased blood flow in the muscular vascular bed, causing a decreased vascular resistance. Flow is increased in the main arteries of the leg, and an adequate oxygen supply is thus provided. The normal muscular metabolism is maintained, as is the flow pattern.

In cases of obstruction, however, exercise results in the same demand for blood in the vascular bed and decreased resistance but the obstructed vessels and collaterals cannot supply enough blood to meet the demand. The pressure in the major arteries (including the ankle arteries) drops, and the waveform diminishes. Metabolic waste products accumulate, causing the pain, cramping, and muscle tiring of claudication.

Doppler treadmill examination

The criteria and examination techniques quoted here are based on information given by Barnes et al.[3]

The Doppler treadmill examination requires a stopwatch, three pressure cuffs, and a treadmill set for a constant load of 2 mph at a 12% grade.

Brachial and ankle systolic pressures are taken, as in the routine examination, and recorded. The patient keeps the ankle cuffs in place and walks on the treadmill for 5 minutes or until claudication forces him to stop. He should tell the examiner where and when pain is noticed and then walk until he would normally stop because of the pain.

At the end of 5 minutes, or when the patient reaches his tolerance limit, the treadmill is stopped and the patient resumes the supine position. The arm with the higher pressure and both ankle pressures are taken and recorded at 1, 2, 4, 6, 10, 15, and 20 minutes following the exercise. Ankle pressures are usually taken until either the preexercise pressure or the time limit is reached (Fig. 38-26).

It should be noted that experience with patients with neuropathic etiologies has shown a return to normal pressures and waveforms within the first minute following exercise, making the first time measurement on the scale of Barnes et al.[3] almost unusable, especially since the patient must be asked to quickly resume a supine position on the examining table. This obviously can take longer than 1 minute, depending on the patient's condition. The severely obstructed or neuropathic patient may take longer than 2 minutes to recover, but the preexercise level is reached usually in less time. Shorter intervals may be required for determining the recovery rate within the first minute after exercise.

If an ECG treadmill examination is also performed, it is often advantageous to do the Doppler treadmill simultaneously; but cardiac and respiratory factors may not allow the patient to lie quickly supine, especially if the heart rate is being evaluated.[3]

Doppler hyperemic postocclusion examination

This method requires the thigh and ankle cuffs and is often performed after the routine Doppler resting examination.

Instead of ambulation, the patient rests supine and the femoral artery is occluded at the upper thigh to simulate exercise and induce metabolic changes. This examination is advantageous when the patient is unable to walk.

Pressure cuffs are placed bilaterally on the ankles and high thighs, and the brachial pressure is taken and recorded. The higher of the two systolic arm pressures is again used for the ankle/brachial indices. One leg is examined at a time.

Before the thigh cuff is inflated, a preocclusive resting waveform and ankle pressure should be taken in the ankle vessels and recorded. The artery with the higher pressure is used for the examination. The probe is held in place, and the thigh cuff is inflated well above the point at which the signal disappears. The pump is then locked off, and

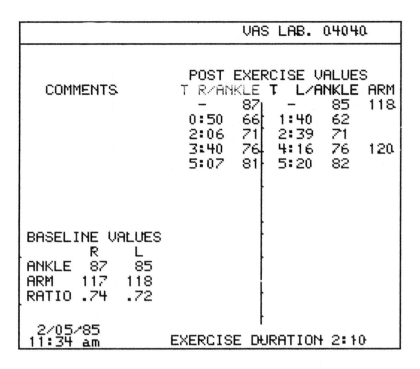

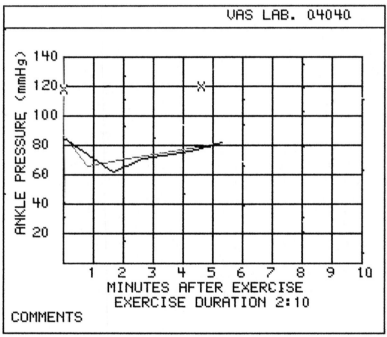

Fig. 38-26. Typical postexercise values and graphic representation.

the stopwatch is started. It is important to monitor the artery and maintain the occlusive pressure for 3 minutes. After that time, the thigh pressure is released all at once and an immediate waveform and ankle pressure are taken and recorded. Waveforms and pressures are continually taken every 15 seconds until the artery reaches its preocclusion pressure and waveform pattern. The technique is repeated for the other extremity.

Most patients will resume normal pressures and waveforms within 30 to 60 seconds. The individual pressures at each interval are divided by the brachial pressure to give sequential ankle/brachial indices up to the preocclu-

sion level. Normal ratios taken immediately after occlusion should be above 0.80. Lower indices or recovery times in excess of 1 minute imply neurologic or obstructive disease.

The disadvantages to this method include possible probe slippage during the occlusive period, intolerance of high thigh cuff pressure by some individuals, and varying results depending on the examiner's ability to take tracings and cuff pressures one after the other every 15 seconds.

This examination also fails to work on patients with obese thighs, noncompressible or calcified arteries, or patients with femoropopliteal bypass grafts.

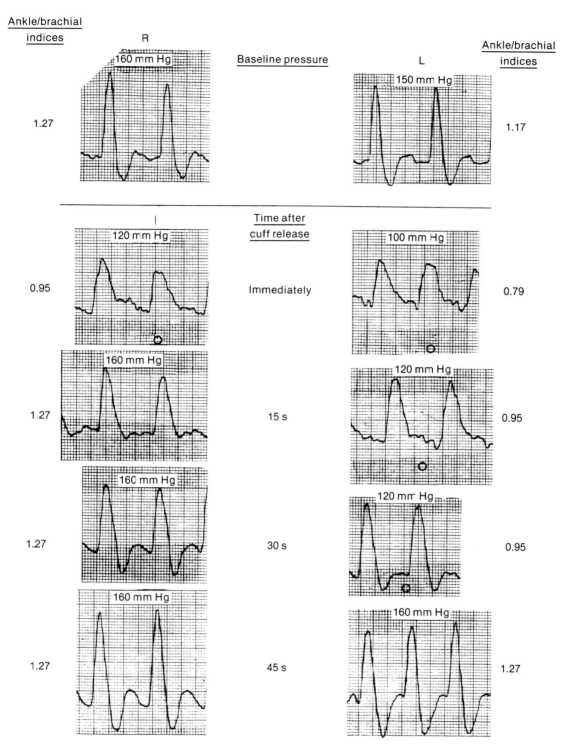

Fig. 38-27. Normal posterior tibial artery signals.

It is not really diagnostic to exercise or perform a hyperemic test on any patient who has an abnormal resting study, especially if moderate to severe occlusive disease is obviously present by waveforms and ankle/brachial index. Doing stress procedures in these cases can cause further discomfort or damage to the patient, and a majority of patients will almost always not tolerate or be able to complete the exam.

There are other methods of hyperemic and treadmill testing as well as studies that have used treadles pumped by the patient in a supine position. However, the results are similar to those reported; reports are available in current journals.[8,11,17,28]

Hyperemia cases. Both patients in the following examples had normal waveforms and indices at rest, but claudication complaints.

CASE 1 (FIG. 38-27): NORMAL. As can be seen at the top of the Fig. 38-27, the resting posterior tibial artery signals are triphasic and normal, with baseline indices of 1.27 on the right and 1.17 on the left. Following thigh occlusion

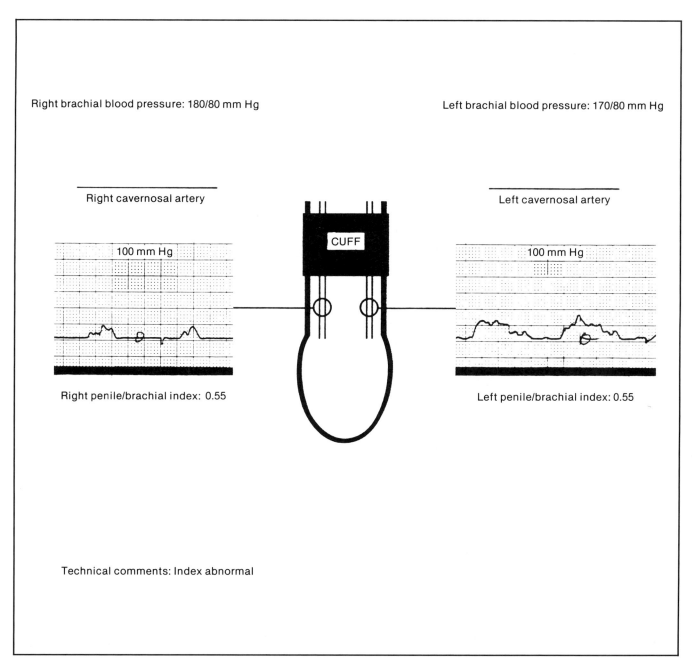

Right brachial blood pressure: 180/80 mm Hg

Left brachial blood pressure: 170/80 mm Hg

Right cavernosal artery

Left cavernosal artery

100 mm Hg

100 mm Hg

Right penile/brachial index: 0.55

Left penile/brachial index: 0.55

Technical comments: Index abnormal

Fig. 38-32.   Bilateral internal iliac or cavernosal artery stenosis.

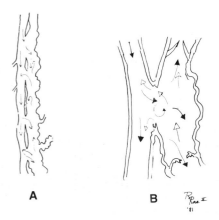

A   B

Fig. 38-33. Arteriovenous fistulas. **A,** Multiple connections in a congenital malformation. **B,** Flow dynamics occurring in an A-V fistula. Arterial flow *(black arrows)* progresses partly through the arterial segment and partly through the fistula to move either antegrade or retrograde in the vein. The pressure can destroy the valves in the distal venous segment and create insufficiency in the veins. Venous flow *(white arrows)* can also enter the arterial segment and disrupt the flow of oxygenated blood to the distal arterial branches.

experience problems, and Doppler and imaging assessment can help localize obstructions, stenoses, defects, hematomas, or other abnormalities. In these shunts, the characteristic turbulence and "hissing" or "burbling" sounds may occur in normal patients; care must be exercised. A beginning vascular technologist can often gain a great deal of experience in learning typical AV fistula sound and flow patterns by examining a shunt patient.

The general technique for Doppler examination of a patient with suspected or known AV fistulas will vary with the individual. When examining a suspected AV fistula patient, follow the normal paths of the arteries and veins and look for specific areas of focal turbulence and abnormally high flow velocities. Bear the following criteria in mind:

1. Collateral channels may exist that shunt flow around a fistula and cause retrograde flow in a given segment immediately distal to the fistula.
2. Venous valves will become incompetent. Thus flow will be reversed in the venous segment *distal* to the fistula and may mimic arterial flow whereas it will be continuous in the *proximal* venous segment.
3. Manual occlusion of the fistula will cause flow in the distal arterial segment to resume normal characteristics.
4. If the standard Doppler extremity examination is performed, there will be a pressure drop distal to the fistula.

Knowledge of these characteristics will facilitate discrimination among AV fistulas.

Arteriovenous fistula cases

CASE 1: CONGENITAL. See case 1 under arterial upper extremity cases, Fig. 38-45.

CASE 2 (FIG. 38-34): ACQUIRED. This patient had had blood drawn from his right arm 2 days prior to his being examined. He presented with a severely painful right arm, which had a hard, slightly swollen area in the antecubital fossa. Examination with a real-time scanner showed a massive acquired AV malformation with encapsulated hematomas apparently connecting the arterial and venous systems in the antecubital region (Fig. 38-34, *A* to *C*). Flow patterns within the visualized masses showed equally bidirectional flow in the venous components (Fig. 38-34, *E* and *G*) and turbulent flow in the arterial components (Fig. 38-34, *F* and *H*). Because of the complexity of the malformation it was difficult to establish which vessels were actually involved, although a definite uninvolved vein was traceable between the masses (Fig. 38-34, *D*). An arteriogram confirmed that the brachial and basilic veins were involved and that the formation had been apparently caused by the phlebotomy needle penetrating both the artery and vein in that area.

DOPPLER UPPER EXTREMITY ARTERIAL EXAMINATION

The Doppler examination of the upper extremities is performed in a manner similar to the examination of the lower extremities. It is not done as frequently as the lower extremity examination, but it is important that the examiner be familiar with these techniques since many of them are used in cooperation with the Doppler cerebrovascular examination.

Arterial anatomy of the upper extremities[14]

This section will cover Doppler-related anatomy in the upper extremity and upper thorax.

The *subclavian artery* is the first major artery to arise from the *aortic arch.* It has a different origin on each side. On the *right* it arises from the *brachiocephalic (innominate) artery,* and on the *left* directly from the aortic arch.

The first branch of the subclavian artery is the *vertebral artery.* Its anatomy will be discussed in more detail in the cerebrovascular anatomy section.

Many other arteries are given off between the arch and the shoulder. At the level of the first rib, the subclavian becomes the *axillary* artery. The axillary artery tends to run superficially through the axilla and then slightly more deeply at the tendon of the teres major. Here it becomes the *brachial* artery (Fig. 38-35).

The brachial artery runs medially along the arm to the elbow. Approximately 1 cm distal to the elbow, it bifurcates into the *radial* and *ulnar* arteries.

These continue on to the wrist on the anterior surface of the arm, the radial on the radial side and the ulnar on the ulnar side. The ulnar artery gives off a *medial interosseus branch,* which may occasionally be heard between the radial and ulnar. Each artery passes into the hand and terminates at respective *radial and ulnar palmar arches,* which are connected by collaterals (Fig. 38-36).

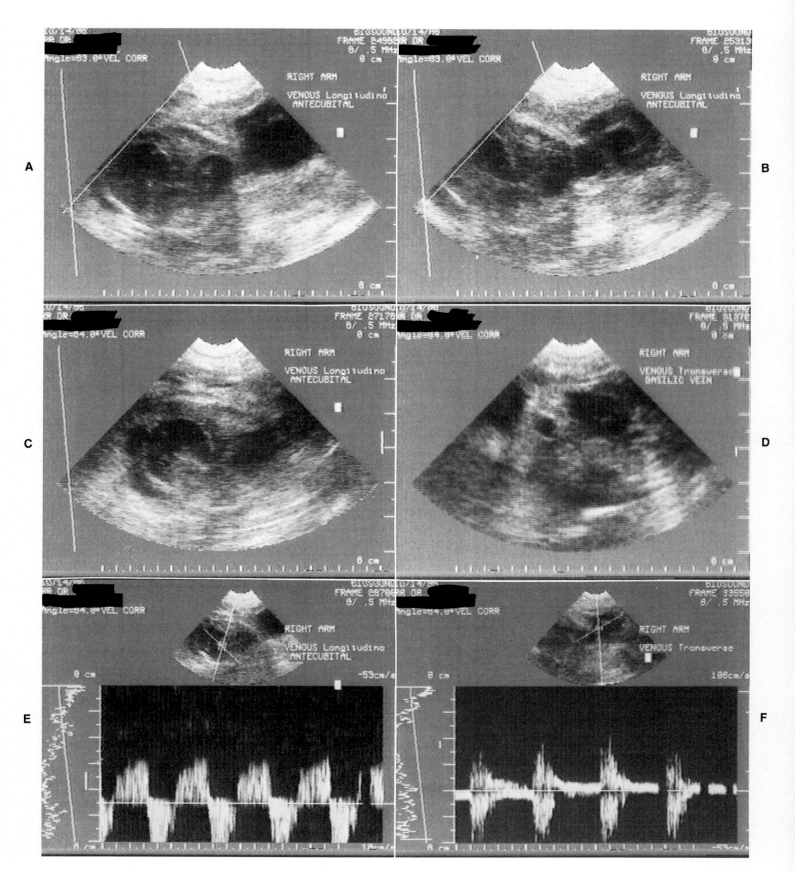

Fig. 38-34. Acquired arteriovenous fistula.

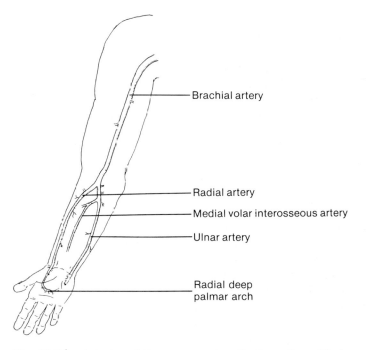

Fig. 38-34, cont'd.   For legend see opposite page.

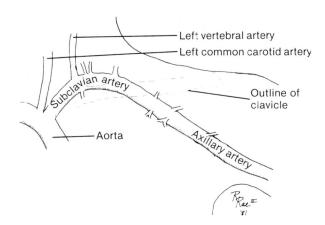

Fig. 38-35.   Arteries of the upper extremity from the aorta to the axilla.

Routine upper extremity arterial examination

The equipment needed for the upper extremity examination is the same as for examination of the lower extremities: a directional Doppler device and pressure cuffs.

A thorough history is obtained once again, with emphasis on upper extremity occlusive disease. The classic symptoms consist of claudication of the arm that occurs with lifting objects or holding the arms raised over the head for short periods.[15] The afflicted arm will also feel colder to the touch than the unobstructed arm, and occasionally numbness and discoloration of the fingers will occur. Systolic blood pressures will usually show a discrepancy between the two sides. Microembolic activity, digital artery or palmar arch stenosis, or vasospastic phenomena can be suspected in cases of digital discoloration when the rest of the arm is normal. Note should be made also of whether the patient notices discoloration with exposure to cold or temperature changes.[7,18]

A patient with dizziness accompanying the extremity problems can be suspected of having a subclavian steal

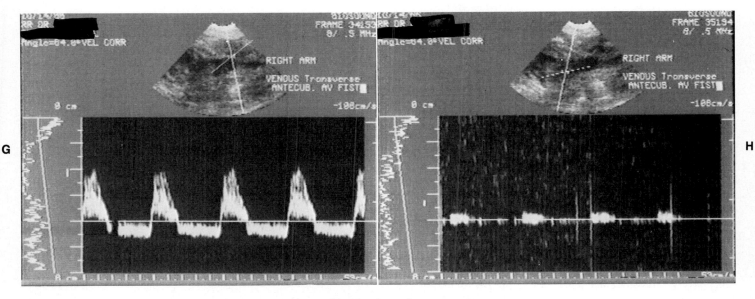

Fig. 38-36.   Arteries of the upper extremity from the axilla to the hand.

syndrome. This is always a possibility when there is a pressure difference of greater than 20 to 40 mmHg between the two arms.[24,27]

After the history is taken, the patient lies supine. Two pressure cuffs are placed on each arm, one on the *forearm* and one on the *upper arm* (Fig. 38-37).

The brachial artery is the first vessel to be checked. A waveform is recorded and the systolic pressure taken. The examiner then moves down to the wrist and monitors the radial artery and takes a tracing. The probe is kept in place and the arm cuff is inflated past the point at which the signal disappears and is then deflated to obtain the systolic pressure at the point where the signal returns.

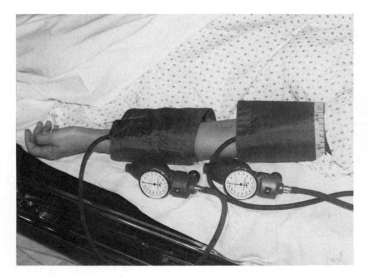

Fig. 38-37.   Pressure cuffs in place for the upper extremity arterial study.

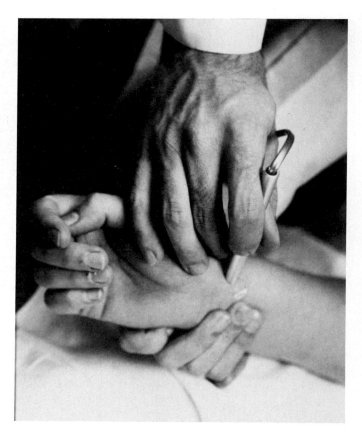

Fig. 38-38.   Performing the Allen's test.

The examiner then follows the same procedure with the forearm cuff and obtains a forearm pressure.

The probe is then moved to the ulnar artery and the same sequence of tracings with arm and forearm pressures is followed.

The examiner next should perform a modified *Allen's test* (Fig. 38-38). The examiner first monitors the radial artery and compresses the ulnar artery on the opposite side of the forearm with his free hand to determine the patency of the palmar arch. Compression is held for four beats and a tracing is made at a slow chart speed to record any changes.

The procedure is repeated, this time monitoring the ulnar artery and compressing the radial artery. The ulnar artery should be recorded for four beats and the radial artery compressed for four beats and then released for four more. Any audible changes should show up on the tracing as an increase in flow.

The other arm is examined the same way, with the brachial signal recorded and the brachial systolic pressure taken. The radial and ulnar arteries are then examined, with pressures taken, and the palmar arch flow is checked.

The cuffs are removed, and the patient's arms are raised. The examiner locates the axillary artery signal in the axilla (Fig. 38-39) and records the signal with the probe angled cephalad. Both axillary arteries are examined.

The examiner then moves to the head of the patient, for ease of examination, and monitors the subclavian and vertebral arteries in the supraclavicular fossa. The subclavian artery is located by angling the probe medially and downward in the fossa until a distinct triphasic signal is heard. The clearest signal is then recorded (Fig. 38-40).

The vertebral artery can be heard in a triangle formed by the inferior border of the sternocleidomastoid muscle, the clavicle, and the lateral side of the neck. Palpate the transverse processes of the cervical spine, then place the probe lateral to the sternocleidomastoid muscle and near

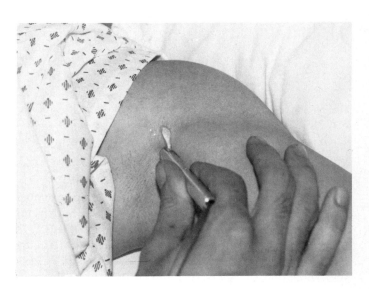

Fig. 38-39.   Examination of the axillary artery.

the processes. The probe should be angled downward and medially slightly, up on the neck but not down in the supraclavicular fossa itself. A distinct low-resistance signal similar to a carotid waveform should be audible in this area but may require a bit of searching to locate (Fig. 38-41). If you think you are on top of a bone, move up or down and aim for the interspaces or the vertebral segment between the subclavian and C-7. A triphasic signal is more than likely the subclavian artery and not the vertebral. A biphasic signal or a signal similar to an external ca-

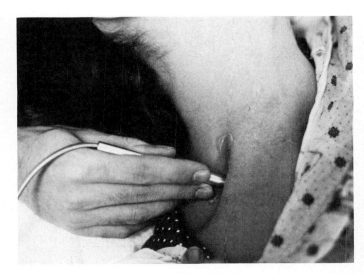

Fig. 38-40. Examination of the subclavian and vertebral arteries.

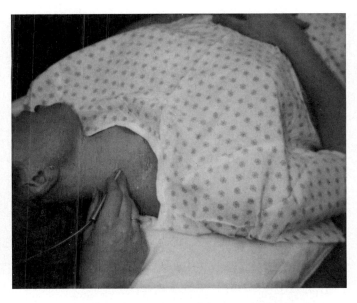

Fig. 38-41. Examination of the vertebral artery.

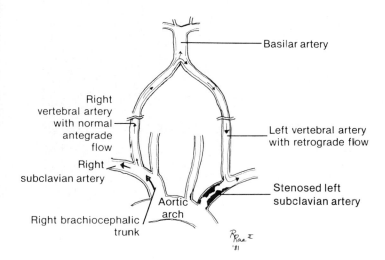

Fig. 38-42. Stenosed left subclavian artery and mechanism of subclavian steal syndrome.

rotid artery may also occur, however. The subclavian and vertebral arteries should be recorded bilaterally.

When a pressure difference of greater than 20 to 40 mm Hg exists between arms, the examiner must pay careful attention to the direction of the vertebral signal on the side that shows evidence of occlusion. This is a definite indication of subclavian steal syndrome.[24,27]

A subclavian steal occurs when an occlusion develops in one of the subclavian arteries proximal to the vertebral artery. If flow is compromised severely enough, flow from the contralateral patent vertebral will be "stolen" around the vertebrobasilar junction *down* the vertebral on the affected side to the patent portion of the subclavian to supply the arm. Flow is therefore *retrograde* in the vertebral artery on the affected side in this condition (Fig. 38-42). (See Chapter 40 for further discussion of vertebrobasilar hemodynamics.)

It is possible that if the proximal innominate artery becomes obstructed that a *carotid steal* can occur. While

this is an extremely rare phenomenon, I personally have encountered this condition twice. Flow travels retrograde in the right carotid system through circle of Willis collaterals to supply the right vertebral and subclavian system. This phenomenon and its hemodynamics will be explained further in the cerebrovascular system, Chapter 40. See also cerebrovascular case 6.

In vertebral reversal, flow may sound similar to the normal vertebral signal but will be retrograde to the expected direction. The examiner should assume that reversal is real if it is heard on the side with an obstructed subclavian artery rather than suspect an incorrectly placed probe.

Examination for suspected subclavian steal syndrome[1,27]

In a patient with vertebral steal, a well-defined reversed vertebral signal on the side with a subclavian stenosis is often more than sufficient to imply a probable steal (Fig. 38-43). In a patient presenting with questionably reversed or weak but antegrade vertebral flow, verification should be made as to whether a steal is present. To check for steal syndrome, the examiner has the patient lie supine and places a pressure cuff on the *arm with the occlusion.* The vertebral artery is monitored, with the cuff inflated to at least 50 mmHg above the systolic pressure to occlude flow to the arm and induce hyperemia. The monitoring continues with the cuff inflated for 3 minutes. At the end of that time, the cuff pressure is released. The chart recorder should be running prior to release of the cuff to show any changes that occur.

In a patient with vertebral steal a *reversed signal* will *augment* for a short period. An antegrade signal will *momentarily reverse* below the zero line for several beats within the first 5 seconds.

Following is a summary of the steps in the upper extremity arterial examination:

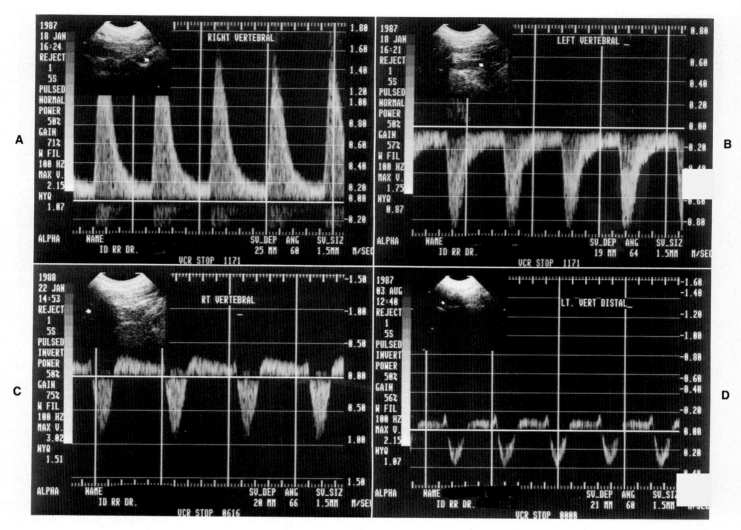

Fig. 38-43. Vertebral steal. **A,** Normal but elevated signal typical of compensatory response from unaffected side. **B,** Strongly reversed signal indicative of frank vertebral steal on affected side in same patient. **C,** Moderate latent vertebral steal (note bidirectional flow and recovery in diastole). **D,** Mild latent vertebral steal.

1. Take the patient's history, with emphasis on claudication and numbness of the arm, and note any discoloration or positional problems.
2. Place cuffs bilaterally on the arms and forearms and take a brachial tracing and blood pressure from one arm.
3. Record the radial and ulnar arteries and take pressures at the arm and forearm in each artery.
4. Evaluate the palmar arch by monitoring the radial artery and ulnar artery and compressing the unmonitored vessel while recording to check for flow changes.
5. Examine the other arm using steps 2, 3, and 4.
6. Record both axillary arteries.
7. Examine and record both subclavian arteries in the supraclavicular fossa.
8. Record both vertebral arteries and check the flow direction.
9. If there is evidence of occlusion and a pressure difference of greater than 20 to 40 mm Hg between the

two arms, do a subclavian steal examination to rule out vertebral steal.
10. Calculate forearm/brachial indices.

Fig. 38-44 shows the probe sites for arterial and venous Doppler examinations.

Interpretation of the upper extremity arterial examination

As in the lower extremity examination, the upper extremity flow status is determined with an index of pressures. In the arms the highest systolic brachial pressure of the two arms is divided into the two systolic forearm pressures of the two arteries examined at the wrist for calculation of the *forearm/brachial* indices. Both the radial and ulnar arteries should have indices calculated, since it is highly probable that one or the other may be more severely stenosed.

The normal patient should have a forearm/brachial index of 1.00 or greater. Indices of less than 1.00 are measured according to the criteria used in the lower extrem-

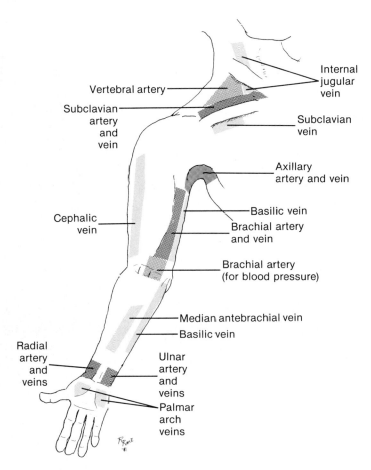

Fig. 38-44. Sites for both arterial and venous examinations of the upper extremity.

ity ankle/brachial index.[3] (See Interpretation of the Lower Extremity Arterial Examination.)

A normal upper extremity examination will have triphasic waveforms in the subclavian, axillary, brachial, radial, and ulnar arteries. The vertebral artery may be triphasic or biphasic. Patency of the palmar arch is shown by an augmentation of flow with compression of the ulnar artery when monitoring the radial and with compression of the radial when monitoring the ulnar.

A patient with distal disease will show decreased waveforms in the radial and ulnar arteries as well as a decreased forearm/brachial index. In addition, a noticeable pressure drop of greater than 40 mm Hg should be present, similar in response to findings in the lower extremity arterial examination. All signals from the brachial to the subclavian artery will be triphasic and normal.

A patient with brachial or low axillary occlusion between the elbow and shoulder will have decreased waveforms at the radial, ulnar, and brachial arteries and a decreased brachial systolic pressure in the affected arm. The axillary, subclavian, and vertebral signals will be normal.

A patient with high axillary occlusion will have reduced waveforms at all sites below the shoulder and a corresponding pressure drop. The subclavian and vertebral arteries will be normal.

A patient with subclavian occlusion will show reduced waveforms at all sites, except for the proximal subclavian

if the occlusion does not extend as far as the vertebral. Otherwise, decreased waveforms and possibly reversed vertebral waveforms can be expected.

It is important to remember that the forearm/brachial index should be calculated to show the degree of occlusion. If *both* arms show evidence of subclavian obstruction, note should be made on the report form that waveforms indicate occlusion and that the forearm/brachial index is ineffective.

Arterial upper extremity cases

CASE 1 (FIG. 38-45): NORMAL LEFT ARM—ABNORMAL RIGHT ARM WITH MULTIPLE CONGENITAL ARTERIOVENOUS FISTULA DEVELOPMENT. This 40-year-old woman had a history of congenital AV fistulas of the right subclavian, brachial, and radial artery-vein systems. She had also had congestive heart failure in 1973 because of the flow problems. A macrofistular area was repaired at the elbow level in 1978.

At the time of this examination she had had intermittent pain and swelling in the right hand for 2 weeks. The right arm itself was swollen, with dilated and tortuous superficial varices, and large purplish green blotches on the right chest, shoulder, and arm. The hand at the base of the thumb was greatly swollen, and the patient could move the fingers only weakly. Amputation had been declined.

The right forearm/brachial index was 1.00, the left 0.92.

On the left side characteristic normal tracings can be seen at the brachial, subclavian, vertebral, axillary, radial, and ulnar arteries. The compression responses show normal flow through the left palmar arch.

On the right side the brachial shows a prominent signal indicative of obstruction and turbulence. The subclavian signal also shows proximal venous connections reducing the flow. The vertebral shows a subclavian steal present, regardless of the normal blood pressure in the arm. The axillary artery also has a turbulent signal, showing flow problems. The radial arterial signal was turbulent and difficult to interpret, for reversed flow in the accompanying vein possibly prevented normal flow to the hand. Compression of the ulnar artery resulted in retrograde flow in the artery, implying a prominent AV connection. The ulnar signal also indicated flow discrepancies, with high-pitched turbulence present. Compression of the radial artery occluded the AV fistula and resulted in resumption of normal flow through the ulnar artery segment.

At surgery the radial artery was ligated and the AV fistula and palmar arch injected and blocked with Ivalon sponge solution. The patient's symptoms subsided, and she was released.

CASE 2 (FIG. 38-46): ABNORMAL—MODERATE SEGMENTAL FOREARM STENOSIS. This patient presented with right forearm and hand numbness after exertion (the left arm had been amputated). Triphasic waveforms can be seen in the subclavian, axillary, and brachial arteries, and monophasic waveforms are present in the radial and ulnar arteries. The Allen's test shows normal augmentation with arterial compressions indicating a normal patent palmar arch system. There is a marked pressure drop between the arm

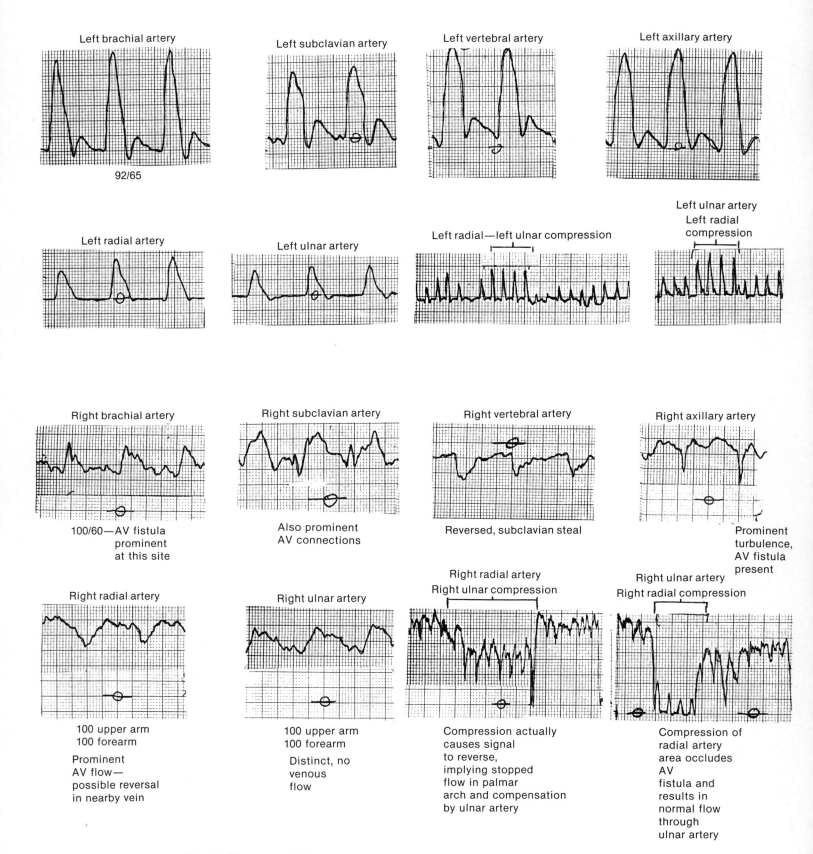

Left brachial artery

92/65

Left subclavian artery

Left vertebral artery

Left axillary artery

Left radial artery

Left ulnar artery

Left radial—left ulnar compression

Left ulnar artery
Left radial compression

Right brachial artery

100/60—AV fistula
prominent
at this site

Right subclavian artery

Also prominent
AV connections

Right vertebral artery

Reversed, subclavian steal

Right axillary artery

Prominent
turbulence,
AV fistula
present

Right radial artery

100 upper arm
100 forearm

Prominent
AV flow—
possible reversal
in nearby vein

Right ulnar artery

100 upper arm
100 forearm

Distinct, no
venous
flow

Right radial artery
Right ulnar compression

Compression actually
causes signal
to reverse,
implying stopped
flow in palmar
arch and compensation
by ulnar artery

Right ulnar artery
Right radial compression

Compression of
radial artery
area occludes
AV
fistula and
results in
normal flow
through
ulnar artery

Fig. 38-45. Normal left arm. Abnormal right arm with multiple congenital AV fistulas.

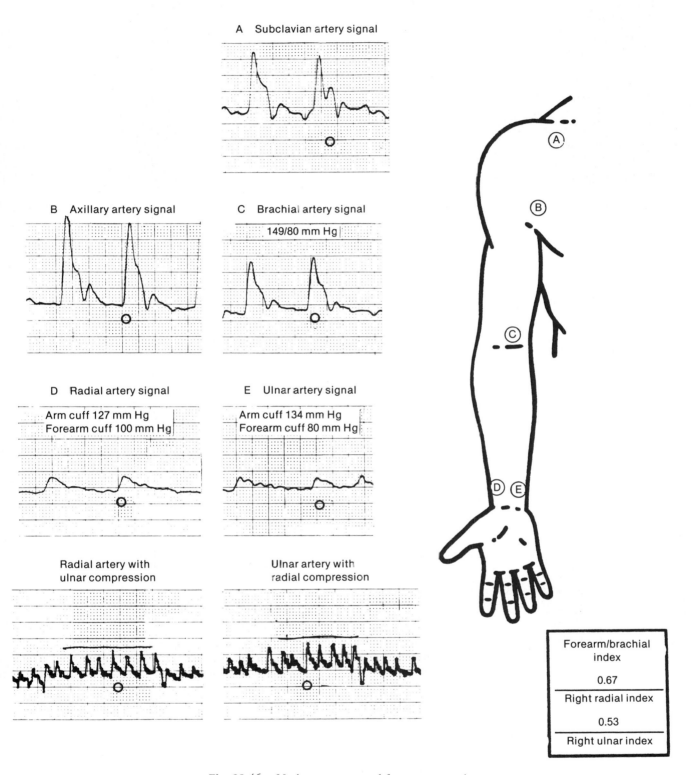

Fig. 38-46.   Moderate segmental forearm stenosis.

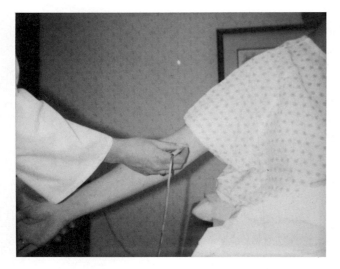

Fig. 38-47. Thoracic outlet examination. Examining the arm at 45-degree angle.

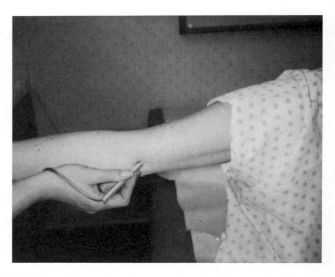

Fig. 38-48. Thoracic outlet examination. Examining the arm at 90-degree angle.

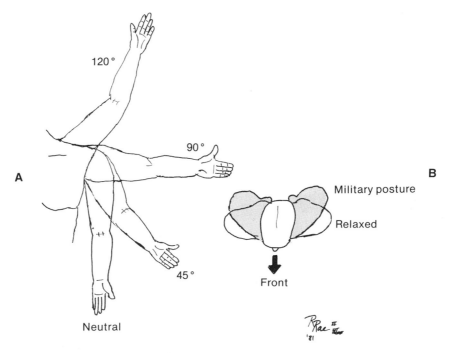

Fig. 38-49. Positions for examination of the patient with thoracic outlet syndrome. **A,** Arm and angles. **B,** Shoulders in relaxed and military postures.

cuff and the forearm cuff, confirming the presence of stenosis implied by the waveforms. In addition, the forearm/brachial indices are 0.67 in the radial and 0.53 in the ulnar, both within the range of moderate impairment.

Thoracic outlet syndrome examination

Many patients will often show completely normal resting upper extremity pressures even though they have difficulty only when their arms are raised or placed at an unusual angle. These patients usually complain of numbness, tingling, and discoloration if the arm is abducted, lain upon, pulled back behind the shoulder, or held over the head. Changing the position of the arm to a more forward or neutral position resolves the symptoms completely.[18] In these patients a routine upper extremity examination

should be performed and then a more specialized examination of the thoracic outlet.

Thoracic outlet syndrome occurs when the arteries, veins, and/or nerves supplying the arm are obstructed by compression between the clavicle and first rib, a cervical rib and the scalene muscles, or the pectoralis minor with hyperabduction of the arm. The vessels usually involved are the subclavian artery and vein and the brachial nerve plexus where it leaves the chest and goes to the arm.[18]

In the thoracic outlet examination the patient should sit either in a chair or on the edge of the examination table with the arms completely relaxed. The examiner takes a tracing from the brachial artery with the arm in a neutral position. Then, with the help of an assistant, the patient's arm is raised to a 45-degree angle (Fig. 38-47). The patient is instructed to let the arm go limp and offer no assistance at all. A tracing is taken from the arm in this position and is marked accordingly. With the arm in this position the patient then is instructed to pull the shoulders back into a military posture and perform a Valsalva maneuver. The examiner keeps the probe in place during the Valsalva and records any changes that occur.

The arm is raised to a 90-degree angle, and the procedure is repeated (Fig. 38-48). A tracing is made both neutrally and with the patient in military posture performing a Valsalva maneuver. The arm is then raised to a 120-degree position and the same steps are repeated. Raising the arm to a 180-degree angle also can be done if symptoms warrant.

Additional maneuvers can include hyperabduction, hyperadduction, and Adson's test. In Adson's test, the patient hyperabducts the arm over the head and turns the head *toward* the side being examined. This position can help reveal the presence of a cervical rib.[18]

Positive findings in thoracic outlet syndrome will be a reduction or cessation of flow at or above a specific degree of elevation or abduction, diminution or cessation with military posturing, and with the application of Adson's test. Any comments the patient makes concerning the onset of symptoms with the assumption of a particular position should be noted on the report form.

The positions for the thoracic outlet examination are shown in Fig. 38-49.

Thoracic outlet cases

CASE 1 (FIG. 38-50): NORMAL RIGHT ARM — ABNORMAL LEFT ARM. This patient suffered pain and numbness in the left arm when it was raised above the shoulder level, following an industrial accident.

On the right side, normal triphasic brachial waveforms are seen that do not diminish or significantly alter as the arm is raised from hanging through 180 degrees. Application of military postures in each position also has no effect with the exception of some mild flow diminution without alteration of the flow pattern when military posturing is applied at 90 degrees.

On the symptomatic left side, there is a normal, triphasic pattern in the brachial artery in the hanging and 45-degree positions with complete compression and loss of signal occurring as the arm is brought to the 90-degree position and is elevated higher. Compression at this level was confirmed by lowering the arm slowly through 90 degrees while continually monitoring the brachial artery. The strip at the bottom shows the gradual return of flow to normal triphasicity during this latter step.

DOPPLER EXAMINATION OF THE DIGITAL ARTERIES

Many patients present with focal ischemia of the fingers and hand resulting from trauma, frostbite, microvascular obstruction, and Raynaud's phenomenon. In these patients often only one or two fingers or even a fingertip will be affected. Vasospasm, whether focal or general, is often corrected microsurgically by digital nerve sympathectomy where the microconnections between the digital artery and nerve are severed, allowing flow to resume.

Carpal tunnel syndrome can also cause a neurologic vasospasm, and a carpal tunnel release can often restore digital flow.

A standard Doppler upper extremity arterial exam will not generally assess the hand, and while photoplethysmographic and temperature-sensing probes may confirm an ischemic problem, these techniques do not pinpoint the level of stenosis or give pressure information.

Angiography is still the best way to show the digital tree and palmar arch, but again there is a noninvasive Doppler technique that, when used as a screening and follow-up tool, can spare the normal patient an angiogram.

Anatomy of the arterial circulation to the hand

The radial and ulnar arteries terminate into the radial and ulnar palmar arches, as shown in Fig. 38-36. The *common digital arteries* arise from the palmar arches, which then terminate into the *proper digital arteries,* one on each side of the finger. Barring a developmental anomaly, the radial arch generally supplies the digital arteries on the radial (lateral) side of the digit, and the ulnar arch the digital arteries on the medial (ulnar) side.

Routine digital artery examination

The protocol below was developed by me based loosely on work done by Thulesius, Nielsen, and Lassen,[22,26] and the developmental study was presented at the 13th Annual Meeting of the SDMS in 1984.[25]

The patient first receives a limited upper extremity arterial examination on the symptomatic side or sides, using segmental pressures and brachial radial ulnar waveforms as outlined previously (see Routine Upper Extremity Arterial Examination) but without axillary, subclavian, and vertebral waveforms being taken. An Allen's test for palmar arch patency is done as well. The examiner then should use an ample amount of gel and monitor the waveforms of the digital arteries on both the lateral and medial sides of the thumb and each finger in turn, (Fig. 38-51). When doing this the examiner should angle the probe caudally and listen between the phalangeal joints of each digit, noting whether a signal is heard. The most distal extent to which a signal is detected in the finger is then mapped out on a report form, using the creases in the fingers as a landmark for the level of patency. If a flow signal is detected at the fingertip or distal phalanx but not in the proximal phalanx on the side being examined, there is likely a technical error. Once the arteries are mapped, the examiner should then place a digit pressure cuff around the proximal phalanx of the digit being examined and record the pressures and a waveform in each digital artery, repeating until the entire hand has been evaluated. Pressures will not likely be obtainable in digits with suspected distal occlusion. Forearm/brachial and digital brachial ratios are calculated.

If the patient shows signs of ischemia only under exposure to cold, a vasospastic phenomenon such as Raynaud's must be suspected and ruled out, using a simple cold stress test.

While sophisticated equipment exists for cold stress of digits, in reality little more is required than a glass of wa-

Right arm UE-TOS

R

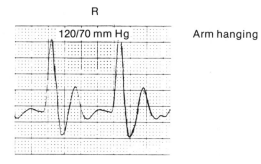

Arm hanging

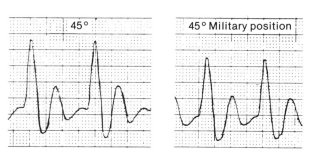

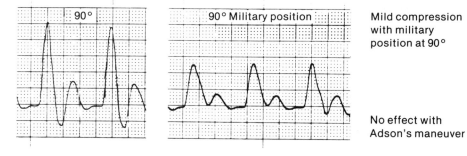

Mild compression
with military
position at 90°

No effect with
Adson's maneuver

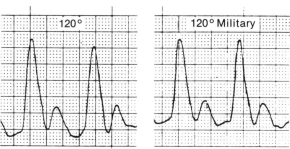

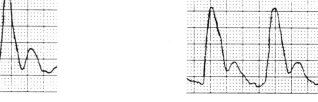

Fig. 38-50.   Normal right arm. Abnormal left arm.

Left arm UE-TOS

L

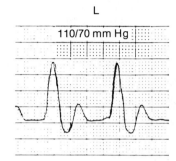

110/70 mm Hg

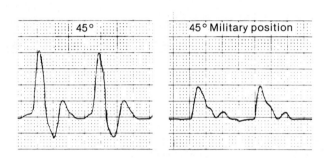

45°   45° Military position

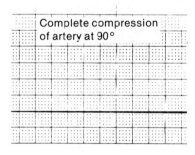

Complete compression
of artery at 90°

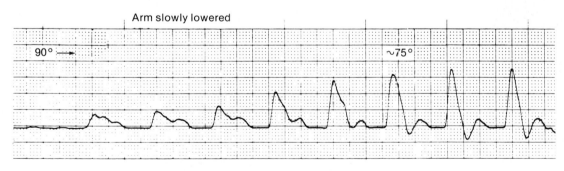

Arm slowly lowered

90° →   ~75°

Fig. 38-50, cont'd.   For legend see opposite page.

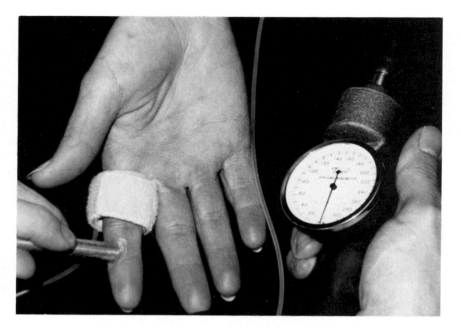

Fig. 38-51.   Recording digital signals and taking digital blood pressures.

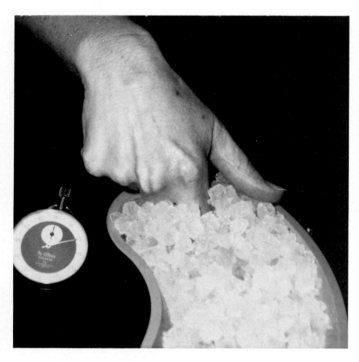

Fig. 38-52.   Digital cold stress using ice water.

ter, ice, and the Doppler to achieve similar results. A pre-immersion signal is obtained in the symptomatic digits, and then the digit is immersed in the ice water for a maximum of 3 minutes or until severe pain occurs (Fig. 38-52). The digits are then removed and are immediately examined with the probe to see whether an audible signal is detected at preimmersion sites. Note: Do not perform cold stress evaluations on any digits with prominent evidence of spastic or occlusive disease (absent distal flow) regardless of symptoms; this may cause further damage to the already ischemic tissue.

Following is a summary of the steps required in the performance of the digital artery evaluation:
1. Obtain a specific history, concentrating on any trauma to the digit or digits of interest, evidence of pain or numbness with exposure to cold, discoloration, ulceration, or ischemic changes.
2. Perform a limited upper extremity examination, taking tracings and segmental pressures from the brachial, radial, and ulnar arteries.
3. Map flow from the base of finger to the fingertip, following the digital artery and noting any areas of absent flow on the mapping form. Use the creases of the fingers on the palmar side to help localize areas of obstruction or spasm as the obstruction usually occurs close to the joint.
4. Take pressures and waveforms from any detectable digital arteries on both sides of each finger using a digit cuff.
5. Calculate the forearm/brachial index and digital/brachial indices for each digital artery recorded.
6. If Raynaud's phenomenon is present, do a cold stress examination.

Interpretation of the Doppler digital examination

As with the routine upper extremity exam, wave morphology and pressure change diagnoses are identical to those listed under Interpretation of the Upper Extremity Arterial Examination.

Flow patterns in the digits tend to be of a lower resistance pattern than those in the arm, and to have higher pressures. Digit/brachial indices from 1.0 to greater than 1.2 are considered normal.

Absence of flow at any distal segment of a digital artery is positive for focal digital artery occlusion at the mapped point.

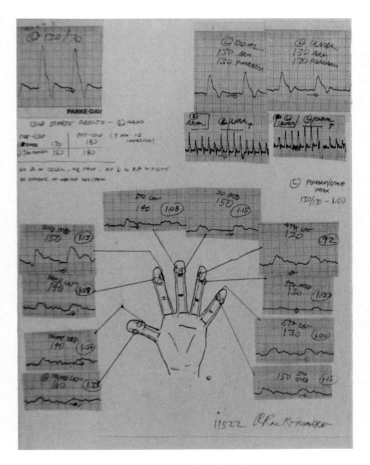

Fig. 38-53. Normal Doppler digital artery study.

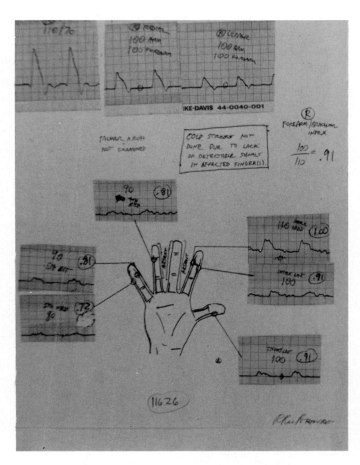

Fig. 38-54. Multiple areas of digital artery occlusion.

Lack of augmentation of either the radial or ulnar artery with opposing compression during the Allen's test is consistent with palmar arch stenosis, occlusion, or congenital incompletion. The arch side affected will often affect its respective digital arteries as well.

Following cold stress, the absence of a signal where one was previously located is positive for cold-induced vasospasm. After warming the digit, the digit signal should be located again to confirm its presence and rule out technical error. The severity of vasospasm is often directly proportional to the amount of time needed for signal recovery.

Digital examination cases

CASE 1 (FIG. 38-53): NORMAL. This is an example of a normal Doppler digital artery study. Brachial, radial, and ulnar waveforms are triphasic and the Allen's test is normal. Note that the digital flow is mapped as patent to the fingertips on both sides of each digit, and representative waveforms are not diminished in appearance. The forearm/brachial indices are 1.00, and digital/brachial indices are not below 0.90

CASE 2 (FIG. 38-54 TO 38-56): MULTIPLE FOCAL DIGITAL ARTERY OCCLUSIONS—PREDIGITAL AND POSTDIGITAL SYMPATHECTOMY. The first examination (Fig. 38-54) shows a patient with

multiple areas of digital artery occlusion occurring in the medial thumb, lateral index finger, distal two thirds of the lateral third finger, and the distal third of the medial fourth and fifth fingers. Brachial, radial, and ulnar arteries are normal, and the Allen's test had no changes with compression. The forearm/brachial indices were normal. The Doppler findings were confirmed by an arteriogram (Fig. 38-55).

Following digital sympathectomy to eliminate vasospastic responses and dilate the digital arteries, a dramatic improvement can be seen as flow is returned to all the digital arteries and normal digital/brachial indices are obtained (Fig. 38-56).

CASE 3 (FIG. 38-57): ULNAR ARTERY OCCLUSION WITH RADIAL GRAFT STENOSIS AND EMBOLIC OCCLUSION OF PALMAR ARCH AND DIGITAL ARTERIES. In this case the ulnar artery signal is absent and a brachioradial graft has occluded at the wrist level. A complete absence of flow was noted in the digital arteries in the medial thumb, lateral artery of the index finger and distal third of the medial artery of the index finger, lateral artery of the third finger and distal third of the medial artery of the third finger, and the medial artery and distal third of the lateral artery on the fourth and fifth fingers. Digital/brachial indices are all abnormal. The DSA confirms the digital obstructions (Fig. 38-58).

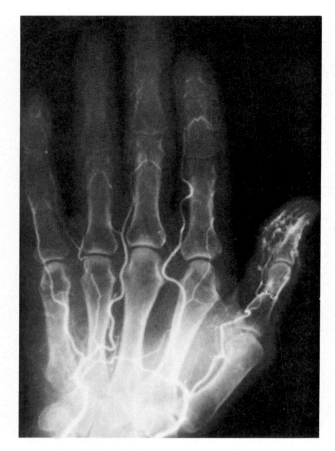

Fig. 38-55. Before digital sympathectomy.

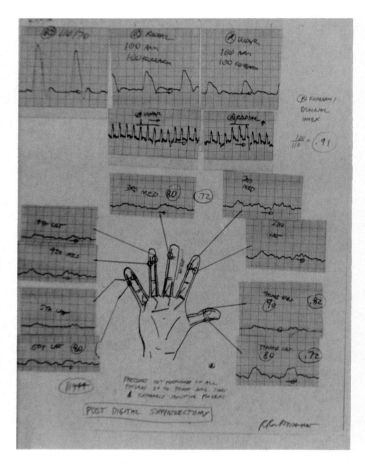

Fig. 38-56. After digital sympathectomy.

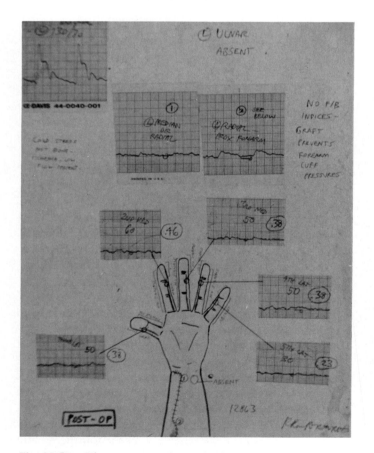

Fig. 38-57. Ulnar artery occlusion with radial graft stenosis and embolic occlusion of palmar arch and digital arteries.

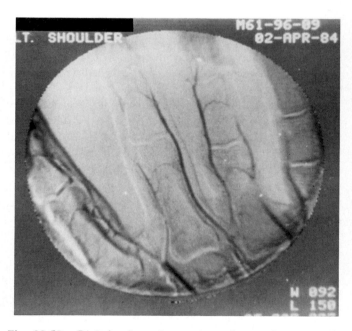

Fig. 38-58. Digital subtraction angiography confirms Doppler findings in Fig. 38-57.

SUMMARY

1. The simplest Doppler examinations to learn and interpret are those pertaining to the arterial system.

2. Arterial occlusive disease and pathoses the examiner is likely to encounter include atherosclerosis, congenital arterial anomalies, Raynaud's phenomenon, Buerger's disease, frostbite, arteritis, mechanical compression syndromes, and entrapment syndrome.

3. Normal arterial Doppler flow signal is evaluated by the chart tracing as well as the audio signals both positive and negative. Chart deflections exist in the arterial signal, with the antegrade flow being positive and retrograde flow being negative. Spectrum analyzers can also be used to further evaluate the arterial Doppler signal.

4. The normal arterial Doppler flow signal in the extremities consists of three components: a large positive deflection with systole, a period of net flow reversal to the negative side of the zero line, and a lesser diastolic positive deflection. This normal arterial flow signal is called triphasic.

5. Abnormal arterial Doppler flow signals are manifested by progressive loss of the diastolic components of the arterial signal, and a decrease in the systolic peak. Waveforms that lose one diastolic component are called biphasic, and waveforms that have lost the second and third diastolic components that have a blunted and rounded systolic peak are classified as monophasic. Triphasic waveforms are found in normal arteries and proximal to a stenosis. Mild to moderate arterial stenoses result in biphasic waveforms distal to the stenosis. Moderate to moderately severe stenoses result in monophasic waveforms distal to the stenosis.

6. As evidenced by Poiseuille's law, a drop in flow pressure will occur distal to a stenosis, which is proportional to the degree of luminal reduction. Segmental pressure measurements enable a pressure drop secondary to a stenosis to be generally localized at a specific level in the leg. The ankle/brachial index, calculated from the systolic pressure at the ankle divided by the highest systolic pressure in the brachial arteries helps to measure this pressure. Indices greater than 1.0 are considered normal. Indices from 0.45 to 1.0 imply mild to moderate disease, and indices from 0.10 to 0.45 imply severe disease.

7. Arterial Doppler examinations are a simple and effective means to follow patients postoperatively or following angioplastic procedures.

8. Patients with claudication who have normal arterial Doppler studies at rest can often benefit from an exercise test or reactive hyperemia test to further evaluate neurologic or physiologic conditions that may be causing the patient's symptoms.

9. Doppler arterial methods can be used to effectively evaluate patients for vasculogenic impotency.

10. Doppler arterial evaluation can be used to assess and localize patients with arteriovenous malformations.

11. In the upper extremity, Doppler waveform analysis and segmental pressure analysis can be used to help localize and measure stenoses. Doppler can also be used to evaluate patients with suspected subclavian steal syndrome, thoracic outlet syndrome, Raynaud's phenomenon, or focal digital ischemia.

REFERENCES

1. Baker JD: Poststress Doppler ankle pressures: a comparison of treadmill exercise with two other methods of induced hyperemia. Arch Surg 113:1171, 1978.

2. Barnes RW: Axioms on acute arterial occlusion of an extremity, Hosp Med 14(6):34, 1978.

3. Barnes RW et al: Doppler ultrasonic evaluation of peripheral arterial disease, Iowa City, 1975, University of Iowa Press.

4. Barnes RW and Garrett WV: Intraoperative assessment of arterial reconstruction by Doppler ultrasound, Surg Obstet Gynecol 146:896, 1978.

5. Baron HC: Chronic arterial insufficiency of the lower limbs, Hosp Med 14(9):33, 1978.

6. Baron HC and Hiesiger E: Significance of ankle blood pressure in the diagnosis of peripheral vascular disease, Am Surg 45:289, 1979.

7. Bergan JJ and Yao JST: Gangrene and severe ischemia of the lower extremities, New York, 1978, Grune & Stratton, Inc.

8. Bernstein EF et al: Noninvasive diagnostic techniques in vascular disease, St Louis, 1978, The CV Mosby Co.

9. Cooperman M et al: Use of Doppler ultrasound in intraoperative localization of intestinal arteriovenous malformation, Ann Surg 190:24, 1979.

10. Corson JD et al: Doppler ankle systolic blood pressure. Prognostic value in vein bypass grafts of the lower extremity, Arch Surg 113:932, 1978.

11. Diethrich EB, editor: Noninvasive cardiovascular diagnosis, Baltimore, 1978, University Park Press.

12. Friedman SA: Guide to diagnosis of peripheral arterial disease, Hosp Med 15(1):87, 1979.

13. Gardner AL et al: Arterial occlusions and stenosis: when should you order a Doppler study? Diagnosis 1(5):87, 1979.

14. Goss CM, editor: Gray's anatomy, ed 29, Philadelphia, 1974, Lea & Febiger.

15. Gross WS and Louis DS: Doppler hemodynamic assessment of obscure symptomatology in the upper extremity, J Hand Surg 3(5):467, 1978.

16. Hill DA et al: Haemodynamic validity of lower limb arterial crossover grafts, J Roy Coll Surg Edin 24:170, 1979.

17. Hummel BW et al: Reactive hyperemia versus treadmill testing in arterial disease, Arch Surg 113:95, 1978.

18. Juergens JL, Spittell JA, and Fairbairn JF: Peripheral vascular diseases, Philadelphia, 1980, WB Saunders, Co.

19. Lee BY et al: Noninvasive hemodynamic evaluation in selection of amputation level, Surg Obstet Gynecol 149:241, 1979.

20. Najem Z et al: Arteriovenous malformations of the cecum: operative localization by Doppler ultrasound, Am Surg 45:538, 1979.

21. Nath RL et al: The multidisciplinary approach to vasculogenic impotence, Surgery 89(1):124, 1978.

22. Nielsen SL and Lassen NA: Finger systolic pressures in upper extremity testing for cold sensitivity (Raynaud's phenomenon). In Bernstein EF, editor: Noninvasive diagnostic techniques in vascular disease, ed 2, St Louis, 1982, The CV Mosby Co.

23. O'Reilly MJ et al: Plasma exchange and Raynaud's phenomenon: its assessment by Doppler ultrasonic velocimetry, Br J Surg 66:712, 1979.

24. Platz M: Doppler ultrasound studies of subclavian steal hemodynamics in subclavian stenosis, J Thorac Cardiovasc Surg 27(6):404, 1979.

25. Rae R: Doppler examination of the digital arteries: a reliable method of evaluating focal ischemic phenomena in the hand, Proceedings of 13th Annual Convention of the Society of Diagnostic Medical Sonographers, J Ultrasound Med 3:186, 1984.

26. Thulesius O: Problems in the evaluation of hand ischemia. In Bernstein EF, editor: Noninvasive diagnostic techniques in vascular disease, ed 2, St Louis, 1982, The CV Mosby Co.

27. von Reutern GM et al: Dopplersonographische diagnostik von Stenosen und Verschlussen der Vertebralarterien und des Subclavian-Steal-Syndroms, Arch Psychiatr Nervenkr 222(2-3):209, 1976.

28. Zicot MJ: Combined study of hyperemia after arterial occlusion and exercise by an isotopic test and a Doppler-ultrasonic method, Angiology 29:534, 1978.

39

Venous Sonography and Doppler Examinations

RICHARD E. RAE II

The incidence of venous disease has been estimated to surpass that of cardiac disease and stroke.[1] Venous thrombosis, varicose veins, and pulmonary embolism are among the most common problems encountered in both outpatients and inpatients.

Pulmonary embolism is among the most dangerous of venous diseases. It occurs as a result of venous thrombosis and can especially affect bedridden, paraplegic or quadriplegic, and/or comatose patients in whom clots develop because of a lack of muscular activity leading to venous stagnation.[4,7,8] An embolus can detach itself from the intimal wall in an area of thrombosis and can travel superiorly or inferiorly through vena cava to the pulmonary arteries, where the thrombus can occlude any portion of the pulmonary vasculature and cause severe damage or death. Thrombi that cause pulmonary embolism very rarely travel from calf veins; the majority of these clots come from the femoral, iliac, or inferior vena cava.

Thrombophlebitis is the main reason for evaluating the venous system. A thrombus or clot can form almost anywhere within the venous system, and usually arises as the result of intimal damage to the vein wall with a subsequent platelet response resulting in a focal coagulation of blood. Inflammation of the vein can result. Stagnant venous flow from insufficient venous return also can compound the problem and enlarge the thrombus. A thrombosis can be of an acute or chronic nature; fresh or new (acute) thrombus tends to be less organized and may be easier to resolve with anticoagulant therapy or lysis. Clot that remains in a vein for a long period of time (chronic) will become more organized and firm. Chronic thrombi also increase the flow pressure required to move blood toward the heart and often force collaterals to develop and shunt the blood around the obstruction. Thromboses also can form in the venous valve sinuses where flow slows or stagnates. Progression of these thrombi can "freeze" the venous valves in an open or partially open position, resulting in venous insufficiency and backflow, as well as damage to the valve cusps themselves from the inflammation and flow pressure. A damaged valve usually becomes incompetent, and the distal portion of the vein may deform and dilate because of increased venous back pressure. When this occurs in a superficial vein, this can result in *varicose veins.* After treatment of a venous thrombosis with anticoagulants or lytic agents, or both, these damaged valves may remain insufficient and cause pooling of blood in the dependent veins and thus swelling or edema. When this occurs following resolution of a prior case of thrombophlebitis, this condition may be termed *postphlebitic syndrome.* If severe valvular incom-

935

petence threatens the deep system, a surgical anastomosis of the superficial femoral vein with proximal great saphenous vein below the valve can restore some sufficiency.

The diagnosis of venous disease has proved to be one of the most difficult areas for the physician, exceeding a 50% error margin.[1,3,4] Fortunately many of the classic methods of diagnosis have now been supplemented with newer techniques designed to rule out venous thrombosis or insufficiency.

Contrast phlebography (venography) is the standard method of diagnosing venous thrombosis or embolism.[1,3,5] This is, again, an invasive technique, with many of the same risks found in arteriography (e.g., contrast media reactions, radiation risks). A further complication is that the patient must support his own weight and attempt to remain immobile while tourniquets are applied and irritating contrast medium is injected. The position may, understandably, be difficult to maintain. Venography can also be performed in the supine position, but this does not often result in satisfactory filling of calf or foot veins since the leg or extremity is not dependent. The examination may also, in rare cases, cause a thrombus to form. Venography remains the "gold standard," however, since small thrombi can be readily detected throughout the superficial and deep venous systems even with no flow obstruction.[1]

Nuclear medicine techniques are also used to diagnose sources of venous emboli (thrombi).[1,3,5] These involve injecting radionuclides, which are either followed through the deep venous system by a gamma camera or absorbed by the thrombus and shown on a static scan. The former method uses technetium-99^m pertechnetate and is more efficient for veins above the knee since discrimination of calf veins is impossible due to the diminished resolution. The latter method, using I-125 fibrinogen, allows discrimination of isolated calf thrombi but is not successful in veins above the knee because of the higher background activity from the radionuclide absorption. Both methods eliminate the irritation of the venographic contrast media and are accurate but are not feasible for routine screening of symptomatic patients. Other methods are indicated in these patients.[9]

Another diagnostic technique is impedance phleboplethysmography. The varying methods under this classification involve the measurement of blood flow in the limb based on volume and circumferential changes in response to respiratory variations or automatic inflation of a pressure cuff on the thigh. These methods are prone to error caused by collateral flow, improper respiratory responses, and poor cooperation by the patient.[1,5,9,11]

Examination of the venous system ultrasonically can be accomplished in two ways: the first and most simple method requires only the use of the Doppler device. Small, pocket-sized instruments can be carried for bedside examination to avoid the need for patient transportation. Strip-chart recording is optional if a record of flow is desired. The use of stethoscope or low-frequency sensitive headphones is imperative, because venous velocity signals tend to be very slow and low pitched and could be

missed if external speakers alone are used. The second, and most thorough, method requires the use of a high-resolution real-time duplex scanner, which is much more accurate than venous Doppler alone, since venous Doppler is inaccurate for assessing calf vein thrombosis and is more accurate above the knee. Venous duplex sonography coupled with flow analysis is proving to be more reliable than contrast venography alone and has resulted in much more accurate and specific diagnoses being made. Venous duplex sonography, unlike venography, shows the full extent of a clot and enables some age determination (acute versus chronic). In addition, long-term follow-up is more practical with venous duplex sonography than by radiographic means and also gives important information about the valves and perforator veins unobtainable with venography. Many clinical centers are beginning to hail venous duplex sonography as the "new gold standard."[10,14]

Because venous duplex sonography is a recent development, there are still clinical centers that rely on the venous Doppler method alone or in combination with impedance phlebography. In addition, some postoperative situations and places where space is at a premium may make venous duplex sonography difficult. It is important that a vascular technologist be able to do both types of venous assessment, depending on the situation. This section will discuss the Doppler venous method and then follow with a detailed discussion of the duplex venous technique for the lower and upper extremities, respectively.

CHARACTERISTICS OF THE NORMAL DOPPLER VENOUS VELOCITY SIGNAL[1]

Physiologically, flow dynamics of the venous and arterial systems differs because of the methods by which the blood is moved through them. In the arterial system, blood is pumped directly by the heart, and a pulsatile pattern of flow corresponding to the cardiac cycle is heard. In the venous system, however, there is no pump to force the blood back toward the heart so there should be no pulsatility.

Unlike the arteries, the veins possess valves along their courses that prevent blood from backing up into the more distal segments and ensure a steady flow of blood. The blood is moved through the veins by respiratory variations in intraabdominal and intrathoracic pressure. During inspiration the pressure is increased, the valves close, and flow stops. During expiration the pressure eases, the valves reopen, and blood flows forward once again (Fig. 39-1).

Familiarity with the normal arterial signal can help the examiner locate the venous signals at their various sites. The venous signal has been described as wind-like; it is of a lower velocity than the arterial signal and rises and falls in pitch with expiration and inspiration, respectively. This quality of variation with respiration is called *phasicity*.

There are six normal qualities in the veins that are checked by an examiner at all probe sites.

The first quality is *patency*. This means that a vein allows blood to flow through it without obstruction of the

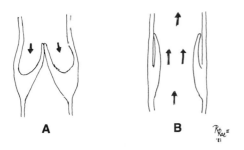

FIG. 39-1. Venous valves. **A,** Closed with inspiration. **B,** Open with expiration.

lumen. Flow heard through a venous segment implies patency of that portion of the vein. Complete absence of a flow signal at any given site implies occlusion of that segment.

The second quality is *spontaneity.* This means that a signal is heard through the vein without manipulation of the limb to force flow through the segment being examined. Spontaneity will not occur in vasoconstricted veins (e.g., those in a cold leg). It will also not occur in veins that are drained of blood, as in an elevated leg. Only the posterior tibial vein may not be normally spontaneous and may require compression of the foot to augment flow.

The third normal quality is *phasicity.* As mentioned earlier, this means that normal variations with respiration should occur in a normal vein. Loss of phasicity will result in a steadily rushing, unchanging, *continuous* flow pattern. This always implies disease.

The fourth normal quality is called *augmentation.* This is the technique of compressing the venous pools in the distal portion of the limb to increase, or augment, the flow. Augmentation can also be created by compressing the segment of the vein proximal to the probe site, holding it for several seconds, and then releasing. This creates a backup of flow, which rushes forward on release. Lack of augmentation implies occlusion between the probe and the compression site.

The fifth quality concerns *competence* of the valves in the limb, or their normal ability to prevent retrograde flow in the venous system. If the valves are destroyed by thrombus or disease, leakage will occur and flow will back up into the distal segment of the vein. Incompetence is often found after treatment of deep vein thrombosis and in varicose veins. Competency is checked by listening for reflux, which may occur with *release of distal* compression or the act of *proximal* compression. Any reflux implies lack of valvular competence between the probe and the compression site. The Valsalva maneuver is also a good test for the valves since it should also stop flow and shut the venous valves.

The sixth and final quality is *nonpulsatility.* It is usually abnormal for the venous system to vary with the cardiac cycle *in the lower extremities.* A patient with congestive or right heart failure may have pulsatility due to increased pressure within the venous system. A patient with an extremely irregular breathing pattern may also show a similar pattern to pulsatility. The veins in the upper extremity thoracic area do not show this quality.

In summary, the six qualities of the normal venous velocity signal are:

1. Patency. Flow can be heard through the venous segment spontaneously or with augmenting.
2. Spontaneity. Flow is heard without manipulation of the limb, except in the posterior tibial vein occasionally.
3. Phasicity. Flow varies with the respiratory cycle.
4. Augmentation. Flow increases normally with distal compression and also with release of proximal compression.
5. Competence. The valves prevent retrograde flow in the vein.
6. Nonpulsatility. The venous flow is not affected by the cardiac cycle.

LOWER EXTREMITY VENOUS EVALUATION
Venous anatomy of the lower extremity[7]

There is usually a corresponding vein for every artery in the Doppler lower extremity examination. The venous system is divided into deep and superficial systems, however.

In the *deep system* various plantar veins anastomose into larger tributaries that unite with the deep venous plantar arch. These veins come together to form the *posterior tibial* vein.

The posterior tibial vein runs on the medial surface of the leg superiorly and is superficially accessible directly posterior to the medial malleolus. Although there are anterior tibial and peroneal veins, they are not examined in the Doppler lower extremity examination.

The posterior tibial vein ascends through the calf and generally forms two venous plexuses. The anterior tibial and peroneal veins also each form two plexuses. These veins join to form the *popliteal* vein.

The popliteal vein runs alongside the popliteal artery behind the knee and continues upward into the thigh, where it becomes the *superficial femoral* vein. The superficial femoral vein continues cephalad and becomes the *common femoral* vein at the point of anastomosis of the *deep femoral (profunda femoris)* vein, which drains the muscles and bone.

The common femoral vein continues cephalad and becomes the *external iliac* vein, which anastomoses with the *internal iliac* vein to form the *common iliac* vein. The common iliacs from each side come together to join with the *inferior vena cava* (Fig. 39-2).

The *superficial system,* for Doppler purposes, consists mainly of the *great* and *small saphenous* veins.

The great saphenous vein arises from the dorsum of the foot and ascends anterior to the medial malleolus. It runs along the medial surface of the leg superficially, outside the knee to the thigh, and anastomoses with the common femoral vein at the saphenofemoral junction. Accessory saphenous veins can occur randomly along the thigh or calf and empty into the great saphenous vein.

The small saphenous vein arises posterior to the lateral malleolus. It progresses superficially up the back of the calf to the knee, where it penetrates the deep fascia and empties into the popliteal vein (Fig. 39-3).

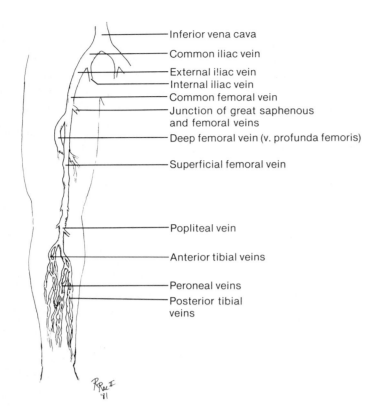

FIG. 39-2.   Deep venous system of the lower extremity.

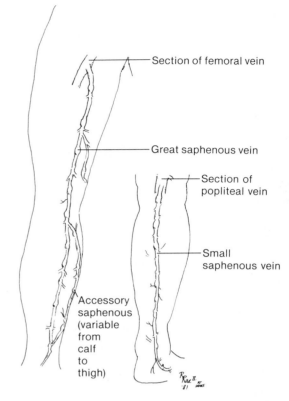

FIG. 39-3.   Superficial venous system of the lower extremity.

Most patients presenting with venous disease will require the examination of the lower limbs. One of the best ways to determine the presence of venous disease is to check for arterial symptoms first and determine whether a pulse is felt.[4] Purplish discoloration and dark areas on the skin usually characterize venous disease, as do swelling and edema of the ankles and legs. The leg will be warm rather than cool as in arterial disease. Pain will occur with dependence of the limb, and relief is obtained by elevation. Swelling will also diminish with elevation of the extremity. Pain will also appear regardless of whether the patient is walking or resting, and walking may actually alleviate the symptoms. Varicosities and red streaks on the limbs also characterize venous disease. Pulling the toes of the foot back toward the leg (dorsiflexion) may cause sharp pain in the calf if calf vein thrombosis is present (Homan's sign),[4] but it should be noted that Homan's sign is positive in 65% of normal patients. These symptoms should aid the examiner in making a differential determination.

Routine lower extremity Doppler venous examination

As in all examinations, the first step is to obtain a thorough history from the patient or the chart. Special attention must be paid to the location of the pain, whether it occurs with walking or rest, and whether elevation relieves the discomfort. Areas of swelling are checked. If unilateral disease is present, one leg will appear larger than the other. Areas of dark almost greenish color are signs of venous insufficiency, as are purple patches and prominent varicose veins. Red streaks imply superficial

disease. The patient should also be questioned about past surgeries, especially if arterial or coronary artery bypasses have been performed. In these cases the saphenous vein is removed in whole or in part and is used for the bypass. A high percentage of post-coronary bypass patients develop venous disease 6 months to 1 year after surgery[12] because of loss of this superficial vein.

Finally, it is helpful to document any past history of phlebitis or deep vein thrombosis and determine whether the patient is currently taking anticoagulants such as heparin or warfarin or is being treated with lytic agents such as streptokinase or urokinase.

The patient should remove all clothing from the lower extremities, including stockings and underwear, and lie supine with the head raised 20 to 30 degrees to ensure venous pooling in the legs.[1,3] The legs should not be elevated and should be relaxed and slightly flexed at the knees to allow good flow dynamics and prevent compression of the popliteal vein against the condyles of the knee joint. The room should be warm to prevent vasoconstriction.

The first vein to be examined is the posterior tibial vein at its site posterior to the medial malleolus. Gel is applied to the site, and the probe is angled caudally. The posterior tibial artery can be used as a landmark for locating the area. The patient is instructed to take in exaggerated breaths to accentuate the phasicity in the veins. A patient with cold feet may have vasoconstriction, and a spontaneous signal may not be heard.

When the site has been determined, the foot may be squeezed to augment flow if spontaneity is not present (Fig. 39-4). The examiner listens for phasicity and nonpul-

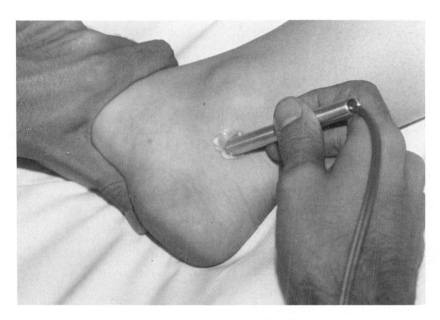

FIG. 39-4.   Posterior tibial vein examination with distal (foot) compression. Note that the probe is angled against the flow.

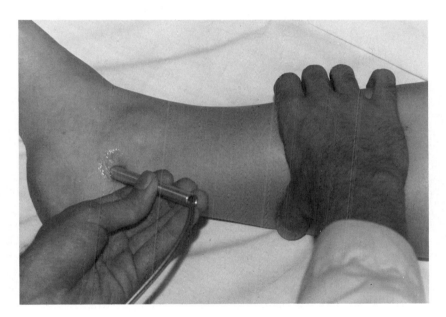

FIG. 39-5.   Examination of the posterior tibial vein, with proximal calf compression.

satility. The amount of augmentation with distal (foot) compression is evaluated; then the leg is grasped at the calf proximally to the probe, compressed for several seconds, and released to elicit augmentation (Fig. 39-5). The flow signal should stop with proximal compression, then resume in a rush, and return to normal with release. Lack of response with either distal or proximal compression implies disease.

The popliteal vein is the next vein to be examined. As with the popliteal artery, there are two ways to position the patient—supine or prone. If the prone method is preferred, examination of the popliteal can be performed as the last step in the examination.

In the supine position the patient's knee should be flexed a bit more, and the probe is placed in the popliteal fossa and angled caudally. (See Fig. 39-6 for relative positioning.) The arterial signal is located, and the probe is angled medially and laterally until a distinct venous signal is heard. The amount of pressure required can vary, for venous collaterals in the fossa should be stopped but the popliteal vein should not be occluded. Gentle pressure usually will not occlude the vein.

When the signal has been found, the examiner checks for patency, spontaneity, phasicity, and nonpulsatility. Augmentation is evaluated by distal compression of the foot and calf (Fig. 39-7) and by proximal compression of the thigh. A Valsalva maneuver may be performed at this point to demonstrate the competence of the proximal venous valves.

In the prone position the patient's feet are elevated ap-

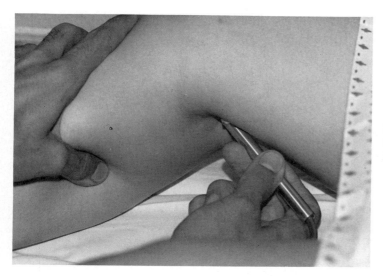

FIG. 39-6. Supine examination of the popliteal vein, with distal calf compression. Note that the transducer is angled against the flow.

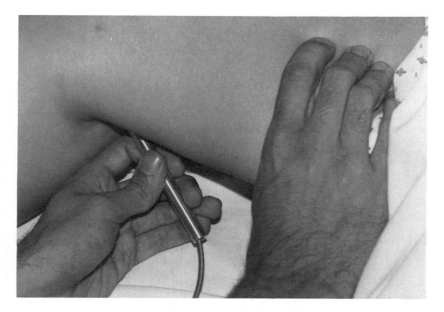

FIG. 39-7. Examination of the popliteal vein with thigh (proximal) compression.

proximately 30 degrees by pillows. With this exception, the examination is performed in the exact sequence as described above for the supine position. (See Fig. 38-13) for positioning.)

The common femoral vein is examined next. The best site to examine the vein is superior to the inguinal ligament. The common femoral artery is first located, and the probe is moved medially and angled caudally to obtain the venous signal. Pressure may be applied to the probe gently to occlude the superficial venous collaterals since the femoral vein will not be as easily compressed. Once again, the signal is evaluated for patency, spontaneity, phasicity, and nonpulsatility. Augmentation is elicited by distal compression (calf, thigh) and proximal compression of the vein superior to the probe site by Valsalva maneuver. Competence is assessed by listening for reflux with compression and by the response to the Valsalva.

If a discrepancy between the groin and knee is noted, the superficial femoral vein may be examined in the groove superior to the vastus medialis and the sartorius on the thigh. The examination should follow the same procedure of signal evaluation, distal and proximal compression, and the Valsalva as used at the other sites. This completes the examination of the deep veins.

The superficial system examination is less involved but requires a finer degree of awareness on the part of the examiner.

The great saphenous vein can be examined anywhere along its course from ankle to the saphenofemoral junction. A light probe pressure is required to avoid compression of the vessel. Flow *may* or *may not* be *spontaneous* or *phasic* through the saphenous systems. It is helpful to position the probe at the site on the inside medial thigh and percuss or milk the distal vein to augment its flow.

Whether the responses obtained by augmentation and the relative flow dynamics signify disease will depend on whether a predisposing factor is suspected. Femoral thrombosis extending into the saphenofemoral junction, varicose veins, and evidence of superficial venous thrombic symptoms are all predisposing factors that will affect the flow and/or occlude the vein. Following the saphenous along its length will often help localize small thrombi.

The small saphenous follows the same criteria and can be examined along its course at the back of the calf from the lateral malleolus to the knee. Be careful when evaluating this vein in the popliteal area to avoid confusing it with the popliteal venous signal; conversely, a patent small saphenous vein in the presence of a thrombosed popliteal vein distal to the small saphenous insertion can also create a false-negative response regarding the popliteal vein's patency. Venous duplex sonography should be ideally used to avoid this occurrence (see below).

The above deep and superficial vein examination is repeated for the other leg.

In summary, these are the steps in the routine lower extremity venous examination:

1. Obtain a history, with emphasis on past phlebitis, graft surgery, pain location, swelling, and discoloration.
2. The patient lies supine with the knees flexed and the head elevated 30 degrees.
3. Examine the posterior tibial vein for flow pattern abnormalities, with distal compression of the foot and proximal compression of the calf to augment flow.
4. Examine the popliteal vein in the supine position. Check the signal for abnormalities and perform distal and proximal compression.
5. Examine the common femoral vein. Check the signal for abnormalities and perform distal compression. Proximal compression and/or Valsalva can also be used for augmentation.
6. Examine the superficial femoral vein if there is evidence of thrombosis between the knee and groin.
7. Check the superficial veins to determine whether thrombosis exists either within or at the points where they anastomose with the deep veins.
8. Repeat steps 1 through 7 for the other leg.
9. If popliteal examination was not performed in the supine position, have the patient turn over, elevate the feet, and examine the vein in the prone position.

See Fig. 38-14 for examination sites in the lower extremity venous study.

Interpretation of the lower extremity venous examination. It may be helpful to reiterate the normal responses obtained in the examination at each site:

1. All deep veins should be patent and phasic, respond well to augmentation, be nonpulsatile, have competent valves, and, with the exception of the posterior tibial vein, be spontaneous.
2. If no spontaneous flow is heard, the vein should be augmented to determine whether flow is present and the vessel patent.
3. Normal distal augmentation will result in an abrupt increase in flow that will then return to normal. Normal proximal augmentation will result in stopping of flow with the act of compression, and a sharp increase in

flow with a return to normal will follow release of compression.
4. The normal superficial venous system may or may not be spontaneous and/or phasic but should augment well and allow patency to be determined.

In *calf vein thrombosis* the posterior tibial signal is less phasic or continuous if it is spontaneous. Distal compression will be normal unless the ankle veins are occluded. There will be decreased augmentation upon release of calf compression.

The popliteal signal will usually be continuous or less phasic depending on whether the thrombus extends into the distal popliteal. The signal may not be spontaneous, and there will be decreased augmentation with foot compression. Foot compression will not result in any augmentation of flow through the calf veins.

Both the superficial and the common femoral signals will be normal, with normal responses to augmentation except by calf compression. It may help to compare the affected leg with the unaffected leg if the disease is unilateral.

In *femoropopliteal vein thrombosis* the posterior tibial vein signal is continuous, with normal distal and decreased proximal augmentation.

The popliteal vein will have either no signal or markedly reduced flow. Usually high-pitched collaterals will be heard in the popliteal fossa. Distal and proximal augmentation maneuvers will result in either extremely reduced or absent augmentation.

The common femoral vein will be continuous or less phasic, again depending on whether the thrombus extends into the proximal femoral segment. The superficial femoral will be absent, or reduced and continuous. Abnormal augmentation responses can be anticipated. An increased flow signal at the femoral may be due to saphenous shunting around the thrombus.

In *iliofemoral thrombosis* the posterior tibial, popliteal, and superficial femoral veins will be continuous, with reduced augmentation at all sites. The common femoral will have absent or reduced continuous flow with poor or absent responses to augmentation maneuvers. Prominent collaterals may exist in the groin.

The diagnosis of superficial vein thrombosis by Doppler alone is often difficult, for there may or may not be spontaneous or phasic flow present. The determination of disease should be based on the predisposing factors mentioned earlier and on reduced or absent augmentation.[3,4]

Occasionally patients will present with diminished-sounding flow or flow that seems continuous where normal responses to compression are noted. The examiner should recheck results for the presence of collaterals, by applying gentle pressure to the probe at the site, and should check the patient's breathing pattern and have him inspire more deeply and exhale more forcibly to be certain that a phasic pattern does not exist in the veins.

Findings in postphlebitic patients and examination additions. Postphlebitic syndrome occurs in patients who have had deep vein thrombosis at one time but have undergone anticoagulation treatments. These patients may have a recurrence of symptoms due to insufficiency resulting from the destruction of the valves by the earlier thrombus. When assessing these patients, the examiner must check their history to help determine whether the insufficiency may be due to a new thrombus or to the destruction of the old valves from the previous phlebitis.

The normal Doppler examination is done with attention given to reflux heard after *proximal* compression or the *release* of *distal* compression. The area of reflux enables one to pinpoint the site of the old thrombus. Valsalva maneuvers will not stop the flow if there are no competent valves proximal to the thrombus site.

In the superficial system, reflux through the saphenous implies destruction of the valves at the saphenofemoral junction.

In evaluations of the perforating venous system between the superficial and deep systems for incompetence, the legs should be elevated and emptied of blood and a tourniquet applied to the calf to prevent superficial reflux. The probe is then moved lightly over the leg, which is covered with couplant, and the thigh is squeezed *above* the tourniquet to determine whether any reflux between the superficial and deep systems is detected. The tourniquet should *not* be tied tightly enough to occlude the calf veins.[1]

Venous lower extremity Doppler cases

CASE 1 (FIG. 39-8): NORMAL RESPONSES AND FLOW IN RIGHT LEG, ABNORMAL RESPONSES IN LEFT LEG. This 23-year-old woman was admitted to the hospital with left leg pain and swelling of 2 weeks' duration. She had recently had hepatitis. There was marked tenderness of the calf and thigh but no red streaking. Thrombophlebitis was suspected.

The right leg showed normal responses and qualities at the posterior tibial, popliteal, and femoral veins.

The left leg had phasic flow at the posterior tibial, with normal responses. At the popliteal, superficial femoral, and femoral sites, however, there was definite continuous flow with only a vague hint of phasicity. Valsalva maneuvers did not stop the flow as they did in the right leg. Iliofemoral thrombophlebitis and valvular incompetence were implied by these findings and confirmed by a subsequent venogram.

The patient was given anticoagulant therapy, which resolved the problem and dissolved the thrombus. Illustrated in Fig. 39-8 are typical normal and abnormal responses in the lower limb.

Venous duplex examination of the lower extremities

Duplex assessment of the lower extremity veins is a relatively recent development, but is one that has shown remarkable diagnostic capabilities and has begun to challenge the ascending contrast venogram as the "gold standard." Techniques for evaluating the venous system by imaging differ considerably from assessment with Doppler alone, but with practice and patience examinations of superb diagnostic quality can be performed.

Venous landmarks. This brief review of the lower extremity venous anatomy may help you locate veins in relationship to nearby bone structures and arteries. Calf veins are usually, but not always, paired and run alongside their respective artery. The posterior tibial vein is accessible on the medial side of the leg posterior to the medial malleolus and runs superiorly along the tibia to its insertion in the deep calf. The peroneal vein runs close to the fibula and lies in the posterior portion of the calf. The anterior vein follows the lateral side of the tibia. The popliteal vein can be found behind the knee in the popliteal fossa and can be traced posteriorly and on the medial side of the leg where it joins the superficial femoral vein. The superficial femoral vein runs medial to the femur and becomes the femoral vein around the pubic crest. Above the pubic crest, the external iliac vein will be seen medial to the iliac artery.

Here is a summary of bone-vein relationships (Fig. 39-9):

- Iliofemoral: above the pubic crest in-line with the medial border of the femur
- Superficial femoral: medial to the femur
- Popliteal: posterior to the condyles of the femur
- Posterior tibial: medial to the tibia
- Anterior tibial: lateral to the tibia
- Peroneal: posterior and medial to the fibula

Veins are usually deep to or flanking the corresponding artery.

For more information, see the venous anatomy section previously discussed.

Preparation. Preliminary procedures are as with the routine lower extremity Doppler venous examination.

Equipment. Use a 7.5 or 8 MHz probe. Linear or sector probes work well, but there may be distortion of the vein caused by the probe shape with a sector scanhead. A 5 MHz probe may be needed in cases where the veins lie very deep. Start at a field depth of 5 cm, but the examiner may need to expand or reduce the field size during the exam in relation to vein depth.

Positioning. The patient should be sitting on the edge of an examination table. The examiner should sit on a chair in front of the patient and rest the foot of the leg being examined on a towel placed on his or her knee. The leg may be easily rotated to various positions for access to the leg veins during the exam. The dependent position helps distend and fill the veins for better visualization and flow determination.

Scanning procedure. For each vein being visualized, look for the following criteria:

1. Compressibility. The vein walls should meet when compressed with the probe (Fig. 39-10). Firm pressure may be required. This can best be seen by doing this in transverse, especially with a sector probe.
2. Valves should coapt (when seen) and should have thin leaflets.
3. Flow should be spontaneous and phasic (augmentation may still be necessary).
4. Perforator veins should not be easily seen.

Remember that veins may be paired in the calf and

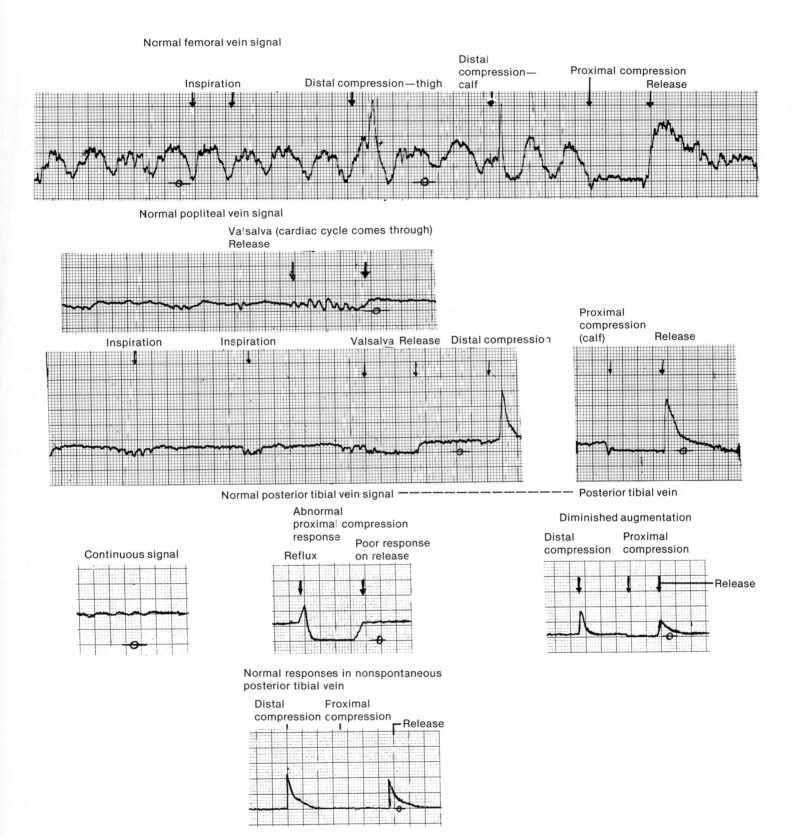

FIG. 39-8.   Normal responses and flow in right leg, abnormal responses in left leg.

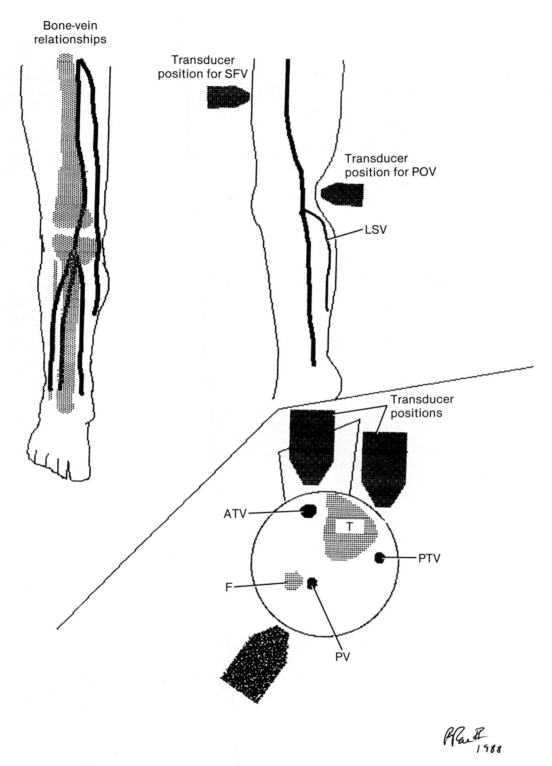

FIG. 39-9.   Diagram showing the relationships of deep and superficial veins to bones, and appropriate examination positions for venous duplex sonography. *SFV,* superficial femoral vein; *POV,* popliteal vein; *LSV,* lesser saphenous vein; *ATV,* anterior tibial vein; *T,* tibia; *PTV,* posterior-tibial vein; *PV,* peroneal vein; *F,* fibula.

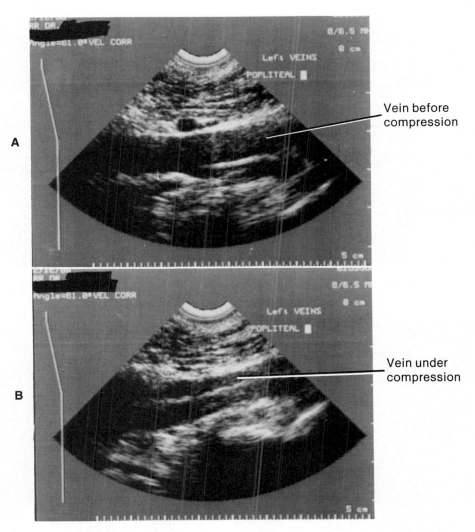

FIG. 39-10.   Normal popliteal vein before, **A,** and during, **B,** compression. Note that the walls meet smoothly, implying an absence of lumen-occupying clot.

may also be doubled even in the popliteal and superficial femoral vein regions. Both sections should be evaluated in these cases to avoid missing a thrombosis that may be in one limb of the vein and not the other. Blood echoes can usually be seen moving through the vein, and phasicity can be assessed visually at times as well as audibly with Doppler.

Start by scanning the *posterior tibial vein* on the medial side of the leg starting at the ankle (Fig. 39-11). Two positions help—one with the probe aiming in *straight and just medial to the tibia,* and with direct scanning *aiming lateroanterior below the malleolus.* Follow the vein up to its insertion at the popliteal vein, compressing along its course with the probe to rule out the presence of clot. Start in the longitudinal position, then look transversely (the compression effect is easier to assess in the transverse view). Use Doppler to assess flow functions (patency, spontaneity, reflux) and to distinguish between arteries and veins. Record any abnormal findings (image or flow) by hardcopy.

Scan *popliteal* area next (Fig. 39-12) to its proximal boundary by placing the probe in the *popliteal fossa and*

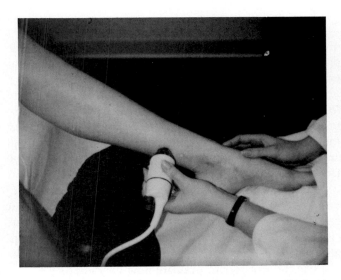

FIG. 39-11.   Duplex examination of the posterior tibial vein.

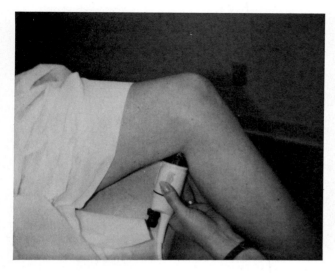

FIG. 39-12.   Duplex examination of the popliteal vein.

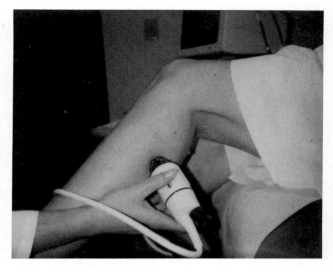

FIG. 39-13.   Duplex examination of the peroneal vein.

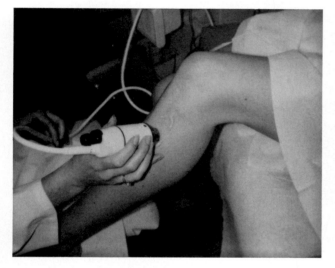

FIG. 39-14.   Duplex examination of the anterior tibial vein.

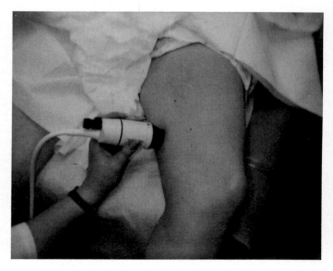

FIG. 39-15.   Duplex examination of the superficial femoral and great saphenous veins.

aiming anteriorly. Scan in longitudinal and transverse planes. Compress the vein area and use the Doppler to evaluate flow characteristics.

Scan the leg caudally and follow the *peroneal* vein by *locating and placing the transducer posterior to the fibula and angling toward the tibia* (Fig. 39-13). Follow the vein(s) down to the malleolus. Scan in longitudinal and transverse planes. Compress the vein area and use the Doppler to evaluate flow characteristics.

Scan the *anterior tibial vein* by placing the probe *medial to the tibia, angling straight back,* then follow it caudally from below the patella to the lateral malleolus (Fig. 39-14). The vein will lie near the bone. Scan in longitudinal and transverse planes. Compress the vein area and use the Doppler to evaluate flow characteristics.

The *superficial femoral vein* is followed up the medial side of the leg from the knee to the groin by *aiming straight in or angling medial to the femur* (Fig. 39-15).

Scan in longitudinal and transverse planes. Compress the vein area and use the Doppler to evaluate flow characteristics. Having the patient lie supine with the upper body elevated may help make this easier.

The *iliac and femoral veins* are best imaged with a sector probe with adequate penetration. The patient should lie supine for this stage, with the upper body flat. Use the inguinal ligament as a landmark, then scan above it in both longitudinal and transverse planes (Fig. 39-16). The external iliac/femoral *artery is lateral to the vein* on each side. Compress the vein area and use the Doppler to evaluate flow characteristics.

The *superficial veins* can be either imaged separately at this point or included during the deep imaging of the femoral and popliteal veins. The *greater saphenous vein* is imaged on the medial side of the leg and lies within 2 cm of the skin. It can be followed from the saphenofemoral junction near the groin to the origin below the knee.

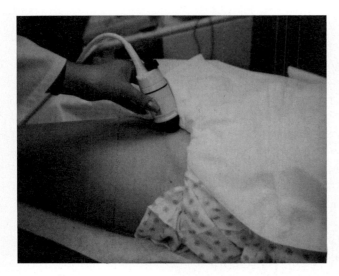

FIG. 39-16. Duplex examination of the iliac and femoral veins.

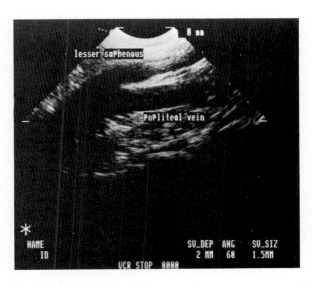

FIG. 39-17. Venous duplex image showing insertion of the lesser saphenous vein into the popliteal vein.

This vessel may split into one or more accessory branches and each branch should be followed. There is a very important valve at the saphenofemoral junction that should particularly be checked. When the patient is supine the saphenofemoral junction is more easily seen. The *lesser saphenous vein* is imaged on the superficial surface of the posterior calf in line with the popliteal vein (Fig. 39-17). It should be followed from its easily seen insertion at the popliteal vein as far distal as possible.

Interpretation of the lower extremity venous duplex examination

NORMAL VEINS

1. Easy compressibility, smoothly meeting walls under compression, (Fig. 39-18 and 39-19).
2. Competent, coapting valves; thin leaflets (when valves are seen) (Fig. 39-20).
3. Phasic and spontaneous Doppler flow.
4. Perforator veins should not be easily seen.

ABNORMAL FINDINGS

1. Veins that do not allow the walls to meet under compression imply the presence of thrombus. Thrombus will appear as an echogenic mass occupying the lumen (Fig. 39-21). The degree of echogenicity increases with the age of the clot. The vein will be dilated distal to an obstruction. Doppler flow may or may not be continuous, depending on the degree of obstruction (Fig. 39-22).
2. Thickened or stiff valves imply disease. Thrombus can often be seen in the valve sinuses that occasionally may be "freezing" the valve open. Doppler flow patterns will demonstrate reflux under standard proximal and distal compression. Valves may occasionally be seen to prolapse with proximal vein compression (Fig. 39-20).
3. Reflux through a venous segment implies proximal valvular insufficiency to that segment, and is easily assessed with duplex Doppler (Fig. 39-23).

CLASSIFICATION OF THROMBUS. The morphology of a thrombus that is visualized may often be a diagnostic indication as to whether the venous disease is of a recent or long-standing etiology. Whether the thrombus is acute or chronic also can make a difference in the type of therapy the patient will receive:

1. Acute
   a. Free-floating or adherent clot; may be slightly compressible
   b. Smooth surface
   c. Soft, homogenous appearance
   d. Distended vein distal to clot
2. Chronic
   a. Firm, stationary clot
   b. Irregular surface
   c. Heterogenous texture, quite prominent echogenicity
   d. Prominent collaterals and perforators seen (Fig. 39-24)
   e. Recanalized flow, often through old clot (see Fig. 39-22)

Technical factor comments. Carefully adjust the TGC and slope as well as the near and far gain and contrast controls to give the best image possible, free of artifact and reverberation. This is important, since inadequate gain settings will prevent the visualization of acute thrombus, and overcompensated gain will create artifacts that may be misinterpreted as thrombus, especially if a vein proves difficult to compress because of improper technique. The ideal setting will allow the intimal linings to be distinctly seen, and there will be some faint specular echoes of moving blood in the veins.

Miscellaneous applications for venous duplex sonography in the lower extremity. In addition to evaluating veins for thrombophlebitis, venous duplex sonography can be used to evaluate the quality of saphenous veins for possible use in coronary or peripheral bypass grafting, or for in situ bypass grafting. The procedures for tracing the saphenous vein above are used. Indelible or

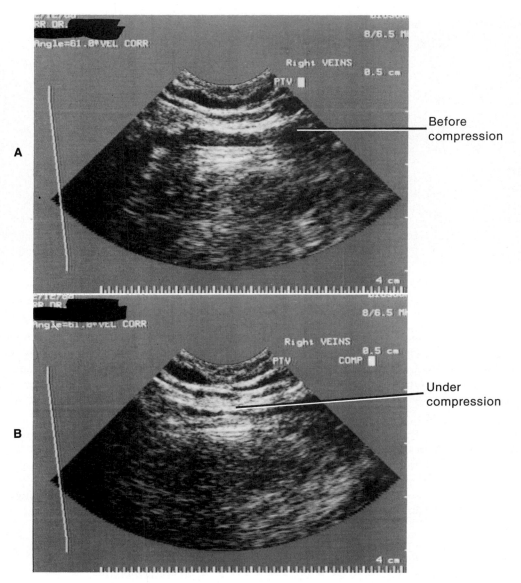

FIG. 39-18.   Compression response of the normal posterior tibial vein. **A,** Before, and **B,** during.

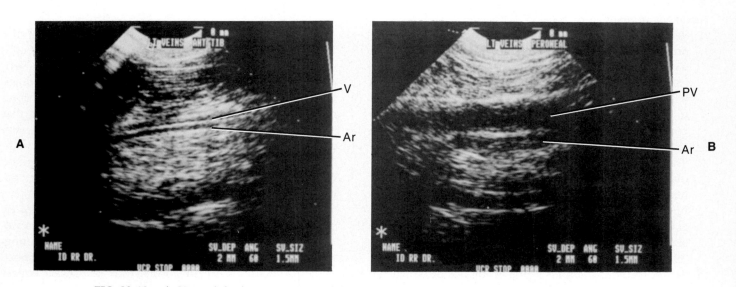

FIG. 39-19.   **A,** Normal duplex appearance of the anterior tibial vein and artery. **B,** Normal duplex appearance of the peroneal vein and artery. *V,* vein; *Ar,* artery; *PV,* peroneal vein.

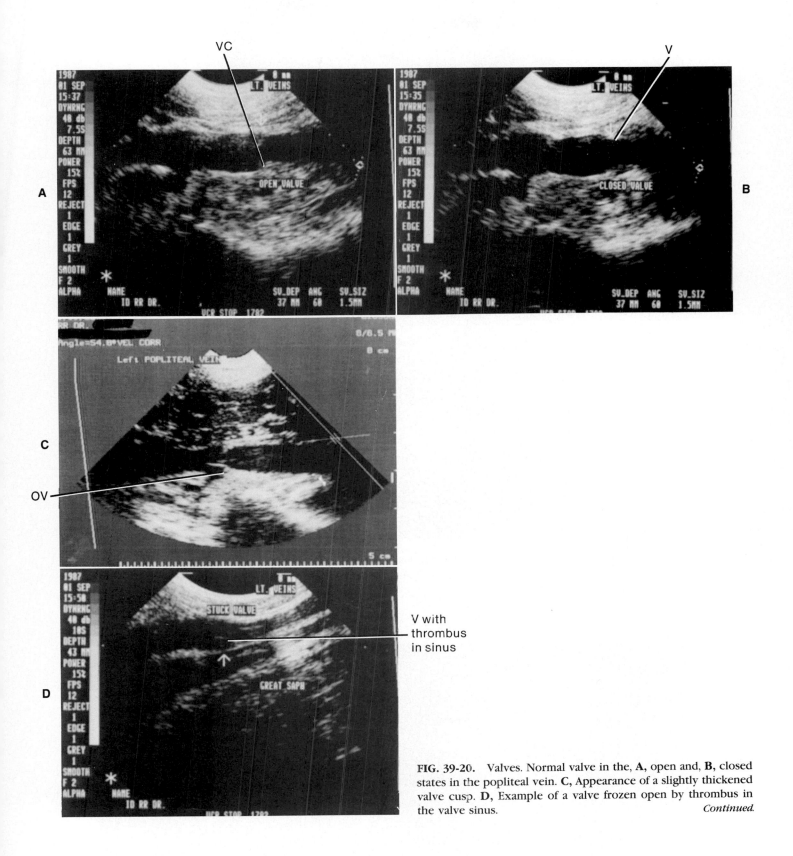

FIG. 39-20.   Valves. Normal valve in the, **A,** open and, **B,** closed states in the popliteal vein. **C,** Appearance of a slightly thickened valve cusp. **D,** Example of a valve frozen open by thrombus in the valve sinus.   *Continued.*

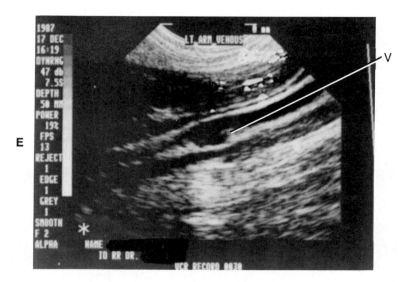

Fig. 39-20, cont'd. **E,** Appearance of a typical valve and valve sinus in a brachial vein. *VC,* valve cusps; *V,* valve; *OV,* open valve.

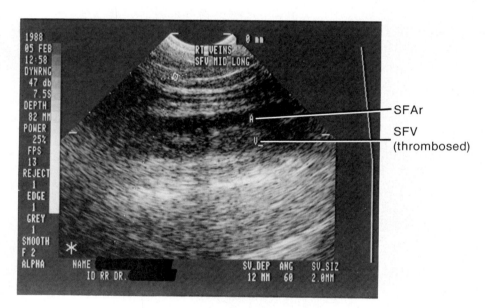

FIG. 39-21. Venous thrombosis. The superficial femoral vein is filled with homogeneous echoes and is noncompressible. Typical sonographic appearance of clot. *SFAr,* superficial femoral artery; *SFV,* superficial femoral vein.

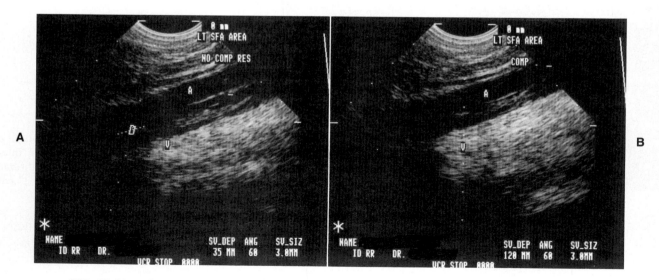

FIG. 39-22. Chronic thrombus. **A,** The clot is only partially obstructive and highly echogenic. Evidence of recanalization through the clot can be seen. **B,** The vein is partially compressible but stops at the border of the clot.

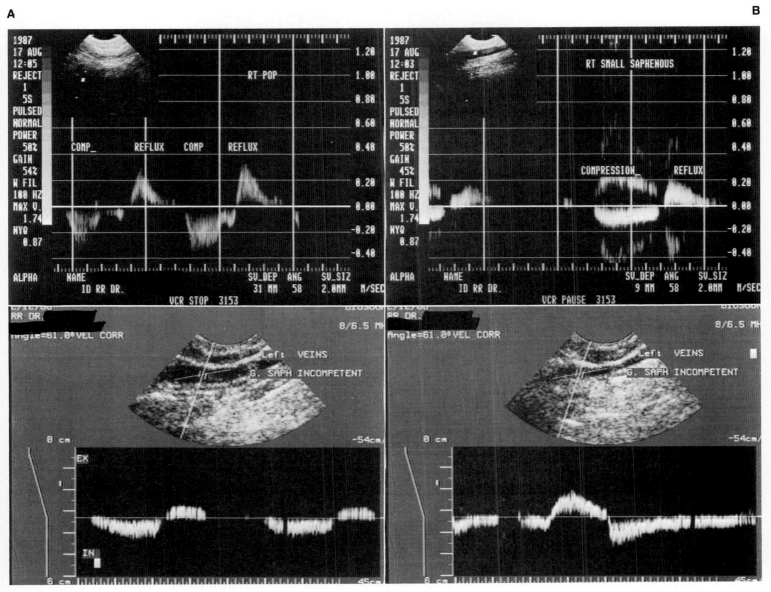

FIG. 39-23. Doppler reflux patterns in the popliteal, **A,** and lesser saphenous, **B,** veins showing venous insufficiency. The great saphenous venous signal in C shows severe incompetence with reflux occurring during simple respiration. With calf compression and release, the signal shows moderate to severe valvular incompetence, **D.**

surgical markers are often used to map the course of the vein for the surgeon and also mark where branches that dump into the saphenous vein are located if ligation is required prior to in situ arterial bypass graft surgery.

Lower extremity venous duplex sonography cases

CASE 1 (FIG. 39-25): THROMBOSED SUPERFICIAL FEMORAL VEIN AND DEEP SYSTEM. This patient presented with a 3-week history of calf pain and swelling. The patient was a wrestling coach and did not comply with the physician's advice when the onset of discomfort was noted. One week later the patient developed a severe calf pain with positive Homan's sign.

Prominent echogenic thrombus was seen to be filling

the entire deep system from calf veins to just below the saphenofemoral junction (Fig. 39-25, A to F). The veins with the thrombus did not compress (Fig. 39-25, G and H). Imaging of the proximal femoral and great saphenous veins showed no thrombus. Doppler signals were absent distal to the thrombus, but normal phasic and spontaneous signals were obtained proximal to the thrombus (Fig. 39-25, I) and throughout the patent great saphenous vein (Fig. 39-25, J), which apparently was now acting as the major conduit shunting flow from the distal limb. Two weeks of heparinization failed to lyse the clot, although swelling diminished. A follow-up duplex exam showed no change in the clot.

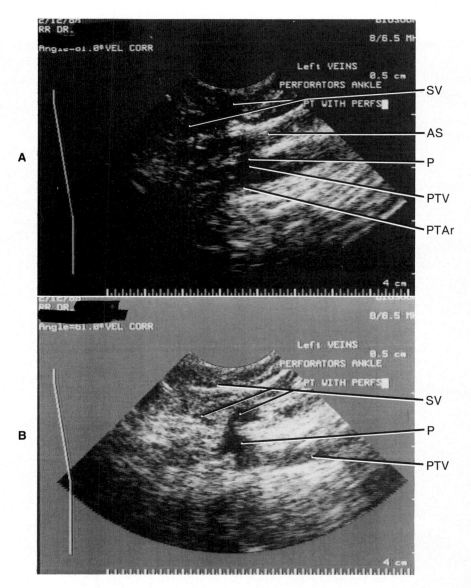

FIG. 39-24.   Perforator veins. **A** and **B,** Prominent perforator vein connecting the posterior tibial and saphenous systems. *SV,* superficial varicosities; *AS,* accessory saphenous vein; *P,* perforator; *PTV,* posterior tibial vein; *PTAr,* posterior tibial artery; *SV,* superficial varicosities; *PTV,* posterior tibial vein.

CASE 2 (FIG. 39-26): THROMBOSED SUPERFICIAL VARICOSE VEIN. This patient had a severely painful and hard dilated tortuous vein on the lateral surface of his thigh. Imaging revealed a chronic, extensively thrombosed varicose vein that appeared to be at least 1 cm or more in diameter and was approximately 15 cm in length.

CASE 3 (FIG. 39-27): SAPHENOUS VEIN ANEURYSM. This patient had a small, dilated area in the great saphenous vein, which distends with dependence, a potential varicosity.

CASE 4 (FIG. 39-28): ACUTE POPLITEAL THROMBOSIS. This 22-year-old woman overdid it during her first aerobics class, presenting with a 3-day history of calf pain. Venous duplex sonography revealed a large thrombosis extending from the distal popliteal vein to the distal superficial femoral vein, obstructing the lesser saphenous vein origin. Calf veins were slightly distended and not spontaneous. The thrombus was not compressible.

UPPER EXTREMITY VENOUS EVALUATION

Though the major incidence of venous disease occurs in the lower extremities, the upper extremities are also the site of venous occlusions that can be just as serious as those found in the legs. Since the introduction of intravenous solution administration, monitoring catheters, and dialysis operations for the patient in renal failure, the incidence of upper extremity phlebitis has increased.[3,4] As in the legs, the upper extremity veins may also thrombose and give off pulmonary emboli.[4,8] The contrast method of venography may not be suitable, especially in the dialysis patient with a surgically produced AV fistula. Determining the patency of veins often becomes a factor in decisions on whether to proceed with venography, to intervene surgically, or to attempt anticoagulant therapy to resolve the problem. Use of Doppler and duplex sonography

Text continued on p. 958.

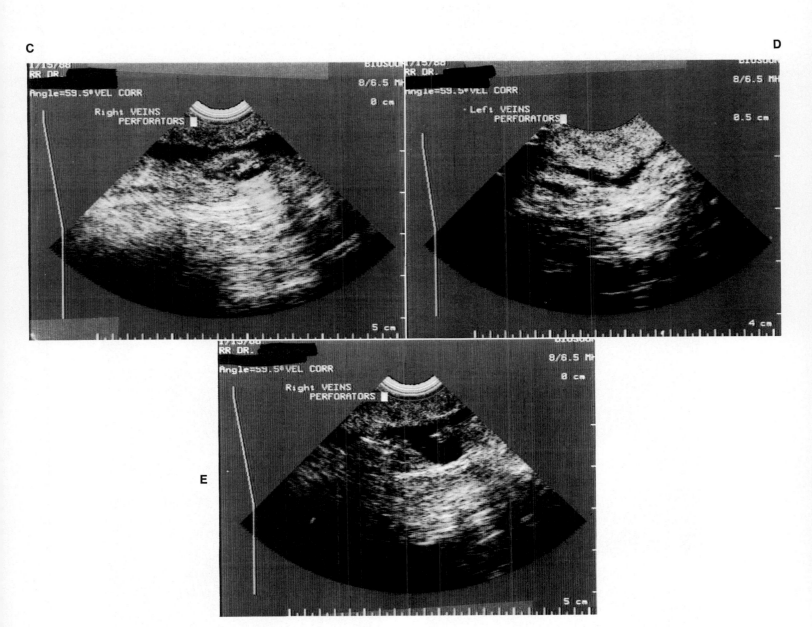

FIG. 39-24, cont'd. C to E, Various appearances of perforators and dilated collateral veins seen in chronic venous insufficiency.

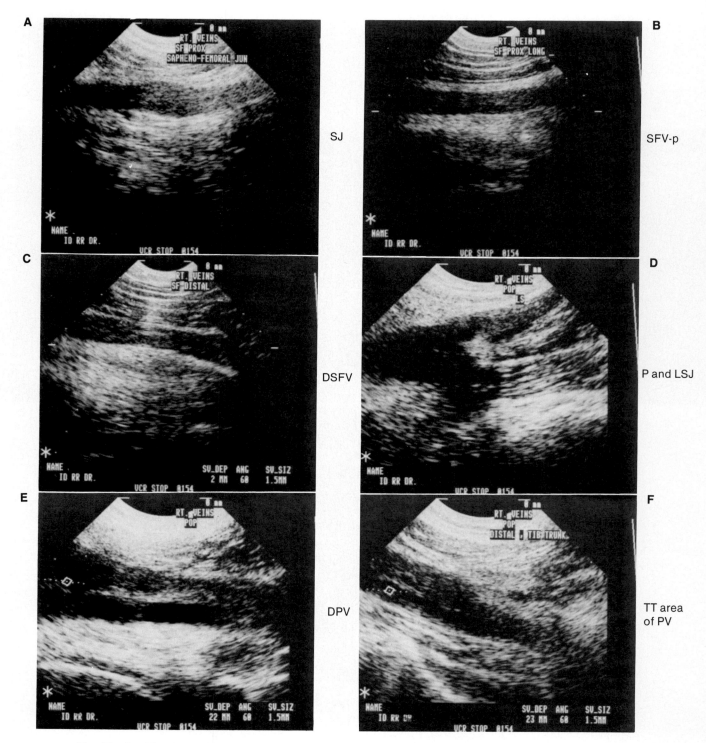

Fig. 39-25. Thrombosed superficial femoral vein and deep system. **A,** Saphenofemoral junction. **B,** Superficial femoral vein, proximal. **C,** Distal superficial femoral vein. **D,** Popliteal and lesser saphenous junction. **E,** Distal popliteal vein. **F,** Tibial trunk area of popliteal vein. **G,** Superficial femoral vein, transverse. **H,** No change with compression. **I** and **J,** See text. *SJ,* saphenofemoral junction; *SFV-p,* superficial femoral vein, proximal; *DSFV,* superficial femoral vein, distal; *P,* popliteal; *LSJ,* lesser saphenous junction; *DPV,* popliteal vein, distal; *TT,* tibial trunk; *PV,* popliteal vein; *Ar,* artery; *V,* vein.

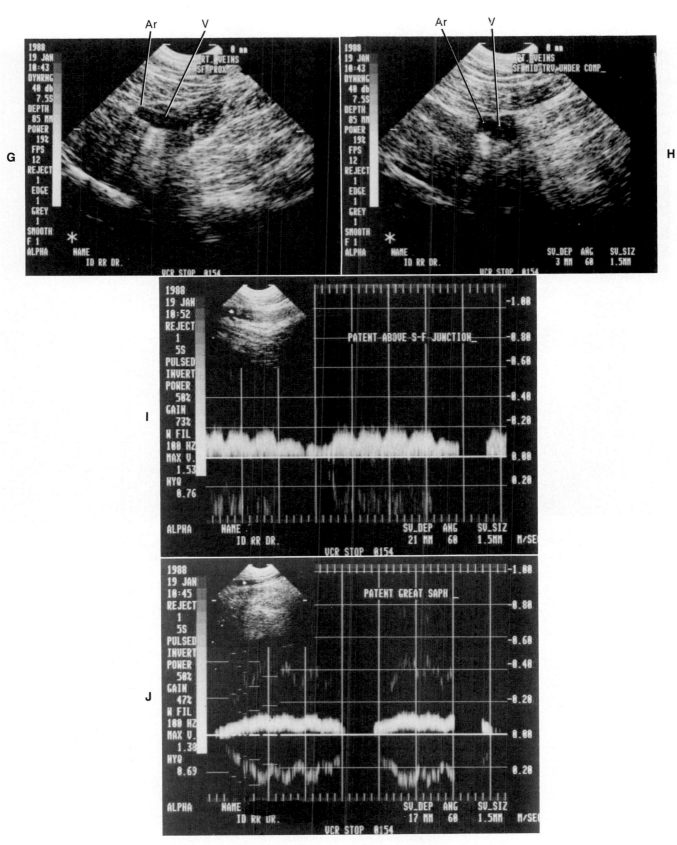

Fig. 39-25, cont'd. For legend see opposite page.

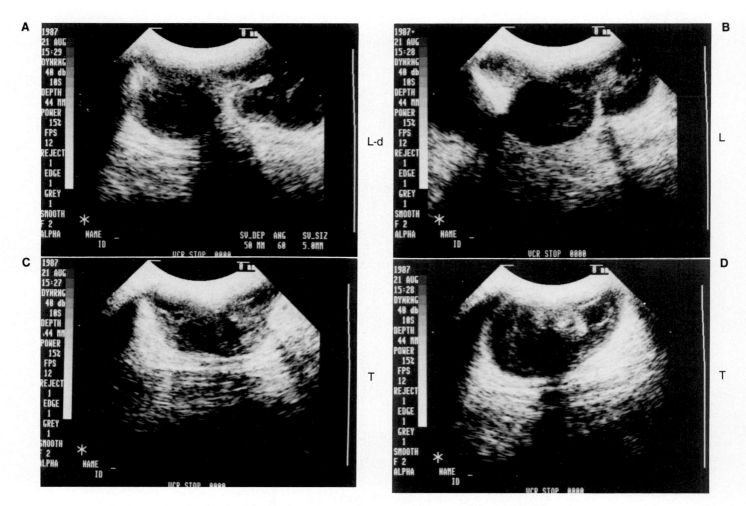

Fig. 39-26. Thrombosed superficial varicose vein. **A,** Distal, longitudinal view. **B,** Longitudinal view. **C** and **D,** Transverse views. *L-d,* longitudinal, distal; *L,* longitudinal; *T,* transverse.

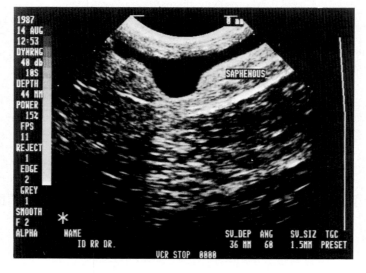

Fig. 39-27. Saphenous vein aneurysm.

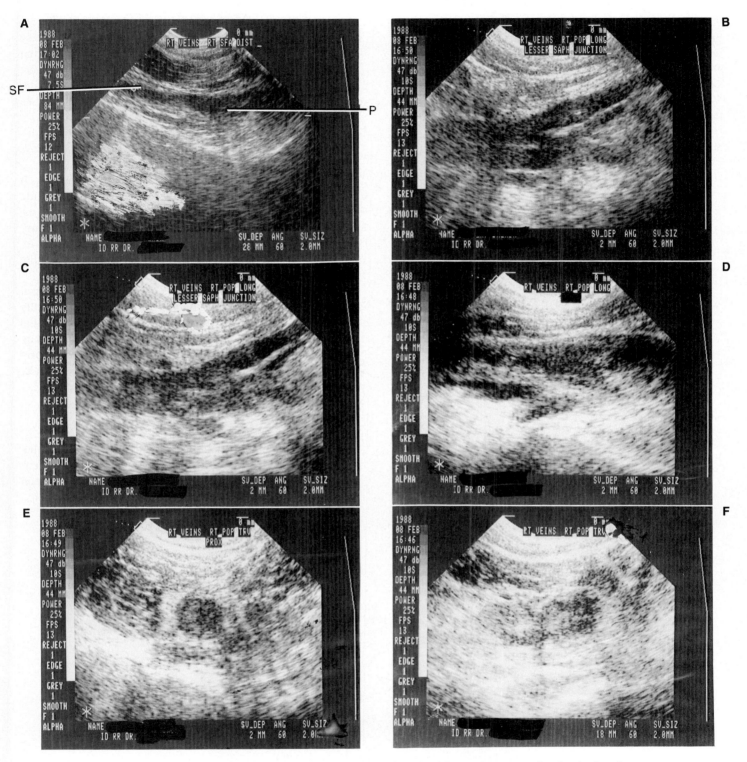

Fig. 39-28. Acute popliteal thrombosis. **A,** Distal superficial femoral vein, popliteal vein, longitudinal view. **B,** Popliteal vein and lesser saphenous vein, longitudinal view. **C,** Popliteal vein and lesser saphenous vein. **D,** Popliteal vein. **E** and **F,** Popliteal vein, transverse view. *SF,* superficial femoral vein; *P,* popliteal vein.

again provides an easily available and accurate method of examination.

Venous anatomy of the upper extremities

Both deep and superficial systems exist in the complex upper extremities.

The *deep* venous system is of somewhat small caliber and difficult to examine in the forearm. A decent signal can occasionally be obtained from the *radial* and *ulnar* veins, which arise from venous plexuses in the venous palmar arches. These veins run superiorly along with their respective radial and ulnar arteries and anastomose at the antecubital fossa to form the *brachial* vein.

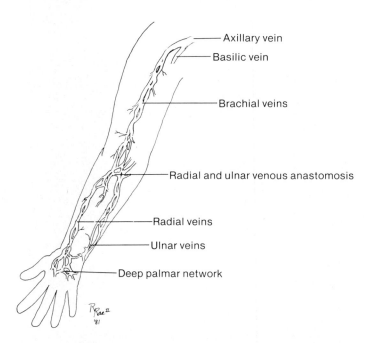

FIG. 39-29. Deep venous system of the upper extremity to the axilla.

The brachial vein runs superiorly along either side of the brachial artery and anastomoses with the *axillary* vein at the junction of the basilic (superficial) vein at the shoulder (Fig. 39-29).

The axillary vein continues superiorly into the thorax, where it becomes the *subclavian* vein at approximately the lateral border of the first rib. The subclavian vein then anastomoses with the *internal jugular* vein to form the *brachiocephalic* vein. The right and left brachiocephalic veins join the *superior vena cava,* which then empties into the right atrium of the heart (Fig. 39-30).

The *superficial* venous system of the upper extremity consists of two major veins, the *basilic* and *cephalic* veins.

The basilic vein begins on the ulnar side of the arm. It runs proximally on the posterior surface of the ulnar side of the arm and continues superiorly along the medial aspect of the arm to the axilla, where it joins the axillary vein. The *median antebrachial* vein lies between the radial and ulnar arteries and anastomoses with the basilic vein approximately 2 cm below the antecubital fossa.

The cephalic vein begins in the radial part of the dorsal venous network of the hand. It extends proximally around the radial border of the forearm to the antecubital fossa, where it anastomoses with the median cubital vein. It then continues up the lateral side of the arm superiorly and enters the shoulder to anastomose with the subclavian vein (Fig. 39-31).

Routine upper extremity Doppler venous examination

The patient's history is once again obtained, with emphasis on pain, discoloration, swelling, and history of recent intravenous infusions; and differentiation is made between arterial and venous disease as in the lower extremity examination.

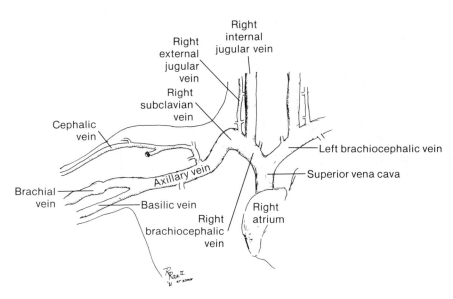

FIG. 39-30. Deep venous system in the thorax to the right atrium.

The patient lies supine in a room with the same environmental conditions as for the lower extremity examination.

First, the deep veins are examined when practicable. The deep veins in the forearm are not as easily assessed due to the complexity of the superficial system in the forearm. General guidelines, however, can be given. The radial and ulnar veins are located at the wrist by locating their companion arteries. The probe is then angled caudally, and the venous signal is distinguished and evaluated by the standard characteristic qualities of the normal venous signal. Note that expansion of the superior vena cava due to negative intrathoracic pressure may increase venous flow in the upper extremity with *inspiration* rather than expiration.

When the flow signal is evaluated, the forearm is compressed and is released after several seconds for proximal augmentation. Distal augmentation may be performed by compression of the fleshy part of the hand. Both the radial and the ulnar veins are evaluated in this manner.

Next, the brachial vein is examined. It is monitored at its site on the medial side of the arm at the intramuscular septum. Locating the artery first may, once again, aid the examiner. The standard signal qualities are used to evaluate the venous flow signal. Distal compression is performed by compression of the forearm (Fig. 39-32), and the Valsalva maneuver is used for proximal compression. Responses should be the same as in the lower extremity venous examination.

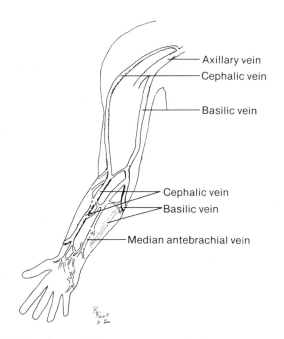

FIG. 39-31. Superficial venous system in the upper extremity.

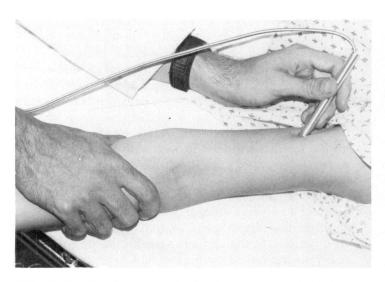

FIG. 39-32. Examination of the brachial vein with distal forearm compression. The transducer is angled against the flow.

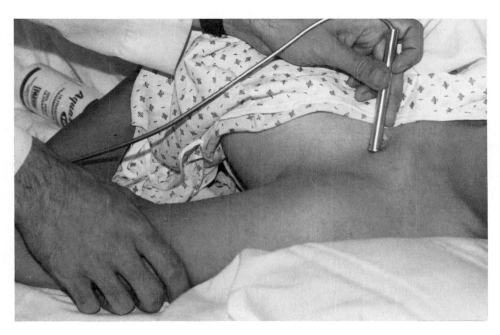

FIG. 39-33. Obtaining the subclavian venous signal.

The axillary vein is then located by angling caudally in the axilla, medial to the axillary artery. The axillary signal may be *pulsatile* and is one of the few exceptions to the rule of nonpulsatility. (All pulsatile signals from this site proximally should be interpreted as normal.) Distal compression of the upper arm and forearm should be performed. Proximal compression consists of the Valsalva maneuver.

The subclavian vein is located by placing the probe either beneath the clavicle and angling superiorly and laterally or in the supraclavicular fossa and angling laterally and inferiorly (Fig. 39-33). This signal is also pulsatile and must be carefully distinguished from the subclavian artery signal. Examination is performed as for the axillary vein.

If axillary or subclavian thrombosis is indicated, the internal jugular vein should be evaluated for determination of the extent of the thrombus.

The internal jugular is located by angling the probe inferiorly and laterally to either the inferior or the superior border of the sternocleidomastoid muscle. The internal jugular signal can be phasic, continuous, or pulsatile and usually is heard as a high-velocity variable hissing sound. The only maneuver performed is a Valsalva. Diminished augmentation on release implies a proximal brachiocephalic venous thrombus.[1]

The superficial veins are examined in a manner similar to that for the veins of the lower extremity. They can, again, be monitored anywhere along their course; and they also require light probe pressure. Usually a slightly phasic or continuous signal is heard, and augmentation is performed by percussion or light compression. Reduced or absent flow may imply a thrombus near the axillobrachial junction in the cephalic vein and in the subclavian vein with diminished basilic vein flow.

In summary, these are the steps in the venous examination of the upper extremity:

1. Obtain the history.
2. Examine the radial and ulnar veins. Distal compression of the hand and proximal compression of the forearm may be performed for augmentation.
3. Examine the brachial vein. Distal compression of the forearm may be performed, and a Valsalva maneuver for proximal compression.
4. Examine the axillary vein, with distal compression of the forearm and Valsalva maneuver.
5. Examine the subclavian vein in the supraclavicular fossa, or underneath the clavicle the same way as the axillary vein.
6. Examine the internal jugular vein if there is a question of thrombus extending into the brachiocephalic vein. A Valsalva maneuver also may be performed.
7. Evaluate the basilic and cephalic veins.

See Fig. 38-44 for upper extremity venous probe site locations.

Interpretation of the upper extremity venous examination. It may be helpful again to reiterate the findings in the upper extremity venous examination.

In *brachial vein thrombosis* there will usually be a continuous signal in the radial and ulnar veins. One or both may be continuous, depending on the level of the thrombus. There will be poor augmentation responses with release of upper arm compression or Valsalva.

The brachial venous signal will be either absent or continuous, with a markedly reduced flow rate.

The axillary and subclavian signals will be normal with normal responses to Valsalva but poor distal augmentation responses will arm compression.

The superficial veins will show changes reflecting the extent of the thrombus, especially if it extends into the axillary.

In both *axillary* and *subclavian venous thrombosis* the radial and ulnar vein signals will be continuous. Poor proximal augmentation can be expected.[13]

The axillary signal may be absent or continuous, depending on the location of the thrombus and collateral circulation. Both distal compression and Valsalva maneuver responses will be poor.

The subclavian vein will reflect the same conditions as in the axillary; but if thrombosis is suspected in the proximal brachiocephalic vein, the jugular signal should be evaluated.

In the internal jugular vein, a reduced Valsalva response will imply a brachiocephalic venous occlusion. Flow may be reduced, depending on the extent of the thrombus.

The use of IV infusions tends to be the greatest cause of superficial phlebitis in the upper extremities.[1] In cases of superficial thrombus in the basilic and cephalic veins, flow will usually be completely absent with poor or limited response to augmentation maneuvers. Evaluation must be based on augmentation and patency, as in the lower extremity veins.

Venous upper extremity Doppler cases

CASE 1 (FIG. 39-34): NORMAL UPPER EXTREMITY VENOUS FLOW— POSTOPERATIVE EXAMINATION. This 68-year-old woman was admitted for a mass felt in the right supraclavicular fossa, which was suspected to be a thrombosed subclavian artery aneurysm. The patient went to surgery, but the mass was found to be a subclavian *vein* aneurysm involving the external jugular and three adjacent veins. It was thrombosed, but fortunately was off one wall of the subclavian vein and did not involve the entire circumference of the vein. It was resected, and the four involved branches were ligated. Determination of flow was performed postoperatively.

Normal waveforms with normal phasicity, pulsatility, and augmentation maneuvers are shown. The internal jugular was checked to ensure that proximal flow was normal. There was a normal response to the Valsalva maneuver.

Venous duplex examination of the upper extremity

Upper extremity evaluation with the duplex real-time scanner uses many of the same criteria as in the lower extremity duplex venous exam, but the flow patterns will be different as mentioned above because of the intrathoracic pressure difference, and a "phasic pulsatility" of the vein

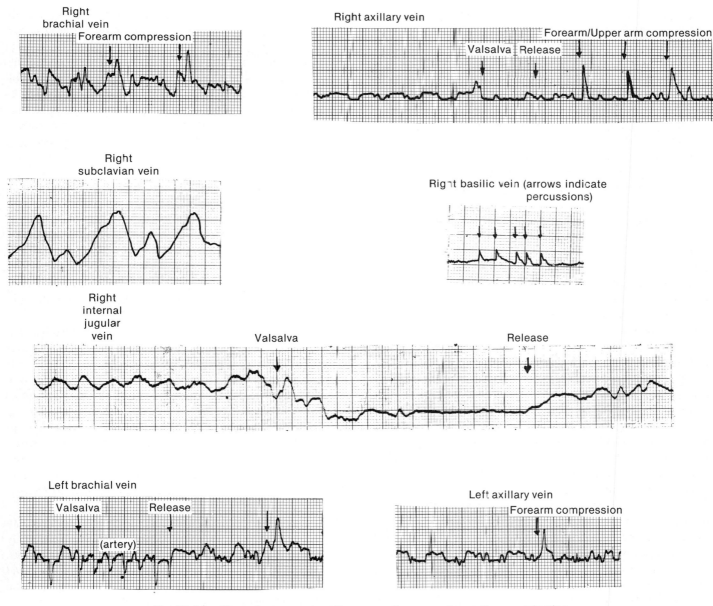

Fig. 39-34.   Normal upper extremity venous flow—postoperative examination.

will be encountered. Thrombosis will retain the same appearances as those mentioned earlier, as will flow augmentation responses. The main differences will be in the examination technique.

Venous landmarks. As in the lower extremity, the examiner can use adjacent bony structures to help locate the deep veins in the arm. The *radial* and *ulnar* veins lie very superficially to the bright echo of the radius and ulna, and adjacent to the arteries. The *brachial* vein runs medial to the humerus, and is again adjacent to the brachial artery. The *axillary* vein is easily located in the axilla and anteromedial to the artery. The *subclavian* vein is also located posterior to the clavicle and may be visualized either from above or below the clavicle. The *internal jugular* vein is easily found lateral to the common carotid artery in the neck.

The course of the superficial veins can vary, as discussed in the previous anatomy section. Some confusion

can result near the basilobrachial junction, since both veins can be of similar dimension. Almost always, the *basilic* vein can be seen to run posterior and medial to the brachial vein when traced. The *cephalic* vein is easier to trace, since it is on the superficial and lateral aspect of the arm.

Preparation. Preliminary procedures are as with the routine upper extremity Doppler venous exam.

Equipment. In the upper extremity and especially in the superficial veins, 10 MHz linear or sector probes work best, since the veins run especially close to the skin. There may be distortion of the vein caused by the probe shape with a sector scanhead, and light pressure is all that is required. Use of a 7.5 MHz probe is indicated in the supraclavicular or axillary areas. Start at a field depth of 4 cm; the examiner may need to expand or reduce the field size during the exam in relation to vein depth.

Positioning. The patient can be either sitting on the

edge of an examination table or lying supine with the upper body elevated, but the examiner should have complete access to the arm, axilla, and supraclavicular area. A dependent position helps distend and fill the veins for better visualization and flow determination.

Scanning procedure. For each vein being visualized, look for the following criteria:

1. Compressibility. The vein walls should meet when compressed with the probe. Firm pressure may be required. This can best be seen by doing this in transverse, especially with a sector probe.
2. Valves should coapt (when seen) and should have thin leaflets.
3. Flow should be spontaneous and phasic (augmentation may still be necessary).

Remember that veins may be paired. Take Doppler readings frequently to ensure that veins and arteries are discriminated. Blood echoes can usually be seen moving through the vein, and phasicity can be assessed visually at times as well as audibly with Doppler.

If the patient is having discomfort in the forearm or hand, examine the *radial* and *ulnar* arteries on the ventral aspect of the arm. Bear in mind that they may not be easily seen as are the arm veins. Scan in longitudinal and transverse planes when practical. Compress the vein area and use the Doppler to evaluate flow characteristics.

Examine the veins in the *antecubital fossa,* and look for any thrombotic areas that may be present. The antecubital fossa has numerous junctures with the superficial system present, so use of the Doppler to discriminate between veins and arteries and to identify the vessels is vital.

Follow the *brachial* vein proximally from the antecubital fossa and do forearm compressions as well as Valsalva manuevers to assess flow patterns and valve function (when seen). Scan in longitudinal and transverse planes. Compress the vein areas and use the Doppler to evaluate flow characteristics.

Continue up into the axilla, examining the *axillary* vein and also examining the junctions of the *basilic* and *cephalic* veins. Scan in longitudinal and transverse planes, compressing as you go and obtaining Doppler flow signals.

Have the patient lie supine; then evaluate the supraclavicular area, examining as much of the *subclavian* vein and thoracic portion of the proximal *axillary* vein as can be seen. Compressibility is very difficult, so assessment of this region primarily centers on visual recognition of thrombus and Doppler flow patterns.

Turn the patient's head to the side away from the side being examined; then examine the *internal jugular* vein by angling the scanhead caudally as far into the supraclavicular area as you can, then moving cephalad. The internal jugular origins, as well as portions of the brachiocephalic vein, can be seen in most cases. Light compression of the jugular is all that is needed, and Doppler signals coupled with a Valsalva manuever can help assess the flow here as in the routine Doppler upper extremity venous exam. The vein is examined in both longitudinal and transverse planes.

The *superficial veins* can be either imaged separately at this point or included during the deep imaging of the arm veins. The *cephalic* vein is best evaluated by starting at its insertion into the *axillary* vein and progressing distally along the lateral arm. The *basilic* vein can be followed from its insertion at the basilobrachial junction distally and medially. These veins are extremely superficial, so a very light touch and ample coupling gel are required. Scan in longitudinal and transverse planes, compressing as you go and obtaining Doppler flow signals.

Interpretation of the upper extremity venous duplex examination

NORMAL VEINS
1. Easy compressibility, smoothly meeting walls under compression.
2. Competent, coapting valves; thin leaflets (when valves are seen).
3. Phasic and spontaneous Doppler flow, some pulsatility normal.

ABNORMAL FINDINGS. The abnormal duplex criteria are identical to those in the lower extremity duplex venous examination:

1. Veins that do not allow the walls to meet under compression imply the presence of thrombus. Thrombus will appear as an echogenic mass occupying the lumen. The degree of echogenicity increases with the age of the clot. The vein will be dilated distal to an obstruction. Doppler flow may or may not be continuous, depending on the degree of obstruction, but flow velocity in the distal segment may increase in nonobstructive thrombus.
2. Thickened or stiff valves imply disease. Thrombus can often be seen in the valve sinuses, which occasionally may be "freezing" the valve open. Doppler flow patterns will demonstrate reflux under standard proximal and distal compression. Valves may occasionally be seen to prolapse with proximal vein compression.

Technical factor comments. Again, carefully adjust the TGC and slope as well as the near and far gain and contrast controls to give the best image possible, free of artifact and reverberation. This is important, since inadequate gain settings will prevent the visualization of acute thrombus, and overcompensated gain will create artifacts that may be misinterpreted as thrombus, especially if a vein proves difficult to compress because of improper technique. Remember, the ideal setting will allow the intimal linings to be distinctly seen, and there will be some faint specular echoes of moving blood in the veins.

See Venous Duplex Examination of the Lower Extremities for thrombus morphology and classification. See also Interpretation of the Upper Extremity Venous Examination.

Upper extremity venous duplex sonography cases

CASE 1 (FIG. 39-35): AXILLARY VEIN THROMBOSIS. This patient presented with a swollen and tender forearm. Duplex imaging revealed a partially occlusive axillary thrombosis at

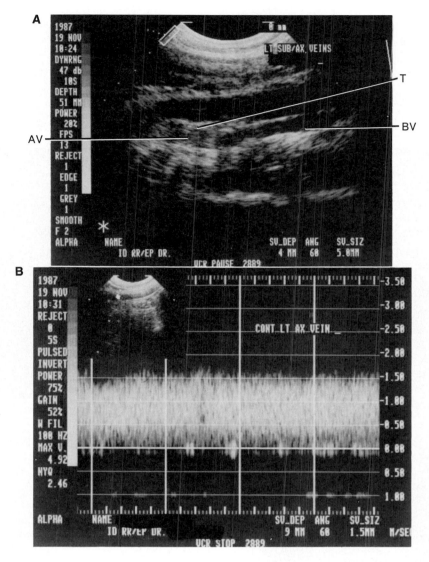

Fig. 39-35. **A,** Axillary vein thrombosis. **B,** Continuous flow pattern. *AV,* axillary vein; *T,* thrombosis; *BV,* brachial vein.

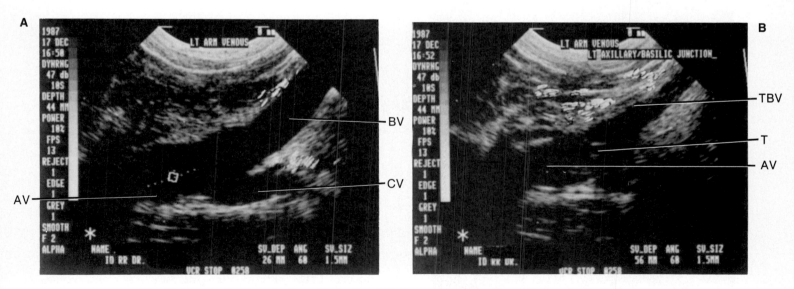

Fig. 39-36. **A,** Basilic vein thrombosis. **B** and **C,** Transverse view. **D** and **E,** Longitudinal view. **F,** Transverse view. **G,** Normal subclavian vein signal. **H,** Normal axillary vein signal. **I,** Normal axillary vein with slight disturbance at basilic axillary junction. **J** and **K,** Absent basilic vein signals. *AV,* axillary vein; *BV,* brachial vein; *CV,* cephalic vein; *TB* and *TBV,* thrombosed basilic vein; *T,* thrombus; *SV,* subclavian vein; *AJ,* axillary junction; *ABV,* absent basilic vein. *Continued.*

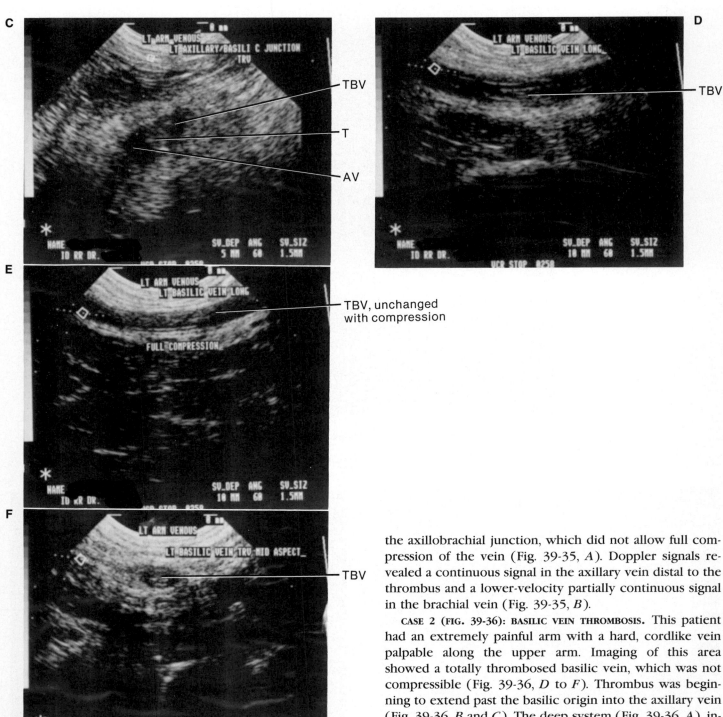

Fig. 39-36, cont'd. For legend see p. 963.

the axillobrachial junction, which did not allow full compression of the vein (Fig. 39-35, *A*). Doppler signals revealed a continuous signal in the axillary vein distal to the thrombus and a lower-velocity partially continuous signal in the brachial vein (Fig. 39-35, *B*).

CASE 2 (FIG. 39-36): BASILIC VEIN THROMBOSIS. This patient had an extremely painful arm with a hard, cordlike vein palpable along the upper arm. Imaging of this area showed a totally thrombosed basilic vein, which was not compressible (Fig. 39-36, *D* to *F*). Thrombus was beginning to extend past the basilic origin into the axillary vein (Fig. 39-36, *B* and *C*). The deep system (Fig. 39-36, *A*), including the brachial, axillary, and subclavian veins, was normal. Flow patterns from the subclavian and axillary veins (Fig. 39-36, *G* to *I*) were normal. No signals were obtainable in the basilic vein (Fig. 39-36, *J* and *K*).

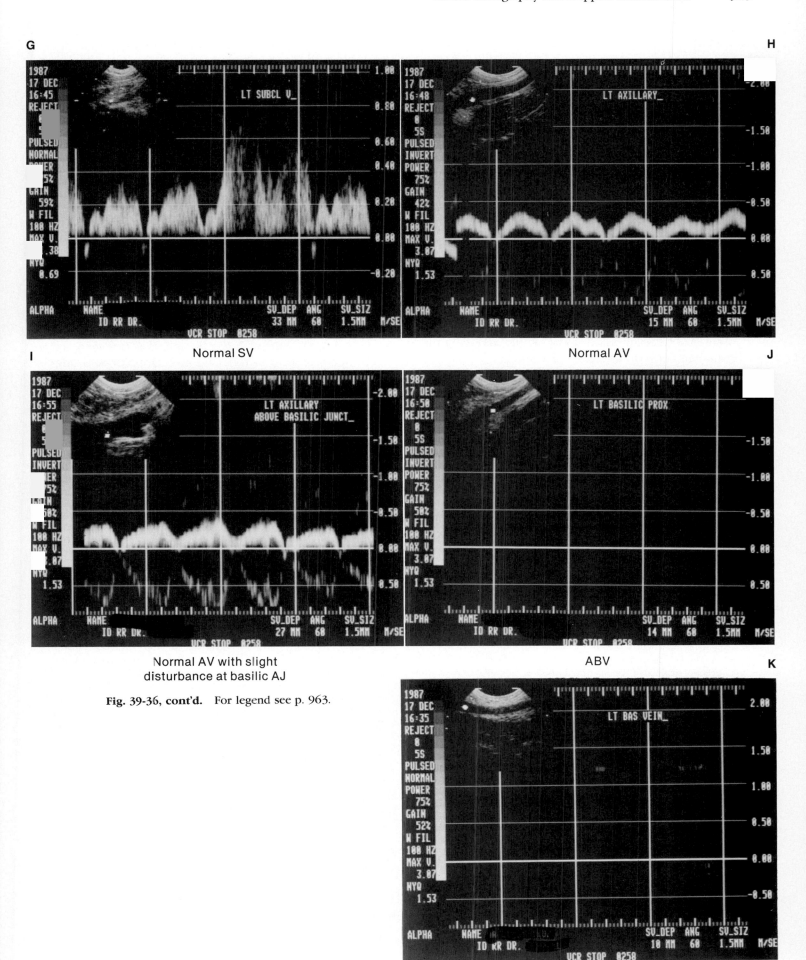

Normal SV

Normal AV

Normal AV with slight
disturbance at basilic AJ

ABV

Fig. 39-36, cont'd. For legend see p. 963.

SUMMARY

1. Both the Doppler venous study and the duplex venous exam are technically demanding yet accurate and convenient methods for evaluating the peripheral venous system noninvasively.

2. Although the venous examination is probably the most difficult to learn and examiner dependent study of all the Doppler techniques, expertise can be gained with practice on normal subjects to determine the correct differentiation of normal and abnormal signals.

3. Careful examination is required for distinguishing collaterals from deep veins and for determining the correct amount of probe pressure to avoid occluding the veins.

4. Careful adjustment of the image factors and gain must be used during the duplex exam to avoid diagnosing image artifact as disease as well as careful application of compression and Doppler usage to discriminate between arteries and veins.

5. False results are almost always due to technical error, so it is important to recheck the results in cases of uncertainty.

6. In conclusion, here are several guidelines to remember:
    a. Arteries and veins are almost always paired, making location of either simple.
    b. Exaggerated breathing will accentuate phasicity.
    c. Continuous flow in a vein is usually significant of a thrombosis. If a patient is receiving anticoagulant therapy, the flow pattern may be of higher velocity; and this should be noted on the report form. Flow will almost always be phasic proximal to an occlusion.
    d. Reflux accompanying release of distal compression in a vein or occurring with proximal compression always implies incompetent valves between the compression site and the probe. In stereophonic headphones this will be heard in the ear opposite the side with antegrade flow.
    e. Absence of flow in a distal ankle vein implies occlusion only if collaterals are prominent and vasoconstriction is not occurring. Lack of response with foot compression may also imply distal occlusion.
    f. Lack of compressibility in a vein during duplex sonography implies that a thrombus may be occupying the lumen. If the thrombus is not seen, adjust technical factors and use Doppler and augmentation techniques to evaluate the area. Remember, fresh clot may not be echogenic enough to see but flow will be affected.

7. Careful examination and thorough knowledge of characteristic responses will ensure accurate examinations. If performed correctly and with confidence, these examinations can be a valuable adjunct to contrast studies or other diagnostic efforts.[6,11]

REFERENCES

1. Barnes RW et al: Doppler ultrasonic evaluation of venous disease, Iowa City, 1975, University of Iowa Press.
2. Barnes RW et al: Doppler ultrasonic spectrum analysis of carotid velocity signals, Richmond, 1980, Medical College of Virginia.
3. Bernstein EF et al: Noninvasive diagnostic techniques in vascular disease, St. Louis, 1978, The CV Mosby Co.
4. Couch NP: Axioms on venous thrombosis, Hosp Med 13(6):68, 1977.
5. Diethrich EB, editor: Noninvasive cardiovascular diagnosis, Baltimore, 1978, University Park Press.
6. Flanigan DP et al: Vascular laboratory diagnosis of clinically suspected deep vein thrombosis, Lancet 2:331, 1978.
7. Goss CM, editor: Gray's anatomy, ed 29, Philadelphia, 1974, Lea & Febiger.
8. Netter FH and Divertie MB, editors: Ciba collection of medical illustrations, vol 7, Respiratory system, Summit, NJ, 1979, Medical Education Division, Ciba Pharmaceutical Co.
9. Pollak EW: The choice of test for diagnosis of venous thrombosis, Vasc Surg 11:219, 1977.
10. Rollins DL, Ryan TJ, et al: Diagnosis of deep venous thrombosis using real-time ultrasound imaging. In Negus D, and Jantet G, editors: Phlebology '85, 1986, John Libbey & Co.
11. Salles-Cunha SX et al: Reliability of Doppler and impedance techniques for the diagnosis of thrombophlebitis, Med Instrum 12(2):117, 1978.
12. Strandness DE and Sumner DS: Hemodynamics for surgeons, New York, 1975, Grune & Stratton, Inc.
13. Schlagenhauff RE et al: The value of Doppler ultrasonography in internal carotid disease, Neurology 27:356, 1976.
14. Semrow C, Friedell M, et al: Characterization of lower extremity venous disease using real-time B-mode ultrasonic imaging, J Vasc Tech 11:187-191, 1987.

40

Examination of the Cerebrovascular System

RICHARD E. RAE II

Cerebral ischemia to the brain secondary to arterial occlusion or rupture, known as stroke, is one of the leading causes of death in the world. Cerebral ischemia may manifest itself with any or all of the following symptoms:

- *Vision changes,* including *amaurosis fugax,* a monocular blindness typically described as "a shade being lowered over my eye" that may obstruct all or part of the patient's sight, *blurry vision,* or frank *blindness*
- *Dizziness,* with or without nausea and vomiting
- *Syncopal or near-syncopal episodes,* which may be described as "blacking out" by the patient
- *Headache*
- *Transient confusion*
- *Hemiparesis,* a unilateral weakness that may affect one or both extremities on one side of the body and may affect the face and tongue as well
- *Numbness,* occurring either by itself or in combination with hemiparesis, affecting limbs, face, and tongue
- *Speech changes,* including slurred speech (dysphasia) or complete loss of functional speech (aphasia) (The patient may know what he or she wants to say but is unable to do so.)

When the episode resolves in less than 12 hours, it is classed as a *transient ischemic attack,* or TIA. If the attack lasts longer than 12 hours but resolves within 24 hours, it may be classed as a *resolving ischemic neuro-*logic deficit, or RIND. Any debilitating ischemic attack that lasts longer than 24 hours and that may show evidence of profound cerebral damage is classed as a *cerebrovascular accident* or CVA. A CVA may or may not resolve with time or therapy, and if symptoms seem to increase in type and severity gradually during the episode, the stroke may be progressing as a result of an intracerebral bleed.

Causes of these ischemic episodes include the following:

1. *Atherosclerotic plaque in the carotid arteries.*[11] Atherosclerosis initially manifests itself as a collection of lipids into the intima, resulting in an intimal thickening process known as the *fatty streak.* Fatty streaks are smooth-surfaced, do not disrupt the intimal lining, and therefore do not obstruct blood flow. This lesion may regress or develop into the *fibrous plaque.* A fibrous plaque is a progression of fatty cells, collagen, and fibrous material that, as it develops, will elevate the intimal lining into the lumen and progress to a point where the lumen is significantly narrowed and may cause flow disturbance. This lesion also may regress or remain the same, but it also can develop into a *complex plaque.* Complex plaques have the most potential for cerebral and arterial damage, since the fibrous and fatty lesions may have calcific changes and internal hemorrhage into the plaque, which can increase the

size of the lesion. *Subintimal neorosis* of the lesion can occur and the smooth intimal continuity can be disrupted, resulting in an *ulceration* of the intima. Ulcerations can collect platelet aggregates, which cause a thrombosis to develop over the ulcer (parts or all of which may detach), or the material within the plaque can be discharged into the bloodstream. Both conditions result in embolic phenomena that can travel distal and occlude intracerebral branches and cause cerebral ischemic changes.

2. *Arterial aneurysm.* An aneurysm of a cerebral artery can eventually rupture and cause an intracerebral hemorrhage. Aneurysms of the internal carotid artery can develop thrombus, as in abdominal or extremity arteries, dissect, or rupture. Thrombotic aneurysms can also embolize distally.

3. *Cardiac emboli.* Emboli of cardiac origin can travel distally through the carotid system to the brain. Some sources for these emboli include valve vegetations, intracardiac thrombi, and myxoma.

4. *Diseases of the intima,* including Takayasu's and giant cell arteritis, can cause the intima to swell and occlude the lumen.

5. *External compression or vascular anomaly* such as carotid body tumor, tortuosity, or kinking can severely reduce blood flow and at times even promote thrombus or plaque formation.

Many syndromes that affect the carotid arteries can remain asymptomatic or clinically silent for years; often the seemingly insignificant dizzy spell or episode of numbness is passed off by the patient until such a time when an episode occurs that does not resolve and may lead to permanent debilitation or death.

Fortunately, many techniques have been developed over the years to help diagnose carotid and cerebral arterial conditions, many times enabling surgeons to intercede before plaques progress to the point of occlusion or imminent stroke. Cerebral and selective carotid arteriography and digital subtraction imaging remain the "gold standard" for the diagnosis of these conditions, but research and studies in recent years are beginning to challenge this view. The true "gold standard" is the findings at surgery, and carotid duplex sonography coupled with spectrum analysis of carotid blood flow is proving to be more accurate than arteriography.[12] Arteriography is open to radiologist variance in interpretation, and many of the fine details of plaque morphology such as intraplaque hemorrhage, intimal ulceration, and soft plaque are impossible to assess with arteriography. Arteriograms depend on localizing filling defects, and when a smooth plaque with little encroachment on the lumen is present, or when it is on a wall obscured by contrast, false interpretations are likely (see Fig. 37-1). Sonography also allows a transverse view of the plaque and lumen unavailable with arteriography. Many vascular surgeons throughout the world are now operating on the basis of duplex sonography findings rather than arteriograms, something unthinkable a few years ago.[9] In addition, carotid duplex sonography and Doppler flow assessment are ideal for

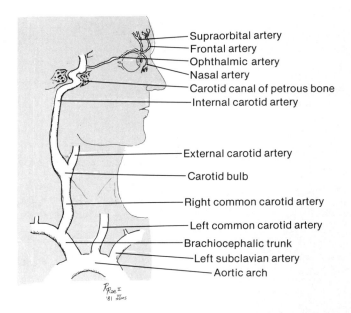

FIG. 40-1.   Aortic branches and the internal carotid arterial system.

screening patients with suspected carotid problems or following up on evolving plaques because they are noninvasive and present virtually no risk to patients. Long-term follow-up of postendarterectomy patients is also practical with sonographic methods. Most patients would be reluctant to consent to arteriography every 6 months!

ANATOMY OF THE CEREBROVASCULAR CIRCULATION[11,15]

The first major vessels involved in the Doppler examination are the *common carotid* arteries. The right common carotid artery arises from the *brachiocephalic (innominate)* artery, and the left common carotid artery arises directly from the aortic arch. Both travel superiorly in the neck to just above the thyroid cartilage. Here the carotids widen into the *carotid bulbs* and bifurcate into the *internal* and *external* carotid arteries.

The internal carotid artery has no branches within the neck. It continues upward to enter the skull through the *carotid canal.* It makes several twists and turns anteriorly and posteriorly and then gives off its first branch intracranially, the *ophthalmic* artery (Fig. 40-1).

The ophthalmic artery continues anteriorly into the orbit, where several branches arise and pass superiorly over the globe and exit the orbit onto the face near the orbital margin. The peripheral branches are the *supraorbital, frontal (supratrochlear),* and *nasal (dorsal nasal)* arteries. These three arteries are the most easily accessible vessels that reflect the hemodynamics of the distal internal carotid.

The supraorbital artery passes through the supraorbital notch or foramen, and branches onto the forehead. The frontal artery exits the orbit at the upper medial angle and also branches onto the forehead. The nasal artery passes out of the orbit at the inferomedial angle and runs alongside the nose to anastomose with the angular artery from the external carotid (Fig. 40-2).

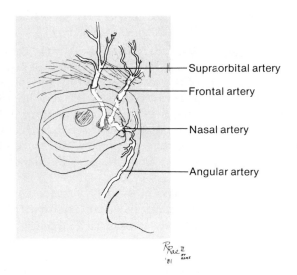

FIG. 40-2. Terminal branches of the ophthalmic artery.

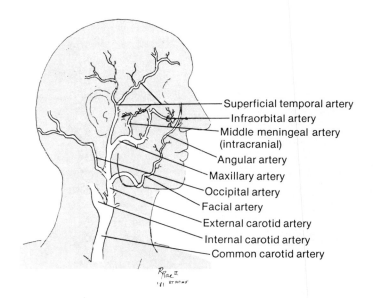

FIG. 40-4. Two views of the vertebral artery.

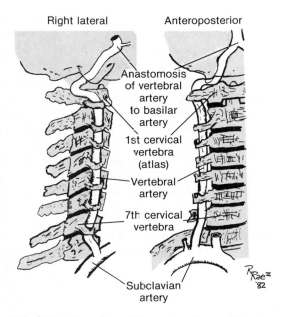

FIG. 40-3. Branches of the external carotid artery.

The external carotid primarily supplies the extracranial structures. It gives off several branches in the neck, beginning with the superior thyroid artery at the bulb and progressing up to the *occipital* artery, which passes posterosuperiorly toward the ear.

The next branch given off is the *facial* artery, at about the same level. It passes anteriorly around the inferior border of the mandible and continues superiorly to the medial corner of the orbit. It becomes the *angular* artery at about the corner of the mouth.

The external carotid then continues superiorly and bifurcates into the *superficial temporal* and the *internal maxillary* arteries just below the ear.

The superficial temporal artery continues upward just in front of the ear and gives off several branches, the anterior of which branches onto the forehead.

The internal maxillary artery gives off the *middle*

meningeal artery, which supplies the dura and floor of the cranium and then gives off deep intramaxillary branches before terminating as the *infraorbital* artery, which exits the skull to the superficial facial muscles through the infraorbital foramen (Fig. 40-3).

The next major arteries are the *vertebral* arteries. Each vertebral artery arises from its respective subclavian artery, and travels superiorly and posteriorly to enter the transverse foramen of the sixth cervical vertebra. The vertebral arteries travel through the transverse foramina of the next five vertebrae until they exit the first cervical vertebra, curve anteriorly and posteriorly, and enter the skull through the foramen magnum.

Upon entering the skull the two vertebral arteries anastomose to form the *basilar* artery (Fig. 40-4).

The vertebral, basilar, and internal carotids service or are serviced by the *circle of Willis*, an arterial circle at the base of the brain. It is formed by the following vessels (Fig. 40-5):

1. The *right and left anterior* and *middle cerebral* arteries (which are the terminal branches of the internal carotids)
2. The *posterior cerebral* arteries (terminal branches of the basilar artery)
3. The *anterior* and *posterior communicating arteries*

The cerebral arterial circle of Willis provides a common collateral pathway in cases of single or multiple arterial obstruction. For example, if one internal carotid artery is diseased or occluded, the other internal carotid artery can supply its needs by shunting flow via the circle of Willis. The basilar artery can also supply either or both carotids in severe obstruction

HEMODYNAMICS AND POSSIBLE ANASTOMOSES IN CEREBRAL ARTERIAL OBSTRUCTIONS[2,3,11]

In the circle of Willis the following routes of shunting occur with obstructive disease of the internal carotid:

1. *One obstructed internal carotid* can be supplied by ei-

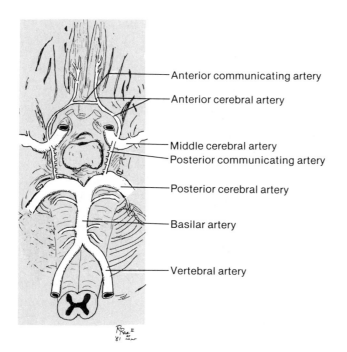

FIG. 40-5.   Circle of Willis.

ther the *opposite internal carotid* via the *anterior cerebral and anterior communicating* arteries or by the *vertebrobasilar* arteries via the *posterior cerebral and posterior communicating* arteries.

2. If *both internal carotids are obstructed,* they are supplied by the *vertebrobasilar* arteries via *both posterior cerebral and both posterior communicating* arteries.

Obstruction in the vertebral or carotid arteries is often masked if excellent flow is maintained in the circle of Willis. I have seen cases in which the patient with bilateral total carotid occlusion was asymptomatic and the condition was discovered during examination for a completely unrelated problem.

Obstructions can also cause anastomoses between the internal and external carotid systems. Potential anastomoses include the following:

1. *Superficial temporal artery* (external carotid)–*supraorbital and/or frontal arteries* (internal carotid)—usually on or across the forehead;
2. *Facial-angular artery* (external carotid)–*nasal artery* (internal carotid);
3. *Infraorbital artery* (external carotid)–*nasal artery* (internal carotid) via the *angular artery;* and
4. Middle meningeal (external carotid)–*ophthalmic artery* (internal carotid) with a direct intracranial connection.

When one subclavian artery is obstructed proximal to the vertebral orifice, the *vertebrovertebral* anastomosis results in a subclavian steal. See Chapter 38 for explanation of the hemodynamics involved, and Fig. 38-42 for illustration.)

On rare occasion, *vertebral artery* anastomoses with the *occipital artery* high in the neck may draw flow from the external carotid to counteract vertebral insufficiencies.

CHARACTERISTICS OF THE DOPPLER ARTERIAL SIGNAL IN THE CEREBRAL EXAMINATION

Unlike the signal in the extremities, the normal Doppler signal in the carotid and cerebral circulation is of high velocity, and because of the low resistance of the intracranial vascular bed it does *not* go below the zero line. The same basic components as in the extremity artery signal exist here, but there is a much shorter secondary component and a larger diastolic component. The secondary component may be absent, depending on disease or vascular resistance.

The only normal exception to low-resistance flow will be in the external carotid artery signal. This signal is still of a higher overall velocity than in an extremity artery; because of the facial branches this artery supplies, the signal is much more like an extremity artery and has a distinctive pattern from the normal common and internal carotid signal (see Fig. 40-27 for normal carotid flow patterns.)

In disease, blunting of systolic flow and diminishing of diastolic flow will occur proximal to a stenosis as disease increases. In cases of a complete internal carotid occlusion, diastolic flow may vanish completely and there may seem to be a reversed flow component as in the extremity artery, since there is major resistance to flow distally (see Fig. 40-33). Prominent bidirectional flow in the carotids may rarely be seen in cases of innominate artery occlusion and carotid steal.

If one is using a zero-crossing chart recorder, turbulence or high-velocity flow disturbances may cause inaccurate readings (see Continuous-Wave Doppler). This can be remedied using a spectrum analyzer.

ROUTINE CEREBROVASCULAR SONOGRAPHIC EVALUATION

In general, examination of the cerebrovascular circulation and carotid arteries is best accomplished using a combination of duplex sonography and continuous-wave Doppler. Some institutions rely on Doppler ultrasonic angiography or duplex sonography alone or in combination with non-Doppler devices such as the oculoplethysmograph (OPG) and photoplethysmograph (PPG). This section will discuss the standard method of evaluating the carotids and periorbital flow with continuous-wave Doppler and spectrum analysis, and the method of evaluating the carotids using a duplex scanner, since these are the most common devices in general use at present. Variations are, of course, possible on the protocols stated here, but these methods are extremely accurate and can result in a quick but accurate assessment of the carotid and cerebral circulation. Following this section, the use of Doppler ultrasonic angiography (Doppler scanning) will be discussed as well as the technique, application, and interpretation of transcranial Doppler, the newest Doppler modality for cerebrovascular evaluation.

Equipment for routine cerebrovascular sonographic examination consists of a duplex scanner, videotape recorder, a continuous-wave directional Doppler, one or two blood pressure cuffs and inflation source, a spectrum analyzer with hard copy, a stethoscope or carotid phonoangiograph (CPA), and a strip-chart recorder (optional).

The first step is to obtain a history from the patient or chart. Emphasis should be placed on typical cerebrovascular symptoms, including dizziness, monocular blindness, nausea, confusion, syncope, headache, personality change, hemiparesis, numbness, and other known symptoms significant for probable carotid stenosis. If the patient has had a frank TIA or CVA, note the number of occurrences, the date of the most recent TIA or onset of CVA, the brain hemisphere affected if a CVA has occurred, whether the symptoms have resolved, and approximately how long it has taken for them to resolve, if at all.

The carotids should be auscultated with a stethoscope or carotid phonoangiograph for the presence of *bruits.* A bruit will be heard as a low-to-high–pitched squirting noise occurring with systole and may range from soft to loud. It results from intraarterial flow turbulence and is usually heard directly over the area of stenosis, although it may be detected in the distal portion of the artery as well. Bruits should be considered significant of disease, especially when they occur in the asymptomatic patient, for they may indicate the presence of severe stenosis and atherosclerotic plaque.

Bruitlike sounds can be heard in patients with systolic blowing murmurs of cardiac origin that radiate through the arch to the carotids. The heart should therefore also be checked to determine whether murmurs that could be radiating are present. Bruits can, of course, be present in the subclavian or vertebral arteries if a severe stenosis exists there, and can radiate distally to the carotid region. Bruits from the vertebral origin can also sound similar to carotid bruits in the cervical area. Simulated bruits can occur in young people or in individuals with low carotid bifurcations due to increased vascular dynamics. As a rule, a bruit in the low carotid region occurring bilaterally and fading in the distal carotid and accompanied by a cardiac murmur is of cardiac origin; bruits high or midway in the neck that can be isolated by the stethoscope with no cardiac murmur are strongly indicative of carotid stenosis.

A severely stenosed external carotid artery can also cause bruits and many times can exist right beside a patent internal carotid. Any time a bruit or bruitlike sound is heard in the high cervical or supraclavicular area, the examiner should apply himself or herself to detecting the cause of the bruit and documenting the area of flow turbulence during the course of the examination.

Doppler direct carotid evaluation

Before reading this section, review the discussion Anatomy of the Cerebrovascular Circulation.

Direct carotid Doppler analysis is often performed after duplex sonography, since imaging allows the examiner to determine how the arteries lie, where the bifurcation is, and how much disease is present. While most individuals can be examined completely with duplex scanners, direct carotid Doppler enables more accurate peak flow measurement in severe cases of stenosis and also allows the examiner to evaluate internal carotids that may lie too deep for adequate assessment with duplex. In addition, the periorbital evaluation allows the examiner to obtain additional indirect information from the intracranial segment of the internal carotid artery and often suggest the presence of intracranial collateralization.

Direct carotid Doppler analysis is discussed first to enable the reader to establish a working knowledge of obtaining carotid flow signals without imaging, since a thorough knowledge of many of the principles used in interpreting carotid flow signals and pathways for collateralization is necessary for optimal use of pulsed Doppler and duplex sonography.

Once the initial patient history has been obtained, if a spectrum analyzer is used it should be connected to the Doppler device and the appropriate signal input level selected on devices that allow the signal input to be amplified or attenuated to prevent signal overload (seen as a dropout in the display) and artifact production (artifacts appear as noise interference). The patient should lie supine with a pillow or bolster placed slightly under the shoulders to extend the head back and expose more of the neck. A pressure cuff is applied to each arm, and the brachial artery signal is monitored and recorded bilaterally. The systolic (and optional diastolic) pressures are then taken from each arm. If there is a greater than 20 to 40 mm Hg difference between arms, with a corresponding reduction of the waveform, evaluation of vertebral flow direction and a subclavian steal evaluation should be done during the course of the procedure on the affected side (see Chapter 38). A blood pressure reading also may be taken with the patient sitting if there is dizziness with positional changes, to help determine whether there is an orthostatic blood pressure drop.

The common carotids are examined next, one at a time. The examiner locates the probe site by having the patient turn his head slightly opposite the side being examined, then palpating the superior or inferior border of the sternocleidomastoid muscle. Gel is applied to the neck, and the probe is placed on the intended site and angled caudally. A gentle amount of pressure may be required to displace tissue (Fig. 40-6).

Two obstacles may interfere with obtaining a clear waveform: the sternocleidomastoid muscle and the internal jugular vein. Ideally the probe position should be on either side of the muscle. Retraction of the muscle by the probe may be necessary when examining the middle section of the common carotid. The vein will usually be heard as a loud phasic or continuous irregular hissing signal—frequently directly over the low common carotid—and may mask the pulsatile signal or dominate the negative side of a zero-crossing circuit (if analog tracings are made) or spectrum analyzer display so as to make recording difficult.

If one is moving the probe medially or laterally and angling around the vein does not work, the vein may be stopped momentarily by having the patient do a Valsalva. The vein may also be manually compressed above the probe site.

When an adequate low or mid–common carotid signal is obtained, the probe should be angled cephalad, and the spectral display or chart tracing inverted so that flow

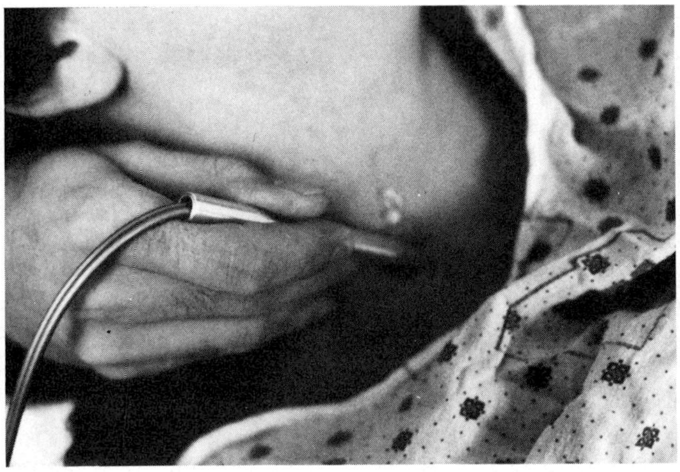

FIG. 40-6.   Examination of the common carotid artery.

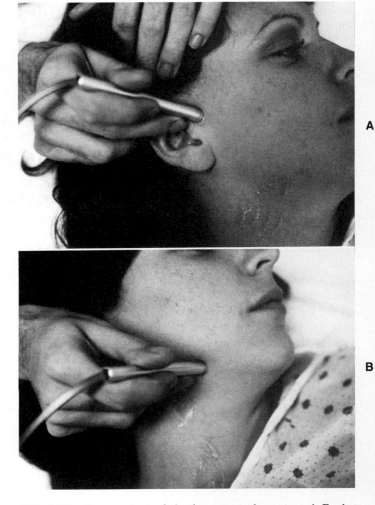

FIG. 40-7.   Examination of, **A,** the temporal artery and, **B,** the facial artery.

moving away from the probe face is interpreted as antegrade flow. The probe is placed lateral to the thyroid cartilage and adjusted so that flow in the bifurcation-carotid bulb area can be evaluated.

The bifurcation level varies in most individuals. It can be found anywhere from the base of the carotid to above the lower angle of the mandible but in the general population is usually found from the thyroid cartilage up. The signals are occasionally obscured if calcified plaque or turbulence is present.

With the probe still angled cephalad, individual spectral recordings of the internal and external carotids are next made.

The external carotid is usually found anteriorly in the neck. It has a distinct signal different from that of the internal carotid. The external signal is much more distinct in the accentuation of the second component and may sound almost like an extremity artery in a patient with a particularly dynamic vascular bed. If the bifurcation area is established, the examiner should move the probe anteriorly while angling cephalad to pick up the signal. If the bifurcation position is not easily located, finding the external carotid signal first and then following the artery proximal until the lower-resistance bulb signal is detected may help.

Moving posteriorly from the bulb will usually bring in the internal carotid. The internal carotid signal usually is of a higher velocity than that of the external carotid, with no second component and diastolic flow well above the zero line. If the takeoff of the internal carotid is severely stenosed, the signal may be almost of a pulsatile high-pitched hissing nature because of the jet effect (see spectral analysis, Chapter 37). Signals should be recorded from the distal segment of the internal carotid when practicable to document any hemodynamic flow disturbances downstream if a proximal internal carotid stenosis is implied.

Doppler periorbital examination

As stated previously, in Poiseuille's law a drop in flow pressure occurs distal to a stenosis. In the internal carotid,

a lack of flow pressure will cause collateralization (see Hemodynamics and Possible Anastomoses in Cerebral Arterial Obstructions) from external carotid branches or the circle of Willis in an attempt to compensate for the deficient flow from the internal carotid. This occurrence is the basis of the *Doppler periorbital examination.*

After the carotids have been evaluated bilaterally, the examiner may wish to take tracings from the *superficial temporal artery* in front of the ear and the *facial artery* at the mandibular notch. These may be of value in determining whether increased flow in either is present, implying possible collateralization, or if there is decreased flow, indicative of external carotid occlusion[6] (Fig. 40-7).

The examiner moves to the head of the examining table, asks the patient to relaxedly close his eyes, and places the probe gently just superior to the inner canthus of the eye within the orbital rim. The probe should be angled medially and cranially until the *frontal artery*[2,7] signal is obtained (Fig. 40-8).

When the signal is located, the chart recorder should be run at slow speed to show the direction of flow. The flow signal is normally antegrade. Retrograde flow implies a greater than 70% internal carotid obstruction.[2,3]

Various compression maneuvers are next performed to

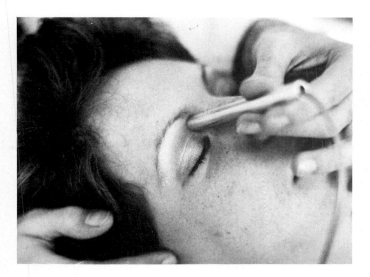

FIG. 40-8. Positioning for the frontal artery.

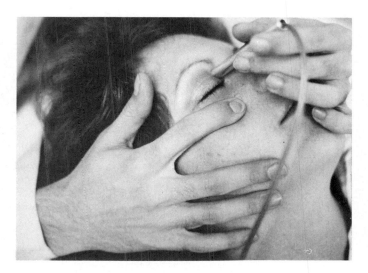

FIG. 40-9. Compression of the infraorbital artery.

determine whether compression of the external carotid branches from the ipsilateral and contralateral sides will cause any increase, decrease, or reversal of the frontal artery signal. The examiner steadies the position of the probe by resting one hand on the patient's chin or by steadying the examining arm in some fashion prior to beginning the compressions. This is to ensure that the probe will not slip off the artery during the time the compression is being attempted.

The first vessel to be compressed is the superficial temporal artery on the side being examined. Normally this either will cause an increase in flow or will not affect the signal. It should be held for at least three beats and then be released.

The facial artery on the same side is then compressed and held for three beats. A normal response to this compression is either an increased or an unchanged signal.

The infraorbital artery on the same side is compressed next. The normal response is an unchanged signal (Fig. 40-9).

With the probe still in place the examiner switches hands and compresses the superficial temporal, facial, and infraorbital arteries of the opposite side of the face in turn. Compression of the contralateral arteries should not affect the frontal artery flow signal.

When the contralateral compressions are completed, the examination procedure is repeated for the remaining frontal artery.

The supraorbital artery should be examined bilaterally by palpating the supraorbital notch and monitoring the artery at that site. This artery should be examined in cases where frontal artery flow may be absent or when directional and collateral determination is difficult from the frontal artery. Compression of the ipsilateral temporal artery usually augments flow.

Summary of steps in the direct carotid and periorbital Doppler examination. To summarize, here are the steps in the routine direct carotid and periorbital Doppler examinations:

1. Take a history with emphasis on cerebral insufficiency and symptoms.

2. Examine the neck with a stethoscope for bruits.
3. Take brachial arterial signals and blood pressures and determine the need for subclavian steal examination.
4. Examine and record both common carotids.
5. Examine and record distal common carotid–bulb-bifurcation area signals from both sides of the neck.
6. Record signals from the internal and external carotid arteries. Record a distal internal carotid signal if a stenosis is implied in the proximal internal carotid.
7. Perform a Doppler periorbital examination. Examine the frontal artery.
8. Compress the superficial temporal on the side being examined. Either an augmented or an unchanged signal results.
9. Compress the facial artery on the same side. It also will either augment or not change the frontal signal.
10. Compress the infraorbital artery on the same side. It should result in an unchanged signal.
11. Compress the contralateral temporal, facial, and infraorbital arteries. This should not change their signals.
12. Check the supraorbital artery for flow direction and possible collateral flow connections.
13. Repeat steps 8 through 13 for the frontal and supraorbital arteries on the other side.

An optional tracing may be made of the vertebral arteries at their bases to reaffirm patent or occluded cerebral flow from all sources. (See Routine Upper Extremity Arterial Examination, Chapter 38, for the technique of obtaining this tracing.)

The sites for monitoring and compression in the cerebrovascular examination are shown in Fig. 40-10.

Interpretation of the direct carotid examination. Basically, the findings discussed under Interpretation of the Spectral Display, Chapter 37, apply to diagnosis of the carotid waveform and hemodynamics. Please review that section for more information. A brief review is presented here.

The normal common carotid waveform and bulb-bifurcation waveform will have a clearly defined envelope and little spectral broadening (under pulsed Doppler); peak

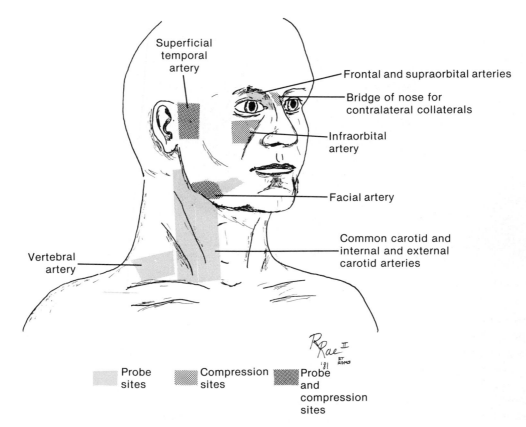

FIG. 40-10. Sites for examination and compression in the cerebrovascular Doppler examination.

frequency will seldom exceed 5 kHz, and peak velocity will not exceed 80 cm/s. A minor degree of turbulence without velocity elevation may occur in the bulb waveform, which is normal. Diastolic flow will be present, and no part of the flow waveform will be below the zero baseline (see Characteristics of the Doppler Arterial Signal in the Cerebrovascular Examination) (see Fig. 40-27).

The normal internal carotid waveform will be a low-resistance signal, with a distinct envelope, well-defined window, little if any spectral broadening, a peak systolic frequency of less than 5 kHz, and flow velocities at or under 90 cm/s (see Fig. 40-27).

The normal external carotid waveform will be a higher-resistance signal of shorter systolic duration and be equally well-defined. Peak systolic frequencies of less than 8 kHz and systolic velocities of less than 120 cm/s are generally seen (see Fig. 40-27).

The following general guidelines in spectral interpretation should help in classifying the presence of carotid disease and the severity of a stenosis. Normal peak systolic frequency and velocity measurements are higher with higher frequency Dopplers; figures given here will assume the use of a 5 MHz continuous- or pulsed-wave Doppler (see also Spectral Analysis of Doppler Signals, Chapter 37).

1. In general, there will be no increase in peak systolic frequency or velocity until a stenosis of 60% occurs. In the internal carotid artery peak systolic velocities greater than 100 cm/s or peak systolic frequencies greater than 5 kHz imply a greater than 60% stenosis.

2. Spectral broadening will increase as the severity of stenosis increases. Spectral broadening without significant velocity elevation (less than 100 cm/s or 5 kHz) implies a stenosis of 50% or less.

3. Marked turbulence and loss of window will occur with a luminal reduction of 70% or greater.

4. *End-diastolic peak frequencies* of less than 5 kHz or 120 cm/s occur below an 80% stenosis. Over 5 kHz or 120 cm/s are highly suggestive of stenosis greater than 80%.

5. In the common carotid, systolic flow may be diminished and diastolic flow may be dampened or absent when a distal common or internal carotid occlusion is present.

Fig. 40-11 shows typical changes occurring with different grades of stenosis in the carotid system.

Interpretation of the periorbital examination and findings in cerebrovascular obstruction. The normal responses mentioned in the preceding section should be memorized so diagnosis during the examination will be facilitated. Discussion of likely collateralization will be discussed in specific occlusion disorders.

The frontal flow signal is an important indicator of intracerebral hemodynamics. Direction of flow is the primary diagnostic finding, but while stenoses generally need to exceed 75% to cause a reversal of the frontal signal, a reversal may not occur if intracranial collaterals are well developed. The *amplitude* of the signal will still visibly *decrease* in severe or subsevere internal carotid stenosis, and a *bidirectional* frontal signal, while not totally re-

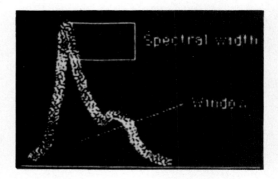

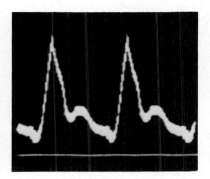

NORMAL

Narrow spectral width
Window clear using
pulsed Doppler
Velocity peak does not
exceed 5 kHz

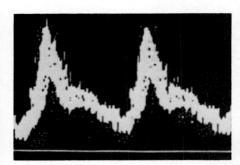

MILD (15%-50%)

Spectral width has increased
Window less clear using
pulsed Doppler
Peak and velocity still within
normal limit

A

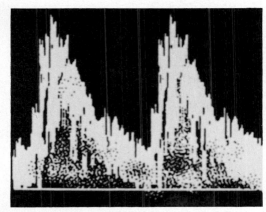

MODERATE (50%-75%)

Width is quite broad
Window fills in more
Noticeable turbulence in
waveform
Systolic velocity > 120 cm/s
Diastolic velocity low
Peak frequency is high but
less than 11 kHz
Diastolic peak under 3 kHz

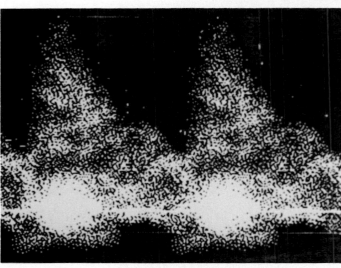

SEVERE (75%-99%)

Severe turbulence with
concentration at baseline
No window
Velocities exceeding 150 cm/s
Peak systolic > 10 kHz frequency
Peak diastolic ≥ 3 kHz frequency
Using pulsed Doppler,
peaks may be cut off or
exceed 9 kHz due to
aliasing

FIG. 40-11.   A, Chart showing appearances in spectral signals that correspond with increases in
the level of stenosis.   *Continued.*

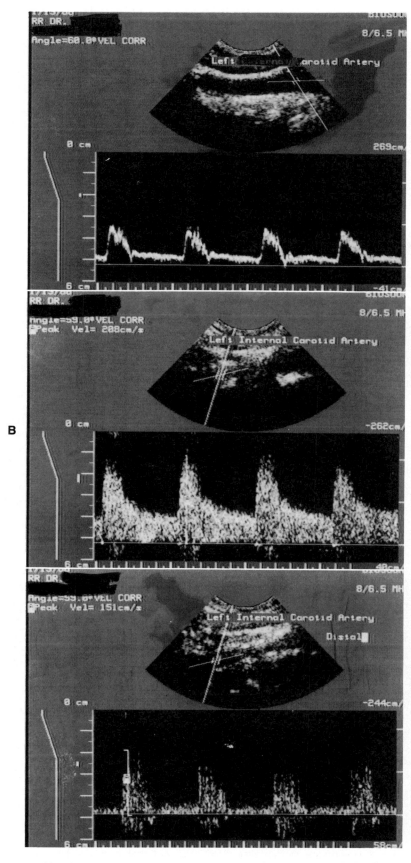

FIG. 40-11, cont'd.   B, Sequential example of changes below, across, and distal to a severe internal carotid stenosis. **B-1,** Pre-stenoses (low common carotid). **B-2,** Across stenosis. **B-3,** Distal to stenosis. *SW,* spectral width; *W,* window.

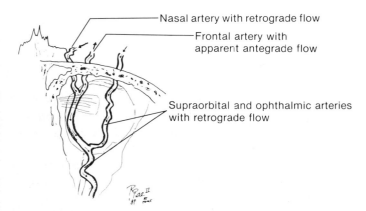

Nasal artery with retrograde flow

Frontal artery with apparent antegrade flow

Supraorbital and ophthalmic arteries with retrograde flow

FIG. 40-12. Diagram of nasal artery flow "stolen" by the frontal artery.

versed, is an indicator that internal carotid pressure has dropped to the point where the signal is going antegrade with systole but pressure in diastole is insufficient to prevent retrograde collateral supply from dominating. It is therefore important to look not only at direction but also at amplitude when a severe stenosis is suspected of decreasing intracranial flow. The comments for interpreting the frontal signal that follow are based on clear-cut directional changes.

In internal carotid obstruction with an *ipsilateral superficial temporal artery collateral:*

1. Frontal flow will be retrograde, since flow travels *into* instead of *out from* the orbit.
2. Compression of the ipsilateral temporal artery will either *stop* or *reverse the flow pattern to antegrade,* provided there is sufficient internal carotid pressure or another intracranial collateral supply to compensate.
3. Same-sided facial and infraorbital compression will not change the signal.
4. Contralateral compressions will have no effect.

When the internal carotid is obstructed with a *contralateral temporal* collateral, compression of the contralateral temporal will have the same effect as in no. 2 above. Other results will be as stated.

In obstruction with a *facial collateral:*

1. Frontal flow may be either antegrade *or* retrograde.
2. Flow will be unchanged with temporal compression.
3. In retrograde flow, ipsilateral facial compression will stop or reverse the signal. If a *contralateral* facial collateral is present, compression of the contralateral facial rather than the ipsilateral facial will cause the change. Since this latter collateral can come across the *bridge of the nose* due to contralateral angular collateral connections, compression at the bridge should have the same effect as direct facial compression.
4. Other compressions will have no effect.

When flow is antegrade, the signal will still change. The apparent antegrade signal may result from retrograde flow in the angular artery entering the nasal artery and making a "U-turn" to come back out the frontal artery (Fig. 40-12). The examiner should check flow in the supraorbital artery to be certain that retrograde flow in the ophthalmic artery is present.

In internal carotid obstruction with *infraorbital artery collaterals:*

1. Frontal artery flow usually will be retrograde.
2. Temporal and facial compressions bilaterally will have no effect on the signal.
3. Either ipsilateral or contralateral infraorbital compression will affect the signal. The contralateral collateral network may also cross the bridge of the nose, as with the facial artery.

Intracranial or *circle of Willis collaterals* may also occur.[1,3,16,17] When the *contralateral internal carotid* is supplying the obstructed artery, the following occurrences will be seen:

1. The frontal artery signal will be *antegrade.*
2. Peripheral external carotid artery branch compressions will cause augmentation or no changes, as in a normal examination.

In this situation it may be necessary to compress the common carotids one at a time, for this is the only definite way to distinguish the abnormality by Doppler.

With a physician, preferably, performing the compression the carotid is located, straddled by the tips of two fingers, and compressed low in the neck for *no more than two beats* while the frontal signal is monitored.

The result of contralateral carotid compression should be *obliteration* or *diminishing* of the signal. Ipsilateral compression will augment flow.

When a *vertebrobasilar collateral* situation exists, contralateral carotid compression will have *no effect.* Having the patient hyperextend the neck may result in successful compression of the vertebrals at their entrance to the foramen, but this is not usually feasible.

Intracranial collaterals are among the hardest to diagnose with Doppler, but proper examination can limit the possibilities of their being missed.

Discussion of false-positive and false-negative conditions[3]. The direct carotid Doppler and periorbital examinations are open to any number of occurrences that can cause diagnostic and interpretive errors to take place. These errors are less likely to occur when carotid duplex sonography is used as an adjunctive procedure or precedes direct Doppler assessment. As transcranial Doppler techniques gain in use, almost all of the problems with the periorbital examination can be eliminated. Some of these errors are technical in nature; some are due to inherent factors related to Doppler ultrasound measurement.

A few of the false-negative conditions will be discussed first:

1. Doppler is a fairly reliable indicator of occlusion when the vessel lumen is obstructed by 70% to 80% of its transverse diameter, but this figure must be attained before a significant pressure drop occurs in the cerebrovascular system. Diagnosis of a false-normal condition may occur when the artery is not occluded enough to reduce flow. This factor can be reduced if the Doppler examination is performed with a carotid high-resolution real-time study as part of the routine examination (see Carotid Duplex Sonography below).

2. Many deep and nonaccessible arteries and collaterals exist that cannot be compressed or heard with the probe. These may also give a false impression of normal flow.

3. There are some nonstenotic soft tissue plaques that do not obstruct flow and therefore cause no audible change in the signal. With carotid duplex sonography these can be seen.

4. Sometimes both the internal and the external carotids can be stenosed or occluded simultaneously. Flow recordings of the facial and temporal arteries may imply that this obstruction is present, and these should be obtained any time a question as to the patency of the external carotid arises.

5. Inaccurate measurement of the frontal and supraorbital arteries can occur if the examiner places the probe outside the orbital rim and catches the flow signal at an incorrect angle or tries to make a reversed signal "antegrade" if unsure of the probe technique.

6. Using a nondirectional Doppler will not show flow direction and may lead an inexperienced examiner to believe a patient has normal flow, especially in postoperative patients.

Following are some false-positive diagnoses. Diagnoses 2 through 6 are false-positive occurrences related to the periorbital examination.

1. A false diagnosis of internal or external carotid stenosis or occlusion can be made if there is transposition of the external and internal carotids (in other words, the internal may occasionally lie anterior and medial to the external), or if when one is using continuous-wave Doppler, a weak signal from one vessel is superimposed over the other because the vessels are lying in the same examination plane. Although real-time duplex sonography can eliminate this problem, an inexperienced examiner can still make this mistake; thus careful examination including the determination of flow patterns and anatomy must be made.

2. Excessive probe pressure may occlude the frontal or supraorbital, making flow seem reduced or absent. The probe can also slip off the artery without the examiner's noticing it during compression maneuvers, occasionally giving one the idea that compression has affected the flow.

3. Flow caught leaving the forehead by an incorrectly angled probe may lead to false diagnosis of flow reversal.

4. Monitoring the palpebral artery in the eyelid instead of the supraorbital may cause confusion, for the palpebral usually stops with temporal compression and this leads to a false diagnosis.

5. Monitoring the nasal artery can cause problems, especially if the patient fits in the category of retrograde flow (45% of normal individuals).[3] This is rarely encountered with good probe technique.

6. If the ophthalmic artery is occluded, flow will be reversed.[8] The patient will usually show signs of blindness without cerebral symptoms, however. Arteriography is indicated to specify this condition.

Common sense, care, and steady probe positioning will usually produce an accurate examination. Research should be done by the examiner if an unusual situation occurs.

Carotid duplex sonography

Carotid duplex sonography is the method of choice for noninvasively evaluating the cerebrovascular system. Again, the arteriographic "gold standard" is being challenged by the many accurate correlations being made when comparing carotid duplex sonography with surgical findings. Carotid duplex sonography does not eliminate arteriography, however, for evaluating structures above the mandible or intracranially, especially regarding the many small cerebral vessels inaccessible to conventional Doppler and imaging, and also since transcranial Doppler use is still not widespread. Arteriography still is too risky and invasive for routine screening of patients with suspected carotid stenosis as well. In general, carotid imaging should never be performed without either duplex or direct carotid Doppler assessment, since imaging alone can miss a surprising number of carotid stenoses.

Description of the carotid duplex real-time image.
Before performing or interpreting an examination, the sonographer must have a thorough knowledge of the appearance and anatomy of the carotid system. This can be reviewed in Anatomy of the Cerebrovascular Circulation and seen in Figs. 40-1 and 40-3.

The *common, internal, and external carotids* appear to have sonolucent fluid-filled lumina bordered by two bright reflections, the arterial walls. The walls are lined with a low-level gray layer bordered by a fine, slightly brighter echo, thought to represent the *intima* of the arteries.

Orientation of the image can vary, depending on the make of duplex scanner, but commonly cephalad is to the left and caudad to the right of the image in the longitudinal axis, with the medial side of the body to the left of the image in transverse.

The *common carotid artery* can be followed superiorly from the supraclavicular area and lies medial to the trachea. The even parallel echoes of the common carotid wall can be traced distally.

Usually an irregular vessel without the thicker-walled characteristics of an artery is seen either anterior to or on one side of the common carotid. This is the *internal jugular vein.* It can be distinguished by its lack of pulsatility, its phasic dilation and collapse with respiration, its tendency to be irregularly shaped and to widen out at the base, and the ease with which it is collapsed by light pressure from the transducer. This is much more apparent when compared with the even diameter, thicker walls, regular pulsatility, and much more stable appearance of the common carotid.

As the transducer moves up the neck, the carotid will be seen to widen out into the area of the *carotid bulb.* The bulb is the most common site of plaque and intimal thickening, which is usually seen to extend into the internal and/or external carotids directly above the bulb.

Contrary to some beliefs, a perfect Y appearance of the

carotid bifurcation is infrequently seen. The bifurcation tends to be rotated differently in certain individuals, and the appearance will depend on the ability to obtain both vessels in the same view. For evaluation the internal and external carotids are best examined individually.

Longitudinally the *internal carotid* can be seen by moving the transducer in a posterior direction from the area of the bulb. It is a vessel generally of slightly larger diameter than the external carotid, tapering into regularly spaced walls that come off the bulb. Locating the distal common carotid and bulb, a *slight* counter-clockwise rotation of the probe (on the right side of the neck) or clockwise rotation (on the left side of the neck) using the fingers should bring in the internal carotid origin.

The *external carotid* is seen by moving anteriorly and rotating the probe axis in a direction opposite to that used to locate the internal carotid. It is usually of smaller diameter without the prominent widening frequently seen at the takeoff of the internal carotid. The superior thyroid artery can often be seen coming off the external carotid or right at the bulb and confirms the external carotid location, since there are no branches off the internal carotid in the neck. (Two rare anomalous branches, the hypoglossal and proatlantal, arise from the internal carotid but are rarely seen on duplex evaluations.) This fact is important in case a large-diameter artery at the bifurcation with a branch next to a smaller-diameter artery is encountered; the examiner can assure himself or herself that the vessel with the branch is the external carotid.

When evaluating transversely, the common carotid will appear as a rounded lumen posterior or lateral to the irregularly shaped jugular vein. The normal carotid retains its round appearance to the level of the bulb, where the diameter of the vessel becomes larger and begins to elongate as the bifurcation approaches.

The internal and external carotids will be seen as two separate round lumina forming from the bulb as the transducer moves superiorly. The internal will be larger than the external and positioned slightly posterior to the smaller round lumen of the external.

Disease in the carotid appears as low-to-moderate gray, soft, and smooth to irregularly edged deformations of the intima extending into the lumen. Calcific plaque is a bright echo with sonic dropout extending past the lesion. Calcific plaque can be incorporated into a "soft" (medium to low echogenic) plaque and is troublesome when the area of dropout obscures the deep wall and a superficial wall plaque is present. Ulcerated plaque can be seen as indentations or erosions in either soft-tissue plaque or the intima. For a detailed discussion of disease appearances, see Interpretation of the Carotid Duplex Examination following the technique section.

Examination technique in carotid duplex sonography. As has been discussed previously, there are a number of different types and configurations of duplex scanners on the market. There are as many ways of holding and guiding the duplex transducer as there are types of transducers the vascular technologist may encounter. In spite of this, the approach to imaging the carotids and vertebrals and obtaining duplex Doppler information from them is basically the same for all machines. This section will discuss these standard scanning techniques, all of which allow room for variation and adaptation as required.

As in direct carotid Doppler, the patient should lie supine with the head and shoulders lying on a pillow and the neck extended back to allow the examiner full access to the neck and supraclavicular area. The examiner requires the duplex scanner, a videotape recorder, a hard-copy printer or camera, and optionally a continuous-wave Doppler for blood pressure measurement, periorbital examination, and to obtain signals from deep or image-inaccessible arteries.

On the majority of duplex scanners the image display should be oriented so that when imaging longitudinally, the head of the patient is to the left of the screen, following standard ultrasound imaging protocol. One duplex scanner (Biosound, Inc. Indianapolis, Indiana), however, orients the image sideways so that the patient's head may be at the top of the screen when the right side is being examined, and inverts the image when the left side is being examined. Some of the images accompanying the text are in this format and are so noted. When imaging transversely, the medial side of the patient should be toward the left as well. The Biosound unit places the medial side at the top of the image when examining the right side and at the bottom when examining the left side.

Initially, the carotids should be examined in the *longitudinal* plane. There are three longitudinal approaches, or *positions,* that afford optimal visualization of the neck vessels and allow almost the entire visible circumference of the carotids to be evaluated. While the technologist should eventually synthesize all these positions into one smooth longitudinal examination, each of the approaches will be discussed individually.

The first position used is the *anterior* position. The patient should turn his or her head to the left side to expose the right side of the neck, and vice versa when examining the left carotid. The sagittal plane of the head should be at about a 45-degree angle to the surface of the bed. The neck is coated with gel, and the transducer is placed on the neck, oriented for long-axis imaging. To obtain as true an anterior view as possible, the examiner should come in directly parallel with the sagittal plane of the neck (Fig. 40-13).

The examiner then examines the common carotid from the base to the bifurcation in long axis, being careful to show the artery continuously. Slight side-to-side motion of the transducer is used to pick up plaque, which may project from a lateral wall parallel with the plane of the examination (Figs. 40-14 and 40-15). It is noted, recorded on the videotape, or photographed for later reference.

Upon reaching the bifurcation, the examiner moves the transducer anteriorly and posteriorly to determine the takeoffs of the external and internal carotids at the bifurcation.

When the position and identification of each artery are

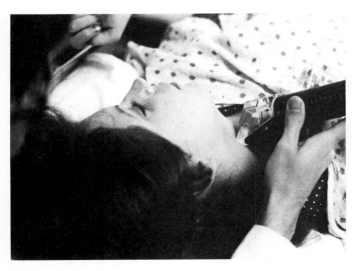

FIG. 40-13. Examination of the carotid artery in the anterior position.

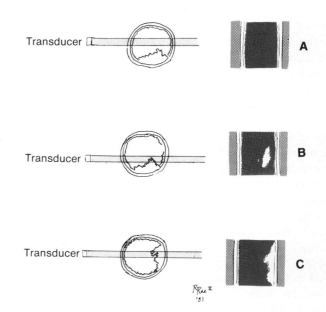

FIG. 40-14. Rocking the transducer. **A,** Plaque on the lateral walls may be missed by the parallel beam. **B,** Slight lateral motion of the transducer enables one to image the peaks of the plaque. **C,** When the transducer is moved to a different examination angle, the plaque is shown in cross section.

determined, the examiner checks to see if any disease is present in the common carotid, bulb, and bifurcation areas. The transducer is moved accordingly to show the extent and degree of occlusion of the disease. Areas of disease are documented and the positioning described.

The examiner then determines the lie of the internal carotid and moves the transducer posteriorly toward the ear while rotating it slightly along the plane of the long axis of the artery. It is followed up as high as practicable.

The transducer next is moved anteriorly and rotated or angled to demonstrate the external carotid. As much of the artery as possible should be seen.

The anterior view is not the best, for the probe will come against the mandible within the area of the bifurcation. It can, however, show disease that is not well seen in the other long axis views.

The patient should turn his head a little more to facilitate the *lateral* position. The transducer is brought around so the beam intersects the artery perpendicular to the sagittal plane of the *head.* The vessels are examined in the fashion described above (Fig. 40-16).

The patient should then turn his head as far as possible. In the *posterior* position the transducer is brought in from behind the sternocleidomastoid muscle and angled toward the anterior side of the patient. The arteries are located and examined as above. The common and bifurcation vessels may be deep in this view and not readily visualized. The Y appearance of the bifurcation tends to be seen in this position more often than in any other (Fig. 40-17).

As stated previously, these three positions can be combined into one smooth scan with the examiner compensating and instinctively turning the transducer, rocking the transducer, and shifting planes. When videotaping, the examiner should be certain to note what position he is in, where the transducer is being moved, what vessels are being imaged, the nature of the plaque and vessel walls, and the orientation of the vessel (e.g., cephalad is to the left of the image).

The carotid should appear as one continuous parallel structure (see Description of the Carotid Duplex Real-Time Image), and it is important to show continuity (i.e., CCA to bulb, ECA connections to bulb, ICA origin and bulb) even in cases of tortuosity, since the jugular vein is so close to the carotid; maladjusted technical factors or a slip of the probe by an inattentive technologist can often make the jugular seem as part of the carotid (or even be mistaken for it).

It is appropriate here to mention some tips that may help when imaging the carotids in the longitudinal plane. A common mistake of novice technologists is to hold the wrist rigid when scanning, which doesn't allow the technologist to follow the natural curves of the carotid. Keep the wrist loose, and use the fingers as pivot joints. Don't try to strangle the transducer. Also, novice technologists forget to rock the transducer or change planes and positions, which often causes them to miss plaque on the lateral walls. In contrast, some technologists move too much, often sweeping past the very structures they are trying to image. Remember that distances in the carotids are very small and that you are imaging a vessel that is less than a centimeter in size, so adjustments involve minimal motions of the transducer.

Once the longitudinal images are obtained, the examiner should turn the probe 90 degrees to image the carotid arteries in the *transverse* plane. While there is only one position here, the transducer can be directed at angles around the circumference of the neck to show the arteries and plaque surfaces optimally (Fig. 40-18).

The transducer should be placed at the clavicle level and slowly moved cephalad, following the common carotid to the bulb and bifurcation. Special attention should

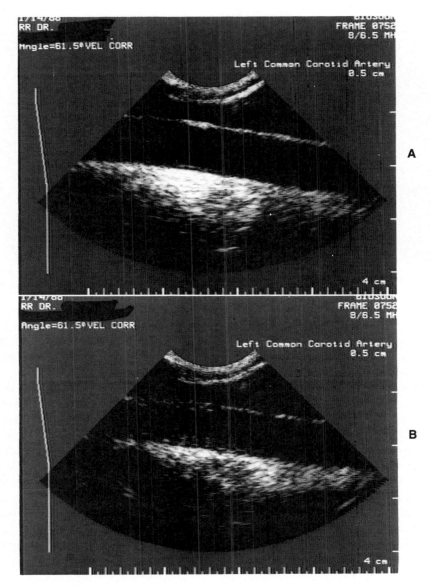

FIG. 40-15. Sonographic example of plaque on a lateral wall. With the carotid centered in the longitudinal image, **A,** the vessel appears normal. "Rocking" the transducer from side to side across the vessel reveals a semi-circumferential plaque along the lateral wall, **B.**

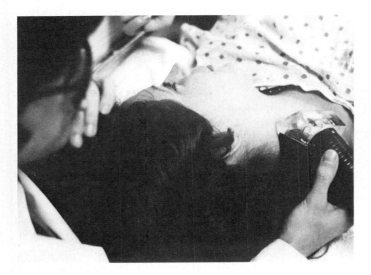

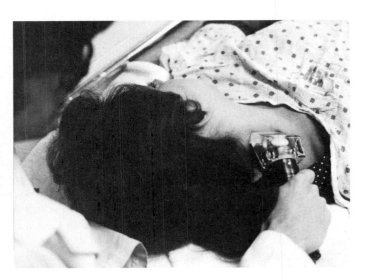

FIG. 40-16. Examination of the carotid artery in lateral position.

FIG. 40-17. Posterior position.

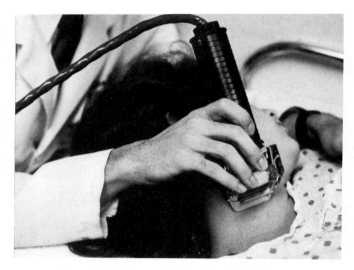

FIG. 40-18.   Transverse position.

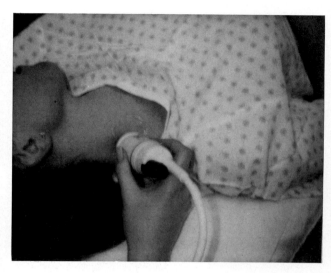

FIG. 40-19.   Positioning for examining the vertebral artery with a duplex imaging transducer.

be given to documenting any plaque formations shown in the longitudinal views.

The area of the bifurcation should be evaluated for circumferential or partly obstructive plaques that may be at the origins but not extended into the internal or external carotids. The transducer can then be moved cephalad further to image the internal and external carotids. They should be followed cephalad as far as practicable. In cases where the internal and external carotids bifurcate at odd angles or run deep to the transducer, accurate transverse evaluation may not be possible.

The internal carotid will be seen posterior to the external. On the right, in machines with the skin surface to the left side of the screen and medial to the top, this means that the uppermost vessel will usually be the external carotid. On the left this position will be reversed. Positioning is less confusing in equipment with the skin surface to the top of the screen.

If there is a question as to whether the vertebrals are stenosed, they also can be evaluated by the duplex scanner. The vertebral origins are the easiest and most complete portion of the arteries to be seen, since the main portion of the artery runs through the transverse processes of the cervical spine and thus is obscured, although sections of the vertebral can be seen between the interspaces.

Vertebral imaging is primarily done only in the longitudinal plane, as few individuals have the optimal body habitus for adequate visualization of the vertebral origins in transverse. The transducer is placed on the neck lateral to the carotid and above the clavicle, then moved laterally and slightly cephalad (Fig. 40-19). Look for regularly spaced areas of shadowing with what appear to be vessel walls between them, then attempt to follow the vessel to its origin at the subclavian. Following the subclavian artery laterally starting at the carotid area and looking for the vertebral origin also works. The vertebral is often easier to find on the right side, since the examiner can trace the origin of the right common carotid to the innominate

artery and then follow the subclavian artery laterally from the innominate-carotid bifurcation to the vertebral origin (Fig. 40-20).

It is usually best to only use the duplex Doppler for vessel orientation and initial flow determination during the imaging portion of the exam; this allows the technologist to concentrate fully on the image and the presence of disease. Once the longitudinal and transverse images have been recorded, the technologist can then use the duplex Doppler in earnest for flow assessment and can concentrate on the Doppler parameters.

Routine duplex signals should be taken at the proximal common carotid, the distal common carotid−bulb area, the proximal internal carotid, and the external carotid. If there is a stenotic signal in the proximal portion of the internal carotid artery, a signal should be recorded distally in the internal to show hemodynamic changes. Each waveform should have at least the peak systolic and end-diastolic velocities or frequencies measured for quantification and diagnosis. Vertebral Doppler signals can be taken by placing the sample between the cervical interspaces into the visualized vertebral. Directional flow orientation and vector angle correction should be carefully monitored.

Since there are a number of duplex scanners that have fixed-angle Doppler, the transducer must be physically moved or angled to obtain an accurate flow measurement. When the Doppler is fixed to sample through the center of the image, the transverse position is often the best position to obtain signals, since the transducer can often be angled more flexibly and without inadvertently digging the corners of the scanhead into the patient's neck. When the Doppler is fixed at an angle and lies parallel with the long axis of the scanhead, the longitudinal plane is the best for Doppler acquisition, but again the fixed angle will often prevent accurate flow measurement of tortuous arteries. Regardless of the positioning of the Doppler the flow measurements should probably be in frequency instead of velocity because of the inability to correct the

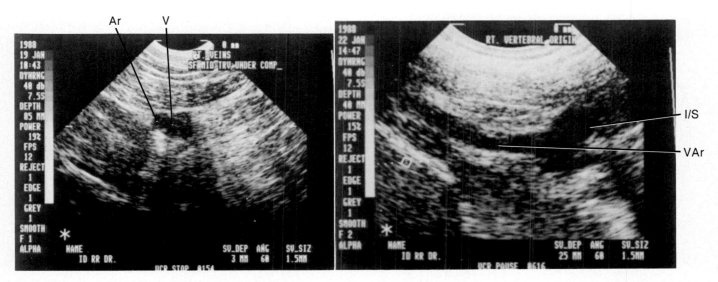

FIG. 40-20. Normal sonographic appearance of the proximal vertebral artery. *VAr,* vertebral artery; *I/S,* innominate/subclavian artery.

flow angle. Velocity *is* available on some fixed-angle duplex machines except that the vector line is also fixed and the transducer must be angled in an often awkward manner to make the vector line parallel with the flow direction.

Once the imaging and duplex assessment is complete, direct carotid or periorbital examination or both can be performed bilaterally for additional diagnostic information.

Interpretation of the carotid duplex examination. Once the examination is completed, the study should be interpreted based on all the data collected. Interpreting the imaging results without taking into consideration the Doppler findings results in only a partial and often inaccurate diagnosis; a patent-appearing internal carotid may be totally occluded with soft plaque or fresh thrombus, or a middle-cerebral artery occlusion in a CVA could be present and causing a distal internal carotid obstruction. Reading the carotid as "normal" in these cases could be potentially dangerous for the patient. In short, *the Doppler flow findings are just as important as the imaging procedure,* and the diagnosis often hinges on the hemodynamic state shown by Doppler when imaging is poor. However, Doppler assessment alone can only imply suspected stenoses or flow conditions that are severe. Without imaging, some conditions cannot be exactly diagnosed, especially if flow is absent, as in total vascular occlusion, or if disease is not hemodynamically significant.

Delayed interpretation of carotid duplex images should always be done from a videotape of the examination. This enables the interpreter to see all changes in the vessel in real time, and ensures that there will be no loss of grayscale resolution or confusion of vessels as may occur with hard copy images. Hard copies, when taken, should always be used in combination with the tape. Duplex Doppler samples can also be recorded during the exam for comparison with visualized stenoses, and the interpreter can also hear the flow changes as well as see the spectral

characteristics. Videotape also provides one of the best teaching tools for education.

Stenoses that are visualized can be measured using *diameter* and *area* calculations and electronic calipers. The calculations are made by first measuring the vessel perimeter and then measuring the residual lumen, which then are averaged together and the difference displayed as a measurement of the relative percent stenosis. They are usually more accurate than a rough visual estimation can be. Diameter stenosis measurements are done on longitudinal images and are usually less accurate than the area stenosis measurements made on transverse images (Fig. 40-21). Comparing the image stenosis measurement with the estimated stenosis by Doppler spectrum analysis can usually result in a very accurate estimation of the true luminal reduction.

We have already covered the changes with disease in carotid flow signals and the appearance of those changes on spectral analysis. Characterizing and categorizing the visual data obtained by sonography is somewhat more involved and highly open to individual interpretation.

Atherosclerotic disease in the carotid arteries adopts the following appearances:

The fatty streak and fatty plaque will appear low-level to moderate-level gray homogenous thickening or elevations of the intima, extending into the lumen from one or both walls (Fig. 40-22). The intima normally follows the vessel walls closely, making intimal thickening or plaqueing dramatically obvious when well visualized. This appearance is also typical of so-called "soft" plaque and thrombus.

The fibrous plaque will appear as a moderate to highly echogenic luminal irregularity or focal plaque, or "mixed plaque" (Fig. 40-23). Low-level gray areas often are found alongside areas of higher echogenicity. These appear as elevations and focal enlargements into the lumen.

The calcified plaque will be bright with high echogenicity and sonic dropout extending deep and parallel with

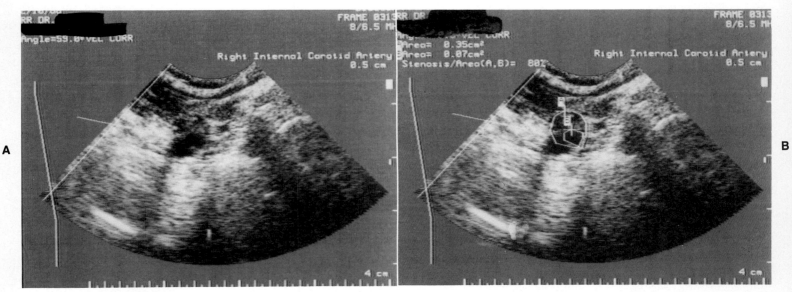

Before area measurement

After area measurement

FIG. 40-21. Area stenosis measurement with electronic calipers. **A,** Before area measurement. **B,** After area measurement.

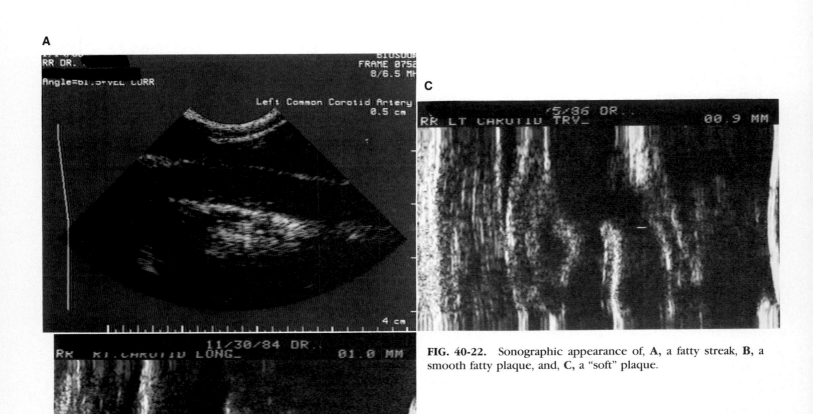

FIG. 40-22. Sonographic appearance of, **A,** a fatty streak, **B,** a smooth fatty plaque, and, **C,** a "soft" plaque.

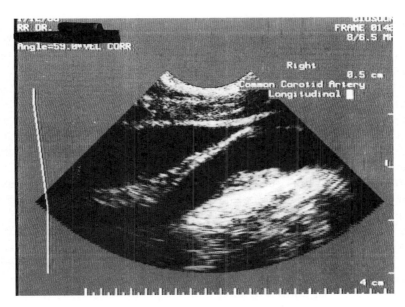

FIG. 40-23. Sonographic appearance of fibrous plaque.

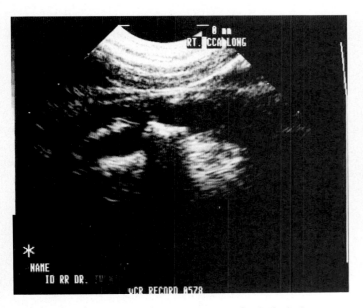

FIG. 40-24. Sonographic appearance of calcified plaque.

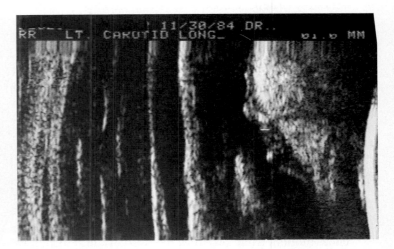

FIG. 40-25. Sonographic appearance of a complex lesion.

the beam path (Fig. 40-24). The inability of the ultrasound beam to penetrate calcific plaque often obscures areas deep to the plaque and can obliterate the lumen, making stenosis calculation almost impossible across the plaque area. Relocation of the transducer may be necessary to look around the area of calcification.

The complex plaque may have a speckled appearance, with areas of calcification within (Fig. 40-25). The calcium and denser-appearing areas are often the result of necrosis or intraplaque hemorrhage. The lesion also may have an extremely irregular and pock-marked appearance on the intimal side; in some cases the fine line of the intimal lining can appear disrupted in places. Ulcerations usually appear in these areas, and deep craters are not infrequently seen. Occasionally these ulcerations can be shown longitudinally, transversely, and axially if the beam

catches the surface correctly when parallel to the plaque surface. All cases of ulceration should be documented thoroughly.

Aneurysm is seen as a widely ectatic, dilated area of the common carotid, bulb, internal and/or external carotids. Plaque, mural thrombus, dissection, and calcification are often seen in combination with an aneurysm. The ectasia will be dramatic when compared to the normal widening of the carotid bulb area or origin of the internal carotid. Aneurysms generally exceed 2 cm in diameter.

Unstable lesions are classed as loose intimal flaps, free-floating thrombus, partially organized plaque ulcers, moving plaque, or any other moving intravascular anomaly that could separate and cause a significant embolic problem. "Bouncing" thrombi, "flapping" plaques, and pseudovalves have been personally encountered. *Intimal flaps* will appear as a flickering or oscillating echo on a wall or in the lumen, moving with each systolic pulse. *Moving thrombus* adopts the appearance of the soft, low-level echogenic plaque but may move up and down within the lumen with each beat. *Pseudovalves* are motile plaques acting like "valves" attached to an adjacent wall at the origin of an artery and have been seen to obstruct lumens either with systole or diastole. *Large ulcerated plaques* can be considered unstable when the ulcer is on the side toward the flow rather than parallel or downstream. Slowed or stagnant blood flow can sometimes be seen entering the ulcer then flowing out, with a dramatic effect of moving flow echoes swirling within the firm, stable portion (Fig. 40-26). Unstable lesions should always be immediately reported to a physician since they can be, in effect, a "time bomb waiting to go off."

Complete occlusion takes on several appearances, all of them distinctive. One appearance may be of a large obstructive plaque formation at the origin with what appears to be a patent artery distal to it. Another, more common appearance, is of a lumen completely filled with soft specular echoes. A border can usually be detected between an echo-free patent lumen and the echo-filled occlusion, which can be enhanced by increasing the gain or power. If there is a suspected total carotid occlusion, comparison with the jugular vein (usually echo free) may help diagnose this. A less frequently seen and potentially confusing appearance is that of an atrophied internal carotid, which may occur after a long-term process. What is confusing is that the external carotid may be considerably larger as a result of compensation and the atrophied internal can easily be missed if the origin of the internal is not traced distally. Usually there will be a collection of organized soft-to-medium gray plaque in the origin with a marked tapering distal to the formation. No detectable flow will be present with Doppler evaluation, although a blip may occasionally be seen that is due to Doppler detection of vascular motion from proximal pressure rather than flow presence.

Extracarotid lesions such as carotid body tumors can be seen as soft-tissue homogenous masses resembling the texture of the thyroid gland but with tumor vasculature seen within. These malignant masses can be seen to surround the internal or external as they increase in size but generally are found between the internal and external since they are outgrowths of the carotid body located in the bifurcation. The walls of the vessels will appear to be incorporated into the mass, although patent lumens can still be seen.

Obstacles to the performance of carotid duplex sonography. There are many variations in anatomy and pathology that can hinder the examination and prevent a complete or accurate study. The following paragraphs will discuss some of these obstacles:

1. The *location of the bifurcation* varies in every individual, even from side to side in some people. Occasionally the bifurcation will be above the lower border of the mandible and will be unreachable by the transducer. Sometimes the proximal areas of the internal and external are visualized, but disease above that level can be missed.

2. *Fat and musculature,* especially in the short-necked patient, will cause the artery to lie deep and be difficult to visualize. The fat and tissue also may attenuate the sound beam, which cannot always penetrate because of the higher frequency at which the transducer operates.

3. *Calcific plaque,* as mentioned earlier, will cause an area of dropout to occur past the lesion that may obscure part or all of the bifurcation if it appears on the superficial wall of the artery. Once again, either rocking the beam through the artery or repositioning may afford better visualization of areas on the wall opposite the plaque.

4. *Congenital anomalies and variations* can cause the most confusion if their presence has not previously

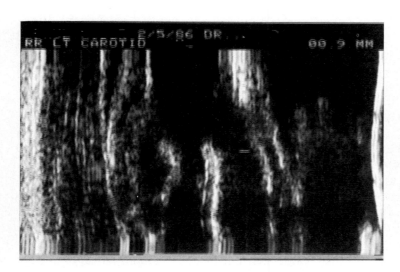
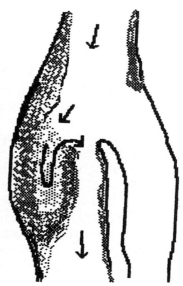

FIG. 40-26. Sonographic appearance of a "turbulent" unstable plaque with a diagram showing the path of blood flow into and out of the ulcer in the plaque that was visualized during duplex evaluation.

been mentioned. *Tortuosity* (usually of the internal or common carotid artery) is a frequently seen condition in which the artery's complex twists and turns make long-axis and transverse visualization extremely difficult. Patience and perseverance are required for a thorough examination. *Coarctation* or *kinking* is not so much an anomaly as a disease state, due to its flow obstruction. *Anomalous vessels* are occasionally seen. Some examples that I have detected by carotid sonography include a separate origin of the external carotid from the subclavian, absence of the bifurcation with separate internal and external carotids, and bilateral low bifurcations at the clavicle level.

5. The *internal jugular vein* has been confused with the common carotid occasionally but can be easily distinguished by the previously mentioned characteristics.

6. *Inversion of the positions of the internal and external carotids* has caused many inaccurate diagnoses. This often happens when a transposed external is diseased and the internal is not. Since disease tends to be found more in the internal carotid, careless interpretation without checking vessel takeoff and internal diameters could lead to a false-positive report. If a Doppler is installed, the flow characteristics of the separate arteries should be readily distinguishable and assist in verifying the individual vessels.

7. *Machine artifacts* will sometimes simulate the appearance or leading edges of plaques. Careful adjustment of gain, periodic transducer maintenance, and regular flushing and replacement of the fluid path medium will resolve most artifacts. If the examiner is in doubt as to whether an area is artifact or disease, the transducer should be moved. Any lines or gray areas that remain in the same location on the screen will be artifactual.

If there is a case in which distal branches or segments of the carotid cannot be visualized, the Doppler cerebrovascular test will help to determine whether a flow obstruction occurs further up the neck. Conversely, the carotid real time examination can be used to confirm areas of turbulence or implications of internal carotid stenosis found with the Doppler examination. One technique therefore can cover the other and make difficult evaluations more simple.

Cerebrovascular Doppler and duplex sonography cases

CASE 1 (FIG. 40-27): NORMAL. These examples are from a 20-year-old man who complained of headaches. The individual scans are labeled as to the normal structures and positions.

A, Normal anterior view of the common carotid. The walls and intima are well seen.

B, Normal lateral view of the bifurcation area, showing the carotid bulb and the internal and external carotid arteries. The jugular vein is anterior.

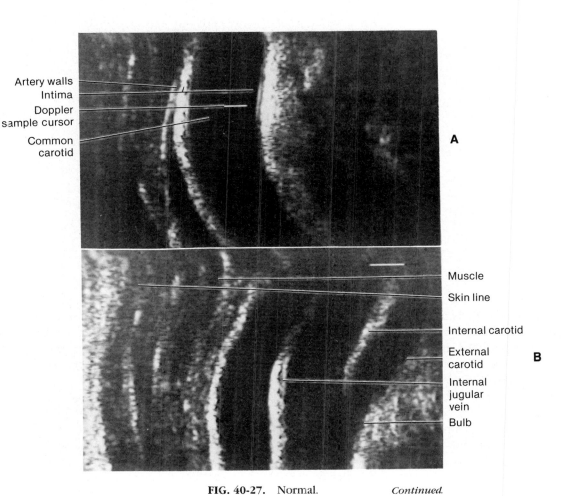

Artery walls
Intima
Doppler sample cursor
Common carotid

A

Muscle

Skin line

Internal carotid

External carotid

B

Internal jugular vein

Bulb

FIG. 40-27. Normal.   *Continued.*

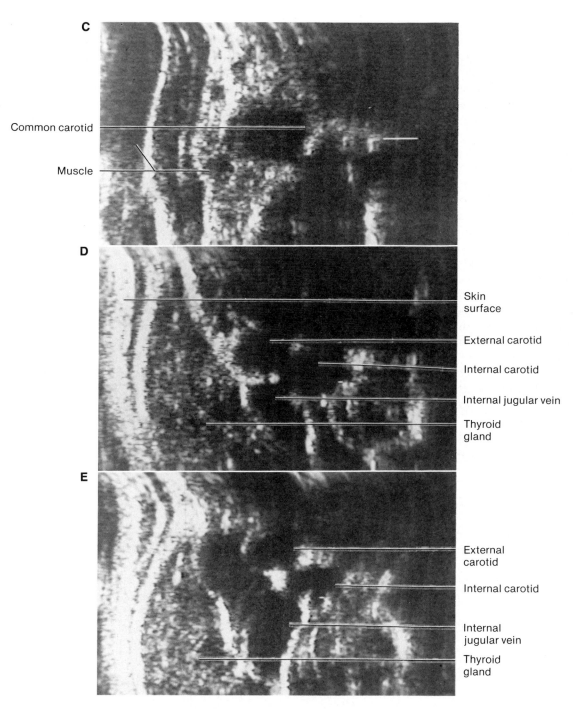

FIG. 40-27, cont'd. Normal.

C, Normal transverse view of the middle common carotid. The medial side is to the top of the screen.

D, Normal transverse view at the bifurcation point showing the figure-8 where the individual vessels join the bulb.

E, Normal transverse view showing the appearance of the internal and external carotids above the bifurcation.

CASE 2 (FIG. 40-28): TOTAL COMMON, INTERNAL, EXTERNAL CAROTID OCCLUSION WITH PROXIMAL FREE-FLOATING ("BOUNCING") THROMBUS. This 56-year-old woman was admitted for a possible coronary artery bypass operation. She had a long history of vascular disease and mitral insufficiency. She also complained of occasional dizziness and had numbness of three fingers of the right hand since an earlier cardiac catheterization. She had bilateral bruits in the carotids, and surgery was to be performed or cancelled, depending on the results of the Doppler examination and carotid sonography.

A, On the right side a normal brachial signal with a pressure of 190/100 was obtained. The common carotid artery at the clavicle had abnormally low, practically nonexistent, flow; and the signal at the bifurcation was barely more than a thump. The right vertebral had normal but reduced antegrade flow. The facial artery sig-

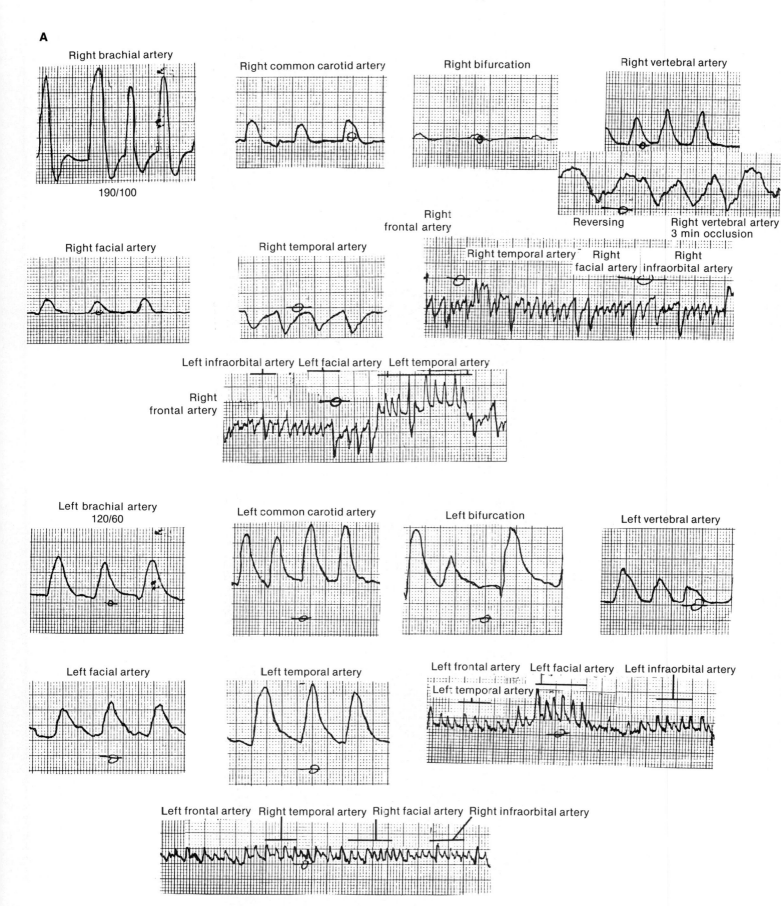

FIG. 40-28. Total common, internal, external carotid occlusion with proximal free-floating ("bouncing") thrombus.

Continued.

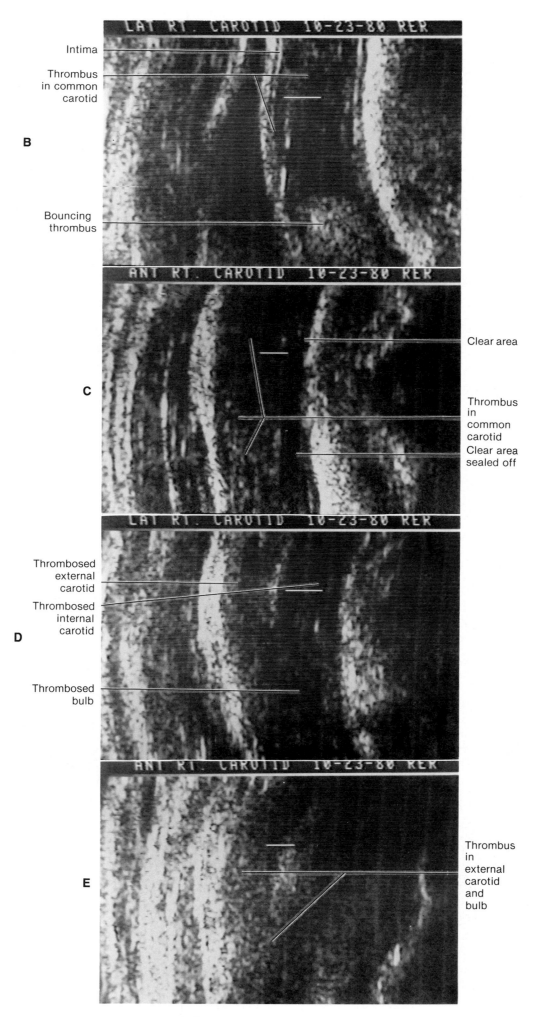

FIG. 40-28, cont'd. For legend see p. 989.

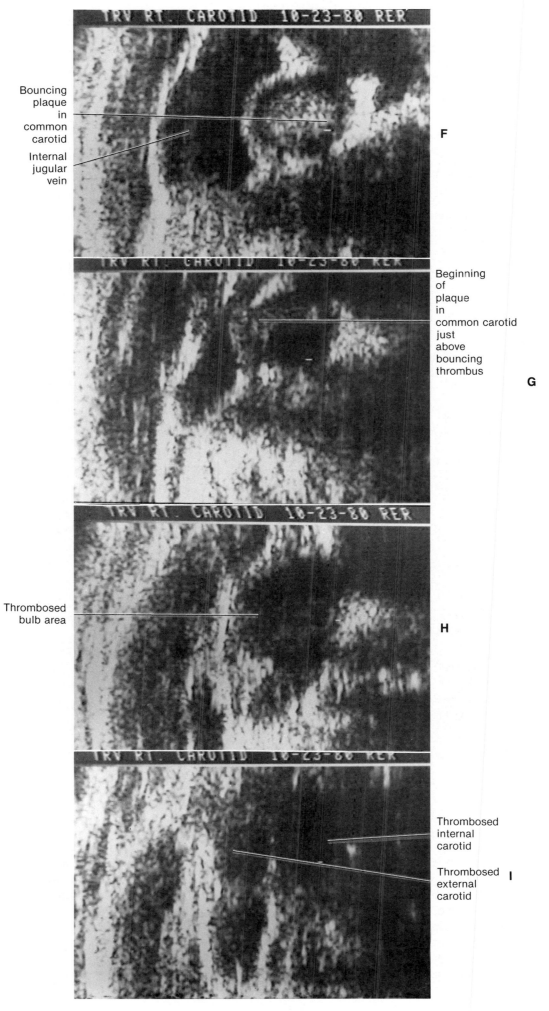

Bouncing
plaque
in
common
carotid

Internal
jugular
vein

F

Beginning
of
plaque
in
common carotid
just
above
bouncing
thrombus

G

Thrombosed
bulb area

H

Thrombosed
internal
carotid

Thrombosed
external
carotid

I

FIG. 40-28, cont'd.   For legend see p. 989.

Continued.

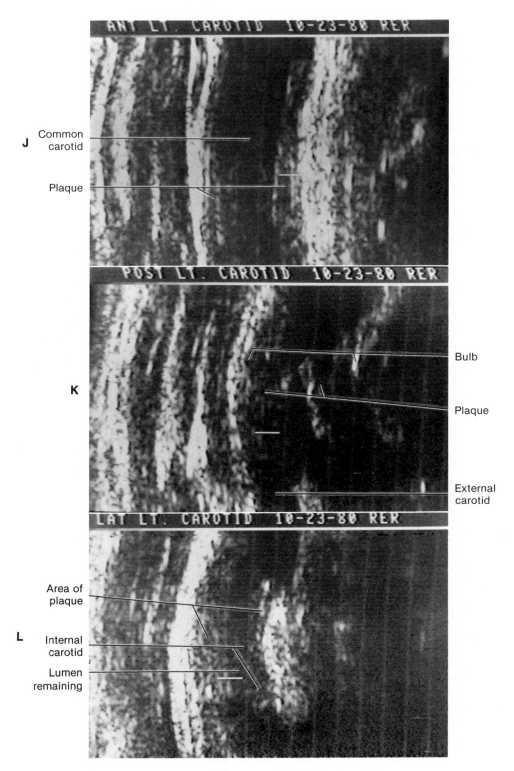

J Common carotid
Plaque

K Bulb
Plaque
External carotid

L Area of plaque
Internal carotid
Lumen remaining

FIG. 40-28, cont'd.   For legend see p. 989.

nal was also reduced. The right temporal artery was actually *reversed,* implying severe collateral compensation. The ophthalmic test showed retrograde flow in the frontal artery, which was not affected by right-sided compressions. Compression of the left temporal, however, caused resumption of antegrade flow in the right frontal, suggesting contralateral collateralization from the left temporal. The other compressions had no

effect. In regard to the apparent occlusion of the right common, it was thought that the frontal flow's becoming antegrade was caused by circle of Willis collateral supplies.

The left side was next examined. The left brachial artery signal was reduced and significant of subclavian stenosis and vertebral steal. A reduced antegrade vertebral signal was seen; however, postocclusive hypere-

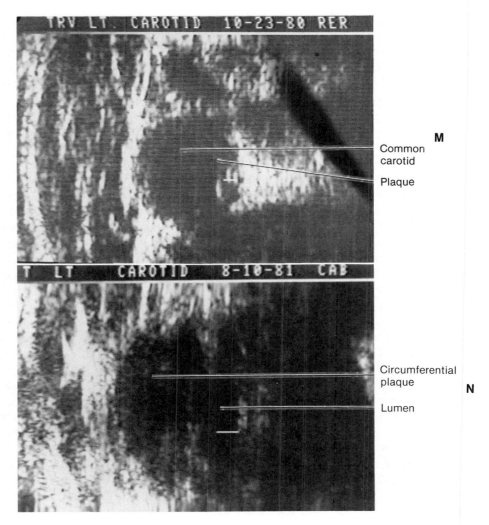

TRV LT. CAROTID 10-23-80 RER

Common carotid

Plaque

M

T LT CAROTID 8-10-81 CAB

Circumferential plaque

N

Lumen

FIG. 40-28, cont'd. For legend see p. 989.

mia caused a flow reversal within 10 seconds, verifying the steal. A much more normal-looking common carotid signal was noted; but throughout the carotid there was roughening of the sound quality, implying flow problems. Bifurcation, facial, and temporal signals were of normal pattern, with some increase in flow in the temporal artery. The ophthalmic test showed an antegrade but decreased frontal signal, which increased markedly with left facial compression. All other compressions were normal. Neither right nor left supraorbital arteries were audible.

Carotid sonography showed a thrombus occluding the right common, internal, and external carotids from the middle of the common carotid up, with a partly congealed clot floating free and moving up and down with each cardiac cycle in the low common carotid. The left side had scattered areas of plaque partly occluding the bulb and internal carotid. (See *B* to *N* for selected examples of this case.)

An arteriogram was obtained and confirmed the level and extent of the occlusion in the right carotid. The right vertebral flow reduction was caused by a stenosis at the takeoff of the vessel. A severe stenosis of the left internal carotid was also shown, as was a con-

firmation of the left subclavian obstruction and subclavian steal.

The patient was observed for 3 months until the loose "bouncing" clot had congealed. At that time the patient was readmitted and had another arteriogram, which showed some collateralization that filled the external carotid. The patient was taken to surgery, and a combination right carotid endarterectomy and mitral commisurotomy and repair were performed. The patient recovered and was released.

B, Lateral view of the right common carotid artery low in the neck. The thrombus, which "bounces" up and down with each cardiac beat, is shown. This thrombus was completely free and unattached to the walls. Above this, the proximal portion of the congealed thrombus lining the carotid is shown. The intima is clearly seen, showing the thrombus to be separate and not a thickened part of the intima.

C, Anterior view taken just above the previous image. A much more extensive view of the thrombus is seen, as is a clear area on the deep wall that had minimal flow. This clear area was sealed off just below the bulb.

D, Lateral view showing the bulb and bifurcation. The same mass of gray echoes fills the entire lumen. Doppler examination here gave an absent signal.

E, Anterior view, giving a better perspective of the filled-in external carotid and bulb.

In the following series of transverse views, levels have been chosen to correspond best with the longitudinal images.

F, View low in the common carotid, showing the transverse appearance of the moving thrombus caught in a freeze-frame image.

G, View of the area of the carotid just above the area with the moving plaque, showing the irregular edges of the thrombus and the decreased lumen.

H, Area of the bulb just below the bifurcation. The bulb is entirely filled in with echoes. No Doppler signals could be heard.

I, Appearance of the internal and external carotid arteries. Once again, they too are filled in, which corresponds with the findings in the long-axis images. No Doppler flow signals could be obtained.

The left side was also diseased and gives good examples of severe disease in the bulb and internal and external carotid arteries. Reference to the Doppler tracings mentioned earlier may be of aid in understanding flow correlations. In all the views on the left side the patient's head now inverts to the *bottom* of the image. All directions will be given in respect to the patient's actual position and not the position of the structure in the image unless otherwise stated.

J, Anterior view of the left common carotid. Areas of plaque and intimal thickening are readily seen.

K, Posterior view of the area of the bulb and external carotid. Highly stenotic soft plaque can be seen on both the superficial and deep walls, with the superficial plaque extending into the origin of the external carotid.

L, Lateral view shows the internal carotid. Plaque areas can again be seen on both walls, extending partly up into the internal carotid. The dark area between the plaque sites is the actual lumen that remains unobstructed.

The two transverse views are oriented so that the medial side of the body is to the bottom of the image.

M, Common carotid just below the bulb. The areas of circumferential plaque are easily seen, corresponding with the areas seen in the long-axis views.

N, Transverse view of the bulb, showing the occluded appearance of the bulb area, as the circumferential soft plaque surrounds the lumen. This is a cross-section through the widest area of bulb plaque; the lumen tended to widen superior to the bulb, as can be seen in the long-axis views.

CASE 3 (FIG. 40-29): SEVERE INTERNAL CAROTID STENOSIS, ULCERATED PLAQUE. These waveforms and images are from a 70-year-old woman who complained of a sudden onset of right leg discomfort and near paralysis of the extremity from the hip down. She also complained of pain and cramping in the limb, with some numbness of the leg below the knee. Her left leg gave her no difficulties. Distal extremity pulses were nonpalpable. She had prominent carotid bruits, the left louder than the right, but denied dizziness, syncope, and other cerebral symptoms. She was referred for a Doppler examination of the lower extremities and the carotid system. Flow in the right leg was within normal limits but in the left leg was diminished, suggesting a CVA or TIA as the source of the right leg paralysis and discomfort.

In all the following images the head of the patient is oriented toward the bottom of the longitudinal sections and the medial side of the body toward the bottom of the transverse sections:

A, Midportion of the common carotid artery. Note the gray soft tissue plaque areas on the superficial and deep walls of the artery.

B, Transverse section across the center of the area in *A*

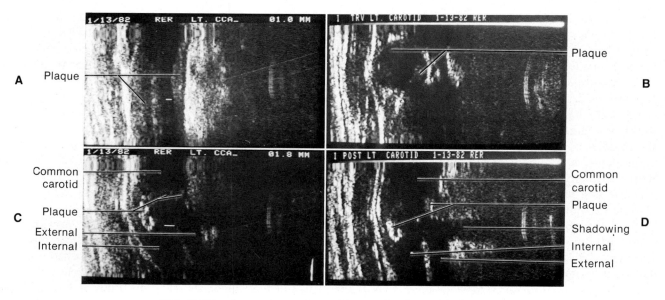

FIG. 40-29. Severe internal carotid stenosis, ulcerated plaque.

showing the vessel with the plaque and the stenosed lumen.

C, and *D,* Carotid bulb, bifurcation, and internal and external carotid arteries. A large, circumferential, complex plaque is obstructing both the internal and the external carotids about 80%. Shadowing is seen from the calcified portion of the lesion. *C* shows part of the circumferential plaque on the lateral wall of the bulb more clearly.

E, Transverse image of the bulb area just below the bifurcation. Note the irregular circumferential plaque lining the artery, of which only a small section could be visualized in the longitudinal views.

F, Transverse view showing the internal carotid artery at its origin. Note the obstructive plaque on the superficial wall (also shown in *C* and *D*) and the reduced size of the remaining lumen.

Fig. 40-29, *G* to *M,* is a series of spectrally analyzed Doppler flow signals of this artery recorded at various levels to show the changes that occurred along the course of the vessel. The scale factors (5, 10, and 20 kHz) are shown at the bottom of each photograph.

G, Tracing taken midway in the common carotid, at approximately the center of the stenotic area. Note that the envelope has begun to take on a ragged appearance and that the window is nearly filled in. The frequencies are fairly evenly distributed, which signifies a moderate stenosis.

H, Signal obtained from the bulb area across the stenotic region. Note the blunting of the waveform and the short clear area signifying some turbulence. The window is absent, and the envelope is still ragged. A strained, burbling sound was heard at this site.

I, Signal obtained immediately distal to the stenosis at the base of the internal carotid and typical of the jet effect. Note the concentration of frequencies at the baseline, indicative of turbulence, along with the extremely high peak, which could barely be shown at the 20 kHz scale setting. A harsh, strained, hissing sound was heard here.

J, Signal obtained more distally from the stenosis, away from the jet area. Flow is markedly reduced (see the 5 kHz scale), with a disrupted envelope and turbulence still present.

K, Signal taken along the clear, well-preserved distal internal carotid. The disrupted envelope and lower-frequency intensities are still evident. The window reappears, but the flow is still uneven. A low-pitched, almost normal, but roughened sound was heard here.

L, Signal of the external carotid immediately distal to the stenotic plaque at its origin. Though the artery is not obstructed enough to give a jet effect, turbulence is still present (as evidenced by the baseline concentration). The roughened envelope and reduced overall frequencies suggest a proximal stenosis. A high-pitched wheezing sound was heard here.

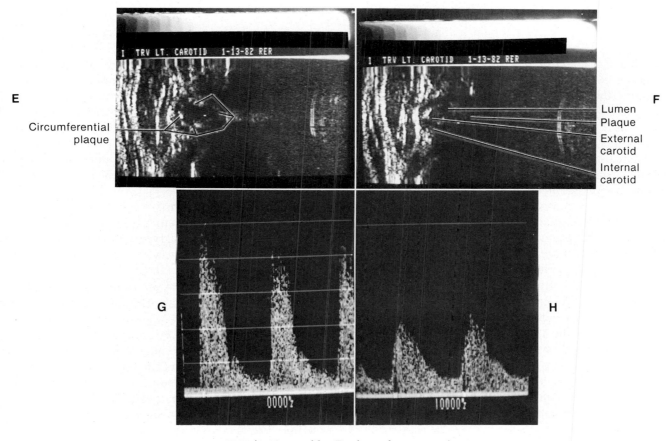

FIG. 40-29, cont'd.   For legend see opposite page.

Continued.

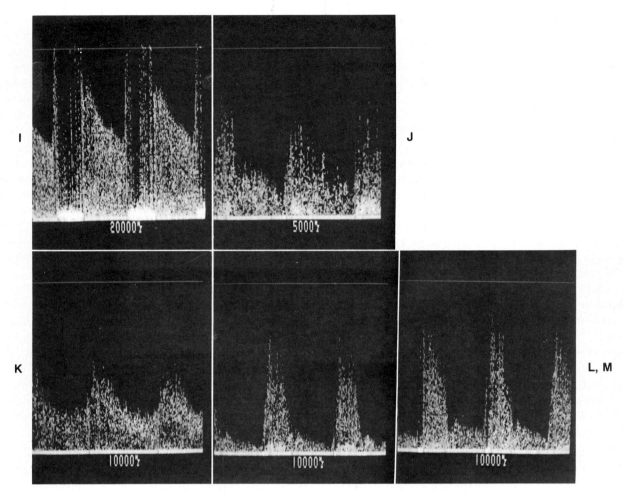

FIG. 40-29, cont'd.   For legend see p. 994.

M, Signal obtained along the clear distal external carotid. Most of the normal waveform features reappear; however, note the widely distributed frequencies and ragged envelope. Some baseline concentrations are still evident. A strained sound was again heard but was a bit smoother overall.

The examinations were interpreted as significant of carotid disease. Frontal artery flow was antegrade, implying enough flow compensation to maintain pressure despite the better than 80% stenosis found by carotid sonography and both arch and digital subtraction arteriography. By all these modalities the plaque was considered ulcerated. The patient had no further problems, and surgery was postponed pending observation.

CASE 4 (FIG. 40-30): CAROTID BODY TUMOR, MODERATE INTERNAL CAROTID STENOSIS. This patient had classic TIA symptoms; in addition to a severe stenosis, a carotid body tumor located between the internal and external carotids was initially implied by DSA.

A shows the internal carotid with a focal stenosis at the origin. *B* shows the tumor, which lies medial to the internal carotid. Note the homogeneous texture typical of chemodectoma. As the scanhead was moved medial to the tumor, the external carotid was seen, *C. D* is a transverse image that shows the relationships of the internal and ex-

ternal carotids to the tumor. The tumor measured approximately 1.52 by 1.69 by 1.82 cm, *E* and *F.*

G shows the moderately turbulent internal carotid waveform, which also shows a moderate velocity increase. *H* shows the external carotid signal. *I* and *J* are signals taken from within the carotid body tumor, which was highly vascularized and had numerous internal collaterals.

The tumor was resected and an endarterectomy was performed.

CASE 5 (FIG. 40-31): CAROTID STEAL SYNDROME — INNOMINATE ARTERY OCCLUSION. This patient presented with dizziness and syncope. Real-time sonography of the carotid systems revealed minimal intimal thickening and no evidence of a significant stenosis.

Doppler findings, however, indicated a more significant problem. There was a 60 mm Hg difference in pressure between the arms, with the right side being lower and having a monophasic waveform. Direct carotid evaluation with a continuous-wave Doppler and spectrum analysis revealed bidirectional flow in the entire right carotid system, with reversal during systole, *A* to *D.* A reversed right vertebral signal was present, *E,* with recovery of an antegrade monophasic subclavian signal, *F.* Arteriography confirmed the presence of innominate artery occlusion.

The patient subsequently received an axillosubclavian

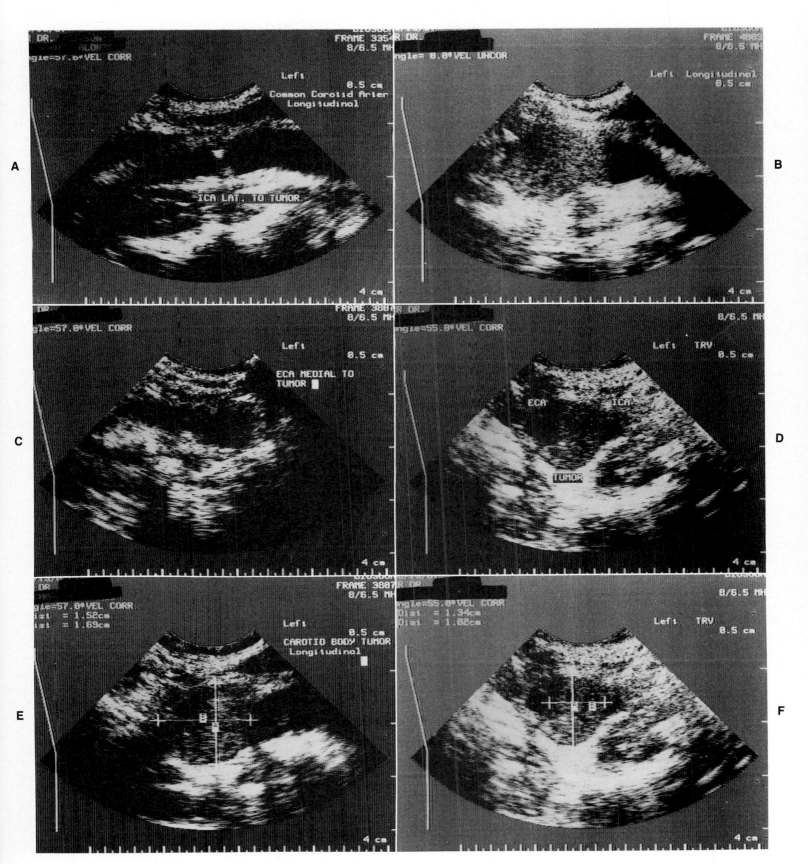

FIG. 40-30.   Carotid body tumor, moderate internal carotid stenosis.   *Continued.*

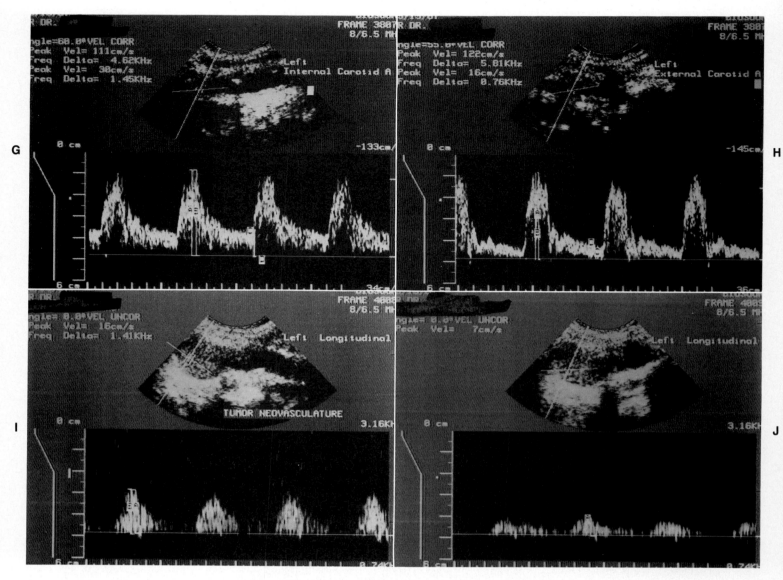

FIG. 40-30, cont'd.   For legend see p. 997.

bypass graft, which shunted flow from the left to the right, and which restored normal flow direction in the carotid and vertebral systems.

CASE 6 (FIG. 40-32): SEVERE FOCAL INTERNAL CAROTID STENOSIS. This patient was asymptomatic, and was referred for bilateral carotid bruit evaluation.

Real-time sonography showed a prominent, shelf-like plaque formation obstructing the right internal carotid artery at the origin approximately 80% to 90%. Whereas the plaque profile is best seen in the longitudinal view, *A,* the transverse view shows the full extent of luminal compromise, *B.* Doppler internal carotid spectra (not shown here) were highly turbulent and peaked at 15 kHz, which helped confirm the severity of the stenosis.

CASE 7 (FIG. 40-33): NEAR OCCLUSION OF INTERNAL CAROTID AND EXTERNAL CAROTID. This patient presented with amaurosis fugax of the left eye.

Real-time sonography of the right side showed a moderate stenosis (not shown here) and relatively normal flow patterns proximally. The left side, however, had a

large area of soft plaque occupying the proximal internal carotid but with poorly defined luminal borders, *A.* The external carotid also appeared filled with fine gray echoes at the origin (see small image in *G*). The effect of this ICA stenosis on the hemodynamics was evident with the duplex Doppler findings. The proximal common carotid signal, *B,* was attenuated (<45 cm/s) and typical of a high-resistance pattern with the abnormal loss of the diastolic component. This appears with a distal obstruction that severely reduces flow. The distal common carotid signal was even more attenuated, barely reaching 20 cm/s, *C.* In direct contrast, there is a severe and dramatic increase in velocity in the internal carotid at the origin, *D,* with a peak velocity of nearly 350 cm/s with severe spectral broadening typical of the jet effect. About 2 cm distal to this, the velocity lessens a bit to 250 cm/s, and turbulence creates strong energy concentrations at the baseline with systole and becomes more disturbed, *E* and *F* (compare velocities between *D* and *F,* which are on the same scale). A markedly reduced and monophasic external carotid sig-

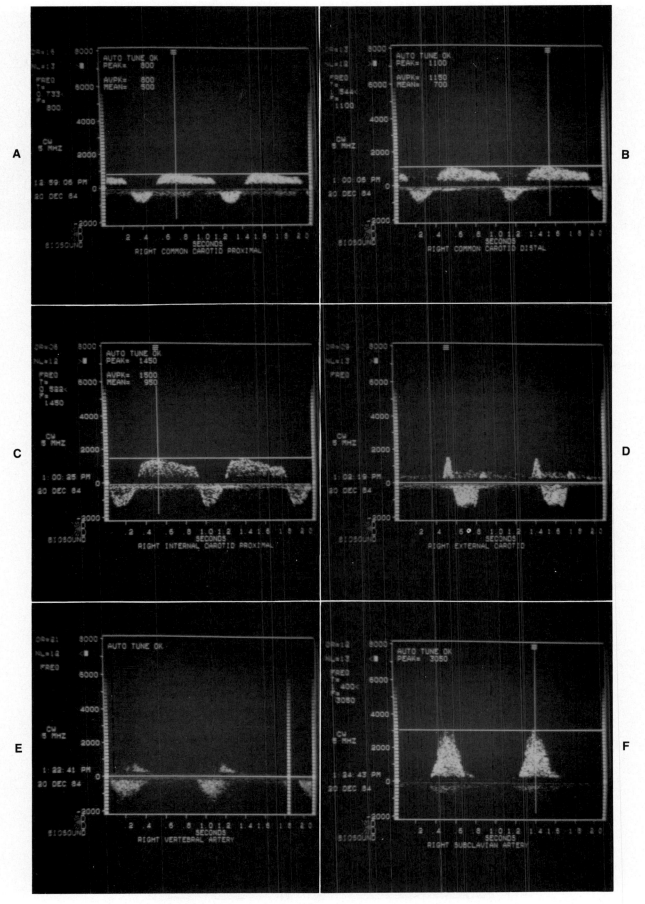

FIG. 40-31.   Carotid steal syndrome—innominate artery occlusion.

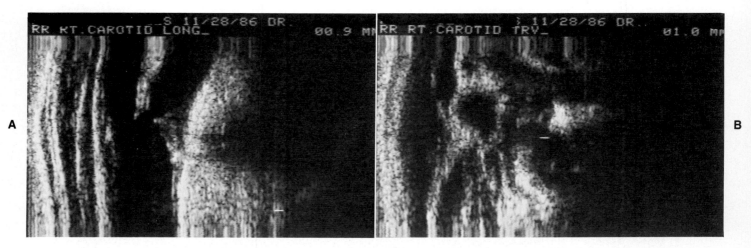

FIG. 40-32.   Severe focal internal carotid stenosis.

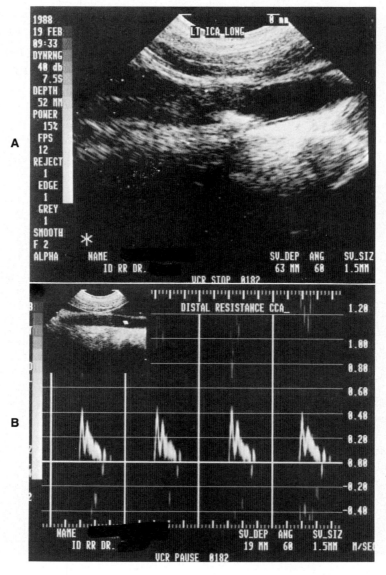

FIG. 40-33.   Near occlusion of internal carotid and external carotid.

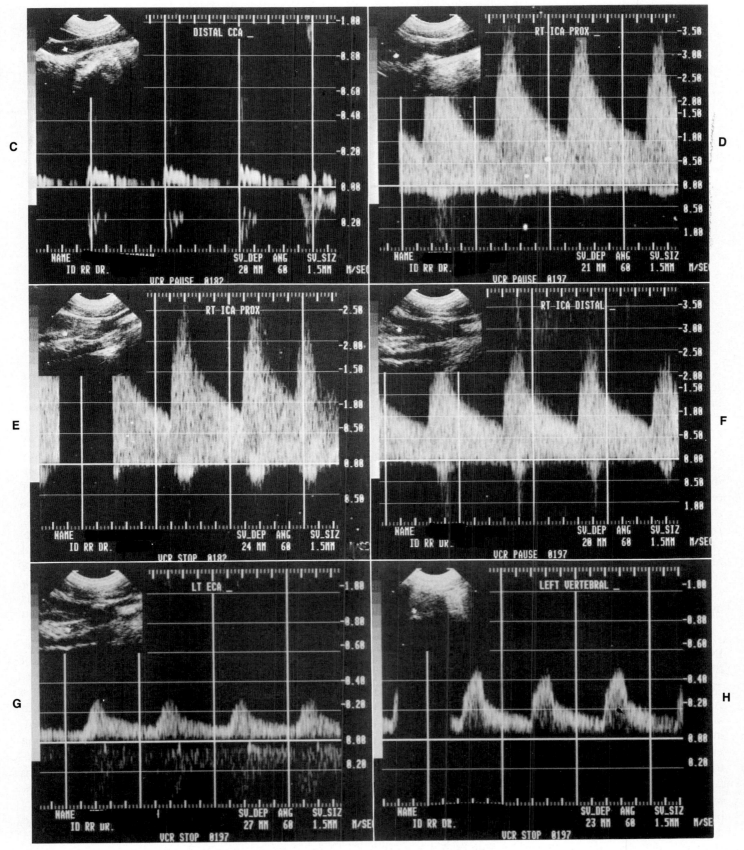

FIG. 40-33, cont'd.   For legend see opposite page.

Continued.

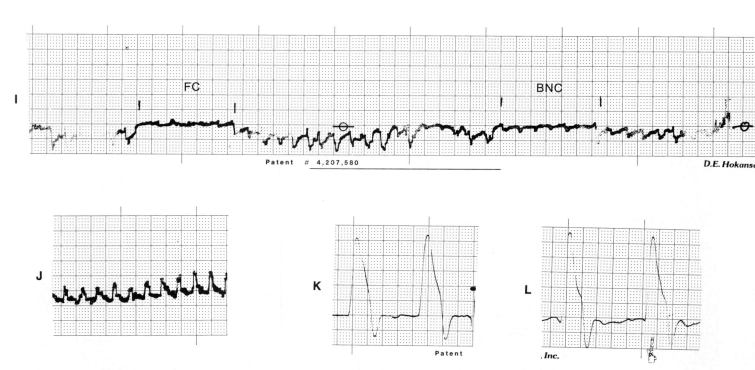

FIG. 40-33, cont'd. **I,** Left frontal artery. **J,** Right frontal artery, no changes. **K,** Right brachial. **L,** Left brachial. *FC,* facial compression; *BNC,* bridge of nose compression.

nal with none of the typical characteristics of a normal external carotid waveform was seen, *G.* A normal left vertebral signal was obtained, *H.*

Frontal artery examination showed a retrograde signal, *I,* which did not change with left-sided branch compressions. *Right* facial artery compression, however, caused a decrease and partial reversal of the frontal signal, showing the presence of a cross-face collateral from the facial artery. The collateral pathway across the lower bridge of the nose was confirmed with compression there. The right frontal signal was antegrade and did not change with bilateral branch compressions, *J.* Brachial artery flow and pressure was normal bilaterally, *K* and *L.*

The overall interpretation was of a severe left internal carotid stenosis of at least 90% to 95% with severe hemodynamic changes.

INTRAOPERATIVE AND POSTOPERATIVE EVALUATION OF THE CEREBROVASCULAR SYSTEM

The most common procedure to alleviate stenoses of the carotid artery system is the *endarterectomy.* In this technique the carotid artery is exposed, then a shunt is placed in the distal common artery below the stenotic area and inserted above the stenosis into the internal carotid artery. This shunt enables the surgeon to divert the carotid flow around the area he or she intends to endarterectomize and avoid any neurologic deficits caused by lack of blood flow. An arteriotomy is made across the area of stenosis. An intimal elevator is used to dissect the intimal layer and area of plaque away from the walls, and this area is cut away. The loose ends of the residual intima are tacked down with sutures, remaining bits of plaque in the area are removed, the area is flushed with saline, and the vessel is closed. The shunt is removed and flow is re-

stored. Although the carotid is carefully examined before closing, emboli or bits of plaque inadvertently left still can detach and reocclude the artery higher up following surgery.

Intraoperative real-time scanning is being used by more and more surgical centers during endarterectomy and can help the surgeon evaluate the stenosis by scanning the exposed carotid directly both before and after endarterectomy has been performed. Duplex Doppler assessment can be used also to document the flow dynamics of the surgical area. The general procedure involves placing the transducer and cable in a sterile sleeve, coupled with gel. A gel-filled cap can be placed over the sleeve where it contacts the transducer face, which helps eliminate air bubbles in the beam path. The surgical area is usually filled with saline, and the vessel is scanned through the water path. Controls and knob adjustments are made either by an attending technologist or by the surgeon through a sterile cover placed over the control panel. The appearance of the artery is similar to that described in the duplex sonography section above except that the walls and intima are always much clearer and well defined. After surgery and before the neck is closed, a second evaluation is made. Bits of plaque and remaining material are extremely easy to detect, and if they are detected, the surgeon can easily reopen and remove the material. Before intraoperative scanning was done, a deficit often was not discovered until the postoperative period, which necessitated taking the patient back to surgery and repeating the entire procedure.

Laser atherectomy and percutaneous transluminal angioplasty are also being investigated as tools for removing carotid lesions, but these procedures still run a strong risk of embolic sequelae and are not in general use at the time of writing.

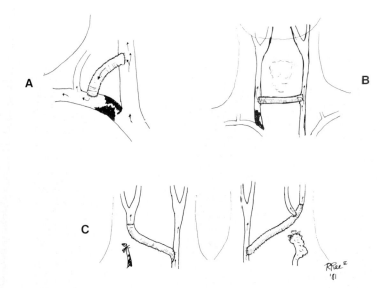

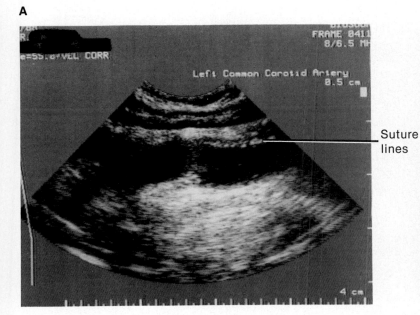

FIG. 40-34. Types of bypass grafts. **A,** Carotosubclavian. **B,** Carotocarotid. **C,** Two examples of cross-carotid reconstruction.

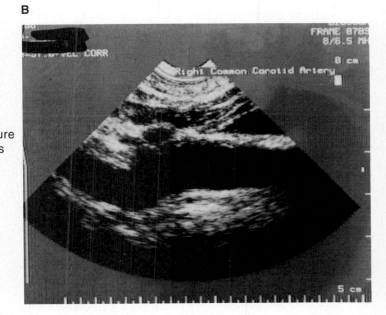

Suture lines

FIG. 40-35. **A,** and **B,** Typical appearances of two different internal carotid arteries postendarterectomy.

Various grafts may be used in severe flow problems for shunting. They are usually synthetic and have a variety of applications. Some typical situations are mentioned below and shown in Fig. 40-34:

1. *Common carotid-subclavian.* This is used either to correct a subclavian steal by shunting flow from the carotid distal to an existing subclavian stenosis and restoring arm and vertebral flow, or to shunt flow from the subclavian to the carotid in cases of proximal carotid occlusion.
2. *Carotocarotid.* This is palpable and can be found usually extending subcutaneously across the lower thyroid cartilage. It supplements a carotid that is kinked or stenosed in the low portion near the base.
3. *Various cross-carotid.* Connections between the contralateral common carotid and ipsilateral bulb and/or internal carotid may be established, depending on the disease and its severity.

Percutaneous transluminal angioplasty has been per-

formed also for stenotic bulb lesions. The risk of embolization, as can be imagined, is much more significant than in the extremities, and the procedure is rarely performed.

The examination procedure in the postop patient is the same as in the routine patient, with the possible exception of direct carotid studies on the operative side. Careful documentation of flow direction and flow changes is extremely important. Preoperative examinations should be compared, and an optional carotid real-time study performed several days after surgery may assist in follow-up evaluation.

Postoperatively, any endarterectomy or graft can be evaluated and followed by carotid duplex sonography and direct carotid Doppler. The procedure for evaluation is the same as that used for the routine direct carotid or duplex carotid examination with the exception that care should be taken around sutures and wound areas during the study. The sonographic appearance of the carotid postendarterectomy is identical to that of a normal carotid

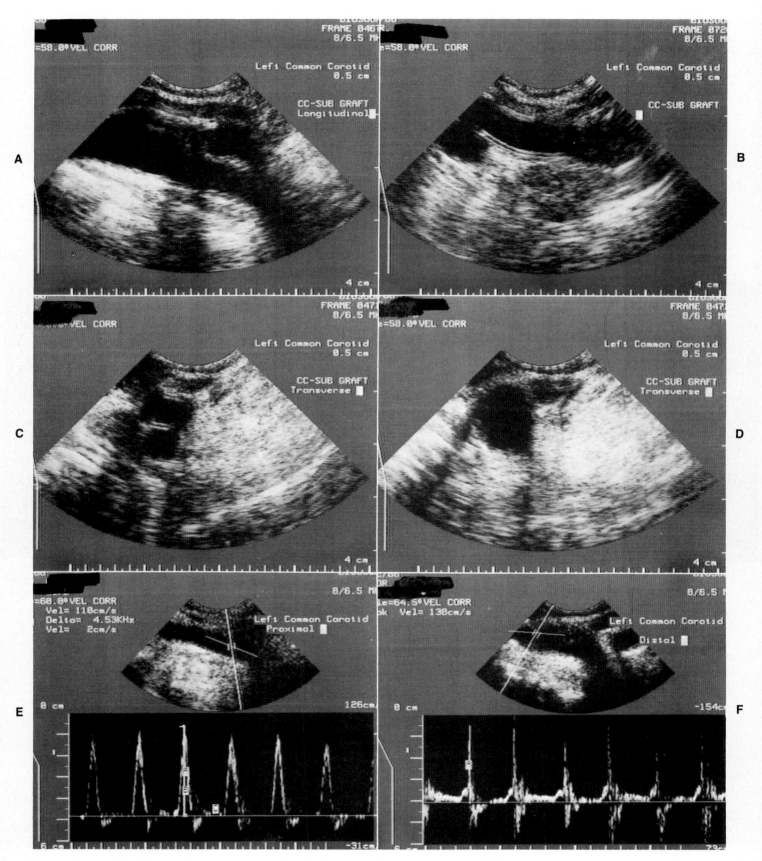

FIG. 40-36. Carotosubclavian graft.

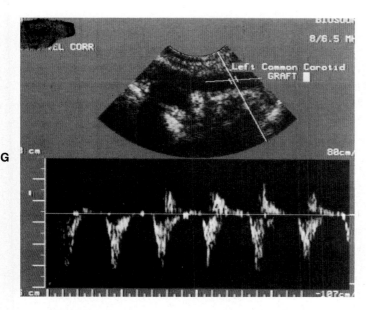

FIG. 40-36, cont'd.   For legend see opposite page.

except that there will be no intimal echoes within the area of surgery, and the walls may appear ectatic or dilated (Fig. 40-35). There may be a distinct "shelf" of intimal lining in the distal common carotid, which marks the lower point of the endarterectomy.

Normal flow dynamics with duplex or direct carotid Doppler assessment are the same as in the routine exam also, but because of decreased resistance and an increase in the elasticity of the carotid wall in the endarterectomy area, a mild increase in flow velocity as well as mild to moderate turbulence may be seen. If used, color-flow imaging demonstrates a swirling flow effect that will be more pronounced if a patch has been used to expand the endarterectomy site. This can be considered normal unless the velocity increase is significant enough to imply a severe restenosis. In general, pulsed Doppler sampling should be taken distal or proximal to the actual area of the endarterectomy. The periorbital exam also may indicate a restenosis if the frontal artery on the repaired side is reversed following surgery.

Postoperative cerebrovascular case

CASE 1 (FIG. 40-36): CAROTOSUBCLAVIAN GRAFT. This patient received a carotosubclavian graft to restore flow to the left subclavian, which was obstructed proximally. The anastomosis of the graft to the common carotid can be seen clearly in the longitudinal plane, A. The highly defined, smooth-walled appearance of the graft was more easily seen lateral and inferior to the anastomosis, B. The graft can be easily distinguished from the less stark-appearing common carotid in the transverse view below the common carotid anastomosis, C, and the dilated, ovoid appearance of the anastomosis is seen in D.

Flow direction and function determination were assessed with the pulsed Doppler. E shows a normal, strong common carotid signal, which displays a high-resistance characteristic because it is proximal to the anastomosis

and is shunting flow through the graft. Turbulence and bi-directionality are seen at the graft anastomosis area, F, and flow is then documented as going through the graft toward the arm, the normal direction in this case, G.

DOPPLER ULTRASONIC ANGIOGRAPHY (DOPPLER SCANNING)

One of the original methods of Doppler assessment of the carotids and one that still finds common usage in certain institutions today is the noninvasive imaging of arteries and veins based on the creation of an image from Doppler signals on a storage cathode ray tube (CRT). This technique uses a Doppler device connected to a signal-processing unit and an X-Y axis scanning arm, similar to that used in conventional B-scan imaging. A directional Doppler probe is used, and current devices either create the image in bistable on a CRT or use a more sophisticated color image system.[13,20] Directions of flow or flow intensities are assigned color levels, as in spectral analysis, and the image of the artery or vein is a composite of colors showing some flow and morphologic information. The Doppler angiograph can also be connected to spectral analyzers or microcomputers for additional information. Some Doppler arteriographs have integral analyzers and computers[5,10,13,19,20] and show several types of information simultaneously on the monitor.

Examination techniques. The Doppler angiograph (Fig. 40-37) can be used for both arteries and veins,[10] but it is most frequently used in scanning the carotid bifurcation. The basic technique involves positioning the patient, immobilizing the area intended for study, and positioning the scanning arm.[13] The examiner coats the area with gel and creates the image by moving the probe back and forth transversely across the artery and/or vein being examined. A Doppler signal received by the probe is heard and shown as a trace on the screen. The examiner steps the arm to another position, thereby building up a series of traces until an image of the vessel is shown on the screen (Fig. 40-38). Lines are also placed on the image to denote the inferior border of the mandible on carotid scans and the skin line on transverse scans. When the image has been created, a hard copy is made photographically.

Further processing is possible at this point. Some devices have a cursor that shows the position of the probe anywhere along the arterial or venous image, which enables simultaneous spectral flow patterns and/or Doppler signals to be recorded showing the point in the artery or vein where the signal is heard (Fig. 40-39). Some devices are equipped with computers to allow beam/vessel angle measurement, measure velocity profiles, and compute blood flow volumes. Flow tracings are also provided.

Either pulsed mode or continuous-wave Doppler is used, with some devices incorporating both. The pulsed Doppler systems tend to provide better resolution of the image (1 mm or more) and, if depth gates are employed, can give a crude form of transverse image. The probe is often detachable to allow hand-held Doppler studies to be performed in addition to imaging.

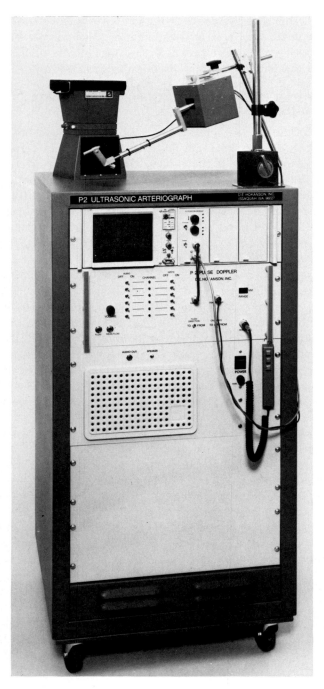

FIG. 40-37. Ultrasonic arteriograph. (Courtesy D.E. Hokanson, Inc.)

Interpretation and discussion. Doppler angiographic images appear as a series of dots or lines making up the profile of a vessel being examined. Areas where no Doppler signal is received appear as gaps or indentations in the profile (Fig. 40-40). In color-coded devices brighter color intensities correspond to higher-frequency flow. Some devices have as few as 3 or as many as 15 color gradients. Others use only red, blue, and yellow, for either frequency categorization or flow direction.

Areas where signals are not received usually correspond to plaques, lesions, or occluded vessels; but calcium deposits may cause false diagnoses of occlusion. Devices coupled with spectral analysis or flow profiling can help in determining the status of flow distal to such areas (Fig. 40-41).

Although these devices have definite benefits, moving plaques (e.g., pseudovalves) may not be detected since unobstructed flow will be received as a normal signal; or if detected on one sweep, they may be obscured on the return sweep of the probe. Some areas (e.g., the carotid bifurcation) may be inaccessible to the probe and prevent accurate flow detection. Prominent branches of the external carotid in internal carotid occlusion may simulate the bifurcation, causing an incorrect image.[13] Vessels lying in the same plane may not be distinguished on longitudinal scans, and external and internal carotids that approximate each other may blend together on transverse images.

Another disadvantage is the length of time required to perform the study. Contrary to some manufacturers' claims, the examination can take from 30 minutes to 1½ hours to perform, even in skilled hands. This, of course, depends on the type of processing to be done on the signal or image, the difficulty of the patient, and the examiner's ability. These devices are extremely operator dependent, and untrained personnel may measurably affect the examination results and performance time. Routine screening can sometimes be impractical.

Summary. Doppler ultrasonic angiography can be beneficial in determining the flow status of arteries and veins and may allow location of some obstructive lesions. Correlating the results with cerebrovascular Doppler studies, carotid real-time sonography, and Doppler spectral analysis will give more thorough coverage of the cerebrovascular circulation; but some redundancy may occur

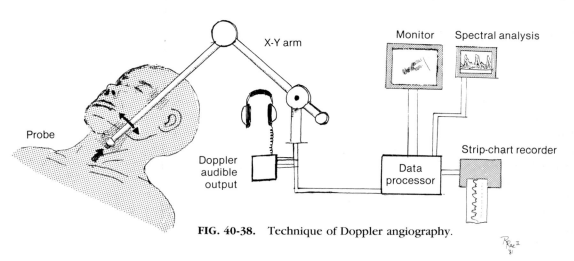

FIG. 40-38. Technique of Doppler angiography.

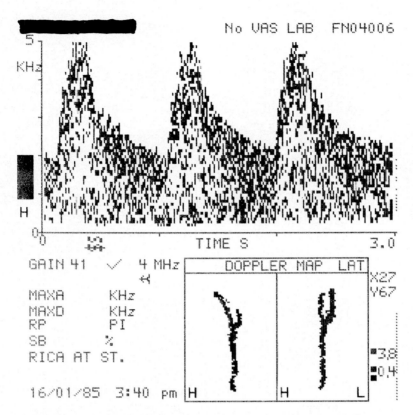

FIG. 40-39.   Ultrasonic arteriographic flow map with spectral analysis.

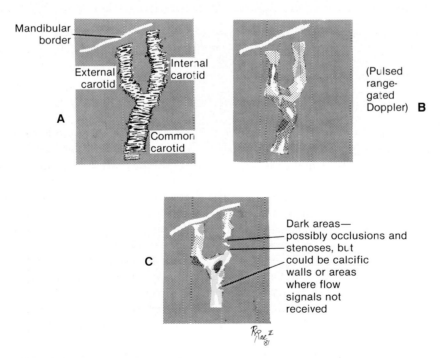

FIG. 40-40.   Typical appearances of Doppler angiographic scans of the carotid bifurcation. **A,** Normal image on a CRT. **B,** Normal image on a gray scale or color-coded system. **C,** Abnormal image showing the appearance of nonvisualized areas indicative of vascular stenosis, occlusion, or calcific vessel walls.

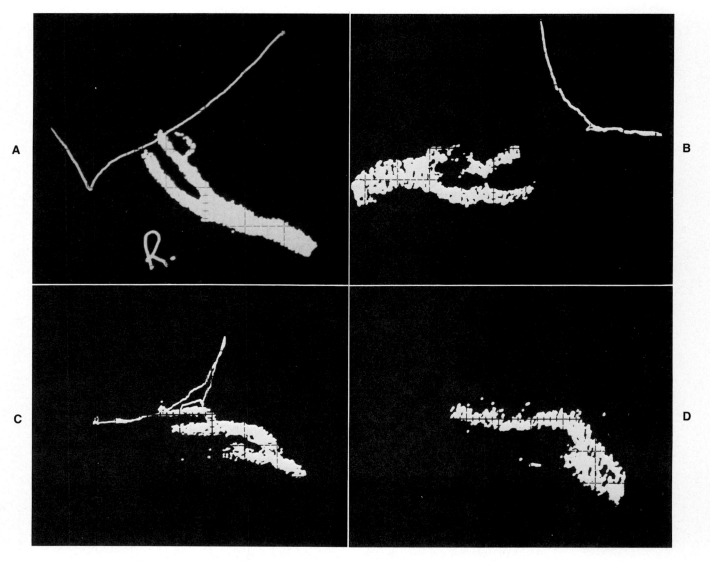

FIG. 40-41. Examples of ultrasonic arteriograms. **A,** Normal carotid. **B,** Mild-moderate internal carotid stenosis or calcified plaque. **C,** Distal internal carotid occlusion. **D,** Total occlusion of internal carotid. (Courtesy D.E. Hokanson, Inc.)

when both carotid real-time scanners and Doppler angiographs exist in the same department, since somewhat more specific information concerning plaque obstruction can be obtained by combined usage of the cerebrovascular Doppler examination, spectral analysis, and a carotid B-mode real-time device. The best deployment of the current Doppler angiographic instrumentation seems to be in determining flow volume measurements and profiles and showing respective flow directions and intensities in arteries and veins. As with most Doppler-related examinations, the best overall results are obtained by correlation with the basic Doppler examination and/or another imaging modality.

TRANSCRANIAL DOPPLER ASSESSMENT[14]
Recently, new developments in Doppler technology have enabled examiners to assess the flow of the intracranial branches indirectly, using thinner areas of the skull as sonic windows to the circle of Willis, basilar artery, middle cerebral, and anterior cerebral arteries. These new techniques, while seeming to bring us back to the days of indirect blind assessment of arteries, are actually quite sensitive[4] and have the potential to allow full, accurate, noninvasive assessment of the entire cerebrovascular state in the right hands. The procedure was introduced by Rune Aaslid in 1982, and has developed since then into a truly diagnostic tool.

Equipment. The device used is a bidirectional pulsed Doppler with a 2 MHz probe, which has sufficient ability to penetrate bony structures at maximum allowable power levels of 100 mW/cm^2. The sample focal depth is variable on these devices since they by necessity must be range-gated, and depth increments range from 2 to 5 mm at a time, to a maximum depth of about 150 mm. Pulse-repetition rates are also adjustable since velocities are inevitably quite high and Doppler velocities assume an an-

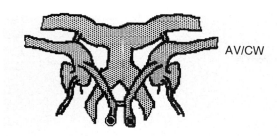

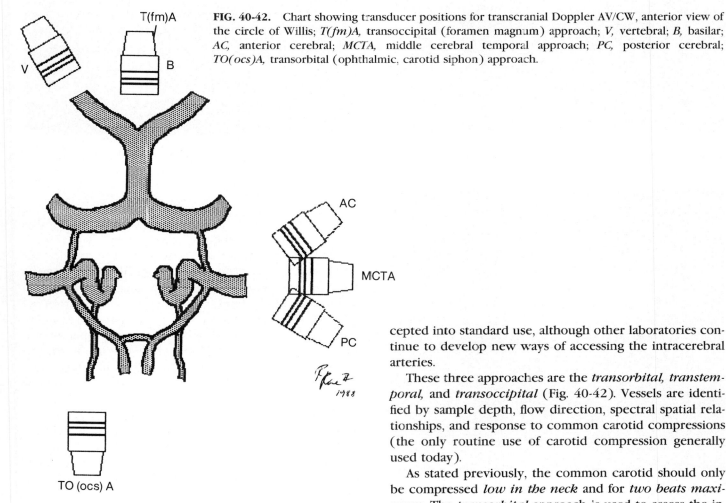

FIG. 40-42. Chart showing transducer positions for transcranial Doppler AV/CW, anterior view of the circle of Willis; *T(fm)A*, transoccipital (foramen magnum) approach; *V*, vertebral; *B*, basilar; *AC*, anterior cerebral; *MCTA*, middle cerebral temporal approach; *PC*, posterior cerebral; *TO(ocs)A*, transorbital (ophthalmic, carotid siphon) approach.

gle of nearly 0 degree because the beam intercepts the arterial flow at nearly that angle because of anatomic restrictions. A spectrum analysis display is incorporated into these units, and focal depth, velocity, and flow direction are displayed as well.

Examination technique. Review the Anatomy of the Intracranial Cerebrovascular Circulation. In summary, the arteries accessible to the transcranial Doppler are the *anterior communicating, anterior cerebral, ophthalmic, intracranial internal carotid, middle cerebral, posterior communicating, posterior cerebral, basilar,* and *distal vertebral arteries.*

Since transcranial Doppler is a recent and evolving procedure, examination approaches have been developed by numerous institutions and authors internationally. Based on their research, three of these approaches have been ac-

cepted into standard use, although other laboratories continue to develop new ways of accessing the intracerebral arteries.

These three approaches are the *transorbital, transtemporal,* and *transoccipital* (Fig. 40-42). Vessels are identified by sample depth, flow direction, spectral spatial relationships, and response to common carotid compressions (the only routine use of carotid compression generally used today).

As stated previously, the common carotid should only be compressed *low in the neck* and for *two beats maximum.* The *transorbital* approach is used to assess the intracranial internal carotid in the area of the carotid siphon. Power levels are set low (about 10 mW/cm^2) to avoid overexposure of the eye to excessive acoustic power levels. The eye is closed and the transducer is placed over the eyelid and coupled with gel. The beam is oriented anterior-posterior with a slight tilt to the midline.

The *ophthalmic* artery is evaluated at a sample depth of 40 to 50 mm (Fig. 40-43). The sample depth is increased slowly as adjustments are made to keep the ophthalmic artery in the Doppler beam. At 55 to 70 mm the *carotid siphon* area is located and is easily discerned by the higher diastolic velocity compared with the ophthalmic signal. The different curved segments of the intracranial internal carotid where it exits the carotid canal and before it joins the circle of Willis (proximal, *parasellar,* curve, *genu,* distal and posterior, *supraclinoid*) are de-

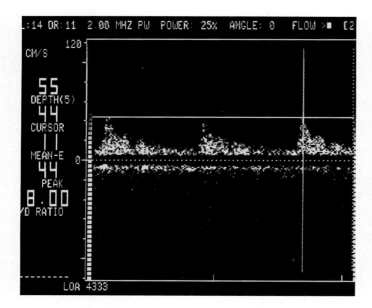

FIG. 40-43. Normal ophthalmic artery spectrum.

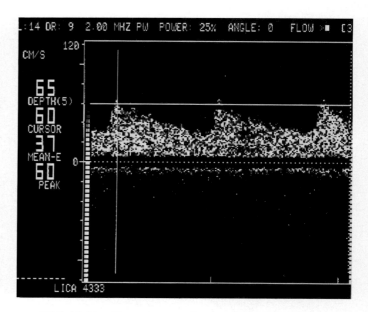

FIG. 40-44. Normal internal carotid siphon spectrum.

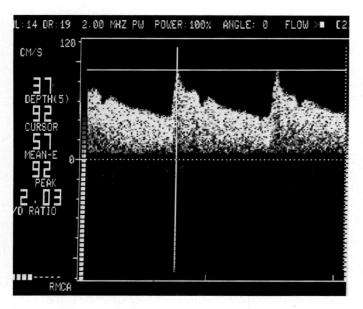

FIG. 40-45. Normal middle cerebral artery spectrum.

tected by flow direction. The parasellar (near the sella turcica) portion is found by angling inferiorly, and flow will be toward the transducer (Fig. 40-44). The flow in the anterior curve (genu section) will be bidirectional (since the beam is entering perpendicular to the flow). Locating the genu section first can help locate the other two segments. The supraclinoid segment is found by angling superiorly, and flow will be away from the transducer.

The *transtemporal* approach is used for evaluating the *middle cerebral artery, anterior cerebral artery, terminal portion of the internal carotid, posterior cerebral artery,* and the *anterior* and *posterior communicating arteries.* This approach is operator dependent, since the examiner must locate an area in the temporal bone that is thin enough to allow an adequate acoustic window where the Doppler can penetrate the bone well. The location for transtemporal insonation is superior to the zygomatic arch, and the probe may need to be aimed anteriorly, posteriorly, or dead center, depending on which "window" allows the best reception of the Doppler signals from the circle of Willis arteries. The best location is found by setting the sample depth at 55 to 60 mm and then moving to obtain a clear Doppler signal from any of the arteries that lie at that depth, usually the anterior, middle, or posterior cerebral arteries and the terminal internal carotid.

The *middle cerebral artery* is located by reducing the sample depth between 25 and 50 mm, which should detect it since it is the most shallow arterial signal (Fig. 40-45). The middle cerebral flow signal is toward the transducer and will diminish with low common carotid compressions.

The *internal carotid bifurcation* into the *middle and anterior cerebral arteries* can be found at a sample depth of 55 to 65 mm and has a bidirectional signal (Fig. 40-46). The bidirectional middle and anterior cerebral bifurcation is a reference point for obtaining signals from the anterior, middle, and posterior cerebral arteries. Common carotid compressions will reverse the anterior cerebral flow component if the anterior communicating artery is patent and will diminish the signal if the anterior communicating artery is obstructed or absent. The middle cerebral component will diminish as mentioned previously.

The *terminal internal carotid* is located by angling inferior to the middle and anterior cerebral bifurcation. Flow velocities are lower than in the middle and anterior cerebral arteries, and the signal is obliterated by common carotid compression.

The middle and anterior cerebral bifurcation is relocated and the sample depth is increased to 70 to 80 mm

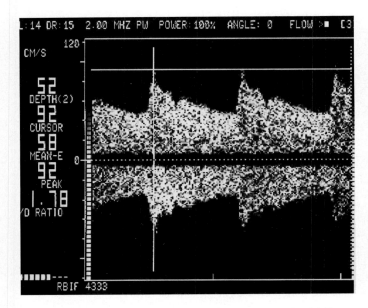

FIG. 40-46. Normal middle cerebral/anterior cerebral bifurcation spectrum.

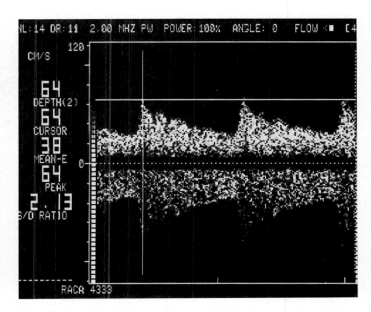

FIG. 40-47. Normal anterior cerebral artery spectrum (inverted).

(brain midline) while adjusting and keeping the *anterior cerebral signal* centered (Fig. 40-47). Flow is normally away from the transducer. Reversed signals imply cross-channel collateral flow from the opposite side, and this may occur when the ipsilateral internal carotid is severely stenosed, and the contralateral anterior cerebral will exhibit increased flow velocities. Common carotid compression will normally reverse the anterior cerebral signal or will diminish flow in the absence of a patent *anterior communicating* artery. The anterior communicating artery is not normally detected unless it is acting as a collateral, when high velocities and turbulence will be noted at the 70 to 80 mm level.

The *posterior cerebral artery* signal is located by beginning at the middle and anterior cerebral bifurcation, increasing the sample depth by about 5 mm then angling posteriorly and inferiorly (Fig. 40-48). Flow is toward the transducer and may occasionally be confused with the middle cerebral, but the posterior cerebral artery cannot be tracked at any depth shallower than 55 mm whereas the middle cerebral artery can. The distal posterior cerebral artery flow signal will appear to travel away from the probe or be bidirectional since the anatomic course of the posterior cerebral changes in relation to the transducer window and the beam "sweeps" across the curve.

The *posterior communicating artery* is seldom located, but will appear as a turbulent, high-velocity signal when acting as a collateral and is found in a manner similar to that used for the posterior cerebral artery.

The *transoccipital* approach is used for the evaluation of the intracranial *vertebral* arteries and *basilar* artery. The head is slightly flexed forward and the probe is placed in the center of the suboccipital area with a sample depth of 60 to 70 mm. The probe is angled laterally right and left of midline to assess the individual vertebrals. The sample depth is then increased until the vertebrobasi-

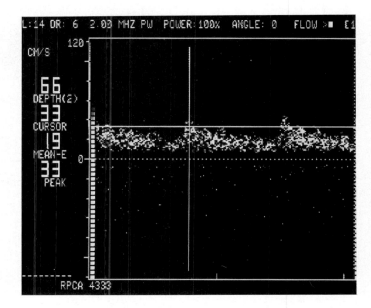

FIG. 40-48. Normal posterior cerebral artery spectrum.

lar junction is located (85 to 100 mm) and the single basilar artery signal is assessed. The probe may need to be elevated superiorly when following the arteries. The flow in the vertebrals and basilar will be away from the transducer normally. A reversed signal in one vertebral or the other with turbulence at the basilar junction is indicative of a subclavian steal, and evidence to this effect should already have been gained from earlier extracranial duplex carotid or direct carotid Doppler assessments.

Characteristics and interpretation of the Doppler intracranial arterial waveform. [14] The normal appearance of the intracranial waveform is similar to that of the extracranial internal carotid artery since the intracranial arteries are a low-resistance system. The diastolic seg-

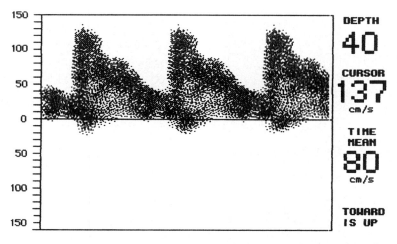

FIG. 40-49.   Typical normal transcranial waveform appearance.

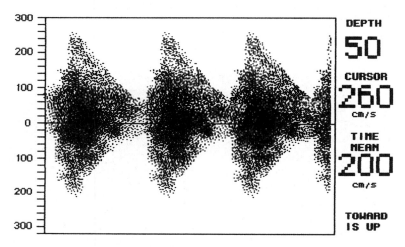

FIG. 40-50.   Typical abnormal stenotic waveform appearance.

ment of the spectral waveform will not normally go below the baseline and the concentration of frequencies will follow the envelope contour, as in the normal internal carotid signal (Fig. 40-49).

The primary factor used in quantifying the intracranial Doppler signal is the peak systolic velocity, which is measured in the same location on the waveform as in the rest of the carotid system. Normal velocities are as follows:

1. The *middle cerebral artery*—94 to 105 cm/s
2. The *anterior cerebral artery*—72 to 85 cm/s
3. The *posterior cerebral artery*—60 cm/s
4. The *basilar* artery—64 cm/s

The internal carotid velocity, as specified earlier, should not exceed 80 cm/s normally, and the vertebral velocity normally does not exceed 100 cm/s.

Flow direction is another diagnostic criterium, as is the presence of turbulence and diminished waveforms. Some spectral broadening occurs naturally in the intracranial arteries because of the many branches and bifurcations and their small caliber; therefore normal spectral broadening criteria do not apply with the exception of turbulence and velocity increase.

Abnormal findings (similar to diagnostic findings in the

duplex and direct carotid Doppler exam) include the following:

1. *Increased velocity shifts* exceeding the normal range. As in other vessels, a jet effect and velocity increase is proportional to the amount of stenosis, although actual percentages are not generally calculated in the intracranial system as of this writing. High velocities are also detectable in collateral arteries.

2. *Flow disturbance and turbulence.* These also are associated with stenoses and velocity increases. Because of the small size of the intracranial arteries, turbulent signals often manifest themselves as "squeaking" or "whining" sounds, almost musical in nature (Fig. 40-50).

3. *Diminished waveforms.* As noted earlier, flow will dampen and the waveform pulsatility will decrease distal to a severe stenosis. Obtaining a notably diminished signal implies a severe stenosis or occlusion proximal to the area being evaluated.

Conditions that can be diagnosed with the transcranial Doppler examination. [14,18] Numerous intracerebral arterial phenomena can be evaluated with transcranial Doppler. Among these are the following:

1. *Vasospasm.* Vasospastic disorders of the middle cerebral or anterior cerebral arteries can be initially evaluated and then followed over a period of time without repeated angiography.
2. *Intracranial stenoses.* Middle cerebral artery stenosis or occlusion, basilar artery stenosis, intracranial or supramandibular internal carotid stenosis inaccessible to duplex scanning, and stenosis of other circle of Willis branches can be identified and evaluated. This modality is proving extremely valuable in cases of high internal carotid occlusion, which is only implied by duplex Doppler signals obtained proximally in the common and proximal internal carotids.
3. *Cross-channel circle of Willis collateralization* following internal carotid stenosis can be truly documented and pathways charted instead of inferred by the results of indirect methods as before.
4. *Distal assessment of vertebrobasilar stenoses* as well as documentation of subclavian or carotid steal syndromes is possible using the transcranial Doppler.

Summary. Transcranial Doppler gives the examiner a direct method of evaluating the circle of Willis and intracranial arterial system noninvasively, and as investigators publish their findings, even more will be known about the ultimate impact of transcranial Doppler's diagnostic capabilities. At present, it seems that the ideal cerebrovascular noninvasive test in the future may consist of duplex evaluation of the carotid arteries in the neck (with or without color-flow mapping) and transcranial Doppler evaluation of the cerebral vasculature. Regardless of the methods employed, this most recent addition to the arsenal of Doppler methods shows great promise for diagnosis.

SUMMARY

1. Cerebral ischemia is one of the leading causes of death in the world. Causes of ischemic episodes include atherosclerotic plaque in the carotid arteries, arterial aneurysm, cardiac emboli, diseases of the intima, and external compression. Many techniques have been developed over the years to help diagnose carotid and cerebral arterial conditions.
2. Carotid duplex sonography coupled with spectrum analysis of carotid blood flow is proving to be more accurate than arteriography to help diagnose carotid and cerebral arterial conditions.
3. In general, examination of cerebrovascular circulation and carotid arteries is best accomplished using a combination of duplex sonography and continuous-wave Doppler.
4. Direct carotid Doppler analysis is often performed after duplex sonography since imaging allows the examiner to determine how the arteries lie, where the bifurcation is, and how much disease is present.
5. The direct carotid Doppler and periorbital examinations are open to any number of occurrences that can cause diagnostic and interpretive errors to take place. These errors are less likely to occur when carotid duplex sonography is used as an adjunctive procedure or precedes direct Doppler assessment.
6. Carotid duplex sonography is the method of choice for noninvasively evaluating the cerebrovascular system. It does not eliminate arteriography, however, for evaluating structures above the mandible or intracranially.
7. Intraoperative real-time scanning is being used by more and more surgical centers during endarterectomy. It helps the surgeon evaluate the stenosis by scanning the exposed carotid directly both before and after endarterectomy. Duplex Doppler assessment can be used also to document the flow dynamics of the surgical area.
8. Postoperatively, any endarterectomy or graft can be evaluated and followed by carotid duplex sonography or direct carotid Doppler. The sonographic appearance of the carotid postendarterectomy is identical to that of a normal carotid except that there will be no intimal echoes within the area of surgery, and the walls may appear ectatic or dilated.
9. Transcranial Doppler assessment enables examiners to assess the flow of the intracranial branches indirectly, using thinner areas of the skull as sonic windows to the circle of Willis, basilar artery, middle cerebral, and anterior cerebral arteries.

REFERENCES

1. Baker W et al: The cerebrovascular Doppler examination in patients with non-hemispheric symptoms, Ann Surg 186:190, 1977.
2. Barnes RW et al: Doppler cerebrovascular examination: improved results with refinements in technique, Stroke 8:468, 1977.
3. Barnes RW et al: Doppler ultrasonic evaluation of cerebrovascular disease, Iowa City, 1975, University of Iowa Press.
4. Bishop CCR, Powell S, et al: Transcranial Doppler measurement of middle cerebral artery blood flow velocity: a validation study, Stroke 17:913, 1986.
5. Blackwell E, Merory J, et al: Doppler ultrasound scanning of the carotid bifurcation, Arch Neurol 34:145, 1977.
6. Budingen HJ et al: Die Differenzierung der Halsgefässe mit der direktionellen Doppler-Sonographie, Arch Psychiatr Nervenkr 222:177, 1976.
7. Burger R et al: Choice of ophthalmic artery branch for Doppler cerebrovascular examination: advantages of the frontal artery, Angiology 28:421, 1977.
8. Corson JD et al: Doppler ankle systolic blood pressure. Prognostic value in vein bypass grafts of the lower extremity, Arch Surg 113:932, 1978.
9. Crew J, Dean M, et al: Carotid surgery without angiography, Am J Surg 184:217, 1984.
10. Day TK, Fish PJ, et al: Detection of deep vein thrombosis by Doppler angiography, Br Med J 1:618, 1976.
11. Fields WS: Aortocranial occlusive vascular disease (stroke), Clin Symp 26(4):3, 1974.
12. Johnson J: Angiography and ultrasound in diagnosis of carotid artery disease: a comparison, Contemp Surg vol 20, March, 1982.
13. Johnston KW, deMorais D, et al: Cerebrovascular assessment using a Doppler carotid scanner and real-time frequency analysis, J Clin Ultrasound 9:443, 1981.
14. Kuehn K, Sola N, et al: Transcranial pulsed Doppler for evaluation of cerebral arterial hemodynamics. Presentation at the 10th Annual Convention of the Society of Noninvasive Vascular Technologists, June 6, 1987, Toronto.

15. Netter FH, Kaplan A, et al: Ciba collection of medical illustrations, Vol 1, Nervous system, Summit NJ, 1953 (1979 printing), Medical Education Division, Ciba Pharmaceutical Co.

16. Towne JB et al: Periorbital ultrasound findings: hemodynamics in patients with cerebrovascular disease, Arch Surg 114:158, 1979.

17. von Reutern GM et al: Diagnose und Differenzierung von Stenosen und Verschlussen der Arteria carotis mit der Doppler-Sonographie, Arch Psychiatr Nervenkr 222(2-3):191, 1976.

18. Wechsler L, Ropper A, et al: Transcranial Doppler in cerebrovascular disease, Stroke 17:905, 1986.

19. Widder B: Ein vereinfachtes Doppler-Angiographie-Gerat zur unblutingen Diagnostik von Karotis-Stenosen, Nervenarzt 48:397, 1979.

20. Wood CPL, and Meire HD: A technique for imaging the vertebral artery using pulsed Doppler ultrasound, Ultrasound Med Biol 6:329, 1980.

41

Miscellaneous Applications of Doppler and Duplex Sonography

RICHARD E. RAE II

DUPLEX SONOGRAPHY OF THE PERIPHERAL ARTERIAL SYSTEM

Real-time duplex sonography has recently been performed on the peripheral arteries in the extremities with a good deal of success. The basic techniques discussed in the carotid duplex sonography section above apply, although the anatomy differs. A brief discussion of duplex evaluation of the extremity arteries will be presented here. Please review the previous appropriate sections on the arterial anatomy in the extremities.

Lower extremity

The best types of duplex imagers for evaluating peripheral arteries are those with linear and/or phased-array transducers since more of the artery can be seen in longitudinal sections with less distortion. All arteries should be imaged in both longitudinal and transverse planes. The techniques used for venous duplex examination also can be used since the arteries and veins will be side by side.

The iliac artery should be examined starting above the inguinal ligament and moving distally, and can be distinguished from the iliac vein as it will lie lateral to the easily compressed vein the be pulsatile. Confirmation by Doppler also can be done. The iliac will become the femoral at the ligament level and can be followed to the profunda bifurcation where the superficial femoral artery begins. The superficial femoral artery is followed down the me-

dial thigh to the level of the kneecap. The popliteal artery is best evaluated with the patient supine and the transducer placed posteriorly behind the popliteal fossa (Fig. 41-1). Imaging of the trifurcation can be accomplished by moving distal to the popliteal and scanning the area of the gastrocnemius muscle, with the anterior tibial takeoff being the first branch visualized. Depth adjustments should be made as needed.

As with the carotid evaluation, duplex Doppler signals should be taken in each artery visualized and proximal and distal to any stenosis that may be seen. Stenoses should be documented in both planes. In cases of possible arterial aneurysm, distance measurements should be made from vessel wall to vessel wall, especially in areas of ectasia. Lower extremity duplex Doppler findings are interpreted by the same criteria previously mentioned (see Interpretation of the Lower Extremity Arterial Examination, Chapter 38, and the discussion of spectrum analysis in Chapter 37).

Duplex applications in the lower extremity involve some of the following:

1. *Evaluation of focal plaque disease* in any visualized arterial segment.
2. *Presurgical and postsurgical or parasurgical procedures.* Duplex sonography can be used for the initial evaluation and follow-up on such procedures as thrombectomy, atherectomy, angioplasty, and endarterectomy.

1015

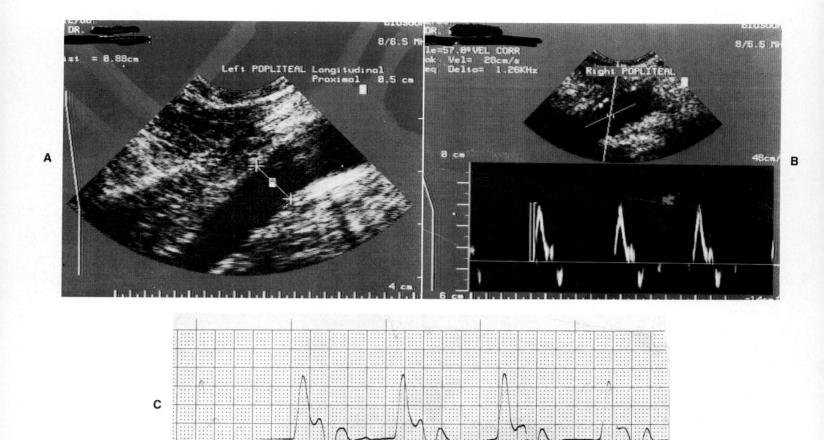

FIG. 41-1. Normal popliteal artery duplex image, **A,** with, **B,** normal pulsed Doppler signal and, **C,** normal analog waveform.

3. *Evaluation of bypass grafts* can be performed to evaluate patency and document areas of stenosis, kinking, or to evaluate the origin and insertion of the graft for pseudoaneurysm or hematoma.

Upper extremity

Using the same types of duplex scanners as described above, the arm arteries can also be examined in longitudinal and transverse sections. Again, the procedure is very similar to that used for evaluating the venous system. The procedure usually involves scanning from distal to proximal. The radial and ulnar arteries can be traced from the wrist to antecubital fossa and the branchial bifurcation, and the bifurcation of the median artery off the ulnar artery can also be seen. This artery often can supply the hand in cases of an occluded distal ulnar artery, making assessment of this vessel important. The brachial artery can next be followed up into the axilla, where the distal axillary artery can be examined. The examiner must direct the probe supraclavicularly or infraclavicularly to visualize the subclavian artery, which can often be seen behind the vein. The origin of the vertebral can also be seen, as has been mentioned previously. Duplex Doppler signals can be obtained at any level, and all flow patterns should be documented.

Duplex signals should be taken in each artery visualized and proximal and distal to any stenosis that may be seen. Stenoses should be documented in both planes. In cases of possible arterial aneurysm, distance measurements should be made from vessel wall to vessel wall, especially in areas of ectasia. Upper extremity duplex Doppler findings are interpreted by the same criteria previously mentioned (see Interpretation of the Upper Extremity Arterial Examination, Chapter 38, and the discussion of spectrum analysis in Chapter 37).

DUPLEX SONOGRAPHY AND DOPPLER EVALUATION OF ABDOMINAL VESSELS

Evaluation of the abdominal vasculature by real-time and B-scan sonography has already been covered in other chapters, and this section will not review those techniques in depth. Duplex Doppler assessment of the abdominal vessels is, however, becoming more and more widespread as high-quality pulsed Doppler is integrated into scanning devices designed for the deep abdomen. Some companies coin the term "deep Doppler" for machines with abdominal capabilities to distinguish them from machines with Doppler that are oriented toward peripheral vessels. These devices routinely operate at imaging and Doppler frequencies from 2.25 to 5 MHz, with 3.5

MHz being the most common. Color-flow and/or phased-array devices that allow simultaneous Doppler and image are almost a must when examining the renal arteries, mesenteric arteries, and portal venous system, since respiratory motion affects the positioning of these vessels the most, and they can move in and out of the Doppler sample continually.

The display of most abdominal duplex machines is identical to those discussed earlier, including the angle line, sample volume, and vectoring controls. Abdominal machines generally are of the mechanical sector, linear, or phased-array type.

Prior to duplex Doppler evaluation, the abdomen should be auscultated with a stethoscope at the midline to the umbilicus, over each kidney, and in the groin over the iliac areas. The presence of an abdominal bruit implies a celiac or mesenteric stenosis; over the kidney, a renal artery stenosis; and an iliac bruit implies a stenosis of the aortic bifurcation or iliac arteries. Scrupulous adherence to standard preps by the patient is required; presence of bowel or stomach gas not only will obscure visualization but will make Doppler assessment impossible. The patient should, when possible, suspend respiration when a Doppler signal is taken.

Routine evaluation of any abdominal vasculature follows standard sonographic technique, except that a Doppler sample is placed in the artery or vein of interest and then appropriate waveforms are taken.

Applications for abdominal Doppler include the following:

1. *Abdominal aorta.* Doppler signals can be obtained in the proximal and distal aorta during aneurysm evaluation and to determine the effect of distal aortic stenoses on the proximal common iliac arteries. Normal abdominal aortic Doppler waveforms are triphasic but less dynamic than those found in the extremities, and normal velocities seldom exceed 40 cm/s. Flow tends to slow within an aneurysm; high aortic velocities are seldom seen.

2. *Mesenteric arteries.* The celiac axis and superior mesenteric arteries are frequent sites of stenosis, and their obstruction can cause gastric and bowel ischemia, which in turn can lead to an infarction and gangrenous bowel. The most common place for sampling is in the longitudinal plane and at the origins of the arteries since stenoses occur most commonly there. The inferior mesenteric is occasionally sampled when visualized. As with other small-caliber arteries, there is often a mild amount of turbulence, and abnormality is documented by excessive turbulence and abnormally high velocities. Some suspected mesenteric artery stenoses can be enhanced by feeding the patient then measuring the postprandial velocity and waveform responses.

3. *Renal arteries.* The renal arteries are probably evaluated with Doppler more often than other vessels, since renal artery stenosis can cause renovascular hypertension. Sampling is best done in the axial or transverse position, and the procedure is extremely time consuming as the arteries move in and out of the field of view with each respiration. Suspended respiration helps, but the timing must often be right and the examiner must have a quick hand to center the sample over the artery, adjust the vector for accurate velocity measurement, and then take the waveform before the patient turns blue! Simultaneous Doppler image duplex probes can reduce this obstacle. The renal artery lies posterior to the renal vein, and samples are best taken close to the origins of the arteries near the aorta. Turbulence and increased velocities are significant for stenosis. For quantifying the amount of stenosis, sometimes a waveform and peak velocity reading is taken from the aorta at the level of the renal takeoffs, and this velocity reading is divided into the peak velocity of the renal artery, giving a figure called the *renal aortic ratio* (RAR). Renal aortic indices greater than 3.00 are considered diagnostic of significant renal artery stenosis.[1]

4. *Hepatoportal venous system.* Venous obstruction and thrombosis of the portal vein and hepatic veins can cause severe liver and digestive dysfunction. Doppler can be used to evaluate the portal system and document flow patterns within the hepatic veins. Porta hepatic venous signals should be phasic and spontaneous as in other veins. Continuous or unusually high flow may imply a venous obstruction.

5. *Inferior vena cava.* The vena cava can be evaluated for thrombosis as in the extremity veins, especially if there is a danger of pulmonary embolism. The iliacs and distal vena cava are commonly evaluated, and incompressibility implies the presence of a lumen-occupying thrombus as in the legs or arms. Continuous or absent flow is also significant for obstruction. Additionally, the status of Greenfield filters inserted in the vena cava to prevent thrombi from traveling superiorly can be periodically evaluated and flow patterns documented.

6. *Renal transplants.* The evaluation of flow to renal transplants is proving to be an important way of determining early rejection and the viability of the transplant. Continuous or high-velocity signals may imply pending rejection. Acute tubal necrosis will present as a high-resistance signal.

∎ ∎ ∎ ∎ ∎

Abdominal Doppler usage is proving to be a vital tool in the noninvasive evaluation of abdominal vasculature. Color-flow devices are proving valid in this area, and while duplex Doppler has not yet supplanted angiography for some of the most sensitive vascular conditions in the abdomen, there are more than enough conditions that benefit from this approach to indicate the need for continued development of "deep Doppler" techniques.

Duplex abdominal cases

CASE 1 (FIG. 41-2): NORMAL ABDOMINAL AORTA, BILATERAL COMMON ILIAC STENOSIS. This patient had a palpable thrill in the femoral arteries bilaterally, with a bruit noted over the umbilical area and distally. A lower extremity arterial Doppler exam had been performed, which had triphasic waveforms but had high thigh pressures lower than the systolic brachial pressures and ankle brachial indices in

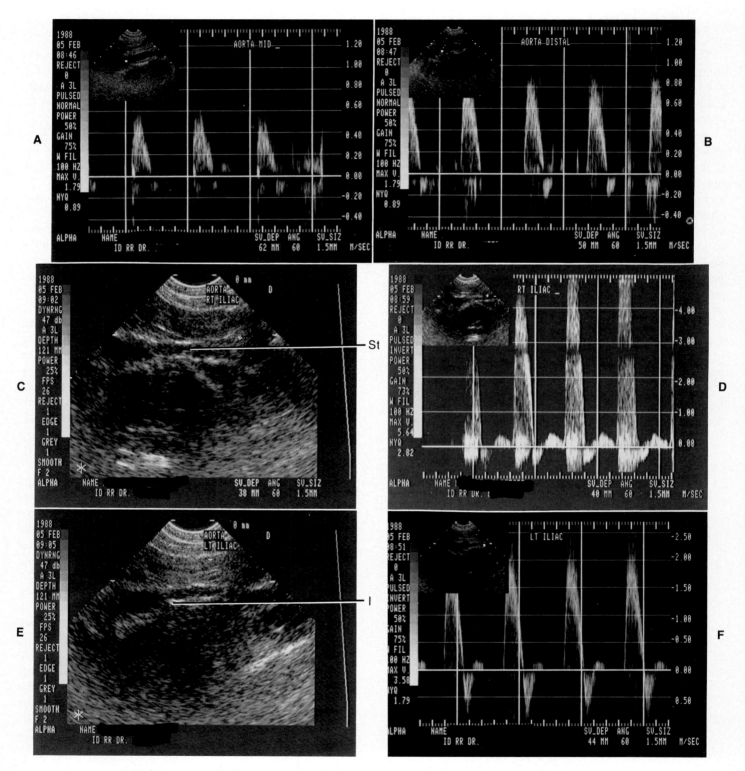

FIG. 41-2. Normal abdominal aorta, bilateral common iliac stenosis. *St,* stenosis; *I,* irregularity.

the mild-moderate impairment range, both findings that implied a proximal iliac or aortic lesion.

Normal aortic Doppler signals were obtained in the normal, nonectatic aorta (Fig. 41-2, *A* and *B*). Evaluation of the common iliacs showed a focal lesion in the right common iliac, *C*, which caused severe turbulence and an abnormally elevated velocity of >400 cm/s on duplex Doppler evaluation, *D*. The left common iliac had circumferential irregularity in the origin, *E*, which caused a moderate velocity shift of about 250 cm/s in the vessel but with minimal spectral broadening, *F*.

Arteriography confirmed the presence of a severe stenosis of the right common iliac with a mild to moderate stenosis of the left common iliac.

SUMMARY

1. Real-time duplex sonography has recently been performed on the peripheral arteries in the extremities with good success.

2. Duplex Doppler assessment of the abdominal vessels is becoming more widespread as high-quality pulsed Doppler is integrated into scanning devices designed for the deep abdomen.

REFERENCE

1. Kohler TR, Zierier RE, et al: Non-invasive diagnosis of renal artery stenosis by ultrasonic duplex scanning, J Vasc Surg 4:450, 1986.

Appendix A

The Diagnostic Sonographer

The diagnostic sonographer is a skilled person qualified by academic and clinical training to provide patient services using diagnostic ultrasound under the supervision of a physician or osteopath responsible for the use and interpretation of ultrasound procedures. The sonographer may be involved with the patients of the physician in any medical setting for which the physician is responsible.

EDUCATION

Individuals admitted for training should have completed high school or the equivalent and should have post-secondary education in the following areas: medical ethics, medical terminology, clinical anatomy and physiology, medical orientation and administration, nursing procedures, general human anatomy, and elementary physics. Individuals in the allied health field of nuclear medicine or radiologic technology are good applicants for diagnostic ultrasound, since they already possess imaging capabilities. Cardiopulmonary technologists and cardiac catheterization technologists have proved to be capable candidates for the echocardiology section of ultrasound.

PERSONAL QUALIFICATIONS

Individuals should be mature, responsible, and able to use initiative and independent judgment when necessary. They should have a high standard of medical ethics and empathy with the patient.

Sonographers must have the ability to establish and maintain effective working relationships with patients, employees, physicians, and the general public. They should be capable of working without supervision within the guidelines set by department heads.

Self-motivation to maintain an increasing level of understanding and knowledge of the field and new procedures is necessary for the development of the sonographer.

SKILLS

The sonographer should have a high degree of technical aptitude with an in-depth knowledge of anatomy and physiology. An ability to improvise the standard of procedure when necessary is essential. The sonographer must be able to supervise the work activities of the backup technologist and ancillary personnel.

Knowledge of ultrasound techniques should be thorough. The number of procedures known will depend on the sonographer's particular interests, background, and training. The general sonographer should have current knowledge of neurology, cardiology, and abdominal, obstetric, and gynecologic applications. In addition, this person must have the ability to deal effectively with patients and to act quickly in an emergency.

A complete knowledge and understanding of the complex instrumentation used to extract the finest-quality performance from the equipment is necessary.

The ability to deviate from normal techniques when necessary and to develop new and better techniques to keep the department up to date is also the responsibility of the sonographer and the physician.

DUTIES
Sonographer I*

QUALIFICATIONS. High school graduate and 2 years of allied health background in an AMA-accredited program.

PERFORMANCE OF DIAGNOSTIC ULTRASOUND PROCEDURES

1. Check the physician's requisition for complete information on the procedure requested; refer any questions to the ultrasound physician before performing the procedure.
2. Review the patient's chart to obtain pertinent clinical history, correlative test results, and laboratory data.
3. Position the patient for examination, explain the procedure, and give necessary instructions for carrying out the procedure.
4. Perform emergency examinations in the department or at the bedside with physician supervision.

OPERATION OF DIAGNOSTIC ULTRASOUND EQUIPMENT

1. Operate ultrasound equipment with a knowledge of A-mode, M-mode, B-mode, Doppler, and real-time techniques.
2. Select the proper transducer frequency and diameter for performance of the examination.
3. Utilize ancillary devices (oscilloscopes, cameras [Polaroid and multiformat], videorecorders) to obtain a permanent record of the examination.
4. Maintain quality control of the equipment.

---

*The roman numeral designates level of training.

1020

INTERPRETATION OF ULTRASOUND PROCEDURES

1. Recognize the significance of all structures that are visualized on the oscilloscope.
2. Be able to differentiate artifacts from anatomic/pathologic structures and to recognize equipment limitations.
3. Be capable of recognizing a diagnostic quality scan.
4. Possess a knowledge of anatomy and physiology and be able to relate this to the ultrasound examination.

PROFESSIONAL DEVELOPMENT

1. Read journals and attend local symposiums to keep abreast of new techniques.
2. Review the pathology, surgery, and delivery reports to follow the patient's progress and provide a means of reviewing the accuracy of ultrasound examinations.
3. Periodically review anatomy, physiology, and pathology as related to ultrasonics.
4. Maintain ethical working relationships and good rapport with all referring physicians, hospital staff, and commercial agencies.

ADMINISTRATIVE RESPONSIBILITIES

1. Maintain supplies for the service or room assigned.
2. Maintain cleanliness of the equipment and a general orderliness of the area assigned.
3. Obtain x-ray film folders from the file room, inscribe the x-ray and ultrasound film folders with the appropriate data, and record the examination performed on a file card.
4. Make copies of teaching or research cases as needed.

Sonographer II

QUALIFICATIONS. Two years' allied health background in an AMA-approved program or 2 years of college. One year in diagnostic ultrasound (either a formal program or 18 months' equivalent experience). Must be ARDMS eligible.

PERFORMANCE OF DIAGNOSTIC ULTRASOUND PROCEDURES

1. Check the physician's requisition for complete information on the procedure requested; refer any questions to the ultrasound physician before performing procedure.
2. Consult with the referring physician regarding the patient's medical history and the appropriate ultrasound procedure required.
3. Review the patient's chart to obtain pertinent clinical history, correlative test results, and laboratory data.
4. Position the patient for examination, explain the procedure, and give necessary instructions for carrying out the procedure.
5. Be able to deviate from normal techniques when necessary and to develop better techniques to keep the department up to date.
6. Perform emergency examinations in the department or at the bedside with physician supervision.

OPERATION OF DIAGNOSTIC ULTRASOUND EQUIPMENT

1. Operate ultrasound equipment with an in-depth knowledge of A-mode, M-mode, B-mode (analog and digital), Doppler, and real-time techniques.
2. Select the proper transducer frequency and diameter for performance of the examination.

3. Utilize ancillary devices (oscilloscopes, cameras [Polaroid and multiformat], videorecorders) to obtain a permanent record of the examination.
4. Maintain quality control of the equipment.
5. Calibrate ultrasound and photographic equipment when necessary.

INTERPRETATION OF ULTRASOUND PROCEDURES

1. Recognize the significance of all structures that are visualized on the oscilloscope.
2. Be able to differentiate artifacts from anatomic/pathologic structures and to recognize electronic equipment limitations.
3. Possess a high degree of technical expertise, with an in-depth knowledge of anatomy and physiology, and be able to improve standard procedures to enhance diagnostic results when needed.
4. Be capable of recognizing a diagnostic scan and rendering an initial interpretation to the referring physician as reported by the staff sonologist.
5. Maintain ethical working relationships and good rapport with all referring physicians, hospital staff, and commercial agencies.

RESEARCH IN AND DEVELOPMENT OF ULTRASOUND TECHNIQUES

1. Evaluate new products and equipment for future use.
2. Read journals and attend annual conventions, seminars, and symposiums to keep abreast of new techniques.
3. Review the pathology, surgery, and delivery reports to follow the patient's progress and provide a means of reviewing the accuracy of ultrasound examinations.
4. Continuously review anatomy and physiology and the effect of disease processes with relation to ultrasonics.

COORDINATION OF ADMINISTRATIVE RESPONSIBILITIES

1. Maintain supplies for the service or room assigned.
2. Obtain x-ray film folders from the file room, inscribe the x-ray and ultrasound film folders with the appropriate data, and record the examination performed on a file card.
3. Record interesting cases for teaching or research purposes.
4. Make copies of teaching or research cases as needed.

Sonographer III

QUALIFICATIONS. Two years' allied health background in an AMA-accredited program or 2 years of college. Two years' experience/training in diagnostic ultrasound. Must have ARDMS in at least two specialty areas (i.e., abdomen, obstetrics, Doppler, or cardiology).

PERFORMANCE OF DIAGNOSTIC ULTRASOUND PROCEDURES

1. Check the physician's requisition for complete information on the procedure requested; refer any questions to the ultrasound physician (sonologist) before performing the procedure.
2. Consult with the referring physician regarding the patient's medical history and the appropriate ultrasound procedure required.
3. Review the patient's chart to obtain pertinent clinical history, correlative test results, and laboratory data as they apply to the ultrasound examination.
4. Position the patient for examination, explain the pro-

cedure, and give necessary instructions for carrying out the procedure.

5. Be able to deviate from normal techniques when necessary and to develop better techniques to keep the department up to date.

6. Perform emergency examinations in the department or at the bedside without physician supervision.

OPERATION OF DIAGNOSTIC ULTRASOUND EQUIPMENT

1. Operate ultrasound equipment with an in-depth knowledge of A-mode, M-mode, and B-mode (analog and digital), Doppler, and real-time techniques.

2. Select the proper transducer frequency and diameter for performance of the examination.

3. Utilize ancillary devices (oscilloscopes, cameras [Polaroid and multiformat], videorecorders) to obtain a permanent record of the examination.

4. Maintain quality control of the equipment. Record results on a regular basis.

5. Calibrate ultrasound and photographic equipment when necessary.

INTERPRETATION OF ULTRASOUND PROCEDURES

1. Recognize the significance of all structures that are visualized on the oscilloscope.

2. Be able to differentiate artifacts from anatomic/pathologic structures and recognize electronic equipment limitations.

3. Possess a high degree of technical expertise, with an in-depth knowledge of anatomy and physiology, and be able to improve standard procedures when needed.

4. Be capable of recognizing a diagnostic scan and rendering an initial interpretation to the referring physician as reported by the staff sonologist.

5. Establish and maintain ethical working relationships and good rapport with all referring physicians, hospital staff, and commercial companies.

RESEARCH IN AND DEVELOPMENT OF ULTRASOUND TECHNIQUES

1. Evaluate new products and equipment for possible future use.

2. Research, develop, and formulate new techniques for ultrasound procedures.

3. Read journals and attend annual conventions, seminars, and symposiums to keep abreast of new techniques.

4. Review the pathology, surgery, and delivery reports to follow the patient's progress and provide a means of reviewing the accuracy of ultrasound examinations.

5. Continuously review anatomy and physiology and the effect of disease processes with relation to ultrasonics.

COORDINATION OF ADMINISTRATIVE RESPONSIBILITIES

1. Maintain a procedures manual.

2. Secure and maintain supplies for the service or room assigned.

3. Keep records on all service calls for equipment and what service was done.

4. Obtain x-ray film folders from the file room, inscribe the x-ray and ultrasound film folders with the appropriate data, and record the examination performed on a file card.

5. Record interesting cases for teaching or research purposes.

6. Make copies of teaching or research cases as needed.

INSTRUCTION AND SUPERVISION OF CLINICAL EXPERIENCE FOR ULTRASOUND STUDENTS AND RADIOLOGIC TECHNOLOGY STUDENTS

1. Teach the techniques and applications of ultrasound to students, visiting sonographers, and physicians, residents, and fellows.

2. Provide impromptu explanations and demonstrations for visitors and students.

Sonographer IV, Chief

QUALIFICATIONS. High school graduate and 2 years' allied health background in an AMA-accredited program or 2 years of college. Three years' experience/training in diagnostic ultrasound. Must have ARDMS in at least three specialty areas (i.e., abdomen, obstetrics, Doppler, or cardiology). Should have extensive experience with available ultrasound equipment in terms of product evaluation, troubleshooting, and quality control. Must be mature and responsible, able to use initiative and independent judgment when necessary, and capable of working without supervision within guidelines established by the director of the division. Self-motivation with regard to increasing one's level of understanding and knowledge of the field is important, as is a background that will qualify one to teach diagnostic ultrasound.

In addition to the duties of Sonographer III, the Sonographer IV candidate is responsible for coordinating the activities of the sonologic staff and ancillary personnel and, under the supervision of the director of ultrasound, performing administrative duties of supervision within the division.

COORDINATION OF STAFF WITHIN THE ULTRASOUND DIVISION

1. Act as coordinating bond for all staff sonographers assigned within the division of ultrasound.

2. Maintain the quality of performance of sonographers as related to skills and duties.

3. Mediate problems relative to staffing, morale, scheduling, salary adjustments, discipline, and other actions regarding personnel.

4. Act as consultant in hiring, promoting, or terminating employees.

5. Assume responsibilities for patient flow and all other matters pertaining to patient care within the division.

6. Ensure patient and employee safety.

OPERATION OF DIAGNOSTIC ULTRASOUND EQUIPMENT

1. Have a knowledge of the correct operation of all divisional equipment, accessories, and procedures (as listed for Sonographer III).

2. Be able to diagnose basic equipment malfunction, communicate with service personnel, and maintain service records.

COORDINATION OF ADMINISTRATIVE RESPONSIBILITIES

1. Review monthly budget reports for accuracy and report discrepancies.

2. Maintain files on revenue analysis and expenditures, trend reports, and store-house charges.

3. Secure supplies for the division.

4. Recommend action necessary for improvement of the overall quality of the department.

5. Assume responsibilities for public relations in intrahospital dealings.

Supervision

The sonographer is under the supervision of the director of diagnostic ultrasound. Working under personal initiative to achieve quality work after initial assignments are received, the sonographer may also supervise other staff sonographers with less experience, students of ultrasound, visiting sonographers and physicians, or visiting house staff, medical students, and fellows.

Line of promotion

The larger medical centers with diagnostic ultrasound programs have a more extensive staff than do community hospital laboratories. The former program may have a staff consisting of an educational coordinator, a clinical coordinator, staff instructors, and staff sonographers specializing in neurology, cardiology, and B-scan techniques. The smaller departments may have one of three sonographers sharing the duties of the department.

Performance

The number of cases a sonographer can perform in a day depends on the type of examination ordered. Although there is usually a protocol established for each examination, the sonographer may take additional views of the area of interest for a more accurate diagnostic interpretation by the physician. Because of the anatomic and acoustic properties of each patient, it is difficult to place a rigid time factor for each examination performed. The experienced sonographer, in most cases, should be able to perform an average of 10 to 12 cases a day.

The approximate time (in minutes) required to complete each ultrasound study is as follows:

- Echocardiography, complete: 30 to 45
- Doppler: 40 to 60
- Abdominal: 20 to 40
- Renal: 15 to 30
- Gynecologic: 30 to 45
- Obstetric: 40 to 45
- Thyroid: 15 to 20

Of course, the number of patients a sonographer can examine depends on ancillary personnel to aid in the function of the ultrasound department. Escort service for the patient, secretarial assistance for the mounting, labeling, and sorting of scans, and telephone assistance for appointments and reports are necessary to increase the number of patients the sonographer is able to examine daily.

AVAILABILITY

The director of the ultrasound laboratory should determine whether 24-hour service is necessary for quality patient care. If it is deemed necessary, the sonographer and physician should provide adequate technical and interpretive skills.

CURRICULUM

The structure of the curriculum for individuals meeting the entrance requirements should be based on a minimum of a calendar year (12 months) of full-time study. This is to provide didactic content of appropriate scope and depth as well as clinical experiences of sufficient variety and quantity to ensure adequate opportunity to acquire the needed knowledge and skills.

The subject matter for a 1-year program would include introduction to basic physics, ultrasound applications of physics and biologic safety, laboratory experiments, instrumentation, biometrics, cross-sectional anatomy, pathology, physiology, cardiology, clinical medicine, differential diagnosis, comparison of other diagnostic modalities, ultrasonic techniques, interpretation, and journal review, research, and clinical experience.

CONTINUING EDUCATION

The sonographer should maintain an active interest in the field of ultrasound. A current library of ultrasound textbooks, videotapes, slide series, and journals should be maintained in the laboratory as a reference for updating current techniques and interpretations. The sonographer should be encouraged to attend local and regional ultrasound seminars. Attendance at the national ultrasound and echocardiography meetings is important for the sonographer to keep abreast of current developments in the field. Experts in ultrasound should be encouraged to visit particular laboratories if special techniques are newly employed.

Guidelines for Establishing an Educational Program

I became interested in educational programs while I was at the University of California–San Diego in the late 1960s. The early stages of sonography offered no formal education for physicians or sonographers, and as a result, numerous short-term courses, seminars, and lecture series were devised to stimulate the growth of ultrasound. I organized several 12-week seminars through the continuing education department at UCSD and discovered that there was an overwhelming quest for education in diagnostic ultrasound that was not yet met on a national basis.

My first real experience in hospital-based formal education was in Philadelphia with Barry Goldberg. We began with three students for a 6-month period and gradually built the program to 14 students for a 1-year period.

The contents of Appendix B reveals the experience I have had over the past 15 years in establishing a hospital-based program in sonography. To maintain a program that is viable year after year, one must meet and overcome several obstacles. Support must be gained from the hospital administrator, department chairman, medical director of the program, technical staff in the department, other departments within the hospital through which the students should rotate, clinical affiliates, and the students themselves.

We have found it very efficient to render all our lecture notes in either outline or text form so that transparencies and copies can be made for the students. We then use the overhead projector in the lecture room and the students are able to follow along with their own copy, making additional notes as the discussion proceeds.

Likewise, the lesson plan can utilize slides or other teaching aids. (In case the lecture has been given by another individual, the material will be ready and class will not have to be cancelled.)

STAGE I

When you have decided to start a program in diagnostic medical sonography, you should consider several things:
1. Do you have a *medical director* who is really interested in an educational program and willing to spend a great deal of time teaching the students? The medical director should have thoughts on education similar to yours (so the program will be effective), should be able to lecture to students and spend time in readout sessions, should provide a stimulus for various student projects, and should be supportive of the program in terms of the entire department's needs.
2. Do you have a *hospital administrator* who is enthusiastic toward starting a program?
3. Do you have a *department administrator* who is enthusiastic about the program? This is extremely important as regards the purchasing of new equipment and teaching aids (audiovisual, phantoms, etc.) or the funding of special projects that may be called for.
4. Is your *clinical staff* in sonography supportive of students? Does it understand exactly your feelings toward having students in the department? Are the members good instructors (can they teach clinical concepts to the students)?
5. What *subject areas* do you plan to cover in your program? Do you have communicative access to other departments (cardiology, ophthalmology, obstetrics, etc.) if necessary to provide adequate experience for the students?
6. Are there *other hospitals* nearby through which the students may rotate for different viewpoints and broader clinical experience?
7. What is your *source of students?* Is there a need for educated sonographers in your area? Are there other hospitals that already offer formal education in sonography?

STAGE II

Your next step is to become familiar with the teaching facilities that your hospital has to offer. Ideally a hospital connected with a larger university or a medical school will offer more teaching aids than will a small community hospital.
1. First, search the library for
   a. Research material

b. Audiovisual material and equipment
c. Individual teaching carrels
d. Journal accessibility
2. Then, locate possible lecturers:
a. Medical school
b. Medical physics
c. Specialty departments
d. Residents
e. Ph.D. candidates
3. Finally, contact other departments:
a. Cardiology
b. Pediatrics
c. Ophthalmology
d. Obstetrics
e. Oncology
f. Vascular surgery
g. Medical physics

You may receive a tremendous amount of support from departments other than your own. Most people involved with sonography are eager to educate others and are very enthusiastic about a program in the specialty.

STAGE III

Now you should have a fairly accurate impression as to the type of program you can offer and the kind of support you will receive from your own department as well as the rest of the hospital. The previous two stages may take some time to establish if you are new to the hospital. If you have been an employee for a few years, you should be familiar with all the politics and personalities within the hospital and thus be able to plan your program fairly easily.

A curriculum should be established. I use the *SDMS Educational Outline* as my starting point and build from that.

In our own program we include
- Physics
- Anatomy (gross and cross-sectional)
- Pathology
- Physiology
- Clinical medicine (differential diagnosis, comparison with other modalities)
- Cardiology
- Abdomen, retroperitoneal
- Obstetrics and gynecology
- Superficial structures
- Doppler
- Breast
- Ultrasonic techniques
- Ultrasound interpretation
- Teaching file, museum cases
- Journal club
- Research papers
- Clinical experience

When you have decided which subjects to offer, you may decide what teaching aids you have and what you should purchase for the program.
- Videotapes
- Slide sets

- Library books
Other teaching aids we have found to be very effective are
- Local ultrasound meetings
- Visiting physicians/sonographers
- Outside seminars
- Affiliate hospitals
- Field trips (other hospitals, commercial companies)
- Commercial teaching aids (lecturers, videotapes)

You will have to decide how many students you can handle with your present equipment, staff, and classroom facilities. We generally plan on one student per piece of equipment (contact scan/real-time or M-mode/real-time). If you have a large classroom, you may find it beneficial to open your lectures to more students. For example, we offer our affiliate hospitals the opportunity to send their personnel for the lecture series at no charge in return for letting our students rotate through their department. This has proved very effective—it promotes good will and good education in the ultrasound community, which in turn benefits the patient. We also allow students to audit the courses for a reduced tuition if they are able to receive their clinical experience at some other institution.

STAGE IV

Publicity about the program:
- Brochure
- Advertisements—*SDMS Newsletter, Journal of Clinical Ultrasound*
- Word of mouth spreads very quickly

STAGE V

In the selection of students we try to make a decision at least 6 months before the starting date; this lets students prepare for the 1-year program without salary. We require a nonrefundable tuition of $100 (which is applied to the tuition) upon acceptance into the program.

It is difficult to make a general statement about the type of student selected. I have found that some radiology students do very well if they have been in a program that stressed anatomy, pathology, and differential diagnosis in their training. I have also found students with a 4-year degree doing extremely well in sonography regardless of their major course of study. Individuals with a particular interest in photography seem to succeed in sonography.

Our selection of students is based upon several items: grade point average, previous medical background, interest in and level of knowledge of the field of ultrasound, letters of recommendation, previous work experience, personal reasons for entering the ultrasound field. It is important to choose a student who has a high scholastic average, for the workload in a comprehensive program is very extensive.

ESTABLISHING A DIAGNOSTIC ULTRASOUND EDUCATIONAL PROGRAM

Since the 1970s, interest in ultrasound has risen geometrically, causing an acute shortage of educated sonographers and physicians. This demand has been the impetus

tinely be assigned to certain students. Each student should be required to copy the pertinent ultrasound articles for reference and discussion in the weekly or bimonthly journal club review. This exposes students to current literature in a uniform manner and encourages them to read and selectively interpret the available information.

Research assignments are an important part of the students' training. The first project should be a review of the literature and/or cases on a particular subject of the student's choice. This paper will be critiqued by and discussed among the other students. The second project should consist of research in which the student actually evaluates one particular aspect of ultrasound. Thus scanning techniques, artifacts, patient data and evaluation, and a review of the pertinent literature are included in this paper.

RESEARCH PAPER FORMAT

Each student will be responsible for completing two research papers during the 1-year program.

The first should be more of a review-type paper that concentrates on a particular subject of the student's choice—e.g., "The Renal Transplant," "Common Artifacts Encountered in Sonography," "Gallbladder Disease," "Vascular Aneurysms."

The second paper should be a research-oriented approach concentrating again on a particular subject with accumulated data compiled by the student to include sonograms, clinical history, and surgical and laboratory results—e.g., "The Sonographic Appearance of Renal Transplant Rejection," "The Echogenicity of the Normal Pancreas," "Patterns of Liver Disease."

For both papers the following format should be utilized:

1. Title page
2. Table of contents
3. Abstract
4. Contents
   a. Introduction
   b. Anatomy
   c. Physiology
   d. Laboratory data
   e. Pathology
   f. Ultrasound patterns and differential diagnoses
   g. Summary
5. Annotated bibliography (should include 10 to 15 current articles [after 1975] and 4 or 5 textbooks)

Some laboratories may find field trips to other laboratories useful. This exposes the students to new or different techniques available to the ultrasonographer. Trips to manufacturers of equipment or transducers may promote understanding and appreciation of ultrasound devices.

Of course, interdepartmental exposure to other diagnostic modalities should be incorporated if the students' acquaintance with these modalities is limited. Thus exposure to cardiac catheterization, phonocardiography, treadmill electrocardiography, cardiac clinic, radiology, and nuclear medicine will add to their understanding of the echographic procedure.

Echocardiographic Measurements and Normal Values (Adult)

Table C-1   Adult normal values

	cm
Body surface area	1.45 to 2.22
Right ventricular dimension (flat)	0.7 to 2.3
Right ventricular dimension (left lateral)	0.9 to 2.6
Left ventricular internal dimension (flat)	3.7 to 5.6
Left ventricular internal dimension (left lateral)	3.5 to 5.7
Posterior left ventricular wall thickness	0.6 to 1.1
Posterior left ventricular wall amplitude	0.9 to 1.4
Interventricular septal thickness	0.6 to 1.1
Interventricular septal amplitude	0.3 to 0.8
Left atrial dimension	1.9 to 4.0
Aortic root dimension	2.0 to 3.7
Aortic cusp separation	1.5 to 2.6
Mean rate of circumferential shortening (Vcf)	1.02 to 1.94 circ./s

From Feigenbaum H: Echocardiography, ed 3, Philadelphia, 1981, Lea & Febiger.

Table C-2   Adult normal values corrected for body surface area

	cm/m^2
Right ventricular dimension/ m^2 (flat)	0.4 to 1.4
Right ventricular dimension/ m^2 (left lateral)	0.4 to 1.4
Left ventricular internal dimension/m^2 (flat)	2.1 to 3.2
Left ventricular internal dimension/m^2 (left lateral)	1.9 to 3.2
Left atrial dimension/m^2	1.2 to 2.2
Aortic root/m^2	1.2 to 2.2

From Feigenbaum H: Echocardiography, ed 3, Philadelphia, 1981, Lea & Febiger.

Appendix D

Congenital Heart Disease: Cardiac Structure Growth Patterns

(Chapter 35)

Roge et al.[2] used M-mode echocardiography to measure the dimensions of the ventricular walls and cavities, great vessels, and left atrium and atrioventricular valve excursions on 93 children and infants without heart disease. The data was analyzed by relating each dimension in millimeters to body surface area (BSA) in square meters, and the 90% tolerance limits for the data was calculated (Fig. D-1).

The right ventricular anterior wall thickness (RVAWD), left ventricular posterior wall thickness (LVPWD), right and left ventricular cavity diastolic dimensions (RVDD and LVEDD), interventricular septal thickness (SEPT D), and mitral valve excursion (MVDE) were measured at the level of the posterior mitral leaflet at end diastole, defined by the peak of the R wave on the ECG. Left ventricular end systolic dimension was measured at the peak upward motion of the posterior left ventricular endocardium. The right ventricular anterior wall thickness was obtained by proper selection of transducer and careful anterior gain control. The right ventricular-septal and left ventricular-septal interfaces were defined by proper damping and reject control. The anterior mitral leaflet excursion was measured from the D point vertically to the E point at maximal excursion. The left atrium and aorta were measured on a continuous sweep from the left ventricle. Left atrial systolic dimension (LAS) was measured at the largest distance between the anterior aspect of the left atrial posterior wall and the inner aortic posterior wall. Aortic end diastolic diameter (AOD) was measured at the beginning of the QRS complex and end systolic diameter (AOS) at the same point used for measuring the left atrium. The aorta was measured from the anterior surface of the anterior root echo to the anterior surface of the posterior root echo.

The pulmonary artery diameter (PAD) was measured at the onset of the QRS complex, whenever possible, or when the anterior echo moved parallel to the posterior pulmonary root at any point in the cardiac cycle. The maximum excursion of the anterior leaflet of the tricuspid valve (TVDE) was measured the same way as for the mitral valve.

The suprasternal view provides visualization of the aortic arch and right pulmonary artery. These normal values are presented in Fig. D-2.

REFERENCES

1. Epstein ML, Goldberg SJ, Allen HD, et al: Great vessel, cardiac chamber and wall growth patterns in normal children, Circulation 51:1124, 1975.
2. Roge CLI, Silverman H, Hart PA, and Ray M: Cardiac structure growth pattern determined by echocardiography, Circulation 57:285, 1978.

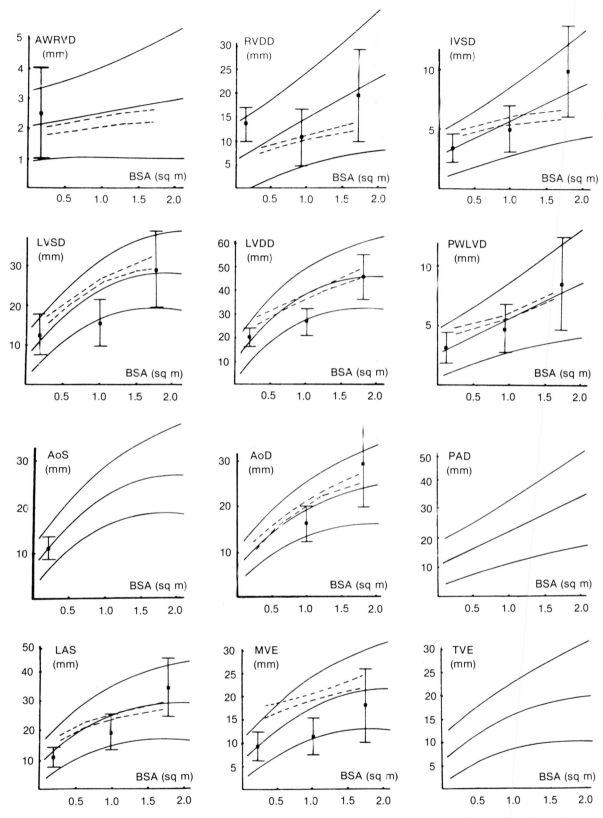

FIG. D-1. The normal range for neonates (mean and two standard deviations) are plotted at 0.2 m², and the normal adult data and the corrected values per square meter BSA are shown at 1.73 and 1 m², respectively. The inner growth curves *(broken lines)* are the 5th and 95th percentile limits of the data from Epstein et al.[1] The outer heavy lines are the 90% tolerance lines from Roge's data.[2]

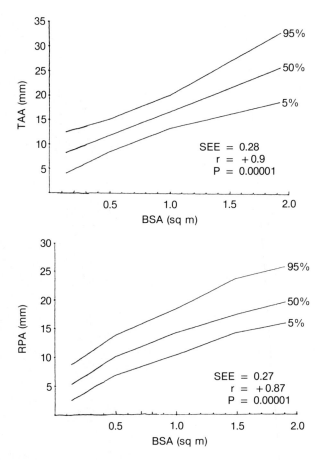

FIG. D-2.   Normal values for transverse aortic arch and right pulmonary artery.

Appendix E

Estimated Fetal Weights

Biparietal diameters	Abdominal circumferences											
	15.5	16.0	16.5	17.0	17.5	18.0	18.5	19.0	19.5	20.0	20.5	21.0
3.1	224	234	244	255	267	279	291	304	318	332	346	362
3.2	231	241	251	263	274	286	299	312	326	340	355	371
3.3	237	248	259	270	282	294	307	321	335	349	365	381
3.4	244	255	266	278	290	302	316	329	344	359	374	391
3.5	251	262	274	285	298	311	324	338	353	368	384	401
3.6	259	270	281	294	306	319	333	347	362	378	394	411
3.7	266	278	290	302	315	328	342	357	372	388	404	422
3.8	274	286	298	310	324	337	352	366	382	398	415	432
3.9	282	294	306	319	333	347	361	376	392	409	426	444
4.0	290	303	315	328	342	356	371	386	403	419	437	455
4.1	299	311	324	338	352	366	381	397	413	430	448	467
4.2	308	320	333	347	361	376	392	408	424	442	460	479
4.3	317	330	343	357	371	387	402	419	436	453	472	491
4.4	326	339	353	367	382	397	413	430	447	465	484	504
4.5	335	349	363	377	393	408	425	442	459	478	497	517
4.6	345	359	373	388	404	420	436	454	472	490	510	530
4.7	355	369	384	399	415	431	448	466	484	503	523	544
4.8	366	380	395	410	426	443	460	478	497	517	537	558
4.9	376	391	406	422	438	455	473	491	510	530	551	572
5.0	387	402	418	434	451	468	486	505	524	544	565	587
5.1	399	414	430	446	463	481	499	518	538	559	580	602
5.2	410	426	442	459	476	494	513	532	552	573	595	618
5.3	422	438	455	472	489	508	527	547	567	589	611	634
5.4	435	451	468	485	503	522	541	561	582	604	627	650
5.5	447	464	481	499	517	536	556	577	598	620	643	667
5.6	461	477	495	513	532	551	571	592	614	636	660	684
5.7	474	491	509	527	547	566	587	608	630	653	677	701
5.8	488	505	524	542	562	582	603	625	647	670	695	719
5.9	502	520	539	558	578	598	619	642	664	688	713	738
6.0	517	535	554	573	594	615	636	659	682	706	731	757
6.1	532	550	570	590	610	632	654	677	700	725	750	777
6.2	547	566	586	606	627	649	672	695	719	744	770	797
6.3	563	583	603	624	645	667	690	714	738	764	790	817
6.4	580	600	620	641	663	686	709	733	758	784	811	838
6.5	597	617	638	659	682	705	728	753	778	805	832	860
6.6	614	635	656	678	701	724	748	773	799	826	853	882
6.7	632	653	675	697	720	744	769	794	820	848	876	905
6.8	651	672	694	717	740	765	790	816	842	870	898	928
6.9	670	691	714	737	761	786	811	838	865	893	922	952
7.0	689	711	734	758	782	807	833	860	888	916	946	976
7.1	709	732	755	779	804	830	856	883	912	941	971	1,002
7.2	730	763	777	801	827	853	880	907	936	965	996	1,027
7.3	751	775	799	824	850	876	904	932	961	991	1,022	1,054
7.4	773	797	822	847	874	901	928	957	987	1,017	1,049	1,081
7.5	796	820	845	871	898	925	954	983	1,013	1,044	1,076	1,109
7.6	819	844	870	896	923	951	980	1,009	1,040	1,072	1,104	1,137
7.7	843	868	894	921	949	977	1,007	1,037	1,068	1,100	1,133	1,167
7.8	868	894	920	947	975	1,004	1,034	1,065	1,096	1,129	1,162	1,197
7.9	893	919	946	974	1,003	1,032	1,062	1,094	1,126	1,159	1,193	1,228
8.0	919	946	973	1,002	1,031	1,061	1,091	1,123	1,156	1,189	1,224	1,259
8.1	946	973	1,001	1,030	1,060	1,090	1,121	1,153	1,187	1,221	1,256	1,292
8.2	974	1,001	1,030	1,059	1,089	1,120	1,152	1,185	1,218	1,253	1,288	1,325
8.3	1,002	1,030	1,059	1,089	1,120	1,151	1,183	1,217	1,251	1,286	1,322	1,359
8.4	1,032	1,060	1,090	1,120	1,151	1,183	1,216	1,249	1,284	1,320	1,356	1,394
8.5	1,062	1,091	1,121	1,151	1,183	1,216	1,249	1,283	1,318	1,355	1,392	1,430
8.6	1,093	1,122	1,153	1,184	1,216	1,249	1,283	1,318	1,354	1,390	1,428	1,467
8.7	1,125	1,155	1,186	1,218	1,250	1,284	1,318	1,353	1,390	1,427	1,465	1,505
8.8	1,157	1,188	1,220	1,252	1,285	1,319	1,354	1,390	1,427	1,465	1,504	1,543
8.9	1,191	1,222	1,254	1,287	1,321	1,356	1,391	1,428	1,465	1,503	1,543	1,583
9.0	1,226	1,258	1,290	1,324	1,358	1,393	1,429	1,456	1,504	1,543	1,583	1,624
9.1	1,262	1,294	1,327	1,361	1,396	1,432	1,468	1,506	1,544	1,584	1,624	1,666
9.2	1,299	1,332	1,365	1,400	1,435	1,471	1,508	1,546	1,586	1,626	1,667	1,709
9.3	1,337	1,370	1,404	1,439	1,475	1,512	1,550	1,588	1,628	1,668	1,710	1,753
9.4	1,376	1,410	1,444	1,480	1,516	1,554	1,592	1,631	1,671	1,712	1,755	1,798
9.5	1,416	1,450	1,486	1,522	1,559	1,597	1,635	1,675	1,716	1,758	1,800	1,844
9.6	1,457	1,492	1,528	1,565	1,602	1,641	1,680	1,720	1,762	1,804	1,847	1,892
9.7	1,500	1,535	1,572	1,609	1,547	1,686	1,726	1,767	1,809	1,852	1,895	1,940
9.8	1,544	1,580	1,617	1,654	1,693	1,733	1,773	1,815	1,857	1,900	1,945	1,990
9.9	1,589	1,625	1,663	1,701	1,740	1,781	1,822	1,864	1,907	1,951	1,996	2,042
10.0	1.635	1,672	1,710	1,749	1,789	1,830	1,871	1,914	1,958	2,002	2,048	2,094

Log (birth weight) = −1.7942 + 0.166 (BPD) + 0.032 (AC) − 2.646 (BPD) × AC/1000.

SD = 106.0 g/kg of body weight.

From Shepard *et al:* Am. J. Obstet. Gynecol. 142:47, 1982.

Abdominal circumferences												
21.5	22.0	22.5	23.0	23.5	24.0	24.5	25.0	25.5	26.0	26.5	27.0	27.5
378	395	412	431	450	470	491	513	536	559	584	610	638
388	405	423	441	461	481	502	525	548	572	597	624	651
397	415	433	452	472	493	514	537	560	585	611	638	666
408	425	444	463	483	504	526	549	573	598	624	652	680
418	436	455	475	495	517	539	562	587	612	638	666	695
429	447	466	486	507	529	552	575	600	626	653	681	710
440	458	478	498	519	542	565	589	614	640	667	696	725
451	470	490	510	532	554	578	602	628	654	682	711	741
462	482	502	523	545	568	592	616	642	669	697	727	757
474	494	514	536	558	581	606	631	657	684	713	743	773
486	506	527	549	572	595	620	645	672	700	729	759	790
498	519	540	562	585	609	634	660	688	716	745	776	807
511	532	554	576	600	624	649	676	703	732	762	793	825
524	545	567	590	614	639	665	692	719	749	779	810	843
538	559	581	605	629	654	680	708	736	765	796	828	861
551	573	596	620	644	670	696	724	753	783	814	846	880
565	588	611	635	660	686	713	741	770	801	832	865	899
580	602	626	650	676	702	730	758	788	819	851	884	919
594	617	641	666	692	719	747	776	806	837	870	903	938
610	633	657	683	709	736	765	794	824	856	889	923	959
625	649	674	699	726	754	783	812	843	876	909	944	980
641	665	690	717	744	772	801	831	863	895	929	964	1,001
657	682	708	734	762	790	820	851	883	916	950	986	1,023
674	699	725	752	780	809	839	870	903	936	971	1,007	1,045
691	717	743	771	799	828	859	891	924	958	993	1,030	1,068
709	735	762	789	818	848	879	911	945	979	1,015	1,052	1,091
727	753	780	809	838	869	900	933	966	1,001	1,038	1,075	1,114
745	772	800	829	858	889	921	954	989	1,024	1,061	1,099	1,139
764	792	820	849	879	911	943	977	1,011	1,047	1,085	1,123	1,163
784	811	840	870	900	932	965	999	1,035	1,071	1,109	1,148	1,189
804	832	861	891	922	955	988	1,023	1,058	1,095	1,134	1,173	1,214
824	853	882	913	945	977	1,011	1,046	1,083	1,120	1,159	1,199	1,241
845	874	904	935	967	1,001	1,035	1,071	1,107	1,145	1,185	1,226	1,268
867	896	927	958	991	1,025	1,059	1,096	1,133	1,171	1,211	1,253	1,295
889	919	950	982	1,015	1,049	1,084	1,121	1,159	1,198	1,238	1,280	1,323
911	942	973	1,006	1,039	1,074	1,110	1,147	1,185	1,225	1,266	1,308	1,352
935	965	997	1,030	1,065	1,100	1,136	1,174	1,213	1,253	1,294	1,337	1,381
958	990	1,022	1,056	1,090	1,126	1,163	1,201	1,241	1,281	1,323	1,367	1,411
983	1,015	1,048	1,082	1,117	1,153	1,190	1,229	1,269	1,310	1,353	1,397	1,442
1,008	1,040	1,074	1,108	1,144	1,181	1,219	1,258	1,298	1,340	1,383	1,427	1,473
1,033	1,066	1,100	1,135	1,171	1,209	1,247	1,287	1,328	1,370	1,414	1,459	1,505
1,060	1,093	1,128	1,163	1,200	1,238	1,277	1,317	1,358	1,401	1,445	1,491	1,538
1,087	1,121	1,156	1,192	1,229	1,267	1,307	1,348	1,390	1,433	1,478	1,524	1,571
1,114	1,149	1,184	1,221	1,259	1,297	1,338	1,379	1,421	1,465	1,511	1,557	1,605
1,143	1,178	1,214	1,251	1,289	1,328	1,369	1,411	1,454	1,499	1,544	1,592	1,640
1,172	1,207	1,244	1,281	1,320	1,360	1,401	1,444	1,487	1,533	1,579	1,627	1,676
1,202	1,238	1,275	1,313	1,352	1,393	1,434	1,477	1,522	1,567	1,614	1,663	1,712
1,232	1,269	1,306	1,345	1,385	1,426	1,468	1,512	1,557	1,603	1,650	1,699	1,749
1,264	1,301	1,339	1,378	1,418	1,460	1,503	1,547	1,592	1,639	1,687	1,737	1,787
1,296	1,333	1,372	1,412	1,453	1,495	1,538	1,583	1,629	1,676	1,725	1,775	1,826
1,329	1,367	1,406	1,446	1,488	1,531	1,575	1,620	1,666	1,714	1,763	1,814	1,866
1,363	1,401	1,441	1,482	1,524	1,567	1,612	1,657	1,704	1,753	1,803	1,854	1,906
1,397	1,436	1,477	1,518	1,561	1,605	1,650	1,696	1,744	1,793	1,843	1,895	1,948
1,433	1,473	1,513	1,555	1,599	1,643	1,689	1,735	1,784	1,833	1,884	1,936	1,990
1,469	1,510	1,551	1,594	1,637	1,682	1,728	1,776	1,825	1,875	1,926	1,979	2,033
1,507	1,548	1,589	1,633	1,677	1,722	1,769	1,817	1,866	1,917	1,969	2,022	2,077
1,545	1,586	1,629	1,673	1,717	1,764	1,811	1,859	1,909	1,960	2,013	2,067	2,122
1,584	1,626	1,669	1,714	1,759	1,806	1,854	1,903	1,953	2,005	2,058	2,113	2,169
1,625	1,667	1,711	1,756	1,802	1,849	1,897	1,947	1,998	2,050	2,104	2,159	2,216
1,666	1,709	1,753	1,799	1,845	1,893	1,942	1,992	2,044	2,097	2,151	2,207	2,264
1,708	1,752	1,797	1,843	1,890	1,938	1,988	2,039	2,091	2,144	2,199	2,255	2,313
1,752	1,796	1,841	1,888	1,936	1,984	2,035	2,086	2,139	2,193	2,248	2,305	2,363
1,796	1,841	1,887	1,934	1,982	2,032	2,083	2,135	2,188	2,242	2,298	2,356	2,414
1,842	1,887	1,934	1,982	2,030	2,080	2,132	2,184	2,238	2,293	2,350	2,407	2,467
1,889	1,935	1,982	2,030	2,080	2,130	2,182	2,235	2,289	2,345	2,402	2,460	2,520
1,937	1,984	2,031	2,080	2,130	2,181	2,233	2,287	2,342	2,398	2,456	2,515	2,575
1,986	2,033	2,082	2,131	2,181	2,233	2,286	2,340	2,396	2,452	2,510	2,570	2,631
2,037	2,085	2,133	2,183	2,234	2,286	2,340	2,395	2,451	2,508	2,567	2,627	2,688
2,089	2,137	2,186	2,237	2,288	2,341	2,395	2,450	2,507	2,565	2,624	2,684	2,746
2,142	2,191	2,241	2,292	2,344	2,397	2,452	2,507	2,564	2,623	2,682	2,743	2,806

Continued.

Biparietal diameters	Abdominal circumferences											
	28.0	28.5	29.0	29.5	30.0	30.5	31.0	31.5	32.0	32.5	33.0	33.5
3.1	666	696	726	759	793	828	865	903	943	985	1,029	1,075
3.2	680	710	742	774	809	844	882	921	961	1,004	1,048	1,094
3.3	695	725	757	790	825	861	899	938	979	1,022	1,067	1,114
3.4	710	740	773	806	841	878	916	956	998	1,041	1,087	1,134
3.5	725	756	789	823	858	896	934	975	1,017	1,061	1,107	1,154
3.6	740	772	805	840	876	913	953	993	1,036	1,080	1,127	1,175
3.7	756	788	822	857	893	931	971	1,012	1,056	1,101	1,147	1,196
3.8	772	805	839	874	911	950	990	1,032	1,076	1,121	1,168	1,218
3.9	789	822	856	892	930	969	1,009	1,052	1,096	1,142	1,190	1,240
4.0	806	839	874	911	949	988	1,029	1,072	1.117	1,163	1.212	1.262
4.1	828	857	892	929	968	1,008	1,049	1,093	1,138	1,185	1,234	1,285
4.2	841	875	911	948	987	1,028	1,070	1,114	1,159	1,207	1,256	1,308
4.3	859	893	930	968	1,007	1,048	1,091	1,135	1,181	1,229	1,279	1,331
4.4	877	912	949	987	1,027	1,069	1,112	1,157	1,204	1,252	1,303	1,355
4.5	896	932	969	1,008	1,048	1,090	1,134	1,179	1,226	1,275	1,326	1,380
4.6	915	951	989	1,028	1,069	1,112	1,156	1,202	1,249	1,299	1,351	1,404
4.7	934	971	1,010	1,049	1,091	1,134	1,178	1,225	1,273	1,323	1,375	1,430
4.8	954	992	1,031	1,071	1,113	1,156	1,201	1,248	1,297	1,348	1,401	1,455
4.9	975	1,013	1,052	1,093	1,135	1,179	1,225	1,272	1,322	1,373	1,426	1,482
5.0	996	1,034	1,074	1,115	1,158	1,203	1,249	1,297	1,347	1,399	1,452	1,508
5.1	1,017	1,056	1,096	1,138	1,181	1,226	1,273	1,322	1,372	1,425	1,479	1,535
5.2	1,039	1,078	1,119	1,161	1,205	1,251	1,298	1,347	1,398	1,451	1,506	1,563
5.3	1,061	1,101	1,142	1,185	1,229	1,276	1,323	1,373	1,425	1,478	1,533	1,591
5.4	1,084	1,124	1,166	1,209	1,254	1,301	1,349	1,399	1,452	1,506	1,562	1,620
5.5	1,107	1,148	1,190	1,234	1,279	1,327	1,376	1,426	1,479	1,534	1,590	1,649
5.6	1,131	1,172	1,215	1,259	1,305	1,353	1,402	1,454	1,507	1,562	1,619	1,678
5.7	1,155	1,197	1,240	1,285	1,332	1,380	1,430	1,482	1,535	1,591	1,649	1,709
5.8	1,180	1,222	1,266	1,311	1,358	1,407	1,458	1,510	1,564	1,621	1,679	1,739
5.9	1,205	1,248	1,292	1,338	1,386	1,435	1,486	1,539	1,594	1,651	1,710	1,770
6.0	1,231	1,274	1,319	1,366	1,414	1,464	1,515	1,569	1,624	1,682	1,741	1,802
6.1	1,257	1,301	1,346	1,393	1,442	1,493	1,545	1,599	1,655	1,713	1,773	1,835
6.2	1,284	1,328	1,374	1,422	1,471	1,522	1,575	1,630	1,686	1,745	1,805	1,868
6.3	1,311	1,356	1,403	1,451	1,501	1,552	1,606	1,661	1,718	1,777	1,838	1,901
6.4	1,339	1,385	1,432	1,481	1,531	1,583	1,637	1,693	1,751	1,810	1,872	1,935
6.5	1,368	1,414	1,462	1,511	1,562	1,615	1,669	1,725	1,784	1,844	1,906	1,970
6.6	1,397	1,444	1,492	1,542	1,594	1,647	1,702	1,759	1,817	1,878	1,941	2,006
6.7	1,427	1,474	1,523	1,574	1,626	1,679	1,735	1,792	1,852	1,913	1,976	2,042
6.8	1,458	1,505	1,555	1,606	1,658	1,713	1,769	1,827	1,887	1,949	2,012	2,078
6.9	1,489	1,537	1,587	1,639	1,692	1,747	1,803	1,862	1,922	1,985	2,049	2,116
7.0	1,521	1,570	1,620	1,672	1,726	1,781	1,839	1,898	1,959	2,022	2,087	2,154
7.1	1,553	1,603	1,654	1,706	1,761	1,817	1,875	1,934	1,996	2,059	2,125	2,193
7.2	1,586	1,636	1,688	1,741	1,796	1,853	1,911	1,971	2,044	2,098	2,164	2,232
7.3	1,620	1,671	1,723	1,777	1,832	1,890	1,948	2,009	2,072	2,137	2,203	2,272
7.4	1,655	1,706	1,759	1,813	1,869	1,927	1,987	2,048	2,111	2,176	2,244	2,313
7.5	1,690	1,742	1,795	1,850	1,907	1,965	2,025	2,087	2,151	2,217	2,265	2,354
7.6	1,727	1,779	1,833	1,888	1,945	2,004	2,065	2,127	2,192	2,258	2,326	2,397
7.7	1,764	1,816	1,871	1,927	1,985	2,044	2,105	2,168	2,233	2,300	2,369	2,440
7.8	1,801	1,855	1,910	1,966	2,025	2,085	2,146	2,210	2,275	2,343	2,412	2,484
7.9	1,840	1,894	1,949	2,006	2,065	2,126	2,188	2,252	2,318	2,386	2,456	2,528
8.0	1,879	1,934	1,990	2,048	2,107	2,168	2,231	2,296	2,362	2,431	2,501	2,574
8.1	1,919	1,975	2,031	2,089	2,149	2,211	2,275	2,340	2,407	2,476	2,547	2,620
8.2	1,960	2,016	2,073	2,132	2,193	2,255	2,319	2,385	2,462	2,522	2,594	2,667
8.3	2,002	2,059	2,116	2,176	2,237	2,300	2,364	2,431	2,499	2,569	2,641	2,715
8.4	2,045	2,102	2,160	2,220	2,282	2,345	2,410	2,477	2,546	2,617	2,689	2,764
8.5	2,089	2,146	2,205	2,266	2,328	2,392	2,457	2,525	2,594	2,665	2,739	2,814
8.6	2,134	2,192	2,251	2,312	2,375	2,439	2,505	2,573	2,643	2,715	2,789	2,864
8.7	2,179	2,238	2,298	2,359	2,423	2,488	2,554	2,623	2,693	2,765	2,840	2,916
8.8	2,226	2,285	2,346	2,408	2,472	2,537	2,604	2,673	2,744	2,817	2,892	2,968
8.9	2,274	2,333	2,394	2,457	2,521	2,587	2,655	2,725	2,796	2,869	2,944	3,021
9.0	2,322	2,382	2,444	2,507	2,572	2,639	2,707	2,777	2,849	2,923	2,998	3,076
9.1	2,372	2,433	2,495	2,559	2,624	2,691	2,760	2,830	2,903	2,977	3,053	3,131
9.2	2,423	2,484	2,547	2,611	2,677	2,744	2,814	2,885	2,958	3,032	3,109	3,187
9.3	2,475	2,536	2,599	2,664	2,731	2,799	2,869	2,940	3,014	3,089	3,166	3,245
9.4	2,527	2,590	2,653	2,719	2,786	2,854	2,925	2,997	3,070	3,146	3,224	3,303
9.5	2,582	2,644	2,709	2,774	2,842	2,911	2,982	3,054	3,129	3,205	3,283	3,362
9.6	2,637	2,700	2,765	2,831	2,899	2,969	3,040	3,113	3,188	3,264	3,343	3,423
9.7	2,693	2,757	2,822	2,889	2,958	3,028	3,099	3,173	3,248	3,325	3,404	3,484
9.8	2,751	2,815	2,881	2,948	3,017	3,088	3,160	3,234	3,309	3,387	3,466	3,547
9.9	2,810	2,874	2,941	3,009	3,078	3,149	3,222	3,296	3,372	3,450	3,529	3,611
10.0	2,870	2,935	3,002	3,070	3,140	3,211	3,285	3,359	3,436	3,514	3,594	3,676

Abdominal circumferences												
34.0	34.5	35.0	35.5	36.0	36.5	37.0	37.5	38.0	38.5	39.0	39.5	40.0
1,123	1,173	1,225	1,279	1,336	1,396	1,458	1,523	1,591	1,661	1,735	1,812	1,893
1,143	1,193	1,246	1,301	1,358	1,418	1,481	1,546	1,615	1,686	1,761	1,838	1,920
1,163	1,214	1,267	1,323	1,381	1,441	1,504	1,570	1,639	1,711	1,786	1,865	1,946
1,183	1,235	1,289	1,345	1,403	1,464	1,528	1,595	1,664	1,737	1,812	1,891	1,973
1,204	1,256	1,311	1,367	1,426	1,488	1,552	1,619	1,689	1,762	1,839	1,918	2,001
1,226	1,278	1,333	1,390	1,450	1,512	1,577	1,645	1,715	1,789	1,865	1,945	2,029
1,247	1,300	1,356	1,413	1,474	1,536	1,602	1,670	1,741	1,815	1,893	1,973	2,057
1,269	1,323	1,379	1,437	1,498	1,561	1,627	1,696	1,768	1,842	1,920	2,001	2,086
1,292	1,346	1,402	1,461	1,523	1,586	1,653	1,722	1,794	1,870	1,948	2,030	2,115
1,315	1,369	1,426	1,486	1,548	1,612	1,679	1,749	1,822	1,898	1,977	2,059	2,145
1,338	1,393	1,451	1,511	1,573	1,638	1,706	1,776	1,849	1,926	2,005	2,088	2,174
1,361	1,417	1,475	1,536	1,599	1,664	1,733	1,804	1,878	1,954	2,035	2,118	2,205
1,385	1,442	1,500	1,562	1,625	1,691	1,760	1,832	1,906	1,984	2,064	2,148	2,236
1,410	1,467	1,526	1,588	1,652	1,718	1,788	1,860	1,935	2,013	2,094	2,179	2,267
1,435	1,492	1,552	1,614	1,679	1,746	1,816	1,889	1,964	2,043	2,125	2,210	2,298
1,460	1,518	1,579	1,641	1,706	1,774	1,845	1,918	1,994	2,073	2,156	2,241	2,330
1,486	1,545	1,605	1,669	1,734	1,803	1,874	1,948	2,024	2,104	2,187	2,273	2,363
1,512	1,571	1,633	1,697	1,763	1,832	1,904	1,978	2,055	2,136	2,219	2,306	2,396
1,539	1,599	1,661	1,725	1,792	1,861	1,934	2,009	2,086	2,167	2,251	2,339	2,429
1,566	1,626	1,689	1,754	1,821	1,891	1,964	2,040	2,118	2,200	2,284	2,372	2,463
1,594	1,655	1,718	1,783	1,851	1,922	1,995	2,071	2,150	2,232	2,317	2,406	2,498
1,622	1,683	1,747	1,813	1,882	1,953	2,027	2,103	2,183	2,266	2,351	2,440	2,532
1,651	1,713	1,777	1,843	1,913	1,984	2,059	2,136	2,216	2,299	2,386	2,475	2,568
1,680	1,742	1,807	1,874	1,944	2,016	2,091	2,169	2,250	2,333	2,420	2,510	2,604
1,710	1,773	1,838	1,906	1,976	2,049	2,124	2,203	2,284	2,368	2,456	2,546	2,640
1,740	1,803	1,869	1,938	2,008	2,082	2,158	2,237	2,319	2,403	2,491	2,582	2,677
1,770	1,835	1,901	1,970	2,041	2,115	2,192	2,272	2,354	2,439	2,528	2,619	2,714
1,802	1,866	1,934	2,003	2,075	2,150	2,227	2,307	2,390	2,475	2,564	2,657	2,752
1,834	1,899	1,966	2,037	2,109	2,184	2,262	2,342	2,426	2,512	2,602	2,694	2,790
1,866	1,932	2,000	2,071	2,144	2,219	2,298	2,379	2,463	2,550	2,640	2,733	2,829
1,899	1,965	2,034	2,105	2,179	2,255	2,334	2,416	2,500	2,588	2,678	2,772	2,869
1,932	1,999	2,069	2,140	2,215	2,291	2,371	2,453	2,538	2,626	2,717	2,811	2,909
1,967	2,034	2,104	2,176	2,251	2,328	2,408	2,491	2,577	2,665	2,757	2,851	2,949
2,001	2,069	2,140	2,213	2,288	2,366	2,446	2,530	2,616	2,705	2,797	2,892	2,991
2,037	2,105	2,176	2,250	2,326	2,404	2,485	2,569	2,656	2,745	2,838	2,933	3,032
2,073	2,142	2,213	2,287	2,364	2,443	2,524	2,609	2,696	2,786	2,879	2,975	3,075
2,109	2,179	2,251	2,326	2,403	2,482	2,564	2,649	2,737	2,827	2,921	3,018	3,117
2,147	2,217	2,290	2,365	2,442	2,522	2,605	2,690	2,778	2,869	2,964	3,061	3,161
2,184	2,255	2,329	2,404	2,482	2,563	2,646	2,732	2,821	2,912	3,007	3,104	3,205
2,223	2,295	2,368	2,444	2,523	2,604	2,688	2,774	2,863	2,955	3,050	3,149	3,250
2,262	2,334	2,409	2,485	2,564	2,646	2,730	2,817	2,907	2,999	3,095	3,193	3,295
2,302	2,375	2,450	2,527	2,607	2,689	2,773	2,861	2,951	3,044	3,140	3,239	3,341
2,343	2,416	2,491	2,569	2,649	2,732	2,817	2,905	2,996	3,089	3,186	3,285	3,388
2,384	2,458	2,534	2,612	2,693	2,776	2,862	2,950	3,041	3,135	3,232	3,332	3,435
2,426	2,501	2,577	2,656	2,737	2,821	2,907	2,996	3,088	3,182	3,279	3,380	3,483
2,469	2,544	2,621	2,700	2,782	2,866	2,953	3,042	3,134	3,229	3,327	3,428	3,531
2,513	2,588	2,666	2,746	2,828	2,912	3,000	3,090	3,182	3,277	3,376	3,477	3,581
2,557	2,633	2,711	2,792	2,874	2,959	3,047	3,137	3,230	3,326	3,425	3,526	3,631
2,603	2,679	2,757	2,838	2,921	3,007	3,095	3,186	3,279	3,376	3,475	3,576	3,681
2,649	2,725	2,804	2,886	2,969	3,056	3,144	3,235	3,329	3,426	3,525	3,627	3,733
2,695	2,773	2,852	2,934	3,018	3,105	3,194	3,286	3,380	3,477	3,577	3,679	3,785
2,743	2,821	2,901	2,983	3,068	3,155	3,244	3,336	3,431	3,529	3,629	3,732	3,838
2,791	2,870	2,950	3,033	3,118	3,206	3,296	3,388	3,483	3,581	3,682	3,785	3,891
2,841	2,920	3,001	3,084	3,169	3,257	3,348	3,441	3,536	3,634	3,735	3,839	3,945
2,891	2,970	3,052	3,135	3,221	3,310	3,401	3,494	3,590	3,688	3,790	3,894	4,000
2,942	3,022	3,104	3,188	3,274	3,363	3,454	3,548	3,644	3,743	3,845	3,949	4,056
2,994	3,074	3,157	3,241	3,328	3,417	3,509	3,603	3,700	3,799	3,901	4,005	4,113
3,047	3,128	3,210	3,295	3,383	3,472	3,565	3,659	3,756	3,855	3,958	4,063	4,170
3,101	3,182	3,265	3,351	3,438	3,528	3,621	3,716	3,813	3,913	4,015	4,120	4,228
3,155	3,237	3,321	3,407	3,495	3,585	3,678	3,773	3,871	3,971	4,074	4,179	4,287
3,211	3,293	3,377	3,464	3,552	3,643	3,736	3,832	3,930	4,030	4,133	4,239	4,347
3,268	3,350	3,435	3,522	3,611	3,702	3,795	3,891	3,989	4,090	4,193	4,299	4,408
3,326	3,409	3,494	3,581	3,670	3,761	3,855	3,951	4,050	4,151	4,254	4,361	4,469
3,384	3,468	3,553	3,641	3,738	3,822	3,916	4,013	4,111	4,213	4,316	4,423	4,532
3,444	3,528	3,614	3,701	3,791	3,884	3,978	4,075	4,174	4,275	4,379	4,486	4,595
3,505	3,589	3,675	3,763	3,854	3,946	4,041	4,138	4,237	4,339	4,443	4,550	4,659
3,567	3,651	3,738	3,826	3,917	4,010	4,105	4,202	4,302	4,404	4,508	4,615	4,724
3,630	3,715	3,802	3,890	3,981	4,074	4,170	4,267	4,367	4,469	4,573	4,680	4,790
3,694	3,779	3,866	3,956	4,047	4,140	4,236	4,333	4,433	4,536	4,640	4,747	4,857
3,759	3,845	3,932	4,022	4,113	4,207	4,303	4,400	4,501	4,603	4,708	4,815	4,924

Glossary

A

absorption conversion of acoustic energy into heat. Absorption is one mechanism leading to ultrasound beam *attenuation* in tissue.

acoustic impedance (characteristic acoustic impedance) the speed of sound in a medium multiplied by its density. Part of the energy of an ultrasound beam is reflected at interfaces between materials that have unequal acoustic impedances.

acoustic power quantity describing the rate at which acoustic energy is emitted by the ultrasound transducer in an ultrasound instrument.

acoustic pressure amplitude the maximum cycle-to-cycle increase (or decrease) in the pressure due to a sound wave, relative to the background pressure.

acoustic wave see **sound wave**.

address a unique number associated with each memory location in a computer or other digital device.

aliasing the production of artifactual, lower-frequency components in a Doppler signal spectrum when the pulse repetition frequency of the Doppler instrument is less than two times the maximum frequency of the Doppler signal.

A-mode (amplitude mode) display method of displaying pulse echo ultrasound signals in which a trace presents the instantaneous echo signal amplitude versus time after transmission of an acoustic pulse. Since the time referred to is synonymous with reflector distance, this trace also is a record of echo signal amplitude versus reflector distance.

amplitude reflection coefficient the ratio of the reflected pressure amplitude (p_r) to the incident pressure amplitude (p_i) at an interface.

analog-to-digital (A/D) converter component or device that accepts analog signals, such as from a transducer or an amplifier, and converts these to a digital format for processing in a computer.

annular array a transducer array consisting of a number of ring-shaped piezoelectric elements arranged concentrically, along with a central disk. An annular array can provide multiple transmit focal zones, dynamic receive focusing, and dynamic aperture. However, scanning must be done by mechanically sweeping the beam. (See also **sequential array** and **electronically sectored array**.)

aperture another name for the active radiating or receiving surface of a transducer assembly.

apodization decreasing the relative excitation near the edges of the radiating surface of a transducer during transmission, or decreasing the relative sensitivity near the edge of the receiving surface of the transducer, to reduce side lobes. Apodization is used in some array transducer assemblies.

array transducer assembly a group of piezoelectric elements, each of which can be excited individually and whose echo signals can be detected and amplified separately.

articulated arm scan (static scan) the transducer is mounted on an immobile arm to produce spatial tomograms of the body part examined. The transducer is manually moved (sectored) in multiple planes to produce A-mode images on an oscilloscope that are persistently maintained to "build up" a two-dimensional image.

artifact (in an ultrasound image or record) any echo signal whose displayed position does not correspond to the actual position of a reflector in the body or whose displayed amplitude is not indicative of the reflecting or scattering properties of the region from which the echo originated.

attenuation reduction in the amplitude and intensity of a sound wave as it propagates through a medium. Attenuation of ultrasound waves in tissue is caused by absorption and by scattering and reflection.

attenuation coefficient the amount of attenuation per unit distance traveled by a wave; typical units are dB/cm.

auto scanner (automatic scanner) another name for a B-mode scanning instrument in which the sweep of the ultrasound beam is done, either mechanically or electronically, by the instrument itself rather than the operator. Real-time scanners are a type of auto scanner.

autocorrelation see **correlation detector**.

axial resolution minimum reflector spacing along the axis of an ultrasound beam that results in separate, distinguishable echoes on the display. The shorter the pulse duration, the better the axial resolution (i.e., the closer the reflectors can be and be distinguished).

B

bandwidth see **frequency bandwidth**.

base plus fog a slight opacity of photographic or x-ray film, found upon developing without any exposure.

beam the directed ultrasound field produced by an ultrasound transducer.

binary number a system of numbers having 2 as its base. In contrast, the decimal number system has 10 as its base.

biplane imaging simultaneously forming and displaying B-mode images of two different planes, usually perpendicular to one another.

bit fundamental unit of information in a computer or other digital system. It is formed by a device that can be in either of two states—"on" or "off."

B-mode (brightness mode) display method of displaying pulse echo ultrasound signals in which echoes are displayed as intensity modulated dots at a position corresponding either to the reflector location, as in B-mode scanning, or to the reflector depth as in M-mode records. When gray-scale processing is used, the brightness of the dot is related to the echo signal amplitude.

B-mode image a two-dimensional image obtained with a pulse-echo scanner and depicting reflectors and scatterers in a region interrogated by a B-mode scan.

B-mode scan process of generating a two-dimensional ultrasound B-mode image by scanning the sound beam over the region to be examined and displaying resultant echo signals at a position corresponding to the reflector location using the B-mode display. The term B-mode scan also is sometimes used to denote a B-mode image.

B-scan another name for a B-mode scan.

byte group of bits in a computer or other digital system; it usually is used to refer to eight bits.

C

cavitation formation of gas- or vapor-filled cavities within a medium due (in the case of ultrasound waves) to the large acoustic pressures accompanying an intense ultrasound beam. Cavitation also refers to gas bubble activity, such as growth and collapse, as in transient cavitation, in the presence of the sound field.

clutter spurious echo signals originating from points outside the main beam of an array transducer assembly and caused by side lobes, grating lobes, and inadequate isolation between elements.

color flow imaging operating mode available on some ultrasound instruments in which a two-dimensional image is generated that portrays moving reflectors using color. Most instruments that provide color-flow images display gray-scale B-mode images simultaneously.

compound position registration accuracy the accuracy with which a manual scanning instrument, or an automatic scanner that does compound scanning, positions echo signals from a single reflector on the display when the reflector is scanned from different transducer orientations in a fixed scanning plane.

compound scan type of transducer and/or sound beam motion used to generate a B-mode image in which two or more basic scanning motions, such as linear and sector scanning, are combined. (See also **linear scan** and **sector scan**.)

compression (acoustic waves) elevations in the density at a location in a medium, accompanying the cyclic pressure elevations during the passage of a sound wave. (See also **rarefaction**.)

compression (electrical signals) reduction in the effective gain of an amplifier for larger amplitude signals with respect to the gain for lower amplitude signals; compression is done so that weak signals can be boosted above the display threshold at the same time that strong signals do not saturate the display. This allows a greater echo dynamic range to be displayed.

console another name for the part of an ultrasound instrument to which the transducer assembly is attached through its interconnecting cable; the console contains the pulser, receiver, scan converter, and display.

continuous-wave (CW) Doppler type of Doppler device and processing involving transmitting a constant amplitude sound wave continuously into the region to be examined and processing echo signals for Doppler-shifted frequencies. Because the transmitter and transducer continuously flood the examined region, there is little or no discrimination of the depth of the moving reflectors.

contrast resolution the smallest variation in echo level that can be distinguished as a shade of gray on a B-mode display. Also, the smallest variation in scattering level between an object and the surrounding material, which results in the object being just noticeable on a B-mode display.

convex array a type of sequential array transducer assembly used in B-mode imaging in which the array elements are arranged in an arc. A convex array does B-mode scanning in a fashion similar to that of a **sequential linear array**.

correlation detector scheme used to measure changes in a signal wave train from one time to another, such as from one transmit pulse to the next in a color-flow instrument. Such devices are used in color-flow imaging instruments to detect phase changes in echo signals from moving reflectors.

cosine (cos) for an angle A in a right triangle, the ratio of the adjacent side to the hypotenuse.

coupling providing a transonic material between two media, such as the transducer assembly and the skin, to assure that sound waves will propagate from one to the other. Coupling gel or oil eliminates air between the transducer assembly and the patient's skin in an ultrasound examination.

critical angle smallest angle of incidence of a sound beam at a refracting interface for which there is total reflection of the incident beam. A critical angle exists when the speed of sound in the material on the transmitted beam side of the interface is greater than that in the material on the incident beam side.

Curie temperature temperature at which a piezoelectric transducer will become depolarized.

D

damping dissipation of energy in motion of any type; here it is the dissipation of vibrational energy of an ultrasonic transducer to reduce the pulse duration.

decibel (dB) unit used to quantitatively express the ratio of two amplitudes or intensities. Decibels are not absolute units, but express one sound level or intensity in terms of another or in terms of a reference. Example: "The amplitude 10 cm from the transducer is 10 dB lower than the amplitude 5 cm from the transducer." The relation between two signal amplitudes, A_1 and A_2, is expressed in decibels as $20\log(A_2/A_1)$.

depth calibration accuracy a measure of the accuracy to which the distance between two point reflectors, separated along the direction of an acoustic beam line, can be determined on the display of a pulse-echo instrument.

diffraction sound beam pattern when waves from different regions of a source or the edges of an obstacle add up at different points in the field.

diffuse reflector a reflecting interface that has an irregular rather than a smooth surface; the sizes of the irregularities are comparable to or greater than the wavelength. Reflected waves from such an interface spread out in all directions.

digital of or relating to data that are stored, manipulated, or read out in discrete units or levels.

digital calipers circuitry for estimating the distance between reflectors displayed on a B-mode image or M-mode display. The operator positions electronic markers or cursors on the display, adjacent to the structures to be measured, and the instrument computes the distance between cursors.

directional discrimination measure of the ability of a directional Doppler instrument to display flow signals in the proper direction only.

directional Doppler Doppler signal processing in which both the reflector speed and direction of motion (i.e., toward the transducer or away from the transducer) are detected and displayed.

displayed beam width the size of the B-mode image of a point or line target, measured perpendicularly to the direction of the sound beam. The displayed beam width varies with the receiver gain, the reflector depth, the acoustic impedance change at the reflector interface, etc.

displayed dynamic range see **local dynamic range**.

Doppler angle   angle between the direction of reflector motion and the direction of propagation of the ultrasound beam.

Doppler effect   phenomenon whereby there is a change in the perceived frequency of a sound source relative to the transmitted frequency when there is relative motion between a sound source and a listener.

Doppler shift   in general, the change in the perceived frequency relative to the transmitted frequency when there is relative motion between a sound source and a listener; in ultrasound, the difference between the frequency of a transmitted pulse and that of an echo signal when there is motion of the reflector relative to the transducer.

Doppler shift frequency (fD)   the difference between the frequency of received echo signals and the frequency of the transmitted ultrasound pulse in a Doppler study.

duplex scanners   real-time B-mode scanners with built-in Doppler reception, processing, and display capabilities.

duty factor   the fraction of time that the transducer is actively producing ultrasound energy. It is often expressed as a percentage. The duty factor is equal to the pulse repetition frequency times the pulse duration.

dynamic aperture   term used to identify a process whereby the number of receiving elements in a transducer array automatically increases (thereby increasing the size of the aperture) with increasing reflector depth. Increasing the receiving aperture size with increasing reflector depth keeps lateral resolution nearly constant over the entire useful range of a transducer.

dynamic focus   process of electronically changing the *receiving* focal distance of an array transducer assembly so that it tracks the acoustic pulse position and reflector depth in real time. Each time a sound pulse is transmitted the instrument initially sets the receiving focal distance at a shallow depth. As the time duration after the transmitted pulse increases, the receiving focal distance increases automatically.

dynamic frequency tracking   varying the center frequency of the amplifier of a pulse-echo instrument so that it gradually changes with time following each transmit pulse. Dynamic frequency tracking sometimes is used to optimize the receiver's sensitivity so that it coincides best with the frequencies available in the echo signal pulses picked up from structures at different depths. The latter frequencies change with increasing reflector distance because of preferential attenuation of higher frequency sound waves by tissues.

dynamic range   the ratio of the largest to smallest signals that an instrument or a component of an instrument can respond to without distortion. In diagnostic ultrasound the dynamic range frequently is expressed in decibels. (See also **local dynamic range**.)

E

echo signal enhancement   see **enhancement**.

effective beam width   the displayed beam width that results from the combined shape of the transmitted beam and the receiving sensitivity pattern of a transducer assembly. In an array transducer assembly the transmitted beam pattern and receiving sensitivity pattern may be quite different.

electronic burst generator   device used for performance tests of ultrasound instruments that provides simulated echo signals of known relative amplitudes and with known times between signals.

electronically sectored (phased) array   an array transducer assembly that has very thin (usually) rectangular elements arranged side by side. It relies upon electronic beam steering to sweep sound beams over a sector-shaped scanned region.

Beam steering is done using electronic time delays in the transmitting and receiving circuits. (See also **sequential array** and **annular array**.)

elevational resolution   the ability to distinguish between reflectors separated along a line that is perpendicular to the ultrasound image plane. (See also **slice thickness**.)

energy   the capacity to do work. (In this context work is formally defined as that which is done when a force acts on matter and moves it.) Units for energy are *joules*.

enhancement   a manifestation of increased echo signal amplitudes returning from regions lying beyond an object in which the attenuation is lower than the average attenuation in adjacent overlying regions. (See also **partial shadowing**.)

epidemiology   the field of science dealing with the relationships of the various factors involved in the frequencies and distributions of an infectious process, a disease, or a physiologic state. Epidemiology is sometimes used to study whether diagnostic ultrasound exposures of humans have led to a measurable effect of some kind.

F

far field (Fraunhofer zone)   that part of the field of an ultrasound transducer that is a large distance from the probe. In the far field the beam diameter generally increases with increasing distance. For an unfocused circular single-element transducer of radius a the far field is usually taken to extend beyond the distance $a^2/$, where is the wavelength.

FFT analyzer (Fast Fourier Transform analyzer)   device for doing frequency analysis of complex signals. FFT analyzers are often used in Doppler instruments to obtain a display of the frequency characteristics of the signal.

focal distance   the distance from a focused transducer assembly to the plane where the effective beam width is narrowest.

focal zone   the region over which the effective width of the sound beam is within some measure of (such as two times) its width at the focal distance.

focusing (receiver)   process of controlling the receiving sensitivity pattern of a transducer to narrow the effective beam width and improve the lateral resolution over some depth range. The receiving focal distance of an array can change dynamically as echoes from along a given beam line are received.

focusing (transmit)   process of controlling the convergence of a transmitted sound beam to narrow the beam and sometimes to increase the intensity over some axial range. Transmit focusing can be done using a concave transducer element, an acoustic lens, or using an array of elements along with electronic time delays. The focal distance of the array may be varied electronically by changing the electronic delay sequence, and thus may be user selectable.

frame rate   the rate at which images are updated on the display of an auto scanning system. Often used synonymously with scan repetition rate.

frequency   the number of cycles per second that a periodic event or function undergoes; the number of cycles completed per unit of time. The frequency of a sound wave is determined by the number of oscillations per second of the vibrating source.

frequency bandwidth   a measure of the spread of frequencies in a pulsed waveform or the range of frequencies a device responds to. The frequency bandwidth of a transducer can be determined by spectral analysis of an echo signal from a plane, smooth reflector. The shorter the pulse duration emitted by a transducer, the wider the frequency bandwidth, and vice versa.

frequency bandwidth of a receiver the range of ultrasound signal frequencies the receiver can amplify with maximum or nearly maximum gain.

G

gain a measure of the amount of amplification of an amplifier. It is the ratio of the output signal amplitude to the input signal amplitude and can be expressed as a simple ratio or in decibels.

grating lobe in the sound beam from an array, energy falling outside the main lobe or main beam as a result of the active transducer aperture being split into elements. Grating lobes are reduced or eliminated by using very small elements.

gray-scale processing signal processing used to modulate the brightness of dots on a B-mode display in accordance with the amplitude of individual echo signals.

H

hertz unit for frequency, equal to 1 cycle per second and abbreviated Hz.

high PRF mode pulsed Doppler instrument operating condition in which the PRF is so high that a transmit pulse is emitted by the transducer before echo signals corresponding to the previous transmit pulse arrive from the sample volume. Ambiguities may result in the range from which Doppler signals originate. High PRF mode is used to avoid aliasing in pulsed Doppler.

horizontal distance accuracy a measure of the accuracy to which the distance between two point reflectors, separated along a line perpendicular to the direction of the central beam line forming a B-mode image, can be determined on the display.

hydrophone a device consisting of a small piezoelectric element mounted on the end of a narrow tube or supported on a thin membrane, commonly used to measure the acoustic pressure and determine the intensity at points in an ultrasound field.

hyperechoic adjective used to describe a region for which the average echo signal amplitude is greater than that in the material surrounding the region.

hypoechoic adjective used to describe a region for which the average echo signal amplitude is lower than that in the surrounding region.

I

image freeze condition in which B-mode image, M-mode, Doppler, and/or color-flow image data are retained in a scan converter's memory for examination and/or photography as well as for video recording.

image texture see **texture** and **speckle**.

impedance matching layers thin layers attached to the outer surface of a piezoelectric element in a transducer to provide efficient transmission of sound waves from the transducer element to soft tissue, and vice versa. Matching layers minimize reflections at the transducer-to-soft tissue interface, improving the sensitivity.

intensity a measure of the strength of a sound wave. It is equal to the power per unit area transmitted through a region and has units of W/cm^2 (watts per square meter). One also sees intensity expressed in mW/cm^2 (milliwatts per square centimeter) and W/cm^2. For many conditions in ultrasonics the intensity at a point in the field is proportional to the square of the pressure amplitude. The following are commonly used intensity terms:

Im spatial peak intensity averaged over the largest half cycle of a pulse.

spatial average (SA) intensity the intensity averaged over the beam area for a stationary sound beam or over the scan-crossed area for a scanning beam. With a stationary transducer it is equal to the acoustic power, P, contained within the beam, divided by the beam area, A.

spatial-average time-average intensity I (SPTA) the time average intensity also averaged over the beam area for a stationary beam or the scan cross-sectional area for a scanning beam.

spatial peak (SP) intensity the intensity at the point in the sound field where this value is the maximum.

spatial-peak pulse-average intensity I (SPPA) the average intensity in an acoustic pulse, measured at the location where this quantity is the largest.

spatial-peak time-average intensity I (SPTA) the resultant measure of intensity, when averaged for a time equal to a scan repetition period in an automatic scanning mode or a pulse repetition period for a stationary beam, at the location in the field where this quantity is the largest.

temporal peak intensity the maximum instantaneous intensity attained during the pulse.

time average intensity the relatively low value obtained when the intensity at any particular spot in the field, such as at the spatial peak location, is averaged over the time between pulses.

intensity reflection coefficient the ratio of the reflected beam intensity to the incident beam intensity at an interface.

interface surface forming the boundary between media having different properties.

interference variation with distance or time of the amplitude of a wave, which results from the addition of two or more waves.

J

joule unit of energy. (See also **watt, acoustic power,** and **energy.**)

K

kilohertz (kHz) 1000 hertz or 10^3 cycles per second.

L

laminar flow flow within a blood vessel in which most blood cells are moving with general uniformity of direction and velocity, and in which there is an organized distribution of velocities across the flow area.

lead zirconate titanate commonly used material for the piezoelectric element(s) in an ultrasound transducer (abbreviated PZT).

leading edge processing type of B-mode processing and display in which any echo signal whose amplitude is above a threshold level established within the instrument appears as a dot. All dots are of the same brightness regardless of the echo signal amplitude.

linear array see **sequential array**.

linear scan a type of scan used to generate a B-mode image in which motion of a transducer or ultrasound beam is along a straight line at right angles to the beam. (See also **sector scan.**)

local dynamic range the echo signal level change causing the display in a pulse-echo instrument to vary from a just noticeable echo signal (e.g., the lowest gray level) to its maximum response (i.e., maximum brightness). This is also referred to as the "displayed dynamic range."

logarithmic compression (log compression) a form of signal compression used in pulse-echo ultrasound. Logarithmic compression is especially useful for allowing amplitude variations

scanning arm   that part of a static B-mode scanner to which is attached the ultrasound transducer; the arm has sensors for tracking the position and orientation of the transducer while it is scanned over the patient surface. The scanning arm also constrains the transducer to a plane so that sectoring may be done to record echo signals from interfaces at different transducer orientations.

scanning speed   the rate at which the sound beam is swept across the scanned region in a B-mode scan and echo signal data are displayed. The maximum scanning speed is limited by the travel time of sound pulses in tissue.

scatter   reflection of a wave in various directions, caused by interfaces that are near the size of the wavelength or smaller.

sector scan   a type of scan used to generate a B-mode image in which the transducer or the ultrasound beam is rotated or swept through an angle, the center of rotation being near or behind the surface of the transducer. (See also **linear scan** and **compound scan**.)

sensitivity   a measure of the weakest echo signal that an instrument is capable of detecting and displaying.

sequential (linear) array   an array transducer assembly used in B-mode imaging and color-flow studies that has many (usually) rectangularly shaped elements arranged side by side. Scanning is done by transmitting sound beams and receiving echo signals with different clusters, or groups, of elements within the array. The center of the element cluster, and hence the sound beam axis, is shifted electronically from one beam line to the next, thereby producing a scan. (See also **electronically sectored array** and **annular array**.)

shadowing   loss of echo signals from distal structures due to attenuation of overlying structures. (See also **partial shadowing**.)

side lobes   energy in a sound beam that falls outside the main lobe or main beam.

simple harmonic motion   a periodic motion that is a sinusoidal function of time; it is characterized by a particular frequency.

sine   for an angle A in a right triangle, the ratio of the opposite side to the hypotenuse.

sine wave   a wave form in which wave variables at a given location, such as the pressure or the particle displacement, vary in proportion to the sine of a constant times the time. Alternatively, at a fixed time the variable may vary in proportion to the sine of a constant times the distance.

slice thickness   a measure of the largest distance, measured perpendicular to the ultrasound scan plane, a reflector at a given depth can be from the scan plane and still be detected on the display. Slice thickness is closely related to elevational resolution. It is also referred to as "scan plane thickness."

Snell's law   used to express the relationship between the directions of the incident and transmitted waves when refraction occurs at an interface. Stated mathematically, if O_t is the angle of the transmitted wave and O_1 the angle of the incident wave, $\sin O_t = (c_2/c_1)\sin O_1$ where c_2 and c_1 are the speeds of sound on the transmitted and incident beam sides of the interface, respectively.

sound frequency   see **frequency**.

sound wave   an alteration of properties of a medium, such as pressure, particle displacement, and density, that propagates through the medium; a mechanical disturbance that propagates progressively through a medium.

speckle   the granular random *texture* pattern produced in an ultrasound B-mode image of a macroscopically uniform region in tissue or a tissue-mimicking phantom.

spectral analysis   a process by which a complex signal is broken down or analyzed into simple frequency components; it is used, for example, to show the distribution of frequencies in a Doppler signal.

spectral display (for a pulse or a complex signal)   a plot of the fraction of signal within a given frequency interval versus the frequency.

spectrum analyzer   instrument used to measure the relative amount of signal at different frequencies in a pulsed waveform or in a complex signal consisting of many frequencies.

specular reflector   a large smooth interface with dimensions that are greater than the size of the incident ultrasound beam.

stable cavitation   the creation of cavitation bubbles that oscillate with the sound beam but do not collapse violently, as in transient cavitation. See also **cavitation**.

standard 100 mm test object   device consisting of a series of stainless steel reflectors arranged as targets immersed in a liquid whose speed of sound is 1540 m/s and mainly used for geometric tests of ultrasound pulse-echo instruments.

static scanner   another name for a manual scanner.

swept gain   a process whereby the receiver amplification is increased with time following the transmit pulse so that echo signals originating from distant reflectors are amplified more than echo signals originating from reflectors close to the transducer. Swept gain compensates for attenuation in the medium. It is also referred to as "time gain compensation (TGC)."

T

tadpole tail sign   colloquial term used to describe the B-mode image pattern that results from scanning through and around a region, such as a walled cyst, where there is higher than average attenuation near the lateral margins of the region and lower than average attenuation across the middle of the region. On the image, the echo enhancement pattern, bordered laterally by patterns with partial or total shadowing, is said to resemble a tadpole's tail.

texture   in a B-mode ultrasound image, refers to the pixel-to-pixel variations in image brightness due to interference when echo signals are obtained simultaneously from many scatterers or due to properties of the tissue.

time gain compensation   see **swept gain**.

tissue-mimicking phantom   a material, often configured in some specified shape, which mimics certain soft tissue in ultrasonic propagation, and sometimes scattering and reflection properties.

transducer   any device that converts signals from one form to another. Examples include pressure sensing transducers that yield an electric signal proportional to the static pressure, and ultrasonic transducers. (See also **ultrasound transducer**.)

transducer assembly   another name for the transducer in an ultrasound instrument; especially used for the transducer, associated housing, and any internal electronic circuitry attached to the console of real-time scanning instruments.

transient cavitation   a process in which cavitation oscillations grow so strong that the bubbles collapse, producing intense localized effects. See also **cavitation**.

transmit focal distance   the distance from the transducer assembly to the plane where the transmitted beam width is narrowest for a given transmit focus setting.

transonic   adjective used to describe a region that is relatively unattenuating to sound waves.

transverse waves   sound wave for which the direction of displacement of particles in the medium is perpendicular to the direction of propagation of the wave. Transverse waves do not propagate effectively in soft tissues.

U

ultrasonic transducer   a device that converts electric signals to mechanical vibrations and high-frequency pressure pulses to electric signals.

V

variance   in Doppler signal processing, a measure of the variation (over a short time interval) of the mean Doppler signal from the volume corresponding to a single pixel in a color-flow image or a single-pulsed Doppler sample volume. The signal variance is used to detect turbulence.

W

wall filter   electronic filter applied to the audio output signal of a Doppler ultrasound instrument to reduce or eliminate low-frequency Doppler signals, such as those due to vessel wall movement. The lower cutoff frequency of the filter usually is operator adjustable.

watt   unit of power, equal to one joule per second. (See **acoustic power** and **energy**.)

wave   see **sound wave**.

wavelength   the distance over which a wave repeats itself; the distance in the line of advance of a wave from one point to the next point of corresponding phase. Also, the distance the wave travels during one period of oscillation of the source.

weakly focused transducers   transducers that have focusing properties such that beam patterns are very dependent on the transducer diameter and frequency as well as the curvature of the element. In contrast, a strongly focused transducer's beam properties are more dependent on the curvature of the element and less so on the frequency and diameter of the transducer.

wide-band amplifier   an amplifier that responds to ultrasound echo signal that covers a large frequency range; usually it responds equally to all frequencies produced by the different transducer assemblies that can be used with the instrument.

PART TWO
ABDOMINAL AND RETROPERITONEAL
CAVITIES

A

acute tubular necrosis (ATN)   a common cause of acute post-transplant failure.

Addison's disease   disease due to hypofunction of the adrenal cortex that is usually fatal. Signs and symptoms include hypotension, general weakness, loss of appetite and weight, and characteristic bronzing of the skin.

adrenal glands   small secretory organs lying along the superomedial border of both kidneys, each composed of two endocrine glands: the cortex, which secretes a range of steroid hormones, and the medulla, which secretes epinephrine and norepinephrine.

adrenal medulla   the core of the adrenal gland in which groups of irregular cells are located amidst veins that collect blood from the sinusoids; it produces epinephrine and norepinephrine.

adrenal neuroblastoma   the most common malignancy of the adrenal glands in childhood and the most common tumor of infancy. It generally arises within the adrenal medulla.

adrenocorticotropic hormone (ACTH)   hormone that controls the adrenal cortex.

adrenogenital syndrome   hyperfunction of the adrenal cortex that results in precocious puberty in boys and masculinization of the external genitalia in girls.

adult polycystic disease   a disease in which a cyst may arise from any portion of a collecting system.

agenesis of the spleen   see **asplenia of the spleen**.

ammonium   a toxic product of nitrogen metabolism.

amylase   an enzyme of the pancreatic juice that causes hydrolysis of starch.

anatomic position   a position of standing erect, the arms by the side with palms facing forward, the face and eyes directed forward, and the heels together with feet pointed forward.

angiomyolipoma   a benign tumor that occurs most often in the kidneys.

anterior (ventral)   toward the front of the body.

aorta   the largest artery in the body. It distributes blood to the lower part of the body as the thoracic aorta and abdominal aorta and sends branches to the upper extremities from the ascending aorta.

aortic arch   a continuation of the ascending aorta. It has three branches: the innominate or brachiocephalic trunk, the left common carotid artery, and the left subclavian artery.

aponeuroses   thin, tendinous sheets attached to flat muscles.

arteriole   a tiny arterial branch.

asplenia of the spleen   complete absence of the spleen

B

bare area   the portion of the liver that rests directly on the diaphragm.

blood urea nitrogen (BUN)   the level of urea in the blood.

Bowman's capsule   see **capsula glomeruli**.

C

calculi   see **gallstones**.

capsula glomeruli   two layers of flat epithelial cells with a space between them contained in each nephron of the kidney.

cardiac muscle   these muscles, which form the conducting system of the heart, are only found in the myocardium of the heart and in the muscle layer of the base of the great blood vessels.

caudal   toward the feet.

celiac trunk   branch of the abdominal aorta that distributes to structures of the gastrointestinal tract. It gives rise to the left gastric, hepatic, and splenic arteries.

cholecystitis   inflammation of the gallbladder punctuated by intermittent acute episodes, which occur when the cystic duct is obstructed by a calculus.

cholelithiasis   the presence of gallstones in the gallbladder.

colic artery   a left, middle, or right branch from either the inferior mesenteric or the superior mesenteric artery that distributes to the colon.

common bile duct   formed by the common hepatic duct and the cystic duct.

common duct   the duct formed by the junction of the cystic duct with the hepatic duct.

common hepatic duct   the united right and left hepatic ducts, approximately 4 mm in diameter, which descends within the edge of the lesser omentum.

congenital agenesis   absence of one kidney and one ureter at birth.

Conn's syndrome   caused by excessive secretion of aldosterone, usually due to a cortical adenoma.

coronal plane   any vertical plane at right angles to the median plane.

Courvoisier's sign (law)   when a gallstone blocks the common bile duct, the gallbladder is smaller than usual; when the duct is obstructed in some other way, the gallbladder is dilated.

cranial   toward the head.

culling   inspection and destruction of abnormal or senescent erythrocytes as they pass through the spleen.

Cushing's disease   one type of oversecretion disease of the adrenal cortex. This is produced by excessive secretion of glucocorticoids due to hyperplasia, a benign tumor, or carcinoma. Symptoms include increased sodium retention, muscle and bone weakness, and secretion of androgens.

cystic artery   right branch of the proper hepatic artery that distributes to the gallbladder and undersurface of the liver.

D

diaphragm   a dome-shaped muscular and tendinous septum that separates the thorax from the abdominal cavity.

distal   away from the point of origin or away from the body.

duct of Santorini   a secondary duct that drains the upper anterior head of the pancreas.

duct of Wirsung (ductus pancreaticus)   the primary excretory duct of the pancreas extending the entire length of the gland.

E

enzymes   protein catalysts used throughout the body in all metabolic processes.

epigastric artery   a branch of the external iliac artery (inferior epigastric), the femoral artery (superficial epigastric), or the internal mammary artery (superior epigastric) that distributes to the abdominal muscles and peritoneum, the abdomen and superficial fascia, or the abdominal muscles and diaphragm, respectively.

epiploic foramen   the opening of the lesser sac.

external   outside

F

false pelvis   see **major pelvis**.

fasciae   thin sheets of tissue that cover muscles and hold them in their place.

floating gallstone   some gallstones are seen to float when contrast material from an oral cholecystogram is present. This is due to the higher specific gravity of the contrast material than of the bile.

foramen of Winslow   see **epiploic foramen**.

G

gallbladder   a pear-shaped sac, with a capacity of 50 ml, in the anterior aspect of the right upper quadrant closely related to the visceral surface of the liver. Its function includes storage of bile for intermittent release in conjunction with eating.

gallbladder sludge   thick, inspissated bile found in the gallbladder.

gallstones   the small crystals of bile salts that precipitate and vary from pinhead size to the size of the gallbladder itself.

gastric artery   a right, left, or short branch of the celiac, hepatic, or splenic artery that distributes to the esophagus and curvatures of the stomach.

gastroduodenal artery   a branch of the hepatic artery that distributes to the stomach, duodenum, and pancreas.

gastroepiploic artery   a left or right branch of either the splenic or gastroduodenal artery that distributes to the stomach and greater omentum.

Geota's fascia   see **renal fascia**.

glomerulus   a cluster of nonanastomosing capillaries.

glucocorticoids   steroids that play a principal role in carbohydrate metabolism. Cortisone and hydrocortisone are the primary glucocorticoids. They diminish allergic response, especially the more serious inflammatory types (rheumatoid arthritis and rheumatic fever).

glucose tolerance test   a test performed to discover whether there is a disorder of glucose metabolism.

H

Hartmann's pouch   created when the gallbladder folds back on itself at the neck.

hemolytic anemia   the general term applied to anemia referable to decreased life of the erythrocytes.

hepatic artery (common)   branch of the celiac artery that distributes to the stomach, pancreas, duodenum, liver, gallbladder, and greater omentum.

hepatic artery (proper)   branch of the common hepatic artery that distributes to the liver and gallbladder.

hepatorenal recess   the lowest point in the peritoneal cavity when the patient is lying supine. It is in the greatest sac just to the right of the epiploic foramen.

horseshoe kidney   a defect that occurs during fetal development with fusion of the upper or lower poles, where the kidney does not ascend to its normal position in the retroperitoneal cavity.

hydronephrosis   distention of the pelvis and calices of the kidney by urine due to an obstruction in a ureter.

hyperglycemia   an effect of severe liver disease where there is an uncontrolled increase in blood glucose.

hypoalbuminemia   a significant lowering of the serum albumin.

hypoglycemic   an effect of severe liver disease where the body becomes glucose deficient.

I

iliac artery   the common iliac artery is a branch of the abdominal aorta and distributes to the pelvis, abdominal wall, and lower limbs. The external iliac artery is a branch of the common iliac artery and distributes to the abdominal wall, external genitalia, and lower limbs. The internal iliac artery is another branch of the common iliac artery and distributes to the visceral walls of the pelvis, buttocks, reproductive organs, and mid-thigh.

infantile polycystic disease   a disease that causes the tubules in the distal collecting systems to dilate and form small cystic structures.

inferior   below

insulin   a hormone secreted by the beta cells of the islands of Langerhans in the pancreas. It is secreted into the blood where it regulates carbohydrate, lipid, and amino acid metabolism.

internal   inside

intestinal artery   branch of the superior mesenteric artery that distributes to the jejunum and ileum.

intravenous pyelogram (IVP)   a roentgenogram of the kidney and ureter after the injection of a radiopaque dye.

J

jaundice   the disease characterized by the presence of bile in the tissues with the resulting yellow-green color of the skin, sclerae, and body secretions.

L

labeling   an orderly procedure that should be used to identify the anatomic position where the transverse and longitudinal scans have been taken.

lateral   farther from the midline or to the side of the body.

left hepatic duct emerges from the right lobe of the liver in the porta hepatis and unites with the right hepatic duct to form the common hepatic duct.

lesser sac an enclosed portion of the peritoneal space posterior to the liver and the stomach.

linea alba a fibrous band that stretches from the xyphoid to the symphysis pubis and forms a central anterior attachment for the muscle layers of the abdomen. It is formed by the interlacing of fibers of the aponeuroses of the right and left oblique and transversus abdominis muscles.

lipase an enzyme secreted by the pancreas and small intestine that is capable of hydrolyzing some fats to monoglycerides and some to glycerol and fatty acids.

lithogenic bile a form of bile supersaturated with cholesterol that is found in some individuals.

lumbar artery a branch of the abdominal aorta that distributes to the abdominal walls, the vertebrae, the lumbar muscles, and the renal capsule.

M

major pelvis the portion of the pelvis found above the brim of the pelvis; its cavity is that portion of the abdominal cavity cradled by the iliac fossae.

malpighian body see **renal corpuscle**.

medial nearer to or toward the midline.

median plane a vertical plane that bisects the body into right and left halves.

mesenteric artery inferior or superior branch of the abdominal aorta that distributes to either the lower half of the colon and rectum (inferior) or the small intestine and proximal half of the colon (superior).

mesentery a double fold of peritoneum connecting an organ to the abdominal wall.

mesothelium a single layer of cells that forms the peritoneum.

metabolism the physical and chemical process whereby food is synthesized into complex elements, complex substances are transformed into simple ones, and energy is made available for use by the organism.

Mickey Mouse sign appearance of the common duct, hepatic artery, and portal vein on a transverse scan. The portal vein serves as Mickey's face, with the right ear the common duct and the left ear the hepatic artery.

mineralocorticoids steroids that regulate the electrolyte metabolism. Aldosterone is the principal mineralocorticoid; it has a regulatory effect on the relative concentrations of mineral ions in the body fluids and therefore on the water content of tissues.

minor pelvis the portion of the pelvis found below the brim of the pelvis. The cavity of the minor pelvis is continuous at the pelvic brim with the cavity of the pelvis major.

multicystic dysplastic kidney a nonfunctioning kidney whose contour and shape are very irregular and which usually contains multiple cysts of varying sizes.

multipennate muscle a muscle that contains a tendon in the center, and the muscle fibers pass to it from two sides.

N

neoplasm any new growth or development, either malignant or benign, of an abnormal tissue.

nephron a tubular excretory unit of the kidney.

O

omentum a double layer of peritoneum running to the stomach.

ovarian artery branch of the abdominal aorta that distributes to the ovary, uterus, uterine tubes, and ureter.

P

pancreatic juice the pancreas' exocrine function is to produce this juice, which enters the duodenum together with bile.

pancreaticoduodenal artery the inferior pancreaticoduodenal artery is a branch of the superior mesenteric artery, and the superior pancreaticoduodenal artery is a branch of the gastroduodenal artery. Both distribute to the pancreas and duodenum.

parietal peritoneum the portion of the peritoneum that lines the abdominal wall but does not cover a viscus.

patient position the position of the patient described in relation to the scanning table (e.g., right decubitus would mean the right side down).

pennate muscles muscles that have fibers running oblique to the line of pull, resembling a feather.

peristalsis the action of smooth muscles propelling material through vessels or the gastrointestinal tract.

peritoneal cavity the potential space between the parietal and visceral peritoneum.

peritoneal gutters passageways that conduct fluid material from one point of the peritoneal cavity to another.

peritoneal recess small, isolated, slitlike parts of the peritoneal cavity without intestine.

pheochromocytoma a tumor that secretes epinephrine and norepinephrine in excessive quantities. They may be large, bulky tumors with a variety of sonographic patterns, including cystic, solid, and calcified components.

phrenic artery the inferior phrenic artery is a branch of the abdominal aorta and distributes to the diaphragm and adrenals. The superior phrenic arteries are branches of the thoracic aorta and distribute to the upper surface of the vertebral portion of the diaphragm.

phrygian cap folding of the fundus of the gallbladder.

pitting a process by which the spleen removes granular inclusions without destroying the erythrocytes.

portal triad the common collagenous sheath that encases the liver parenchyma, the portal venous and hepatic arterial branches.

posterior (dorsal) the back of the body, or in back of another structure.

pouch of Morrison see **hepatorenal recess**.

prone lying face down.

proximal closer to the point of origin or closer to the body.

R

real time the dynamic "real-time" presentation of sequential images at varying frame rates (depending on frequency and depth).

rectus sheath a sheath formed by the aponeuroses of the muscles of the lateral group.

renal artery branch of the abdominal aorta that distributes to the kidney.

renal corpuscle Bowman's capsule and the glomerulus.

renal fascia the tissue that surrounds the true capsule and perinephric fat.

renal parenchyma the area from the renal sinus to the outer renal surface in which are found the arcuate and interlobar vessels.

renal pyramids the portion of the kidney that is composed of medullary substance, which consists of a series of striated conical masses.

renal sinus fibrolipomatosis sinus fat and fibrous tissue.

retroperitoneal fibrosis   a disease of unknown etiology characterized by thick sheets of fibrous tissue in the retroperitoneal space.

retroperitoneal space   the area between the posterior portion of the parietal peritoneum and the posterior abdominal wall muscles.

right hepatic duct   emerges from the right lobe of the liver in the porta hepatis and unites with the left hepatic duct to form the common hepatic duct.

S

sagittal plane   any plane parallel to the median plane.

septation, complete   double gallbladder.

skeletal muscle   muscle, composed of striped muscle fibers and having two or more attachments, that produces movements of the skeleton.

smooth muscle   muscle composed of long, spindle-shaped cells closely arranged in bundles or sheets.

spermatic artery, internal   branch of the abdominal aorta that distributes to the scrotum and testis.

sphincter of Oddi   the circular muscle fibers that surround the end part of the common bile duct, the main pancreatic duct, and the ampulla; located at the junction of the common bile duct and the duodenum.

splenic artery   branch of the celiac artery that distributes to the spleen, stomach, pancreas, and greater omentum.

superficial inguinal ring   a triangular opening in the external oblique aponeuroses that lies superior and medial to the pubic tubercle.

superior   above.

supernumerary kidney   a rare defect where there is a complete duplicate of the renal system.

supine   lying face up.

T

tendons   the cords of tough, fibrous tissue that attach the ends of muscles to bones, cartilage, or ligaments.

thyroid artery, lowest   branch of the aortic arch as well as the innominate and right carotid arteries that distributes to the thyroid gland.

thyroid artery, superior   branch of the external carotid artery that distributes to the hyoid muscles, larynx, thyroid gland, and pharynx.

transverse plane   any plane at right angles to both the median and coronal planes.

true capsule   the fibrous capsule surrounding the kidney.

true pelvis   see **minor pelvis**.

trypsin   a pancreatic enzyme that may hydrolyze protein molecules to peptides.

tubular secretion   the process in which acids and other substances the body does not need are secreted into the distal renal tubules from the bloodstream.

U

unipennate muscle   a muscle in which the tendon lies along one side of the muscle and the muscle fibers pass oblique to it.

urinoma   a walled-off collection of extravasated urine that develops spontaneously after trauma, surgery, or a subacute or chronic urinary obstruction.

uterine   branch of the internal iliac artery that distributes to the uterus.

V

veins

azygos   front and right side of the lumbar vertebrae.

colic   right, medial, and left veins of intestines.

common iliac   union of external veins draining the sacroiliac and lower lumbar region and emptying into the inferior vena cava.

cystic   gallbladder.

dorsalis penis   vein lying in the midline of the penis between the dorsal arteries.

ductus venosus   a fetal vein that connects the umbilical vein with the inferior vena cava.

duodenal   duodenum.

epigastric   homonymous with epigastric artery; inferior, superficial, and superior.

gastric   short, right, and left veins of the stomach and surrounding area.

gastroepiploic   right and left veins of the stomach and omentum.

hepatic   liver region.

hypogastric   lower and middle abdomen, extending from the greater sciatic notch to the brim of the pelvis, where it joins the external iliac to form the common iliac vein.

ileocolic   ileum and colon.

intercostal   ribs and chest region.

interlobular   renal and hepatic veins of the kidney and liver.

mammary   internal vein of the breast.

mesenteric   superior and inferior vein of the intestines.

ovarian   ovary and broad ligament.

pancreatic   pancreas.

pancreaticoduodenal   pancreas and duodenum.

phlebo   combining form referring to vein.

phrenic   anterior and superior veins of the diaphragm.

plexus   network of veins. (May also refer to nerves and lymphatics.)

portal   liver, eventually forming sinusoids of liver.

pudendal   internal and external genitalia.

pyloric   pylorus and area.

renal   kidney.

sacral   lateral and medial veins of the sacral and coccygeal areas.

spermatic   spermatic cord and surrounding area.

splenic   spleen.

superior and inferior vena cava   large veins that return blood to the heart. The superior vena cava returns blood from the upper extremities, and the inferior vena cava returns it from the lower extremities.

suprarenals   adrenals.

thyroid   inferior and superior veins of the thyroid gland and adjacent structures.

uterine   uterus.

venae vasorum   small veins that return blood from the walls of blood vessels themselves.

veno   term referring to vein.

venules   small veins.

vesical   bladder.

visceral peritoneum   that portion of the peritoneum that covers an organ.

voluntary muscle   the movements of the skeleton produced by the skeletal muscles.

W

Waterhouse-Friderichsen syndrome   malignant form of epidemic cerebrospinal meningitis characterized by the sudden onset of fever, cyanosis, petechiae, and collapse from massive bilateral adrenal hemorrhage.

PART THREE
SUPERFICIAL STRUCTURES

A

adenosis hyperplasia and proliferation of the epithelial component of ducts in the breast characterizing the second stage of fibrocystic disease.

aneurysm dilatation of the venous wall due to high venous pressure or repeated dialysis traumas.

B

breast a differentiated apocrine sweat gland with a functional purpose of secreting milk during lactation.

C

carcinoma breast breast tumors that arise from the epithelium, in the ductal and glandular tissue, usually having tentacles.

  infiltrating infiltration of the breast tissue beyond the basement membrane and into adjacent tissue.

  noninfiltrating carcinoma of the lactiferous ducts that has not infiltrated the basement membrane but is proliferating within the confines of the ducts and its branches.

chronic hypocalcemia a disease caused by renal failure, ricketts, or malabsorption syndromes and induces PTH secretion.

Comedomastitis the dilation of ducts in the breast filled with a secretion produced by desquamated cells from the duct wall.

congenital ureteropelvic junction obstruction (UPJ) obstruction of the renal pelvis with variable degrees of calycectasis occurring.

Cooper's ligaments the supporting structures of the breast that provide the shape and consistency of the breast structure.

cretinism congenital hypothyroidism.

cystic disease the third stage of fibrocystic disease characterized by the involution of lobules and hyperplasia of the surrounding stoma, leading to the formation of cysts.

cystic masses lumps in the breast much like a balloon of water, well delineated but not as mobile as fibroadenomas.

cystosarcoma phyllodes an uncommon breast neoplasia and the most frequent sarcoma of the breast.

E

epididymis the first portion of the duct of the testis and its excretory system.

epididymitis the most common intrascrotal inflammation, appearing sonographically as uniform enlargement of the epididymis and most evident in the globus major.

F

fibroadenoma one of the most common benign breast tumors, the most common in childhood, and occurring primarily in young adult women.

fibrocystic disease breast syndrome with histologic changes occurring on the terminal ducts and lobules of the breast in both the epithelial and connective tissue. General symptoms are pain, nodularity, a dominant mass, cysts, and occasional nipple discharge.

G

goiter enlargement of the thyroid gland as a result of hyperplasia or neoplasia, inflammatory processes, or colloid distention of the follicles.

Graves' disease hyperthyroidism associated with diffuse goiter.

H

hydrocele of the cord the encasement of fluid in a sac of peritoneum within the spermatic cord. It can also present as a cystic mass cephalad to the testis.

hydroceles a fluid collection surrounding the testis that can be associated with infectious processes or tumors.

hyperparathyroidism

  primary a state of increased function of the parathyroid glands characterized by hypercalcemia, hypercalciuria, and low serum levels of phosphate. It occurs when increased amounts of PTH are produced by an adenoma, primary hyperplasia, or, rarely, carcinoma.

  secondary results from chronic hypocalcemia that induces PTH secretion.

hyperthyroidism a hypermetabolic state in which increased amounts of thyroid hormones are produced as a result of pituitary-thyroid regulatory system failure. Manifestations of this condition are weight loss, nervousness, and increased heart rate.

hypothyroidism a hypometabolic state resulting from inadequate secretion of thyroid hormones. It is usually caused by an abnormality of the gland that restricts production of the hormones. Lethargy, sluggish reactions, and a deep husky voice are manifestations.

I

in situ a condition where a carcinoma is contained and has not invaded the basal membrane structure.

iodine metabolism the mechanism for production of thyroid hormones.

M

mammary one of the three well-defined layers of the breast found between the superficial and the deep connective tissue layers.

mammography the most accurate, noninvasive method for the detection of breast lesions, especially in tissue that is predominantly fatty.

mastodynia see **mazoplasia**.

mazoplasia the first stage of fibrocystic disease characterized by an increased proliferation of the stroma and by the small number of lobules or acini.

P

Paget's disease a relatively rare tumor occurring in older women, characterized by changes in the nipple and areola.

parathyroid glands the calcium-sensing organs in the body that produce parathormone (PTH) and monitor the serum calcium feedback mechanism.

polytetrafluoroethylene a material that has become popular for use in vascular access.

precancerous mastopathy apocrine metaplasia with atypia, which carries a similar but slightly decreased risk factor compared to fibrocystic disease.

R

retromammary one of the three well-defined layers of the breast consisting of fat lobules separated anteriorly from the mammary layer by the deep connective tissue plane and posteriorly by the fascia over the pectoralis major.

S

sarcoma breast tumors that arise from the supportive or connective tissues.

decidua capsularis   endometrial membrane covering the gestational sac.

decidua parietalis   membrane that lines the endometrial cavity during pregnancy.

dermoid cyst   one of the more common ovarian tumors with mixed components.

dolichocephaly   fetal head shape that is flattened in the antero-posterior plane and elongated in the frontal-occipital plane. Dolichocephaly is determined by the cephalic index. When present, the biparietal diameter is erroneous for predicting fetal age.

double set-up exam   examination performed at delivery in a patient with vaginal bleeding and suspected placenta previa, whereby a digital exam is performed in the operating room. When previa is confirmed, a cesarean delivery is immediately performed.

dyzygotic twinning   twinning resulting from fertilization of two separate ova (fraternal twins). Each fetus will have a separate placenta and chorionic and amniotic sacs.

E

endometriosis   a common condition in which ectopic endometrium can occur throughout the body. It is usually found on the ovaries, external uterus, and scattered over peritoneal surfaces, especially in the dependent .

epignathus   teratoma arising from the oral cavity and pharynx.

estimated date of confinement (EDC)   the estimated day of delivery as determined by the last missed menstrual period.

ethmocephaly   form of holoprosencephaly in which a rudimentary proboscis-like nose is located between two closely spaced orbits with partial or complete absence of the ethmoid structures.

eventration   abnormal thinning of the diaphragm due to elevation of portions of the diaphragm. May resemble a diaphragmatic hernia sonographically.

F

femur length (FL)   measurement of diaphysis of femur used to determine fetal age and limb growth.

fetal acrania   abnormal brain development with an associated cranial defect in the skull.

fetal microcephalus   a condition marked by an abnormally small fetal calvarium.

fetoscopy   ultrasound-guided fetal surgical procedure performed using a fiberoptic fetoscope to aspirate fetal blood from umbilical cord vessels, for examination of minute anatomic structures, or to biopsy fetal tissue. Certain blood and biochemical disorders can be detected.

fibroids   the most common gynecologic tumor; also termed "leiomyomas" or "myoma."

fundus   the dome-like top of the uterus.

G

Gartner's duct cysts   large, broad ligament cysts that are continuous with the lateral walls of the vagina.

gastroschisis   paraumbilical abdominal wall defect in which uncontained abdominal organs protrude into the amniotic cavity. Frequent association with intrauterine growth retardation and gastrointestinal complications.

genetic scan   see **level II scan**.

gestational sac   the first structure to be identified on early obstetrical ultrasound examination, it is a cystic ring-like structure that occupies the fundus or mid-portion of the uterus.

growth adjusted sonar age   the growth interval compared to average growth using two measurements of the fetus, one between 20 and 26 weeks, the next between 31 and 33 weeks.

H

head circumferene (HC)   measurement of cranial circumference obtained at level of thalamus. Measurement used to assess fetal age and cranial growth.

hemolysis   breakdown of red blood cells in response to an Rh antibody, resulting in fetal anemia.

hemoperitoneum   blood within the peritoneal cavity.

heterozygous achondroplasia   short-limbed dysplasia that manifests in the second trimester of pregnancy. Conversion abnormality of cartilage to bone affecting the epiphyseal growth centers. Extremities are markedly shortened at birth with a normal trunk and frequent enlargement of the head.

holoprosencephaly   cranial abnormality in which the forebrain (prosencephalon) fails to divide or partially divides into cerebral hemispheres or lobes. Alobar, semi-lobar, and lobar forms may occur. Varying facial anomalies may affect orbital spacing (varying degrees of hypotelorism) and formation of the nose, lips, and palate.

homozygous achondroplasia   short-limbed dwarfism affecting fetuses of achondroplastic parents.

human chorionic gonadotropin (HCG)   hormone manufactured by the trophoblastic cells that supply estrogen and progesterone for the pregnancy. HCG is detected in the urine of pregnant women.

hydranencephaly   congenital absence of the cerebral hemispheres due to an occlusion of the carotid arteries. Midbrain structures are present, while fluid replaces cerebral tissue.

hydrocele   congenital collection of serous fluid within the scrotal sac.

hydrocephalus   ventriculomegaly in the neonate. Abnormal accumulation of cerebrospinal fluid within the cerebral ventricles, resulting in compression and frequent destruction of brain tissue.

hydrometrocolpos   abnormality of female genital tract in which there is an abnormal collection of fluid within the uterus and vagina. Frequent association with malformations of the genital tract.

hydrops   condition marked by excessive accumulation of fluid (serous) in the fetal tissues (characterized according to location: ascites, edema, anasarca). Associated with fetuses with severe immune sensitization (RH isoimmunization) or from nonimmune conditions.

hyperstimulation syndrome   a condition that occurs when the ovaries continue to enlarge after ovulation.

hypertelorism   abnormally wide-spaced orbits usually found in conjunction with congenital anomalies and mental retardation.

hypophosphatasia   congenital condition characterized by decreased mineralization of the bones resulting in "ribbon-like" and bowed limbs, underossified cranium, and compression of the chest. Early death often occurs.

hypotelorism   abnormally closely spaced orbits. Association with holoprosencephaly, chromosomal and central nervous system disorders, and cleft palate.

I

immune   resistance to a disease or condition.

implantation bleed   bleeding as a result of implantation of the gestational sac.

incomplete abortion   incomplete expulsion of the products of conception from the uterus.

inevitable abortion   abortion destined to occur due to rupture of the membranes and dilatation of the cervix.

insulin-dependent diabetic   diabetic pregnancy that requires insulin control in patients who have diabetes mellitus prior to conception.

intrapartum period of time during labor and delivery.

intrauterine growth retardation (IUGR) a decreased rate of fetal growth, usually a fetal weight below the 10th percentile for a given gestational age.

isoimmunization blood group incompatibility that occurs when fetal red blood cells enter the maternal blood. Maternal antibodies cross the placenta and destroy fetal red blood cells.

L

level II scan comprehensive sonographic examination of the fetus for exclusion, confirmation, or follow-up of a congenital anomaly. Systematic study of fetal organ systems.

leioyomata see **fibroids**.

M

macrocephaly enlargement of the fetal cranium as a result of ventriculomegaly.

macrosomia abnormally large fetus above the 90th percentile for weight at any given gestational age. Macrosomia results from maternal diabetes mellitus and nonendocrine syndromes.

macrosomia index chest diameter—biparietal diameter.

mean a statistical description of the average value of a given parameter.

Meigs syndrome a benign condition consisting of massive ascites and pleural effusion.

meningocele open spinal defect characterized by the protrusion of the spinal meninges.

meningomyelocele open spinal defect characterized by the protrusion of meninges and spinal cord through the defect, usually within a meningeal sac.

menometrorrhagia irregular menstrual bleeding.

menorrhagia heavy menstrual bleeding.

microcephalus abnormally small fetal cranium with frequent association with mental retardation.

micrognathia abnormally small chin. Commonly associated with other fetal anomalies.

missed abortion pregnancy in which there is death of the fetus. In missed abortion, the products of conception remain within the uterus for at least 8 weeks.

monozygotic twinning twinning that occurs when a single fertilized egg divides (identical twins).

myomata see **fibroids**.

N

nabothian cysts cysts consisting of inspissated secretions along the canal and margin of the portio vaginalis.

neonatal period of time, in terms of the infant, immediately after birth and to the 28th day of life.

nonimmune hydrops condition in which fetal hydrops occurs, which is unassociated with fetomaternal blood group compatibility.

non-insulin-dependent diabetic diabetes that presents during pregnancy in patients without a history of diabetes (gestational diabetes). These pregnancies are most often regulated by diet, although insulin may be required to maintain blood glucose levels.

non-stress test (NST) electronic fetal heart rate monitoring that studies the ability of the fetal heart to accelerate with fetal movements. The NST is used to screen for fetal distress. Abnormal NST tests are typically followed by an oxytocin challenge test (OCT).

O

oculodentodigital dysplasia disorder marked by craniosynostosis, hypertelorism, dental abnormalities and fusion of the digits.

oligohydramnios reduction in amniotic fluid within the uterine cavity which is commonly associated with severe renal disease, intrauterine growth retardation, premature rupture of the membranes, and post-term gestation.

omphalocele anterior abdominal wall defect in which abdominal organs (liver, bowel, stomach) are atypically located within the umbilical cord. Highly associated with cardiac, central nervous system, renal, and chromosomal anomalies.

osteogenesis imperfecta metabolic disorder affecting the fetal collagen system leading to varying forms of bone disease. Intrauterine bone fractures, shortened long bones, poorly mineralized calvaria and compression of the chest may be found in Type II forms.

oxytocin challenge test (OCT) electronic fetal heart rate monitoring which evaluates the fetal heart rate during uterine contractions (induced by administration of oxytocin or using nipple-stimulation method).

P

placenta previa implantation of the placenta close to or over the internal cervical os. Types include complete or total, partial, marginal, or low-lying.

    complete or total previa placenta completely covers the cervical os.

    low-lying placenta placenta implants in the lower uterine segment but does not approach the os.

    marginal previa placental edge is at the margin of the os.

    partial previa placenta partially covers the cervical os.

placental abruption the placenta separates from its site of implantation in the uterus before delivery of the fetus.

polydactyly anomalies of the hands or feet in which there is an addition of a digit. May be found in association with certain skeletal dysplasias.

polyhydramnios excessive amount of amniotic fluid, which may be associated with fetal anomalies, diabetic pregnancies, and Rh incompatibility.

prolapsed cord occurs after the rupture of amniotic membranes. The umbilical cord falls down into the vagina through the cervix. The cord is then susceptible to complete occlusion.

pseudogestational sac (decidual cast) accumulation of fluid within the endometrial cavity in ectopic gestations.

pubic symphysis a palpable midline landmark immediately anterior to the bladder, which is anterior to the uterine corpus.

pyosalpinx a pus-filled tube resulting from an infection in the tubes most commonly from vaginal contamination and cervical ascent of bacteria.

R

renal agenesis congenital absence of one or both kidneys. Bilateral renal agenesis results in Potter's malformations and death of the newborn.

S

septic abortion an infected abortion.

serous cystadenomas simple cystic tumors usually occurring in cycling women.

shoulder dystocia delivery complication that can occur when a macrosomic fetus is delivered vaginally. There is difficulty in delivering the large shoulders after the head has passed through the vagina. Brachial plexus nerve injuries can occur.

spina bifida neural tube defect of the spine in which the dorsal vertebra (vertebral arches) fail to fuse together, allowing the protrusion of meninges and/or spinal cord through the defect. Spina bifida occulta (skin-covered defect of the spine without protrusion of meninges or cord) and spina bifida cystica (open spinal defect marked by sac containing protruding meninges and/or cord).

spina bifida occulta   closed defect of the spine without protrusion of meninges or spinal cord. Alpha-fetoprotein analysis will not detect these lesions.

standard deviation (SD)   degree to which a given value deviates from the mean. Measures the variability of a distribution of parameters. In ultrasound, 2 standard deviations above or below the mean are considered outside of the normal range of error.

struma ovarii   a teratoma composed of thyroid tissue.

symmetrical IUGR   an infant small in all parameters caused by low genetic growth potential, intrauterine infection, severe maternal malnutrition, chromosomal aberration, and severe congenital anomalies.

T

tachyarrhythmia   rapid beating of the heart, with rates in excess of 160, usually in the 200 to 240 range.

thanatophoric dysplasia   lethal short-limbed dwarfism characterized by a marked reduction in the length of the long bones, pear-shaped chest, soft-tissue redundancy, and frequent clover-leaf skull deformity and ventriculomegaly.

threatened abortion   pregnancy of less than 20 weeks complicated by bleeding or cramping. Expulsion of the products of conception may or may not occur.

tocolysis   regimen using medications to stop premature labor.

transverse presentation   fetus assumes a transverse orientation within the uterus.

tubo-ovarian abscess   the loculation of pus resulting from the adhesive, edematous, inflamed serosa becoming further adhered to the ovary.

twin-to-twin transfusion   the arterial blood of one twin is pumped into the venous septum of the other twin due to an arteriovenous shunt within the placenta.

U

urethral atresia   absence of the normal opening of the urethra resulting in massive enlargement of the urinary bladder.

V

ventriculomegaly   abnormal accumulation of cerebrospinal fluid within the cerebral ventricles resulting in dilatation of the ventricles. Compression of developing brain tissue and brain damage may result. Commonly associated with additional fetal anomalies.

version   manual attempt to convert a breech fetus to a cephalic presentation to allow vaginal delivery. External cephalic version is performed through the abdomen wall using ultrasound as a guide. Version is also used to convert the second twin (breech) during the delivery of twin fetuses.

Y

yolk sac (Vittleline duct)   sac-like structure of early pregnancy, which provides nutrition for the embryo.

**PART SIX
CARDIOLOGY**

A

accessory veins   intercepting veins.

aneurysm   a sac formed by the dilatation of the walls of an artery or a vein and filled with blood. Aneurysms may occur in any major blood vessel and include the following varieties: *berry,* a small saccular aneurysm of a cerebral artery, which

may rupture and cause a subdural hemorrhage; *cardiac,* which may follow coronary occlusion; *dissecting,* in which blood is in between the coats of an artery; *endogenous,* which is due to disease of the coats of a vessel; *exogenous,* which is due to a wound; *false,* in which all the coats of the vessel are ruptured and blood is retained in the surrounding tissues; *intramural,* in which the blood is within the wall of the vessel; *mycotic,* which is produced by the growth of microorganisms in a blood vessel wall; *true,* in which the sac is formed by the arterial walls, one of which is unbroken (also called circumscribed); *valvular,* which is an aneurysm between the layers of a heart valve; and *ventricular,* which is dilatation of a ventricle of the heart.

angialgia   pain in a vessel; also known as angiodynia.

angina pectoris   paroxysmal thoracic pain characterized by a feeling of suffocation and radiation of pain down the arm.

anonyma   one of two large veins (right and left) that unite to form the superior vena cava. (The innominate artery is sometimes referred to as the anonyma).

aorta   the largest artery in the body. It distributes blood to the lower part of the body as the thoracic aorta and abdominal aorta and sends branches to the upper extremities from the ascending aorta.

aortic arch   a continuation of the ascending aorta. It has three branches: the innominate or brachiocephalic trunk, the left common carotid artery, and the left subclavian artery.

aortic arch, hypoplasia   underdevelopment of the aortic arch.

aortic arch, persistent, right   aorta develops from the fourth right embryonic aortic arch; may be associated with dextroposition of the aorta as in tetralogy of Fallot.

aortic insufficiency   impairment of the aorta with insufficient circulation of the blood.

aortitis   inflammation of the aorta.

apex   the rounded extremity of the heart pointing forward and downward and to the left. The plural form is apices.

arrhythmia   variation from normal rhythm of heartbeat. This may be sinus arrhythmia; extrasystole; gallop rhythm; heart block; atrial or ventricular fibrillation and flutter; or paroxysmal tachycardia.

arterial valves   semi-lunar valves of the aorta and pulmonary trunk.

arteriole   a tiny arterial branch.

arteritis   inflammation of an artery.

atrial appendage   a continuation of a part of the left and right upper part of the atria. (Older literature refers to these appendages as auricular appendages).

atrio   a term referring to the atrium.

atrioventricular node   a node at the base of the interatrial septum. It is made up of a mass of Purkinje's fibers and forms the beginning of the bundle of His. This node is also called Aschoff's and Tawara's.

atrioventricular valve   valve between the atrium and ventricle of the heart. The left valve is called the bicuspid or mitral valve, and the right valve is called the tricuspid valve.

atrium   the upper chamber on either side of the heart. The right atrium receives blood from the inferior and superior vena cava; the left receives arterial blood from the pulmonary veins. The plural form is atria.

axillary artery   branch of the subclavian artery that distributes to the axilla, chest, shoulder, and upper extremity.

axillary vein   continuation of the basilic vein in the upper extremity.

azygos   front and right side of the lumbar vertebrae.

B

bacteremia   bacteria in the blood.

bacterial endocarditis   bacterial infection of the endocardium.

bicuspid valve   a valve made up of two cusps, the anterior (aortic) and posterior (mural). Actually there are four cusps, including the two small commissural cusps, which are never complete in that they do not reach the anulus, or fibrous ring, around the valve and are incompletely separated from each other. This valve is also known as the mitral valve. It is located between the left atrium and left ventricle.

block   this may be atrioventricular, sinoatrial, bundle-branch, or interventricular. In all cases there is a blockage or obstruction to circulation.

brachial artery   branch of the axillary artery that distributes to the arm. The deep brachial distributes to the inner arm structures.

bradycardia   slow pulse or heartbeat.

bronchial artery   a branch of either the aorta or the intercostal artery that distributes to the lungs.

bundle of His   a muscular band containing nerve fibers. It arises from the atrioventricular node and connects the atria with the ventricles. It conveys stimuli from the atria to the ventricle and is sometimes called the atrioventricular bundle, or the AV bundle.

C

card- and cardio-   terms referring to the heart.

cardiac arrest   stoppage of the heartbeat.

cardiac hypertrophy   enlargement of the heart.

cardiac murmurs   any adventitious sound heard over the region of the heart; may be blowing, cardiorespiratory, diastolic, harsh, presystolic, rough, or systolic.

cardiac sounds   these may be diminished, intensified, reduplicated.

cardiac veins   referred to as small, great, middle, and anterior veins of the heart; also known as venae cordis, magna, media, minimae, and parva.

cardialgia   heart pain; another name is cardiodynia.

cardiectasis   dilatation of the heart.

carditis   inflammation of the heart.

carotid artery   branch of the innominate artery (right common carotid) or the aortic arch (left common carotid) that distributes to the right or left side of the head. The common carotid further divides into the internal, distributing to the inner structures of the head, and the external, distributing to the external structures of the head.

chordae tendineae   tendinous strings resembling cords that act like the shrouds of a parachute to keep the cusps in position when closed. They extend from the cusps of valves to the papillary muscles of the heart.

coarctation of aorta   diffuse involvement of the aortic isthmus with narrowing and constriction of the aorta.

congestive heart failure   sudden fatal cessation of the heart's action.

conus arteriosus   upper and anterior angle of the right ventricle from which the pulmonary trunk arises superiorly and passes backward and slightly upward.

cor   Latin term for heart.

cor pulmonale   heart disease produced by disease of the lungs or of their blood vessels; pulmonary heart disease.

coronary arteries and veins   blood vessels of the heart.

coronary artery   a left or right artery that arises from a coronary sinus in the heart and distributes to either the left ventricle and atrium or the right ventricle and atrium.

coronary heart disease   disease of the heart with involvement of the coronary vessels.

coronary vein   great cardiac vein of the heart and its branches.

cusp   a triangular segment of the cardiac valve; also called leaflet. Cusp means point.

D

dextrocardia   the heart is displaced to the right side of the thoracic cavity.

dextroposition, aorta   the aorta is displaced to the right.

diastole   dilatation or stage of dilatation of the heart, especially that of the ventricles.

ductus arteriosus   a channel in the fetus for circulation from the pulmonary artery to the aorta. This should close after birth, but if it does not, it creates a patent ductus arteriosus, a congenital anomaly.

ductus venosus   a fetal vein that connects the umbilical vein with the inferior vena cava.

E

Eisenmenger's complex   defects of the interventricular septum with dilatation of the pulmonary artery, hypertrophy of the right ventricle, and dextroposition or dextrolocation of the aorta.

electrocardiogram   a graphic tracing of the electric current produced by contraction of the heart muscle.

embolism   the sudden blocking of an artery or vein by a clot or obstruction that has been brought to its place by the bloodstream. The embolus can also be air.

endarteritis   inflammation of the tunica intima of an artery.

endarteritis deformans   chronic endarteritis characterized by fatty degeneration of the arterial tissues, with the formation of deposits of lime salts.

endarteritis obliterans   endarteritis followed by collapse and closure of smaller branches.

endocarditis   infection or inflammation of the endocardium. It may be acute bacterial, subacute bacterial, mycotic (caused by a fungus), verrucous, rheumatic, or septic (malignant).

endocardium   inner lining of the heart.

epicardium   external covering of the heart; it is a portion of the pericardium.

F

fibroma   a tumor made up of fibrous connective tissue.

foramen ovale   opening between the atria in fetal life. It is normally closed after birth.

H

hemangioma   a blood tumor.

hematemesis   vomiting blood.

hematopericardium or hemopericardium   effusion of blood within the pericardium.

hematoperitoneum   effusion of blood within the peritoneum.

hemothorax   collection of blood in the thoracic cavity.

hypertensive heart disease   high blood pressure.

I

infarction   the formation of an infarct (i.e., an area of coagulation necrosis in a tissue caused by local anemia resulting from the obstruction of circulation to the area); may be embolic or thrombotic.

innominate artery   branch of the aortic arch that distributes to the right side of the head, neck, and upper limbs; also called brachiocephalic trunk.

innominate vein   a vein corresponding to the innominate artery; also called anonyma.

intercostal   ribs and chest region.

Interventricular   between ventricles.

Interventricular artery   a branch of the left or right coronary artery that distributes to the heart ventricles or their septa.

M

mammary artery   an internal artery that is a branch of the subclavian artery and distributes to the anterior abdominal wall and mediastinal structures.

mammary vein   internal vein of the breast.

mediastinal   mediastinum.

mitral insufficiency   impairment of mitral valve with malfunctioning.

mitral valve   see **bicuspid valve**.

myocarditis   inflammation of heart muscle.

myocardium   middle muscular layer of the heart.

N

nodes   see **sinoatrial** and **atrioventricular nodes**.

O

oblique, left atrium   atrium.

occlusion   obstruction of a blood vessel; may be caused by a thrombus or an embolus.

P

pacemaker   sinoatrial node that initiates the heartbeat and regulates the rate of contraction.

palpitation   rapid action of the heart felt by the patient.

panarteritis   inflammation of several arteries.

patent ductus arteriosus   an open duct in the heart, which in fetal life was a channel from the pulmonary artery to the aorta and should have closed at birth.

periarteritis nodosa   inflammation of the coats of small- and medium-sized arteries with changes around the vessels and symptoms of systemic infection.

pericardiac   heart.

pericarditis   inflammation or infection of a membrane containing the heart.

pericardium   membrane surrounding the heart.

phlebitis   inflammation of a vein.

phlebo-   combining form referring to vein.

phrenic arteries   the inferior phrenic artery is a branch of the abdominal aorta and distributes to the diaphragm and adrenals. The superior phrenic arteries are branches of the thoracic aorta and distribute to the upper surface of the vertebral portion of the diaphragm.

phrenic veins   anterior and superior veins of the diaphragm.

plexus   network of veins. (May also refer to nerves and lymphatics).

polyarteritis   inflammation of several arteries.

polyserositis   inflammation of the serous membranes with serous effusion.

portal   liver, eventually forming sinusoids of liver.

pulmonary   arteries that originate in the conus arteriosus and distribute to the lungs.

pulmonary, right and left   vessels that return blood to the heart from the lungs.

pulmonary stenosis   narrowing of the opening between the pulmonary artery and the right ventricle. The stenosis may be at the site of the valve, just prevalvular, or postvalvular (arterial); also called pulmonic stenosis.

pulmonary valve   valve at the base of the pulmonary artery; also called semi-lunar valve.

pulse variation   may be alternating (pulsus alternans); bigeminal (occurring in two's); bounding; bradycardiac, irregular; plateau (a pulse that slowly rises and is sustained); running; tachycardiac; thready; trembling; undulating; and vibrating (jerky).

R

rhabdomyoma   a malignant tumor composed of myoma and sarcoma combined.

S

semi-lunar valve   pulmonary or aortic valve.

septal defects, atrial or ventricular   these may be interatrial, with defects located between the atria, or interventricular, with defects located between the ventricles.

septicemia   presence of pathogenic bacteria or toxins in the blood.

sinoatrial node   a well-defined collection of cells at the junction of the superior vena cava with the terminal band of the right atrium. It is called the pacemaker of the heart.

subclavian arteries   branch of the innominate artery (right subclavian) or the aortic arch (left subclavian) that distributes to the neck, upper limbs, thoracic wall, spinal cord, brain, and meninges.

subclavian veins   right and left veins of the arms and upper extremity.

subcostal   branch of the thoracic aorta that distributes to the region below the twelfth rib in the abdominal wall.

superior and inferior vena cava   large veins that return blood to the heart. The superior vena cava returns blood from the upper extremities, and the inferior vena cava returns it from the lower extremities.

systole   a period of heart contraction, especially of the ventricles. Atrial systole precedes the true, or ventricular, systole.

T

tachycardia   characterized by a fast pulse or heartbeat.

teratoma   a tumor composed of disorderly arrangement of tissue, the result of an embryonic defect. Teratomas also occur in the ovary.

tetralogy of Fallot   this includes four anomalies as follows: pulmonic stenosis; dextroposition of the aorta; a large interventricular septal defect; and marked hypertrophy of the right ventricle; also called Fallot's tetrad.

thromboangiitis   inflammation of the intima of a blood vessel with thrombi or clots. When obliterans is added, it means inflammatory and obliterative disease of the blood vessels.

thrombophlebitis   inflammation or infection of a vein with clot formation.

transposition of the aorta and pulmonary artery   aorta arising from the right ventricle and the pulmonary artery from the left ventricle; also called transposition of the great vessels.

tricuspid incompetency   impairment of the tricuspid valve, with incompetent functioning.

tricuspid valve   a valve between the right atrium and the right ventricle, consisting of an anterior, a medial (septal), and one or two posterior cusps. The depth of the commissures between cusps is variable, never reaching the anulus (fibrous ring). Cusps are only incompletely separated from each other.

V

valves   structures in a canal or passage that prevent the reflux of contents. The valves in the heart are the aortic (semi-lunar); the atrioventricular (mitral and tricuspid); and pulmonic (semi-lunar). Valves also occur in veins.

varicose veins   swollen veins.

varicose veins   clotted blood in the veins, usually in the lower extremities.

venae vasorum small veins that return blood from the walls of blood vessels themselves.

veno term referring to vein.

venules small veins.

PART SEVEN
PERIPHERAL VASCULAR AND VASCULAR
SONOGRAPHY

A

angle correction a method of electronically compensating for the curvature of a vessel when using a steerable pulsed Doppler to obtain an accurate angle and accurate blood flow velocity.

antegrade flow flow toward the Doppler transducer face.

D

Doppler (equipment) a sonographic device that allows the measurement of moving media such as blood by measuring the Doppler shift of the reflected ultrasound beam.

Q

quadrature interface a Doppler feature that electronically isolates antegrade and retrograde signals and that allows displaying directional signals simultaneously in their respective directions and respective strengths.

R

retrograde flow flow away from the Doppler transducer face.

S

sample depth the variable depth at which a pulsed Doppler sample can be taken.

sample volume a Doppler gate on a pulsed Doppler that allows a specific area of the flow in a blood vessel to be sampled. The sample volume can be varied by the user from a small size to a large size.

spectral analysis a method of analyzing and displaying the frequency and flow components of a Doppler signal.

spectral broadening a change in the spectral width, which increases with flow disturbance. It can be fairly narrow with a prominent spectral window in a normal waveform, or it can be spread out and widened with filling in or absence of the window when flow is turbulent or disturbed.

spectral width during peak systole, the distance between the outer border at the peak of the waveform and the upper border of the spectral window.

spectral window a relatively clear area within the Doppler spectral waveform indicating a lack of slow-moving blood cells.

V

vector line an adjustable line seen at the sample volume, which is adjusted to obtain a Doppler vessel angle correction with a pulsed Doppler.

W

window see **spectral window**.

Z

zero-crossing circuit a Doppler circuit that averages antegrade and retrograde flow signals into a net flow readout on a chart recorder.

Bibliography

PHYSICS OF DIAGNOSTIC ULTRASOUND

Goldstein A: Range ambiguities in real-time ultrasound, J Clin Ultrasound 9:85, 1981.

Morgan CL, Trought WS, Clark WM, et al: Principles and applications of a dynamically focused array real time ultrasound system, J Clin Ultrasound 6:385, 1978.

Schwenker RP: Film selection for computed tomography and ultrasound video imaging. In Haus AG, editor: The physics of medical imaging, 1979, AAPM.

Winsberg F: Real-time scanners: a review, Med Ultrasound 3:99, 1979.

CROSS-SECTIONAL AND SAGITTAL ANATOMY

Anderson PD: Clinical anatomy and physiology for allied health sciences, Philadelphia, 1976, WB Saunders Co.

Crafts KC: A textbook of human anatomy, ed 2, New York, 1979, John Wiley & Sons.

Hagen-Ansert SL: The anatomy workbook, Philadelphia, 1986, JB Lippincott Co.

Lyons EA: A color atlas of sectional anatomy, St Louis, 1978, CV Mosby.

Snell RS: Clinical anatomy for medical students, Boston, 1973, Little, Brown & Co.

Thompson JS: Core textbook of anatomy, Philadelphia, 1977, JB Lippincott Co.

ABDOMINAL DOPPLER

Arima M, Takahara S, Ihara H, et al: Predictability of renal allograft prognosis during rejection crisis by ultrasonic Doppler flow technique, Urology 19:389-394, 1982.

Athey PA and Tamez L: Lateral decubitus position for demonstration of the aortic bifurcation, J Clin Ultrasound 7:154-155, 1979.

Berland LL, Lawson TL, Adams MB, et al: Evaluation of renal transplants with pulsed Doppler duplex sonography, J Ultrasound Med 1:215, 1982.

Berland LL, Lawson TL, and Foley WD: Porta hepatis: sonographic discrimination of bile ducts from arteries with pulsed Doppler with new anatomic criteria, AJR 138:833, 1982.

Cooper RA, Picker RH, Fulton AJ, et al: The ultrasonic appearance of the liver in hepatic venous outflow obstruction (Budd-Chiari syndrome), J Clin Ultrasound 10:35, 1982.

Cooperman M, Martin EW Jr, Keith LM, et al: Use of Doppler ultrasound in intestinal surgery, Am J Surg 138:856, 1979.

Derchi LE, Biggi E, Cicio GR, et al: Aneurysms of the splenic artery: noninvasive diagnosis by pulsed Doppler sonography, J Ultrasound Med 3:41, 1984.

DiCandio G, Campatelli A, Mosca F, et al: Ultrasound detection of unusual spontaneous portosystemic shunts associated with uncomplicated portal hypertension, J Ultrasound Med 4:297, 1985.

Fleischer AC, James AE Jr, MacDonnell RC Jr, et al: Sonography of renal transplant patients, CRC Crit Rev Diag Imaging 18:197, 1981.

Foley WD, Gleysteen JJ, Lawson TL, et al: Dynamic computed tomography and pulsed Doppler ultrasonography in the evaluation of splenorenal shunt patency, J Comput Assist Tomogr 7:106, 1983.

Foley WD, Varma RR, Lawson TL, et al: Dynamic computed tomography and duplex ultrasonography: adjuncts to arterial portography, J Comput Assist Tomogr 7:77, 1983.

Garg AK, Houston AB, Laing JM, et al: Positioning of umbilical arterial catheters with ultrasound, Arch Dis Child 58:1017, 1983.

George L, Waldman JD, Cohen ML, et al: Umbilical vascular catheters: localization by two-dimensional echocardio/aortography, Pediatr Cardiol 2:237, 1982.

Gill RW: Measurement of blood flow by ultrasound: accuracy and sources of error, Ultrasound Med Biol 11:625, 1985.

Hobson RW, Wright CB, O'Donnell JA, et al: Determination of intestinal viability by Doppler ultrasound, Arch Surg 114:165, 1979.

Hobson RW, Wright CB, Rich NM, et al: Assessment of colonic ischemia during aortic surgery by Doppler ultrasound, J Surg Res 20:231, 1976.

Kane RA and Katz SG: The spectrum of sonographic findings in portal hypertension: a subject review and new observations, Radiology 142:453, 1982.

Loh CL, Atkinson P, and Halliwell M: The differentiation of bile ducts and blood vessels using a pulsed Doppler system, Ultrasound Med Biol 4:37, 1978.

Miller VE, and Berland LL: Pulsed Doppler duplex sonography and CT of portal vein thrombosis AJR 145:73, 1985.

Mintz GS, Kotler MN, Parry WR, et al: Real-time inferior vena caval ultrasonography: normal and abnormal findings and its use in assessing right-heart function, Circulation 64:1018, 1981.

Oppenheimer DA and Carroll BA: Ultrasonic localization of neonatal umbilical catheters, Radiology 142:781, 1982.

Oppenheimer DA, Carroll BA and Garth KE: Ultrasonic detection of complications following umbilical arterial catheterization in the neonate, Radiology 145:667, 1982.

Pasto ME, Kurtz, AB, Jarrell BE, et al: The Kimray-Greenfield filter: evaluation by duplex real-time/pulsed Doppler ultrasound, Radiology 148:223, 1983.

Reinitz ER, Goldman MH, and Sais J: Evaluation of transplant renal artery blood flow by Doppler sound-spectrum analysis, Arch Surg 118:415, 1983.

Rifkin MD, Pasto ME, and Goldberg BB: Duplex Doppler examination in renal disease eval

Sigel B, Flanigan DP, Schuler JJ, et al: Imaging ultrasound in the intraoperative diagnosis of vascular defects, J Ultrasound Med 2:337, 1983.

Smith DF and Lawson TL: Abdominal applications of Doppler ultrasound. In Vascular and Doppler ultrasound, New York, 1984, Churchill Livingstone.

Taylor KJW and Burns PN: Duplex Doppler scanning in the pelvis and abdomen, Ultrasound Med Biol 11:643, 1985.

Taylor KJW, Burns PN, Woodcock JP, et al: Blood flow in deep abdominal and pelvic vessels: ultrasonic pulsed-Doppler analysis, Radiology 154:487, 1985.

Thuroff JW, Frohneberg D, Riedmiller R, et al: Localization of segmental arteries in renal surgery by Doppler sonography, J Urol 127:863, 1982.

ABDOMEN AND VASCULAR

Ackroyd N et al: Duplex scanning of the portal vein and portasystemic shunts, Surgery 99(5):591, 1986.

Anderson PD: Clinical anatomy and physiology for allied health sciences, Philadelphia, 1976, WB Saunders Co.

Athey PA and Tamez L: Lateral decubitus position for demonstration of the aortic bifurcation, J Clin Ultrasound 7:154, 1979.

Carlsen EN and Filly RA: Newer ultrasonographic anatomy in the upper abdomen. I. The portal and hepatic venous anatomy, J Clin Ultrasound 4:85, 1976.

Creagh-Barry M et al: The value of oblique scans in the ultrasonic examination of the abdominal aorta, Clin Radiol 37(3): 239, 1986.

Falkoff GE et al: Hepatic artery pseudoaneurysm: diagnosis with real-time and pulsed Doppler ultrasound, Radiology 158(1):55, 1986.

Filly RA and Goldberg BB: Abnormal vessels. In Abdominal gray scale ultrasonography, New York, 1977, John Wiley & Sons.

Filly RA and Goldberg BB: Normal vessels. In Abdominal gray scale ultrasonography. New York, 1977, John Wiley & Sons.

Gansbeke D et al: Sonographic features of portal vein thrombosis, AJR 144(4):749, 1985.

Gooding GA et al: Obstruction of the superior vena cava or subclavian veins: sonographic diagnosis, Radiology 159(3):663, 1986.

Gooding GAW: Ultrasonography of the iliac arteries, Radiology 135:161, 1980.

Gooding GAW and Effeney DJ: Ultrasound of femoral artery aneurysms, AJR 134:477, 1980.

Hill MC et al: Ultrasonography in portal hypertension, Clin Gastroenterol 14(1):83, 1985.

Huhta JC et al: Cross-sectional echocardiographic diagnosis of azygos continuation of the inferior vena cava, Cathet Cardiovasc Diagn 10(3):221, 1984.

Imura T et al: Noninvasive ultrasonic measurement of the elastic properties of the human abdominal aorta, Cardiovasc Res 20(3):208, 1986.

Isikoff MB and Hill MC: Sonography of the renal arteries: left lateral decubitus position, AJR 134:1177, 1980.

Jager K et al: Measurement of mesenteric blood flow by duplex scanning, J Vasc Surg 3(3):462, 1986.

Kidambi H et al: Ultrasonic demonstration of superior mesenteric and splenoportal venous thrombosis, J Clin Ultrasound 14(3):199, 1986.

King PS et al: The anechoic crescent in abdominal aortic aneurysms: not a sign of dissection, AJR 146(2):345, 1986.

Laing FC et al: Ultrasound identification of portal vein gas, J Clin Ultrasound 12(8):512, 1984.

Leopold GR: Ultrasonic abdominal aortography, Radiology 96:9, 1970.

Leopold GR, Goldberger L, and Bernstein E: Ultrasonic detection and evaluation of abdominal aortic aneurysms, Surgery 72:939, 1972.

Needleman L et al: Vascular ultrasonography: abdominal applications, Radiol Clin North Am 24(3):461, 1986.

Qamar MI et al: Transcutaneous Doppler ultrasound measurements of superior mesenteric artery blood flow in man, GUT 27(1):100, 1986.

Rahim N et al: Ultrasound demonstration of variations in normal portal vein diameter with posture, Br J Radiol 58(688):313, 1985.

Smith HJ et al: Ultrasonic assessment of abdominal venous return. II. Volume blood flow in the inferior vena cava and portal vein, Acta Radiol 27(1):23, 1986.

LIVER

Albarelli JN, and Springer GE: A technical approach to evaluating the jaundiced patient, Semin Ultrasound 1:96, 1980.

Bree RL and Silver TM: Differential diagnosis of hypoechoic and anechoic masses with gray scale sonography: new observations, J Clin Ultrasound 7:249, 1979.

Broderick TW, Gosink BB, Menuck L, et al: Echographic and radionuclide detection of hepatoma, Radiology 135:149, 1980.

Callen PW, Filly RA, and DeMartini WJ: The left portal vein: a possible source of confusion on ultrasonograms, Radiology 130:205, 1979.

Cave-Bigley DJ et al: The value of preoperative ultrasound of the liver in colonic and gastric neoplasm, Br J Radiol 58(685):13, 1985.

Cooper D et al: Ultrasound in the diagnosis of jaundice—a review, Med J Aust 143(9):381, 1985.

Del Torso S et al: Echocardiographic findings in the liver in total anomalous pulmonary venous connection, Am J Cardiol 57(4):374, 1986.

Filly RA and Carlsen EN: Newer ultrasonographic anatomy in the upper abdomen. 2. The major systemic veins and arteries, with a special note on localization of the pancreas, J Clin Ultrasound 4:91, 1976.

Filly RA and Laing FC: Anatomic variation of portal venous anatomy in the porta hepatis: ultrasonographic evaluation. J Clin Ultrasound 6:83, 1978.

Freeman MP et al: Regenerating nodules in cirrhosis: sonographic appearance with anatomic correlation, AJR 146(3):533, 1986.

Gosink BB and Leymaster CE: Ultrasonic determination of hepatomegaly, J Clin Ultrasound 9:37, 1981.

Green D et al: Ultrasonography in the jaundiced infant: a new approach, J Ultrasound Med 5(6):323, 1986.

Hillman BJ, D'Orsi, CJ, Smith EH, et al: Ultrasonic appearance of the falciform ligament, AJR 132:205, 1979.

Holm J et al: Accuracy of dynamic ultrasonography in the diagnosis of malignant liver lesions, J Ultrasound Med 5(1):1, 1986.

Hussain SJ: Diagnostic criteria of hydatid disease on hepatic sonography, J Ultrasound Med 4(11):603, 1985.

Ingis DA: Pathophysiology of jaundice—a primer, Semin Ultrasound 1:143, 1980.

Itoh K et al: Acoustic intensity histogram pattern diagnosis of liver diseases, J Clin Ultrasound 13(7):449, 1985.

Kamin PD, Bernadino ME, and Green B: Ultrasound manifestations of hepatocellular carcinoma, Radiology 131:459, 1979.

Kane RA: Ultrasonographic anatomy of the liver and biliary tree, Semin Ultrasound 1:87, 1980.

Kanematsu T et al: The value of ultrasound in the diagnosis and treatment of small hepatocellular carcinoma, Br J Surg 72(1):23, 1985.

Leopold GR: Ultrasonography of jaundice, Radiol Clin North Am 17(1):1979.

Leyton B, Halpern S, Leopold GR, and Hagen SL: Correlation of ultrasound and colloid Scintiscan studies of normal and diseased liver,

Li DK et al: Pseudo perisplenic "fluid collections": a clue to normal liver and spleen echogenic texture, J Ultrasound Med 5(7):397, 1986.

Livraghi T et al: Focal fatty liver change by sonography, Diagn Imaging Clin Med 53(5):226, 1984.

Machi J et al: Detection of unrecognized liver metastases from colorectal cancers by routine use of operative ultrasonography, Dis Colon Rectum 29(6):405, 1986.

Marchal G et al: Correlation of sonographic patterns in liver metastases with histology and microangiography, Invest Radiol 20(1):79, 1985.

Marchal GJ et al: Anechoic halo in solid liver tumors: sonographic, microangiographic and histologic correlation, Radiology 156(2):479, 1985.

Marks WM, Filly RA, and Callen PW: Ultrasonic anatomy of the liver: a review with new applications, J Clin Ultrasound 7:137, 1979.

Menu Y et al: Budd-Chiari syndrome: ultrasound evaluation, Radiology 157(3):761, 1985.

Menu Y et al: Sonographic and computed tomographic evaluation of intrahepatic calculi, AJR 145(3):579, 1985.

Needleman L et al: Sonography of diffuse benign liver disease: accuracy of pattern recognition and grading, AJR 146(5):1011, 1986.

Neiman HL: Hepatocellular causes of jaundice, Semin Ultrasound 1:118, 1980.

Netter F: The digestive system vol 3, Summit NJ, Liver, gallbladder, and pancreas, 1972, Ciba Pharmaceutical Co.

Prando A, Goldstein HM, Bernardino ME, et al: Ultrasonic pseudolesions of the liver, Radiology 130:403, 1979.

Quinn SF et al: Characteristics of sonographic signs of hepatic fatty infiltration, AJR 145(4):753, 1985.

Riddlesberger MM Jr: Diagnostic imaging of the hepatobiliary system in infants and children, J Pediatr Gastroenterol Nurt 3(5):653, 1984.

Sample WF: Normal abdominal anatomy defined by gray scale ultrasound, Radiol Clin North Am 17(1):1979.

Sample WF, Sarti DA, Goldstein LI, et al: Gray scale ultrasonography of the jaundiced patient, Radiology 128:719, 1978.

Scheible W, Gosink BB, and Leopold GR: Gray scale echographic patterns of hepatic metastatic disease, AJR 129:983-987, 1977.

Schkolnik A: Applications of ultrasound in the neonatal abdomen, Radiol Clin North Am 23(1):141, 1985.

Scott WW, Sanders RC, and Siegelman SS: Irregular fatty infiltration of the liver, AJR 135:67, 1980.

Sheu JC et al: Early detection of hepatocellular carcinoma by realtime ultrasonography: a prospective study, Cancer 56(3):660, 1985.

Sheu JC et al: Hepatocellular carcinoma: ultrasound evolution in the early stage, Radiology 155(2):463, 1985.

Simjee AE et al: Serial ultrasound in amoebic liver abscess, Clin Radiol 36(1):61, 1985.

Sukov RJ, Cohen LJ, and Sample WF: Sonography of hepatic amebic abscesses, AJR 134:911, 1980.

Swobodnik W et al: Multiple regular circumscript fatty infiltrations of the liver, J Clin Ultrasound 13(8):577, 1985.

Taylor KJW, editor: Diagnostic ultrasound in gastrointestinal disease, Clin Diagn Ultrasound 1:1979.

Teefey SA et al: Computed tomography and ultrasonography of hepatoma, Clin Radiol 34(4):339, 1986.

Toni R et al: Accessory ultrasonographic findings in chronic liver disease: diameter of splenic and hepatic arteries, fasting gallbladder volume, and course of left portal vein, J Clin Ultrasound 13(9):611, 1985.

Weill F, Eisenscher A, Aucant D, et al: Ultrasonic study of venous patterns in the right hypochrondrium: an anatomical approach to differential diagnosis of obstructive jaundice, J Clin Ultrasound 3:23, 1979.

GALLBLADDER AND THE BILIARY SYSTEM

Albarelli JN, and Springer GE: A technical approach to evaluating the jaundiced patient, Semin Ultrasound 1(2):1980.

Allen-Mersh TG: Does it matter who does ultrasound examination of the gallbladder? Br Med J (Clin Res) 291(6492):389, 1985.

Arger PH: Obstructive jaundice of malignant origin, Semin Ultrasound 1(2):1980.

Behan M and Kazam E: Sonography of the common bile duct: value of the right anterior oblique view, AJR 130:701, 1978.

Chang VH et al: Sonographic measurement of the extrahepatic bile duct before and after retrograde cholangiography, AJR 144(4):753, 1985.

Colletti PM et al: Hepatobiliary imaging in choledocholithiasis: a comparison with ultrasound, Clin Nucl Med 4(7):482, 1986.

Fink-Bennett D et al: The sensitivity of hepatobiliary imaging and real time ultrasonography in the detection of acute cholecystitis, Arch Surg 120(8):904, 1985.

Glancy JJ, Goddard J, and Pearson DE: In vitro demonstration of cholesterol crystals' high echogenicity relative to protein particles, J Clin Ultrasound 8:27, 1980.

Harbin W and Ferrucci JT: Nonoperative management of malignant biliary obstruction: a radiographic alternative, AJR 135:103, 1980.

Herline P et al: Contrast tomography of the gallbladder wall and ultrasonography in the diagnosis of acute cholecystitis, Br J Surg 7(11):850, 1984.

Hopman WP et al: Gallbladder contraction: effects of fatty meals and cholecystokinin, Radiology 157(1):37, 1985.

Ingis DA: Pathophysiology of jaundice, Semin Ultrasound, 1(2):1980.

Kane RA: Ultrasonographic anatomy of the liver and biliary tree, Semin Ultrasound 1(2):1980.

Kane RA: Ultrasonographic diagnosis of gangrenous cholecystitis and empyema of the gallbladder, Radiology 134:191, 1980.

Krook PM, Allen FH, Bush WH et al: Comparison of real time cholecystosonography and oral cholecystography, Radiology 135:145, 1980.

Lafortune M et al: The V-shaped artifact of the gallbladder wall, AJR 147(3):505, 1986.

Laing FC: Biliary dilatation: defining the level and cause by real time ultrasound, Radiology 160(1):39, 1986.

Laing FC et al: Improved visualization of choledocholelithiasis by sonography, AJR 143(5):949, 1984.

Leopold GR, Amberg J, Gosink BB, et al: Gray scale ultrasonic cholecystography: a comparison with conventional radiographic techniques, Radiology 121:445, 1976.

Mindell JJ and Ring BA: Gallbladder wall thickening: ultrasonic findings, Radiology 133:699, 1979.

Norrby S et al: Intravenous cholecystography and ultrasonography in the diagnosis of acute cholecystitis: a prospective comparative study, Acta Chir Scand 151(3):255, 1985.

Sample WF, Sarti DA, Goldstein LI, et al: Grey scale ultrasonography of the jaundiced patient, Radiology 128:719, 1978.

Scheske GA, Cooperberg PL, Cohen MM, et al: Dynamic changes in caliber of the major bile ducts related to obstruction, Radiology 135:215, 1980.

Simeone JF et al: The bile ducts after a fatty meal: further sonographic observations, Radiology 154(3):763, 1985.

Sukov RJ, Sample WF, Sarti DA, et al: Cholecystosonography—the junctional fold, Radiology 133:435, 1979.

Taylor KJW and Rosenfield AT: Grey scale ultrasonography in the differential diagnosis of jaundice, Arch Surg 112:820, 1977.

Weeks LE, McCune BR, Martin JF, et al: Unusual echographic appearance of a Courvoisier gallbladder, J Clin Ultrasound 5:341, 1977.

Weinstein DP, Weinstein BJ, and Brodmerkel GJ: Ultrasonography of biliary tract dilatation without jaundice, AJR 132:729, 1979.

Wing VW et al: Sonographic differentiation of enlarged hepatic arteries from dilated intrahepatic bile ducts, AJR 145(1):57, 1985.

Yum HY and Fink AH: Sonographic findings in primary carcinoma of the gallbladder, Radiology 134:693, 1980.

Zeman R, Taylor KJW, Burrell MI, et al: Ultrasound demonstration of anicteric dilatation of the biliary tree, Radiology 134:689, 1980.

PANCREAS

Alpern MB et al: Chronic pancreatitis: ultrasonic features, Radiology 155(1):215, 1985.

Arger PH, Mulhern CB, Bonavita JA, et al: Analysis of pancreatic sonography in suspected pancreatic disease, J Clin Ultrasound 7:91, 1979.

Burrell M, Gold J, Simeone J, et al: Liquefactive necrosis of the pancreas, Radiology 135:157, 1980.

Cadet J et al: Combination of ultrasonography and computed tomography in the diagnosis of hemorrhagic pseudocyst of the pancreas, J Clin Ultrasound 13(8):591, 1985.

Carroll B and Sample WF: Pancreatic cystadenocarcinoma; CT body scan and gray scale ultrasound appearance AJR 131:339, 1978.

Eisenscher A and Weill F: Ultrasonic visualization of Wirsung's duct: dream or reality? J Clin Ultrasound 7:41, 1979.

Filly RA and Carlsen E: Newer ultrasonic anatomy in the upper abdomen. II. The major systemic veins and arteries, with a special note on localization of the pancreas, J Clin Ultrasound 4:91, 1976.

Filly RA and Freimanis AK: Echographic diagnosis of pancreatic lesions, Radiology 96:575, 1970.

Filly RA and London SS: The normal pancreas: acoustic characteristics and frequency of imaging, J Clin Ultrasound 7:121, 1979.

Gerzof SG, Robbins AH, Birkett DH, et al: Percutaneous catheter drainage of abdominal abscesses guided by ultrasound and CT, AJR 133:1, 1979.

Goldstein HM and Katragadda CS: Prone view ultrasonography for pancreatic tail neoplasms, AJR 131:231, 1978.

Gooding GAW: Pseudocyst of the pancreas with mediastinal extension: an ultrasonographic demonstration J Clin Ultrasound 5:121, 1977.

Gosink BB and Leopold GR: The dilated pancreatic duct: ultrasonic evaluation, Radiology 126:475, 1978.

Grose-Brown M, Mitchell MA, and Hagen-Ansert SL: Echographic noninvasive clinical assessment of the upper abdomen using various contrast media in the stomach, Med Ultrasound 3:60, 1979.

Hagen-Ansert SL and Manich B: Echographic visualization of normal pancreatic tissue patterns, Med Ultrasound 1:11, 1977.

Jeffrey RB Jr et al: Extrapancreatic spread of acute pancreatitis: new observations with real time, Radiology 159(3):707, 1986.

Kairaluoma MI et al: Impact of new imaging techniques on survival in cancer of the head of the pancreas and the periampullary region, Acta Chir Scand 151(1):69, 1985.

Laing FC, Gooding GAW, Brown T, and Leopold GR: Atypical pseudocysts of the pancreas: an ultrasonographic evaluation, J Clin Ultrasound 7:27, 1979.

Lawson TL: Sensitivity of pancreatic ultrasonography in the detection of pancreatic disease, Radiology 128:733, 1978.

Lees WR: Pancreatic ultrasonography, Clin Gastroenterol 13(3):763, 1984.

Leopold G: Pancreatic echography: a new dimension in the diagnosis of pseudocyst, Radiology 104:365, 1972.

Leopold GR, Berg RN, and Reinke RT: Echographic-radiological documentation of spontaneous rupture of a pancreatic pseudocyst into the duodenum, Radiology 120:699, 1972.

Macmahon H, Bowie JD, and Beezhold C: Erect scanning of pancreas using a gastric window, AJR 132:587, 1979.

Marks WM, Filly RA, and Callen PW: Ultrasonic evaluation of normal pancreatic echogenicity and its relationship to fat deposition, Radiology 137:475, 1980.

McCain AH et al: Pancreatic sonography: past and present, J Clin Ultrasound 12(6):325, 1984.

McGaham JP: The posterior gastric wall: a possible source of confusion in the identification of the pancreatic duct, J Clin Ultrasound 12(6):366, 1984.

Ohto M, Sastome N, Saisho H, et al: Real time sonography of the pancreatic duct, AJR 134:647, 1980.

Paivansalo M et al: Ultrasonography of the pancreatic tail through spleen and through fluid-filled stomach, Eur J Radiol 6(2):113, 1986.

Raymond HW and Zwiebel WJ, editors: The pancreas, Semin Ultrasound 1(3):1980.

Rifkin MD et al: Interoperative sonographic identification of nonpalpable pancreatic masses, J Ultrasound Med 3(9):409, 1984.

Sample WF: Techniques for improved delineation of normal anatomy of the upper abdomen and high retroperitoneum with grey scale ultrasound, Radiology 124:197, 1977.

Sarti DA: Rapid development and spontaneous regression of pancreatic pseudocysts documented by ultrasound, Radiology 125:789, 1977.

Shawker TH et al: The spectrum of sonographic findings in pancreatic carcinoma, J Ultrasound Med 5(3):169, 1986.

Slovis TL, Vonberg VJ, and Mikelic V: Sonography in the diagnosis and management of pancreatic pseudocysts and effusions in childhood, Radiology 135:153, 1980.

Smith EH, Bartrum RJ, and Chang YC: Ultrasonically guided percutaneous aspiration biopsy of the pancreas, Radiology 112:737, 1974.

Sokoloff J et al: Pitfalls in the echographic evaluation of pancreatic disease, J Clin Ultrasound 2:321, 1974.

Swobodnik W et al: Ultrasound characteristics of the pancreas in children with cystic fibrosis, J Clin Ultrasound 13(7):469, 1985.

Warren PS, Garrett WJ, and Kosoff G: The liquid-filled stomach: an ultrasonic window to the upper abdomen, J Clin Ultrasound 6:295, 1978.

Weighall SL, Wolfman NT, and Watson N: The fluid-filled stomach: a new sonic window, J Clin Ultrasound 7:353, 1979.

Weinstein BJ, Weinstein DP, and Brodmerkel GJ: Ultrasonography of pancreatic lithiasis, Radiology 134:185, 1980.

Weinstein DP and Weinstein BJ: Ultrasonic demonstration of the pancreatic duct, Radiology 130:729, 1979.

Wright CH, Maklad F, and Rosenthal S: Grey scale ultrasonic characteristics of carcinoma of the pancreas, Br J Radiol 52:281, 1979.

KIDNEYS

Arger PH, Mulhern CB, Pollack HM, et al: Ultrasonic assessment of renal transitional cell carcinoma, AJR 132:407, 1979.

Beretsky I et al: Sonographic differentiation between the multicystic dysplastic kidney and the ureteropelvic junction obstruction in utero using high resolution real time scanners employing digital detection, J Clin Ultrasound 12(7):429, 1984.

Bree RL and Silver TM: Differential diagnosis of hypoechoic and anechoic masses with gray scale sonography; new observations, J Clin Ultrasound 7:249, 1979.

Brown JM: The ultrasound approach to the urographically nonvisualizing kidney, Semin Ultrasound 11:44, 1981.

Dinkel E et al: Kidney size in childhood: sonographical growth charts for kidney length and volume, Pediatr Radiol 15(1):38, 1985.

Elyaderani MK and Gabriele OF: Ultrasound of renal masses, Semin Ultrasound 11:21, 1981.

Ervin BC et al: A sonographic assessment of neonatal renal parameters, J Ultrasound Med 4(5):217, 1985.

Finberg H: Renal ultrasound: anatomy and technique, Semin Ultrasound 11:7, 1981.

Goldberg BB and Pollack HM: Ultrasonically guided renal cyst aspiration, J Urol 109:5, 1973.

Goldberg BB and Ziskin MC: Echo patterns with an aspiration ultrasonic transducer, Invest Radiol 8:78, 1973.

Goldstein HM, Green B, and Weaver RM: Ultrasonic detection of renal tumor extension into the IVC, AJR 130:1083, 1978.

Han BK et al: Sonographic measurements and appearance of normal kidneys in children, AJR 145(3):611, 1985.

Jeffrey RB et al: Sensitivity of sonography in pyelonephrosis: a reevaluation, AJR 144(1):71, 1985.

Kay CJ, Rosenfield AJ, and Armm JM: Gray-scale ultrasonography in the evaluation of renal trauma, Radiology 134:461, 1980.

Lang EK: Comparison of dynamic and conventioanl computed tomography, angiography, and ultrasonography in the staging of renal cell carcinoma, Cancer 54(10):2205, 1984.

Lee JKT, McClennan BL, Melson GL, and Stanley RJ: Acute focal bacterial nephritis: emphasis on gray scale sonography and computed tomography, AJR 135:87, 1980.

Lewis E and Ritchie WGM: A simple ultrasonic method for assessing renal size, J Clin Ultrasound 8:417, 1980.

Maklad NF, Chuang VP, Doust BD, et al: Ultrasonic characterization of solid renal lesions: echographic, angiographic, and pathologic correlation, Radiology 123:733, 1977.

McDonald DG: The complete echographic evaluation of solid renal masses, J Clin Ultrasound 6:402, 1978.

Melson GL et al: The spectrum of sonographic findings in infantile polycystic kidney disease with urographic and clinical correlations, J Clin Ultrasound 13(2):113, 1985.

Merran S et al: Interoperative localization of renal calculi by real time ultrasonography, Urology 24(4):393, 1984.

Morin ME and Baker DA: The influence of hydration and bladder distention on the sonographic diagnosis of hydronephrosis, J Clin Ultrasound 7:192, 1979.

Norris CS et al: Noninvasive evaluation of renal artery stenosis and renovascular resistance: experimental and clinical studies, J Vasc Surg 1(1):192, 1984.

Patriquin H et al: Urinary milk of calcium in children and adults: use of gravity dependent sonography, AJR 144(2):407, 1985.

Prees GA et al: Papillary renal cell carcinoma: CT and sonographic evaluation, AJR 143(5):1005, 1984.

Ralls P, Esensten ML, Boger D, and Halls JM: Severe hydronephrosis and severe renal cystic disease: ultrasonic differentiation, AJR 134:473, 1980.

Ralls PW and Halls J: Hydronephrosis, renal cystic disease, and renal parenchymal disease, Semin Ultrasound 11:49, 1981.

Resnick MI and Sanders RC: Ultrasound in urology, Baltimore, 1979, The Williams & Wilkins Co.

Rittgers SE et al: Detection of renal artery stenosis: experimental and clinical analysis of velocity waveforms, Ultrasound Med Biol 11(3):523, 1985.

Rosenfield AT, Glickman MG, and Hodson J: Diagnostic imaging in renal disease, New York, 1979, Appleton-Century-Crofts.

Rosenfield AT, Taylor KJW, Crade M, and DeGraaf CS: Anatomy and pathology of the kidney by gray scale ultrasound, Radiology 128:737, 1978.

Rosenfield AT, Taylor KJW, Dembner AG, and Jacobson P: Ultrasound of renal sinus: new observations AJR 133:441, 1979.

Sanders RC, Scott W, Conrad MR, and Kuhn J: The sonographic pattern of infantile polycystic disease, Ultrasound Med 4:251, 1977.

Scheible W and Talner LB: Gray scale ultrasound and the genitourinary tract: a review of clinical applications, Radiol Clin North Am 17:281, 1979.

Scheible W, Ellenbogen PH, Leopold GR, et al: Lipomatous tumors of the kidney and adrenal: apparent echographic specificity, Radiology 129:153, 1978.

Shawker TH et al: Ultrasonography of Turner's syndrome, J Ultrasound Med 5(3):125, 1986.

Steinhardt GF et al: Simple renal cysts in infants, Radiology 155(2):349, 1985.

Talmont C: Renal ultrasonography. In Taylor K et al, editors: Manual of ultrasonography, New York, 1980, Churchill Livingstone, Inc.

Turner PA et al: Renal parenchyma in infancy and childhood: ultrasound characteristics (letter), Radiology 157(3):837, 1985.

Zappasodi F et al: Small hyperechoic nodules of the renal parenchyma, J Clin Ultrasound 13(95):321, 1985.

RENAL TRANSPLANT

Alley K and Geelhoed GW: The use of ultrasonography and renal scanning in renal transplant patients, Am Surg 46:55, 1980.

Anthony CP and Thibodeau GA: Textbook of anatomy and physiology, ed 10, St Louis, 1979, The CV Mosby Co.

Bartrum R Jr, Smith E, D'Orsi C, and Tilney L: Evaluation of renal transplants with ultrasound, Radiology 118:405, 1976.

Bergren CT et al: The role of ultrasound in the diagnosis of cyclosporine toxicity in renal transplantation, Bol Assoc Med PR 78(2):50, 1986.

Brenbridge AN, Buschi A, Cochrane JA, and Lees R: Renal emphysema of the transplanted kidney: sonographic appearance, AJR 132:656, 1978.

Conrad M, Dickerman R, Love I, et al: New observations in renal transplants using ultrasound, AJR 131:851, 1978.

Cook J III, Rosenfield A, and Taylor K: Ultrasonic demonstration of intrarenal anatomy, AJR 129:831, 1977.

Garel L et al: Transplanted kidney in children: comparative value of various echographic signs of acute rejection, Ann Radiol (Paris) 28(3-4):329, 1985.

Guttmann RG: Renal transplantation. 1, N Engl J Med 301:975, 1979.

Guttman RG: 2, N Engl J Med 301:1038, 1979.

Hillman B, Birnholz J, and Busch G: Correlation of echographic and histologic findings in suspected renal allograft rejection, Radiology 132:673, 1979.

Hricak H, Pereyra LT, and Eyler W: Evaluation of acute post-transplant renal failure by ultrasound, Radiology 133:443, 1979.

Hricak H, Pereyra LT, Eyler W, et al: The role of ultrasound in the diagnosis of kidney allograft rejection, Radiology 132:667, 1979.

Kurtz A, Rubin C, Cole-Beuglet CB, et al: Ultrasound evaluation of renal transplant, JAMA 243:2429, 1980.

LaMasters D, Katzberg RW, Confer D, and Slaysman M: Ureteropelvic fibrosis in renal transplants: radiographic manifestations AJR 135:79, 1980.

Maklad N, Wright C, and Rosenthal S: Gray scale ultrasonic appearances of renal transplant rejection, Radiology 131:711, 1979.

Netter FH: Kidneys, ureters, and urinary bladder, vol. 16, Ciba collection of medical illustrations, Summit NJ, 1975, Ciba.

Ostrovsky PD et al: Ultrasound findings in renal transplant rupture, J Clin Ultrasound 13(2):132, 1985.

Rosenfield A: Ultrasonography in renal transplantation, Genitourinary ultrasonography, vol 12, Clin Diag Ultrasound, 1979.

Rosenfield A, Glickman M, and Hodson J: Diagnostic imaging in renal disease, New York, 1979, Appleton-Century-Crofts.

Singh A and Cohen WN: Renal allograft rejection: sonography and scintigraphy, AJR 135:73, 1980.

Slovis TL et al: Renal transplant rejection: sonographic evaluation in children, Radiology 153(3):659, 1984.

ADRENAL GLANDS

Bernardino ME, Goldstein HM, and Green B: Gray scale ultrasonography of adrenal neoplasms, AJR 130:741, 1978.

Forsythe JR, Gosink BB, and Leopold GR: Ultrasound in the evaluation of adrenal metastases, J Clin Ultrasound 5:31, 1977.

SPLEEN

Bhimji SD, Cooperberg PK, Naiman S, et al: Ultrasound diagnosis of splenic cysts, Radiology 122:787, 1977.

Gooding GAW: The ultrasonic and CT appearance of splenic lobulations: a consideration in the ultrasonic differential of masses adjacent to the left kidney, Radiology 126:719, 1978.

Shirkhoda A, McCartney WH, Staab EV, and Mittelstaedt CA: Imaging of the spleen: a proposed algorithm, AJR 135:195, 1980.

Talmont CA: Spleen. In Taylor K et al, editors: Manual of ultrasonography, New York, 1980, Churchill Livingstone, Inc.

RETROPERITONEUM

Doust BD, Quiroz F, and Stewart JM: Ultrasonic distinction of abscesses from other intra-abdominal fluid collections, Radiology 125:213, 1977.

Filly RA, Marglin S, and Castellino RA: The ultrasonographic spectrum of abdominal and pelvic Hodgkin's disease and non-Hodgkin's lymphoma, Cancer 38:2143, 1976.

Harbin WP, Wittenberg J, Ferrucci JT, et al: Fallibility of exploratory laparotomy in detection of hepatic and retroperitoneal masses, AJR 135:115, 1980.

Hillman BJ, and Haber K: Echographic characteristics of malignant lymph nodes, J Clin Ultrasound 8:213, 1980.

Kaftori JK, Rosenberger A, Pollack S, et al: Rectus sheath hematoma: ultrasonographic diagnosis, AJR 128:283, 1977.

McCullough DL and Leopold GR: Diagnosis of retroperitoneal fluid collections by ultrasonography: a series of surgically proved cases, J Urol 115:656, 1976.

Rochester D, Bowie JD, and Kunzmann A: Ultrasound in the staging of lymphoma, Radiology 124:483, 1977.

Smith EH and Bartrum RJ: Ultrasonically guided percutaneous aspiration of abscesses, AJR 122:308, 1974.

HIGH-RESOLUTION ULTRASONOGRAPHY OF SUPERFICIAL STRUCTURES

Albert NE: Testicular ultrasound for trauma, J Urol 124:558, 1980.

Anson BJ: Morris' human anatomy, ed 12, New York, 1966, McGraw-Hill Book Co.

Baker CRF: Complications and management of methods of dialysis access for renal failure, Am Surg 42:859, 1976.

Basmajian JV: Primary anatomy, ed 5, Baltimore, 1964, The Williams & Wilkins Co.

Blum M, Passalaque AM, Sackler JP et al: Thyroid echography of subacute thyroiditis, Radiology 125:795, 1977.

Blumhagen JD and Coombs JB: Ultrasound in the diagnosis of hypertrophic pyloric stenosis, J Clin Ultrasound 9:289, 1981.

Crocker EF, Bautovich GJ, and Jellins J: Grayscale echographic visualization of a parathyroid adenoma, Radiology 126:233, 1978.

Davies AG: Thyroid physiology, Br Med J 2:206, 1972.

Edis AJ: Surgical treatment for thyroid cancer, Surg Clin North Am 57:533, 1977.

Favus MJ, Schneider AB, Stachura ME, et al: Thyroid cancer occurring as a late consequence of head-and-neck irradiation, N Engl J Med 294:1019, 1976.

Forsham PH: Endocrine system and selected metabolic diseases, ed 3, Summit NJ, 1974, Ciba Pharmaceutical Co.

Frigolette FD, Birnholz JC, and Driscoll SG: Ultrasound diagnosis of cystic hygroma, Am J Obstet Gynecol 136:962, 1980.

Guyton AC: Function of the human body, ed 3, Philadelphia, 1969, WB Saunders Co.

Haimou M, Baez A, Neff M, et al: Complications of arteriovenous fistulas for hemodialysis, Arch Surg 110:708, 1975.

Haimou M and Jacobson JH: Experience with the modified bovine arterial heterograft in peripheral vascular reconstruction and vascular access for hemodialysis. Ann Surg 180:291, 1974.

Hammill FS, Johnston CG, Collins GM, et al: A critical appraisal of the changing approaches

to vascular access for chronic hemodialysis, Dial Transpl 19:325, 1980.

Kangarloo H and Sample WF: Ultrasound of the pediatric abdomen and pelvis, Chicago, 1980, Year Book Medical Publishers, Inc.

Leopold G: Ultrasonography of superficially located structures, Radiol Clin North Am 18:161, 1980.

Leopold G, Woo VC, Scheible RW et al: High-resolution ultrasonography of scrotal pathology, Radiology 131:719, 1979.

Massry S and Sellers A: Clinical aspects of uremia and dialysis, Springfield Ill, 1976, Charles C Thomas, Publisher.

Miller FN Jr: Pathology, ed 3, Boston, 1978, Little, Brown & Co.

Miskin M, Rosen IB, and Walfish PG: Ultrasonography of the thyroid gland, Radiol Clin North Am 13:479, 1975.

Oakes DD, Spees ED, Light JA, et al: A three-year experience using modified bovine arterial heterografts for vascular access in patients requiring hemodialysis, Ann Surg 187:423, 1978.

O'Brien WF, Cefalo RC, and Bair DB: Ultrasonic diagnosis of fetal cystic hygroma, Am J Obstet Gynecol 138:464, 1980.

Oppenheimen E: Reproductive system, ed 5, Summit NJ, 1974, Ciba Pharmaceutical Co.

ReMine WH and McConahey WM: Management of thyroid nodules, Surg Clin North Am 57:523, 1977.

Robbins SL and Lotran RS: Pathologic basis of disease, ed 2, Philadelphia, 1979, WB Saunders Co.

Rohr MS, Browder W, Freutz GD, et al: Ateriovenous fistulas for long-term dialysis, Arch Surg 113:153, 1978.

Sackler JP, Passalaque AM, Blum M, et al: A spectrum of diseases of the thyroid as imaged by gray scale water bath sonography, Radiology 125:467, 1977.

Sample WF, Gottesman JE, Skinner DG, et al: Gray scale ultrasound of the scrotum, Radiology 127:225, 1978.

Sample WF, Mitchell SP, and Bledsoe RC: Parathyroid ultrasonography, Radiology 127:485, 1978.

Scheible W: Pediatric applications of high resolution real time ultrasonography, Clin Diagn. Ultrasound 1981.

Scheible W, Deutsch AL, and Leopold GR: Parathyroid adenoma: accuracy of preoperative localization by high resolution real-time ultrasonography, J Clin Ultrasound 9:325, 1981.

Scheible FW and Leopold GR: Diagnostic imaging in head and neck disease: current applications of ultrasound, Head Neck Surg 1:1, 1978.

Scheible FW, Leopold GR, Woo VL, et al: High-resolution real-time ultrasonography of thyroid nodules, Radiology 133:413, 1979.

Scheible W, Skram C, and Leopold GR: High-resolution real-time sonography of hemodialysis vascular access complications, AJR 134:1173, 1980.

Spencer R, Brown MC and Annis D: Ultrasonic scanning of the thyroid gland as a guide to the treatment of the clinically solitary nodule, Br J Surg 64:841, 1977.

Tellis VA, Kohlberg WI, Bhat DJ, et al: Expanded polytetrafluorothylene graft fistula for chronic hemodialysis, Am Surg 189:101, 1979.

Walfish PG, Hazain E, Strawbridge HTG, et al: A prospective study of combined ultrasonography and needle aspiration biopsy in the assessment of the hypofunctioning thyroid nodule, Surgery 82:474, 1977.

Young LW: Radiology case of the month, Am J Dis Child 134:311, 1980.

BREAST

Calderson D, Vilkomerson D, Mezrich R, et al: Differences in the attenuation of ultrasound by normal, benign, and malignant breast tissue, J Clin Ultrasound 4:249, 1976.

Ezo ME: Tissue compression for the optimization of images in water-path breast scanning, Med Ultrasound, October 1981.

Harper P et al: Ultrasound visualization of the breast symptomatic patients. Radiology 137(2):1980.

Kelly-Fry E, Fry FJ, and Gardner GW: Recommendations for widespread application of ultrasound visualization techniques for examination of the female breast. In White D and Brown RE, editors: Ultrasound in medicine, vol 3A, New York, 1977, Plenum Publishing Corp.

Kelly-Fry E, Fry FJ, Sanghvi NT, et al: A combined clinical and research approach to the problem of ultrasound visualization of breast. In White D, editor: Ultrasound in medicine, vol 1, New York, 1975, Plenum Publishing Corp.

Kobayashi T: Gray-scale echography for breast cancer, Radiology 122:207, 1977.

Kossoff G, Kelly-Fry E, and Jellins J: Average velocity of ultrasound in the human female breast, J Acoust Soc Am 53:1730, 1973.

Pilnik S and Leis HP Jr: Clinical diagnosis of breast lesions. In Gallager HS et al: The breast, St Louis, 1978, The CV Mosby Co.

Pilnik S and Leis HP Jr: Nipple discharge. In Gallager HS et al, editors: The breast, St Louis, 1978, The CV Mosby Co.

Rubin CS, Kurtz AB, Goldberg BB, et al: Ultrasound mammographic parenchymal patterns: a preliminary report, Radiology 130:515, 1979.

CARDIAC ANATOMIC AND PHYSIOLOGIC RELATIONSHIPS

Anderson PD: Clinical anatomy and physiology for allied health sciences, Philadelphia, 1976, WB Saunders Co.

Clemente CD: Anatomy, a regional atlas of the human body, Philadelphia, 1975, Lea & Febiger.

Crafts RC: A textbook of human anatomy, New York, 1979, John Wiley & Sons, Inc.

DeBakey M and Gotto A: The living heart, New York, 1977, Grosset & Dunlap, Inc.

Foale R et al: Echocardiographic measurement of the normal adult right ventricle, Br Heart J 56(1):33, 1986.

Graettinger WF: The cardiovascular response to chronic physical exertion and exercise training: an echocardiographic review, Am Heart J 108:1014, 1984.

Green JH: Basic clinical physiology, New York, 1969, Oxford University Press, Inc.

Hauser A et al: Symmetric cardiac enlargement in highly trained endurance athletes: a two-dimensional echocardiographic study, Am Heart J 109:1038, 1985.

Hollinshead WH: Textbook of anatomy, New York, 1979, Harper & Row, Publishers.

Introduction to medical sciences for clinical practice. A self-instructional/tutorial curriculum. Physician's assistant program, Bowman Gray School of Medicine (Winston-Salem NC), Chicago, 1976, Year Book Medical Publishers, Inc.

Keren A et al: Echocardiographic recognition and implications of ventricular hypertrophic trabeculations and aberrant bands, Circulation 70(5):836, 1984.

Maron BJ: Structural features of the athlete heart as defined by echocardiography, J Am Coll Cardiol 7(1):190, 1986.

Ryan T et al: An echocardiographic index for separation of right ventricular volume and pressure overload, J Am Coll Cardiol 5(4):918, 1985.

Snell RS: Clinical anatomy for medical students, Boston, 1973, Little Brown & Co.

Sokolow M and McIlroy MB: Clinical cardiology, Los Altos Calif. 1977, Lange Medical Publications.

Tilkian AG and Conover MB: Understanding heart sounds and murmurs, Philadelphia, 1979, WB Saunders Co.

Wang Y et al: Atrial volume in a normal adult population by two-dimensional echocardiography, Chest 86(4):595, 1984.

Zema MJ et al: Echocardiographic appearance of the Chiari network, J Clin Ultrasound 13(9):671, 1985.

ECHOCARDIOGRAPHIC TECHNIQUES AND EVALUATION

Allen H, Goldberg S, Sahn D, et al: Suprasternal notch echocardiography: assessment of its clinical utility in pediatric cardiology, Circulation 55:605, 1977.

Borer JS, Henry WL, and Epstein SE: Echocardiographic observations in patients with systemic infiltrative disease involving the heart. Am J Cardiol 39:184, 1977.

Cooper R and Leopold G: Diagnostic ultrasound in cardiology, Med Ann DC 41:748, 1972.

DeMaria AN, Neumann A, Schubart PJ, et al: Systemic correlation of cardiac chamber size and ventricular performance determined with echocardiography and alterations in heart rate in normal persons, Am J Cardiol 43:1, 1979.

Feigenbaum H: Clinical applications of echocardiography, Prog Cardiovasc Dis 14:531, 1972.

Feigenbaum H: Echocardiography, Philadelphia, 1972, Lea & Febiger.

Feigenbaum H: Educational problems in echocardiography, Am J Cardiol 34:741, 1974. [Editorial]

Feigenbaum H: Hazards of echocardiographic interpretation, N Engl J Med 289:1311, 1974. [Editorial.]

Gehrke J et al: Non-invasive left ventricular volume determination by two-dimensional echo, Br Heart J 37(9):911, 1976.

Gilbert BW et al: Mitral valve prolapse, two-dimensional echo and angiographic correlation, Circulation 54:716, 1976.

Gilbert BW et al: Two-dimensional echo assessment of vegetative endocarditis, Circulation 55:346, 1977.

Goldberg S, Allen H, and Sahn D: Pediatric and adolescent echocardiography: a handbook, Chicago, 1975, Year Book Medical Publishers, Inc.

Gramiak R, Shah P, and Kramer D: Ultrasound cardiography: contrast studies in anatomy and function, Radiology 92:939, 1969.

Harbold N Jr, and Gau G: Echocardiographic diagnosis of right atrial myxoma, Mayo Clin Proc 48:284, 1973.

Henry WL, DeMaria A, Gramiak R, et al: Report of the American Society of Echocardiography Committee on Nomenclature and Standards in Two-dimensional Echocardiography, 62:212, 1980.

Henry WL, Ware J, Gardin JM, et al: Echocardiographic measurements in normal subjects; growth-related changes that occur between infancy and early childhood, Circulation 57:278, 1978.

Kerber R: Errors in performance and interpretation of echocardiograms, J Clin Ultrasound 1:330, 1973.

Kisslo J et al: Cardiac imaging using a phased array ultrasound system: clinical technique and application, Circulation 53:262, 1976.

Kisslo JA et al: A comparison of real time, two-dimensional echo and cineangiography in detecting left ventricular asynergy, Circulation 55(1):134, 1977.

Kisslo JA et al: Dynamic cardiac imaging using a focused, phased array ultrasound system, Am J Med 63(1):61, 1977.

Lange LW, Sahn DJ, Allen HD, and Goldberg SJ: The utility of subxiphoid cross-sectional echocardiography in infants and children with congenital heart disease, 59:513, 1979.

Lappe DL et al: A two-dimensional echo diagnosis of left atrial myxomas, Chest 74(1):55, 1978.

Lieppe W et al: Two-dimensional findings in atrial septal defect, Circulation 56:447, 1977.

Martin RP et al: Reliability and reproducibility of two dimensional echocardiographic measurement of the stenotic mitral valve orifice area, Am J Cardiol 1979.

Mintz GS et al: Two-dimensional echo recognition of ruptured chordae tendineae, Circulation 57:244, 1978.

Nichol PM et al: Two-dimensional echo assessment of mitral stenosis, Circulation 55:120, 1977.

Nishimura K et al: Real time observation of cardiac movement and structures in congenital and acquired heart diseases employing high-speed ultrasonocardiotomography, Am Heart J 92:340, 1976.

Popp RI et al: Cardiac anatomy viewed systematically with two-dimensional echocardiography, Chest 75:579, 1979.

Ports TA et al: Two-dimensional echo assessment of Ebstein's anomaly, Circulation 58:336, 1978.

Roberts WC: Valvular, subvalvular, and supravalvular aortic stenosis: morphologic features, Cardiovasc Clin 5:98, 1973.

Roeland J et al: Ultrasonic two-dimensional analysis of the mitral valve. In Kalmanson D, editor: The mitral valve, Acton Mass, 1976, Publishing Science Group.

Rossen RM, Goodman DJ, Ingham RE, and Popp RL: Ventricular systolic septal thickening and excursion in idiopathic hypertrophic subaortic stenosis, N Engl J Med 291:1317, 1974.

Sahn DJ, DeMaria A, Kisslo J, and Weyman A: Recommendations regarding quantitation in M-mode echocardiography; results of a survey of echocardiographic measurements, Circulation 58:1072, 1978.

Sahn DJ et al: The comparative utilities of real time cross-sectional echo imaging systems for the diagnosis of complex congenital heart diseases, Am J Med 63(1):50, 1977.

Sahn DJ et al: Real time cross-sectional echo diagnosis of coarctation of the aorta, a prospective study of echo-angiographic correlations, Circulation 56:762, 1977.

Sahn DJ et al: Real time cross-sectional echo imaging and measurement of the patent ductus arteriosus in infants and children, Circulation 58:327, 1978.

Schieken RM and Kerber RE: Echocardiographic abnormalities in acute rheumatic fever. Am J Cardiol 38:458, 1976.

Shah P et al: Echocardiographic assessment of the effects of surgery and propranolol on the dynamics of outflow obstruction and hyperpranolol on the dynamics of outflow obstruction and hypertrophic subaortic stenosis, Circulation 45:516, 1972.

Silverman NH and Schiller NB: Apex echocardiography. A two-dimensional technique for evaluating congenital heart disease, Circulation 57:503, 1978.

Stack R and Kisslo J: Evaluation of the left ventricle with two-dimensional echocardiography, Am J Cardiol 46:1117, 1980.

Tajik AJ et al: A two-dimensional real time ultrasonic imaging of the heart and great vessels: technique, image orientation, structure, identification, and validation, Mayo Clin Proc 53:271, 1978.

Von Ramm OT et al: Cardiac imaging using a phased array ultrasound system: system design, Circulation 53:258, 1976.

Weaver WF et al: Mid-diastolic aortic valve opening in severe acute aortic regurgitation, Circulation 55:145, 1977.

Weyman A et al: Cross-sectional echocardiography in evaluating patients with discrete subaortic stenosis, Am J Cardiol 37:358, 1976.

Weyman A et al: Mechanism of abnormal septal motion in patients with right ventricular volume overload: a cross-sectional echocardiographic study, Circulation 54:179, 1976.

MITRAL VALVE

Barlow JB, Pocock WA, Marchand P, and Denny M: The significance of late systolic murmurs, Am Heart J 66:443, 1963.

Botvinick EH, Schiller NB, Wickramasekaren R, et al: Echocardiographic demonstration of early mitral valve closure in severe aortic insufficiency: its clinical implications, Circulation 51:836, 1975.

Burgess J, Clark R, Kamigaki M, et al: Echocardiographic findings in different types of mitral regurgitation, Circulation 48:97, 1973.

Chung K, Manning J, and Gramiak R: Echocardiography in coexisting hypertrophic subaortic stenosis and fixed left ventricular outflow obstruction, Circulation 49:673, 1974.

DeMaria A, Lies JE, King JF, et al: Echographic assessment of atrial transport, mitral movement, and ventricular performance following electroversion of supraventricular arrhythmias, Circulation 51:273, 1975.

DeMaria AN, King JF, Bogren HG, et al: The variable spectrum of echocardiographic manifestations of the mitral valve prolapse syndrome, Circulation 50:33, 1974.

Dillon JC, Feigenbaum H, Konecke LL, et al: Echocardiographic manifestations of valvular vegetations, Am Heart J 86:698, 1973.

Dillon JC, Haine CL, Chang S, et al: Use of echocardiography in patients with prolapsed mitral valve, Circulation 43:503, 1971.

Dodd M and Wilcken D: Echocardiography in left atrial myxoma: relation to the findings in mitral stenosis, Aust NZ J Med 2:124, 1972.

Duchak JM Jr, Chang S, and Feigenbaum H: The posterior mitral valve echo and the echocardiographic diagnosis of mitral stenosis, Am J Cardiol 29:628, 1972.

Finegan R and Harrison D: Diagnosis of left atrial myxoma by echocardiography, N Engl J Med 282:1022, 1970.

Flaherty J, Livengood S, and Fortuin N: Atypical posterior leaflet motion in echocardiogram in mitral stenosis, Am J Cardiol 35:675, 1975.

Fortuin N and Craige E: Echocardiographic studies of genesis of mitral diastolic murmurs, Br Heart J 35:75, 1973.

Goodman D Harrison D, and Popp R: Echocardiographic features of primary pulmonary hypertension, Am Heart J 86:847, 1973.

Gramiak R and Waag RC: Cardiac ultrasound, St Louis, 1975, The CV Mosby Co.

Henry WL, Clark CE, Glancy DL, et al: Echocardiographic measurement of the left ventricular outflow gradient in idiopathic hypertrophic subaortic stenosis, N Engl J Med 288:989, 1973.

Hernberg J, Weiss B, and Keegan A: The ultrasonic recording of aortic valve motion, Radiology 94:361, 1970.

Johnson A, Lonky S, and Carleton R: Combined hypertrophic subaortic stenosis and calcific aortic valvular stenosis, Am J Cardiol 35:706, 1975.

Johnson ML, Holmes JH, Spangler RD, et al: Usefulness of echocardiography in patients undergoing mitral valve surgery, J Thorac Cardiovasc Surg 64:922, 1972.

Kamigaki M and Goldschlager N: Echocardiographic analysis of mitral valve motion in atrial septal defect, Am J Cardiol 30:343, 1972.

King JF, DeMaria AN, Miller RB, et al: Markedly abnormal mitral valve motion without simultaneous interventricular pressure gradient due to uneven mitral-septum contact in idiopathic hypertrophic subaortic stenosis, Am J Cardiol 34:360, 1974.

Konecke LL, Feigenbaum H, Chang S, et al: Abnormal mitral valve motion in patients with elevated left ventricular diastolic pressures, Circulation 47:989, 1973.

Levisman JA and Abbasi AS: Abnormal motion of the mitral valve with pericardial effusion: pseudo-prolapse of the mitral valve, Am Heart J 91:18, 1976.

Meyer JF, Frank MJ, Goldberg S, and Cheng TO: Systolic mitral flutter, an echocardiographic clue to the diagnosis of ruptured chordae tendineae, Am Heart J 93:3, 1977.

Nanda NC, Gramiak R, Shah PM, et al: Echocardiography in the diagnosis of idiopathic hypertrophic subaortic stenosis coexisting with aortic valve disease, Circulation 50:752, 1974.

Nanda NC, Gramiak R, Shah PM, et al: Mitral commissurotomy versus replacement: preoperative evaluation by echocardiography, Circulation 51:263, 1975.

Nasser WK, Davis RH, Dillon JC, et al: Atrial myxoma. I. Clinical and pathologic features in nine cases, Am Heart J 83:694, 1972.

Nichol PM, Gilbert BW, and Kisslo JA: Two-dimensional echocardiographic assessment of mitral stenosis, Circulation 55:120, 1977.

Parisi A and Milton B: Relation of mitral valve closure to the first heart sound in man: echocardiographic and phonocardiographic assessment, Am J Cardiol 32:779, 1973.

Popp R and Levine R: Left atrial mass simulating cardiomyopathy, J Clin Ultrasound 1:96, 1973.

Popp R et al: Echocardiographic abnormalities in the mitral valve prolapse syndrome, Circulation 49:428, 1974.

Pridie RB, Beham R, and Oakley CM: Echocardiography of the mitral valve in aortic valve disease, Br Heart J 33:296, 1971.

Quinones M et al: Reduction in the rate of diastolic descent of the mitral valve echogram in patients with altered left ventricular diastolic pressure-volume relations, Circulation 49:246, 1974.

Rubenstein J et al: The echocardiographic determination of mitral valve opening and closure: correlation with hemodynamic studies in man, Circulation 51:98, 1975.

Shah P et al: Echocardiographic assessment of the effects of surgery and propranolol on the dynamics of outflow obstruction and hypertrophic subaortic stenosis, Circulation 45:516, 1972.

Shah P et al: Role of echocardiography in diagnostic and hemodynamic assessment of hypertrophic subaortic stenosis, Circulation 44:891, 1971.

Spangler R and Okin T: Echocardiographic demonstration of left atrial thrombus, Chest 67:716, 1975.

Spangler RD, Johnson, ML, Holmes JH, et al: Echocardiographic demonstration of bacterial vegetations in active infective endocarditis, J Clin Utrasound 1:126, 1973.

Sweatman T et al: Echocardiographic diagnosis of mitral regurgitation due to ruptured chordae tendineae, Circulation 46:580, 1972.

AORTA AND LEFT ATRIUM

Brown O, Harrison D, and Popp R: An improved method for echographic detection of left atrial enlargement, Circulation 50:58, 1974.

DeMaria AN, King JF, Salel AF, et al: Echography and phonography of acute aortic regurgitation in bacterial endocarditis, Ann Intern Med 82:329, 1975.

Feizi O, Symons C, and Yacoub M: Echocardiography of the aortic valve: studies of normal aortic valve, aortic stenosis, aortic regurgitation and mixed aortic valve disease, Br Heart J 36:341, 1974.

Francis GS et al: Echocardiographic criteria of normal left atrial size in adults, Cathet Cardiovasc Diagn 2:69, 1976.

Glasser S: Late mitral valve opening in aortic regurgitation, Chest 70:70, 1976.

Gramiak R and Shah P: Echocardiography of the aortic root, Invest Radiol 3:356, 1968.

Gramiak R and Shah P: Echocardiography of the normal and diseased aortic valve, Radiology 96:1, 1970.

Henry WL, Morganroth J, Pearlman AS, et al: Relation between echocardiographically determined left atrial size and atrial fibrillation, Circulation 53:273, 1976.

Hirata T, Wolfe SB, Popp RL, et al: Estimation of left atrial size using ultrasound, Am Heart J 78:43, 1969.

Johnson AD, Alpert JS, Francis GS, et al: Assessment of left ventricular function in severe aortic regurgitation, Circulation 54:975, 1976.

Johnson ML, Warren SG, Waugh RA, et al: Echocardiography of the aortic valve in non-rheumatic left ventricular outflow tract lesions, Radiology 112:677, 1974.

Millward D, Robinson N, and Craige E: Dissecting aortic aneurysm diagnosed by echocardiography in a patient with rupture of the aneurysm into the right atrium, Am J Cardiol 30:427, 1972.

Nanda N, Gramiak R, and Shah P: Diagnosis of aortic root dissection by echocardiography, Circulation 48:506, 1973.

Nanda NC, Gramiak R, Manning J, et al: Echocardiographic recognition of the congenital bicuspid aortic valve, Circulation 49:870, 1974.

Popp RL, Silverman JF, French JW, et al: Echocardiographic findings in discrete subvalvular aortic stenosis, Circulation 49:226, 1974.

Pratt RC, Parisi AF, Harrington JJ, et al: The influence of left ventricular stroke volume on aortic root motion: an echocardiographic study, Circulation 53:947, 1976.

Rothbaum DA, Dillon JC, Chang S, et al: Echocardiographic manifestations of right sinus of Valsalva aneurysm, Circulation 49:768, 1974.

Strunk BL, Fitzgerald JW, Lipton M, et al: The posterior aortic wall echocardiogram, its relationship to left atrial volume change, Circulation 54:744, 1976.

TenCate F et al: Dimensions and volumes of left atrium and ventricle determined by single beam echocardiography, Br Heart J 36:737, 1974.

Vredevoe L, Creekmore S, and Schiller N: The measurement of systolic time intervals by echocardiography, J Clin Ultrasound 2:99, 1974.

Weyman AE, Feigenbaum H, Dillon JC, et al: Noninvasive visualization of the left main coronary artery by cross-sectional echocardiography, Circulation 54:179, 1976.

TRICUSPID VALVE

Ainsworth RP, Hartmann AF, Aker U, and Schad N: Tricuspid valve prolapse with late systolic tricuspid insufficiency, Radiology 107:309, 1973.

Chandraratna P et al: Echocardiographic detection of tricuspid valve prolapse, Circulation 51:823, 1975.

Gooch AS, Maranhao V, Scampardones G, et al: Prolapse of both mitral and tricuspid leaflets in systolic murmur-click syndrome, N Engl J Med 287:1218, 1972.

Lundstrom N: Echocardiography in the diagnosis of Ebstein's anomaly of the tricuspid valve, Circulation 47:597, 1973.

Nanda N, Gramiak R, and Manning J: Echocardiography of the tricuspid valve in congenital left ventricular-right atrial communication, Circulation 51:268, 1975.

Seides SF, DeJoseph RI, Brown AE, and Damato AN: Echocardiographic findings in isolated, surgically created tricuspid insufficiency, Am J Cardiol 35:679, 1975.

Tavel ME, Baugh D, Fisch C, and Feigenbaum H: Opening snap of the tricuspid valve in atrial septal defect: a phonocardiographic and reflected ultrasound study of sounds in relationship to movements of the tricuspid valve, Am Heart J 80:550, 1970.

Waxler EB, Kawai N, and Kasparian H: Right atrial myxoma: echocardiographic phonocardiographic and hemodynamic signs, Am Heart J 83:251, 1972.

Wolfe SB, Popp RL, and Feigenbaum H: Diagnosis of atrial tumors by ultrasound, Circulation 39:615, 1969.

PULMONARY VALVES

Chung KJ, Alexson CG, Manning JA, and Gramiak R: Echocardiography in truncus arteriosus: the value of pulmonic valve detection, Circulation 48:281, 1973.

Goldberg S, Allen H, and Sahn D: Pediatric echocardiography, Chicago 1974, Year Book Medical Publishers, Inc.

Goodman D, Harrison D, and Popp R: Echocardiographic features of primary pulmonary hypertension, Am J Cardiol 33:438, 1974.

Gramiak R, Nanda NC, and Shah PM: Echocardiographic detection of the pulmonary valve, Radiology 102:153, 1972.

Nanda N et al: Echocardiographic evaluation of pulmonary hypertension, Circulation 50:575, 1974.

Wann LS et al: Premature pulmonary valve opening, Circulation 55:128, 1977.

Weyman A et al: Premature pulmonic valve opening following sinus of Valsalva aneurysm rupture into the right atrium, Circulation 51:556, 1975.

Weyman AE, Dillon JC, Feigenbaum H, and Chang S: Echocardiographic patterns of pulmonary valve motion in valvular pulmonary stenosis, Am J Cardiol 36(1):21, 1975.

Weyman AE, Dillon JC, Feigenbaum H, and Chang S: Echocardiographic patterns of pulmonic valve motion with pulmonary hypertension, Circulation 50:905, 1974.

RIGHT VENTRICLE

Brown OR, Harrison DC, and Popp RI: Echocardiography study of right ventricular hypertension producing asymmetrical septal hypertrophy (abstract), Circulation 48(suppl IV):47, 1973.

Diamond MA, Dillon JC, Haine CL, et al: Echocardiographic features of atrial septal defect, Circulation 43:129, 1971.

Popp RL, Wolfe SB, Hirata T, and Feigenbaum H: Estimation of right and left ventricular size by ultrasound. A study of the echoes from the interventricular septum, Am J Cardiol 24:523, 1969.

INTERVENTRICULAR SEPTUM AND INTERATRIAL SEPTUM

Abbasi A et al: Echocardiographic diagnosis of idiopathic hypertrophic cardiomyopathy without outflow obstruction, Circulation 46:897, 1972.

Devereux RB and Reichek N: Echocardiographic determination of left ventricular mass in man: anatomic validation of the method, Circulation 55:613, 1977.

Dillon J et al: Cross-sectional echocardiographic examination of the interatrial septum, Circulation 55:115, 1977.

Epstein SE, Henry WL, Clark CE, et al: Asymmetric septal hypertrophy, Ann Intern Med 81:650, 1974.

Henry WL, Clark CE, and Epstein SE: Asymmetric septal hypertrophy: echocardiographic identification of the pathognomonic anatomic abnormality of IHSS, Circulation 47:225, 1973.

Henry WL, Clark CE, and Epstein SE: Asymmetric septal hypertrophy (ASH): the unifying link in the IHSS disease spectrum. Circulation 47:827, 1973.

Henry WL, Clark CE, Roberts WC, et al: Difference in distribution of myocardial abnormalities in patients with obstructive and nonobstructive asymmetric septal hypertrophy (ASH): echocardiographic and gross anatomic findings, Circulation 50:447, 1974.

Kerber R et al: Effects of acute coronary occlusion on the motion and perfusion of the normal and ischemic interventricular septum, Circulation 54:928, 1976.

King JF, DeMaria AN, Miller RR, et al: Markedly abnormal mitral valve motion without simultaneous intraventricular pressure gradient due to uneven mitral-septal contact in idiopathic hypertrophic subaortic stenosis, Am J Cardiol 34:360, 1974.

Popp RL and Harrison DC: Ultrasound in the diagnosis and evaluation of therapy of idiopathic hypertrophic subaortic stenosis, Circulation 40:905, 1969.

Pridie R and Oakley C: Mechanism of mitral regurgitation in hypertrophic obstructive cardiomyopathy, Br Heart J 32:203, 1970.

LEFT VENTRICLE

Abbasi A et al: Paradoxical motion of interventricular septum in LBBB, Circulation 49:423, 1974.

Bergeron GA, Cohen MV, Teichholz LF, and Gorlin R: Echocardiographic analysis of mitral valve motion after acute myocardial infarction, Circulation 51:82, 1975.

Burch GE, Giles TD, and Martinez E: Echocardiographic detection of abnormal motion of the interventricular septum in ischemic cardiomyopathy, Am J Med 57:293, 1974.

Chang S, Feigenbaum H, and Dillon J: Condensed M-mode echocardiographic scan of the asymmetrical left ventricle, Chest 68:93, 1975.

Diamond M et al: Echocardiographic features of atrial septal defect, Circulation 43:129, 1974.

Dillon J, Chang S, and Feigenbaum H: Echocardiographic manifestations of left bundle branch block, Circulation 49:876, 1974.

Fortuin N et al: Determinations of left ventricular volumes by ultrasound, Circulation 44:575, 1971.

Goldstein S and Willem de Jong J: Changes in left ventricular wall dimension during regional myocardial ischemia, Am J Cardiol 34:56, 1974.

Gramiak R and Nanda N: Echocardiographic diagnosis of ostium primum septal defect, Circulation 45(suppl 2):46, 1972.

Hagan A et al: Ultrasound evaluation of systolic anterior septal motion in patients with and without right ventricular volume overload, Circulation 50:248, 1974.

Karliner J et al: Mean velocity of fiber shortening: a simplified measure of left ventricular myocardial contractility, Circulation 44:323, 1971.

Kerber RE and Abboud FM: Echocardiographic detection of regional myocardial infarction: an experimental study, Circulation 48:997, 1973.

Kraunz R and Kennedy J: Ultrasonic determination of left ventricular wall motion in normal man: studies at rest and after exercise, Am Heart J 79:36, 1970.

Kraunz R and Ryan T: Ultrasound measurements of ventricular wall motion following administration of vasoactivity drugs, Am J Cardiol 27:464, 1971.

Kreamer R, Kerber R, and Abbound F: Ventricular aneurysm: use of echocardiography, J Clin Ultrasound 1:60, 1973.

Layton C et al: Assessment of left ventricular filling and compliance using an ultrasound technique, Br Heart J 35:559, 1973.

Levitsky S and Merchani F: Non-invasive methods of measuring myocardial contractility, Surg Annu 5:205, 1973.

Ludbrook P, Karliner JS, London A, et al: Posterior wall velocity: an unreliable index of total left ventricular performance in patients with coronary artery disease, Am J Cardiol 33:475, 1974.

Ludbrook P, Karliner JS, Paterson K, et al: Comparison of ultrasound and cineangiographic measurements of left ventricular performance in patients with and without wall motion abnormalities, Br Heart J 35:1026, 1973.

McDonald I: Assessment of myocardial function by echocardiography, Adv Cardiol 12:221, 1974.

Morganroth J et al: Comparative left ventricular dimensions in trained athletes, Ann Intern Med 82:521, 1975.

Payvandi M et al: Echocardiography in congenital and acquired absence of the pericardium: an echocardiographic mimic of right ventricular volume overload, Circulation 53:86, 1976.

Pombo J et al: Comparison of stroke volume and cardiac output determination by ultrasound and dye dilution in acute myocardial infarction, Am J Cardiol 27:630, 1971.

Pombo J , Troy B, and Russell R Jr: Left ventricular volumes and ejection fraction by echocardiography, Circulation 43:480, 1971.

Popp R et al: Effect of transducer placement on echocardiographic measurement of left ventricular dimensions, Am J Cardiol 35:537, 1975.

Popp R et al: Sources of error in calculation of left ventricular volumes by echography, Am J Cardiol 31:152, 1973.

Popp R et al: Ultrasonic cardiac echography for determining stroke volume and valvular regurgitation, Circulation 41:493, 1970.

Ratshin R et al: The accuracy of ventricular volume analysis by quantitative echocardiography in patients with coronary artery disease with and without wall motion abnormalities, Am J Cardiol 33:164, 1974.

Ratshin R et al: Quantitative echocardiography: correlations with ventricular volumes by angiography in patients with coronary artery disease with and without wall motion abnormalities, Circulation 48(suppl 4):48, 1973.

Ratshin R, Rackley C, and Russel R: Serial evaluation of left ventricular volumes and posterior wall movement in the acute phase of myocardial infarction using diagnostic ultrasound, Am J Cardiol 29:286, 1972.

Ratshin R, Rackley C, and Russell RL: Determination of left ventricular preload and afterload by quantitative echocardiography in man, Circ Res 34:711, 1974.

Redwood D, Henry W, and Epstein S: Evaluation of the ability of echocardiography to measure acute alterations in left ventricular volume, Circulation 50:901, 1974.

Stack R et al: Left ventricular performance in coronary artery disease evaluated with systolic time intervals and echocardiography, Am J Cardiol 37:331, 1976.

Weyman S et al: Localization of left ventricular outflow obstruction by cross-sectional echocardiography, Am J Med 60:33, 1976.

GENERAL DOPPLER TECHNIQUES IN ECHOCARDIOGRAPHY

Currie PJ et al: Continuous wave Doppler determination of right ventricular pressure: a simultaneous Doppler-catheterization study in 127 patients, J Am Coll Cardiol 6(4):750, 1985.

Gramiak R et al: Left coronary arterial blood flow: noninvasive detection by Doppler ultrasound, 159(3):657, 1986.

Hatle L: Maximal blood flow velocities—haemodynamic data obtained noninvasively with CW Doppler, Ultrasound Med Biol 10(2):225, 1984.

Hatle L: Noninvasive assessment of valve lesions with Doppler ultrasound, Herz 9(4):213, 1984.

Jacoby SS et al: Two-dimensional and Doppler echocardiography in the evaluation of penetrating cardiac injury, Chest 88(6):922, 1985.

Kostucki W et al: Pulsed Doppler regurgitant flow patterns of normal values, Am J Cardiol 58(3):309, 1986.

Martin-Duran R et al: Comparison of Doppler-determined elevated pulmonary arterial pressure with pressure measured at cardiac catheterization, Am J Cardiol 57(10):859, 1986.

Nicolosi GL et al: Analysis of interobserver and intraobserver variation of interpretation of the echocardiographic and Doppler flow determination of cardiac output by the mitral orifice method, Br Heart J 55(5):446, 1986.

Nishimura RA et al: Doppler echocardiography: theory, instrumentation, technique, and application, Mayo Clin Proc 60(5):321, 1985.

Roelandt J: Colour-coded Doppler flow imaging: what are the prospects? Eur Heart J 7(3):184, 1986.

Stewart WJ et al: Variable effects of changes in flow rate through the aortic, pulmonary and mitral valves on valve area and flow velocity: impact on quantitative Doppler flow calculations, J Am Coll Cardiol 6(3):653, 1985.

Teirstein PS et al: The accuracy of Doppler ultrasound measurement of pressure gradients across irregular dual and tunnel-like obstructions to blood flow, Circulation 72(3):577, 1985.

ECHOCARDIOGRAPHIC MEASUREMENTS

Chang S: M-mode echocardiographic techniques and pattern recognition, Philadelphia 1976, Lea & Febiger.

ACQUIRED VALVAR HEART DISEASE

Abbasi AS, Allen MW, DeCristofaro D, et al: Detection and estimation of the degree of mitral regurgitation by range-gated pulsed Doppler echocardiography, Circulation 61:143, 1980.

Cope GD, Kisslo JA, Johnson ML, et al: A reassessment of the echocardiogram in mitral stenosis, Circulation 52:664, 1975.

DeMaria AN, Bommer W, Joye J, et al: Value and limitations of cross-sectional echocardiography of the aortic valve in the diagnosis and quantification of valvular aortic stenosis, Circulation 62:304, 1980.

Henry WL Griffith JM, Michaelis LL, et al: Measurement of mitral orifice area in patients with mitral valve disease by real time, two-dimensional echocardiography, Circulation 51:827, 1975.

Kotler MN, Mintz GS, Parry WR, et al: M-mode and two dimensional echocardiography in mitral and aortic regurgitation: pre- and postoperative evaluation of volume overload of the left ventricle, Am J Cardiol 46:1144, 1980.

Levisman JA, Abassi AS, and Pearse ML: Posterior mitral leaflet motion in mitral stenosis, Circulation 51:511, 1975.

Naito M, Morganroth J, Mardelli TJ, et al: Rheumatic mitral stenosis: cross-sectional echocardiographic analysis, Am Heart J 100:34, 1980.

Nichol PM, Gilber BW, and Kisslo JA; Two-dimensional echocardiographic assessment of mitral stenosis, Circulation 55:120, 1977.

Popp RL, Rubenson DS, Tucker CR, et al Echocardiography: M-mode and two-dimensional methods, Ann Intern Med 93:844, 1980.

Wise JR: Echocardiographic evaluation of mitral stenosis using diastolic posterior left ventricular wall motion, Circulation 61:1037, 1980.

ECHOCARDIOGRAPHY AND DOPPLER TECHNIQUES IN VALVULAR DISEASE

Ascah KJ et al: A Doppler two-dimensional echocardiographic method for quantitation of mitral regurgitation, Circulation 72(2):377, 1985.

Fioretti P et al: Postoperative regression of left ventricular dimensions in aortic insufficiency: a long-term echocardiographic study, J Am Coll Cardiol 5(4):856, 1985.

Gardin JM et al: Effect of imaging veiw and sample volume location on evaluation of mitral flow velocity by pulsed Doppler echocardiography, Am J Cardiol 57(915):1335, 1986.

Goldberg SJ et al: Quantitative assessment by Doppler echocardiography of pulmonary or aortic regurgitation, Am J Cardiol 56(1):131, 1985.

Goldman AP et al: The complementary role of magnetic resonance imaging, Doppler echocardiography, and computed tomography in the diagnosis of dissecting thoracic aneurysms, Am Heart J 111(5):970, 1986.

Goldman ME et al: Intraoperative echocardiography for the evaluation of valvular regurgitation: experience in 263 patients, Circulation 74(3 Pt 2):143, 1986.

Grayburn PA et al: Detection of aortic insufficiency by standard echocardiography, pulsed Doppler echocardiography, and auscultation, Ann Intern Med 104(5):599, 1986.

Harrigan P et al: Diastolic indentation of the interventional septum: a new cross-sectional echocardiographic sign of aortic regurgitation, Am Heart J 111(2):425, 1986.

Holmvang G et al: Noninvasive determination of valve area in adults with aortic stenosis using Doppler echocardiography, Cathet Cardiovasc Diagn 12(1):9, 1986.

Iliceto S et al: Dynamic intracavitary left atrial echoes in mitral stenosis, Am J Cardiol 55(5):603, 1985.

Khandheria BK et al: Doppler color flow imaging: a new technique for visualization and characterization of the blood flow jet in mitral stenosis, Mayo Clin Proc 61(8):623, 1986.

Krafcheck J et al: A reconsideration of Doppler assessed gradients in suspected aortic stenosis, Am Heart J 110(4):765, 1985.

Martinez FF et al: Echocardiographic and hemodynamic features of severe aortic regurgitation with diastolic opening of the aortic valve, Clin Cardiol 9(5):225, 1986.

Otto CM et al: Determination of the stenotic aortic valve area in adults using Doppler echocardiography, J Am Coll Cardiol 7(3):509, 1986.

Panidis IP et al: Diastolic mitral regurgitation in patients with atrioventricular conduction abnormalities: a common finding by Doppler echocardiography, J Am Coll Cardiol 7(4):768, 1986.

Panidis IP et al: Value and limitations of Doppler ultrasound in the evaluation of aortic stenosis: a statistical analysis of 70 consecutive patients, Am Heart J 112(1):150, 1986.

Perez JE et al: Usefulness of Doppler echocardiography in detecting tricuspid valve stenosis, Am J Cardiol 55(5):601, 1985.

Quinones MA: Assessment of valvular lesions with M-mode, two-dimensional and Doppler echocardiography, Herz 9(4):200, 1984.

Rasmussen S et al: Clinical echocardiography in acquired heart disease, Cardiol Clin 2(4):507, 1984.

Richards KL: Doppler echocardiographic diagnosis and quantification of valvular heart disease, Curr Probl Cardiol 10(2):1, 1985.

Richards KL et al: Calculation of aortic valve area by Doppler echocardiography: a direct application of the continuity equation, Circulation 73(5):964, 1986.

Rubler S et al: The role of aortic valve calcium in the detection of aortic stenosis: an echocardiographic study, Am Heart J 109(5 Pt 1):1049, 1985.

Saal AK et al: Noninvasive detection of aortic insufficiency in patients with mitral stenosis by pulsed Doppler echocardiography, J Am Coll Cardiol 5(1):176, 1985.

Simpson IA et al: Clinical value of Doppler echocardiography in the assessment of adults with aortic stenosis, Br Heart J 53(6):636, 1985.

Smith MD et al: Comparative accuracy of two-dimensional echocardiography and Doppler pressure half-time methods in assessing severity of mitral stenosis in patients with and without prior commissurotomy, Circulation 73(1):100, 1986.

Smith MD et al: Systematic correlation of continuous-wave Doppler and hemodynamic measurements in patients with aortic stenosis, Am Heart J 111(2):245, 1986.

Stewart WJ et al: Prevalence of AV prolapse with BAV and its relation to aortic regurgitation: a cross-sectional echocardiographic study Am J Cardiol 54(10):1277, 1984.

Takenaka K et al: A simple Doppler echocardiographic method for estimating severity of aortic regurgitation, Am J Cardiol 57(15):1340, 1986.

Teague SM et al: Quantification of aortic regurgitation utilizing continuous wave Doppler ultrasound, J Am Coll Cardiol 8(3):592, 1986.

Vacek JL et al: The inaccuracy of aortic valve systolic flutter as a screening test for significant aortic stenosis, Clin Cardiol 7(4):229, 1984.

Voyles WF et al: Doppler ultrasound in noninvasive cardiac evaluation: the growing range of applications, Postgrad Med 78(6):151, 1985.

Wilansky S et al: Valve-like intimal flap: a new echocardiographic finding of aortic dissection, Am Heart J 111(6):1204, 1986.

Yock PG et al: Noninvasive estimation of right ventricular systolic pressure by Doppler ultrasound in patients with tricuspid regurgitation, Circulation 70(4):657, 1984.

PROSTHETIC VALVES

Alderman EL, Rytand DA, Crow RS, et al: Normal and prosthetic atrioventricular valve motion in atrial flutter, Circulation 45:1206, 1972.

Assad-Morell J et al: Malfunctioning tricuspid valve prosthesis: clinical, phonocardiographic, echocardiographic and surgical findings, Mayo Clin Proc 42:443, 1974.

Belenkie I, Carr M, Schlant RC, et al: Malfunction of a Cutter-Smeloff mitral ball valve prosthesis: diagnosis by phonocardiography and echocardiography, Am Heart J 86:399, 1973.

Brodie BR, Grossman W, McLaurin L, et al: Diagnosis of prosthetic mitral valve malfunction with combined echo-phonocardiography, Circulation 53:93, 1976.

Burgraff GW and Craige E: Echocardiographic studies of left ventricular wall motion and dimensions after valvular heart surgery, Am J Cardiol 35:473, 1975.

Douglas J and Williams G: Echocardiographic evaluation of the Bjork-Shiley prosthetic valve, Circulation 50:52, 1974.

Gold H and Hertz L: Death caused by fracture of Beall mitral prosthesis, Am J Cardiol 34:371, 1974.

Horowitz M, Goodman D, and Popp R: Echocardiographic diagnosis of calcific stenosis of a stented aortic homograft in the mitral position, J Clin Ultrasound 2:179, 1974.

Johnson ML: Echocardiographic evaluation of prosthetic heart valves. In Gramiak R and Waag RC, editors: Cardiac ultrasound, St Louis, 1975. The CV Mosby Co.

Johnson ML, Holmes JH, and Paton BC: Echocardiographic determination of mitral disc valve excursion, Circulation 47:1274, 1973.

Johnson ML, Paton BC, and Holmes JH: Ultrasonic evaluation of prosthetic valve motion, Circulation 41(suppl 2):3, 1970.

Miller H, Gibson D, and Stephens J: Role of echocardiography and phonocardiography in the diagnosis of mitral paraprosthetic regurgitation with Starr-Edwards prostheses, Br Heart J 35:1217, 1973.

Miller H, Stephens J, and Gibson D: Echocardiographic features of mitral Starr-Edwards paraprosthetic regurgitation, Br Heart J 35:560, 1973.

Nanda NC, Gramiak R, Shah PM, and DeWeese JA: Mitral commissurotomy versus replacement: preoperative evaluation by echocardiography, Circulation 51:263, 1975.

Nanda NC, Gramiak R, Shah PM, et al: Echocardiographic assessment of left ventricular

is echocardiography accurate enough to guide surgical palliation? J AM Coll Cardiol 7(3):610, 1986.

Belkin RN et al: Interatrial shunting in atrial septal aneurysm, Am J Cardiol 57(4):310, 1986.

Bierman FZ: Two-dimensional echocardiography in the older child, J Am Coll Cardiol 5(1 suppl):37S, 1985.

Bricker JT et al: Echocardiographic evaluation of infective endocarditis in children, Clin Pediatr (Phila) 24(6):312, 1985.

Cabrera A et al: Congenital aortic atresia with intact ventricular septum and normal left ventricle: diagnosis by cross-sectional echocardiography, Int J Cardiol 8(3):339, 1985.

Caldwell RL et al: Right ventricular outflow tract assessment by cross-sectional echocardiography in tetralogy of Fallot, Circulation 59:395, 1979.

Candan I et al: Cross-sectional echocardiographic appearance in presumed congenital absence of the left pericardium, Br Heart J 55(4):405, 1986.

Carminati M: Transposition of the great arteries—diagnosis, Ala J Med Sci 23(2):155, 1986.

Casta A: Diastolic atrial compression in a premature infant, J Am Coll Cardiol 4(5):1069, 1984.

Casta A et al: Left ventricular bands (false tendons): echocardiographic and angiocardiographic delineation in children, Am Heart J 111(2):321, 1986.

Chesler E, Joffee HS, Beck W, and Schrire V: Echocardiographic recognition of mitral-semilunar valve discontinuity: an aid to the diagnosis of origin of both great vessels from the right ventricle, Circulation 43:725, 1971.

Chesler E, Joffe HS, Vecht R, et al: Ultrasound cardiography in single ventricle and the hypoplastic left and right heart syndromes, Circulation 42:123, 1970.

Chin AJ et al: Accuracy of prospective 2-D echocardiographic evaluation of left ventricular outflow tract in complete transposition of the great arteries, Am J Cardiol 55(6):759, 1985.

Come PC: Doppler detection of acquired ventricular septal defect, Am J Cardiol 55(5):586, 1985.

Deal BJ et al: Subxyphoid 2DE identification of tricuspid valve abnormalities in transposition of the great arteries with ventricular septal defect, Am J Cardiol 55(9):1146, 1985.

Diamond MA, Dillon JC, Haine CL, et al: Echocardiographic features of atrial septal defect, Circulation 43:129, 1971.

Dillon JC, Weyman AE, Feigenbaum H, et al: Cross-sectional echocardiographic examination of the interatrial septum, Circulation 55:115, 1977.

DiSessa TG, Hagan AD, Pope C, et al: Two-dimensional echocardiographic characteristics of double outlet right ventricle, Am J Cardiol 44:1146, 1979.

Ebels T et al: Anatomic and functional "obstruction" of the outflow tract in AV septal

defects with separate valve orifices (ostium primum atrial septal defect): an echocardiographic study, Am J Cardiol 54(7):843, 1984.

Forfar JC et al: Functional and anatomical correlates in atrial septal defect: an echocardiographic analysis, Br Heart J 54(2):193, 1984.

Fraker TD, Harris PJ, Behar VS, and Kisslo JA: Detection of exclusion of interatrial shunts by two-dimensional echocardiography and peripheral venous injection. Circulation 59:379, 1979.

French JW and Popp R: Variability of echocardiographic discontinuity in double outlet right ventricle and truncus arteriosus, Circulation 51:848, 1975.

Freund M et al: Ultrasound assessment of ductal closure, pulmonary blood flow velocity, and systolic pulmonary arterial pressure in healthy neonates, Pediatr Cardiol 6(5):233, 1986.

Fripp RR: Pulsed Doppler and 2D echo findings in aortico-ventricular tunnel, J Am Coll Cardiol 4(5):1012, 1984.

Fyfe DA et al: Continuous wave Doppler determination of the pressure gradient across pulmonary artery bands: hemodynamic correlation in 20 patients, Mayo Clin Proc 59(11):744, 1984.

Gibbs JL et al: Doppler echocardiography after anatomical correction of transposition of the great arteries, Br Heart J 56(1):67, 1986.

Goldberg SJ: A review of pediatric Doppler echocardiography, Am J Dis Child 138(11):1003, 1984.

Gutgesell HP: Echocardiographic assessment of cardiac function in infants and children, J Am Coll Cardiol 5(1 suppl):955, 1985.

Gutgessel HP et al: Accuracy of two dimensional echocardiography in the diagnosis of congenital heart disease, Am J Cardiol 55(5):514, 1985.

Gutgesell HP et al: Two-dimensional echocardiographic assessment of pulmonary artery and aortic arch anatomy in cyanotic infants, J Am Coll Cardiol 4(6):1242, 1984.

Hagler DJ: Functional assessment of the Fontan operation: combined M-mode, 2D and Doppler studies, J Am Coll Cardiol 4(4):756, 1984.

Hagler DJ, Tajik AJ, Seward JB, et al: Wide-angle two-dimensional echocardiographic profiles of conotruncal abnormalities, Mayo Clin Proc 55:73, 1980.

Hammerman C et al: Prostaglandins and echocardiography in the assessment of patent ductus arteriosus, Crit Care Med 14(5):462, 1986.

Haugland H et al: Echocardiographic characteristics of pulmonary and aortic valve motion in the Eisenmenger's syndrome from ventricular septal defect, Am J Cardiol 54(7):927, 1984.

Houston AB et al: The severity of pulmonary valve or artery obstruction in children estimated by Doppler ultrasound, Eur Heart J 6(9):786, 1985.

Huhta JC: Two dimensional echo spectrum of univentricular atrioventricular connection, J Am Coll Cardiol 5(1):149, 1985.

Huhta JC et al: Cross-sectional echocardio-

graphic diagnosis of total anomalous pulmonary venous connection, Br Heart J 53(5):525, 1985.

Jureidini SB et al: Two-dimensional echocardiographic assessment of adequacy of pulmonary artery banding, Pediatr Cardiol 6(5):239, 1986.

Kansal S et al: Two-dimensional echocardiography of congenital absence of pericardium, Am Heart J 109(4):912 1985.

King DH et al: Mitral and tricuspid valve annular diameter in normal children determined by two dimensional echo, Am J Cardiol 55(6):787, 1985.

Lam J: Two dimensional echo of total anomalous pulmonary venous return of the infradiaphragmatic type, Eur Heart J 5(10):842, 1984.

Lambertz H et al: Visualization of superior vena cava by subcostal two-dimensional echocardiography, Am Heart J 109(6):1401, 1985.

Mahoney LT et al: The newborn transitional circulation: a two-dimensional Doppler echocardiographic study, J Am Coll Cardiol 6(3):623, 1985.

Marino B: Right oblique subxyphoid view for two dimensional echo visualization of the right ventricle in congenital heart disease, Am J Cardiol 54(8):1064, 1984.

Marino B et al: Anatomical-echocardiographic correlations in pulmonary atresia with intact ventricular septum: use of subcostal cross-sectional views, Int J Cardiol 11(1):103, 1986.

Marino B et al: Complete transposition of great arteries: visualization of left and right outflow tract obstruction by oblique subcostal two dimensional echo, Am J Cardiol 55(9):1140, 1985.

Marino B et al: Two-dimensional echocardiographic anatomy in crisscross heart, Am J Cardiol 58(3):325, 1986.

Marx GR et al: Accuracy and pitfalls of Doppler evaluation of the pressure gradient in aortic coarctation, J Am Coll Cardiol 7(6):1379, 1986.

Marx GR et al: Doppler echocardiographic estimation of systolic pulmonary artery pressure in patients with aortic-pulmonary shunts, J Am Coll Cardiol 7(4):880, 1986.

Marx GR et al: Doppler echocardiography estimation of systolic pulmonary artery pressure in pediatric patients with interventricular communications, J Am Coll Cardiol 6(5):1132, 1985.

Mauran P et al: Value of respiratory variations of right ventricular dimension in the identification of small atrial septal defects (secundum type) not requiring surgery: an echocardiographic study, Am Heart J 112(3):548, 1986.

Meissner MD et al: Corrected transposition of the great arteries: evaluation by two-dimensional and Doppler echocardiography, Am Heart J 111(3):599, 1986.

Meyer RA: Echocardiography in assessing cardiac anatomy: summary and discussion, J Am Coll Cardiol 5(1 suppl):445, 1985.

Meyer RA and Kaplan S: Echocardiography in the diagnosis of hypoplasia of the left or right ventricles in the neonate, Circulation 46:55, 1972.

Meyer RA, Schwartz DC, Benzing G, and Kaplan S: Ventricular septum in right ventricular volume overload: an echocardiographic study, Am J Cardiol 30:349, 1972.

Moro E et al: Doppler and two-dimensional echocardiographic observations of systolic anterior motion of the mitral valve in d-transposition of the great arteries: an explanation of the left ventricular outflow tract gradient, J Am Coll Cardiol 7(4):889, 1986.

Murphy DJ Jr et al: Continuous wave Doppler in children with ventricular septal defect: noninvasive estimation of interventricular pressure gradient, Am J Cardiol 57(6):428, 1986.

Nakano H et al: Doppler detection of tricuspid regurgitation following Kawasaki disease, Pediatr Radiol 16(2):123, 1986.

Orsmond GS, Ruttenberg HD, Bessinger FB, and Moller JH: echocardiographic features of total anomalous pulmonary venous connection to the coronary sinus. Am J Cardiol 41:597, 1978.

Paquet M and Gutgesell H: Echocardiographic features of total anomalous pulmonary venous connection, Circulation 51:599, 1975.

Pieroni DR, Homcy E, and Freedom RM: Echocardiography in atrioventricular canal defect: a clinical spectrum, Am J Cardiol 35:54, 1975.

Radtke WE, Tajik AJ, Gau GT, et al: Atrial septal defect: echocardiographic observations, Ann Intern Med 84:246, 1976.

Redel DA: Diagnosis and follow up of congenital heart disease in children with the use of two dimensional Doppler echo, Ultrasound Med Biol 10(2):249, 1984.

Reeder GS: Extracardiac conduit obstruction: initial experience in the use of Doppler echo for noninvasive estimation of pressure gradient, J Am Coll Cardiol 4(5):1006, 1984.

Reeder GS et al: Use of Doppler techniques (continuous wave, pulsed wave, and color flow imaging) in the noninvasive hemodynamic assessment of congenital heart disease, Mayo Clin Proc 61(9):725, 1986.

Rein AJ et al: Cardiac output estimates in the pediatric intensive care unit using a continuous wave Doppler computer: validation and limitations of the technique, Am Heart J 112(1):97, 1986.

Reller MD et al: Hemodynamically significant PDA: an echocardiographic and clinical assessment of incidence, natural history, and outcome in very low birth weight infants maintained in negative fluid balance, Pediatr Cardiol 6(1):17, 1985.

Rice MJ et al: Straddling AV valve: two dimensional echocardiographic diagnosis, classification and surgical implications, Am J Cardiol 55(5):505, 1985.

Robinson PJ: Continuous wave Doppler velocimetry as an adjunct to cross-sectional echo in the diagnosis of critical left heart obstruction in neonates, Br Heart J 52(5):552, 1984.

Robinson PJ: Left ventricular outflow tract obstruction in complete transposition of the great arteries with intact ventricular septum: a cross sectional echocardiography study, Br Heart J 54(2):201, 1985.

Sahn DJ: Real-time two-dimensional Doppler echocardiographic flow mapping, 7(5):849, 1985.

Sahn DJ: Resolution and display requirements for ultrasound Doppler evaluation of the heart in children, infants and the unborn fetus, J Am Coll Cardiol 5(1 suppl):12S, 1985.

Sahn DJ et al: New advances in two-dimensional Doppler echocardiography, Prog Cardiovasc 28(5):367, 1986.

Satomi G et al: Blood flow pattern of the inter-atrial communication in patients with complete transposition of the great arteries: a pulsed Doppler echocardiographic study, Circulation 73(1):95, 1986.

Seward JB et al: Internal cardiac crux: two-dimensional echocardiography of normal and congenitally abnormal hearts, Ultrasound Med Biol 10(6):735, 1984.

Seward JB, Tajik AJ, Hagler DJ, and Ritter DG: Echocardiographic spectrum of tricuspid atresia, Mayo Clin Proc 53:100, 1978.

Silverman NH, Snider AR, and Rudolph AM: Evaluation of pulmonary hypertension by M-mode echocardiography in children with ventricular septal defects, Circulation 61:1125, 1980.

Smallhorn JF et al: Combined noninvasive assessment of the PDA in the preterm infant before and after indomethacin treatment, Am J Cardiol 54(10):1300, 1984.

Smallhorn JF et al: Noninvasive recognition of functional pulmonary atresia by echocardiography, Am J Cardiol 54(7):925, 1984.

Smallhorn JF et al: Pulsed Doppler assessment of pulmonary vein obstruction, Am Heart J 110(2):483, 1985.

Smallhorn JF et al: Pulsed Doppler echocardiographic assessment of the pulmonary venous pathway after the Mustard or Senning procedure for transposition of the great arteries, Circulation 73(4):765, 1986.

Snider AR: Use and abuse of the echocardiogram, Pediatr Clin North Am 31(6):1345, 1984.

Snider AR et al: Comparison of high pulse repetition frequency and continuous wave Doppler echocardiography for velocity measurement and gradient prediction in children with valvular and congenital heart disease, J Am Coll Cardiol 7(4):873, 1986.

Snider AR et al: Doppler evaluation of left ventricular diastolic filling in children with systemic hypertension, Am J Cardiol 56(15):921, 1985.

Steeg CN et al: "Bedside" balloon septostomy in infants with transposition of the great arteries: new concepts using two-dimensional echocardiographic techniques, J Pediatr 107(6):944, 1985.

Stevenson JG: Experience with qualitative and quantitative applications of Doppler echocardiography in congenital heart disease, Ultrasound Med Biol 10(6):771, 1984.

Stevenson JG: Noninvasive estimation of peak pulmonary artery pressure by M-mode echo, J Am Coll Cardiol 4(5):1021, 1984.

Suzuki Y et al: Detection of intracardiac shunt flow in atrial septal defect using a real-time two-dimensional color-coded Doppler flow imaging system and comparison with contrast two-dimensional echocardiography, Am J Cardiol 56(4):347, 1985.

Tajik AJ, Gau GT, Ritter DJ, and Schattenberg TT: Echocardiographic pattern of right ventricular diastolic volume overload in children, Circulation 46:36, 1972.

Vargas-Barron J: Differential diagnosis of various causes of systolic-diastolic murmurs using pulsed Doppler echo, Am Heart J 108(6):1507, 1984.

Vick GW et al: Assessment of ductus arteriosus in preterm infants utilizing suprasternal two-dimensional Doppler echocardiography, J Am Coll Cardiol 5(4):973, 1985.

Vick GW III and Serwer GA: Echocardiographic evaluation of the postoperative tetralogy of Fallot patient, Circulation 58:842, 1978.

Vitarelli A et al: Evaluation of total anomalous pulmonary venous drainage with cross-sectional colour-flow Doppler echocardiography, Eur Heart J 7(3):190, 1986.

Walther FJ et al: Echocardiographic measurement of left ventricular stroke volume in newborn infants: a correlative study with pulsed Doppler and M-mode echocardiography, J Clin Ultrasound 14(1):37, 1986.

Watanabe K: Evaluation of right ventricular pressure by two dimensional Doppler, Jpn Heart J 25(4):523, 1984.

Wessel A: Normal values of two-dimensional echocardiographic evaluation of left and right ventricular geometry in children, Herz 10(4):248, 1985.

Weyman AE, Wann S, Feigenbaum H, and Dillon JC: Mechanism of abnormal septal motion in patients with right ventricular volume overload—a cross-sectional echocardiographic study, Circulation 54:179, 1976.

Williams RG: Echocardiography in the neonate and young infant, J Am Coll Cardiol 5(1 suppl):305, 1985.

Williams RG and Tucker CR: Echocardiographic diagnosis of congenital heart disease, Boston, 1977, Little, Brown & Co.

Yanagisawa M et al: Coronary aneurysms in Kawasaki disease: follow up observation by two-dimensional echocardiography, Pediatr Cardiol 6(1):11, 1985.

FETAL ECHOCARDIOGRAPHY

Allan L, Joseph M, Boyd E, et al: M-mode echocardiography in the developing human fetus, Br Heart J 47:573, 1982.

Allan L, Tynan M, Campbell S, and Anderson R: Normal fetal cardiac anatomy—a basis for the echocardiographic detection of abnormalities, Prenat Diagn 1:131, 1981.

Comstock C: Normal fetal heart axis and position, Obstet Gynecol 70:2, 87.

Copel J, Pilu G, and Kleinman CS: Congenital heart disease and extracardiac anomalies: associations and indications for fetal echocardiography, Am J Obstet Gynecol 154:1121, 1986.

Cyr D, Guntheroth W, Mack L, and Shuman W: A systematic approach to fetal echocardiography using real-time/two-dimensional sonography, J Ultrasound Med 5:343, 86.

DeVore G, Donnerstein R, Kleinman C, et al: Fetal echocardiography: normal anatomy as determined by real-time–directed M-mode ultrasound, Am J Obstet Gynecol 144:249, 1982.

Reed K, Meijboom E, Sahn D, et al: Cardiac Doppler flow velocities in human fetuses, Circulation 73:41, 1986.

Reed K, Sahn D, Marx G, et al: Cardiac Doppler flows during fetal arrhythmias: physiologic consequences, Obstet Gynecol 70:1, 1987.

Sahn DJ, Lange L, Allen H, et al: Quantitative real-time cross sectional echocardiography in the developing normal human fetus and newborn, Circulation 62:3, 1980.

Shime J, Bertrand M, Hagen-Ansert S, and Rakowski H: Two-dimensional and M-mode echocardiography in the human fetus, Am J Obstet Gynecol 1983.

Index